LEADERSHIP
AND NURSING CARE MANAGEMENT

SEVENTH EDITION

LEADERSHIP AND NURSING CARE MANAGEMENT

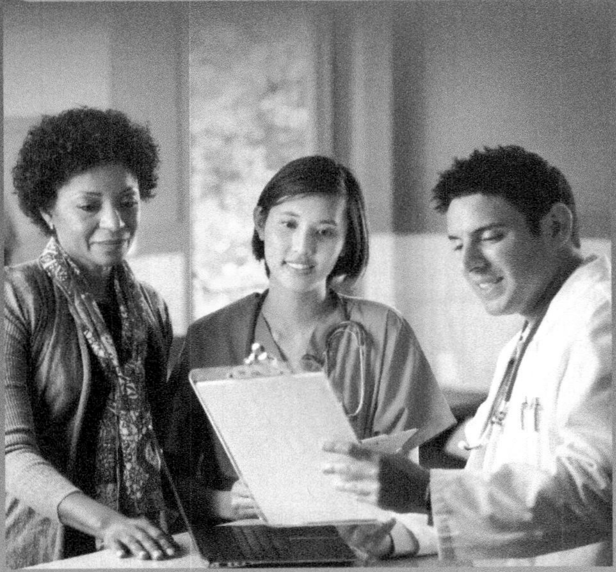

DIANE L. HUBER
PHD, RN, NEA-BC, FAAN
Professor Emeritus
College of Nursing and College of Public Health
The University of Iowa
Iowa City, Iowa

M. LINDELL JOSEPH
PHD, RN, FAONL, FAAN
Clinical Professor,
Director, Health Systems/Administration Program
College of Nursing
University of Iowa
Iowa City, Iowa

ELSEVIER

ELSEVIER

3251 Riverport Lane
St. Louis, Missouri 63043

LEADERSHIP AND NURSING CARE MANAGEMENT, SEVENTH EDITION ISBN: 978-0-323-69711-8

Library of Congress Number: 2020952283

Senior Content Strategist: Yvonne Alexopoulos
Senior Content Development Manager: Lisa Newton
Publishing Services Manager: Shereen Jameel
Senior Project Manager: Umarani Natarajan
Designer: Amy L. Buxton

Printed in the United States of America

Last digit is the print number: 9 8 7 6 5 4 3 2 1

CONTRIBUTORS

Kupiri "Piri" Ackerman-Barger, PhD, RN, CNE, FAAN
Associate Dean for Health Equity, Diversity, and Inclusion
University of California Davis
Betty Irene Moore School of Nursing
Sacramento, California

Mary Jo Assi, DNP, RN, NEA-BC, FAAN
Senior Vice President, Clinical Excellence Solutions and Associate Chief Nursing Officer
Press Ganey,
Dallas, Texas

Jennifer Bellot, PhD, RN, MHSA, CNE
Associate Dean of Academic Practice Integration
Jefferson College of Nursing
Thomas Jefferson University
Philadelphia, Pennsylvania

Michele A. Berg, MSHI, RN-NIC
Nursing Informaticist
Rush University Medical Center
Chicago, Illinois

Richard J. Bogue, PhD, FACHE
Associate Clinical Professor, University of Iowa College of Nursing,
Iowa City, Iowa
President, Courageous Healthcare, Inc.
Bryan, Texas

Debra V. Craighead, PhD, RN, CNL
Associate Professor, CNL Track Leader
Kitty DeGree School of Nursing
University of Louisiana at Monroe
Monroe, Louisiana

Laura Cullen, DNP, RN, FAAN
Evidence-Based Practice Scientist
Office of Nursing Research and EBP
University of Iowa Health Care
Iowa City, Iowa

Cindy J. Dawson, MSN, BSN
Chief Nurse Executive and Associate Director,
University of Iowa Health Care
Iowa City, Iowa

Bob Dent, DNP, MBA, RN, NEA-BC, CENP, FACHE, FAAN, FAONL
Vice President, Chief Nursing Officer
Emory Decatur Hospital, Decatur, Georgia
Emory Hillandale Hospital
Lithonia, Georgia
Emory Long-Term Acute Care Hospital
Lithonia, Georgia

Christina Dempsey, DNP, MBA, MSN, RN, CNOR, CENP, FAAN
Chief Nursing Officer, President for Clinical Excellence Solutions
Springfield, Missouri

Karen Dunn-Lopez, PhD, MPH, RN
Associate Professor and Director of the Center for Nursing Classification & Clinical Effectiveness
College of Nursing
University of Iowa
Iowa City, Iowa

Cole Edmonson, DNP, RN, NEA-BC, FACHE, FAONL, FNAP, FAAN
Chief Experience and Clinical Officer,
AMN Healthcare
Dallas, Texas

Michele Farrington, BSN, RN-BC
Program Manager
University of Iowa Health Care
Iowa City, Iowa

Ellen Fink-Samnick, MSW, ACSW, LCSW, CCM, CRP, DBH(s)
Principal/Owner, EFS Supervision Strategies, LLC
Burke Virginia
Adjunct Faculty: George Mason University
College of Health and Human Services Social Work Department
Part-time Faculty: University of Buffalo, School of Social Work
EFS Supervision Strategies, LLC
Burke, Virginia

Therese A. Fitzpatrick, PhD, RN, FAAN
Senior Vice President, Kaufman Hall and Associates
Assistant Professor, University of Illinois–Chicago
Chicago, Illinois

Betsy Frank, PhD, RN, ANEF
Professor Emerita
School of Nursing
Indiana State University
Terre Haute, Indiana

Mary Louanne Friend, PhD, MN, RN
Assistant Professor, Community Medicine and Population Health
The University of Alabama
College of Community Health Science/Rural Health Research
Tuscaloosa, Alabama

Kirsten Hanrahan, DNP, ARNP, CPNP-PC, FAAN
Director, Nursing Research and Evidence-Based Practice
Department of Nursing and Patient Care Services
University of Iowa Health Care
Iowa City, Iowa

Kimberly K. Hatchel, DNP, MHA, MSN, RN, CENP
Chief Nursing Officer
Blake Medical Center
Bradenton, Florida

Melinda Hirshouer, DNP, RN, MBA, MHSM
Director of Nursing, Cardiovascular and Neurosciences,
Texas Health Dallas
Dallas, Texas

Diane L. Huber, PhD, RN, NEA-BC, FAAN
Professor Emeritus
College of Nursing and College of Public Health
The University of Iowa
Iowa City, Iowa

Palma D. Iacovitti, DNP, MBA, RN
Program Director Surgical Oncology Clinics
Baptist MD Anderson Cancer Center
Jacksonville, Florida

Lisa Janeway, DNP, MSN, RN-BC, CPHIMS
Nursing Informaticist
Northwestern Memorial Healthcare
Resurrection University (Adjunct Faculty)
Chicago, Illinois

(Carol) Susan Johnson, PhD, RN, NPD-BC, NE-BC, FAAN
Founder & Principal
RN Innovations, LLC
Fort Wayne, Indiana

M. Lindell Joseph, PhD, RN, FAONL, FAAN
Clinical Professor,
Director, Health Systems/Administration Program
College of Nursing
University of Iowa
Iowa City, Iowa

Susan R. Lacey, PhD, RN, FAAN
Kitty DeGree Eminent Scholars
Professor and Endowed Chair for Nursing
Kitty DeGree School of Nursing
University of Louisiana Monroe
Monroe, Louisiana

Lyn Stankiewicz Losty, PhD, MBA, MS, RN
Contributing Faculty
Walden University
Minneapolis, Minnesota

Christopher J. Louis, PhD, MHA
Clinical Associate Professor of Health Law, Policy and Management
Boston University School of Public Health
Boston, Massachusetts

Joy Parchment, PhD, RN, NEA-BC
System Director, Nursing Strategy Implementation & Magnet® Program
Orlando Health
Orlando, Florida

Luc R. Pelletier, MSN, APRN, PMHCNS-BC, FAAN, CPHQ, FNAHQ
Clinical Nurse Specialist
Sharp Caster Institute for Nursing Excellence
San Diego, California

Beverly Quaye, EdD, RN, NEA-BC, FACHE
Assistant Professor
California State University
Fullerton, California

Veronica Rankin, DNP, RN-BC, NP-C, CNL
Director of Nursing Excellence—Magnet Program Director
Clinical Nurse Leader Program Administrator
Atrium Health
Charlotte, North Carolina

Barbara Seifert, PhD, LCSW, CPC
President/Owner, Committed to Your Success Coaching & Consulting
President, Elite Leadership Success Institute
Associate Adjunct Professor – Webster University
Adjunct Professor – Florida Institute of Technology
Orlando, Florida

Erin M. Steffen, MSN, RN
Assistant Nurse Manager, Procedure and Imaging Suite, Pediatric APEC
University of Iowa Stead Family Children's Hospital
University of Iowa Health Care
Iowa City, Iowa

Sandra Lynne Swearingen, PhD, RN, MSN, MHA
Director Leadership Development
Courageous Healthcare, Inc.
Bryan, Texas

Linda B. Talley, MS, RN, NE-BC, FAAN
Vice President and Chief Nursing Officer
Children's National Hospital,
Washington, DC

Diane H. Thorgrimson, MHSA, BS
Advisor to the CNO
Children's National Hospital
Washington, DC

Teresa M. Treiger, RN-BC, MA, CCM, CHCQM, FABQAURP
Principal
Ascent Care Management
Quincy, Massachusetts

ANCILLARY WRITERS

Stephanie C. Evans, PhD, APRN, CPNP-PC
Assistant Professor
The Houston J. and Florence A. Doswell College of Nursing
T. Boone Pickens Institute of Health Sciences
Texas Woman's University
Dallas Texas
Test Bank; NCLEX® Review Questions

Charla K. Hollin, RN, BSN
Allied Health Division Chair
University of Arkansas Rich Mountain
Mena Arkansas
TEACH for Nurses, PowerPoint Slides

REVIEWERS

Rebecca Davidson, PhD, MSN, RN
Assistant Professor of Nursing
Caylor School of Nursing
Lincoln Memorial University
Harrogate Tennessee

Kari Lynn Koenig, MS, RN
Associate Degree Nursing Program Director
Nursing
Northland Community and Technical College
East Grand Forks MN

Judy Kay Ogans, DNP, RN, CNE
BSN Program Director and Assistant Professor of Nursing
Nursing
The University of Oklahoma Health Sciences Center College of Nursing
Oklahoma City Oklahoma

Judith T. Pfriemer, RN, MSN
Assistant Professor of Nursing
School of Nursing
Arkansas State University
Jonesboro Arkansas

PREFACE

With the publication of the seventh edition of *Leadership and Nursing Care Management*, we start a new and exciting phase of incorporating Dr. M. Lindell Joseph as coeditor of the book. The history of this book began with the publication of the first edition in 1996, when Dr. Diane Huber wrote the whole first edition. She rewrote the whole second edition but invited chapter authors for the third edition in 2006, making it an edited book. The new phase means that a broader range of chapter authors were solicited, and there is double the editorial expertise. Welcome Lindell!

The development of the seventh edition occurred at a time of change and uncertainty in health care. This has reverberated within health care organizations and systems, in nursing professional organizations, and in the work life of nurses in leadership and administration. Hospitals and health care organizations are struggling with financial and workforce pressures. Nursing professional organizations, such as the American Organization of Nurse Executives (AONE) [now: American Organization for Nursing Leadership (AONL)] and the Council on Graduate Education for Administration in Nursing (CGEAN) [now: Association for Leadership Science in Nursing (ALSN)], have changed their names, as did the Institute of Medicine [now: the National Academies of Sciences, Engineering, Medicine, Health and Medicine Division] in 2016.

It is clear that nurses matter to health care delivery systems. Yet the United States is in the midst of a continuing and projected nurse shortage. Strong nurse leaders and managers are important for clients (and their safety), delivery systems (and their viability), and payers (and their solvency). Pressures remain to balance cost and quality considerations in a complex, chaotic, and turbulent health care environment.

Although society's need for excellent nursing care remains the nurse's constant underlying reason for existence, nursing is much more than that. Because nurses offer cost-effective expertise in solving problems related to the coordination and delivery of health care to individuals and populations in society, they have become a crucial linchpin in health care delivery and are highly valued for their clinical judgment. Nurses are well prepared to lead clinical change strategies and effectively manage the coordination and integration of interdisciplinary teams, population needs, and systems of care across the continuum. This has been increasingly important following implementation of the 2010 Patient Protection and Affordable Care Act (ACA), and nurses are needed to address care coordination and integration across the health care delivery system.

It can be argued that nursing is a unique profession in which the primary focus is caring—giving and managing the care that clients need. Thus, nurses are both health care providers and health care coordinators; that is, they have both clinical and managerial role components. Beginning with the first edition of *Leadership and Nursing Care Management*, it has been this text's philosophy that these two components can be discussed separately but in fact overlap. Because all nurses are involved in coordinating client care, leadership and management principles are a part of the core competencies they need to function in a complex health care environment.

Nurses need a strong background in nursing leadership and care management to be prepared for contemporary and future nursing practice. As nurses mature in advanced practice roles and as the health care delivery system restructures, nurses will become increasingly pivotal to cost-effective health care delivery, and research is bearing this out. This also is seen in the national trend to determine the most optimal organizational structure to effectively use and deploy large numbers of advanced practice providers such as nurse practitioners. Leadership and management are crucial skills and abilities for complex and integrated community and regional networks that employ and deploy nurses to provide health care services to clients and communities.

Today's nurses are expected to be able to lead and manage care across the health care continuum—a radically different approach to nursing from what has been the norm for hospital staff nurses. The COVID-19 pandemic in 2020 showed how critical it is to have nurses' expertise in care management. In all settings, including both nurse-run and interdisciplinary clinics, nursing leadership and management are complementary skills that add value to solid clinical care and patient- and client-oriented practice. Thus there is an urgent need to advance nurses' knowledge and skills in leadership and management. In addition, nurses who are expected to make and implement day-to-day management decisions need to know how these precepts can be practically applied to the organization and delivery of nursing care in a way that conserves scarce resources, reduces costs, and maintains or improves quality of care. This is the emphasis on adding value, innovation, and prevention interventions.

The primary modality for health care in the United States has moved away from acute care hospitalization. As prevention, wellness, and alternative sites for care delivery become more important, nursing's already rich experiential tradition of practice in these settings is emerging. This text reflects this contemporary trend by blending the hospital and non-hospital perspectives with an eye toward systems leadership and management.

PURPOSE AND AUDIENCE

The intent of this text is to provide both a broad introduction to the field and a synthesis of the knowledge base and skills related to both nursing leadership and nursing care management. It is an evidence-based blend of practice and theory that breaks new ground by explaining the intersection of nursing care with leading people and managing organizations and systems. It highlights the evidence base for care management. It combines traditional management perspectives and theory with contemporary health care trends and issues and consistently integrates leadership and management concepts. These concepts are illustrated and made relevant by practice-based examples.

The impetus for writing this text comes from teaching both undergraduate and graduate students in nursing leadership and management and from perceiving the need for a comprehensive, evidence- and practice-based textbook that blends and integrates leadership and management into an understandable and applicable whole.

Therefore the main goal of *Leadership and Nursing Care Management* is twofold: (1) to clearly differentiate traditional leadership and management perspectives and (2) to relate them in an integrated way with the evidence base, contemporary nursing trends, and practice applications. This textbook is designed to serve the needs of nurses and nursing students who seek a foundation in the principles of leading and coordinating nursing services in relation to patient care, peers, superiors, and subordinates.

ORGANIZATION AND COVERAGE

This seventh edition continues the format first used with the third edition. The first two editions were Dr. Huber's single-authored texts. The edited book approach draws together the best thinking of experts in the field—both nurses and non-nurses—to enrich and deepen the presentation of core essential knowledge and skills. Beginning with the first edition, a hallmark of *Leadership and Nursing Care Management* has been its depth of coverage, its comprehensiveness, and its strong evidence-based foundation. This seventh edition continues the emphasis on explaining theory in an easily understandable way to enhance comprehension and is an easy-to-understand bridge to the evidence-based management practices from AONL.

The content of this seventh edition integrates leadership and care management topics with the nurse executive leadership competencies of the 2015 American Organization of Nurse Executives (AONE)/American Organization for Nursing Leadership (AONL). AONL has identified the evidence-based core competencies in the field, and this book has been aligned accordingly to reflect the knowledge underlying quality management of nursing services, thereby synthesizing theory, evidence-based management principles, and application exercises. This will help the reader develop the crucial skills and knowledge needed for core competencies.

The organizational framework of this book groups the 26 chapters into the following five parts:

Part I: Leadership aligns with the AONL competency category of the same name and provides an orientation to the basic principles of both leadership and management. Part I contains chapters on Leadership and Management Principles, Change and Innovation, and Organizational Climate and Culture, and Managerial Decision-Making.

Part II: Professionalism aligns with the AONL competency category of the same name and addresses the nurse's role and management of professional nursing practice. The reader is prompted to examine the role of the nurse leader and manager. Part II discusses the content areas of Managing Time and Stress, Role Management, and Legal and Ethical Issues.

Part III: Communication and Relationship Building aligns with the AONL competency category of the same name. Part III focuses on Communication Leadership, Team Building and Working with Effective Groups, Power and Conflict, and Workplace Diversity. These are essential knowledge and skill areas for nurse leaders and managers as they work with and through others in care delivery.

Part IV: Knowledge of the Health Care Environment covers the AONL competency category of the same name and features a broad array of chapters. Part IV encompasses Organizational Structure, Decentralization and Shared Governance, Strategic Management, Professional Practice Models, Case and Population Management, Evidence-Based Practice: Strategies for Nursing Leaders, Quality and Safety, and Measuring and Managing Outcomes. This discussion highlights the importance of understanding the health care organizational structures within which nursing care delivery must operate. This section includes information on traditional organizational theory, professional practice models, and the dynamics of decentralized and shared governance.

Part V: Business Skills aligns with the AONL competency category on business skills and principles and contains an extensive grouping of chapters related to Prevention of Workplace Violence; Nursing Workforce Staffing and Management; Budgeting, Productivity, and Costing Out Nursing; Performance Appraisal; Emergency Management and Preparedness; Data Management and Clinical Informatics; and Marketing. These chapters discuss the opportunities and challenges for the nurse leader-manager when dealing with the health care workforce. The wide range of human resource responsibilities of nurse managers is reviewed, and resources for further study are provided. The significant share of scarce organization budgets consumed by the human resources of an institution makes this area of management a key challenge that requires intricate skills in leadership and management. This section examines some of the important factors that nurse leader-managers must consider in the nursing and health care environment. Also in this section are chapters that build on organizational theory and demonstrate the importance of integrating organizations and systems with the current technology and theory applications, including data management and informatics, strategic management, and marketing.

The 26 chapters in this text are organized in a consistent format that highlights the following features:

- Concept definitions
- Theoretical and research background
- Leadership and management implications
- Current issues and trends
- Case Studies and Critical Thinking Exercises
- Research Notes

This format is designed to bridge the gap between theory and practice and to increase the relevance of nursing leadership and management by demonstrating the way in which theory translates into behaviors appropriate to contemporary leadership and nursing care management. Case Studies and Critical Thinking Exercises offer opportunities for synthesis, application, and active learning.

TEXT FEATURES

This book contains several interesting and effective aids to readers' comprehension, critical thinking, and application.

CRITICAL THINKING EXERCISES

Found at the end of each chapter, this feature challenges readers to inquire and reflect, analyze critically the knowledge presented, and apply it to the situation.

RESEARCH NOTES

These summaries of current research studies are highlighted in every chapter and introduce the reader to the liveliness and applicability of the available literature in nursing leadership and management.

CASE STUDIES

Found at the end of each chapter, these vignettes introduce the reader to the "real world" of nursing leadership and management and demonstrate the ways in which the chapter concepts operate in specific situations. These vignettes show the creativity and energy that characterize expert nurse administrators as they tackle issues in practice.

NEXT-GENERATION NCLEX® (NGN) EXAMINATION CONTENT

The National Council of State Boards of Nursing (NCSBN) administers the national licensure exam for registered nurses (RNs), called NCLEX®. In 2013–2014 the NCSBN conducted a Strategic Practice Analysis that highlighted the complexity of decisions new nurses make while doing patient care. That prompted the question: Is the NCLEX® measuring the right things? To answer this question, the NCSBN launched the Next Generation NCLEX® (NGN), a research project to determine whether clinical judgment and decision making in nursing practice can reliably be assessed (https://www.ncsbn.org/next-generation-nclex.htm). They have developed a Clinical Judgment Measurement Model and analyzed the current NCLEX® item bank for clinical judgment domain distribution. The conclusion was a need for more research and the use of new item types on the NCLEX®. The research and development continue. As this text goes to press, it is projected that a revised NCLEX® exam will be rolled out in 2023.

The imperative for nursing students preparing to take the licensure exam and for nurse educators is to move into high gear with preparations for NCLEX®'s assessment of clinical decision-making testing even as the new test is in the development phase. New item types include enhanced multiple response, extended drag and drop, cloze items, enhanced hot spots, and matrix/grid. Layer 3 of the NCSBN's Clinical Judgment Measurement Model is focused on patient care and how the nurse recognizes cues, analyzes cues, prioritizes hypotheses, generates solutions, takes actions, and evaluates outcomes.

Leadership and Nursing Care Management, seventh edition, is not primarily focused on individual patient care (one nurse with one patient), but rather on the leadership and management of patient care delivery and the work of nurses. The content is most directly aligned with Layer 4 of the NCSBN's Clinical Judgment Measurement Model (https://www.ncsbn.org/14798.htm): Environmental Factor Examples. There are eight Environmental Factor Examples: (1) environment, (2) client observation, (3) resources, (4) medical records, (5) consequences and risks, (6) time pressure, (7) task complexity, and (8) cultural considerations. Layer 4 is concerned with the context within which a nurse is making clinical judgments and taking action. This is the realm of leadership and management of patient care. For example, the environment, situation, time pressures, resources, and cultural factors all have an influence on the nurse's clinical judgment and subsequent choice of action. The NGN focus is on what the nurse should do. This also applies to leadership and management in clinical practice.

Although NGN is still in development, and we are not informed as to how contextual/environmental content will be tested, we have addressed the NGN initiative in three ways: (1) ever since the first edition of *Leadership and Nursing Care Management*, each chapter has had a case study and a critical thinking exercise feature that promotes the analysis and integration of the application of the content and provides practice in managerial decision-making; (2) there is a dedicated chapter (Chapter 4) on managerial decision-making; and (3) as a new feature in this seventh edition, we have composed an NGN-type single episode case study for five selected chapters. Following the American Organization for Nursing Leadership's (AONL, 2015) Nurse Executive Competencies, which forms the broad structure of five parts of the content, the chapters chosen highlight the core of the five competencies: (1) leadership (Chapter 1), (2) professionalism/managing time and stress (Chapter 5), (3) communication (Chapter 8), (4) knowledge of the health care environment/decentralization and governance (Chapter 13), and (5) business skills/nursing workforce staffing and management (Chapter 21).

Students using this book may begin to prepare for NCLEX® (NGN) by using the NGN case studies. In addition, practice leaders or colleagues of future nurses can use these new case studies to foster their clinical imagination and model high-level thinking to help new graduate nurses prepare for NCLEX® (NGN).

LEARNING AND TEACHING AIDS

For Students

The Evolve Student Resources for this book include the following:

NCLEX® Review Questions, including rationales and page references

For Instructors

The Evolve Instructor Resources for this book include the following:

- *TEACH for Nurses* lesson plans, based on textbook chapter Learning Objectives, serve as ready-made, modifiable lesson plans and a complete road map to link all parts of the educational package. These concise and straightforward lesson plans can be modified or combined to meet your particular scheduling and teaching needs.

- *Test Bank* in ExamView format, featuring over 650 test items, complete with correct answer, rationale, cognitive level, nursing process step, appropriate NCLEX label, and corresponding textbook page references. The ExamView program allows instructors to create new tests; edit, add, and delete test questions; sort questions by NCLEX® category, cognitive level, and nursing process step; and administer and grade tests online.
- *Next-Generation NCLEX® (NGN)-Style Case Studies for Leadership and Nursing Care Management:* Four NGN-style case studies focused on Leadership and Management.
- *PowerPoint Presentations* with more than 650 customizable lecture slides.
- *Audience Response Questions* for i-clicker and other systems with two to three multiple-answer questions per chapter to stimulate class discussion and assess student understanding of key concepts.

ACKNOWLEDGMENTS

This book is dedicated to my children, Brad Gardner and Lisa Witte, and their spouses, Nonalee Gardner and John Witte, for their enthusiasm, caring support, and love. I am forever privileged that they are in my life. I thank them for the gifts of Kathryn Anne Gardner, Anthony James Gardner (A.J.), Logan Thomas Witte, and Olivia Morgan Witte. I love being Grandma to these wonderful people.

To my professional colleagues who inspired me and served as examples of excellence in nursing, I am grateful that you came alongside me and engaged in my life. I also am most grateful for my interdisciplinary health care colleagues who have taught me, role-modeled caring behaviors, and offered invaluable opportunities to learn and grow. To my nursing students, my thanks for being a source of continual intellectual stimulation and challenge. To all of you who have read and used this book, thank you. It is so very humbling and heartwarming when you mention this to me as we intersect on professional pathways. I am glad it is of use to you.

This book's first two editions evolved under the tender care of Thomas Eoyang, former editorial manager at W.B. Saunders Company, whose guidance, support, and caring were invaluable. To the editors in the Elsevier Nursing Division who worked so hard to facilitate everything related to the seventh edition, and to the excellent staff at Elsevier, a sincere thank you.

No acknowledgement is complete without an expression of sincere appreciation to Lindell Joseph for taking on the coeditor role. This textbook is truly enriched by your special talents. Together, all is better.

Diane L. Huber

My contributions in this book are dedicated to Dr. Diane L. Huber, an unbelievable mentor, colleague, and friend. I will always be thankful for her belief and support in my abilities. I am grateful to God, my mother Mary Madelina Joseph, husband Hector Guadalupe, daughter Geneva Guadalupe, cousin Caroline Norbal, aunts Albertha Corneille, Christine Corneille, Tenose Corneille, and Nicholina Felix, extended family members, friends, and Drs. Rose Sherman (Chief Editor of *Nurse Leader*) and Robyn Begley (CEO of AONL) for their ongoing support.

Recently, I had the privilege of observing the care management of my deceased nephew Kimani Joseph. During his battle with lupus, I observed many opportunities where the content in this book would have been useful. I hope that aspiring and current leaders could use this book as a resource to develop or improve care management practices.

I am truly honored and grateful to be the coeditor of the seventh edition of *Leadership and Nursing Care Management*. I am thankful to my colleagues who were invited to provide their expertise on specific content areas. Diane and I are hopeful that readers will find new insights for future leadership and care management practices. Once again, I am thankful to the selfless acts that Dr. Huber has demonstrated toward my personal and professional development.

M. Lindell Joseph

CONTENTS

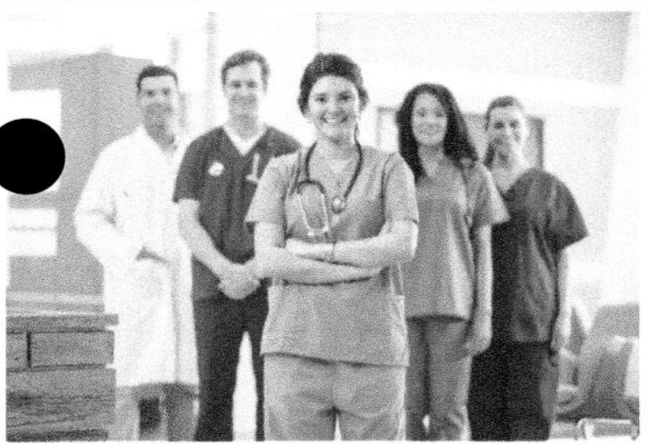

1

Leadership and Management Principles

Diane L. Huber

http://evolve.elsevier.com/Huber/leadership

Health care is a challenging sector to lead and manage. Both the practice of health care professionals and the effectiveness of health care organizations are affected by change, complexity, and environmental turbulence. The twin skills of leadership and management are crucial to nurses' effectiveness and organizational survival. Fortunately there is an evidence base of knowledge about leadership and management, and both can be learned.

Issues of cost, access, methods, and structures of care delivery, human capital management, and quality surround the broader context of health care. The effect on nursing is an urgent need for leadership and management at all levels and places where nurses work. With approximately 3 million licensed registered nurses (RNs) in the United States (US Bureau of Labor Statistics, 2019), RNs are the largest segment of the health care workforce. Strong and prepared leaders are needed to guide their practice. Leading and managing are essential skills, made more acutely urgent given health care system characteristics of rapid change, complexity, and chaos.

Ongoing health care reform, integration of new technologies, and patient-centered care influence the health care delivery system by redefining both how care is delivered and the role of the nursing workforce (The National Academies of Sciences, Engineering, Medicine; Health and Medicine Division, 2020). Emerging care delivery models, with a focus on managing health status and preventing acute health issues, will likely contribute to new growth in demand for nurses as they assume new and/or expanded roles in preventive care and care coordination. An example is the explosion in the growth of roles for Advanced Practice Providers, including nurse practitioners. Supply and demand for nurses will continue to be affected by numerous factors, including population growth, increases in chronic conditions, the aging of the nation's population, overall economic conditions, aging of the nursing workforce, and changes in health care reimbursement.

Leaders guide and motivate nurses to achieve their care provision goals as they practice nursing. Managers organize and guide nurses' work in organizations where they practice. Together the result is structures and processes that deliver desired outcomes. For the health care system, there are two predominant sets of desired outcomes. The first is the six aims for the health care system (Agency for Healthcare Research and Quality, 2018): health care needs to be safe, effective, patient centered, timely, efficient, and equitable. The second is the Institute for Healthcare Improvement's (IHI) (2020) Triple Aim: health care needs to simultaneously improve the health of the population, enhance the experience and the outcomes of the patient, and reduce per capita cost of care to benefit communities. The Triple Aim has been extended to a fourth element ("Quadruple Aim") that focuses on the workforce and is aimed at improving the experience of providing care (Sikka et al., 2015).

The major national leadership initiatives in nursing are the Institute of Medicine's (IOM, now called The National Academies of Sciences, Engineering, Medicine; Health and Medicine Division) (IOM, 2011) report *The Future of nursing: Leading change, advancing health* and the Magnet Recognition Program® (American Nurses

Photo used with permission from FatCamera/Getty Images.

Credentialing Center [ANCC], n.d.). As nurses seek to embed themselves and grow in jobs and careers within health care services, leadership and management knowledge, skills, and abilities are important to overall effectiveness.

In nursing, leadership is studied to increase the knowledge, skills, and abilities that nurses need to facilitate clinical and administrative outcomes while working with people across a variety of situations, settings, and sites. Effective leadership can also increase understanding and control of nurses' professional work settings. *Effective* leadership is important in nursing, specifically because of its impact on the quality of nurses' work lives, because it functions as a stabilizing influence during constant change, and because it underpins nurses' productivity and quality of care delivery.

Nurse leaders and managers are responsible for designing, developing, implementing, and sustaining the organizational infrastructure and environment that enable both large- and small-scale interventions for quality and safety. Research has shown that there are organizational and cultural factors that mediate hospital or system-wide interventions. These include the prevailing culture, such as being patient-centered and having available effort and resources; human relationships, including leadership styles and teamwork; and an approach used for routine monitoring of systems and services (Clay-Williams et al., 2014; Stetler et al., 2014).

This chapter presents definitions and a detailed overview of both leadership and management. Theories are reviewed and important elements are discussed. There is a long history, rich literature, and evidence base regarding leadership theories, much of it from outside of nursing. Nursing has drawn from both classic and contemporary thinkers, especially from business management.

DEFINITIONS

There are a variety of definitions of **leadership**, one of which is the process of influencing people to accomplish goals. It has been described as "the art of motivating a group of people to act toward achieving a common goal" (Ward, 2020). Key concepts related to leadership are influence, vision, communication, group process, goal attainment, and motivation. Hersey et al. (2013) defined leadership as a process of influencing the behavior of either an individual or a group, regardless of the reason, to achieve goals in a given situation. Leaders mobilize others so that they want to make extraordinary things happen (Kouzes & Posner, 2017).

Most leadership definitions incorporate the two components of an interaction among people and the process of influencing. Thus leadership is a social exchange phenomenon. At its core, leadership is about influencing people. In contrast, management involves influencing employees to meet an organization's goals and is focused primarily on organizational goals and objectives. Thus the leader focuses on people, whereas the manager focuses on systems, processes, and structures. A leader innovates; a manager administers.

Management is defined as the coordination and integration of resources through planning, organizing, coordinating, directing, and controlling to accomplish specific institutional goals and objectives. Hersey et al. (2013) defined management as a process of working with and through individuals and groups, using resources (such as equipment, capital, and technology) to accomplish organizational goals. They identified management as a special kind of leadership that concentrates on the achievement of organizational goals.

Followership is defined as "a process whereby an individual or individuals accept the influence of others to accomplish a common goal" (Northouse, 2019, p. 295).

LEADERSHIP AND CARE MANAGEMENT DIFFERENTIATED

Leadership theory is often discussed separately from management theory. Some say leadership and management are two very different things. Yet clearly there is overlap in that an individual can be *both* leading and managing simultaneously in some cases. The area of overlap may not be clear or explained. The premise of this book is that leadership and management are not identical ideas. This can be seen in their distinct definitions, yet sometimes they occur together or via multitasking. Northouse (2019) differentiated leadership and management on elements of activities and outcomes: management produces order and consistency; leadership produces change and movement.

If the delivery of nursing services involves the organization and coordination of complex activities in the human services realm, then both leadership and management are important elements. Both are used to accomplish goals; each has a different focus. Management is focused on task accomplishment, and leadership is focused on human relationship aspects. They may be sequential, and they are interrelated. Clearly, a balance of the two is necessary. Leadership and management have some shared characteristics. There is a "gray area" in which the focus of their outcomes overlaps. In this area of overlap, the processes and strategies look similar and may be employed for a similar outcome or blended together to accomplish goals. This overlap occurs where the two processes are integrated or synthesized to accomplish goals and where the same strategies are employed even though the goals may differ. For example, a nurse may use leadership strategies or management strategies to motivate others, but the desired outcome of the motivation is likely to be different. For example, leadership may be used to empower nurses and management to reduce costs.

Leadership and management are equally important processes. Because they each have a different focus, their importance varies according to what is needed in a specific situation. Hersey et al. (2013) thought that leadership was a broader concept than management. They described management as a special kind of leadership. This view would position management as a part of leadership, not as a distinct concept. However, according to the definitions, characteristics, and processes, the concepts of leadership and management are different; but at the area of overlap they look similar. For example, directing occurs in both leadership and management activities (the area of overlap), whereas inspiring a vision is clearly a leadership function. Both leadership and management are necessary. Leadership occurs in an interactive mode rather than through a stepwise linear process. The interactive nature makes relationships and relationship building fundamental elements. "Transformational change happens one relationship at a time" (Koloroutis, 2004).

Jennings et al. (2007) took an evidence-based approach to differentiating nursing leadership from management to identify discrete competencies through an integrative content analysis of the literature base. In 140 articles reviewed, they found 894 competencies, of which 862 (96%) were common to both leadership and management. Thus the overlap area appeared to be larger than previously thought. However, leadership and management do serve distinct purposes. Perhaps it is time to apply leadership and management concepts and competencies by setting, level of role responsibility, career stage, and social context to more fully apply the evidence base to practice. For example, the American Organization for Nursing Leadership (AONL, formerly AONE) (2015) promulgated two levels of administrative competencies: nurse manager and nurse executive.

LEADERSHIP OVERVIEW

Leadership is an activity of human engagement and a relationship experience founded in trust, communication, inspiration, action, and "servanthood". The four essential dimensions of leadership are process, influence, group setting (context), and vision (Miles & Scott, 2019). Leadership has elements of process, personalities, power relationships, actions, transformation, and skills, all of which are designed to influence. Ideally, for effectiveness, styles are matched. Northouse (2019, p. 5) found five core leadership components: (1) leadership is a process, (2) leadership involves influence, (3) leadership occurs in groups, and (4) leadership involves common goals. The leadership role is so important because it embodies commitment and forward-reaching action. Arising from a drive to make things better, leaders use their power to bring teams together, spark innovation, create positive communication, and drive forward toward group goals.

Leadership is important to study, learn, and practice in today's complex, rapidly changing, turbulent, and chaotic health care work environment. Such an environment generates challenges to the nurse's identity, coping skills, and ability to work with others in harmony. It also presents the opportunity to lead, challenge assumptions, consolidate a purpose, and move a vision forward. Leadership is important for nurses because they need to possess knowledge and skills in the art and science of solving problems in work groups, systems of care, and the environment of care delivery. The effectiveness of an individual nurse depends partly on that individual's competence and partly on the creation of a facilitating environment that contains sufficient resources to accomplish goals. This is an underappreciated reality when it is assumed that results occur from only individual competence and effort. However, health care delivery is a team effort.

The nurse leader combines clinical, administrative, financial, and operational skills to solve problems in the care environment so that nurses can provide cost-effective care in a way that is satisfying and health promoting for patients and clients. Such an environment does not simply happen; it requires special skills and the courage and motivation to move a vision into action. For example, it may be easier to continue on the way things have always been done, but this strategy would not capture the advantages of new innovations. Thus the study of nursing leadership and care management directs critical thinking toward what it takes to be a nursing "environment architect," transition leader, and administrator of care delivery services.

Strong evidence for the nurse leader's critical role both in the business of a health care organization and in the quality and safety of service delivery can be found in influential documents by the IOM (2004), the ANCC's Magnet Recognition Program® (ANCC, n.d.a), and the AONL (2015). The IOM emphasized evidence-based management practice and focused on the following five areas of management practice:

- Implementing evidence-based management
- Balancing tensions between efficiency and reliability
- Creating and sustaining trust
- Actively managing the change process through communication, feedback, training, sustained effort and attention, and worker involvement
- Creating a learning environment

The ANCC's Magnet program acknowledges excellence in nursing services and leadership based on five components: transformational leadership, structural empowerment, new knowledge, exemplary professional practice, and empirical outcomes (ANCC, n.d.a). The Magnet Recognition Program® focuses specifically on nursing, is considered the "gold standard" in nursing, and is addressed in several chapters in this book because of its centrality to the evidence-based management practice called for by the IOM (2004). AONL's (2015) nurse executive competencies are described as falling within the following five domains of skill: communication and relationship management, leadership, business skills and principles, knowledge of the health care environment, and professionalism. Taken together, these source documents overlap and converge on the primary attributes, knowledge domains, abilities, and skills that nurse leaders need to lead people and manage organizations in health care.

The Two Roles of a Nurse

Nursing is a service profession, the core mission of which is the care, restoration of health, and nurturing of human beings in their experiences of health and illness. This is the role of the nurse as a direct care provider. The nurse's care provider or "doing" role is sometimes seen as the most important and valued aspect of nursing. The nurse's second role, the coordinator/integrator role, is a complementary function that arises from nursing's central positioning in the day-to-day coordination of service delivery and central location at the hub of information flow regarding care and service delivery. This linkage relationship is shown visually in Fig. 1.1.

With the shift to primary care and care coordination, the nurse's care management role has become more prominent, needed, and valued. The delivery of nursing services involves the organization and coordination of complex activities. Nurses use managerial and leadership skills to facilitate delivery of quality nursing care. A current example is the shift to population health management (PHM), which is in concert with the Quadruple Aim. Nurses have emerged as well-prepared practitioners, especially at the clinical nurse leader (CNL) and nurse practitioner levels of preparation (Joseph & Huber, 2015).

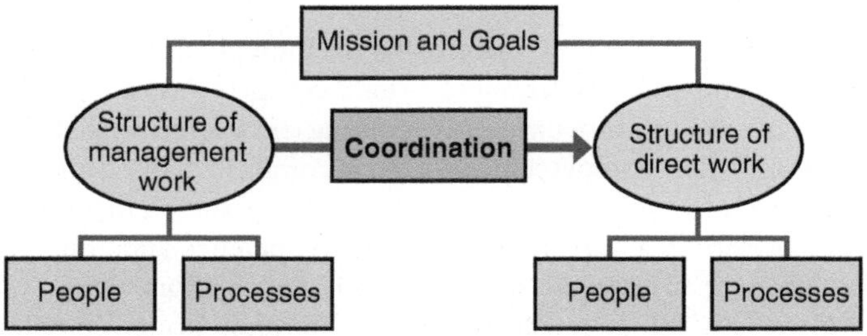

Fig. 1.1 Linkage of clinical and management domains.

The Leadership Role

Leadership is a unique role and function. It can be part of a formal organizational managerial position, or it can arise spontaneously in any group. Certain characteristics, such as being motivated by challenge, commitment, and autonomy, are thought to be associated with leadership. Effectiveness is a key outcome of leadership efforts in health care. It has been suggested that there is a scarcity of leaders and a crisis in leadership in nursing. In times of chaos, complexity, and change, leadership is essential to provide the guidance, direction, and sense of stability needed to ensure followers' effectiveness and satisfaction. Nurses are challenged to respond with leadership and can best respond by demonstrating vision, using innovativeness (Joseph, 2015; Joseph et al., 2016), adapting to changes, seeking new tools for dealing with the new health care environment, and leading the way with client-centered strategies. Effective leaders are change agents and promote innovation. Innovation is seen as a viable mechanism to address care delivery complexity and is further discussed in Chapter 2.

Leadership Skills

Leadership is a natural element of nursing practice because the majority of nurses practice in work groups or units. Possessing the license of an RN implies certain leadership skills and requires the ability to delegate and supervise the work of others. Leadership can be understood as the ability to inspire confidence and support among followers, especially in organizations in which competence and commitment produce performance.

Leadership is an important issue related to how nurses integrate the various elements of nursing practice to ensure the highest quality of care for clients. Every nurse needs two critical skills to enhance professional practice. One is a skill with interpersonal relationships. This is fundamental to leadership and the work of nursing. The second is skill in applying the problem-solving process. This involves the ability to think critically, identify problems, and develop objectivity and a degree of maturity or judgment. Leadership skills build on professional and clinical skills. Hersey et al. (2013) identified the following three skills needed for leading or influencing:

1. *Diagnosing:* Diagnosing involves being able to understand the situation and the problem to be solved or resolved. This is a cognitive competency.
2. *Adapting:* Adapting involves being able to adapt behaviors and other resources to match the situation. This is a behavioral competency.
3. *Communicating:* Communicating is used to advance the process in a way that individuals can understand and accept. This is a process competency.

Emotional Intelligence

Relational and emotional integrity are hallmarks of good leaders. Among the important personal leadership skills for nurses is **emotional** intelligence (EI). EI traits are emotional factors consisting of five defining attributes: self-awareness, self-regulation or discipline, motivation, social awareness, and relationship management. EI can be understood as a constellation of self-perceptions of the person's empathy, impulsivity, and assertiveness, also including elements of social and personal intelligence. EI is seen as an intellectual skill helping to understand and assess the meaning of emotions, to reason, and to problem solve. EI has a strong and positive impact on organizational climate. A positive organizational climate is less likely to contain counterproductive work behaviors or unethical dysfunctional organizational behavior (Al Ghazo et al., 2019). EI has been studied in nursing and shown to be related to transformational leadership (Spano-Szekely et al., 2016), nursing team performance and cohesiveness (Quoidbach & Hansenne, 2009), quality of care (Adams & Iseler, 2014), and as a moderator of **stress** and **burnout** (Görgens-Ekermans & Brand, 2010). Spano-Szekely and colleagues recommended that EI characteristics be considered during the hiring of nurse managers.

Adaptive thinking abilities are needed for leadership in the complex, volatile, and unpredictable environment of health care (Spano-Szekely et al., 2016). This is because the leader operates in a crucial cultural and contextual influencing mode within the organizational environment. The leader's behavior, patterns of actions, attitude, and performance have a special impact on the team's attitude and behaviors and on the context and character of work life. Followers observe and respond to all aspects of what leaders say and do (or do not do). Followers need to be able to depend on role consistency, balance, and behavioral integrity from the leader. The four EI skill sets needed by good leaders are as follows:

1. *Self-awareness:* Ability to read one's own emotional state and be aware of one's own mood and how this affects staff relationships

2. *Self-management:* Ability to take corrective action so as not to transfer negative affect to staff relationships
3. *Social awareness:* An intuitive skill of empathy and expressiveness in being sensitive and aware of the emotions and moods of others
4. *Relationship management:* Use of effective communication with others to disarm conflict and the ability to develop the emotional maturity of team members

Relationship Management and Relational Coordination

High performance, organizational health, and effectiveness are organizational goals. Relationship-based care has been proposed as a model for nursing care that promotes organizational health, thus resulting in positive outcomes (Koloroutis, 2004). Relationship-based care focuses on the care provider's three crucial relationships: relationship with patients and families, with self (nurtured by self-knowing and self-care), and with colleagues (commitment to healthy interpersonal relationships) (Creative Health Care Management, 2020).

Gittell (2016) emphasized the centrality of relationship management because patient care is a coordination challenge. She noted that relational coordination drives quality and efficiency outcomes and health care performance. Relational coordination is defined as "… coordinating work through relationships of shared goals, shared knowledge, and mutual respect" (p. 13). Relational coordination focuses on *relationships among roles* rather than between individuals.

Interpersonal relationship skills are crucial to the work of leadership. Leaders are pivotal for connecting the efforts of followers to organizational goals in order to produce outcomes. However, good leaders manage relationships and are anchors to the vision and the larger mission, guides to coping and being productive, and champions of energy and enthusiasm for the work.

BACKGROUND RELATED TO LEADERSHIP

Terms related to leadership are *leadership styles, followership*, and *empowerment.* **Leadership** styles are defined as different combinations of task and relationship behaviors used to influence others to accomplish goals. **Followership** is defined as an interpersonal process of participation: "a process whereby an individual or individuals accept the influence of others to accomplish a common goal" (Northouse, 2019, p. 295). **Empowerment** means giving people the authority, responsibility, and freedom to act on their expert knowledge and skills.

Self-awareness is an important aspect of both leadership and followership. This means that nurses can assess themselves to better understand their own style and leadership characteristics. Self assessment tools are available to assist nurses in awareness of both leadership and followership behaviors. Examples are the LEAD instruments developed by Hersey et al. (2013), the Multifactor Leadership Questionnaire (MLQ) (Bass & Avolio, 2019), and multiple training instruments. Leadership related research instruments were identified, compared, and evaluated by Huber and colleagues (2000). Some instruments are useful for research and others for leadership training or self-diagnosis. A wide variety of tools are available to help individuals increase their effectiveness through greater awareness and subsequent honing of both their leadership and followership skills.

Leadership can be best understood as a process. Much attention has been focused on leadership as a group and organizational process because organizational change is heavily influenced by the context or environment. Nurses need to have a solid foundation of knowledge in leadership and care management at all levels, although the depth and focus of care management roles and skills may vary by level. For example, the clinical nurse care provider or direct care ("bedside") nurse concentrates on the coordination of nursing care to individuals or groups and is a leader and manager within his or her scope of practice. This may include such activities as arranging access to services, providing direct care, doing referrals, and supporting a patient's family.

Nurses without formal positional authority are **informal leaders**. They influence peers and administrators and function in an influence sphere within interdisciplinary teams. They have varying forms of power, but they are a part of the shadow organization that operates behind the scenes of the formal chain of command in informal networks of people and influence. They serve as advocates for the work being done and heighten the contributions of themselves and others through influence, relationship building, knowledge, and expertise. These nurses can be developed and empowered to affect unit performance and culture.

At the next level, the nurse manager concentrates on the day-to-day administration and coordination of services provided by a group of nurses. The nurse executive's role and functions concentrate on long-term administration of an institution or program that delivers nursing services, focusing on integrating the system and building a culture. CNLs and advanced practice registered nurses (APRNs) provide leadership in the care and care transitions of individuals and populations while providing expertise to the organization in specialty areas.

LEADERSHIP: FIVE INTERWOVEN ASPECTS

Hersey et al. (2013) noted that the leadership process is a function of the leader, the followers, and other situational variables. The leadership process includes five interwoven, connected but distinct, aspects: (1) the leader, (2) the follower, (3) the situation, (4) the communication process, and (5) the goals. Fig. 1.2 shows how these components relate to one another. All five elements interact within any given leadership circumstance.

Process Part 1: The Leader

The values, skills, and style of the leader are important. His or her internalized pattern of basic behaviors influences actions and the ability to lead. Leaders' perceptions of themselves, their roles, and their expectations also have an impact on their followers. Self-awareness is crucial to leadership effectiveness and is an EI skill. Among the internal forces in leaders that impinge on leadership style are values, energy level, confidence in employees, leadership inclinations, motivation for leadership, and sense of security in uncertainty. Interpersonal, emotional, and social intelligence skills also contribute to effective leadership.

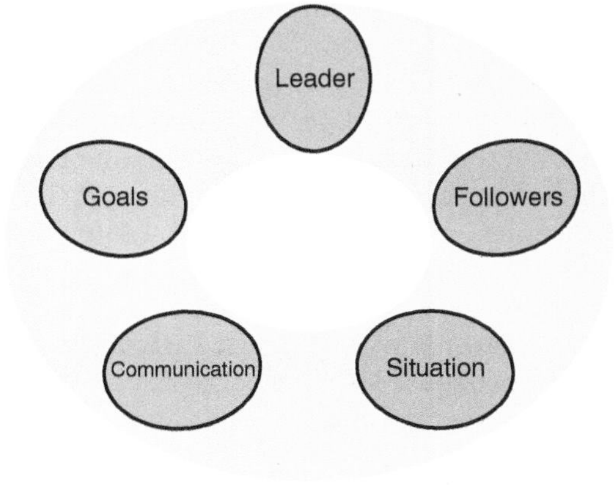

Fig. 1.2 Components of a leadership moment.

Self-awareness is an important aspect of both leadership and followership. This means that nurses can assess themselves to better understand their own style and leadership characteristics. Self-assessment tools are available to assist nurses in awareness of both leadership and followership behaviors. Examples are the LEAD instruments developed by Hersey et al. (2013), the Multifactor Leadership Questionnaire (MLQ) (Bass & Avolio, 2019), and multiple training instruments. A wide variety of tools are available to help individuals increase their effectiveness through greater awareness and subsequent honing of both their leadership and followership skills.

Process Part 2: The Follower and Followership

Followership is the flip side of leadership. It is likely that without followers there is no leadership. Followers are vital because they accept or reject the leader and determine the leader's personal power (Hersey et al., 2013). Followership skill is underappreciated. Grossman and Valiga (2017) suggested that leaders are only leaders if they have followers. Followership can be learned and consciously developed. Northouse (2019) differentiated followership based on roles or positions within an organizational structure versus based on relationships in an interpersonal context.

Types of Followers

There are several typologies that distinguish types of followers. Styles can be plotted along the two axes of passive to active and dependent to independent. Grossman and Valiga (2017) identified types of followers on dimensions of activity and independence: effective or exemplary, alienated, yes people, and sheep.

Understanding types of followers is as important as understanding types of leaders: it creates the ability to match leadership style to effectiveness in care delivery. Effective followers are an asset to be nurtured, developed, and valued. Effective followers contribute to success in organizations because they contribute motivation, enthusiasm, expertise, energy, innovation, and goal-orientation. Nurses can and should examine their own behavior and ask themselves the question, "In this situation, what kind of follower am I?"

There are types of followers, ranging from being vital to the success of the group to being passive and unthinking. Using the variables of performance initiative (high to low) and relationship initiative (high to low), Grossman and Valiga (2017) developed a grid of four followership styles: subordinate, contributor, partner, and politician. Effective followers show characteristics of assertiveness, determination, willingness to challenge ideas, an ability to act, and openness to new ideas. Followers also need self-awareness to know themselves and their expectations. Situations in which members of a group are not accustomed to working together or do not hold shared expectations frequently lead to conflict. Followership is based on trust. Groups have personalities that include a discernible level of trust. The wise leader assesses the trust and readiness to change levels of the group. Northouse (2019) discussed four typologies of followership. For example, Kelley's Typology plots active/passive and independent/dependent critical thinking into five types: passive, conformist, alienated, pragmatic, and exemplary. Other typologies plot dominance versus passivity, support versus challenge, and followers' levels of engagement.

Followership is not as simple as it seems. Followership can be assessed similar to leadership style and becomes a part of self-awareness (e.g., Followership Questionnaire in Northouse, 2019).

Leaders do not operate in isolation. Instead, leadership involves cooperation and collaboration. The basic nature of leadership is interactive; it revolves around the interpersonal relationships among leaders and followers. Therefore cooperation and collaboration between the leader and followers enhance the group's effectiveness. Although it may seem obvious, followership quality is important. There is a dynamic relationship between leaders and followers, and both are important.

Followership is an interpersonal process of participation. It implies an engagement of the follower with the leader, and possibly a group, by which the follower takes guidance and direction from the leader to accomplish group goals. The importance of followership is emphasized because leadership requires the presence of followers. The relationship between the leader and the followers defines leadership. The corollary to leadership is followership, which is helping to get the job done. A good leader clearly needs good followers, and this relationship is based on giving direction, trust, and hope. Kouzes and Posner (2017) noted that for people to follow willingly, they need to believe the leader is honest, forward looking, competent, and inspiring. With these three elements in place, followers are empowered in their participation efforts. Any situation can be analyzed to determine whether the desired leader attributes are present and to what extent.

Process Part 3: The Situation

The specific circumstances surrounding any given leadership situation will vary. Elements such as work demands, control systems, amount of task structure, degree of interaction, amount of time available for decision-making, and external environment shape the differences among situations (Hersey et al., 2013). For example, in acute care hospitals, staffing levels and policies strongly influence many aspects of a nurse's work life. Organizational culture and ethos are also important factors in the situation. For example, in one setting the culture may resemble one big happy family, with an emphasis on teamwork and morale boosting. The cultural aspects of that leadership situation are different from those of an organization where there is a fast-paced tempo and people seem too busy and/or in a bullying environment. Environmental or cultural differences also cause the leadership situation to vary. The leadership situation in a group that is knowledgeable and experienced in solving problems is very different from the leadership situation in a group that is not experienced at the task or at working together. The personality styles of both superiors and subordinates have an influence on the situation, the work demands, and the amount of time and resources available.

Process Part 4: Communication

Communication processes vary among groups regarding the patterns and channels used and the degree to which the communication flow is open or closed. Communicating is basic to the process of influencing and thus to leadership (see Chapter 8). Almost every issue or problem contains a communication aspect. Through communication, the leader's vision and message are received by the followers. After choosing a channel, the sender transmits a message, but the message is filtered through the receiver's perception. Communication is transmitted through both verbal and nonverbal modes. Organizations include a variety of communication structures and flows. These may be downward, upward, horizontal, grapevines, or networks. Communication may be formal or informal (Hersey et al., 2013). Certain acts performed by leaders have positive effects and make people feel more respected; listening and informal chatting are prime examples because they foster interpersonal and relational trust and social cohesion.

Process Part 5: Goals

Organizations have goals, and individuals working in organizations also have goals. These goals may or may not be congruent. For example, the goal of the organization may be to decrease costs or increase revenue. In contrast, the goal of the individual nurse may be to spend time counseling and teaching clients because that is what is seen by the nurse as the most important activity. Goals may thus be in conflict, in which case there is tension and a need for leadership.

Clearly, leadership is a complex and multidimensional process. Nurses need to be aware of the interacting elements in any leadership situation. Critical thinking can be applied to diagnosing and analyzing the five elements, adapting to the situation, and communicating for effectiveness. For example, if a nurse works in a situation in which there is a high level of frustration, it may be time to step back and analyze the basic five elements. Doing so sets the stage for better decision-making about change strategies and strategic management.

LEADERSHIP THEORIES

Leadership is so critical that it has been studied for a very long time, especially in the business literature. There are numerous theories and extensive research. The condensation here will highlight core concepts and common theories.

Leadership is fundamentally about the two basic elements of tasks and relationships. **Tasks** are the job aspects that must be done to produce the product (e.g., nursing care). Human **relationships** are the "people element": the interpersonal workings of humans in a job environment.

Hersey et al. (2013) have done a thorough overview of leadership and organizational theory up through the situational leadership school of thought. From an early awareness of the leader's need to be concerned about both tasks and human relationships (output and people) sprang a long history of leadership theories that can be grouped as *trait, attitudinal*, and *situational* (Hersey et al., 2013). The trait approach focuses on identifying specific characteristics of leaders. The attitudinal approach measures attitudes toward leader behavior. The situational approach focuses on observed behaviors of leaders and how leadership styles can be matched to situations.

Trait Theories: Characteristics of Leadership

Leadership theories have evolved away from an early focus on the traits or characteristics of the leader as a person because it was found that it is not possible to predict leadership from clusters of traits, yet interest remains in the characteristics to look for in good leaders. In the trait approach, theorists have sought to understand leadership by examining the characteristics of leaders, leading to multiple lists of traits proposed to be essential to leadership. One result was the awareness that leadership skills can be both taught and learned. It is important for nurses to recognize that they can learn, practice, and improve their personal leadership competencies.

Leaders are active, not passive. Leaders engage their environment with behaviors of doing, influencing, and moving. These are action terms that need to be melded with expertise and empathy. Leaders are those who talk about adventures into new territory and take the risks inherent in innovation (Kouzes & Posner, 2017). Leadership means giving guidance and using a focused vision.

Characteristics such as knowledge, motivating people to work harder, trust, communication, enthusiasm, vision, courage, ability to see the big picture, and ability to take risks are associated with important leadership qualities in research findings. Kouzes and Posner (2017) found that for people to be willing followers, the leader needs to be honest, forward-looking, competent, and inspiring. They identified the Five Practices of Exemplary Leadership that correlate with leadership excellence:

1. *Model the way*: Leaders set an example and structure events so that incremental progress is celebrated as small wins.
2. *Inspire a shared vision*: Leaders envision the future and enlist others in sharing the dream.
3. *Challenge the process*: Leaders go beyond the status quo to search for opportunities, experiment, and take risks to achieve lofty goals.
4. *Enable others to act*: Leaders foster collaboration and develop and strengthen others so that the whole team performs well.
5. *Encourage the heart*: Leaders appreciate and recognize individual contributions and formally celebrate accomplishments.

This model of leadership has been used in nursing research looking at staff nurse clinical leadership (Patrick et al., 2011).

Vision and Trust

Although the lists of leadership characteristics and competencies vary somewhat, the functions of visioning, setting the direction, inspiration, motivation, and enabling systems and followers are at the core of leadership activity. The one specific defining quality of leaders is vision: the ability to create a vision and put it into operation.

Leadership is founded on trust: "Trust is the emotional glue that binds leaders and employees together and is a measure of the legitimacy of leadership" (Malloch, 2002, p. 14). Organizations that focus on sustaining a healing culture rebuild organizational trust by focusing on trust in relationships with employees. Behaviors that build trust include sharing relevant information, reducing controls, and meeting expectations. Trust-destroying behaviors include being insensitive to beliefs and values, avoiding discussion of sensitive issues, and encouraging competition via winners and losers. Trust goes both ways and needs to be nurtured. Nurses can start by examining their own behaviors and then taking deliberative actions to strengthen trust in the environment.

Leadership Styles Theories

As leadership theories evolved, leadership came to be viewed as a dynamic process and an interaction among the leader, the followers, and the situation. Leadership theory began to move beyond a focus on traits to explore the concept of leadership styles. Styles of leadership range from authoritarian to permissive to democratic and from transactional to transformational. The individual nurse's task is to determine in which environments he or she functions best and is most comfortable or where he or she most likely will succeed. This facilitates placement for success and a better match between leader and follower.

Leadership styles are defined as different combinations of task and relationship behaviors used to influence others to accomplish goals. They are sets or clusters of behaviors used in the process of effecting leadership. Hersey et al. (2013) defined these terms as follows:

- *Task behavior*: The extent to which leaders organize and define roles; explain activities; determine when, where, and how tasks are to be accomplished; and endeavor to get work accomplished
- *Relationship behavior*: The extent to which leaders maintain personal relationships by opening communication and providing psycho-emotional support and facilitating behaviors

Hersey et al. (2013) said that leadership styles are the consistent behavior patterns exhibited in influencing the activities of others by working with and through them, as perceived by those others. Different styles evoke variable responses in different situations. A leader's leadership style is some combination of task and relationship behavior. A style may range from democratic to authoritarian (or subordinate centered to leader centered) (Fig. 1.3). Schooley (2019) identified nine different leadership styles:

1. **Autocratic leadership:** The leader primarily uses directive behaviors. Decisions of policy are made solely by the leader, who tends to dictate tasks and techniques to followers. Leaders tell the followers what to do and how to do it. This style emphasizes a high concern for task. Authoritarian leaders are

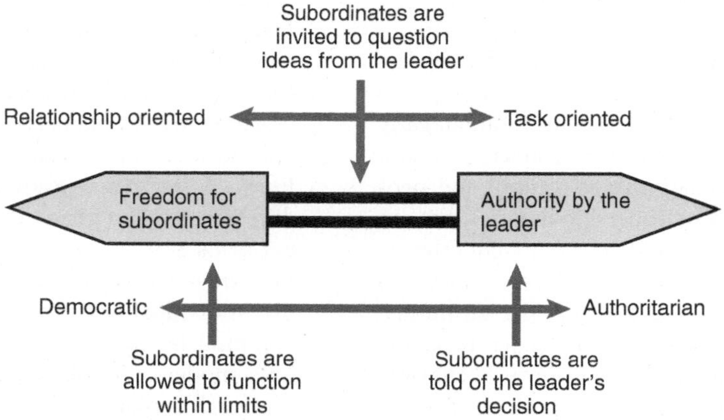

Fig. 1.3 Continuum of leader behavior.

characterized by giving orders. Their style can create hostility and dependency among followers; this may also stifle creativity and innovation. On the other hand, this style can be very efficient, especially in a crisis or during a code situation.

2. **Bureaucratic leadership:** Although not as strict as autocratic leaders, bureaucratic leaders tend to strictly enforce regulations and statuses in the hierarchy. They strive to maintain the status quo. They carry out policies and procedures. This leadership style can be effective in complex healthcare and safety environments or where there is high risk and stability is desired.
3. **Charismatic leadership:** Charismatic leaders have an infectious presence that attracts followers and motivates their team to follow their lead. Their likability helps achieve success. This leadership style can be effective in high-energy work environments that need a lot of positive motivation and team morale. The danger arises in following the "cult of personality" instead of using critical thinking.
4. **Democratic leadership:** A democratic leader often welcomes subordinate participation in decision-making. This approach implies a relationship and person orientation. Policies are a matter of group discussion and decision. The leader encourages and assists discussion and group decision-making. Human relations and teamwork are the focus. The leader shares responsibility with the followers by involving them in decision-making. In nursing, interdisciplinary teamwork is a major element in effectiveness. The democratic style may appear to move more slowly and is thought to take longer than using an authoritarian style. This is because group consensus needs time and facilitation to be fostered. Furthermore, the needs of disenfranchised minority groups must be balanced. Intergroup cohesion is a focus with this style. The challenge of the democratic style is to get people with different professional backgrounds, personal biases, and psychological needs together to focus on the problem and next action steps. Motivating participation is a constant challenge. This leadership style is often admired and can be effective in creative work environments that do not require quick decisions.
5. **Laissez-faire leadership:** Laissez-faire leaders have a hands-off approach and let their employees assume responsibility in the decision-making process, although they must still set expectations and monitor performance. This style promotes complete freedom for group or individual decisions. There is a minimum of leader participation. A leader using this style may seem to be apathetic. Because the style is based on noninterference, a clear decision may never be formulated. The laissez-faire style results in a decision, conscious or otherwise, to avoid interference and let events take their own course. The leader is either permissive and fosters freedom or is inept at guiding a group. Followers may need greater structure than the leader gives them. Despite its potential drawbacks, this style has advantages when used with some circumstances involving groups of fully independent care providers or professionals working together. This leadership style is seen as effective when working with highly experienced and confident employees.
6. **Servant leadership:** Servant leaders are those who share power and decision-making with their subordinates and direct the organization based on the interests of the team. Servant leaders put others first. They choose to make sure that other people's highest-priority needs are being served in a way that promotes personal growth and helps others become freer and more autonomous. This leadership style can be effective for humanitarian organizations, nonprofits, and teams that need to create diversity, inclusion, and morale.
7. **Situational leadership:** Situational leaders see the use of leadership style as situational or contingent based on what produces effectiveness. They first do a specific assessment of all aspects of the situation and then modify their style to match the situation based on the needs of their employees and the environment. Because of its versatility, this type of leadership can be effective in most organizations.
8. **Transactional leadership:** A transactional leader is focused on day-to-day operations and uses a reward/consequence system to motivate employees to achieve success or discourage them from failure. Transactional leadership is a social exchange (this for that). This leadership style can be effective for teams or individuals who are motivated by rewards or immediate needs.
9. **Transformational leadership:** Similar to charismatic leaders, transformational leaders use their inspiring energy and personality to create a magnetic workplace. They engage with others so that leaders and

followers raise each other to higher levels of motivation. The transformational type is often more effective than charismatic leadership, because it also is centered on the followers', not the leader's, needs and goals and motivates teams to build confidence, skills, achievement, and accountability. Transformational leadership can be effective in organizations with intellectual team members who thrive in interactive environments.

There is no one "right" style. Each has its strengths. Effectiveness comes from pairing leadership styles with organizational fit, timing, and needs. There are situational and contextual factors to consider when choosing a style. Styles should vary according to the appropriateness of the situation with reference to an evaluation of effectiveness. Flexibility is important. For example, if a nurse prefers to operate in a democratic style yet suddenly a code situation occurs, then the nurse must rapidly switch from a democratic to an authoritarian style. Some democratic leaders cannot vary their style sufficiently to handle crises. On the other hand, in a staff meeting, an authoritarian leader may be ineffective with a group of professionals and would need to be flexible enough to switch to a democratic or laissez-faire style, depending on the circumstances. The basic needs are for leader self-awareness and knowledge of the group's ability and willingness levels before examining the situational elements and choosing a leadership style. Self-awareness is key to strategically using leadership styles.

Feminist Leadership Perspective

Leadership styles appear to have a gender component. The feminist perspective on leadership was presented originally by Helgeson (1995a, 1995b). She identified female leadership as a web-like structure that is dynamic and continuously expanding and contracting. It is characterized by a concern for family, community, and culture. The inclination is for a democratic power style, and the emphasis is on the importance of establishing relationships, maintaining connections with others, and deriving strength from empowering others. By contrast, leadership approaches described by men, as a generalization, tend to be influenced by the military and participating in team sports. Men tend to spend their time on meetings and tasks requiring immediate attention, focusing on completion of tasks and achievement of goals. Women tend to focus on process; men tend to focus on achievement and closure. Women tend to be more flexible and value cooperation, connectedness, and relationships. Exploring the feminist perspective on leadership is valuable in that it provides food for thought as health care organizations and the predominantly female nurses working in them struggle with not wanting to let go of the familiar hierarchical management style yet needing to reconfigure to the circular or web structure to be effective. It is not known whether gender differences are permanent characteristics or are culturally mediated artifacts that blur with time.

Reynolds (2011) explored the thesis that servant leadership is a gender-integrative, partnership-oriented approach to leadership, using the feminist ethic of care. Leadership is a system for organizing activity, and gender is a system for organizing meaning. Yet mainstream leadership theory has ignored gender-related aspects of power. Scholars of communication and leadership have identified the management of meaning as one of the significant acts of leadership.

Situational Leadership Theories

A group of leadership contingency theories posit that organizational behavior is contingent on the situation or environment. This means that which theory or style is the best all depends on the situation at hand. What is needed by the leader is diagnostic ability. The leader observes and analyzes which abilities and motives are present in the followers. With sensitivity, cues in the environment can be identified and used to make choices regarding leadership style. One choice a leader has is to alter his or her own behavior and the leadership style used. Personal flexibility and leadership skills are needed to vary one's style when the followers' needs and motives change or vary. The ability to diagnose, choose, and alter behavior to implement a leadership style best matched to the situation is a critical skill needed for effective leadership (Hersey et al., 2013).

In situational leadership theories, leadership in groups is never a static circumstance. The situation is dynamic and subject to change. In a very difficult situation, relationships may be the leader's preferred emphasis. However, if interpersonal relationships are not an immediate problem or if the group is on the verge of collapse, then strong authoritative direction is needed to get the group moving and accomplishing. For this situation, the task-oriented leader is a more effective match between leader and job. However, groups do not remain static; they move back and forth through stages. When the problem is no longer just the need to get the group moving but also includes solving numerous interpersonal conflicts, a relationship-oriented leader is better matched to the situation. Eventually, as the situation progresses, a relationship-oriented leader can become less effective. This occurs because once the group has less conflict, individuals may begin to coast along, and positive motivation may be lost as individuals become apathetic. Once again, a task-oriented style is called for to challenge individuals by using the motivation they need to continue to produce. Because of the factor of constant change, maintaining good leadership is complicated for any group.

The Situational Leadership® Model

The Situational Leadership® Model of Hersey et al. (2013; The Center for Leadership Studies, 2020) focuses on the interplay among three elements: the amount of guidance and direction (task behavior) a leader gives; the amount of socioemotional support (relationship behavior) a leader provides; and the Performance Readiness® Level that individuals or teams (followers) exhibit in performing specific activity, task, or job. Using a grid that results from task and relationship axes ranging from high to low, task behavior is plotted on the horizontal axis, and relationship behavior is plotted on the vertical axis. See the grid on The Center for Leadership Studies' (2020) website: https://situational.com/situational-leadership/. This makes it possible to describe leader behavior in four quadrants: (1) high task, low relationship (S1, telling); (2) high task, high relationship (S2, selling); (3) high relationship, low task (S3, participating); and (4) low task, low relationship (S4, delegating). As applied to the continuum of authoritarian versus democratic styles, telling would be authoritarian and participating would be democratic.

To choose an appropriate style, the leader needs to be knowledgeable about the Performance Readiness® level of the followers. This leads to the third dimension of effectiveness: the situation, or environment, which determines the effectiveness of a leader's behavior style (Hersey et al., 2013). Thus the difference between effective and ineffective styles often will not be the actual behavior of the leader but rather the appropriateness of the leader's behavior as matched to the environment in which it is used.

Found below the basic grid is a continuum of Performance Readiness® ranging from low to high. The Performance Readiness® level of an individual or group is determined by both ability and willingness. The first consideration regarding readiness is the followers' ability. *Ability* is the demonstrated knowledge, experience, and skill that a follower brings to a task or activity. *Knowledge* is demonstrated understanding of the task. *Skill* is the demonstrated proficiency in the task. *Experience* is the demonstrated ability gained from performing a task (Hersey et al., 2013).

The other part of readiness is *willingness*. Willingness is the extent to which a follower has demonstrated confidence, commitment, and motivation to accomplish a specific task. *Confidence* is demonstrated self-assurance in the ability to perform a task. *Commitment* is demonstrated dedication to perform a task. *Motivation* is demonstrated desire to perform a task (Hersey et al., 2013). Both ability and willingness need to be assessed; then they can be plotted on the grid to determine readiness.

Hersey et al. (2013) combined the aspects of ability and willingness and showed them displayed on the grid in four levels of readiness: (1) R1: both unable and unwilling or insecure; (2) R2: unable but willing or confident; (3) R3: able but unwilling or insecure; and (4) R4: both able and willing or confident. The Situational Leadership® Model correlates the four different levels of Performance Readiness® to the four basic leadership styles. The result is a visual display and model that provides the opportunity for the leader to assess a follower's behavior and identifies a way to understand and select the leadership style that has the highest probability of effectively influencing a specific person for a specific task.

Thus at the Situational Leadership® Model's core, Hersey et al. (2013) emphasized the importance of the readiness of followers. Any leader behavior is predicted to be more or less effective depending on the Performance Readiness® of the followers that the leader is attempting to influence. The leader's chosen leadership style would have to consider where the followers are in terms of their Performance Readiness® level. The principles of the Situational Leadership® Model can be applied to a work group. The leader begins with assessment and analysis. Have the members worked together for a long time in the job, or are they new employees? The culture is more solidified in a work group that has worked together for many years on a unit. Using the Situational Leadership® Model, leaders (1) identify the specific job, task or activity, (2) assess current Performance Readiness®, and (3) match and communicate by selecting and exhibiting the appropriate leadership style: S1, S2, S3, or S4 (Hersey et al., 2013). For example, telling is an appropriate leadership style to use with followers who are at the novice level and with followers who are unable, unwilling, or insecure. An example is when a nurse is appointed as chair of a committee. The nurse needs to assess and then adapt his or her leadership style to match the Performance Readiness® level of the followers in order to be most effective.

Thus in this view of leadership, it is situational or contingent and concerned with what produces effectiveness. Hersey et al. (2013) noted that the common themes include the following: the leader needs to be flexible in behavior, able to diagnose the leadership style appropriate to the situation, and able to apply the appropriate style given the Performance Readiness® of followers.

Transactional and Transformational Leadership

Another way of looking at leadership is how leaders produce quantum results. The concept of leadership styles broadened over time to include two types of leaders: the transactional leader and the transformational leader.

A *transactional leader* is defined as a leader or manager who functions in a caretaker role and is focused on day-to-day operations. Such leaders survey their followers' needs and set goals for them based on what can be expected from the followers. A transactional leader is focused on the maintenance and management of ongoing and routine work. Transactional leadership is a social exchange: one thing is exchanged for another, generally to accomplish daily work (Steaban, 2016).

A *transformational leader* is defined as a leader who motivates followers to perform to their full potential over time by influencing a change in perceptions and by providing a sense of direction. Transformational leaders use charisma, individualized consideration, and intellectual stimulation to produce greater effort, effectiveness, and satisfaction in followers. Transformational leaders grow and develop others by empowering them (Steaban, 2016). Fig. 1.4 distinguishes between transactional and transformational leadership.

The transactional leader is more common. This type of leader approaches followers in an exchange posture, with the purpose of exchanging one thing for another,

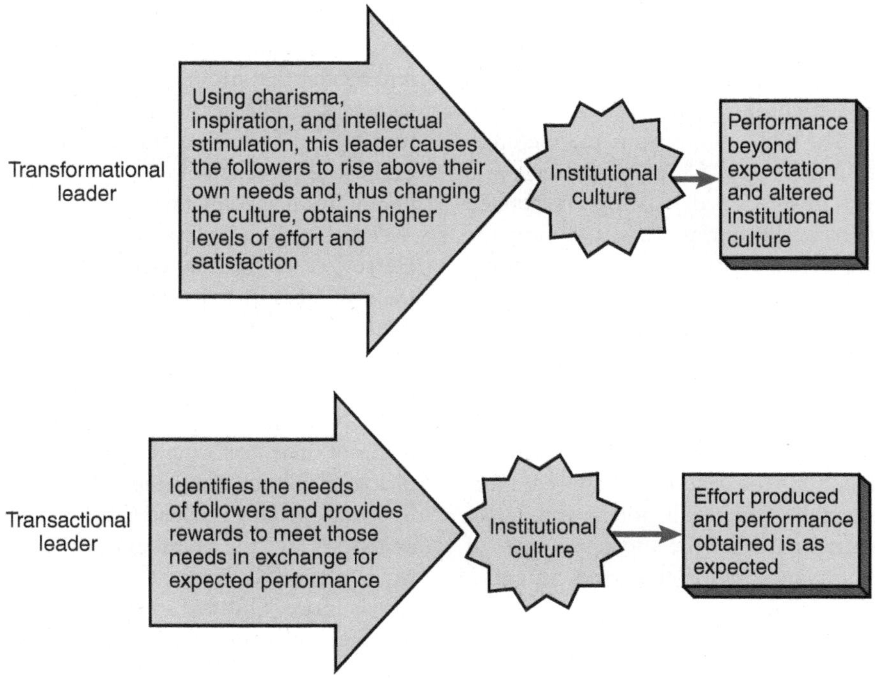

Fig. 1.4 Transactional and transformational leadership.

such as a politician who promises jobs for votes. Transactional leadership is about the exchange of valued things. Therefore transactional leadership is comparable to a bargain or contract for mutual benefits that aids both the leader and the follower. The transactional leader works within the existing organizational culture and is an essential component of effective leadership at the level of task accomplishment. Examples would be the exchange of a salary for the services of a nurse to provide care or when a leader offers release time or paid time to entice staff members to do project or committee work. Continuous or incremental change, the first order of change, can be handled well at the transactional level.

Transformational leadership occurs when persons engage with others so that leaders and followers raise each other to higher levels of motivation. Instead of emphasizing differences between the leader and the followers, transformational leadership focuses on collective purpose and mutual growth and development. Transformational leadership augments transactional leadership by being committed, having a vision, and empowering others to heighten motivation in a way that attains extra effort beyond performance expectations. Transformational leadership is used for higher-order change and to change the organization's culture. Circumstances of growth, change, and crisis call forth transformational leaders, and transformational leadership has been studied regarding successful change management (Deschamps et al., 2016).

There is nursing research to demonstrate the positive outcomes of transformational leadership. The American Nurses Credentialing Center's (ANCC, n.d.a) Magnet Recognition Program® has emphasized transformational leadership approaches. For example, the chief nursing officer of Magnet-designated organizations' transformational leadership style has been shown to have a positive impact on the work environment (Buck & Doucette, 2015). Transformational leadership was the type of leadership most often reported in early Magnet research studies (Upenieks, 2003a; 2003b). A transformational leadership style has been shown to generate greater follower commitment, follower satisfaction, and overall effectiveness (Kleinman, 2004). In nursing homes, the most transformative style of top managers (consensus managers) was found to be associated with better quality outcomes (Castle & Decker, 2011). Deschamps et al. (2016) found that leadership is an important factor in implementing changes, but justice is also a crucial factor. The positive impact of transformational leadership is mediated by organizational justice.

Transformational leaders have been shown to have an impact on both organizations and individuals. Organizational impacts include increased organizational citizenship, stronger organizational culture, and clearer organizational vision (Thomson et al., 2016). Improvements in outcomes for individuals, including empowerment, job satisfaction, commitment, trust, self-efficiency, beliefs, and motivation, have also been linked to transformational leadership (Givens, 2008). Transformational leadership is also associated with a decrease in staff turnover (Weberg, 2010). Overall, transformational leadership qualities appear to be better suited to the work of professionals and important for leadership in nursing.

CONTEMPORARY LEADERSHIP: INTERACTIONAL AND RELATIONSHIP-BASED

In this information age there has been a metamorphosis in health care organizations as they transform into knowledge or learning organizations. Nurses are knowledge workers who use expertise and specialized knowledge in the care of patients. They need matching organizational structures that will value, nurture, and foster the acquisition of the data, information, and knowledge needed for effectiveness. Today's health care environments demand that frontline workers such as nurses have and maintain the expertise and have the information necessary (e.g., evidence-based practice) to take action to solve problems. They need leadership that is interactional, relational, and transformational at all levels.

Arising in conjunction with the application of complexity theory and chaos theory (as discussed under Contemporary Management Theories), leadership was described by Wheatley (2006) as having important elements of connectedness and relationships within self-organizing systems. Nursing has a natural niche within interactional and relationship leadership theories. Optimal health care delivery is truly interdisciplinary, holistic, and highly team based. When connections and relationships are strong, patients benefit. Contemporary definitions of leadership describe leadership as being the result of a relationship between leaders and followers where a distinct set of competencies is used to allow the relationship to achieve shared goals. This is complex and requires nurses to be creative and flexible. It is proposed that "quantum" leadership is needed to produce results in today's health care environment. Quantum leadership is about discovering using an ongoing process of exploration, curiosity, and asking questions. Driven by organizational stress and the feeling that something more and different in work life is needed, quantum leadership is one type of leadership strategy that helps nurses focus on the future, stretch and break boundaries, and encourage breakthrough thinking to solve problems in a complex and fluid care environment. Quantum approaches build on feminist and transformational leadership perspectives and dive more deeply into the behavioral, relational, and interactional elements that form the activities and functions of a leader. Innovation is desired and encouraged.

Complexity Leadership

Traditional leadership theories were developed during the industrial era and describe traits, situations, and a role with power concentrated in a position in the organization. The focus is on maximizing production and reducing variance. Linear models assume input will yield a proportional output (linear processes). Weberg (2012) argued that a focus on linear systems requires management, not leadership, because it removes the capacity for the system to change and innovate. Using complexity science principles and systems thinking, Weberg advocated for complexity leadership because it gives a context for organizational operations whereby the behaviors of leadership foster interaction, increase network strength, and generate stability in order to create the energy for constant change, growth, and adaptation. Interconnectedness and change become normal operating conditions. Complexity leadership is a type of leadership "based on adaptive capacity, understanding the external environment and connecting with the internal organizational culture and thriving in situations where groups need to learn their way out of unpredictable problems" (Weberg, 2012, p. 271). In health care, this will require a shift toward complexity behaviors that embrace complex systems and continually search for value-added innovations. Leaders need to develop innovation competence.

Servant Leadership

Another popular contemporary leadership concept is called *servant leadership*. Greenleaf (2002) originally used the term to describe leaders who choose first to serve others and then to be a leader, as opposed to those who are leaders first (often because of a power drive or need to acquire material possessions) and later choose to serve. When applied to health care, servant leadership is an attractive alternative to the traditional bureaucratic environment experienced by nurses. The servant leadership model draws attention to the necessity for leaders to be attentive to the needs of others and is a model that enhances the personal growth of nurses, improves the quality of care, values teamwork, and promotes personal involvement and caring behavior. Reynolds (2011) melded the feminist and servant leadership perspectives, calling servant leadership gender-integrative leadership that values equally the masculine and feminine dualities, qualities, activities, and behaviors. Hanse et al. (2016) studied the impact of servant leadership dimensions on leader–member exchange among health care professionals and found that servant leadership dimensions are likely to help develop stronger exchange relationships between nurse managers and individual subordinates. A servant leader culture involves interpersonal interaction and promotes strong relationships and trust between leaders and followers.

Authentic Leadership

Following from the IHI's Triple Aim and moving to the Quadruple Aim, focus has now turned to the importance of employees thriving in organizations for organizational performance. Thriving at work is defined as a state where individuals at work experience both a sense of vitality and a sense of learning (Mortier et al., 2016) and is an aspect of work life and nurse vitality. Mortier and colleagues found that nurse managers' authentic leadership enhances nurse thriving.

Authentic leadership was described by Avolio and Gardner (2005) as a leadership style rooted in the concept of authenticity ("to thine own self be true"), where the leader is a fully functioning person in tune with themselves and their basic nature, self-actualizing, and having strong ethical convictions. Authentic leaders are "those who are deeply aware of how they think and behave and are perceived by others as being aware of their own and others' values/moral perspectives, knowledge, and strengths; aware of the context in which they operate; and who are confident, hopeful, optimistic, resilient, and of high moral character" (Avolio & Gardner, 2005, p. 321).

There are four aspects of authentic leadership:

- Self-awareness: how the leaders perceive themselves in comparison with the world and with their understanding of their own strengths and weaknesses
- An internal moral perspective: leaders align their beliefs with their actions and are not often persuaded by external pressures
- Balanced processing: their decision-making is based on analyses of all relevant data, being positive or confirming information or negative clues
- Relational transparency: how openly the leader presents him- or herself to others

The authentic leadership style is seen as fair and supportive and one that provides a healthier and more ethical work environment (Avolio & Gardner 2005; Mortier et al., 2016). This style has been studied in nursing and shown to have a positive effect on nurse job satisfaction and performance (Wong & Laschinger, 2013).

Clinical Leadership

All nurses in all positions exhibit leadership. For example, the "bedside" nurse uses informal leadership to influence high quality care delivery. Mannix et al. (2013) used an integrative review of literature on clinical leadership to elicit defining attributes of contemporary clinical leadership in nursing. The technical and practical skills necessary for competent clinical practice and leading a team emerged. The data were grouped into three categories of clinical leadership with either a clinical, follower/team, or personal qualities focus. "Clinical leaders who demonstrate clinical competence, possess effective communication and are supportive of colleagues have been linked to building healthy workplaces" (Mannix et al., 2013, p. 19). For example, one staff nurse who worked on a surgical and neuroscience intensive care unit recognized that there was incomplete and incorrect spinal cord injury/surgical patient assessment and documentation, which is critical when a patient's condition declines so that the degree of change is known. She took the initiative and contacted the nurse manager, invited other staff nurses to join her, set up a small committee, updated and simplified the assessment tool, and led the education of the staff on the revised tool with positive outcomes. This is clinical leadership.

There is a renewed focus on clinical leadership models at the point of care. Typically aimed at a hospital unit where care is delivered, the crucial role played by nurses in quality, safety, care coordination, and related aims of the IOM and IHI are the centerpiece. Nursing roles of care coordinator, CNL, and APRN have emerged and show continued growth. Joseph and Huber (2015, p. 56) defined clinical leadership as "the process of influencing point-of-care innovation and improvement in both organizational processes and individual care practices to achieve quality and safety of care outcomes." Patrick et al. (2011) viewed every registered staff nurse as a clinical leader and used Kouzes and Posner (2017) model of transformational leadership as a framework to describe and measure clinical leadership practices. Their review of literature identified five key aspects of clinical leadership: clinical expertise, effective communication, collaboration, coordination, and interpersonal understanding. Empowering work environments create a supportive structure for staff nurses as clinical leaders to achieve the best outcomes of care. "Clinical leadership uses the skills of the RN and adds components of general leadership skills, skills in management of care delivery at the point of care, and focused skills in using evidence-based practice for problem solving and outcomes management. There is clearly a need for clinical leadership in nursing because of the many and varied point-of-care implementation problems that arise" (Joseph & Huber, 2015, p. 56).

EFFECTIVE LEADERSHIP

Effective leadership is an integrated blend of leadership principles and characteristics with management principles and techniques. Nurses can grow such skills by knowledge and awareness (e.g., through assessment tools) and then may put knowledge and skills to work through guided exercises and mentored experiences. This is especially true for succession planning and the development of nurse managers (Mackoff et al., 2013).

Leadership effectiveness is based on the ability to adapt in a complex and chaotic environment. Adaptive problems arise from change and chaos and are often systems problems that affect people, planning, institutional operations, or work processes. Effective leaders first have strong self-awareness of their leadership strengths and weaknesses as well as preferred or most comfortable leadership styles and flexibility. Then they expand this to a grasp of themselves, their team, their goals, nursing and health care, and important evaluative data for "dashboards." They use their personal style, vision, and energy to focus on goal attainment and group satisfaction. Starting with whatever natural talent a nurse possesses, essential leadership skills can be practiced over time for greater effectiveness. Effective leadership uses empowerment. For nurses, empowering means that the power over clinical practice decisions is invested in staff nurses, enabling them to do what they do best and make decisions related to their practice. This process is similar to nurses empowering clients. Leadership involves elements of vigor and vision and can be understood as a dynamic combination of competence, willingness to take responsibility, and strength of character to do what is right because it is the right thing to do. See Chapter 10 for further discussion of sources of power.

MANAGEMENT OVERVIEW

Along with an array of opportunities such as instantaneous communication across vast distances, health care organizations and the people in them struggle with an ever-accelerating rate of change, knowledge explosion, technology, and information flow. The recruitment, development, deployment, motivation, and leveraging of human capital (nurses) as scarce resources and prime assets are critical management issues for service industries in general and specifically for nursing and health care. At the core, managers manage people and organizations. People's time and effort—as well as organizations' money, facilities, and supplies—need to be directed in a coordinated effort to achieve best results and meet objectives. Managers focus on the needs of the organization and on getting the work done.

Because nurses are the central hub of care delivery and information flow, it is helpful to think of the work of nurses as having both care delivery and care coordination aspects. Although the coordination of care has always been a key nursing function, it is becoming more visible and valued in health care and as nurses assume care coordination roles that focus on integrating clinical care. However, the relative proportion of the nurse's role that is devoted to management and coordination functions varies within nursing according to the job category. Nurse managers balance two competing needs: the needs of the staff related to growth, efficiency, motivation, morale, and accomplishment with the outcome of staff satisfaction and the needs of the employer for productivity, quality, and cost effectiveness with the outcome of productivity.

DEFINITIONS

Management is defined as the process of coordination and integration of resources through activities of planning, organizing, coordinating, directing, and controlling to accomplish specific institutional goals and objectives. Management has been viewed as an art and a science related to planning and directing both human effort and scarce resources to attain established organizational goals and objectives.

Management, then, applies to organizations. The definition of leadership emphasizes actions that influence toward group goals; the definition of management focuses on organizational goals. The achievement of organizational goals through leadership and manipulation of the environment is management. In a systems approach to management, the inputs would be represented by human resources and physical and technical resources. The outputs would be the realization of goals through task accomplishment, culture development, removal of barriers, and efficiency optimization.

Thus management is a separate function with a specific purpose and related roles but one that is focused on organizations and operations. It is associated with important day-to-day functions geared toward maintenance and stability and associated with transactional leadership or "doing things right" via task accomplishment. To achieve organizational goals, managers are involved in activities such as analyzing issues, establishing goals and objectives, mapping out work plans, organizing assets and supplies, developing and motivating people, communicating, managing technology, handling change and conflict, measurement, analysis, and evaluation. Without talent and attention to these functions, effectiveness and morale drop. This affects quality. In addition, it is important to do the background work needed to keep the organization functioning ("making the trains run on time") so that services are delivered seamlessly. Effective managers are thought to be those who can weave strategy, execution, discipline, inspiration, and leadership together as they unite an organization toward achieving its goals.

BACKGROUND: THE MANAGEMENT PROCESS

Drucker (2004) suggested that effective executives do not need to be leaders. "Great managers may be charismatic or dull, generous or tightfisted, visionary or numbers oriented. But every effective executive follows eight simple practices" (Drucker, 2004, p. 59). These eight practices are divided into the following three categories:

A. Practices That Give Executives the Knowledge They Need
   1. They asked: "What needs to be done?"
   2. They asked: "What is right for the enterprise?"
B. Practices That Help Executives Convert Knowledge to Action
   3. They developed action plans.
   4. They took responsibility for decisions.
   5. They took responsibility for communicating.
   6. They were focused on opportunities, not problems.
C. Practices That Ensure That the Whole Organization Feels Responsible and Accountable
   7. They ran productive meetings.
   8. They thought and said "we" not "I."

Effective management also appears to be a result of artful balancing, because managers need to function at the point at which reflective thinking combines with practical doing. This is described as managerial mind-sets within the bounds of management practice. Managers interpret and deal with their world from the following five perspectives (Gosling & Mintzberg, 2003):

1. *Reflective mind-set*: Managing self
2. *Analytic mind-set*: Managing organizations
3. *Worldly mind-set*: Managing context
4. *Collaborative mind-set*: Managing relationships
5. *Action mind-set*: Managing change

These five mind-sets were described as being like threads for the manager to weave. The process is as follows: analyze, act, reflect, act, collaborate, reanalyze, articulate new insights, and act again.

Management is central to the work of nursing. **Nursing management** is defined as the coordination and integration of nursing resources by applying the management process to accomplish nursing care and service goals and objectives.

It is important to recognize that managers perform unique and discrete functions: they plan, organize, coordinate, and control. Nurses work to deliver care (produce the product); managers manage organizations toward goal achievement. Someone needs to monitor financial indicators; hire, train, and evaluate personnel; improve quality; coordinate work and effort; fix systems problems; and ensure that goals are met. In nursing, this means that nurses do the work of providing nursing care while nurse managers coordinate and integrate the work of individual nurses with the larger system and solve problems for them so they can deliver high quality care. These are distinctly different activities.

The four steps of the management process are planning, organizing, directing/leading, and controlling. These functions make up the scope of a manager's major effort. Planning involves determining the long-term and short-term objectives and the corresponding actions that must be taken. Organizing means mobilizing human and material resources to accomplish what is needed. Directing/leading relates to methods of motivating, guiding, and leading people through work processes. Controlling has a specific meaning closer to the monitoring and evaluating actions that are familiar to nurses. The management process can be compared with an orchestra performing a concert or a team playing a football game. There is a plan and an organized group of players. A director manages the performance and controls the outcome by making corrections and adjustments along the way but does not play an instrument or a position. The management process is a rational, logical process based on problem-solving principles.

Planning

Planning is the managerial function of selecting priorities, results, and methods to achieve results; setting the direction for a system; and then guiding the system. It is decision-making and determining courses of action. **Planning** is defined as "[a] basic management function involving formulation of one or more detailed plans to achieve optimum balance of needs or demands with the available resources. The planning process (1) identifies the goals or objectives to be achieved, (2) formulates strategies to achieve them, (3) arranges or creates the means required, and (4) implements, directs, and monitors all steps in their proper sequence" (BusinessDictionary.com, 2020a). Planning can be detailed, specific, and rigid, or it can be broad, general, and flexible. Planning is deciding in advance what is to be done and when, by whom, and how it is to be done. It is traditionally thought of as a linear process. Hersey et al. (2013) described planning as involving the setting of goals and objectives and developing "work maps" to show how they are to be accomplished. Planning activities include identifying goals, objectives, methods, resources, responsible parties, and due dates. There are two types of planning: strategic and tactical.

Strategic planning: More broad-ranged, this approach means determining the overall purposes and directions of the organization. This is often focused on mission, vision, and major goal identification (see Chapter 14).

Tactical planning: More short-ranged, this type means determining the specific details of implementing broader goals. Examples are project planning, staffing planning, and marketing plans.

Planning heavily depends on the decision-making process. Part of planning is choosing among a number of alternatives. Thus in nursing, the manager often must balance the needs of patients, staff, administrators, and physicians under conditions of limited resources.

Planning involves considering systems inputs, processes, outputs, and outcomes. The process of planning in its larger context means that planners work backward through the system. Starting with the results, outcomes, or outputs desired, they then identify the processes needed to produce the results and the inputs or resources needed to carry out the processes. Typical planning phases include the following:

- Identify the mission.
- Conduct an environmental scan.
- Analyze the situation (e.g., SWOT analysis of strengths, weaknesses, opportunities, and threats).
- Establish goals.
- Identify strategies to reach goals.
- Set objectives to achieve goals.
- Assign responsibilities and timelines.
- Write a planning document.
- Celebrate success and completion.

The nurse is engaged in a constant mental planning operation when deciding what specific things are to be accomplished for the patient. The same is true for the nurse manager who is deciding how to devise, implement, and maintain a positive and productive work environment for nurses. Planning is a function that assumes stability and the ability to predict and project into the future. A turbulent environment makes planning difficult. Learning and adapting are important abilities in a changeable environment.

Organizing

Organizing is a management function related to allocating and configuring resources to accomplish preferred goals and objectives. It is the activities done to collect and configure resources to implement plans effectively and efficiently and involves coordination. **Organizing** can be defined as "assembling required resources to attain organizational objectives" (BusinessDictionary.com, 2020b). It is the mobilizing of the human and material resources of the institution to achieve organizational objectives. The organizing function is focused on building up material and human structures into a working infrastructure. Authority, power, and structure are used for influence. The goal is to get the human, equipment, and material resources mobilized, organized, and working effectively. Organizing so that the goals and objectives can be accomplished includes forging and strengthening relationships between workers and the environment. The first step is to organize the work, then the people are organized, and finally the environment is organized. The essence of organizing is the integration and coordination of resources (Hersey et al., 2013).

There are a wide variety of topics related to organizing, which is considered to be one of the major functions of management. For example, organizing can be thought of as a process of identifying roles in relationship to one another. Thus organizing involves activities related to establishing a structure and hierarchy of jobs and positions within a unit or department. Responsibilities are assigned to each job. The complexity of this aspect of organizing is related to the size of the organization and the number of employees and jobs. Organizing in nursing also relates to the activities of budget management, staffing, and scheduling and to other human resources and personnel functions such as developing committees and bylaws, orientation, and staff in-service. Institutions organize by establishing a structure, such as a hierarchy with divisions or departments, and by developing some method for division of labor and subsequent coordination among subunits.

Directing/Leading

Directing/leading is the managerial function of establishing direction and then influencing people to follow that direction. This involves managing, motivating, and directing people/teams to carry out desired actions. Directing is defined as "a basic management function that includes building an effective work climate and creating opportunity for motivation, supervising, scheduling, and disciplining" (BusinessDictionary.com, 2020c).

Along with communicating and leading, motivation is often included with the description of the activities of directing others. Motivating is a major strategy related to determining the followers' level of performance and thereby to influencing how effectively the goals of the organization will be met. The amount of employee effort that can be influenced by motivation is thought to be from 20% to 30% at the low end and as high as 80% to 90% for highly motivated people (Hersey et al., 2013). A wide range of effort can be affected through motivation.

On a day-to-day basis, coaching is used as a technique to direct and motivate followers. The manager delegates activities and responsibilities when making assignments. The function of directing involves actions of supervising and guiding others within their assigned duties. The use of interpersonal skills is required to delicately balance the need to direct and supervise for task accomplishment with the need to create and maintain a motivational climate with high participation and positive outcomes.

Within nursing there is a legal aspect to the managerial directing function. Under some state licensing laws, supervision is a defined and regulated legal element of nursing practice. Because delegation and supervision are viewed legally as a part of the practice of nursing, nurses have a specific need to know and understand this area of nursing responsibility within their scope of practice. Nurses carry responsibility and accountability for the quality and quantity of their supervision, as well as for the quality and quantity of their own actions regarding care provision. Nurse managers carry the added responsibility and accountability for the coordination of groups of nurse providers and assistive or ancillary personnel, sometimes across settings and sites of care. Nurse managers also have an overall responsibility to monitor and provide surveillance or vigilance regarding situations that can lead to failure to rescue, patient safety errors, or negligence. Too many hours worked, nurse fatigue from stress, too heavy a patient workload, and other systems problems are situations to monitor regarding legal accountability.

Controlling

Controlling is the management function of monitoring and adjusting the plan, processes, and resources to effectively and efficiently achieve goals. It is a way of coordinating activities within organizations by systematically figuring out whether what is occurring is what is wanted. It is the activities focused on monitoring and evaluating what is occurring. The controlling aspect of the managerial process may seem at first to carry a negative connotation. However, when used in reference to management, the word *control* does not mean being negatively manipulative or punitive toward others. Managerial controlling means ensuring that the proper processes are followed. In nursing, the term *evaluation* is used to refer to similar actions and activities. Control or evaluation means ensuring that the flow and processes of work, as well as goal accomplishment, proceed as planned. **Controlling** is defined as "the basic management function of (1) establishing benchmarks or standards, (2) comparing actual performance against them, and (3) taking corrective action, if required" (BusinessDictionary.com, 2020d). Thus it is concerned with comparing the results of work with predetermined standards of performance and taking corrective action when needed by taking some action to modify, remediate, or reverse variances.

The coordination of activities of a system is one aspect of managerial control, along with financial management, compliance, quality and risk management, feedback mechanisms, performance management, policies and procedures, and research and trend analysis. Ongoing, careful review using standardized documents, informatics systems, and standardized measures prevents drift and the waste of time and resources that occur when direction is vague. Well-exercised, managerial control is flexible enough to allow innovation yet present enough to effectively structure groups and organizations toward goal attainment. This is an artful balance.

The management function of controlling involves feeding back information about the results and outcomes of work activities, combined with activities to follow up and compare outcomes with plans. Appropriate adjustments need to be made wherever outcomes vary or deviate from expectations (Hersey et al., 2013). For example, when a standardized clinical practice protocol is used in nursing to track client care, the variances are analyzed and corrected as a function of managerial control. The controlling function of management is a constant process of internal reevaluation.

CONTEMPORARY MANAGEMENT THEORIES

Human organizations are complex in nature. It is tricky to provide overall direction for an organization in times of rapid environmental change. The recent focus of leadership theory has been on interactional, relational, and transformational leadership to guide organizations through successful change and chaos. However, less attention has been focused on how to advise managers who are working toward the organization's goals and trying to use resources effectively and efficiently under conditions of change, scarcity, and complexity. Forces such as technology, the Internet, social media, increasing diversity, and a global marketplace create pressure to be more sensitive, flexible, and adaptable to stakeholders' expectations and demands. This is like a fine dance on a balance beam.

The result has been a push toward reconfiguration or restructuring of many organizations from the classic hierarchical, top-down, rigid form to a more fluid, organic, team-based, collaborative structure. Health care is evolving toward multidisciplinary team-based care. This has had an impact on how managers manage. Managers cannot control continued rapid change. Old familiar plans and behaviors no longer provide clear direction for the future. Managers now need to focus on two major aspects of management: managing change through constant assessment, guidance, and adaptation and managing employees through worker-centered teams and other self-organizing and self-designing group structures. Bureaucratic management is out; organic and virtual management is in.

A variety of contemporary theories of management have arisen to help organize management thought. Four major management theories now predominate: contingency theory, systems theory, complexity theory, and chaos theory. Each one contributes principles useful for nursing management and administration and for nurse managers working to coordinate and integrate health care delivery.

Contingency Theory

Contingency theory is considered a leadership theory, but it also applies to management. The basic principle is that managers need to consider the situation and all its elements when making a decision. Managers need to act on the key situational aspects with which they are confronted. Sometimes described as "it all depends" decision-making, contingency theory is most often used for choosing a leadership or management style. The "best" style depends on the situation. This relates to concepts of situational leadership theory.

Systems Theory

Systems theory has helped managers to recognize their work as being embedded within a system and better understand what a system is. Managers have learned that changing one part of a system inevitably affects the whole system. General systems theory is a way of thinking about studying organizational wholes. A system is a set of interrelated and interdependent parts that are designed to achieve common goals. Systems contain a collection of elements that interact with each other in some environment. The elements of an open system and related examples in health care are shown in Table 1.1.

A key principle of systems theory is that changes in one part of the system affect other parts, creating a ripple effect within the whole. Using systems theory implies a rational approach to common goals, a global view of the whole, and an emphasis on order rather than chaos. The input–throughput–output model exemplifies this linear thinking aspect of general systems theory.

Systems theory is easy to understand but difficult to apply in bureaucratic systems or organizations with strong departmental "silos." This is because coordinators and integrators with sufficient organizational power to cross the system are needed but often not deployed. Without integrators, systems parts tend to make changes

TABLE 1.1 Open System Elements and Health Care Examples

Open System Elements	Health Care Examples
Inputs to the system (resources)	Money, people, technology
Transforming processes and interactions (throughputs)	Nursing services, management
Outputs of the system	Clinical outcomes, better quality of life
Feedback	Customer and nurse satisfaction, government regulation, accreditation, lawsuits

without consideration of the whole system. Shifting to systems theory thinking helps managers view, analyze, and interpret patterns and events through the lens of interrelationships of the parts and coordination of the whole.

In health care, concepts such as interrelatedness and interdependence fit well with multidisciplinary teamwork and shared governance professional models (see Chapter 13). However, concepts of attaining a steady state and equilibrium are difficult to reconcile with the reality of uncertainty, risk, change, and ambiguity that characterize the turbulence of the change occurring in the health care delivery environment. An example of the use of systems theory is basing an analysis of a planned change, such as implementing a new program, on systems concepts by identifying inputs, throughputs, outputs, and feedback loops to more effectively plan how the new program fits into the existing system. Sometimes this process is used for short time frame or rapid response team projects.

Complexity Theory

Complexity theory is a more general umbrella theory that encompasses chaos theory. Arising in scientific fields such as astronomy, chemistry, biology, geology, and meteorology and involving disciplines such as engineering, mathematics, physics, psychology, and economics, the body of literature on the behavior of complex adaptive systems has been growing since the late 1980s. Complexity theory explains the behavior of the whole system. Complex systems are networks of people exchanging information and are self-organizing. Complexity theory core concepts are self-organization, interaction, emergence, system history, and temporality (Chandler et al., 2015). The focus of complexity theory is the behavior over time of certain complex and dynamically changing systems. The concern is about the predictability of the behavior of systems that perform in regular and predictable ways under certain conditions but in other conditions change in irregular and unpredictable ways, are unstable, and move further away from starting conditions unless stopped by an overriding constraint. What is most intriguing is that almost undetectable differences in initial conditions will lead to diverging reactions in these systems until the evolution of their behavior is highly dissimilar?

Stable and unstable behavior can be thought of as two zones. In the stable zone, a disturbed system returns to its initial state. In the unstable zone, any small disturbance leads to movement away from the starting point and further divergence. Which subsequent type of behavior will occur depends on environmental conditions? The area between starting and divergence is called *chaotic behavior*. This refers to systems that have behavior with certain regularity yet defy prediction based on that regularity. This unpredictability was puzzling.

Complexity theory has informed classical management theories. Previous management theories heavily emphasized rationality, predictability, stability, setting a mission, determining strategy, and eliminating deviation. Discoveries from complexity and chaos theories include the fact that the natural world does not operate like clockwork machinery.

Managers need to alter their reflexive behaviors, put an emphasis on "double-loop learning" that also examines the appropriateness of operating assumptions, foster diversity, be open to strategy based on serendipity, welcome disorder as a partner, use instability positively, provoke a controlled ferment of ideas, release creativity, and seek the edge of chaos in the complex interactions that occur among people. Change management takes on a noticeably different form when complexity theory is used. Complexity theory is being used in health care to explain the complexity of the social context in order to better explain the organization of health care and patterns of professional behavior (Chandler et al., 2015). "A new style of leadership is required in complex adapting organizations. This style is one in which the leader serves their people with vision and guidance to see the interconnectedness of the whole system. The leaders must first gain and communicate a shared identity and then be able to allow the organization ownership of that identity" (Berry, 2006, p. 2).

Chaos Theory

Most would agree that one characteristic of nursing is its unpredictability and its chaos and complexity. To use a theory about chaos and complexity is intuitively attractive. Sometimes no matter how hard nursing leaders try to maintain consistency and control, things do become chaotic. Projects seem to take off on their own and defy direction. Chaos is commonly known as disorganization and disorderliness, but the meaning for this concept in chaos theory is quite different. It refers to behavior that is unpredictable despite certain regularities.

Randomness and complexity are two principal characteristics of chaos. There is a paradox in the fact that even in the simplest of systems, it is extraordinarily difficult to accurately predict the course of events, yet some order arises spontaneously even in these simple systems. Patterns form in nature. Some are orderly, and some are not. Concepts of nonlinearity and feedback help explain situations of complexity without randomness (with order). Chaos theory suggests that simple systems may give rise to complex behavior, and complex systems may exhibit simple behavior. At the essence of chaos is a fine balance between forces of stability and those of instability. Two examples are snowflake formation and the behavior of the weather.

Chaos has become one concept of complexity theory. Over the past three or four decades, complexity theory has been the focus of scientific disciplines such as astronomy, chemistry, physics, evolutionary biology, geology, and meteorology. Systems studied in these disciplines have phenomena in common, which seem to pass from an organized state through a chaotic phase and then emerge or evolve into a higher level of organization. There are examples from sciences such as pharmacology, where chaos theory and complexity theory seemed relevant to some patients' unpredictable responses to drugs. The field of research called pharmacogenomics has emerged as a part of precision medicine to address this chaos by studying how a patients' genes affect how they respond to medications.

In management, the traditional focus for leaders is to identify organizational goals and to make decisions facilitating goal achievement. Control is central to logical management processes, but in complexity theory, the idea of control is considered a delusion because uncertainty and deviations would be denied and disregarded. The natural world, according to this theory, does not operate this way and is continually evolving to a higher level of complexity. In complexity theory, the future is so unpredictable that long-term planning is not helpful. Rather, it is suggested that managers need to look for instability and complex interactions among people so that learning occurs and the best result "emerges." The idea of the interconnectedness of the parts (people) of the whole suggests that communication among the parts (people) is a key feature of complexity theory.

Chaos, as used in complexity theory, is not utter confusion and disorder but rather a system that defies prediction despite certain regularities. Chaos is the boundary zone between stability and instability, and systems in chaos exhibit bounded instability and unpredictability of specific behavior within a predictable general structure of behavior. At first, this seems to make no sense. However, chaos theory principles can be applied in health care. For example, managerial planning for an evidence-based practice change such as bedside reporting can produce chaos and unpredictable results. An example of chaos theory in action is when a seemingly small change, such as using assistive personnel instead of professionals, in effect creates ripples and larger impacts on the system than preplanning would seem to indicate. This is why organizations use small tests of change.

As many health care organizations move away from bureaucratic models and recognize organizations as whole systems, more organic and fluid structures are replacing the older ones. Sometimes referred to as "learning organizations," these structures are tapping into the inherent capacity for individuals to exhibit self-organization. In the transition, experiences of change, information overload, entrenched behaviors, and chaos reflect human reactions to organizations as living systems that are adapting and growing (Wheatley, 2006). Complexity and a sense of things being beyond one's control create a search for a simpler way of understanding and leading organizations.

The manager's job is to reveal and handle the mostly hidden dynamics of the system and forge a direction for the organization as a complex adaptive system. The goal is for a self-managed system with people capable of engaging in cooperative behavior, using feedback to learn and adapt, self-organizing, and operating with flexibility.

LEADERSHIP AND MANAGEMENT IMPLICATIONS

It can be argued that all nurses are managers. Staff nurses are the employees at the most critical point in fulfilling the purpose of health care organizations: They are in close and frequent contact with the patient at the point of care, and they coordinate the delivery of health care services.

As nurses work in a rapidly changing practice environment, leadership is important because it affects the climate and work environment of the organization. It affects how nurses feel about themselves at work and about their jobs. By extension, leadership affects organizational and individual productivity. For example, if nurses feel goal-directed and think that their contributions are important, they are more motivated to do the work. Important for the professional practice of nurses is how they feel about themselves and how satisfied they are with their jobs. Both aspects have implications for how well nurses are retained and recruited. Leadership cannot be overlooked because leaders' function as problem finders and problem solvers. They are people who help everyone else overcome obstacles. The leadership role is one of bridging, integrating, motivating, and creating organizational "glue."

Leadership in nursing is crucial. *First*, it is important to nurses because of the size of the profession. Nurses make up the largest single health care occupation and one that is experiencing critical shortages. Pressures in the health care environment, including costs, thrust nurses into leadership roles in highly complex and stressful work situations.

Given the challenges of cost containment, increased chronic conditions, an aging population needing more health care services, and issues of access and quality of care, nurse leaders are experiencing greater pressure to perform and produce more effective alignment of key processes, functions, and resources. Organizations have underinvested in nursing leadership skill development. Thus there is a call for structured transition management and leadership development programs for nurses assuming leadership and management responsibilities in organizations (Campbell, 2016).

Second, nursing's work is complex, often conducted in complex and chaotic settings. Tremendous changes in nursing have occurred. Leadership is needed to guide and motivate nurses and health care delivery systems toward positive achievements for better patient care. Leadership in nursing is needed to influence the organizational context of care for greater effectiveness and productivity because leaders establish norms and values, define expectations, reward behaviors, and reinforce culture. Authenticity and caring are valued in nurse leaders as are people who are genuine, trustworthy, reliable, and believable and who create a positive environment.

Third, nurses are knowledge workers in an information and high-tech age. Knowledge workers respond to inspiration, not supervision. Nurses as functioning professionals in complex systems need protection and support from leaders and managers in order to be creative and innovative followers and deliver care in complex environments. Leaders need to model what they want. Nurses can read, learn, and practice effective leadership and followership.

CURRENT ISSUES AND TRENDS

Current issues and trends that have significance for leadership in nursing include the dramatic US demographic data related to both the aging of the baby boom generation and the demographic profile of nursing in the United States. A major societal and public policy issue related to the aging of a large demographic bulge of baby boomers is beginning to reach a critical point. Called the "2030 problem" (Bahrampour, 2013), this socioeconomic and demographic phenomenon is real, looming, urgent, and fraught with health care challenges. Statistics show that there are approximately 49.2 million Americans ages 65 years and older, representing 15.2% of the population, or one in seven Americans (Administration on Aging, 2018). The percentage of Americans 65 years of age and older has tripled since 1900. Issues related to health burdens and chronic illness are characteristic of older adults. In fact, persons 85 years of age and older may spend up to half of their remaining lives inactive or dependent.

US population and health trends are assessed and monitored by governmental agencies such as the US Census Bureau, Administration on Aging, Centers for Disease Control and Prevention, Bureau of Labor Statistics, and Health Resources and Services Administration. The statistics related to the baby boom generation are impressive. Born between 1946 and 1964, baby boomers in 2030 will be between the ages of 66 and 84 years, are projected to include 60 million people, thus one in five (20%) Americans will be 65 or older. In addition to baby boomers, the US population in 2030 is projected to also include 9 million people born before 1946. By 2029, all of the baby boomers will be 65 years or older, making more than 20% of the population over the age of 65 years. The projected population of people 65 years and older in 2050 is 88.5 million (US Census Bureau, 2014). This predictable tidal wave will make chronic illness and long-term care a huge economic burden. Medical costs and the costs of long-term care loom large. An overwhelming economic burden could occur if tax rates need to be raised dramatically, economic growth is retarded because of high service costs, or future generations of workers have worse general well-being because of service costs or income transfers. Nurses and the health care system will be challenged to find evidence-based care delivery and service systems models and strategies that address the projected growth industry in chronic illness care. One response has been the emphasis on prevention and wellness, targeting behavior change upstream from the development of chronic illness.

Leadership is considered key to the success of health care organizations. Nurses are pressed to demonstrate the outcomes of their care and provide evidence of the effectiveness of their service delivery. The link between leadership style and staff satisfaction highlights the importance of leadership in times of chaos. A nurse leader needs to be dynamic, show interpersonal skills, and be a visionary for the organization and the profession. The ability to inspire and motivate followers to carry out the vision is crucial. Effective leadership has a profound impact on nurse recruitment and retention.

The classic notions of management and managerial work were developed in a sociopolitical era of industrialization and bureaucratization. Competitive pressures and economic forces now are compelling organizations to adopt new flexible strategies and structures. Organizations are being urged to become leaner, more entrepreneurial, and less bureaucratic. This trend has created levels of complexity and interdependency that challenge nurse leaders and managers.

Current and emerging issues in health care are complex and ethically challenging for managers. The "big three" issues of access, cost, and quality continue to be persistent themes that affect any organization's internal operations. Medical insurance coverage is an issue of access, as is the geographical location of facilities, providers, and services. Increased complexity and technology prompt provider specialization and affect cost. Consumer preferences and increased health care awareness affect both cost and quality. Critical medical errors and patient safety issues create pressure related to the need for quality. Complexity, randomness, and chaos created by change call for new management and leadership strategies.

As health care reconfigures, health care delivery settings will likely be knowledge-based organizations composed primarily of specialists whose performance is directed by organized feedback from colleagues, patients, and data analytics. Nurses are positioned at the care coordination intersection and have needed skills for facilitating flow and integrating care delivery. Nurses' roles may change, but their need for leadership inspiration and managerial competence will remain. Nurses are well prepared to serve as leaders, care providers, integrators, and facilitators of patient care. This is the age of the nurse as leader and manager.

RESEARCH NOTE

Source

Shaughnessy, M.K., Quinn Griffin, M.T., Bhattacharya, A., & Fitzpatrick, J.J. (2018). Transformational leadership practices and work engagement among nurse leaders. *Journal of Nursing Administration*, 48(11), 574–579.

Purpose

Transforming the work environment is important to support the work of nurses and meet the challenges of a complex health care system. The purpose of this study was to identify and describe transformational leadership (TL) characteristics and work engagement (WE) by clinical nurse leaders in the United States. The research question asked about the relationship between TL and WE among nurse leaders.

Discussion

Transformational leadership has been shown to inspire followers and create an environment that enhances nurse satisfaction, recruitment, and retention. Work engagement has been shown to be connected to organizational outcomes such as lower levels of burnout and sustaining a culture of professional nursing practice. To explore the relationship between TL and WE, a descriptive correlational study was done with a convenience sample of clinical nursing leaders such as Chief Nurse Officers (CNOs), nurse managers, and educators, who attended the American Nurses Credentialing Center's National Magnet Conference in October 2016. The Leadership Practices Inventory (LPI) by Posner and Kouzes, the Utrecht WE Scale (UWES), and a demographic questionnaire were administered to 218 RNs. Of note, half of the sample was master's prepared, and about 75% were certified. Descriptive statistics were computed, including correlation analyses. A statistically significant positive relationship of moderate strength was shown between LPI and UWES total scores.

RESEARCH NOTE—cont'd

Application to Practice

This study sample was different regarding the level of education and job titles (higher than comparison studies). Nurse leaders' lowest scores were on future vision, taking risks, and supporting innovation, with "inspiring a shared vision" being the weakest leadership behavior. In the literature, an adapted clinical leadership program on leadership competencies was found to create significant improvement. TL can be learned. Leaders play a crucial role in infusing followers with a shared vision and by taking risks and supporting innovation. Nursing practice benefits from greater WE that fosters autonomy and professional growth.

NEXT-GENERATION NCLEX® EXAMINATION-STYLE CASE STUDY

The medical/surgical units at St. Helens Community Hospital are busy with a complex mix of patient diagnoses and conditions and have a staff of 88 employees, with a few nurses of long tenure, but mostly new graduates and nurses with less than 2 years of experience. They have 4 very different leaders:

1. Nurse Manager Dan has 3 years of experience as a nurse manager. He prefers to tell the followers what to do and how to do it in order to get tasks done.
2. Nurse Manager Maria has 3 years of experience as a nurse manager. She prefers to use her outgoing personality and likability to achieve success, using positive motivation and team morale.
3. Nurse Manager Jorge has 3 years of experience as a nurse manager. He prefers to have a hands-off approach and let his employees assume responsibility in the decision-making process.
4. Nurse Manager Olivia has 3 years of experience as a nurse manager. Her unit is busy with a complex mix of patient diagnoses and conditions. She prefers to use her inspiring energy and personality to create a magnetic workplace by engaging with others, centering on followers' needs and goals, and thus raising each other to higher levels of motivation.

Use the numbered scenarios above, to indicate the best approach and priority area to lead the unit.

Nursing Situation	Best Approach
The entire facility has a power outage in a storm. Backup generators do not come on in the ICU.	
Nurses complain about being understaffed for Christmas vacation.	
Nurses have organized a shared governance committee.	
The bariatric unit does not have an adequate number of Hoyer lifts, and the NM is concerned about future back injuries.	

CRITICAL THINKING EXERCISE

Nurse manager Mike Catney has a problem. He has detected angry venting and counterproductive work behavior affecting the morale of the clinic. He goes to observe and assess. It was the end of another long, hectic, and frustrating day in Ambulatory Clinic A for Nurse John Folkrod. There were daily issues with sluggish patient flow and long wait times for patients in the waiting room. John's usual reaction was to bottle up the frustration, causing personal health issues, or to vent it by complaining to colleagues. Neither method influenced a positive change in the situation. Fortunately, the nurse manager is a visionary, authentic leader. However, John has not approached him, assuming that the situation was obvious to the manager and not desiring to "make waves" or be seen as a troublemaker. In the meantime, Nurse Catney evaluates the organizational climate (how the surroundings are perceived by the staff) and reviews principles of EI. He consults the literature (Al Ghazo et al., 2019).

1. What is the problem?
2. Whose problem is it?
3. What are John's followership role and options for followership strategies to resolve the situation?
4. What leadership behaviors and styles might be effective? What should nurse manager Catney do?
5. How might the situation be analyzed using relationship-based care and EI principles?

REFERENCES

Adams, K. L., & Iseler, J. I. (2014). The relationship of bedside nurses' emotional intelligence with quality of care. *Journal of Nursing Care Quality, 29*(2), 174–181.

Administration on Aging (AoA), Administration for Community Living, US Department of Health and Human Services. (2018). *2017 Profile of older Americans*. Washington, DC: Author. Retrieved from https://acl.gov/sites/default/files/Aging%20and%20Disability%20in%20America/2017OlderAmericansProfile.pdf.

Agency for Healthcare Research and Quality. (2018). *Six domains of healthcare quality*. Retrieved from https://www.ahrq.gov/talkingquality/measures/six-domains.html.

Al Ghazo, R. H., Suifan, T. S., & Alnuaimi, M. (2019). Emotional intelligence and counterproductive work behavior: The mediating role of organizational climate. *Journal of Human Behavior in the Social Environment, 29*(3), 333–345. https://doi.org/10.1080/10911359.2018.1533504.

American Nurses Credentialing Center (ANCC). (n.d.). *ANCC Magnet Recognition Program*. https://www.nursingworld.org/organizational-programs/magnet/.

American Organization for Nursing Leadership (formerly AONE). (2015). Nurse executive competencies. Chicago, IL. https://www.aonl.org/resources/nurse-leader-competencies.

Avolio, B. J., & Gardner, W. L. (2005). Authentic leadership development: Getting to the root of positive forms of leadership. *The Leadership Quarterly, 16*(3), 315–338.

Bahrampour, T. (2013). Huge shortage of caregivers looms for baby boomers, report says. https://www.washingtonpost.com/national/health-science/huge-shortage-of-caregivers-looms-for-baby-boomers-report-says/2013/08/25/665fb2aa-0ab1-11e3-b87c-476db8ac34cd_story.html.

Bass, B. M., & Avolio, B. J. (2019). *Multifactor Leadership Questionnaire™*. *Mind Garden*. https://www.mindgarden.com/16-multifactor-leadership-questionnaire.

Berry, B. L. (2006). There is a relationship between systems thinking and W. Edwards Deming's theory of profound knowledge. The Berrywood Group. https://pdfs.semanticscholar.org/a090/48ae9c5cd2efbe90f3feb8a2b9ca57a9f6e9.pdf?_ga=2.49216102.1570324709.1578433890-316060041.1578433890.

Buck, S., & Doucette, J. N. (2015). Transformational leadership practices of CNOs. *Nursing Management, 46*(9), 42–48.

BusinessDictionary.com. (2020a). Planning. http://www.businessdictionary.com/definition/planning.html.

BusinessDictionary.com. (2020b). Organizing. http://www.businessdictionary.com/definition/organizing.html.

BusinessDictionary.com. (2020c). Directing. http://www.businessdictionary.com/definition/directing.html.

BusinessDictionary.com. (2020d). Controlling. http://www.businessdictionary.com/definition/controlling.html.

Campbell, G. (2016). Growing and developing our future nurse leaders. *Voice of Nursing Leadership, 14*(4), 4–6.

Castle, N. G., & Decker, F. H. (2011). Top management leadership style and quality of care in nursing homes. *The Gerontologist, 51*(5), 630–642.

Chandler, J., Rycroft-Malone, J., Hawkes, C., & Noyes, J. (2015). Application of simplified complexity theory concepts for healthcare social systems to explain the implementation of evidence into practice. *Journal of Advanced Nursing, 72*(2), 461–480.

Clay-Williams, R., Nosrati, H., Cunningham, F. C., Hillman, K., & Braithwaite, J. (2014). Do large-scale hospital- and system-wide interventions improve patient outcomes: A systematic review. *BMC Health Services Research, 14*, 369. https://doi.org/10.1186/1472-6963-14-36.

Creative Health Care Management. (2020). Relationship-based care. https://chcm.com/solutions/relationship-based-care/.

Deschamps, C., Rinfret, N., Lagace, M. C., & Prive, C. (2016). Transformational leadership and change: How leaders influence their followers' motivation through organizational justice. *Journal of Healthcare Management, 61*(3), 194–22.

Drucker, P. F. (2004). What makes an effective executive. *Harvard Business Review, 82*(6), 58–63.

Feather, J., McGillis Hall, L., Trbovich, P., & Baker, G. R. (2018). An integrative review of nurses' prosocial behaviours contributing to work environment optimization, organizational performance and quality of care. *Journal of Nursing Management, 26*(7), 769–781.

Gittell, J. H. (2016). *Transforming relationships for high performance: The power of relational coordination.* Stanford, CA: Stanford University Press.

Givens, R. J. (2008). Transformational leadership: The impact on organizational and personal outcomes. *Emerging Leadership Journeys, 1*(1), 4–24.

Görgens-Ekermans, G., & Brand, T. (2010). Emotional intelligence as a moderator of the stress-burnout relationship: A questionnaire study on nurses. *Journal of Clinical Nursing, 21*(15–16), 2275–2285.

Gosling, J., & Mintzberg, H. (2003). The five minds of a manager. *Harvard Business Review, 81*(11), 54–63.

Greenleaf, R. K. (2002). *Servant leadership: A journey into the nature of legitimate power and greatness* (25th anniversary ed). Mahwah, NJ: Paulist Press.

Grossman, S. C., & Valiga, T. M. (2017). *The new leadership challenge: Creating the future of nursing* (5th ed.). Philadelphia, PA: F.A. Davis Company.

Hanse, J. J., Harlin, U., Jarebrant, C., Ulin, K., & Winkel, J. (2016). The impact of servant leadership dimensions on leader-member exchange among health care professionals. *Journal of Nursing Management, 24*, 228–234.

Helgeson, S. (1995a). *The web of inclusion: A new architecture for building organizations.* New York, NY: Doubleday.

Helgeson, S. (1995b). *The female advantage: Women's ways of leadership* (2nd ed.). New York, NY: Doubleday.

Hersey, P. H., Blanchard, K. H., & Johnson, D. E. (2013). *Management of organizational behavior: Leading human resources* (10th ed.). Upper Saddle River, NJ: Pearson Education.

Institute for Healthcare Improvement (IHI). (2020). Triple aim for populations. http://www.ihi.org/Topics/TripleAim/Pages/default.aspx.

Institute of Medicine (IOM). (2004). *Keeping patients safe: Transforming the work environment of nurses.* Washington, DC: National Academies Press.

Institute of Medicine (IOM). (2011). *The future of nursing: Leading change, advancing health.* Washington, DC: National Academies Press.

Jennings, B. M., Scalzi, C. C., Rodgers, J. D. III., & Keane, A. (2007). Differentiating nursing leadership and management competencies. *Nursing Outlook, 55*, 169–175.

Joseph, M. L. (2015). Organizational culture and climate for promoting innovativeness. *Journal of Nursing Administration, 45*(3), 172–178.

Joseph, M. L., & Huber, D. L. (2015). Clinical leadership development and education for nurses: Prospects and opportunities. *Journal of Healthcare Leadership, 2015*(7), 55–64.

Joseph, M. L., Rhodes, A., & Watson, C. A. (2016). Preparing nurse leaders to innovate: Iowa's innovation seminar. *Journal of Nursing Education, 55*(2), 113–117.

Kleinman, C. (2004). The relationship between managerial leadership behaviors and staff nurse retention. *Hospital Topics, 82*(4), 2–9.

Koloroutis, M. (2004). *Relationship-based care: A model for transforming practice.* Minneapolis, MN: Creative Health Care Management.

Kouzes, J. M., & Posner, B. Z. (2017). *The leadership challenge: How to make extraordinary things happen in organizations* (6th ed.). Hoboken, NJ: John Wiley & Sons, Inc.

Mackoff, B. L., Glassman, K., & Budin, W. (2013). Developing a leadership laboratory for nurse managers based on lived experiences: A participatory action research model for leadership development. *Journal of Nursing Administration, 43*(9), 447–454.

Malloch, K. (2002). Trusting organizations: Describing and measuring employee-to-employee relationships. *Nursing Administration Quarterly, 26*(3), 12–19.

Mannix, J., Wilkes, L., & Daly, J. (2013). Attributes of clinical leadership in contemporary nursing: An integrative review. *Contemporary Nurse, 45*(1), 10–21.

Miles, J. M., & Scott, E. S. (2019). A new leadership development model for nursing education. *Journal of Professional Nursing, 35*(1), 5–11.

Mortier, A. V., Vlerick, P., & Clays, E. (2016). Authentic leadership and thriving among nurses: The mediating role of empathy. *Journal of Nursing Management, 24*, 357–365.

Northouse, P. G. (2019). *Leadership: Theory and practice* (8th ed.). Thousand Oaks, CA: Sage.

Patrick, A., Laschinger, H. K. S., Wong, C., & Finegan, J. (2011). Developing and testing a new measure of staff nurse clinical leadership: The clinical leadership survey. *Journal of Nursing Management, 19*, 499–460.

Quoidbach, J., & Hansenne, M. (2009). The impact of trait emotional intelligence on nursing team performance and cohesiveness. *Journal of Professional Nursing, 25*(1), 23–29.

Reynolds, K. (2011). Servant-leadership as gender-integrative leadership: Paving a path for more gender-integrative organizations through leadership education. *Journal of Leadership Education, 10*(2), 155–171.

Schooley, S. (2019). What kind of leader are you? 9 leadership types and their strengths. Business News Daily. https://www.businessnewsdaily.com/9789-leadership-types.html.

Shaughnessy, M. K., Quinn Griffin, M. T., Bhattacharya, A., & Fitzpatrick, J. J. (2018). Transformational leadership practices and work engagement among nurse leaders. *Journal of Nursing Administration, 48*(11), 574–579.

Sikka, R., Morath, J. M., & Leape, L. (2015). The Quadruple Aim: Care, health, cost and meaning in work. *BMJ Quality & Safety, 24*(10), 608–610.

Spano-Szekely, L., Quinn Griffin, M. T., Clavelle, J., & Fitzpatrick, J. J. (2016). Emotional intelligence and transformational leadership in nurse managers. *Journal of Nursing Administration, 46*(2), 101–108.

Steaban, R. L. (2016). Health care reform, care coordination, and transformational leadership. *Nursing Administration Quarterly, 40*(2), 153–163.

Stetler, C. B., Ritchie, J. A., Rycroft-Malone, J., & Charns, M. P. (2014). Leadership for evidence-based practice: Strategic and functional behaviors for institutionalizing EBP. *Worldviews on Evidence-Based Nursing, 11*(4), 219–226. https://doi.org/10.1111/wvn.12044.

The Center for Leadership Studies. (2020). Situational leadership. https://situational.com/situational-leadership/.

The National Academies of Sciences, Engineering, Medicine; Health and Medicine Division. (2020). The future of nursing 2020–2030. http://www.nationalacademies.org/hmd/Activities/Workforce/futureofnursing2030.aspx.

Thomson, N. B., Rawson, J. V., Slade, C. P., & Bledsoe, M. (2016). Transformation and transformational leadership: A review of the current and relevant literature for academic radiologists. *Academic Radiology, 23*(5), 592–599.

Upenieks, V. (2003a). Nurse leaders' perceptions of what compromises successful leadership in today's acute inpatient environment. *Nursing Administration Quarterly, 27*(2), 140–152.

Upenieks, V. (2003b). What constitutes effective leadership? *Journal of Nursing Administration, 33*(9), 456–467.

US Bureau of Labor Statistics. (2019). Occupational employment statistics: Occupational employment and wages, May 2018, 29-1141 Registered Nurses. https://www.bls.gov/oes/current/oes291141.htm.

US Census Bureau. (2014). The baby boom cohort in the United States: 2012 to 2060: Population estimates and projections. https://www.census.gov/prod/2014pubs/p25-1141.pdf.

Ward, S. (2020). The definition of leadership. https://www.thebalancesmb.com/leadership-definition-2948275.

Weberg, D. (2010). Transformational leadership and staff retention: An evidence review with implications for healthcare systems. *Nursing Administration Quarterly, 34*(3), 246–258.

Weberg, D. (2012). Complexity leadership: A healthcare imperative. *Nursing Forum, 47*(4), 268–277.

Wheatley, M. J. (2006). *Leadership and the new science: Discovering order in a chaotic world* (3rd ed.). San Francisco, CA: Berrett-Koehler.

Wong, C. A., & Laschinger, H. K. S. (2013). Authentic leadership, performance, and job satisfaction: The mediating role of empowerment. *Journal of Advanced Nursing, 69*(4), 947–959.

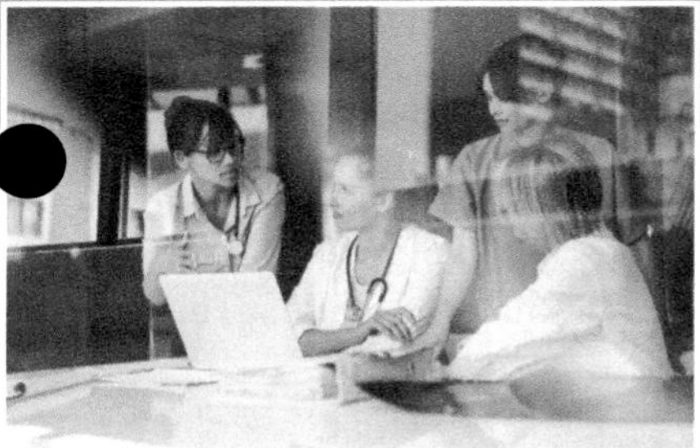

2

Change and Innovation

Beverly Quaye

http://evolve.elsevier.com/Huber/leadership

As we enter our third decade of the 21st century, we reflect on significant health care changes in the United States since 2000. These include national health care reform with provider incentives for Medicare and Medicaid, and an option for purchasing insurance on state exchanges as a result of the Patient Protection and Affordable Care Act (ACA, 2010). ACA incorporates individual mandates, accompanying subsidies, tax credits, health benefits, and discrimination protections, such as preexisting conditions (Department of Health and Human Services [DHHS], 2018, p. 19432). There is more emphasis on coordination across the full care delivery continuum, and an increase in evidence about health promotion, disease prevention, and early detection of disease. Other achievements are more emphasis on increasing alternatives to traditional medicine, significant growth in retail and urgent care clinics (Heath, 2017), and rapid expansion in telemedicine. ACA has driven reform and innovation needs by health care leaders due to economic, quality, access to care, and service implications as a result of this new direction.

Care delivery has shifted from health care institutions that were individualized to collaboration across organizations and expanding and strengthening networks (Raus et al., 2018). There is also a shift from a business to a person-centered model that may also be due to changing demographics, that is, senior and diverse population growth, an information-driven society, social media in real-time, and global communication. Additionally, the use of personal health devices in telemedicine for monitoring and sharing data such as blood sugar, cardiac rhythms, blood pressure, and weight with providers (Centers for Medicare & Medicaid Services [CMS], 2019) is proliferating. Lastly, physician networks' use of health care professional extenders, telemedicine, and hospitalists is on the rise and is resulting in economic efficiencies, better access to care, evidence-based and quality services, improved patient safety and enhanced experiences, and maximization of technology (Raus et al., 2018).

It is imperative that mastering change and innovation calls for preparing our future nurse administrative *and* clinical leaders to (1) comprehend an idealized future state, and (2) acquire skills that will positively impact nursing practice, care delivery, patient outcomes, and health care policy. Changes in 21st century health care have been described as "revolutionary" (Longenecker & Longenecker, 2014). Today's frontline nurses are accustomed to changing processes, systems, roles, and responsibilities. Those at the point of care are often charged with leading, implementing, and evaluating the effects of change. As professionals, nurses frequently desire to maintain their emphasis on humanism and healing in the face of ongoing and perpetual change (Perregrini, 2019). This may be stressful for nurses, often leading to change fatigue resulting in lowered job performance and satisfaction, as well as health issues (Sherman, 2018).

Change is complex and disruptive. Initiating, following through, and sustaining change is challenging, whether on a personal or organizational level. Even planned personal "healthy" changes, such as smoking cessation, weight loss, a new exercise program, or continuing education, can be challenging and contribute to stress. In the work setting, when change is directive, not understood, or threatens nurse autonomy and security, it can result in conflict and resistance. To facilitate the change process, nursing management and leadership need to follow evidence-based practice grounded in change theory, research, and successful process and systematic outcomes to support nurses in accepting and adapting to change and creating a culture of innovation.

DEFINITIONS

Consistency in language via definitions will contribute to better understanding in acquiring new knowledge, skills, and the ability to translate this information into practice.

Change—an alteration to make something become different (Cambridge Dictionary, 2020a). Change is a complex process that occurs over time and is influenced by any number of unpredictable variables.

Planned change—"any kind of alternation or modification which is done in advance and differently for the improvement of present position into brighter one is called planned change" (Bank of Information, 2014, p. 1).

Emergent change assumes that change is a continuous, open-ended, and unpredictable process of aligning and realigning an organization to its changing environment (Burnes, 2009).

Transformation—"a complete change in the appearance or character of something or someone, especially so that thing or person is improved" (Cambridge Dictionary, 2020b).

Resistance—to refuse to accept or be changed by something, a force that acts to stop the progress of something or make it slower (Clarke, 2013).

Change agent—a person who encourages people to change their behavior or opinions and who may function as a change facilitator (Cambridge Dictionary, 2020c).

THEORETICAL FRAMEWORK

There are multiple change theories and models in the literature that impact how change in organizations is accomplished. Shanley's (2007) seminal work on planned or emergent change was selected as framework throughout this chapter because it addresses planned and emergent change and remains highly relevant today. Although planned change is critical in operationalizing organizational goals and strategies, modifications of Shanley's original work to meet the needs of our current health care environment often are needed. Critics of Shanley's traditional approach object to sequential and linear methods employed in his planned change work in most current situations. Due to the complexity of health care operations requiring multidimensional perspectives and flexibility, there is more demand for emergent change methods.

Shanley's classic model was characteristic of a top-down leadership approach and a strong role of managers that needs adaptation in most contemporary scenarios. The dominant role of management has shifted to a more participatory and collaborative one in planning, managing, and executing change projects, with benefits from diverse views and skills from other professional and support staff, affiliated partners, and external suppliers. Principles and processes of change become central especially when there has been limited or no time for planning, strategizing, and supporting what is needed to be effective (Longenecker & Longenecker, 2014; Shanley, 2007) in emerging change. Shanley's model will be demonstrative in the understanding of both planned and emerging change needs as well as the associated roles and responsibilities, including change agents and recipients, in creating and sustaining change.

BACKGROUND

For the past three decades, a 70% failure rate in organizational change outcomes (Hammer, 1990; Kotter, 1995) frequently has been reported and has produced negative attitudes and beliefs about change by both change experts and the lay public. It can be said this has become a self-fulfilling prophecy in organizational change and remains commonplace today. Curious about how to break some of these long-standing assumptions, Hughes (2011) critically reviewed five separate publications that identified a 70% failure rate and concluded there was no valid and reliable empirical evidence to support this claim. Participants who experience emergent problems in the change process often revert to this negative and toxic bias, resulting in disengagement and eventual failure in their change process. Klein and O'Brien (2017) found that people assume failure as a more likely expected result of a change process compared with success, and attribute positive outcomes as luck and negative results as undeniable proof that change is difficult and often escapes us. Despite the effort required to ward off this issue, their research also discovered that most people who commit to change initiatives do eventually succeed. Studies have found that people do successfully improve with minimal effort and are quicker to notice improved changes versus setbacks. Based on this evidence, Tasler (2017) believed that it is timely to change our thinking, and an opportunity exists to write a new story by reminding us that "adaptation is the rule of human existence, not the exception."

Structurally, too often organizational change initiatives are initiated and based on top-down planned change tactics. Too frequently the focus is on the role of administrators and top managers in the change process. The reasons for this are generally pressure from decision makers desiring fast change, noncompliance from regulatory and accrediting bodies requiring immediate corrective action, health system directives, an overall lack of infrastructure to support change management and sustainability, and a lack of leadership acumen in evidence-based proven results. Table 2.1 displays contrasting views of change.

Research supports that not only is top-down change undesirable, but it does not result in successful outcomes and sustainability (Balogun, 2006; Longenecker & Longenecker, 2014). Porter-O'Grady and Malloch (2015) conceptualized this as "moving from the center, or the point of service (POS), outward." Staff and other "recipients" of change at the POS must be viewed as assets rather than barriers who are integral to the process. Representatives from all levels and parts of the system need to participate in all steps of the process: readiness, justification of need, assessment, planning, implementation, measurement, evaluation, and sustaining goals. In addition, when considering the processes of change, issues of power and how individuals make sense of the change are essential.

Little evidence is available in the literature on the success of specific approaches to planned change (Hallencreutz & Turner, 2011). Current evidence supports an emergent view of change (Shanley, 2007) that is more likely to produce positive outcomes (Balogun, 2006; Packard & Shih, 2014). The literature points to a shift in the roles and responsibilities of executives to those affected at the frontline when change needs have been identified and needs to be executed. The traditional planned approach has often been too simplistic, made too many assumptions, and has not allowed for the analysis of the increased complexity of the aspects of change over time. Leadership needs to acknowledge that improved technology, fast-paced information technology, and increased use of personal mobile devices have accelerated access to real-time information and communication, resulting in a consumer-driven society. Today, change efforts need to be localized and incorporate a variety of approaches (Hallencreutz & Turner, 2011), since organizations have become more complex, need to keep pace with competition in services and care delivery, and accommodate consumer needs and choices.

Organizational Change

A current definition of organizational change is "a change in organizational structure, its system/subsystems, employees and relationships between them in a planned or non-planned way" (Bejinariu et al., 2017, p. 322). Management efforts are employed to transition

TABLE 2.1 Contrasting Views of Change

	Planned Change (Traditional View)	Emergent View
Direction	Top-down, linear	Multidirectional, multidimensional
Initiator	Leader initiated	Diffuse
Process	Planned, step-by-step process	Principles to guide process
Organizational culture	May be considered	Essential to consider
Power issues	Not considered or not spoken	Essential to consider
Role of staff/recipients of change	Resisters	Participants in change process
View of the change recipients	May be assessed so they can be changed or manipulated	Essential to process

an organization from a current state to a desired future state to increase organizational functioning when there is an identified need for this type of change. Suddaby and Foster (2017) theorized that organizational change was positively influenced by the capacity of leadership to develop a historical consciousness. He suggested that leaders should aim for a heightened self-awareness of feelings, reactions, and appreciation of how their assumptions about the past may influence their understanding of the organization's current state and an envisioned future state. By reframing attitudes and preconceived notions about the past, successful change can occur (Suddaby, 2016). Organizational change is recognized in today's context as a complex process that is not necessarily linear (Jansson, 2013), and innovative approaches to organizational change that are consistent with emergent views are common in the evidence.

Nursing's Contribution

The role of nurses in change management is a critical leadership competency for nurses and is congruent with the human side of change. Nurses take part in most patient/client health care needs in a multitude of settings, and also have the most direct contact with them. Nurses' education is comprehensive, their scope of practice and span of control is broad, their practice ranges from general to highly specialized, and roles, functions, and responsibilities are immense. Because of this variety and scope, registered nurses have outstanding knowledge and expertise in working within organizations and fully engaging in change management.

The *Nurse Executive Competencies* of the American Organization of Nurse Executives (AONE), now the American Organization for Nursing Leadership (AONL) (2015), emphasized the need for change management knowledge, skills, and abilities. The ground-breaking report *The future of nursing: Leading change, advancing health* of the Institute of Medicine (IOM), now the National Academies of Sciences, Engineering, and Medicine, Health and Medicine Division (HMD 2010), called on nurses to use their expertise and influence to act in leading roles that support and promote health care change and innovation.

CHANGE THEORIES/MODELS

Nurse leaders, from the frontline to the executive suite, need to understand and be able to apply a variety of change theories, individualizing them to their organization and situation. Theories of change that focus on the human side of change are person-centered, align with consumer demand, and support leader–collaborator relationships that are desirable. Nurse leaders who assess and respect participants' responses to change, are mindful of political and power issues, and are sensitive to departmental and organizational values and culture will be more successful at facilitating and sustaining change (Longenecker & Longenecker, 2014). Nurse leaders are called upon to focus on the importance of human relationships in the change process.

Anderson and Anderson's (2009) work examined traditional hierarchical mind-sets of relying on power and control and top-down, manager-driven approaches, determining these were unsuccessful. They learned that when leaders focused on the process of change and human relationship aspects, better outcomes in change projects were achieved. The researchers identified the emerging mind-set, like other complexity views, as one grounded in wholeness and relationship, embracing co-creation and participation. By utilizing relationship-based change methods, an industrial mind-set used by organizational leaders shifted to an emerging mind-set. The industrial mind-set had a mechanistic worldview that relied on power and control, certainty, and predictability. A component of the emerging mind-set is that leaders need to move to what they call *conscious change* leadership.

Conscious change leaders are aware of the dynamics of change (Carson, 2016) and are more apt to lead from the principles of an emerging mind-set. Conscious change leaders need to be willing to look internally to transform their own mind-set (Carder, 2015) by expanding their thinking about process and systems and evolve their own unique leadership style.

Other models or worldviews that influence organizational change, that is, systems theory, complexity theory, and chaos theory, are also consistent with the foundations of the emerging mind-set (see Chapter 1). The focus of these theories is on interrelationships, processes, and systemic behavior. These models are congruent with the behaviors of complex systems characterized by nonlinearity, spontaneity, and self-organization. Small changes can often lead to larger dynamic changes and effects that are often unintentional. Systems, complexity, and chaos theories help

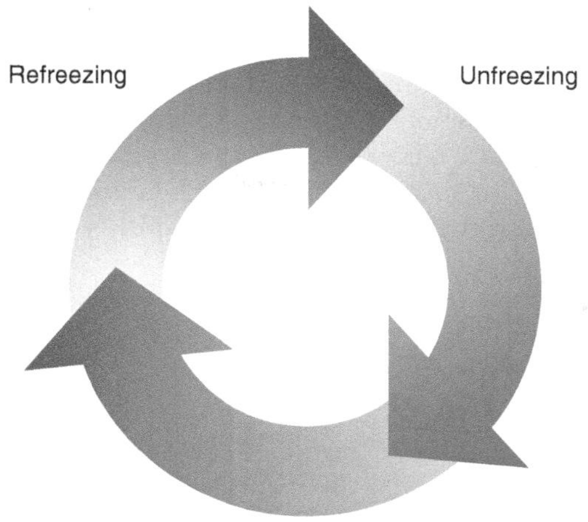

Fig. 2.1 Elements of a successful change. Data from Lewin, K. (1947). Frontiers in group dynamics: Concept, method, and reality in social science; social equilibrium and social change. *Human Relations, 1*(1), 5–41; Lewin, K. (1951). *Field theory in social science: Selected theoretical papers*. New York, NY: Harper & Row.

navigate changes in complex systems and understand how to enable systems to adapt to change (Porter-O'Grady & Malloch, 2015).

The majority of change theories originated or were influenced by Kurt Lewin (1947; 1951) and his seminal work on the three elements for successful change processes: (1) unfreezing, (2) moving, and (3) refreezing (Fig. 2.1). Some view his ideas as more consistent with traditional views of planned change (Burnes, 2004); however, his model is currently and frequently used to frame how groups and organizations change and also serves as the basis for many newer theories.

Lewin's Change Process

Lewin coined the term *planned change* to distinguish the process from accidental or imposed change (Burnes, 2004). Lewin's (1947, 1951) theory of change used ideas of equilibrium within systems. *Unfreezing*, the first stage of change, is characterized as a process of "thawing out" the system. Unfreezing creates an awareness of the need for change and defines motivation and readiness for change. This first stage solicits a cognitive exposure to the change idea, diagnosis of the problem, and work to generate alternative solutions. When those involved in the change process understand and generally accept the necessity of change the unfreezing stage is complete.

Moving, the second stage of change, demonstrates proceeding to a new level of behavior, evidenced by the occurrence of the actual visible change. After the individuals involved collect adequate information that clarifies and identifies the problem, the change itself can be planned and initiated. Lewin (1951) observed that a process of "cognitive redefinition"—or looking at the problem from a new perspective—happens. As a first step to launch a change, a pilot test may be performed so that the change can be pretested, and a transition period launched.

Refreezing, the final change stage, is when new changes are integrated and stabilized. Behavioral reinforcement is crucial as individuals integrate the change into their own value system and organizational culture. Leadership strategies to recognize and reward new behaviors and change, such as *positive feedback, encouragement*, and *constructive criticism* are effective means of reinforcement. Refreezing is a significant step in the sustainability plan for lasting change.

Lewin's (1947, 1951) planned change process stages can be compared with the nursing process and the generic problem-solving process (Table 2.2). *Unfreezing* is like assessing in the nursing process and like problem identification and definition in the problem-solving process. *Moving* is similar to planning and implementing in the nursing process and similar to problem analysis and seeking alternative solutions in the problem-solving process. *Refreezing* is like evaluation in the nursing

TABLE 2.2 Similarities of Change, Nursing Process, and Problem Solving

Change	Nursing Process	Problem Solving
Unfreezing	Assessing	Problem identification and definition
Moving	Planning and implementing	Problem analysis and seeking alternatives
Refreezing	Evaluation	Implementation and evaluation

Data from Workman, R., & Kenney, M. (1988). The change experience. In S. Pinkerton, & P. Schroeder (Eds.), *Commitment to excellence: Developing a professional nursing staff* (pp. 17–25). Rockville, MD: Aspen.

process and like implementation and evaluation in the problem-solving process.

Individuals and systems are like organisms in that they naturally strive for equilibrium. Lewin (1951) saw this as a balance between driving forces that promote change and restraining forces that inhibit change. Both driving and restraining forces exist within any change situation. To create change, the equilibrium is broken by altering the relative strengths of driving and restraining forces. The relative strengths of these forces may be analyzed. A force field analysis facilitates the identification and analysis of driving and restraining forces in any situation. *Unfreezing* occurs when disequilibrium is introduced into the system to disrupt the status quo. *Moving* is the change to a new status quo. *Refreezing* occurs when the change becomes the new status quo and new behaviors are frozen. The process of change may flow back and forth among stages. It is not a simple linear process in which one step follows the preceding one. The process may move rapidly or may stall in any of its stages. The goal of planned change is to manage the planning, and control and evaluate the change. Lewin's theory (1947, 1951) depicted a classic foundation for other change theories. Successive theorists were inspired and created new change theories based on further understanding and application of Lewin's theory.

Lippitt (1973) refined and expanded Lewin's (1947, 1951) work to identify seven phases of change that more fully supported planned change in dynamic and complex situations. The first three steps correlate to Lewin's unfreezing, steps 4 and 5 to moving, and steps 6 and 7 to refreezing Lewin's (1947, 1951). Lippitt's model consists of the following seven steps:

Kotter (1995) introduced his change management model based on his experiences as a consultant with businesses undergoing change. Like other change models, Kotter's has not been empirically tested, but its popularity seems to derive both from its direct and practical format and its successful utilization in multiple settings (Appelbaum et al., 2012). His model consists of the following eight steps:

1. Establish a sense of urgency.
2. Create a guiding coalition.
3. Develop a vision and strategy.
4. Communicate the change vision.
5. Empower employees for broad-based action.
6. Generate short-term wins.
7. Consolidate gains and produce more change.
8. Anchor new approaches in the culture.

Kotter's model is inclusive of employees and focuses on both engaging them in the change process and empowering them to be involved. Its emphasis is on helping others to see the need for the change and to embrace it. One potential shortcoming is that Kotter (2012) insisted that the eight steps be implemented in order, without substantial overlap. Because studies have suggested that organizations prefer to use change strategies that best fit their culture, such strict adherence to the plan may be harder to adapt. After reviewing the work of Lewin, Lippitt, and Kotter, it is evident that the various conceptualizations of the stages of the process of change bear similarity to one another but vary in emphasis (Table 2.3).

Lippitt's model consists of the following seven steps:

1. Diagnosis of the problem 2. Assessment of motivation and capacity to change 3. Assessment of the change agent's motivation and resources	Unfreezing
4. Selecting progressive change objectives 5. Choosing an appropriate role for the change agent	Moving
6. Maintaining the change once it is started 7. Termination of the helping relationship with the change agent	Refreezing

TABLE 2.3 Comparisons of the Process of Change Theories

Lewin	Rogers	Lippitt	Kotter
Unfreezing	Awareness, interest, evaluation	Steps 1, 2, 3	Stages 1–6
Moving	Trial	Steps 4, 5	Stage 9
Refreezing	Adoption	Steps 6, 7	Stage 10

THE PROCESS OF CHANGE

Change in health care has been continuous, rapid, and accelerating. It may appear to be like a continuum from haphazard drift at one end to a structured, planned change at the other. Van Woerkum et al. (2011) acknowledged that "change happens" and that there are three ways by which it happens: (1) the emergence of events—essentially change by chance; by the use of language—how we arrive at new interpretations and ideas, (2) talking with one another about them, and (3) the development of practices—the result of a chain of activities, purposeful and planned.

Within nursing and health care, change is often circumstantial, whether it be updating policies and procedures because of lessons learned from a natural disaster, or changes in practice needed for new regulatory, accreditation, or licensing requirements. Through language, which may include information from meetings, investigations, reports, other documents, and records, nurses make conscious efforts to change and meet the latest requirements for quality improvements or safety standards. The development of modified and/or new practices in response to new evidence or best practices (evidence-based practice [EBP]) occurs regularly and falls under planned change. One example is the broad adoption of evidence-based protocols and practices as a way of making sure that desirable outcomes are achieved.

Readiness Assessment

Assessment of organizational readiness for change (ORC) may be helpful when preplanning the management of change and can empower leaders with a greater understanding of how increased levels of readiness may positively affect change outcomes. The ORC definition most widely accepted today is "the extent to which organizational members are psychologically and behaviorally prepared to implement change" (Weiner et al., 2008, p. 381). However, readiness for change assessments has been mostly measured on individuals and less on organizations. Several tools are available in publications, from consultants, and on the Internet that purport to capture employees' opinions on readiness for change. However, like so many other areas in the study of organizational change, there continues to be limited evidence of reliability and validity of most of the published tools for assessing readiness for change (Weiner et al., 2008; Weiner, 2009).

Collecting data on organizational readiness includes how employees consume, process, and interpret information related to change within their work setting (Petrou et al., 2016). There are many methods that have been tried for data collection utilizing different approaches: manual or electronic surveys, focus groups, open forums, mailers, and interviews, yet reliability and validity have been problematic. According to Shea et al. (2014), as a result of their testing, psychometric evidence supports a newly created theory-based tool of ORC named "Organizational Readiness for Implementing Change" (ORIC). Phillips (2017) compared the laboratory-tested results of ORIC to a field-proven scenario using the same tool. His study found change valence and informational assessment were positive and significantly associated with increased ORC scores ($\beta = 1.778$, $P < .001$, and $\beta = 1.392$, $P < .001$, respectively). In a principal components analysis of the ORC score, change commitment and efficacy were both favorable.

Another valid and reliable tool available is the "Organizational Readiness for Knowledge Translation" (OR4KT) (Puchalski Ritchie & Straus, 2019), based on the framework of Holt et al. (2010). The OR4KT includes individual and organizational psychological and structural factors and levels of analysis. There are some limitations to the OR4KT tool, such as its length, average time for completion of 15–20 minutes, and limited use in high-income country settings based on its testing (Gagnon et al., 2018). Therefore, the change agent/leader needs to proceed with caution in selecting and using a tool, selecting one that is consistent with organizational culture and using judgment in the application of the findings. Open communication within the change process, early involvement of staff, listening to their input and concerns, and engaging them in the change may continue to be the most effective means to assess readiness for change.

Change Fatigue

To ensure that the process of change is effective, it is important to understand how unintended consequences can result in change fatigue from ineffective communication and top-down planning. The focus needs to change from one of top-down control to one of participation and communication. Five strategies to help staff manage change fatigue are to (1) utilize effective communication using common language to frame people, situations, and events that staff will find logical and believable, (2) show support and meet staff where they are in the acceptance of the change process by listening and not being indifferent, (3) forfeit control and involve staff in the change process by empowering them on how to implement the change in their department, (4) identify where and how staff can fit into the change process to alleviate anxiety and build staff optimism, and (5) give them hope by modeling a positive outlook and energy that will mobilize and energize staff (Sherman, 2018).

Emergent Process Methods

With the emphasis on patient safety and quality goals in today's health care environment, there is a need to make small rapid changes to improve care. Two related models can be used: (1) rapid cycle change, and (2) Transforming Care at the Bedside (TCAB) (Robert Wood Johnson Foundation [RWJF], 2018). Both use the plan-do-study-act (PDSA) model (Agency for Healthcare Research and Quality [AHRQ], 2015), originated by W. Edwards Deming, as a foundation (Leis & Shojana, 2016). Rapid cycle change is based on the idea that changes should first be piloted on a small scale to see how they work. TCAB was a program created by RWJF that ran from 2003 through 2008. Its goal was to improve quality and safety on medical–surgical acute care units by engaging in changes to improve practice. The idea was to create a small test, evolve the idea, get feedback, make modifications based on feedback, and proceed with the next cycle of change, until the best outcome was achieved. Once the process reached that level, it was approved, and the process continued its use by replication based on the evidence of achievement of positive outcomes and sustainability. RWJF has a downloadable toolkit on its website (RWJF, 2018) to help organizations use the process. Numerous projects were implemented and carried out between 2003 and 2008. They included the creation of rapid response teams, the initiation of multidisciplinary rounds at the bedside, and planned interventions to prevent or decrease patient falls. One of the key features of TCAB is that it was not a top-down approach, but engaged clinicians at the bedside in the design and implementation of new work practices and systems (RWJF, 2018). TCAB also emphasized that the improvement process was continuous, not a one-time occurrence.

Rapid cycle change, a methodology adapted from Toyota Production System principles, uses a small, focused, rapid process to make process improvements (AHRQ, 2015). Rather than initiating long research studies, in rapid cycle change staff are encouraged to brainstorm new ideas, try a potential change, and test its effectiveness. This can be done with one nurse, one shift, and one patient. Demonstrating the effectiveness of small change encourages nurses to try others. Rapid cycle change is often discussed and used in conjunction with TCAB but has broad application for most process changes (Valente, 2011).

Resistance

Where there is change, there is *resistance*. Resistance is inevitable, and of concern because it impacts the change process. If resistance is anticipated as a naturally occurring phenomenon in the process of change, and treated as such, the results of working through it collaboratively can be a growth experience for individuals, groups and the organization at large. Historically in some change situations, nurses have been characterized as the targets or victims of change, irrational resisters, and problems to overcome rather than as co-creators of change. Nurses are the largest group of health care providers and are central to change within health care and are influential in success, failure, and sustenance of change depends on the commitment to the change by those on the frontline. Their resistance is typically rooted in fear, anxiety, anger, and egos. Reducing and/or eliminating resistance in the work setting is not just a management and leadership function, but a disruption that needs to be identified, opened, and embraced by those involved in the change process.

According to Caruth and Caruth "change produces uncertainty, threatens stability, elicits defensive reactions, triggers feelings of angst and prompts thoughts of failure" (Caruth & Caruth, 2018, p. 21). The authors' definition of resistance is three-fold: (1) observable behavior in response to the challenge or disagreement as a result of the introduction of new ideas, methods, or devices, (2) the degree to which those within the department or organization oppose the idea of anything new, and (3) the external orientation toward an implemented change.

Interpreting change and resistance as two opposing forces may also result in *stereotyping* one group as irrational resisters rather than as partners in and co-creators of change. Strategies for disseminating information about the change and intervening when resistance is identified so that individuals and groups can achieve adoption of the change process should be integrated into the plan.

The repercussions of not identifying or taking action on employees' overt and covert resistant actions intended to prevent, interrupt, or damage the change process is problematic for the organization. It is disruptive to operations, fosters a lack of commitment, erodes loyalty, contributes to turnover, is costly, and may be irreparable if not detected or addressed. From an individual point of view, some may have a vested interest in the status quo, others may believe that change diminishes their informal/formal power and negatively affects their personal network of interpersonal relationships. Change can threaten employees' sense of control, income/benefits, and employment. Delayed, inaccurate, or absent communication regarding change fuels resistance efforts. When resistance is perceived as a warning to management or the change agent(s), it can be a wake-up call. It creates an opportunity to understand their perspective, and to reevaluate the change, clarify the purpose, and improve messaging. It is a time for leadership to take pause and reconceptualize their approach to the change. Using a strategy to reconceptualize frontline nurses as assets and problem solvers is critical. Vos and Rupert (2018) found that when change agents created space to enable employees to think and act differently by employing creative behavior, this actually resulted in higher levels of resistance. However, when the change agents used positive framing to facilitate an emotional connection between the employees and the change, resistance significantly improved.

Leaders also need to understand that resistance is an adaptive response to power (Thomas & Hardy, 2011). When those affected by change have played a part in negotiating the process of change, there is more likelihood they will buy into the change. In addition, when it is understood that power and resistance act together, the focus can change. It shifts the question to: how do relations of power and resistance operate together in producing change? (Thomas & Hardy, 2011). Leaders who understand the power–resistance relationship will be more equipped to guide change in their settings.

Nurses live with change daily. The common belief that nurses resist change is just not accurate. One way to reframe perceptions of resistance is to consider the positive effect that resisters and resistance have played in history and in US development. Examples include rebels in the Boston Tea Party, antislavery abolitionists, passive Civil Rights protestors, and me-too protestors. These resisters led and inspired others to work for change. Just as the resisters reconceptualized a future state for others as the co-creators of change by providing an alternative view, so can health care leaders reconceptualize a new vision that they share with staff and create new strategies collaboratively for moving organizations toward change.

Managing Responses to Change

Dealing with change evokes emotional responses for all involved. Although individuals must devote personal resources and energy to accomplish change, organizations may also consider creative options. Krügel and Traub (2018) did an experimental study to determine if employees would increase change approval if the employees engaged in reciprocity towards the employer. The intervention was for the employees to play a combination of a gift exchange and a threshold contribution game. Employees were grouped, and in each group of five, one employer chooses a wage and then each group decides on their effort. If the employees exert at least a minimum threshold of effort, it is conceived as an increase in change approval. The authors found that uncertainty over payoffs does not necessarily lead to resistance, and if the employer is able to trigger reciprocal behavior in employees by offering a fair wage, employee resistance was significantly reduced. The likelihood of reform approval is especially high if the employer is able to trigger reciprocal behavior in employees by offering a fair wage, which confirms the authors' hypothesis.

Mid-level managers can provide emotional support to staff in periods of stress and change. Some effective strategies to consider are active listening, promoting action steps and solutions, keeping staff informed of decisions, soliciting input and encouraging participation, and reframing difficult messages. The meaning that a change has for the individual and/or department is important and influences how the staff view the change. The meaning that the initiator of change intends is not always what the recipient of change perceives. For example, a hospital implementing professional shared governance saw this as an opportunity for increased empowerment for the staff, yet many of those on the receiving end saw it as an increase in workload. Any perceived positive gain was negated by the personal feelings of added work. Additional factors influencing this implementation were the role of emotional contagion and staff perception of inadequate, infrequent, and poorly timed education. Emotions can play a strong role in change effort, and the associated emotional contagion was due to the staff influencing one another. Although most people inherently distrust change, change can be viewed either positively or negatively. To facilitate the change process, leaders or change agents need to actively involve the recipients of change, work to understand their view, and plan adequate, timely education on the change. An additional intervention might be to monitor unit-level reactions and understanding, because individuals who understand change better tend to view it more positively. It is helpful for leaders of change and change agents to identify early adopters of the change processes and other participants who can contribute to enthusiastically spread the work.

Transtheoretical Stages of Change Model (TTM)

This classic biopsychosocial model introduced by Prochaska and DiClemente (1983) defined self-change stages for individuals in need of behavioral change, specifically smoking cessation. Since the original work there has been widespread application inclusive of behavioral health, physical rehabilitation, weight loss, and alcoholism and other substance disorders. This model was ground-breaking in that it took an integrative process approach to intentional behavior change. Individuals could be successful at deciding on and incrementally changing personal behavior by working through a series of stages to modify behavior. The time an individual spends in each stage is variable; the tasks in each stage are not. The five stages are (1) precontemplation, (2) contemplation, (3) preparation, (4) action, and (5) maintenance. Patient stages have correlated to specific health care provider actions (stage-matched interventions) and facilitated desired behavior change. Although TTM has been used extensively to guide health promotion changes in care delivery since the advent of the ACA's goal of improving population health, its stages may also be used to positively impact individual, team, and organizational behavior during periods of significant change and innovation.

LEADERSHIP AND CHANGE

Never doubt that a small group of thoughtful, committed citizens can change the world.
Indeed, it is the only thing that ever has.

Margaret Mead

Nurse leaders are an essential part of the change process, and their values, approaches, and skills brought to change efforts are integral to success outcomes. Change is so critical to this systematic process that Burns (1978) introduced a novel model he termed *transformational leadership* (TL), emphasizing a central concept that embodied change over 40 years ago. Hindsight is 20/20, but we can all appreciate how TL has evolved into the most popular model used in nursing leadership today. In 1994, Rost conceived leadership as no longer positional but as an active process that inspired people to work collaboratively within organizational structures (Rost, 1994). The value of Rost's definition is that there was no longer a need to depend on positional structure but to re-define the leader's role and responsibilities as adaptable and driven by the needs of the organizational entity and its desired change. As these classic theories and leadership methods evolved, they were consistent with the external changes in the US healthcare arena engendering a paradigm shift to managing from an emergent change perspective. As leaders tailored their roles during these transitional times, they often struggled with their own intense emotions and likened them to feelings associated with disasters, catastrophes, and even abuse (Shanley, 2007). Managing stress for self-care as well as supporting direct reports in the work environment posed risk for negative morale, disengagement, motivational issues, and low self-esteem to grow if the management of change and human reactions was not effective.

Nurse executives and administrators are responsible for providing and sharing the vision of a preferred future, initiating change, and helping guide the direction of change that is aligned with the organization's mission, vision, values, and philosophy. As a member of the executive team, they are the colleague and liaison to effectively communicate, influence, and collaborate, garnering support for high-value patient care needs for change. Members of the change team are inclusive of middle-level and first-level managers, educators, clinical specialists, nurse practitioners, case managers, navigators, frontline staff, and other non-clinical nursing support roles, as well as other health care providers; and recipients of change take on roles as change agents, opinion leaders, and early adopters of innovations. Change agents can follow several steps in the process of change:

- Articulate a clear need and justification for change.
- Group participation in details at the point-of-service changes.
- Provide reliable information and details to the implementers of the change.
- Motivate through rewards and benefits to maintain engagement and progress.
- Do not promise anything that cannot be delivered.

For example, when implementing a planned change to a new care delivery system, the change agent's clarity and consistent messaging regarding the benefits of the change is critical throughout its inception and the entire change process. Benefits might include greater nurse autonomy, patient/staff safety, higher quality outcomes, improved patient experience, staff satisfaction, improved process effectiveness, and an overall healthy work environment with joy in the work setting. After reliable and detailed evidence is presented to the change team, the details of implementation should be arrived at by consensus of group members. Specific, realistic, and achievable goals should be the foundation for the motivation for change, reinforced by rewards and benefits—not demands or threats about performance scrutiny. High performing teamwork itself may be motivating, provide a high degree of internal satisfaction, and contribute to career development within the organization.

POWER AND POLITICS

When planning for change, power issues and politics are often overlooked and need to be incorporated into change management plans. Shanley (2007) suggested that change initiators ask, "Whose needs are being met by the change, and whose interests are being served by the change?" If hierarchical managerial practices and top-down directives are unavoidable, understanding power may assist the leadership in this scenario to reframe their views of resistors and engage them as co-creators of change. For example, powerful change can occur through professional shared governance mechanisms that bolster empowerment and sustainability, such as developing a unit-based council or integrating this project into one that already exists. Also, creating incentives for meeting criteria for career ladder advancement, or acquiring other skills related to change projects, that is, Six Sigma, STEPPS, or nursing informatics, can build competencies and proficiencies in areas that may prepare nurses for other organizational opportunities.

The business aspects of health care, running the gamut from organizational ownership changes, physician practice changes, contractual loses, shifting demographics, and reimbursement reductions, to a whole host of other non-controllable issues and often unpredictable events, can have downstream negative effects on employees, services, and the community at large.

These types of changes are usually externally imposed and require cost reductions and/or containment to survive. Top-down decisions and actions often result in negative consequences for those affected based on increased demands, fewer resources, bigger workloads, reductions in force, less benefits, changes in positions, and reporting relationships. The impact can be demoralizing and instill feelings of loss, anger, depression, disloyalty, and increased turnover contributing to lowered performance, increased sick time, reduced quality, higher risk and safety issues, shortages in labor, and more. These economic or political forces may pressure nurse leaders to make organizational changes or enact restructuring to alleviate immediate or short-term problems. Unfortunately, the long-term effects of these changes may be difficult to foresee or to quantify. There are unintended consequences. Nurses at all levels must learn to speak up, articulate, and support the value of their role and evaluate change for the long term. As nurses assume more leadership responsibilities in the health care system, as suggested in the *Future of nursing* report (IOM, 2011), they can use their own positional power and influence to chart nursing's own destiny and, hopefully, prevent further destructive practices that do not necessarily serve the better good.

INNOVATION THEORY

Change and *innovation* are companion terms, but many authors differentiate innovation from change. An *innovation* is defined as something new, the introduction of a new process or new way of doing something. Innovation implies creativity and doing things differently. According to Hernandez et al. (2013, p. 167), innovation is "a process involving several steps from the creation of a novel idea to its adoption, implementation, and spread (diffusion) within and/or across organizations." Research has determined that leaders in practice and academia experience significant gaps in innovation competencies in formal and continuing education (White et al., 2016). Leaders need to develop skill proficiency that promotes innovation and contributes to a culture that incorporates the most effective evidence-based practices. This will help to meet needs of patients and for providers to gain or maintain a competitive advantage in health care service delivery.

Research on innovation in nursing began to emerge (Joseph, 2015) to solve complex problems by adopting behaviors, processes, and systems that foster innovation. A good example is how Kaiser Permanente created their Innovation Model to develop, test, improve, transform, and spread new ideas, equipment, products, care procedures, and services. The Innovations Unit was designed as an inpatient unit where operational and process innovations are trialed.

The Deloitte Center for Healthcare Solutions (DCHS) has developed a framework based on expected fundamental changes to the health care industry, driven by consumerism, data availability and use, and scientific innovation (Batra & Shukla, 2020). DCHS is tracking progress on innovations made by several public and private entities. The Centers for Medicare & Medicaid Services (CMS) has Blue Button 2.0 application (Verdict Medical Devices, 2018) that allows 53 million Medicare beneficiaries to access health information on their mobile devices. Access to their personal data (i.e., prescriptions, coverage, and costs) can also be shared with other health care providers to support decision-making. Apple Health Records® has an application that allows over 100 million Apple iPhone® consumers to link personal health data from several different sources on conditions, medications, claims and utilization, genomics, and wellness, and can also share it with other health care providers to support decision-making (Muoio, 2019; Terry, 2019).

The first step to innovation for leaders is to realize forces of innovation and change have mobilized. In order to change mindsets, learned ways of thinking, communication, and decision-making, leaders must be open to increase knowledge of what is happening apart from the current setting and comfort level. Considerations to include in a personal development plan for innovation are (1) share data, (2) review analyses and transformative work in data architecture, (3) continue to improve access to health care, (4) empower the consumer with convenience and transparency, and (5) support care and services that integrate digital tools, such as artificial intelligence, remote devices, and sensors, and (6) stay abreast of the scientific communities' innovative work (Batra & Shukla, 2020).

Rogers' Innovation Theory

First published in 1962 by the late Everett M. Rogers, Innovation Theory is the best-known theory on innovation (Kapoor et al., 2014). Known as the "inventor" of innovation, Rogers produced multiple editions of his book, with the 5th edition published in 2003. Rogers (2003) described a cognitive innovation-decision process that individuals and groups go through. He delineated five stages of the innovation-decision process: (1) first knowledge of an innovation's existence and functions, (2) persuasion to form an attitude toward the innovation, (3) decision to adopt or reject, (4) implementation of the new idea, and (5) confirmation to reinforce or reverse the innovation decision (Rogers, 2003). The innovation-decision process is a sequence of actions, behaviors, and choices beginning with the evaluation of a new idea and ending with a decision to accept or reject the incorporation of the innovation into practice. The perceived newness and associated uncertainty are distinctive aspects of the innovation.

Individuals need to be interested in the innovation and committed to making change occur. Hersey et al. (2013) suggested that effective change must involve people in four levels of change: (1) knowledge, (2) attitude, (3) individual behavior, and (4) group or organizational behavior. Typically to test out an innovation, the change agent would begin to work on awareness-knowledge, then address attitudes and emotions, but a focus on the development of how-to skills is the driver of creating sustainable behavioral change. Most change agents concentrate on creating knowledge and raising awareness, but Rogers (2003) believed that concentrating on practical how-to information was more critical when adopters needed to change individual, group, and organizational behaviors. Once the innovation has been tested, a knowledge-attitude-practice gap (KAP-gap) emerges. This is when individuals have gained awareness knowledge and how-to knowledge about an innovation, have formed a favorable attitude towards it, but have not acted upon it. The KAP-gap informs and influences a reevaluation of the new idea, product, or practice (Singer, 2019), and, based on the level(s) of change the individuals/group members are falling out at, will determine what modifications to make to fill the gap.

Individual members of a group or social system will adopt an innovation at different rates. This time element of the adoption of an innovation usually follows a normal, bell-shaped curve when plotted over time on a frequency basis. However, if the cumulative number of adopters is plotted, an S-shaped curve appears (Rogers, 2003). The normal adopter frequency distribution was segmented into the following five categories of innovators, early adopters, early majority, late majority, and laggards (Rogers, 2003).

Change agents can anticipate these five categories as an expected phenomenon, identify followers as to early adopter category, and target interventions accordingly. This means that for effective change, nurse leaders can recognize that there will be individual variance in acceptance of an innovation, plan for this with targeted strategies to decrease resistance, and capitalize on the power of innovations and early adopters.

Individuals need to be interested in the innovation and committed to making change occur. The outcomes of change are that the change is either accepted, adopted, or rejected. If the change is accepted, it can be either continued or eventually dropped. If the change is rejected, it can remain rejected or be adopted later in some other form. Rogers' theory (Rogers, 2003) described change as more complex than Lewin's (1947, 1951) three stages. Rogers (2003) identified the following five factors as determinants of successful planned change:

1. *Relative advantage*: The degree to which change is thought to be better than the status quo.
2. *Compatibility*: The degree to which change is compatible with values of the individuals/group.
3. *Complexity*: The degree to which a change is perceived as difficult to use and understand.
4. *Trialability*: The degree to which a change can be tested out on a limited basis.
5. *Observability*: The degree to which the results of a change are visible to others.

Kapoor et al. (2014) conducted an extensive meta-analysis of research on innovation. They found that of the five factors that Rogers (2003) identified, only *relativity* and *compatibility* could be positively correlated with successful change and that complexity was *negatively* correlated. None of the other factors were found significant in those studies. Simply stated, if members of an organization perceive a change to be better than the status quo, consistent with their values and relatively easy to understand, there will be a much better chance of adoption.

Rogers (2003) did the initial research on how acceptance of a new idea spread and was the original creator of the *Diffusion of Innovations* model. Innovators need tools to test whether their new ideas, products, or practices will be used.

Singer (2019, p. 1) defined diffusion as "the process by which an innovation is communicated through certain channels over time among the members of a social system." When leaders determine what level of change the people are in, they must communicate with the members of the social system with enthusiasm, new information, and authority about the likelihood of adoption. It also raises questions for ongoing steps toward dissemination of the innovation, such as should we conduct user research to make sure we solve actual problem(s)? What metrics are the most important ones to track? What advertising strategies should we use so we attract people who will be interested in our offering?

Innovation in Health Care

For nurses to be equipped to participate and/or lead in viable improvements in health care, they need to be open and mindful of new methods to try out via innovation. Innovation in health care requires creativity and ownership of practice solutions. Two government agencies, CMS (n.d.) and Agency for Healthcare Research and Quality (AHRQ)(n.d.), and private organizations such as the Center for Creative Leadership (CCL, 2014) have developed resources useful to nurses and health care providers wishing to innovate. In CCL's white paper, *Innovation leadership: How to use innovation to lead effectively, work collaboratively, and drive results,* they noted that underlying the pressure on individuals and organizations to adapt is the need to innovate. Their six innovative thinking skills are paying attention, personalizing, imaging, serious play, collaborative inquiry, and crafting. To begin experimenting with innovation they recommend reframing the challenge, focusing on the customer experience, and rapid prototyping. Nurses can use these resources to apply innovative thinking to the solution of problems.

AHRQ (n.d.) has a Health Care Innovations Exchange (https://innovations.ahrq.gov/) that offers Innovation Profiles and quality tools, articles and collections, and sponsored learning communities on high-priority patient care delivery topic areas.

CMS (n.d.) has an Innovation Center (https://innovation.cms.gov/) that supports development and testing of innovative health care payment and service delivery models. The website offers webinars, forums, reports, and datasets to the community of health care innovators, data researchers, and policy analysts.

Recognizing innovations created by nurses promotes a better understanding of the nurse role in innovation. Johnson & Johnson Nursing (2019) shared the stories of five nurse innovators at https://nursing.jnj.com/nursing-news-events/nurses-leading-innovation/5-nurses-making-waves-in-healthcare-innovation.

How might leaders best identify, support, and promote innovators? First, they need to seek out people who are not afraid to take risks (Cullen, 2015). Cullen characterized innovators as having the following assets: questions common beliefs and practices, comfort level with uncertainty and failures, expert knowledge, identifies innovations that may apply in their organization, and connects with other innovators through their professional network.

Nurse leaders need to create plans to add or develop existing innovation groups within their organization. Producing environments that support innovation empowers nurses to generate creative ideas and design the way of our future. Providing opportunities for frontline nurses to share ideas with colleagues both within and outside the organization and health care environment, can inspire clinical and administrative solutions that embrace ambiguity and reinforce the art of possibilities (Cullen, 2015). Innovation-promoting behaviors are relatively new considering other professions have been studying and developing evidence for a long time. To keep pace with the rapid and changing demands in health care, the value to the organization of having frontline caregivers contribute to meaningful innovation is immeasurable.

Disruptive Innovation

In contrast to system-related views of innovation, it is important to understand the history behind another type, *disruptive innovation.* Christensen and colleagues from Harvard Business School described disruptive innovation as a process wherein a simplifying technology takes root and displaces more established technologies or business practices that are slower to change, rooted in tradition, or constrained by regulation and the status quo (Christensen et al., 2000). Disruptive innovations were defined by Christensen et al. (2000, p. 104) as: "*disruptive innovations*—cheaper, simpler, more convenient products or services that start by meeting the needs of less-demanding customers."

As an example, Christensen et al. identified a portable low-intensity x-ray machine designed to be used in clinics, doctors' offices, and in the field. The technology was estimated to cost 10% of traditional x-rays, but it did not gain acceptance in the market at that time. The assumption was that this was because it threatened current business models. Further analysis suggested that regulators were encouraged not to approve the technology; insurance companies would not approve the reimbursement because they could charge more in other radiology settings; and hospitals were driven to reap a return on investment in newly purchased equipment, radiologists in their medical staff, and radiology centers. Christensen et al. (2000) also identified other disruptive innovations that held promise to improve health care in the United States, that is, increasing use of nurse practitioners in primary care, and further expanding the care continuum by increasing ambulatory services and home care. An example of a disruptive innovation is shown in Box 2.1. Christensen et al. (2000) had evidence and vision for health care reform, creative leaders, and flexible organizations to incorporate new ideas and innovations, yet the business and economics of health care appears to have thwarted progress in some areas.

BOX 2.1 Example of Disruptive Innovation in Health Care

Disruptive innovations were described by Christensen et al. (2000) as simplifying "technology" that takes root. One such innovation that fits his definition was a barber-based blood pressure control program for African American men (AHRQ, n.d.). In this innovation, "trained barbers in African American owned shops provided ongoing monitoring of blood pressure to African American male patrons during each haircut, along with printed educational materials and feedback designed to encourage those with elevated blood pressure to visit the doctor." African American men suffer higher rates of hypertension than the rest of the population and often have higher rates of disability because of it. By providing this screening and educational materials at every haircut, the program significantly improved treatment rates and blood pressure control in hypertensive patrons. This outside-the-box innovation was a low-cost approach that was successful in meeting a community health need.

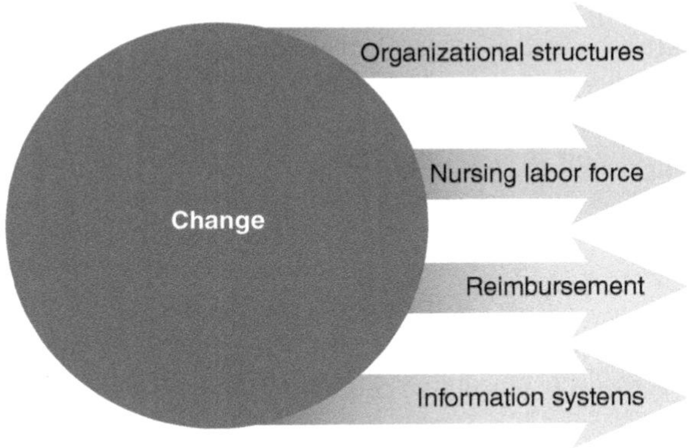

Fig. 2.2 Areas of major change in health care and nursing.

LEADERSHIP AND MANAGEMENT IMPLICATIONS

Change is a current expectation of leadership by envisioning future states as a necessity and mastering skills to develop achievable processes that are mutually agreeable to the frontline. The essentials of leadership are the ability to communicate and share the vision, collaborate on issues inherent in the change, support inclusivity from all key stakeholders in the change process, and incorporate into the organization's culture. Role modeling leader access, visibility at all levels, and support of creative and innovative ideas that translate into change initiatives will inspire and gain commitment from the change team.

Emblematic of transformational leaders, strategic change work includes being able to ignite a vision and have the ability to support changes in structure, mindsets, and power structures, and empowers others to fully participate in change initiatives (Robbins & Davidhizar, 2007). When trust and cooperation are achieved between the frontline and administration, a high performance is the norm.

Because of a current state of continuous change, the nursing perspective has also adapted to include four key areas signifying major change areas in nursing practice: (1) organizational structure, (2) nursing labor force, (3) reimbursement, and (4) information systems (Fig. 2.2). First, organizational structures have been modified and reconfigured in response to changes in health care reimbursement and other external and internal environmental factors. Population-based care, insurance and contractual reform, patient- and family-centered care, and patient safety initiatives are examples of redesigns in patient care systems to accommodate the aforementioned environmental factors.

After a decade, the ACA has resulted in more integrated networks, advancements of technological support across care settings, increased remote care improving patient access to care, a rise in digital personal devices providing real-time clinical information to providers, and consumer ownership of health care information, options, and care decisions. The complexion of the nurse workforce has experienced exponential change, and a new wave of leaders from all generations and at all career levels is emerging and rising to the challenges in health care.

Learning Organizations

An organization committed to keeping pace with health care needs and demands needs to embrace continuous lifelong learning principles from a systems perspective. Porter-O'Grady and Malloch (2015) endorsed four practices for current workplaces that foster learning organizations:

(1) empowerment, (2) shared decision-making, (3) self-direction, and (4) shared governance.

Senge popularized the concept of a learning organization based on his belief that "every organization is a product of how its members think and interact" (Senge et al., 1994, p. 48). A learning organization requires an infrastructure that supports ongoing learning and knowledge acquisition by using systems thinking, mental models, personal mastery, team learning, and shared vision. Its aim is to transform behaviors within an organization resulting in a learning culture that is adaptable and responsive. Essentially the creation, acquisition, and transference of knowledge are used to adapt behavior to establish new evidence, new knowledge, and new insights at all levels.

CURRENT ISSUES AND TRENDS

At the end of the last century, multiple authors identified future trends in health care. They predicted that these amounted to major paradigm shifts. In 1996, Issel and Anderson identified the following six interconnected transformations that are major areas of change still influencing health care today:

1. From person-as-customer to the population-as-customer
2. From illness care to wellness care and prevention
3. From revenue management to cost management
4. From autonomy of professionals to their interdependence
5. From client as non-consumer to consumer of cost and quality information
6. From continuity of provider to continuity of information.

There have been continual shifts toward those changes. For example, the ACA (2010) is not just a payment or insurance program; its aims are to guide the United States to shift health care priorities from a disease and illness mindset to wellness and prevention.

Another area of important change in health care is reimbursement. For example, reimbursement (payment) for physicians has changed, driven previously by the federal government's relative value units' determinations, pay for performance, pay based on outcomes, and now value-based purchasing and population health management. Reimbursement for nurse practitioners is allowed now under Medicare/Medicaid. Payment reforms are likely to continue and change. The cost areas include physician payment, already being ratcheted down; pharmaceutical costs; and equipment and technology costs. The government will continue to review and analyze health care expenditures to reduce a huge national budget deficit fueled partly by health care costs.

A massive transformation in computerized information systems occurred with the upgrade from manual medical records to electronic health records (EHR) and meaningful use initiatives. Powerful computers and sophisticated software programs have a pattern of frequently undergoing updates and generational changes, which creates challenges of compatibility, archival retrieval, maintaining currency, and staff training. Compatibility among systems, such as relational databases, remains challenging.

These changes have and will continue to alter the health care delivery system. They present both opportunities and challenges, and nurses need to be able to anticipate and monitor trends for their immediate and long-term effects on practice. Nurses can participate in and even lead some of these trends, as they create new environments or establish new organizational documents to shape the direction of health care. It is a question of which courses of action are the best and what is the best way to direct the transformations.

The health care environment has been described as turbulent because of the rapid rate of change and the perceived constancy of change. However, change can be growth producing, renewing, and invigorating for individuals and organizations. This occurs as individuals and organizations enlist creativity to derive an innovation that improves the environment or client care delivery. Believe in the impossible.

> *"There is no use trying," said Alice. "One can't believe impossible things." "I daresay you haven't had much practice," said the Queen. "When I was your age, I always did it for half an hour a day. Why, sometimes I've believed as many as six impossible things before breakfast."*
>
> **Lewis Carroll**

BEST PRACTICE SUGGESTIONS FOR NURSE LEADERS

There are multiple models and approaches to change, but little evidence on what works or what will work for a particular setting. This is understandable, as organizational change is decidedly difficult to research. There are multiple confounding variables and differences in settings (from systems to specific units to individual nurses). Here are a few "take-aways" for best practice in considering the information presented in this chapter:

- Assess your particular setting and the type of change proposed.
- There is no ONE best theory or model to follow; find a model or process (or combination) suited to your specific setting.
- Communicate the vision for the change.
- Avoid top-down implementation.
- Involve the frontline and those who are at the point of care.
- Engage the "early adopters"; have them help you to influence others.
- Remember that power and resistance go hand-in-hand.
- Reassess and reevaluate frequently, and modify the strategy when needed.
- Maintain the change by making it part of the new culture.
- Communicate, communicate, communicate.
- Listen, listen, listen.

Change and innovation is a complex process with multiple approaches and models. The transfer of this knowledge coupled with applying new skills and managing the change process will determine the "best way" for a nurse to proceed in implementing and mastering change as a leader.

RESEARCH NOTE

Source

"Nursing innovation is a fundamental source of progress for healthcare systems around the world."

Joseph, M.L. (2015). Organizational culture and climate for promoting innovativeness. *Journal of Nursing Administration*, 45, 172–178. https://doi.org/10.1097/NNA.0000000000000178.

Purpose

This qualitative study had dual purposes: (1) to find out more about the experiences of nurses and nurse leaders in a hospital with a mission to support innovation, and (2) to generate a thematic map of the experience.

Discussion

Because nurses are critical in developing innovations that impact patient care, it is important to understand how you, as leader, can best create a healthy work environment that supports innovation. This study consisted of two phases: the first phase was based on semi structured interviews of six staff nurses and six nurse leaders, and the second phase involved focus groups to validate the model. The qualitative data were analyzed using content analysis methods, which entails reviewing and analyzing the data, immersion in the data to gain a sense of the whole, identifying commonalities that led to coding and labeling, and sorting into categories. A model demonstrating innovativeness in nursing was developed from newly acquired evidence from the analysis (see Fig. 2.3).

Results

Joseph identified:

Five concepts as preconditions for innovativeness:

(1) organizational values, (2) workplace relationships, (3) organizational identification, (4) organizational support, and (5) relational leadership.

Six additional concepts emerged that revealed a social process for innovativeness:

(1) trust, (2) inquiry, (3) idea generation, (4) support, (5) trialing, and (6) learning.

Three key concepts related to innovativeness in nursing:

(1) relationships, (2) leadership style, and (3) context.

Application to Practice

Study results support the need for the leader to build a strong relationship with staff aligned with organizational values and to create an innovative climate that positively affects the organization's culture. Leaders need to have an impact at all staff and organizational levels that fosters consistency across departments and sustainability.

continued

RESEARCH NOTE—cont'd

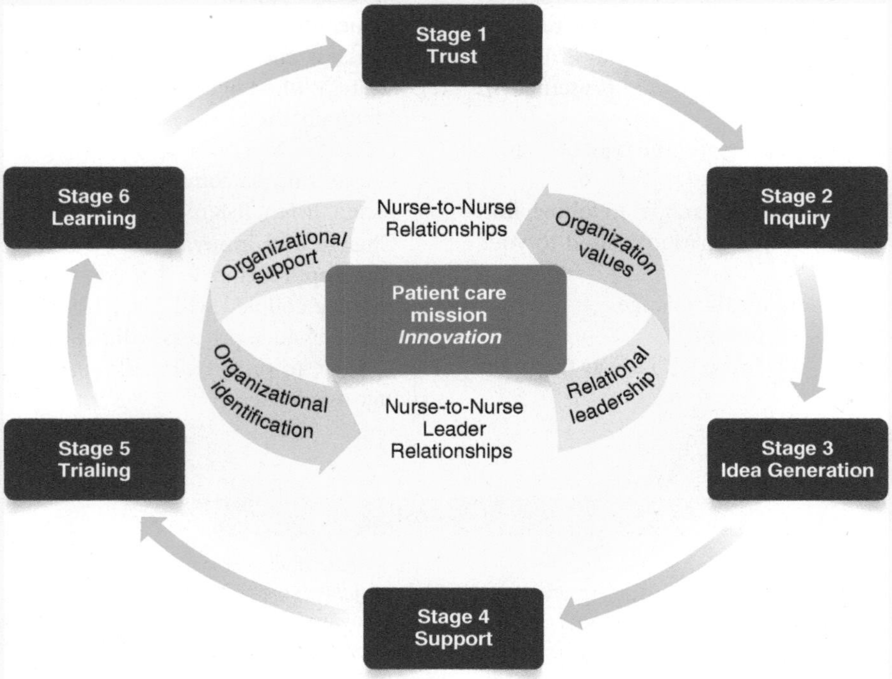

Fig. 2.3 Innovativeness in nursing. (Reprinted with permission from Joseph, M.L. [2015].)

CASE STUDY

Amanda Gonzalez, RN and Gus Lopez, RN work as diabetic case managers (DCMs) who support the family practice and internal medicine areas in a large community health care system. The case management and education departments are charged with restructuring some of the processes to improve efficiency and comply with the National Committee for Quality Assurance.

In the midst of these changes, researchers from the local university approached departmental administrators to seek assistance in recruiting qualified patients for a blood pressure research study. The administrators decided that the DCMs should be the ones to take on the recruitment responsibilities, but Amanda and Gus were not consulted about the change, nor was their workload discussed. This responsibility to recruit participants for the research study was presented to the DCMs in addition to their current responsibilities, which include contacting patients post hospital discharge, monitoring an assigned case load, educating diabetic patients, and monitoring their diet, activity, blood sugars, and medications.

The DCMs believe the additional responsibility has a negative impact on the quality of their patient education. They are concerned that because of the increased workload, they may increase risk for omissions or errors in care and jeopardize patient safety. Since this change was initiated, the DCMs are not able to meet all patient care needs due to these unrealistic additions to their workload.

CASE STUDY—cont'd

They are stressed and confused about the expectations they were not consulted on prior to this decision. There was a lack of discussion and collaboration within the work unit regarding this new responsibility. The DCMs are receiving more patient applications for the study than they can accommodate. The result so far has been slow recruitment to the research protocol, potential patient safety issues, and poor patient and staff satisfaction.

1. What type of change would you call this? How was it initiated?
2. Has this been a successful change so far?
3. Where do you think the leaders went wrong in approaching this change?
4. List three strategies that the administrators might have used to increase the possibility of a positive change.

CRITICAL THINKING EXERCISE

Carol Butterworth, RN, is a staff nurse in a 22-bed critical care unit within a large health care organization for over 10 years. She returned to school for a master's degree in nursing last year and would like to do her graduate project in her clinical area. Carol identified the rate for hospital-acquired ventilator associated pneumonia (VAP) was higher than local, state, and national benchmarks. She gathered information about sedation and intubation in her intensive care unit (ICU) and decided that an evidence-based nurse-directed sedation protocol could improve patient outcomes. She plans to enlist the support of the VAP committee that includes members of the interdisciplinary team and frontline health care workers. She first seeks consultation from the Advanced Practice Provider, who is a nurse practitioner.

Carol wants to develop and implement policies, procedures, physician order sets, and establish a sedation protocol based on national clinical guidelines. She has identified key stakeholders, that is, physicians, frontline nurses, clinical nurse specialists (CNS), ICU mid-level managers, pulmonary technicians, and directors of intensivists, critical care, and pharmacy. She is contemplating how to gain support for this project that will be piloted on this one unit. Critical care nurses as well as the intensivists will receive sufficient education on this evidence-based guideline and its protocol.

1. Analyze some of the issues that Carol must anticipate.
2. Explain what theory or model might be useful and why?
3. Who should be recruited for the committee and why?
4. Describe Carol's first step in the innovation process and why it is a priority?
5. How might Carol and the committee problem-solve staff resistance?

REFERENCES

Agency for Healthcare Research and Quality (AHRQ). (n.d.). *AHRQ health care innovations exchange*. https://innovations.ahrq.gov/.

Agency for Healthcare Research and Quality (AHRQ). (2015). *Plan-Do-Study-Act (PDSA): Directions and examples.* https://www.ahrq.gov/health-literacy/quality-resources/tools/literacy-toolkit/healthlittoolkit2-tool2b.html.

American Organization for Nursing Leadership (AONL). (2015). AONE nurse executive competencies. *Nurse Leader, 3*(1), 15–21.

Anderson, L. A., & Anderson, D. (2009). *Awake at the wheel: Moving beyond change management to conscious change leadership*. http://www.beingfirst.com/.

Appelbaum, S. H., Habashy, S., Malo, J., & Shafiq, H. (2012). Back to the future: Revisiting Kotter's 1996 change model. *Journal of Management Development, 31*(8), 764–782. https://doi.org/10.1108/02621711211253231.

Balogun, J. (2006). Managing change: Steering a course between intended strategies and unanticipated outcomes. *Long Range Planning, 39*, 29–49.

Bank of Information. (2014). *Planned change*. http://bankofinfo.com/definition-of-planned-change/.

Batra, N., & Shukla, M. (2020). *Six assumptions for measuring health disruption: The future of health is further along than some might think.* The Deloitte Center for Health Solutions. https://www2.deloitte.com/content/dam/Deloitte/ec/Documents/life-sciences-health-care/DI_Six-assumptions-for-measuring-health-disruption.pdf.

Bejinariu, A. C., Jitarel, A., Sarca, I., & Mocan, A. (2017). Organizational change management: Concepts definitions and approaches inventory, 321–331. Paper presented at the "Management Challenges in a Network Economy" conference, *Management, Knowledge and Learning International Conference Technology, Innovation and Industrial Management*. Lublin, Poland. http://www.toknowpress.net/ISBN/978-961-6914-21-5/papers/ML17061.pdf.

Burnes, B. (2004). Kurt Lewin and complexity theories: Back to the future? *Journal of Change Management, 4*(4), 309–325.

Burnes, B. (2009). Reflections: Ethics and organizational change—time for a return to Lewinian values. *Journal of Change Management, 9*(4), 359–381. https://doi.org/10.1080/14697010903360558.

Burns, J. (1978). *Leadership*. New York, NY: Harper & Row.

Cambridge Dictionary. (2020a). *Change*. https://dictionary.cambridge.org/us/dictionary/english/change.

Cambridge Dictionary. (2020b). *Transformation*. https://dictionary.cambridge.org/us/dictionary/english/transformation.

Cambridge Dictionary. (2020c). *Change agent*. https://dictionary.cambridge.org/us/dictionary/english/change-agent.

Carder, B. (2015). A psychological theory of culture: Balancing the conscious and unconscious mind to improve leadership. *The Journal for Quality & Participation, 38*(3), 18–22.

Carson, F. (2016). Why personal change is important for a conscious leader. *Industrial and Commercial Training, 48*(6), 300–302 https://doi.org/10.1108/ICT-12-2015-0085.

Caruth, D. L., & Caruth, G. D. (2018). Managing workplace resistance to change. *Industrial Management, 60*(4), 21.

Center for Creative Leadership (CCL). (2014). *Innovation leadership: How to use innovation to lead effectively, work collaboratively, and drive results.* https://www.ccl.org/openenrollmentprograms/?keyword=center%20for%20creative%20leadership&matchtype=e&gclid=CjwKCAiA7t3yBRADEiwA4GFlI57-kAETFU6yLk0Ht4ozCG6eJUYHkqgYyP-eMrdEPUVlP4sqUe6hU8hoCI0EQAvD_BwE.

Centers for Medicare & Medicaid Services (CMS). (2019). *Telemedicine*. https://www.medicaid.gov/medicaid/benefits/telemedicine/index.html.

Centers for Medicare & Medicaid Services (CMS). (n.d.). *CMS Innovation Center*. https://innovation.cms.gov/.

Christensen, C. M., Bohmer, R., & Kenagy, J. (2000). Will disruptive innovations cure health care? *Harvard Business Review, 78*(5), 102–112.

Clarke, C. S. (2013). Resistance to change in the nursing profession: Creative transdisciplinary solutions. *Creative Nursing, 19*, 70–76 https://doi.org/10.1891/1078-4535.19.2.70.

Cullen, L. (2015). Evidence into practice: Awakening the innovator in every nurse. *Journal of PeriAnesthesia Nursing, 30*, 430–435.

Department of Health and Human Services. (2018). Clarification of final rules for grandfathered plans, preexisting condition exclusions, lifetime and annual limits, rescissions, dependent coverage, appeals, and patient protections under the Affordable Care Act. *Federal Register, 83*(86), 19431–19436.

Gagnon, M. P., Attieh, R., Dunn, S., Grandes, G., Bully, P., Estabrooks, C. A., et al. (2018). Development and content validation of a transcultural instrument to assess organizational readiness for knowledge translation in healthcare organizations: The OR4KT. *International Journal of Health Policy Management, 7*(9), 791–797.

Hallencreutz, S. S., & Turner, D. (2011). Exploring organizational change best practice: Are there any clear-cut models and definitions? *International Journal of Quality and Service Sciences, 3*, 60–68.

Hammer, M. (1990). Reengineering work: Don't automate—obliterate. *Harvard Business Review, 68*(4), 104–112.

Heath, S. (2017). *What is the difference between urgent care, retail health clinics?* https://patientengagementhit.com/news/what-is-the-difference-between-urgent-care-retail-health-clinics.

Hernandez, S. E., Conrad, D. A., Marcus-Smith, M. S., Reed, P., & Watts, C. (2013). Patient-centered innovation in health care organizations: A conceptual framework and case study application. *Health Care Management Review, 38*(2), 166–175. https://doi.org/10.1097/HMR.0b013e31825e718a.

Hersey, P., Blanchard, K. H., & Johnson, D. E. (2013). *Management of organizational behavior: Leading human resources* (10th ed.). Upper Saddle River, NJ: Pearson Education.

Holt, D. T., Helfrich, C. D., Hall, C. G., & Weiner, B. J. (2010). Are you ready? How health professionals can comprehensively conceptualize readiness for change. *Journal General Internal Medicine, 25*(Supplement 1), 50–55. https://doi.org/10.1007/s11606-009-1112-8.

Hughes, M. (2011). Do 70 per cent of all organizational change initiatives really fail? *Journal of Change Management, 11*(4), 451–465. https://doi.org/10.1080/14697017.2011.630506.

Institute of Medicine (IOM). (2011). *The future of nursing: Leading change, advancing health*. Washington, DC: National Academies Press.

Issel, L. M., & Anderson, R. A. (1996). Take charge: Managing six transformations in healthcare delivery. *Nursing Economic$, 14*(2), 78–85.

Jansson, N. (2013). Organizational change as practice: A critical analysis. *Journal of Organizational Change Management, 26*, 1003–1019. https://doi.org/10.1108/JOCM-09-2012-0152.

Johnson & Johnson Nursing. (2019). *Five nurses making waves in healthcare innovation*. https://nursing.jnj.com/nursing-news-events/nurses-leading-innovation/5-nurses-making-waves-in-healthcare-innovation.

Joseph, M. L. (2015). Organizational culture and climate for promoting innovativeness. *Journal of Nursing Administration, 45*, 172–178. https://doi.org/10.1097/NNA.0000000000000178.

Kapoor, K. K., Dwivedi, Y. K., & Williams, M. D. (2014). Rogers' innovation adoption attributes: A systematic review and synthesis of existing research. *Information Systems Management, 31*, 74–91. https://doi.org/10.1080/10580530.2014.854103.

Klein, N., & O'Brien, E. (2017). The power and limits of personal change: When a bad past does (and does not) inspire in the present. *Journal of Personality and Social Psychology, 113*(2), 210–229. https://doi.org/10.1037/pspa0000088.

Kotter, J. P. (1995). Leading change: Why transformation efforts fail. *Harvard Business Review, 73*(2), 59–67.

Kotter, J. P. (2012). *Leading change*. Boston, MA: Harvard Business Review Press.

Krügel, J. P., & Traub, S. (2018). Reciprocity and resistance to change: An experimental study. *Journal of Economic Behavior & Organization, 147*, 95–114. https://doi.org/10.1016/j.jebo.2017.12.017.

Leis, J. A., & Shojana, K. G. (2016). A primer on PDSA: executing plan-do-study-act cycles in practice, not just in name. *BMJ Quality & Safety, 26*(7), 572–577. https://doi.org/10.1136/bmjqs-2016-006245.

Lewin, K. (1947). Frontiers in group dynamics: Concept, method, and reality in social science; social equilibrium and social change. *Human Relations, 1*(1), 5–41.

Lewin, K. (1951). *Field theory in social science: Selected theoretical papers*. New York, NY: Harper & Row.

Lippitt, G. (1973). *Visualizing change: Model building and the change process*. La Jolla, CA: University Associates.

Longenecker, C. O., & Longenecker, P. D. (2014). Why hospital improvement efforts fail: A view from the front line. *Journal of Healthcare Management, 59*, 147–157.

Muoio, D. (2019, June 28). Apple Health Records now available to all US providers with compatible EHRs. *Mobihealthnews*. https://www.mobihealthnews.com/news/north-america/apple-health-records-now-available-all-us-providers-compatible-ehrs.

National Academies of Sciences, Engineering, and Medicine, Health and Medicine Division (HMD). (2010). *The future of nursing: Leading change, advancing health*. http://www.nationalacademies.org/hmd/Reports/2010/The-Future-of-Nursing-LeadingChange-Advancing-Health.aspx.

Packard, T., & Shih, A. (2014). Organizational change tactics: The evidence base in the literature. *Journal of Evidence-Based Social Work, 11*, 498–510. https://doi.org/10.1080/15433714.2013.831006.

Patient Protection and Affordable Care Act [ACA]. (2010). https://www.dpc.senate.gov/healthreformbill/healthbill04.pdf.

Perregrini, M. (2019). Mitigating resistance to change in the workplace. *Creative Nursing, 25*(2), 154–156. https://doi.org/10.1891/1078-4535.25.2.154.

Petrou, P., Demerouti, E., & Schaufeli, W. B. (2016). Crafting the change: The role of employee job crafting behaviors for successful organizational change. *Journal of Occupational Health Psychology*. https://doi.org/10.1177/0149206315624961.

Phillips, J. E. (2017). *Effects of change valence and informational assessment on organizational readiness for change*. Minneapolis, MN: Walden University. https://scholarworks.waldenu.edu/cgi/viewcontent.cgi?article=5119&context=dissertations.

Porter-O'Grady, T., & Malloch, K. (2015). *Quantum leadership: Building better partnerships for sustainable health* (4th ed.). Sudbury, MA: Jones and Bartlett.

Prochaska, J. O., & DiClemente, C. C. (1983). Stages and processes of self-change of smoking: Toward an integrative model of change. *Journal of Consulting and Clinical Psychology, 51*(3), 390–395.

Puchalski Ritchie, L. M., & Straus, S. E. (2019). Assessing organizational readiness for change. *International Journal of Health Policy Management, 8*(1), 55–57. https://doi.org/10.15171/ijhpm.2018.101.

Raus, K., Mortier, E., & Eeckloo, K. (2018). The patient perspective in health care networks. *BMC Medical Ethics*, 19–52. https://doi.org/10.1186%2Fs12910-018-0298-x.

Robert Wood Johnson Foundation (RWJF). (2018). *The transforming care at the bedside (TCAB) toolkit*. Princeton, NJ: Robert Wood Johnson Foundation. https://www.rwjf.org/en/library/research/2008/06/the-transforming-care-at-the-bedside-tcab-toolkit.html.

Robbins, B., & Davidhizar, R. (2007). Transformational leadership in healthcare today. *The Healthcare Manager, 26*, 234–239.

Rogers, E. M. (2003). *Diffusion of innovations* (5th ed.). New York, NY: Free Press.

Rost, J. C. (1994). Leadership: A new conception. *Holistic Nursing Practice, 9*(2), 1–8.

Senge, P., Kleiner, A., Roberts, C., Ross, R., & Smith, B. (1994). *The fifth discipline fieldbook*. New York, NY: Doubleday.

Shanley, C. (2007). Management of change for nurses: Lessons from the discipline of organizational studies. *Journal of Nursing Management, 15*, 538–546. https://doi.org/10.1111/j.1365-2834.2007.00722.x.

Shea, C. M., Jacobs, S. R., Esserman, D. A., Bruce, K., & Weiner, B. J. (2014). Organizational readiness for implementing change: A psychometric assessment of a new measure. *Implementation Science, 9*(7), 1–15. https://doi.org/10.1186/1748-5908-9-7.

Sherman, R. (2018). Managing change fatigue. *Emerging Nurse Leader*. https://www.emergingrnleader.com/managing-change-fatigue/.

Singer, L. (2019). *Thoughts on human behavior and making software (blog). On the diffusion.* https://leif.me/2016/12/on-the-diffusion-of-innovations-how-new-ideas-spread/.

Suddaby, R. (2016). Toward a historical consciousness: Following the historic turn in management thought. *M@n@gement, 19*(1), 46–60.

Suddaby, R., & Foster, W. M. (2017). History and organizational change. *Journal of Management, 43*(1), 1–20. https://doi.org/10.1177/0149206316675031.

Tasler, N. (2017). *Stop using the excuse "Organizational change is hard"*. https://hbr.org/2017/07/stop-using-the-excuse-organizational-change-is-hard.

Terry, K. (2019, July 3). *Apple opens iPhone EHR feature to all healthcare organizations. Medscape.* https://www.medscape.com/viewarticle/915208.

Thomas, R., & Hardy, C. (2011). Reframing resistance to organizational change. *Scandinavian Journal of Management, 27*, 332–331.

Valente, S. (2011). Rapid cycle change projects improve quality of care. *Journal of Nursing Care Quality, 26*(1), 54–60.

Van Woerkum, C., Aarts, N., & Van Herzele, A. (2011). Changed planning for planned and unplanned change. *Planning Theory, 10*, 144–161. https://doi.org/10.1177/1473095210389651.

Verdict Medical Devices. (2018, December 19). Heavily promoted Medicare Blue Button 2.0 will speed up machine learning in healthcare. *eClinicalWorks*. https://www.medicaldevice-network.com/comment/heavily-promoted-medicare-blue-button-2-0-will-speed-up-machine-learning-in-healthcare/.

Vos, J. F. J, & Rupert, J. (2018). Change agent's contribution to recipients' resistance to change: A two-sided story. *European Management Journal, 36*(4), 453–462. https://doi.org/10.1016/j.emj.2017.11.004.

Weiner, B. J., Amick, H., & Lee, S. Y. (2008). Conceptualization and measurement of organizational readiness for change: A review of the literature in health services research and other fields. *Medical Care Research Review, 65*(4), 379–436. https://doi.org/10.1177/1077558708317802.

Weiner, B. J. (2009). A theory of organizational readiness for change. *Implementation Science, 4*(1), 67–76. https://doi.org/10.1186/1748-5908-4-67.

White, K. R., Pillay, R., & Huang, X. (2016). Nurse leaders and the innovation competence gap. *Nursing Outlook, 64*(3), 255–261. https://doi.org/10.1016/j.outlook.2015.12.007.

Workman, R., & Kenney, M. (1988). The change experience. In S. Pinkerton, & P. Schroeder (Eds.), *Commitment to excellence: Developing a professional nursing staff* (pp. 17–25). Rockville, MD: Aspen.

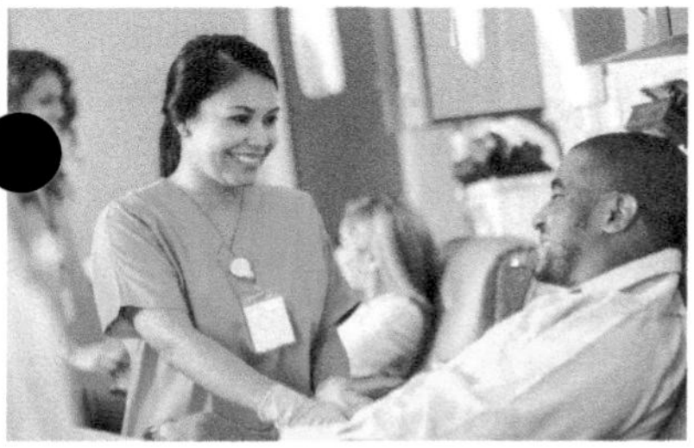

3

Organizational Climate and Culture

Jennifer Bellot

http://evolve.elsevier.com/Huber/leadership

Since the 1960s, health care organizations have systematically responded to economic, social, and financial challenges that have ultimately caused a transformation in health care delivery. Health care organizations now compete in a marketplace based on their ability to demonstrate lean performance, increased efficiency, and quality health outcomes. Particularly since the implementation of the Affordable Care Act (ACA) in the United States, the payment structure for health care has largely shifted from fee-for-service to prospective payment to pay-for-performance and outcomes.

Crossing the quality chasm (IOM, 2001), a landmark report of the Institute of Medicine (IOM, now called the National Academies of Sciences, Engineering, and Medicine, Health and Medicine Division), described the challenge of care provision in the 21st century and was one of the first publications to detail the shift from provider-centered care to patient-centered care. Inclusion of patient and family values, norms, customs, and family/caregiver participation are now dominant factors in treatment decisions. Furthermore, recent inquiry regarding patient safety has emphasized patient outcomes as well as the processes and behaviors that lead to safe care. An explosion in information technology capacity is altering the speed and transparency of communication and information delivery. Interprofessional care is gaining prominence, showing mixed to positive evidence that teamwork leads to better patient outcomes (Reeves et al., 2013). The impact of a nurse shortage, the increasing demand for nursing care, and the drive to incorporate evidence-based practice are changing the face of nursing care. Taken together, these issues have transformed health care structures and delivery, creating a fast-paced and ever-changing practice environment for nurses to negotiate. There is an inevitable impact on organizational climate and culture.

An appreciation for workplace culture is critical for today's nurse leader. In the perfect storm, nurses may wonder how the issues detailed here link with organizational culture, the professional role of the nurse, and nurse leaders. Nurses' insight into organizational culture enables them to understand staff behaviors and relationships, norms, change processes, expectations, and communications. This holds true for all levels of nurses—from novice to expert practitioner and from direct care provider to administrator. This chapter provides an overview of culture, focusing on the factors that affect the culture within an organization. This chapter also discusses organizational culture and climate and their relationship to the nursing work environment, workforce, and practice.

DEFINITIONS

Culture

Organizational culture is rooted in anthropology, psychology, sociology, and management theory. It first appeared in the academic literature in 1952. **Culture** is the set of values, beliefs, and assumptions that are shared by members of an organization. An organization's culture provides a common belief system among its members. Culture provides a common bond so that members know how to relate to one another and how to show others who are outside of the organization what is valued. For example, organizational culture can encompass things like the mission statement, policies, procedures, organizational positions, the way people dress, and the language they use. Additionally, culture encompasses what is implicit in the organization, such as the unwritten rules and customs that pervade the work environment. Collectively, these variables define the character and norms of the organization.

Culture is represented in several ways. One example is that the care delivery model that guides nursing practice helps interpret the culture. For instance, when a relationship-based nursing care model is used, it represents an underlying belief in patient-centered care. Open visiting hours in the intensive care unit convey the importance of family as partners in care delivery. How new nurses are oriented expresses values about the socialization of new nurses. Many visible aspects of culture reflect the underlying values of the organization.

Culture is a multifaceted phenomenon, difficult to comprehend and unravel. The health care system is incredibly complex. High-quality health care delivery is dependent on good communication and collaboration between providers, patients, and their families. One way to better understand such relationships is to appreciate how the hospital culture affects nursing units, nursing practice, and patient outcomes. For a nurse to function effectively in an organization, a solid grasp of organizational culture, characteristics, and operations is essential.

Culture has been measured both quantitatively and qualitatively. Initially it was thought that something as diffuse and intangible as culture could only be measured using qualitative techniques. Bellot (2011, p. 33) stated that "early culture researchers believed that standardized, quantitative instruments were inappropriate for cultural assessment because they would be unable to capture the subjective and unique aspects of each culture." A strictly qualitative approach to cultural assessment can be time consuming, expensive, less generalizable, and difficult to interpret. Thus, various quantitative tools have been developed to more quickly assess culture and allow for comparison across different work environments. In reality, it is likely that a combination of qualitative and quantitative measures are best for capturing organizational culture (Bellot, 2011). As with any selection of a measurement tool, the choice of a measurement instrument should be directed by definition, purpose, and context for cultural assessment.

Because of the confusion around the tendency to use organizational culture and climate interchangeably and definitional confusion, measuring these two can be difficult. Gershon et al. (2004) searched the literature and identified and described 12 organizational climate and culture instruments. They described the dimensions and subconstructs of each instrument and then displayed five major dimensions of leadership, group behaviors and relationships, communications, quality of work life, and health care worker outcomes by instrument. Recommendations for use were presented. A rigorous assessment of the organizational culture and climate sets the stage for planned change. Choosing the right instrument is important.

Climate

Organizational climate is a concept that is closely linked to the organization's culture and is often confused with it. Although many people use *culture* and *climate* interchangeably, the terms are not the same. **Climate** is an *individual* perception of what it feels like to work in an environment (Snow, 2002). It is how nurses perceive and feel about practices, procedures, and rewards (Sleutel, 2000). People form perceptions of the work environment because they focus on what is individually important and meaningful to them. This explains why some aspects of culture may be interpreted differently. A key feature of culture is its *group* orientation.

Climate can be easier to identify than culture. Researchers who study climate describe various components of the work environment that influence behaviors (Sleutel, 2000). Some characteristics that are used to study climate are decision making, leadership, supervisor support, peer cohesion, autonomy, conflict, work pressure, rewards, feeling of warmth, and risk (Stone et al., 2005). Within organizations, it is common to identify sub-climates that focus on specific aspects of the organizations (e.g., climates related to patient safety, ethics, and learning). For example, some organizations have adopted principles of a learning organization to establish an organizational culture change using knowledge and learning.

Culture–Climate Link

Climate research has formed the basis for the definition and research surrounding organizational culture, and the two are closely linked (Bellot, 2011). Regardless of the practice setting, a link exists between culture and climate. That link is what is important to understanding attitudes, motivations, and behavior among nurses (Stone et al., 2005). Culture and climate can be described as the interaction of shared values about what things are important, beliefs about how things work, and behaviors about how things get done.

Nurse Practice Environment

Although organizations usually have a single, overarching culture, many climates can exist within that culture—from unit to unit, for instance. Groups and organizations exist within society and develop a culture that has a significant effect on how members think, feel, and act. Culture becomes a learned product of the group experience. In general, nurses work together in a group such as on a nursing unit, in home care, in long-term care, or in communities. The nursing unit is a small geographical area within the larger organization where nurses work interdependently to care for patients. Nursing work groups naturally spend time together and set up their own norms, values, and ways to communicate with each other. These factors contribute to that work group having its own climate, or perception of what it feels like to work within a geographical area, contributing to the **nurse practice environment**. The nurse practice environment is also often referred to as the "professional practice environment."

Climate is evident in staff perceptions of policies, practices, and goal achievement. Some authors have described this as an organizational subculture (Hatch & Cunliffe, 2013). Understanding organizational culture from the perspective of individual nurse practice environments can offer an unprecedented view of nurses' work. Creating an environment with a culture and climate that empowers nurses to practice in ways that support a positive professional practice environment can maximize both nurse and patient outcomes.

Using strict social science definitions, the predominance of nursing organizational research focuses on *organizational culture*—or employs the more general term *work environment*—rather than climate. For the purposes of the everyday nurse leader, the terms are interchangeable, although "organizational culture" or "work environment" are typically distinguished more precisely in the research literature.

BACKGROUND

The business focus on culture is as the means to achieve organizational success and competitive advantage. Industry leaders in the corporate world quickly realized that the philosophy and values of an organization could determine success and secure market advantage (Wooten & Crane, 2003). The health care industry has been slower than the corporate world to embrace culture as a means to optimize organizational performance.

Organizational culture is defined as "the set of shared assumptions that relate to the core values of the organization" (Levine et al., 2020, p. 131). These shared assumptions guide members on how to problem solve, adapt to the external environment, and manage relationships. The mission statement for an organization offers a snapshot of strategic priorities and is an important way to get a sense of organizational values.

Organizational culture affects the quality of nursing care and patient outcomes. Shared meanings—the taken-for-granted practice and assumptions of a work group—can exert a significant effect on performance and outcomes. Basic underlying assumptions are those that are never questioned and make up an integral part of the fabric of an organization that extends to the unit work level, such as a commitment to excellence and to the surrounding community. Each organizational unit and work group has cultural norms and values that blend the social realities and features that shape interactions among staff, patients, and families. The manner in which the staff perceives organizational culture, manages boundaries, and translates implied values to the unit level has a direct effect on patient care (Carthon et al., 2015).

RESEARCH

Since the mid-1990s a growing body of research has confirmed that the relationship between nurse staffing and patient outcomes is influenced by culture or climate and the organizational characteristics of the structure in which nurses practice (Wong et al., 2013). More recently, studying the impact of culture has shifted from the organizational level to the unit level, where caregiver relationships, communication, and autonomy intersect to inform care decisions that affect individual outcomes. To understand how the culture of the organization and climate of a unit are related to professional practice, five contemporary trends in achieving a culture/climate of quality are discussed here: the Magnet Recognition Program®, the professional practice environment, patient safety culture, healthy work environments, and just culture.

Magnet Recognition Program®

In 1983, the American Academy of Nursing's Task Force on Nursing Practice in Hospitals studied nursing service best practices by surveying 163 hospitals. The goal was to identify and describe those factors that, when present, created an environment that attracted and retained qualified RNs who delivered quality care. The 41 best hospitals were called "Magnet hospitals" because of their clear ability to attract professional nurses. The 14 original characteristics they displayed were identified and called "Forces of Magnetism." Now administered by the American Nurses Credentialing Center (ANCC, n.d.), the Magnet Recognition Program® has become the gold standard for excellence in nursing.

Magnet hospitals are an example of a positive culture that affects nurse and patient outcomes. Today, hospitals and long-term care facilities wanting to achieve Magnet Recognition Program® status must meet five key components identified by the ANCC (n.d.): transformational leadership; structural empowerment; exemplary professional practice; new knowledge, innovations, and improvements; and empirical outcomes. In 1998 Magnet recognition was expanded to include long-term care facilities, although Magnet designation still largely applies to the acute care, hospital environment.

In Magnet-designated organizations, a strong visionary nurse leader nurtures a professional nursing environment and advocates for, and is supportive of, excellence in nursing practice. Magnet-designated hospitals have been recognized over the years for excellence in patient care, strong nursing practice environments, and the ability to attract and retain nurses. The advancement of professionalism, autonomy, and nursing's knowledge base are hallmarks. Periodically, the ANCC queries Magnet-designated facilities to establish an official national research agenda that is current and germane to ongoing professional development.

Aiken and colleagues have transformed the initial Magnet hospital work into a program of research congruent with quality of care and organizational effectiveness through study of the links between hospital organizational culture and care outcomes. Magnet hospitals were conceptualized as those institutions that have a specific organizational culture with characteristics of autonomy, practice control, and collaboration. In a seminal work, Aiken et al. (1994) examined mortality rates in 39 Magnet hospitals and 195 control hospitals using multivariate matched control sampling. Magnet hospitals had a significantly lower mortality rate (4.6% lower) for Medicare patients than did control hospitals. The Magnet-designated hospitals' cultures provided higher levels of autonomy and control of practice for nurses and fostered stronger professional relationships among nurses and physicians than did non–Magnet-designated hospitals. In one study RNs had significantly lower work engagement after the loss of Magnet designation (Wonder et al., 2017).

Magnet research and an organizational framework developed by Aiken et al. (1997) provide the means to better understand the link between unit culture characteristics and adverse events. A nursing unit culture that supports and values nurse autonomy and the provision of adequate resources and effective communication among providers most likely constitutes an environment where practice excellence is the norm. Examples of research regarding Magnet-designated hospitals show associations with lower central-line-associated bloodstream infections (Barnes et al., 2016), lower selected-cause readmissions (McHugh & Ma, 2013), lower rates of hospital-acquired pressure ulcers (Ma & Park, 2015), more positive patient experiences (McCaughey et al., 2020), and multiple other nurse and patient outcomes (Kutney-Lee et al., 2015). A repository of research references on Magnet research can be found at https://www.nursingworld.org/organizational-programs/magnet/program-resources/research-materials/

Professional Practice Environment

In the journey toward Magnet designation, research and evidence-based practice become important in meeting the core criteria and representing a culture and climate of learning that is supportive of a professional practice environment that involves continuous learning and professional nursing development. A **professional practice environment** is characterized by a shared and positive perception of the value of learning to enhance practice, quality, and outcomes. This may be reflected in principles of a learning organization.

Cultures in which continuous learning is valued are less likely to become outdated and stale. In the past, it was not unusual to hear nurses say in relation to their practice, "We have always done it this way." Today, a professional practice environment encourages nurses to propose new ideas and adopt and implement evidence-based practices to promote clinical excellence. Moving new research findings into practice has historically taken many years. In a culture that supports professional practice, nurses are challenged to ask, "How can this be done better?" Nurses interact with many patients on a daily basis. Patients are experts about themselves, and nurses are experts about nursing practice. Blending these areas of expertise puts nurses in the best position to ask the question, "How can practice and the environment in which practice occurs be improved?" Nursing practice then becomes a vehicle for generating questions that are important to practice. This idea, along with creating a culture of lifelong learning, is one cornerstone of the IOM report *The future of nursing: Leading change, advancing health* (IOM, 2011). Progress in nursing recognition and positive workforce culture has led to the Robert Wood Johnson Foundation commissioning a second Future of Nursing study (2020–2030), currently in production, and focusing on the nurses' role in addressing social determinants of health and health equity.

The formation of the team at the unit level creates a collective vision for continuous learning and professional practice. In turn, the norm for learning intersects with the desire for good practice and forms a cohesive unit that shares a value for learning that generates excitement for moving beyond traditional practice. Cultures in which knowledge is freely shared can have a groundswell effect. Examples of outward and visible signs that support nurses' shared values for professional practice include activities such as journal clubs, unit presentations, poster displays, and participation in evidence-based practice teams.

Patient Safety Culture and Climate

An emphasis on an organization's patient safety culture and climate has driven an avalanche of research and change in hospital practices since the publication of the IOM's (1999) report *To err is human: Building a safer health system*, which suggested that 98,000 persons die annually in hospitals because of errors. A safety culture is an outgrowth of the larger organizational culture and emphasizes the deeper assumptions and values of the organization toward safety, whereas the safety climate is the shared perception of employees about the importance of safety within the organization (DeJoy et al., 2004). Like organizational climate, the safety climate has a number of different components, including leadership, involvement, blameless culture, communication, teamwork, commitment to safety, beliefs about errors and their cause, and others (Blegen et al., 2005).

Safety climate refers to keeping both patients and nurses safe. Strong surveillance skills regarding patients are at the heart of safety. Because they are on the front line of patient care, nurses are in an optimal position to monitor patients to prevent adverse events or near misses of adverse events. The ability of nurses to understand a patient's baseline status and recognize early, critical warning signs or changes in health status is a skill derived from having a strong nursing knowledge base. It is not simply task application. Astute recognition of deviations from normal and timely interventions signify that nurses understand the patient's baseline status and are capable of intervening to prevent or remediate an adverse event. Knowledge of the patient and the patient's baseline status is derived through subjective, objective, and intuitive observations that are honed as nurses develop a level of expertise in working with specific patient populations. Factors that influence a nurse's ability to watch over patients to avoid errors and adverse events include managerial leadership, communication style and clarity, staffing levels, excess fatigue, and lack of education and experience (Higgins, 2015; McHugh et al., 2016; Van Bogaert et al., 2014). Other aspects of a safety climate and culture, such as Six Sigma and lean health care organizations, are techniques related to creating quality.

Healthy Work Environments

Included in the concept of a safety culture/climate is a focus on nurses' health and safety. Nurses working in hospitals have one of the highest rates of work-related injuries, including back injury, needle sticks, and chemical exposures (Stokowski, 2014). When fewer nurses are working, less help is available to provide care to patients. This results in more work needing to be done in a shorter time and can lead to taking shortcuts, also known as workarounds, which can result in injury to the nurse and/or poor patient outcomes. To address these issues, the American Nurses Association (2016) has created a variety of resources, position papers, and compiled research on a healthy work environment (HWE) (https://www.nursingworld.org/practice-policy/work-environment/). The ANA has defined an HWE as one that is safe, empowering, and satisfying. Paramount is a culture of safety for both patients and health care workers. General workplace improvements such as in decision making, communication, and collaboration, along with provision of authentic leadership and meaningful recognition are needed. In addition, an HWE would have programs in place to address specific workplace issues such as fatigue management, safe handling of patients, bullying and violence, infection control and prevention, sharps injury, environmental health, and disaster preparedness to demonstrate the organization's commitment to partnership with nurses.

Regardless of whether the focus of safety is on the patient or the nurse, the likelihood of injury can be lessened where there is a cohesive team. When there is a shared perception among a group of care providers about the value and importance of safety, they are more likely to work together effectively toward common goals. Espousing the values of a safety climate and endeavoring to prevent, detect, and mitigate the effect of errors and injuries increases the likelihood of improved outcomes. As nurses work together as a team, they share information, can anticipate events, and are more likely to respond appropriately to unanticipated events.

Just Culture

One major shift in an organization's safety culture/climate is the move from a punitive and reactive culture to a fair and just culture. The concept of a **just culture** was first developed by John Reason in 1997. A just culture represents the middle ground between patient safety and a culture that supports error reduction (Reason, 1997). In a fair and just culture, expectations for system and individual learning and accountability are transparent. Underlying these beliefs, the overall organizational strategy must effectively implement a fair and just culture. When an organization can freely discuss mistakes with the intention of learning from them, and when it takes the time and resources needed to understand the mistakes using root cause analysis, the organizational culture changes from punitive to respectful and open to learning. For example, within a systems-oriented approach, learning from adverse events can encourage error reporting, rather than concealment, and lead to new wisdom and improved ways of doing things. This is called a just culture. In 2010 the American Nurses Association published a position statement, formally endorsing the creation of a just culture for nurses across the health care work environment (American Nurses Association, 2010).

LEADERSHIP AND MANAGEMENT IMPLICATIONS

Nurses work in a wide variety of health care organizations, such as clinics, educational organizations, health insurance organizations, health care associations, home health care, hospitals, long-term care facilities, physician practices, mental health organizations, public health departments, rehabilitation centers, and research institutions. These organizations vary as to their business configuration, ownership, and mission, such as for-profit, not-for-profit, or governmental. The type of organization in which the nurse works has an impact on the differences seen in organizational culture and climate.

Culture is characterized by complexity and is relatively enduring, making it hard to change. Climate, on the other hand, can be easier to change. Regardless, the basic elements that constitute culture and climate must be understood before any change. Change that begins at the unit level may be most influenced by nursing leadership. Nurses have the ability to create or change a work culture, climate, or environment to accomplish a change that may affect productivity and satisfaction and promote safe, high-quality, patient-centered care. For example, units experiencing high turnover can make strategic and evidence-based decisions about processes and relationships in order to convert to a more satisfying work environment that attracts and retains nurses.

A key role of a nursing leader is to influence the culture and the climate. A primary task of the leader is to create a convincing vision that inspires and engages the entire team to move it forward. Values drive behaviors. The leader communicates this vision by influencing norms and values and creating a shared perception through role modeling and ensuring role clarity, accountability, and a nurse practice environment that promotes safe patient- and family-centered care.

Unit-based nurse managers serve as bridges between the senior nursing leadership and direct care nursing staff. Nurse Managers are instrumental in shaping and managing the core values of their staff. There are a multitude of tools available to document the relationship between nursing management behavior and registered nurse (RN) job satisfaction (Feather et al., 2015). Professional organizations such as the American Organization for Nursing Leadership and the American Nurses Association have long campaigned for healthy work environments that reflect positive nurse management. Increasingly, studies are showing that the nurse manager is important in retention (Al-Hamdan et al., 2016), stress management (Parry et al., 2014), and work environments (D'Ambra & Andrews, 2014).

Key areas within the leader's scope of control are recruiting and retaining staff, welcoming new staff, providing orientation, celebrating and recognizing staff accomplishments, facilitating change, and promoting a just culture and professional practice environment. Climate is evident in how policies are enacted, unit norms, dress code and appearance, environment, communication, and teamwork. The nurse manager can articulate the vision, mission, and goals of the organization and work with staff to translate them into unit-level values for performance, thus linking the context of the organization to clinical practice.

Values drive the way resources are distributed. They contribute to a general attitude and sense about the quality of work life and reflect the organization's core goals. Clues can be gleaned from organizational documents such as philosophy statements and meeting minutes. Caring values of the organization are reflected in the way the organization treats its staff. Organizational values may not mirror professional values. The leader's role is to bridge such values with the values of individual team members to shape the individual unit climate. Values support the mission and the related vision, which, in turn, support strategies and action plans. The key platform is shared values. Given the complexity and diversity of the nursing workforce, developing and sustaining a set of shared values is no easy task and requires leadership skill.

Leaders are expected to chart a clear course for change and mobilize staff to accomplish organizational goals. This means implementing change effectively. Effective cultural change requires communication, passion, and clear understanding of the existing culture. The nurse manager can create such opportunities by using focus groups, holding team meetings, coaching and mentoring, posting minutes from staff meetings, using clear and directive communication, and empowering staff by soliciting their input. The value of communication cannot be overstated.

In their landmark organizational behavior research, Peters and Waterman (1982) stressed that the greatest professional need people have is to find meaning in their work life. Finding meaning at work is a fundamental motivational strategy related to job satisfaction. The job of managers is to help create meaning through the use of stories, slogans, symbols, rituals, legends, and myths that convey the values, beliefs, and meanings shared among the staff. Managers should function as passionate leaders to motivate staff.

The challenges of leadership belong to every nurse, not just those in formal administrative or management roles. Leadership at the staff level may be informal and simply take a different form. For example, a staff nurse adapting to a challenging patient assignment, taking initiative to change practice through performance improvement, or challenging the status quo is participating in unit culture construction. Informal clinical leadership is manifested among peers, for example, when a staff nurse sees an area for improvement and mobilizes peers or the unit-based council to pursue a solution. This can create a positive unit climate with a "can do" attitude. Further, staff nurses are critical to founding and maintaining a Magnet-designated organization.

Nurse leaders with an accurate and comprehensive assessment of culture and climate can identify strategic areas for change. A thorough understanding of organizational culture and climate is a powerful diagnostic tool that may be used to identify both troubled and high-performance areas. An effective organizational culture empowers nurses to practice to the full extent of their education and training (IOM, 2011). The culture of a nursing unit practice environment may exert a significant and independent effect beyond that of staffing and skill mix by enhancing or impeding interventions once problems are detected. Nurses serve as the surveillance system for early detection of adverse events.

Culture and Strategy

> *"Culture eats strategy for breakfast."*
>
> ***—attributed to Peter Drucker***

A principal responsibility for nursing leadership and management is short- and long-term planning, creating a strategy for the unit and organization as a whole. Organizational culture is a key component to consider when creating strategy. Having a thorough baseline assessment of organizational culture and current resources (workforce, technology, financial, etc.) will inform the nurse leader if the desired vision, goals, and outcomes included in a strategic plan are appropriate given the characteristics of the organization/unit.

Regardless of the organization's or leader's priorities for a strategic plan, they will be unsuccessful in realizing those goals unless there is cultural congruence, employee buy-in, and sufficient resources to support the strategic plan.

CURRENT ISSUES AND TRENDS

At the beginning of the chapter, a number of forces were identified that have had significant influence in changing the culture of health care delivery. Several of these forces have particular impact on nursing care, and a brief discussion of patient- and family-centered care, generational diversity, and the Quality and Safety Education for Nurses (QSEN, 2020) initiative follows to exemplify current issues and trends related to organizational climate and culture.

Patient-Centered Care and the Patient-Centered Medical Home

Beginning in 2001 with the IOM's landmark report *Crossing the quality chasm*, it has been widely promulgated that the culture of patient care must transition from care that is driven by providers to care that is patient centered and family centered, in which patient and family norms, values, and preferences are respected. Shortly thereafter, the Agency for Healthcare Research and Quality (AHRQ) agreed with these recommendations and discussed four other features of optimal primary care to create national recognition for the patient-centered medical home (PCMH) model of primary care delivery.

First introduced in the 1960s as a means to coordinate primary and specialty care for children, the PCMH model evolved to include other areas of primary care. In this model, nurses work as part of an interprofessional team to deliver care that helps to improve patient outcomes, the patient experience, and value. There is a large body of research that supports the success of the PCMH model, and it has since been advocated for as a best practice for primary care by the AHRQ and many major payers.

There are five core functions and attributes in the PCMH model: comprehensive care, patient-centered, coordinated care, accessible services, and quality and safety. Comprehensive care is providing care that is inclusive of both physical and mental health care, wellness, prevention, and illness care. Comprehensive care requires a team of providers, and this is where the nurses' role is central. Patient-centered care is relationship-based, inclusive of the whole person, and respectful of the patient's values, culture, and preferences. Coordinated care coordinates information across all levels and sites of care. For example, this would include primary and specialty care, inpatient, outpatient, home, subacute, and long-term care. Accessible services refer to providing care that is easiest for patients to obtain such as offering telephonic access, shorter wait times, and hours conducive to the patients' needs. Finally, quality and safety refers to a provider employing evidence-based care and clinical decision support tools. For more information about the PCMH model, including the wide base of supportive research, see the AHRQ website at www.pcmh.ahrq.gov.

Beginning research on the PCMH model showed small to moderate effects on nurse outcomes and experiences (Jackson et al., 2013). It has been noted in some studies that the transition to this model inherently results in a conflict with how a nurse traditionally organizes and structures the workday (Bellot, 2012; Stewart et al., 2015). Although the PCMH model is an admirable way to encourage comprehensive, holistic patient care that is informed by interprofessional, team-based communication, it is also important to consider the practice and cultural transformation that must occur to facilitate its implementation.

Culture Change in Long-Term Care

After the passage of the Nursing Home Reform Act legislation (OBRA, 1987, https://www.congress.gov/bill/100th-congress/house-bill/3545) a series of quality improvement programs were implemented in nursing homes. By the mid-1990s the culture change movement had begun to gain popularity and continues to spread today. Culture change is distinguished from typical quality improvement activities in its attempt to simultaneously alter multiple aspects of care and caregiving in the nursing home. Culture change is so named because of its aim to adopt an entirely new philosophy in long-term elder care. There is no universal operational definition of what specific elements constitute culture change programming. Instead, culture change refers to the movement to reorganize nursing home care completely. Included under this umbrella are several different initiatives that address staff, resident, environmental, or behavioral outcomes or some combination of these factors. Most culture change initiatives are focused upon resident-directed (patient-centered) care, providing services that are directed by the strengths and preferences of the individual resident and/or family.

Research has been done to evaluate various culture change initiatives, but some models have been promulgated and replicated more than others. Early culture change initiatives, although generally dedicated to the same principles of resident-directed care and homelike social structures, were unique from organization to organization. Despite the wide range of programming, research has found that nursing homes that have engaged in culture change activities report declines in avoidable hospitalizations and 30-day hospital readmissions (Zimmerman et al., 2016), declines in bedfast residents (Afendulis et al., 2016), and decreased Medicare spending (Grabowski et al., 2016).

In 1995, at a meeting of the National Citizens' Coalition for Nursing Home Reform (NCCNHR), a panel of administrators whose nursing homes were engaged in culture change initiatives was convened. This group grew in size and strength and became known as the Pioneer Network. Today, the Pioneer Network is an organization of facilities engaged in many diverse culture change initiatives dedicated to a common set of values. These values include returning the locus of control to residents, enhancing the capacity of frontline staff to be responsive, and establishing a homelike environment that values choice, dignity, respect, self-determination, and purposeful living (https://www.pioneernetwork.net/). Some of the most prominent culture change models include the Eden Alternative, the Green House Project, and the Wellspring Program.

Development of a new model or culture change must be preceded by comprehensive assessment of the organization culture, an understanding of the patient population, what members of the staff need to care for them, and what roles are required to form the change team. There is no one right model, nor does one size fit all settings. The work entails a deliberative process to facilitate change that will improve outcomes. Culture development must be an essential component of any new culture change. Transparency and frequency of clear communication is critical for cultural transformation and buy-in from all staff (Bellot, 2012).

Engagement

Nurse engagement is a term of growing interest and emphasis in nursing leadership, quality and outcomes research. Nurse engagement is defined as "nurses' commitment to and satisfaction with their jobs...nurses' level of commitment to the organization that employs them and their commitment to the nursing profession itself" (Dempsey & Reilly, 2016, p. 1). Some regard nurse engagement as the opposite of burnout. It is a burgeoning area of nursing research and a major area of focus for initiatives such as Press Ganey surveys, the National Database of Nursing Quality Indicators (NDNQI) and other sources of key data that drive the Magnet Recognition Program®. Nurse engagement has been found to correlate with safety, quality and patient experience outcomes (Day, 2014; Laschinger & Leiter, 2006; Nishioka et al., 2014; Press Ganey, 2013).

The nurse leader needs to consider culture as a key ingredient to stimulate employee engagement. The Advisory, Conciliation and Arbitration Service (ACAS) has identified four factors that lead to a more satisfied and productive workforce. These factors are:

- Leaders with a vision who value how individuals contribute
- Managers who empower, rather than control their staff
- Values that are lived, not just spoken, leading to a sense of trust and integrity
- Employees who have the chance to voice their views and concerns (ACAS, n.d.)

These four factors are important for the nurse leader to consider when creating a work environment that engages and rewards its employees.

There are a number of other ways the nurse leader can promote positive nurse engagement in the workplace. For example, Kutney-Lee et al. (2016) found increased nurse engagement when the professional practice environment incorporates higher levels of shared governance. As ACAS promotes, it is intuitive for a nurse leader to posit that employees who have the chance to voice their views and concerns (shared governance) will enjoy higher satisfaction and commitment to the workplace (engagement). Other strategies for nurse leaders to promote nurse engagement include recognition and empathy for the difficulty of work and talent required to do the job of a nurse, adequate resources in areas ranging from emotional support to safe staffing levels, trust and delegation so that the nurse feels valued and respected, and encouragement for and modeling of a work/life balance. When these values are promoted in the professional practice environment *and* modeled by nurse leaders, it sends a clear signal to nurses that they are valued contributors.

Predictive Analytics

The use of predictive analytics in nursing management and leadership is a new application of an old method. Predictive analytics, broadly, refers to using statistical or data-driven modeling to determine outcomes based on current or historical data. Predictive analytics have been applied in various aspects of the professional practice environment including determining if a potential nurse employee is a good cultural match for the unit, modeling safe staffing in uncertain conditions and determining risk for 30-day readmissions and undesirable patient outcomes given nursing workforce resources. As sources of big data such as the electronic medical record become more robust, it is expected that predictive analytics will be used increasingly to modulate the professional practice environment.

Generational Differences

The importance of a positive work climate on organizational, patient, and nurse outcomes is firmly established and evidence-based. However, creating a work environment for nurses that meets their personal and professional values can be a challenge. In 2008, for the first time since the inaugural National Sample Survey of RNs, the numbers of nurses working who were under age 30 years and over age 60 years were almost equal (US Department of Health and Human Services, 2010). Because nurses from each of these generations were raised with a different set of priorities and values, a work environment supportive to each generation is an important retention strategy. For example, baby boomer nurses value rewards. Recognition and pay may be motivators for them. In contrast, Generation X nurses are concerned with a better balance of work and life. Further, Generation Y (sometimes called Millennials) have shown indications of increased mobility and higher willingness to move to another job when dissatisfied with the work environment and culture (Tourangeau et al., 2013). Tailoring the work environment to meet generational and life-stage needs is a recurrent theme in being able to address successfully the impending nursing shortage.

As Generations X and Y become a larger proportion of the nursing workforce, a marked shift in values has been noted. Research from the Pew Research Center (2018) has indicated that younger workers place a higher emphasis on finding a professional practice environment that promotes work/life balance, flexible working arrangements, and values-driven work. Younger generations tend to place less value on material items like pay and more value on time and flexibility. A 2019 survey of 20,000 RNs discussed how care is becoming more complex, demand for services is increasing, and there is a wave of Baby Boomer retirements (Edmonson & Marshall, 2020). These forces generate rising consumer demand coupled with a limited nursing workforce supply. Issues from the 2019 survey highlighted that there is a growing burden on the nursing workforce as reflected in (Edmonson & Marshall, 2020, p. 131):

- The significant percentages of nurses working second jobs
- The reality that many nurses are unable to spend the time they need with patients
- Concerns that their jobs are affecting their health
- Plans to leave their current jobs within a year
- The need for greater work-life balance

Professional practice environments and policies that support well-being, making healthy choices, and clear communication and expectations are highly desired by new nurses. Nurse leaders may want to consider, although the physical work of the bedside nurse cannot be made remote, perhaps other things required of the job such as evaluations or professional development can be more flexible regarding where they occur. Perhaps a more meaningful recognition than a chair massage or tote bag during Nurses Week would be a demonstrated commitment from nursing leadership to creating a sustainable year-round professional practice environment and considering recognition and rewards in the form of a day off or preferred/discounted parking. Taking these generational preferences into account is important as nurse leaders consider recruitment strategies as well as retention. Younger generations have shown greater mobility and intent to leave when they are dissatisfied with the work environment. As evidenced by the #metoo movement, younger generations typically have a much lower tolerance for hostile work environments and will simply leave for a workplace more suitable to their needs.

Quality and Safety Education for Nurses

In 2005, Quality and Safety Education for Nurses (QSEN, 2020), a joint project of the Robert Wood

Johnson Foundation and the National League for Nursing, was announced. The purpose of QSEN is "to address the challenge of preparing future nurses with the knowledge, skills and attitudes (KSAs) necessary to continuously improve the quality and safety of the health care systems in which they work" (QSEN, 2020, Project Overview page). Widespread rollout of the QSEN program has resulted in extensive nursing faculty education that is designed to create nursing curriculum that emphasizes organizational culture attributes such as the implementation of patient-centered care, emphasis on teamwork and collaboration, integration of evidence-based practice, and creation of a culture that supports quality improvement, safety, and informatics. To this end, QSEN's key tenets are geared toward teaching nursing students the competencies they will need to affect organizational culture and create an environment that maximizes patient safety and health outcomes.

By incorporating these elements into nursing education, it is believed that nurses will enter the workforce with the tools necessary to help create an organizational culture that fosters high-quality nursing care. QSEN has now expanded to target nurses both prelicensure and at the advanced practice level and is permeating into practice at the direct care level. This initiative is an example of how to make large-scale cultural change in nursing.

RESEARCH NOTE

Source

Levine, K.J., Carmody, M., & Silk, K.J. (2020). The influence of organizational culture, climate and commitment on speaking up about medical errors. *Journal of Nursing Management, 28*(1), 130–138.

Purpose

To make patient safety a priority, nurse managers have an important role in creating the communication culture that fosters speaking up. However, there is high variability with regard to whether medical errors are reported. The purpose of this study was to understand how a hospital's culture and climate impact nurses' active behavior of speaking up about medical errors.

Discussion

Using an online survey given to 162 medical professionals and support staff at one Midwestern hospital, data were collected about organizational commitment, importance of reporting medical errors, consequences for reporting medical errors, supervisory responsiveness, and ease of reporting medical errors to determine their impact on intentions to speak up about medical errors. Organizational commitment used an existing scale. Data gathered from focus groups and one-on-one interviews were used to develop the remaining scales.

Organizational commitment, culture, and climate to understand why medical errors go unreported. Organizational commitment is an established measure of the relative strength of a person's identification and involvement in an organization. Organizational responsiveness and the importance of reporting medical errors measure the culture. Organizational climate is measured by ease of reporting medical errors and interpersonal consequences of reporting. The results of the study showed a strong culture in this hospital: if people feel that reporting is important, then they have a great likelihood of reporting. However, findings suggest that the culture reflects one value but the climate makes fulfilling that value difficult. The perception of reporting an error is that this is like writing up a co-worker or "tattling." The existing culture is one of fear, mistrust, and intimidation. By contrast, in a culture where near misses and errors are commonly reported, there is a greater focus on quality of care. The bottom line is a confusing set of messages coming from upper management about speaking up about medical errors.

Application to Practice

In this study employees reported high levels of organization and group/unit commitment. However, the organization's culture and climate worked against an overarching organizational goal of effective and proactive patient care. Thus the major organizational goal is over-shadowed by working environment realities. Nurse Managers need to be assertive in communications about the problem of speaking up to assure patient safety. The literature indicates that teaching strategies for assertive communication were linked to higher levels of reporting medical errors by residents and interns. Nurse Managers are crucial to affecting change; they can be a pivotal force in changing organizational culture and climate by realizing the connection between organizational culture and patient safety.

CASE STUDY

Several months ago, a sentinel event occurred on an acute rehabilitation unit in which the mother of a high-profile community member suffered severe anoxic brain injury by becoming trapped between her mattress and the bed rails. This event was heavily reported by the media and a competing rehabilitation hospital in the neighboring county decided to tout their image as the "safest, most alert rehab for your loved one." The competitor hospital then required its nurses to take five different measurements of the gap between the bed frame and mattress at the beginning of each shift. Nurses, already stretched tightly for staffing, were upset because obtaining these measurements was time-consuming when they felt they could be providing more important patient care. There were no tape measurements provided for this task; nurses had to take paper rulers from wound care kits. Further, nurses were not advised what was an acceptable versus dangerous gap, nor what to do if the gap was deemed "too big." Some nurses placed pillows between the mattress and bed frame to lessen the gap...which angered other nurses, who felt pillows should be reserved for therapeutic positioning. One nurse refused to take measurements at all, loudly stating that it was a useless activity since every time the bed was adjusted or sheets were changed, the measurements would change anyway. After a week of this new policy, most of the nurses simply copied over the measurements from the previous shift and did not perform any new measurements.

At the monthly management meeting, all staff were re-advised of the original policy and several nurses were informed that they were being placed on disciplinary probation for falsifying their charting by using previous measurements. Tension was high. Nurses claimed they were not consulted in the initial policy, that it was not evidence-based, and that they were given no direction on how to interpret measurements or rectify a gap that was "too big." Management thought that nurses were being lazy and inflexible, but they were sure that using the threat of disciplinary probation would convince the nurses that they were "serious about safety." Several people left the meeting in tears and two considered finding another job.

1. What are the problems?
2. Identify challenges faced by nurses and by management.
3. What steps would you take to define a culture of safety?
4. How would you define the culture of this facility? How would you change it?
5. What can the nurses do? What can management do?

CRITICAL THINKING EXERCISE

The Magnet Recognition Program's® website offers case studies about Magnet designation that showcase culture change. One example of multiple Magnet designations is the Carle Foundation Hospital/Carle Physician Group of Urbana, Illinois (https://www.nursingworld.org/organizational-programs/magnet/program-resources/case-studies/).

In presenting their case study, the Carle Foundation Hospital noted that it launched its first Magnet® journey as a strategy to improve nurse recruitment and retention. The process involved nursing leaders reviewing the Magnet standards. They realized that Magnet is focused on doing the right thing, including for nurses, the organization, and patients. They achieved their initial designation with great pride of accomplishment in 2009.

This pride drove their re-designation journey four years later. Because Magnet status put the hospital among the nation's elite, everyone was determined to maintain Magnet designation at the time of re-designation. However, there was a new environmental and cultural change to account for: the recent integration with Carle Physician Group. The integration of a hospital with a physician group posed some challenges. The climate and culture of the physician's group clinic differed from the hospital. For example, certification rates in the ambulatory clinic were low, and nurses showed little enthusiasm to pursue specialty credentials. To address this situation, nursing leaders developed and implemented a policy of paying the certification fee in advance for RNs. Rates for certification skyrocketed from 14% to 36% in just 8 weeks.

Other benefits to Carle from Magnet designation include a bolster to its mission to provide high-quality, world-class health care that garners national recognition. It is an important recruitment and retention tool. Physicians and nurses cite the hospital's Magnet status when choosing to work for Carle. Employees are proud to say they work for a Magnet organization.

Magnet appraisers named their New Nurse Residency Program an exemplar during their most recent site visit because the program boasted a 96% retention rate its first year.

Pursuit of Magnet standards improved outcomes. For example, implementation of Chlorhexidine gluconate (CHG) (basinless) bathing in the cardiovascular intensive care unit significantly reduced surgical site infection rates, with no deep/organ space infections for more than a year. This successful program has been expanded to other surgical areas.

Evidence of a culture of Magnet, with resources and programs to support nurses in enhanced competence, is seen in providing tuition assistance (rather than reimbursement) to nurses to pursue educational goals. This initiative produced a steady increase in Bachelor of Science in nursing (BSN) rates since the hospital's first designation in 2009. Now 46% of nurses have BSNs, and there is a clear plan to get to 80% by 2020 as recommended by the IOM (2011).

Carle's nursing leaders call Magnet an "indispensable roadmap" for success because it directs the organization to where they need to focus and pinpoints what they need to do to achieve desired outcomes. The Magnet journey is seen as a continuous, evolving process. Clearly, their pursuit of excellence is not a once-every-4-year goal, but rather it is an integral part of the organization's daily work.

1. What are three examples of a professional practice environment for nurses at Carle Foundation Hospital/ Medical Group?
2. Based on the information provided in the case study, what are likely some prominent features of Carle's culture? Climate?
3. Based on the information provided in the case study, how might Carle continue to capitalize on their successes innovatively?
4. What steps would you take to implement one of Carle's programs in your own work environment?
5. What are some barriers you might anticipate to culture change in your work environment?
6. How might you think about planning proactively to address barriers to culture change in your work environment?

REFERENCES

Advisory, Conciliation and Arbitration Service (ACAS). (n.d.). *Employee engagement: Happy and productive people equals growth*. https://archive.acas.org.uk/engagement.

Afendulis, C. C., Caudry, D. J., O'Malley, A. J., Kemper, P., & Grabowski, D. C. for the THRIVE Research Collaborative. (2016). Green house adoption and nursing home quality. *Health Services Research, 51*(1 Pt 2), 454–474.

Aiken, L. H., Lake, E. T., Sochalski, J., & Sloane, D. M. (1997). Design of an outcomes study of the organization of hospital AIDS care. *Research in the Sociology of Health Care, 14*, 3–26.

Aiken, L. H., Smith, H. L., & Lake, E. T. (1994). Lower Medicare mortality among a set of hospitals known for good nursing care. *Medical Care, 32*, 771–785.

Al-Hamdan, Z., Nussera, H., & Masa'deh, R. (2016). Conflict management style of Jordanian nurse managers and its relationship to staff nurses' intent to stay. *Journal of Nursing Management, 24*(2), E137–E145.

American Nurses Association. (2010). *Position statement: Just culture*. https://www.nursingworld.org/practice-policy/nursing-excellence/official-position-statements/id/just-culture/.

American Nurses Association. (2016). *Healthy work environment*. https://www.nursingworld.org/practice-policy/work-environment/.

American Nurses Credentialing Center (ANCC). (n.d.). *ANCC Magnet Recognition Program®*. https://www.nursingworld.org/organizational-programs/magnet/.

Barnes, H., Rearden, J., & McHugh, M. D. (2016). Magnet® hospital recognition linked to lower central line-associated bloodstream infection rates. *Research in Nursing & Health, 39*(2), 96–104.

Bellot, J. (2011). Defining and assessing organizational culture. *Nursing Forum, 46*(1), 29–37.

Bellot, J. (2012). Nursing home culture change: What does it mean to nurses? *Research in Gerontological Nursing, 5*(4), 264–273.

Blegen, M. A., Pepper, G. A., & Rosse, J. (2005). *Safety climate on hospital units: A new measure*. http://www.ncbi.nlm.nih.gov/books/NBK20592/.

Carthon, J. M. B., Lasater, K. B., Sloane, D. M., & Kutney-Lee, A. (2015). The quality of hospital work environments and missed nursing care is linked to heart failure readmissions: A cross-sectional study of US hospitals. *BMJ Quality & Safety, 24*(4), 255–263.

D'Ambra, A. M., & Andrews, D. R. (2014). Incivility, retention and new graduate nurses: An integrated review of the literature. *Journal of Nursing Management, 22*(6), 735–742.

Day, H. (2014). Engaging staff to deliver compassionate care and reduce harm. *British Journal of Nursing, 23*(18), 974–980. https://doi.org/10.12968/bjon.2014.23.18.974.

DeJoy, D. M., Schaffer, B. S., Wilson, M. G., Vandenbert, R. J., & Butts, M. M. (2004). Creating safer workplaces: Assessing the determinants and role of safety climate. *Journal of Safety Research, 35*, 81–90.

Dempsey, C., & Reilly, B. A. (2016). Nurse engagement: What are the contributing factors for success? *OJIN, 21*(1), 2. https://doi.org/10.3912/OJIN.Vol21No01Man02.

Edmonson, C., & Marshall, J. (2020). Keeping the human in health care human capital: Challenges and solutions for RNs in the next decade. *Nurse Leader, 18*(2), 130–134.

Feather, R. A., Ebright, P., & Bakas, T. (2015). Nurse manager behaviors that RNs perceive to affect their job satisfaction. *Nursing Forum, 50*(2), 125–136.

Gershon, R. R. M., Stone, P. W., Baaken, S., & Larson, E. (2004). Measurement of organizational culture and climate in healthcare. *Journal of Nursing Administration, 34*(1), 33–40.

Grabowski, D. C., Afendulis, C. C., Caudry, D. J., O'Malley, A. J., & Kemper, P. for the THRIVE Research Collaborative. (2016). The impact of green house adoption on Medicare spending and utilization. *Health Services Research, 51*(1 Pt 2), 433–453.

Hatch, M. J., & Cunliffe, A. L. (2013). *Organization theory: Modern, symbolic and postmodern perspectives*. New York: Oxford University Press.

Higgins, E. A. (2015). The influence of nurse manager transformational leadership on nurse and patient outcomes: Mediating effects of supportive practice environments, organizational citizenship behaviours, patient safety culture and nurse job satisfaction. *Electronic Thesis and Dissertation Repository*. Paper 3184. vhttp://ir.lib.uwo.ca/cgi/viewcontent.cgi?article=4453&context=etd.

Institute of Medicine (IOM). (1999). *To err is human: Building a safer health system*. Washington, DC: National Academies Press.

Institute of Medicine (IOM). (2001). *Crossing the quality chasm*. Washington, DC: National Academies Press.

Institute of Medicine (IOM). (2011). *The future of nursing: Leading change, advancing health*. Washington, DC: National Academies Press.

Jackson, G. L., Powers, B. J., Chatterjee, R., Bettger, J. P., Kemper, A. R., Hasselblad, V., et al. (2013). The patient-centered medical home: A systematic review. *Annals of Internal Medicine, 158*(3), 169–178.

Kutney-Lee, A., Germack, H., Hatfield, L., Kelly, S., Maguire, P., Dierkes, A., Del Guidice, M., & Aiken, L. (2016). Nurse engagement in shared governance and patient and nurse outcomes. *Journal of Nursing Administration, 46*(11), 605–612. https://doi.org/10.1097/NNA.0000000000000412.

Kutney-Lee, A., Stimpfel, A. W., Sloane, D. M., Cimiotti, J. P., Quinn, L. W., & Aiken, L. H. (2015). Changes in patient and nurse outcomes associated with Magnet hospital recognition. *Medical Care, 53*(6), 550–557.

Laschinger, H. K., & Leiter, M. P. (2006). The impact of nursing work environments on patient safety outcomes. *The Journal of Nursing Administration, 36*(45), 259–267.

Levine, K. J., Carmody, M., & Silk, K. J. (2020). The influence of organizational culture, climate and commitment on speaking up about medical errors. *Journal of Nursing Management, 28*(1), 130–138. https://doi.org/10.1111/jonm.12906.

Ma, C., & Park, S. H. (2015). Hospital Magnet status, unit work environment, and pressure ulcers. *Journal of Nursing Scholarship, 47*(6), 565–573.

McCaughey, D., McGhan, G. E., Rathert, C., Williams, J. H., & Hearld, K. R. (2020). Magnetic work environments: Patient experience outcomes in Magnet versus non-Magnet hospitals. *Health Care Management Review, 45*(1), 21–31.

McHugh, M. D., & Ma, C. (2013). Hospital nursing and 30-day readmissions among Medicare patients with heart failure, acute myocardial infarction, and pneumonia. *Medical care, 51*(1), 52.

McHugh, M. D., Rochman, M. F., Sloane, D. M., Berg, R. A., Mancini, M. E., Nadkarni, V. M., et al. (2016). Better nurse staffing and nurse work environments associated with increased survival of in-hospital cardiac arrest patients. *Medical Care, 54*(1), 74–80.

Nishioka, V. M., Coe, M. T., Hanita, M., & Moscato, S. R. (2014). Dedicated education unit: Student perspectives. *Nursing Education Perspectives, 35*(5), 301–307. https://doi.org/10.5480/14-1380.

Parry, J. S., Calarco, M. M., & Hensinger, B. (2014). Unit-based interventions: De-stressing the distressed. *Nursing Management, 45*(8), 38–44.

Peters, T., & Waterman, R. H. (1982). *In search of excellence*. New York, NY: Warner Communications.

Pew Research Center. (2018). *Millennials are the largest generation in the U.S. labor force*. https://www.pewresearch.org/fact-tank/2018/04/11/millennials-largest-generation-us-labor-force/.

Press Ganey Associates, Inc. (2013). *Every voice matters: The bottom line on employee and physician engagement*. South Bend, IN. http://healthcare.pressganey.com/2013-PI-Every_Voice_Matters.

Quality and Safety Education for Nurses (QSEN). (2020). *QSEN Institute*. https://qsen.org/.

Reason, J. (1997). *Managing the risks of organisational accidents*. London, UK: Ashgate Publishing.

Reeves, S., Perrier, L., Goldman, J., Freeth, D., & Zwarenstein, M. (2013). Interprofessional education: Effects on professional practice and healthcare outcomes (update). *Cochrane Database of Systematic Reviews, (3)*, Article CD002213.

Sleutel, M. R. (2000). Climate, culture, context, or work environment? Organizational factors that influence nursing practice. *Journal of Nursing Administration, 30*, 53–58.

Snow, J. (2002). Enhancing work climate to improve performance and retain valued employees. *Journal of Nursing Administration, 33*(2), 111–117.

Stewart, K. R., Stewart, G. L., Lampman, M., Wakefield, B., Rosenthal, G., & Solimeo, S. L. (2015). Implications of the patient-centered medical home for nursing practice. *Journal of Nursing Administration, 45*(11), 569–574. https://doi.org/10.1097/NNA.0000000000000265.

Stokowski, L. A. (2014). The risky business of nursing. *Medscape*. January 14, 2014 http://www.medscape.com/viewarticle/818437.

Stone, P. W., Harrison, M. I., Feldman, P., Linzer, M., Peng, T., Roblin, D., et al. (2005). *Organizational climate of staff working conditions and safety: An integrative model.* http://www.ncbi.nlm.nih.gov/books/NBK20497/.

Tourangeau, A. E., Thomson, H., Cummings, G., & Cranley, L. A. (2013). Generation-specific incentives and disincentives for nurses to remain employed in acute care hospitals. *Journal of Nursing Management, 21*(3), 473–482.

US Department of Health and Human Services: Health Resources and Services Administration. (2010). *The registered nurse population: Findings from the 2008 National Sample Survey of Registered Nurses.* https://bhw.hrsa.gov/sites/default/files/bhw/nchwa/rnsurveyfinal.pdf.

Van Bogaert, P., Timmermans, O., Weeks, S. M., van Heusden, D., Wouters, K., & Franck, E. (2014). Nursing unit teams matter: Impact of unit-level nurse practice environment, nurse work characteristics, and burnout on nurse reported job outcomes, and quality of care, and patient adverse events—A cross-sectional survey. *International Journal of Nursing Studies, 51*(8), 1123–1134.

Wonder, A. H., York, J., Jackson, K. L., & Sluys, T. D. (2017). Loss of Magnet® designation and changes in RN work engagement: A report on how 1 hospital's culture changed over time. *Journal of Nursing Administration, 47*(10), 491–496.

Wong, C. A., Cummings, G. G., & Ducharme, L. (2013). The relationship between nursing leadership and patient outcomes: A systematic review update. *Journal of Nursing Management, 21*(5), 709–724.

Wooten, L. P., & Crane, P. (2003). Nurses as implementers of organizational culture. *Nursing Economic$, 21*, 275–279.

Zimmerman, S., Bowers, B. J., Cohen, L. W., Grabowski, D. C., Horn, S. D., & Kemper, P. (2016). New evidence on the green house model of nursing home care: Synthesis of findings and implications for policy, practice, and research. *Health Services Research, 51*(Suppl.), 475–496.

4

Managerial Decision-Making

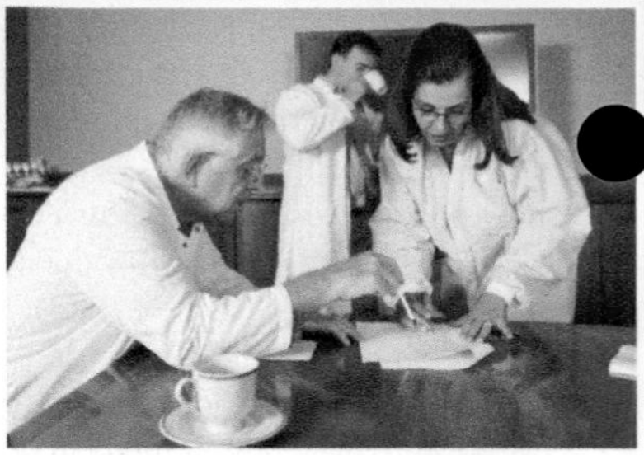

Betsy Frank

http://evolve.elsevier.com/Huber/leadership

All nurses make decisions. Decisions can be categorized as clinical, involving direct care, or managerial. Decision-making is central to all managerial roles (Clark-Burg & Alliex, 2017). Managerial decisions range from managing groups of patients at the unit level to the organization or community or health care delivery system levels (see Fig. 4.1). In order for nurses to make effective decisions, they need the analytical skills that account for individual staff and patient care needs and an understanding of ethical frameworks and human resource and financial considerations. Whether at the point-of-care, unit, or organizational level, all decisions affect the level of quality and safe care that is delivered and the climate of the work environment in which nurses and other health professionals work. Furthermore, all decisions need to be made with the entire system in mind.

In an era of corporate mergers, changing reimbursements, value-based purchasing, and expanded roles for nursing in the health care delivery system, decision-making is an important skill for nurses caring for patients and for nurse leaders and managers. Both the American Nurses Association's (2016) and the American Organization for Nursing Leadership (2015) standards for practice and competencies for nurse managers support the fact that in a fast-paced health care delivery environment, staff nurses, leaders, and managers all must be able to analyze and synthesize a large array of information, make decisions to deliver effective day-to-day patient care, and solve multifaceted problems that occur in complex health care delivery systems. Furthermore, the Magnet Recognition Program® (American Nurses Credentialing Center, 2020) and the *Future of nursing* report (2011) of the Institute of Medicine (IOM, now called the National Academies of Sciences, Engineering, and Medicine, Health and Medicine Division) highlighted the need for nurses to be able to be fully involved and even take the lead in decision-making from the unit level to the larger health care delivery system, including on health care institution governing boards (Thew, 2019).

DEFINITIONS

Decision-making is the process of making the best evidenced-informed choice, while taking into the context of the decision (Krishnan, 2018; Spiers et al., 2016). For example, if a nurse calls in sick, staff coverage decisions have to be made immediately. However, a union contract may influence how the manager adjusts the unit's staffing model in the short run, as well as the long term, if the unit is chronically understaffed. Decisions about staffing assignments greatly affect nurses' work life and patient outcomes. These include skill mix, patient-to-nurse ratios, and specific patient assignments.

The process of selecting one course of action from alternatives forms the basic core of the definition of decision-making. Nibbelink and Brewer (2018) noted that decisions made at the unit level are influenced by a unit's culture, patient acuity, and nursing staff expertise. In a chaotic health care delivery environment, where regulations and standards of care are always changing, any decision may cause unanticipated consequences. For example, a decision may be made to implement team-based delivery of care. However, if this new staffing model is made without considering availability of staff of various skill levels, the model might fail.

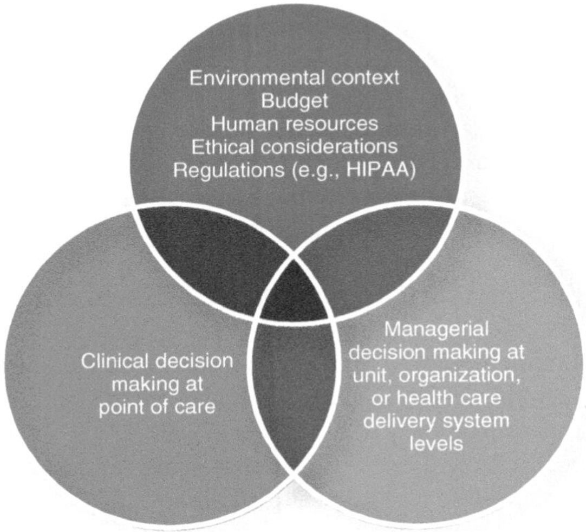

Fig. 4.1 The relationship between clinical and managerial decision-making.

Decision-making environment is the context in which decisions are made. The complexity of patient care needs, staffing expertise, budget allotted to care for patients, union contracts, reimbursement regulations, and leadership styles all affect the decisions that are made. Ultimately all these factors affect the quality of the patient care that is delivered.

Clinical judgment involves forming, refining, and evaluating hypotheses based upon recognizing and analyzing cues (National Council of State Boards of Nursing, 2019).

Clinical reasoning is the decision-making process that is grounded in the professional thought process (Gummesson et al., 2018).

Clinical decision-making involves clinical judgments that result in interventions at the point of patient care (Johansen & O'Brien, 2016; Razieh et al., 2018).

Managerial and organizational decision-making involves decisions for groups of patients at the unit, organizational, or health system levels.

BACKGROUND

Decision-Making Models

All nurses, whether managers or not, use models to help them make decisions. Many of the models include step-by-step frameworks that can guide decision-making. In reality, however, decision-making is an iterative process that may include an intuitive component (Benner, 1984; Tanner, 2006). Yet models can help the staff nurse and manager make some sense of the complex environment in which all decisions are made.

Such models are more than just for immediate problem solving. Decision-making may also be the result of opportunities, challenges, or more long-term leadership initiatives, as opposed to being triggered by an immediate problem. In any case, the processes are virtually the same, but their purposes may be slightly different. Nurse managers use decision-making in managing resources and the environment of care delivery. All decision-making involves an evaluation of the effectiveness of the outcomes that result from the decision-making process itself.

The nursing process is an example of one well-known model for clinical decision-making. However, the nursing process does not truly capture the important component of how the staff nurse or nurse manager makes the choice between competing alternatives for action. Other models may be more appropriate.

Moving beyond the nursing process, Tanner's (2006) model has formed the basis for understanding how clinical decisions are made. Her clinical judgment model involves noticing patient cues, interpreting those cues and responding to (acting on) them, and finally reflecting on the course of action chosen so that clinical learning occurs. The National Council of State Boards of Nursing (2019) published a model of clinical judgment that takes into account not only individual patient assessment but also environmental factors including resources, task complexity, and cultural considerations when making decisions about patient care. Furthermore, this model considers the nurse's knowledge and experience.

Nurse managers consider the environment and their own knowledge and experience when making decisions as well. For example, a nurse manager might want to implement a mentorship program for all new staff on the unit. However, the budget might cause the manager to only assign mentors to new graduates, not all new staff.

Guo's (2008) DECIDE Model is a model that is useful for managerial as well as clinical situations (Aitamaa et al., 2019b; Esan et al., 2016). Using this model can help prevent cognitive bias in high-stress environments because it can help prevent the missing of cues and thus choosing the wrong course of action.

Nurse managers also can use the decision-making dependency (DMD) model to assist in their decision-making processes (Chisengantambu-Winters et al., 2020). This model emphasizes the importance of consulting with personnel at all levels of an organization when a manager makes a decision.

The model outlined here is a combination of the models of Guo (2008) and Chisengantambu-Winters et al. (2020):

- Define the problem or need and its urgency. Does the problem require immediate action (Chisengantambu-Winters et al., 2020)?
- Establish desirable criteria for what you want to accomplish. What should stay the same and what can be done to avoid future problems? Predict how long it will take to respond to the changing environment.
- Consider all possible alternative choices that will accomplish the desired goal or criteria for problem solution. In other words, what is a desirable outcome?
- Identify the best choice or alternative based on experience, intuition, and experimentation while considering what human and material resources and time are needed to implement the choice. Consider what impact the decision will have.
- Develop and implement an action plan for problem solution taking into account policies that influence the decision-making process. Consider does the decision have to made immediately or can it be made when the manager can carefully consider all the criteria in the process such ethical and financial factors.
- Evaluate decision through monitoring, troubleshooting, and feedback. This step involves the reflective process emphasized by Tanner (2006).

Notice how these steps are somewhat similar to the nursing process well known to all nurses.

Thus decision-making is used to solve problems. Table 4.1 displays the use of the DECIDE model to

TABLE 4.1 Possible Formation of an Inpatient Hospice Unit Using the DECIDE Model

D—Define the Problem	E—Establish the Criteria	C—Consider All the Alternatives and Steps to Be Taken	I—Identify the Best Alternatives	D—Develop and Implement the Action	E—Evaluate and Monitor the Solution
The Federal government mandates inpatient hospice care. Nurses on med-surg units are not equipped to provide hospice level of care. Therefore a non-profit hospice agency must decide how to provide inpatient care when needed.	The inpatient unit must meet all Federal and State regulations for operation, and census has to be high enough to meet costs. Death certificates must be analyzed to determine which deaths have a hospice diagnosis in order to determine potential census. The competition must be determined. An assessment showed no other inpatient hospice unit is within 60 miles.	Two alternatives exist. One is to construct a free-standing inpatient hospice facility. The second alternative is to remodel a vacant unit at a local hospital and share services such as dietary and maintenance, but rent must be paid to the hospital.	The inpatient hospice unit in the existing local hospital was chosen because total cost was less than a free-standing unit	The Board of Directors of the hospice agency, patients, families, and the medical director must all agree on the plan for the hospice unit. The hospital's architect must be hired to design the unit. Fund raising to remodel the vacant unit for hospice services must occur.	The State Board of Health must give approval to open the unit. Costs must not exceed revenue if the unit is to remain viable. If costs exceed revenue, the hospice agency must determine how to make up for the difference through fundraising and other means.

Acknowledgement: Trudy Rupska MSN, RN, CEO of VNA Homecare and Hospice of the Wabash Valley.

analyze whether to establish an inpatient hospice unit. The DECIDE model depicted in Table 4.1 shows information to consider in making a decision regarding the inpatient unit.

The person at the next level may look at the chosen alternative in a different context. For example, the chief executive officer may frame issues as a competitive struggle not unlike a sports event. The marketing staff may interpret problems as military battles that need to be won. Nurse executives may view concerns from a care or family frame that emphasizes collaboration and working together. Learning and understanding which analogies and perspectives offer the best view of a problem or issue are vital to effective decision-making. It may be necessary for nurse managers to expand their frame of reference and be willing to consider even the most outlandish ideas. Effectiveness is tied to mirroring and messaging language that fosters shared understanding.

Chisengantambu et al. (2018) developed a sandwich support model that can be integrated into the DECIDE and DMD model (Chisengantambu-Winters et al., 2020). Both models demonstrate the importance of having environmental support for the nurse manager from staff as well as the executive level. The models define support in terms of environmental, technical, and financial resources. With support, nurse managers can implement organizational policies while at the same time supporting the staff nurses who work within the organization. Nurse executives can guide the nurse manager in how to effectively support staff during the decision-making process. With support work performance is enhanced and ultimately quality and safe patient care can be delivered.

One note of caution is that no matter the model used or the organizational level where the decision is made, cognitive bias can occur. Fig. 4.2 is an illustration of what can happen in a faulty decision process when data are ignored or biases are present in the process. According to Sherman (2015), by allowing others to question your thinking you can avoid cognitive bias.

DECISION-MAKING PROCESS

Decisions are the visible outcomes of the leadership and management process. Decision-making is essentially the process of selecting one course of action from alternatives. Decisions are made at all levels, but it is important to know who the decision maker is and what the process and timeline of decision-making is. Nurses' control over decision-making may vary as to amount of control and where in the process they can influence decisions. The basic elements of decision-making are identifying the goal for decision-making and making the decision.

The process follows the basic problem-solving process but also involves an evaluation of the effectiveness of the outcomes that result from the decision-making process itself. The seven steps of the problem solving process are (1) define the problem, (2) gather information, (3) determine the overall goal or desired outcome, (4) develop solutions, (5) consider the consequences, (6) make a decision, and (7) implement and evaluate

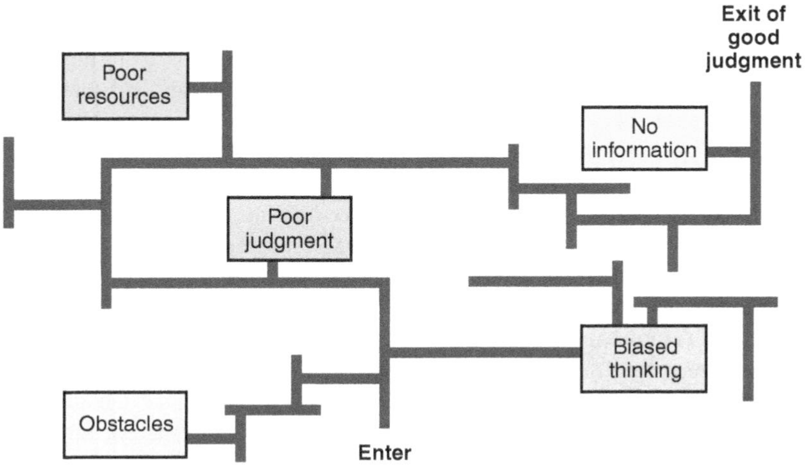

Fig. 4.2 Decision-making maze.

the solution. The decision-making process adds a final step of testing or assessing the solution and the decision-making process itself. Nurses may be sole decision makers or may facilitate group decision-making. Decisions are often made within the structure of shared governance or by using interprofessional teams for problem solving and decision-making.

CLINICAL DECISION-MAKING

Clinical decision-making is the heart of nursing practice. Point-of-care decisions ultimately have an impact on the total organization's performance and, consequently, its financial viability. Delivering quality and safe patient care is a goal for all health care organizations. Thus effective clinical decisions must be made.

Clinical reasoning is a career-long development process. This process must carry over from skills learned during a nurse's education to the workplace. Nurse residency programs are one way to help newly licensed nurses develop their clinical decision-making abilities. Kramer et al. (2012) found that newly licensed nurses identified that autonomous decision-making and prioritization were challenging for them. New graduates often felt that they needed to verify their decisions with others more competent than themselves. The graduates noted they could identify what care needed to be implemented but needed support to develop confidence in making the right decisions regarding care. The use of preceptors and/or coaches and didactic presentations in the residency program helped the new graduates develop their confidence to make autonomous decisions. Staff nurses must continually make autonomous decisions regarding patient care delivery. Therefore nurse residency programs could promote the new graduate's ability to make the necessary decisions when delivering nursing care autonomously. Some examples of decisions nurses make involve such day-to-day activities as documentation, medication administration, intravenous drug therapy, and prioritization for what care is delivered to a group of patients such as by triage.

In the course of their day, nurses make many decisions from what to chart, how and when to give medications, or when to call a rapid response team. All these decisions have consequences for patient safety.

Medication administration involves many decisions. All nurses know that giving medications involves giving the right patient the right medication, the right dose, the right route, at the right time. If anyone of these rights is wrong, the nurse must take appropriate action. For example, if the dose is wrong, the nurse must contact the prescriber for a new medication order. Medication administration takes place in an environment prone to interruptions which can disturb the nurse's decision-making processes. In fact, Reed et al. (2018) found that medication administration, including preparation of the medication to be administered, was interrupted 39% of the time. Such interruptions have the potential to compromise patient safety.

In addition to distractions other factors can contribute to medication errors ultimately caused by faulty decision-making during medication administration (Keers et al., 2018). Keers and colleagues interviewed 20 nurses who described medication errors, including near misses. They found that a stressful work environment that includes short staffing, improper skill mix, and multitasking all impact decision-making during medication administration. The five "rights" of medication administration are just the beginning of a complex decision-making process.

Triage decisions occur in a very complex environment, and a computerized system can assist in this process (Chang et al., 2017). Using a computerized system, the nurse can enter assessment data to determine the level of triage or urgency. Chang and colleagues interviewed 15 Taiwanese emergency department triage nurses in order to gain an understanding of the clinical decision-making process during triage. Although the computerized data assessment was used, the nurse's experience, the patients' overall health status, and environmental factors such as available equipment and conflict with staff and patients also affected the triage decision. For example, if a patient required a procedure that might indicate a lower level of triage as determined by the computer, but the nurse thought the procedure was more urgent, the nurse would "up" the level of triage.

Prioritization occurs not only in triage situations but also across the care spectrum. Nurses take care of more than one patient at a time. Thus decisions have to be made regarding what care has to be delivered and what care can possibly be omitted (Harvey et al., 2018). Ethical frameworks may be unconsciously used when making decisions (see Chapter 7). Some patient care activities can be delegated, but on a busy day even thinking about delegation can be challenging.

Clinical decision-making is complex and step-by-step processes are helpful, but not all situations lend themselves to such processes. A more holistic approach is often needed as priorities can rapidly change (Benner et al., 2010). Therefore leaders and managers at all levels of an organization need to foster a culture where effective, evidence-based clinical decision-making can occur.

MANAGERIAL AND ORGANIZATIONAL DECISION-MAKING

All nurse managers and leaders need to consider the implications of their decisions. Each decision made involves financial, ethical, and human resources. Furthermore, reimbursement and other regulations must be considered. Nurse managers, for example, make staffing decisions and thus commit financial resources for the purpose of delivering patient care. Hospital administrators may decide to add additional services to keep up with external forces. These decisions subsequently have financial implications related to reimbursement, staffing, and human resources deployment.

Nurse managers work in a complex environment that causes stress that may ultimately hamper their cognitive decision-making abilities (Shirey et al., 2013). In any situation, a nurse manager's experience, level of work complexity, and situation factors such as uncertainty and role overload influence how he or she recognizes environmental patterns and cues and the subsequent questions asked. The decisions that result have wide impact on the organization. If a manager is stressed, important factors in the cognitive decision-making process may be missed and organizational outcomes adversely affected. Not only does stress impact organizational outcomes, but the nurse manager's own mental and physical health can be impacted (Udon et al., 2017). Lack of autonomy in decision-making is one stressor that can adversely impact a manager's health (Fallman et al., 2019). On the other hand, support from staff and upper level management can mitigate some of the stress in the work environment (Chisengantambu et al., 2018).

Ethical decision-making is inherent in the role of the nurse manager. When decisions involve an ethical dilemma, nurse managers may experience stress (Ganz et al., 2015). Aitamaa et al. (2016) interviewed nine nurse managers and found that ethical dilemmas occur in four areas: conflicts with staff, patients, and administration; lack of appreciation for the value of nursing as a profession; disregard of problems that had to be ignored because the problems were considered "normal" in the organization; inability to carry out the job due to obstacles such as financial and limited power within the organization. How the nurse manager deals with these dilemmas has an effect on the quality of the work environment.

One way to deal with ethical dilemmas is through moral case discussions between staff and managers (Weidema et al., 2015). In an open and safe environment, a case study is presented for full debate, analysis, and sharing of possible action steps for resolution. However, using this participatory management technique is hard to incorporate in the workflow when there is a heavy day-to-day workload. Furthermore, conducting case discussions between staff and managers could inhibit free discussion between the two groups just because of the presence of hierarchal relationships (Weidema et al., 2015). Weidema and colleagues suggested that if staff nurses feel empowered to make autonomous decisions, then communication in the case discussions could actually occur without the presence of the manager.

Nurse managers need to develop ways of being that strengthen their ability to make ethical decisions (Roshanzadeh et al., 2019). Nineteen nurse managers were interviewed, and data analysis showed that assertiveness, commitment, and insight promoted sound decision-making. If a nurse manager is assertive, then the manager has confidence in their ethical decision-making ability. A nurse manager who has commitment takes responsibility for decision-making and aims to prevent errors. A manager who has insight is self-aware, logical, intelligent and is fair in the decision-making process.

On an organizational level, Aitamaa et al. (2019a) suggested that a values-based organization can mitigate the severity of ethical problems. They also stated that ethics education could enhance the nurse manager's ability to make ethical decisions.

A nurse manager's leadership style may affect how decisions are made throughout the organization. Leadership style influences decision-making by promoting structural empowerment and engagement in the work (Garcia-Sierra & Fernández-Castro, 2018).

Praising employees affects a nurse's job satisfaction (Sveinsdóttir et al., 2016). This in turn contributes to a healthy work environment wherein nurses are free to make autonomous decisions that contribute to positive patient outcomes. Dans and Lundmark (2019) noted that autonomy is one of the most important influences on patient outcomes. Furthermore, Kowalski et al. (2020) integrative literature review confirms that autonomy in decision-making is a key component of a practice environment that promotes positive patient outcomes. Transformational leaders are the key to achieving these positive outcomes (Moon et al., 2019).

Patient Acuity and Staffing: An Example of Decision-Making

An example of decision-making in nursing practice is staffing and assignment decisions. Patients need nursing care. Needs for care are not uniform. The need severity (physical and psychological) is called *patient acuity*, which is a rating of the complexity of the patient's condition. The degree of work needed for any patient is called *nursing intensity* and is a combination of the severity of illness, the patient's dependency, the complexity of care, and the amount of time needed. The organization staffs a set number of nurses and assistants to deliver care to patients. Both patients' needs for nursing care and the amount of nurse time that is required to meet patients' needs for care must be matched up and caregivers deployed, sometimes 24/7.

Frontline nurses are responsible for the decision-making about patient acuity and nursing intensity. Managers are responsible for the decision-making about staffing and scheduling. The individual nurse experiences this decision-making as workload (nursing work activities), nurse-to-patient ratios, and patient assignments. In theory, the nursing interventions required to support the patients' needs should be in proportion to the levels of severity and degrees of intensity (Gray & Kerfoot, 2016). However, for a variety of reasons, decision-making around staffing, scheduling, patient assignments is imprecise and creates tension and stress for both nurses and managers. For example, data-driven acuity systems often do not consider experience levels of staff, and the systems, themselves, often rely on subjective data when calculating the acuity score (Gray & Kerfoot, 2016).

Allen (2015) interviewed 14 charge nurses in order to explore how staffing decisions were made. Findings showed that nurse-patient assignments involved a complex process that included not only patient factors, such as acuity; the nurse, including expertise; and the environment, including nurse patient ratios and location of patients on the unit. Given the complexity of staffing decisions, the nurse manager needs to think about what unanticipated and adverse consequences could occur as a result of staffing decisions.

DECISION-MAKING TOOLS

Both nurses at the point of care and nurse managers need a variety of tools to facilitate effective decision-making. For example, there are a variety of clinical decision-making tools such as algorithms, policies, procedures, clinical protocols, standard order sets, and smart alerts.

Although trial and error or a shoot-from-the-hip approach can work, direct patient care nurses and managers have a variety of other approaches that can be used to make decisions that promote quality and safe care. For example, by analyzing the data in Table 4.2, the nurse can help decide if an additional medical assistant should be hired in a small rural health clinic. The nurse must also decide if the assistant should be hired full or part-time.

Shared Governance

Another decision-making approach is shared governance. Although this topic is discussed more fully in Chapter 13, a brief discussion is warranted here. Shared governance is an organizational structure that promotes empowerment and autonomous decision-making at the point of care, accountability that is shared among all parties in a decision, and organizational processes that promote an egalitarian environment in decision-making processes. Shared governance promotes staff nurses' responsibility and accountability for patient outcomes (Medeiros, 2018). For example, a committee within a shared governance organization could develop and test a new fall-prevention protocol, exhibiting nursing practice empowerment. Nurse leaders have a critical role in promoting the success of the decisions that arise out of shared governance. They can use their expertise to coach staff on how to implement their decisions, as well as facilitate effective group functioning when group process within the governance structure goes awry.

Evidence-Informed Decision-Making

Nurses are familiar with evidence-based practice for clinical standards of practice. In the management realm, using evidence to make decisions is as important as is using evidence for clinical decisions. One example is the evidence-based protocol that is widely used by staff

TABLE 4.2 Desired Objectives Analysis

Objective	Alternative A Full-time Hire	Alternative B Part-time Hire	Alternative C No Hire
Increases workflow	5	4	1
Enables more examination rooms to be filled at one time	5	3	1
Decreases patient wait time	4	3	1
Increases the number of patients seen in a day	4	3	1
Revenue minus personnel costs increase	4	5	5
Total score	22	18	9

1, Does not meet objective; *2*, meets some aspects of objective; *3*, meets objective; *4*, exceeds objective; *5*, significantly exceeds objective.

nurses to prevent catheter acquired urinary infections (American Nurses Association, 2017). But what about managers? Jansson and Forsberg's study (2016) revealed that nurse managers have a critical role in facilitating the use of evidence at the point of care.

Specific interventions at the organizational level can promote better decision-making. Thomson and colleagues (2017) conducted an educational program for primary health providers in Britain's national health care system (NHS). Participants were divided into three groups: Group 1 attended a full day educational session, Group 2 a half-day session, and Group 3 six 2.5-hour sessions. All groups found a self-reported increase in understanding of the theory of decision-making following the educational sessions. The educational intervention appeared to have little impact on application to practice. The researchers posited that perhaps the self-reported questionnaire could not detect small differences in improvement in decision-making in practice (Thomson et al., 2017). Another factor may have accounted for this finding. Perhaps a longer term follow-up using observations of clinical practice rather than self-report may have more precisely captured any changes in decision-making following the educational program.

Pilot Projects

Pilot projects are critical for implementation for evidence-informed decision-making. Pilot projects or carefully defined trials are used to try out a solution alternative on a small or restricted basis to reduce risk and to see whether major problems will occur. Pilot project strategies may resemble research projects, and these projects may also be linked to quality improvement initiatives. One example of a pilot quality improvement project was reported by Massarweh and colleagues (2017). An eAssignment sheet for nurse staffing was developed at a California multi-hospital system to replace multiple paper records of assignments. This decision support tool for staffing considered such things as union contract requirements, legislated nurse-patient ratios, and nurse competency. If a less experienced nurse was assigned to a complex patient, the system alerted the nurse manager who reached out to that nurse to assist in problem solving when necessary. The system also alerted the nurse manager if care hours assigned did not conform with the expected care hours based on acuity. Nurse managers agreed that patient care assignments were more data-driven and took less time than did the paper system. Furthermore, the data collected through the eAssignment system was used for financial management.

SBAR

SBAR is a communication technique that helps members of the health team communicate effectively so that appropriate decisions can be made. Because hand-off communication is so crucial to decision-making about patient care, SBAR is used to clarify and organize essential but complex patient care information (see Chapter 2). The acronym stands for **S**ituation, **B**ackground, **A**ssessment, **R**ecommendation (Stewart & Hand, 2017). Teaching SBAR to students helps them to develop their clinical judgment skills and can also be used to help new nurses further develop their autonomous decision-making.

SBAR has been demonstrated to be particularly useful in a rapid paced emergency department where incomplete reporting can result in errors being made (Campbell & Dontje, 2019). Therefore all providers need a way to communicate in order to guide effective clinical decision-making. When SBAR was used as a framework for bedside reporting at change of shift in the emergency department, as part of a quality improvement project, nurses reported that SBAR helped to reduce the number of poor patient outcomes that were due to incomplete communication between shifts (Campbell & Dontje, 2019).

Simulation

Simulation is a well-known technique for developing and maintaining clinical decision-making. It is used to teach skills and verify competencies. Simulation could also be used to improve management decision-making. A meta-analysis conducted by Orique and Phillips (2018) showed that simulation was effective in improving knowledge and skills in recognizing clinical deterioration. Likewise, simulation is a useful strategy for practicing interprofessional collaboration (Blondon et al., 2017).

Simulation is also useful for nurse leaders to practice skills particular to their role. Junious (2020) used simulation in a master's in nursing administration program to help future nurse leaders learn root cause analysis for errors that could "lead to a sentinel event" (Junious, 2020, p. 57). Students had to work through the root cause analysis procedure and identify flaws in the system of care. Debriefing is an important and necessary part of instruction using simulation. Junious (2020) described this post-simulation evaluation by debriefing as all students and faculty participating in a roundtable debriefing discussion done immediately after completing the scenario and focused on students' initial thoughts and feelings. Faculty critiques included positive and negative feedback and advice. Students used this to develop a presentation on the process.

Data Analytics and Decision Support Systems

Decisions need to be data driven. Nurses and nurse managers have a wide array of data—including electronic health records, human resource data, and financial data—available to them for use in making decisions (Murphy et al., 2013). Making sense of these data is necessary but often a challenge.

By analyzing big data sets, nurse managers can improve staff performance. For example, Loresto and colleagues (2019) studied patterns of medication delivery to individual patients. The data were used to look, in particular, at delays in medication administration. Over a million medications were given to over 29,000 by patients by 704 nurses on 18 hospital units. Although nurse and patient characteristics had little effect on the delays, Loresto and colleagues (2019) suggested that patient mix and nurse staffing could have affected the medication delays.

Data analytics can also be used to promote financial success across the health care delivery system. Polancich and colleagues (2017) described how data analytics helped to improve the financial performance of nurse-led clinics that served patients with diabetes and heart failure. The measure of success was the number of inpatient days avoided and the resultant cost avoidance, or costs that did not occur. The clinic that served the patients with diabetes avoided $300,000 in annualized costs through decreasing inpatient days by 50%. For the patients with heart failure, inpatient days decreased by 18% after the nurse-led clinic was instituted. Cost avoidance was over $47,600. By analyzing data such as these, nurse managers can justify their return on investment for new or continuing patient care delivery models.

In addition to the use of data analytics to help decide if a particular patient care delivery system is justified, nurse managers can use decision support systems to make day-to-day decisions concerned with patient care unit operation. Staffing is one of the primary decisions that managers make. In addition, determining supply availability and patient flow are other uses for decision support systems. Peltonen and colleagues (2019) surveyed nurse managers in Finland to determine whether or not the information systems in their hospitals assisted them in day-to-day decision-making. Results showed that respondents were fairly satisfied with access to information, but the information was not always useful in decision-making. The respondents noted that multiple systems of information had to be accessed in order to make decisions. In another study by Peltonen and colleagues (2018), respondents noted the need for information to be shared with all stakeholders in the decision-making process. For decision supports systems to be useful, all stakeholders, including nurse managers, need to have a say in the systems' design.

Using a personal device such as a smartphone has the potential for assisting nurse managers and beside clinicians in making decisions. Martinez and colleagues (2017) interviewed 10 Canadian nurse managers for the purpose of studying the acceptance of personal devices, such as smartphones and tablets, in the clinical setting. One advantage was ready access to evidence-based information to use in patient care decisions. One big disadvantage identified was concerns for patient privacy and data security. As the use of mobile technology expands, nurse managers and leaders will need to take the lead in determining how best to use this rapidly expanding information system.

Artificial intelligence also has possibilities for improving decision-making for clinicians and nurse leaders (Clancy, 2020). Artificial intelligence could help analyze patterns of data and suggest courses of action. Robots could deliver supplies, saving human resources for more important tasks (Clancy, 2020).

Six Sigma is a quality and decision support technique that uses data to build process-improvement models. The goal is to eliminate defects in safety and quality in health care delivery (American Society for Quality, n.d.). Essentially Six Sigma is a variant of the plan-do-study-act (PDSA) cycle promoted by the Institute for Healthcare Improvement (n.d.). For example, data may be used to identify ways to decrease health care acquired infections. Improta and colleagues (2018) used an interprofessional team to investigate how Six Sigma could be used to decrease infections. Through the Six Sigma process, needed corrections in processes were identified, which led to a decreased infection rate across a variety of patient care units. Thus Six Sigma and Lean quality improvement techniques can be used for clinical and managerial decision-making as well (see Chapter 18).

Data analytics are most useful in assisting in decision-making, and an expanded discussion of the use of data analytics is found in Chapter 25. However, use of data to make decisions can have unintended consequences. Aron and colleagues (2019) examined data from Veteran's Affairs hospitals and discovered that many patients with diabetes were overtreated. However, when reduction in overtreatment was promoted, an increase in patients who were undertreated occurred. Nurse managers and leaders need to recognize that decision based on data analysis can lead to better or worse organizational outcomes.

LEADERSHIP AND MANAGEMENT IMPLICATIONS

All health care is delivered in complex and sometimes chaotic organizations. Decisions made using a variety of tools and strategies can lead to safer care delivery environments. However, the rapid pace of decision-making may hamper the use of available evidence to assist in that decision-making. Furthermore, the time for reflection about clinicians' and managers' actions may hamper development of clinical judgment and managerial decision-making abilities.

Strategies for Decision-Making

The focus of leadership and management decision-making is more closely related to the nurse's role as care coordinator and systems problem solver. Some decisions, such as those requiring disciplinary action, do require the manager's *direct intervention*. In conflicts between staff members or between family and staff members, the manager might use negotiation and other forms of conflict management that could be viewed as *indirect intervention* because the manager does not actually decide what should be done to deal with an issue but rather persuades others to solve the problem themselves. The nurse manager might *delegate* the decision-making to others. For example, a unit manager might ask a team of staff nurses and the unit secretary to figure out when the best time is to order supplies for the unit.

Sometimes the nurse manager might choose *watchful waiting*. A particular staff member might be causing some interpersonal difficulties. If the staff member has submitted his or her resignation, dealing with the behavior might not be worth the energy.

Most decision-making should take place within the confines of *collaboration and consultation*. That collaboration often takes place within an interprofessional context. Patient care requires a team approach among nursing, medicine, and other disciplines such as physical therapy. Working in an interprofessional context is an essential skill for both clinicians and managers (Interprofessional Education Collaborative, 2016).

Shared governance initiatives have shown that collaboration and consultation result in high-quality patient care delivery systems (Dans & Lundmark, 2019). Therefore a critical role for nurse managers and leaders is *facilitation* by fostering a climate that encourages creativity and interdependence.

Modeling desired decision-making behaviors is also important. For example, in hospitals, nurse leaders and managers can use change-of-shift reports to promote deep clinical reasoning using the Socratic method and asking who, what, when, and where questions such as "What nursing interventions have been effective?" or "What will happen if this course of action is chosen?" An organizational climate that fosters patient safety can enhance nurses' clinical reasoning skills. Fig. 4.3 summarizes global strategies used for decision-making that contribute to quality and safe patient care.

Clearly all nurses are on information overload. Ways to capture the available data and use it for effective problem solving and decision-making are critical. The use of computerized informatics applications to aid decision-making is on the rise. For example, hospital information systems can be used to capture data such as length of stay, skill mix, case mix, patient and employee job satisfaction, and other variables that can be important when decisions need to be made (Peltonen et al., 2019). Refinements such as smart alerts show promise to ease the complexity and information overload of care delivery and thus reduce errors.

Nurse managers and leaders solve problems in complex systems where all decisions carry some amount of risk (Shirey et al., 2013). Understanding a manager's cognitive workflow has the potential for use in decision support tools (Effken et al., 2011). Cognitive workflow analysis includes work domain, decision-making procedures, personnel skill level, and social organization and collaboration patterns.

Braaten (2015) used qualitative methods to investigate barriers to workflow using the example of when to call a Rapid Response Team (RRT). The results indicated that human resources in the form of appropriate staffing helped to identify patients in need of an RRT. Nonhuman resources included the electronic medical record and policies related to the RRT. Respondents had to justify calling the RRT within the framework of policies and enough staffing to recognize the change, which was often subtle, in the patient's condition as observed and not from data in the medical record. If policies were unclear, the nurse's decision-making was hampered. Based on the findings of this study, Braaten noted the critical importance of managerial support so that appropriate decisions could be made.

Just like complex patient-care scenarios, complex social organizations such as hospitals can produce the best outcomes when creativity and ability of the staff at all levels of the organization are enabled (Belrhiti et al., 2018). Expert nurse leaders need to understand the system they work in is often unordered and rapidly changing. Because change is occurring so rapidly, nurse managers may feel stressed when past practices no longer apply. Therefore decentralized decision-making is essential.

Inevitably some mistakes will be made, but nurse managers and leaders who view mistakes as learning opportunities help promote effective organizations. Such an attitude fosters the concept of a learning organization (see Chapter 2), where organizations stay vital by learning and growing. Leaders can foster a climate wherein new communication patterns emerge, bottom-up communication changes the organization, and differences in talents, structures, and communication networks come forth and promote high-performing organizations.

CURRENT ISSUES AND TRENDS

Creativity and innovation will be the cornerstone of nurses' participation in the health care system of the future. An IOM report (2011) and the 2015 update (Altman et al., 2015) noted that nurses should and must take the lead in providing care for patients in a complex, rapidly changing health care system. An additional role for all nurses, including leaders, is to get nurses on various health care and community boards of directors (Nurses on Boards Coalition, 2020). New roles have

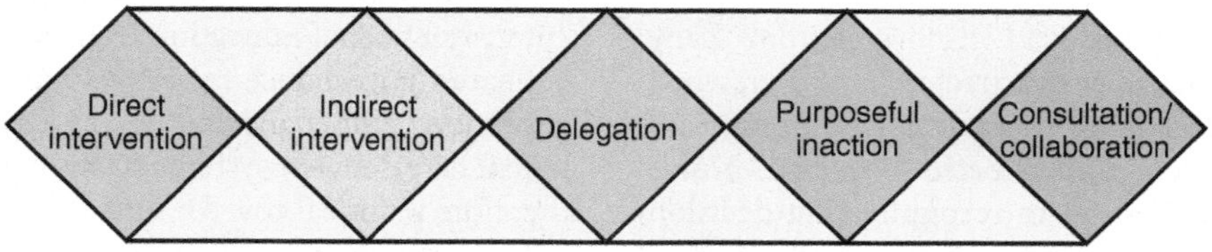

Fig. 4.3 Global decision-making strategies that contribute to quality and safe patient care.

emerged, such as the clinical nurse leader, who is a bedside leader and coordinator of complex care. Nurse leaders are in a unique position in the implementation of Accountable Care Organizations (ACOs), which will coordinate primary care for groups of patients. These leaders understanding and skills necessary to coordinate the continuum of care across the full spectrum of the health care delivery system will be critical to the success of the ACOs (Morrison, 2016). Cost savings will be critical, therefore nurse managers need to take the lead in delivering quality, cost efficient care.

The emphasis on quality and safety will be the focus of much of nurse managers' and leaders' planning and resultant decision-making. The seminal report *To err is human* (IOM, 1999), pointed out that human error was rampant in the health care system, causing lives lost and increasing health costs. Makary and Daniel (2016) and many others have pointed out that medical errors are the third leading cause of death in the United States. However, Mazer and Nabhan (2019) questioned the accuracy of these statistics. Nevertheless, nurse leaders and managers can foster team decision-making in a shared governance environment in order to improve processes of care delivery and mitigate errors (Fischer et al., 2018).

Although financial considerations in an organization are important, quality and safe care that is patient- and family-centered is equally important. The Quality and Safety Education for Nurses (QSEN, 2020) competencies will continue to serve as a guide for clinicians and managers alike as they strive to increase personal and organization performance.

Changing reimbursement patterns as a result of the attempts to modify the Patient Protection and Affordable Care Act (2010) and changing reimbursement regulations from the Centers for Medicare & Medicaid Services (CMS) (2020) will challenge nurse leaders and managers to find creative ways to facilitate the delivery of safe and quality care. More than likely costs will go up, but reimbursements may not keep pace with costs.

Despite the need for creativity, a certain amount of standardization must occur if safe patient care is to happen in complex care environments. Evidence-based management is the ideal, but barriers to implementation do exist, including communication gaps between those who develop guidelines and decision makers (Hasanpoor et al., 2019). Nurse managers have a critical role in incorporating evidence along with patient-centered care and clinical experience in their decision-making (Karlsson et al., 2019).

Nurse leaders need to advocate for a preferred future for nursing and evaluate the effectiveness of decision-making in practice. Both are aimed at making careful projections about what decisions to make—given uncertainty—to improve organizational and system performance. In times of change, nursing has an opportunity to make decisions that proactively direct the future. Nursing has demonstrated its value to the health care system. Therefore nurse leaders must be a party to all decisions regarding how care is delivered in health care organizations via shared governance arrangements (Medeiros, 2018).

Many hospitals are applying for Magnet recognition from the American Nurses Credentialing Center (ANCC, 2020). One of the 14 Forces of Magnetism from the old model that is incorporated in the new model of five domains involves management style and another promotes interdisciplinary collaboration. These two elements—a management style that is collaborative and the promotion of interdisciplinary staff input in decision-making—are evidence-based "best practices" (ANCC, 2020).

The efficiency, efficacy, and effectiveness of health care decisions will continue to enjoy a strong focus in nursing, with shifts toward outcomes specification. As performance improvement specialists, nurses will be challenged to make decisions that directly affect quality, access, cost, productivity, and the "bottom line." Effective approaches to decision-making are needed when care is delivered in a complex system in which multiple stakeholders need to be served, time is constrained, and the amount of information is overwhelming. The decisions that nurse managers and leaders make must be translated from the corporate "lingo" into terms that the clinicians understand if true buy-in is to be achieved (Porter-O'Grady, 2015). Furthermore, all nurses need to have leadership competencies, including the ability to make effective decisions (IOM, 2011). Nurses need to be at the forefront of all decision-making in health care, including at the governing board level.

RESEARCH NOTE

Source

Fischer, S. A., Horak, D., & Kelly, L. A. (2018). Decisional involvement: Differences related to characteristics, role, and shared leadership participation. *Journal of Nursing Care Quality, 33*(4), 354–360.

Purpose

The purpose of this study was to investigate the relationship between nurse attributes, role, and shared leadership participation in their perceptions of decisional involvement that affect their practice (p. 356).

Discussion

Staff nurses and managers from one health system in seven states responded to the Decisional Involvement Scale. Over 1900 nurses and managers responded to the survey, Decisional involvement scale scores were positively correlated with participation in shared leadership councils and years of experience. Managers, however, had higher decisional involvement scores than did staff nurses. Nurse managers perceived that staff nurses had more decisional involvement than did the staff nurses themselves.

Application to Practice

As nurses gain more years of experience, they become more comfortable with sharing their ideas for practice improvement. However, all front-line nurses need to be mentored in the shared leadership model. When decisions are shared by staff and managers, patient care quality improves.

CASE STUDY

Effective decision-making relies, in part, on analyzing alternative levels of uncertainty or risk. Staffing and scheduling decisions exemplify this. In addition to making "apples to apples" comparisons through such tools as staffing matrices recommended by professional bodies, daily and monthly patient census data, and patient acuity and nursing intensity data can guide unit managers in their analysis, which might precede a request for more staffing. In addition, the nurse manager needs to have an awareness of the environment in which care is delivered in order to make the analysis complete.

Fig. 4.4 is an example of a decision tree. A nurse manager in a home care agency could use a decision tree to justify hiring more licensed practical nurses or more registered nurse case managers. The tree has several branches, and, depending on the end point, an increase in needed personnel could be handled in several ways. Diagrams such as decision trees can be invaluable in understanding complicated alternative solutions. These diagrams are useful in assessment and problem definition and in considering the available alternatives for dealing with a problem. Once the alternative is chosen, a plan needs to be formulated for implementing the chosen approach. The choice implemented must be evaluated. Note, however, that the decision tree in Fig. 4.4 only lists three alternatives. A more complex tree could be constructed that includes more alternatives based on a different combination of tree branches.

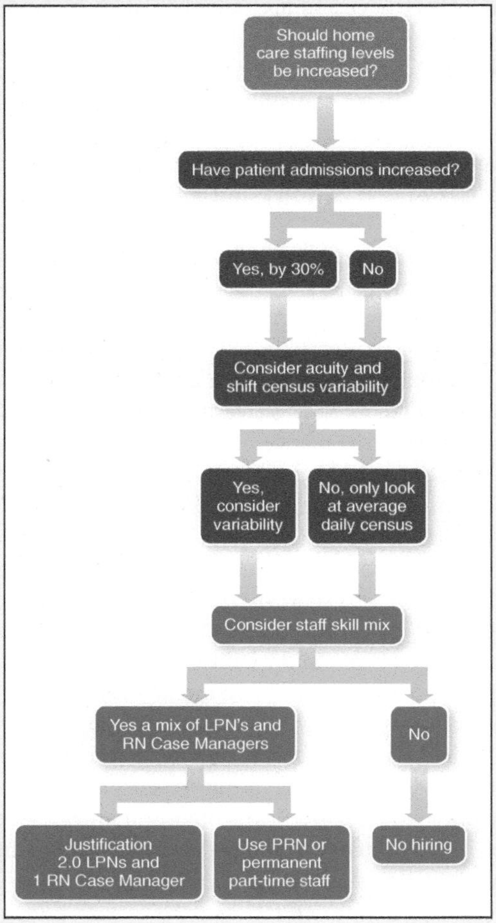

Fig. 4.4 Decision tree for home care staffing.

Acknowledgement: Jessica Wilson, BSN, RN, Clinical Coordinator, VNA Homecare and Hospice of the Wabash Valley.

CRITICAL THINKING EXERCISE

Adam Dean is a new nurse manager on a med-surg unit. One nurse on the night shift is ill and cannot come to work. He contacts the area director, and the director floats a nurse from the mental health unit to his unit to assist. This nurse did work on a med-surg unit until 6 months ago. She and another nurse each have a patient receiving blood transfusions. The float nurse needs another unit of blood, and while the other nurse covers, she goes to the blood bank and signs out the unit of blood. Upon returning to the unit, her colleague is tied up in a procedure and says she will be out in about 20 minutes. After briefly conferring with her colleague, the float nurse hangs the blood on her patient. When her colleague completes her procedure, the two of them are in the process of checking the blood and discover that the blood obtained from the Blood Bank was for the other patient. The blood is stopped, the supervisor is notified as is the patient's physician, and an incident report completed. As it turns out, the patient is a universal recipient. When Adam interviews each nurse individually, the nurse who administered the blood shows no remorse and tells Mr. Dean she cannot understand what the issue is because nothing happened. Adam Dean reviews with her the issue and related policies. She insists that Mr. Dean is upset over nothing. When speaking with the other nurse, she is overwrought, in tears, and asks if Mr. Dean wants her to resign. What actions does Mr. Dean, the manager, take for each nurse and why?

Using the SBAR framework identify:

1. What was the situation?
2. What was the background information?
3. What information does Mr. Dean need to assess the situation?
4. What disciplinary action should Mr. Dean take for each nurse, if any? Should the action be different for each nurse?

As you consider the SBAR scenario, think about what organizational policies you need to consider. What departments in the hospital could assist Mr. Dean in his decision-making process?

Acknowledgement: A. Christine Delucas, DNP, MPH, RN, NEA-BC, Associate Professor and DNP Program Director, University of New Mexico College of Nursing.

REFERENCES

Aitamaa, E., Leino-Kilpi, H., Iltanen, S., & Suhonen, R. (2016). Ethical problems in nursing management: The views of nurse managers. *Nursing Ethics, 23*(6), 646–658. https://doi.org/10.1177/0969733015579309.

Aitamaa, E., Suhonen, R., Iltanen, S., Puukka, P., & Leino-Kilpi, H. (2019a). Ethical problems in nursing management: Frequency and difficulty of the problems. *Health Care Management Review*, Advance online publication. https://doi.org/10.1097/HMR.0000000000000236.

Aitamaa, E., Suhonen, R., Iltanen, S., Puukka, P., & Leino-Kilpi, H. (2019b). Ethical problems in nursing management: A cross-sectional survey about problem solving. *BMC Health Services Research, 19*(417). https://doi.org/10.1186/s12913-019-4245-4.

Allen, S. B. (2015). The nurse patient assignment: Purposes and decision factors. *Journal of Nursing Administration, 45*(12), 628–635. https://doi.org/10.1097/NNA.0000000000000276.

Altman, S., Gubrud, P., Phillips, B., & Salsberg, E. (2015). *Assessing progress on the institute of medicine report: The future of nursing*. Washington, DC: The National Academies Press.

American Nurses Association. (2016). *Nursing administration: Scope and standards of practice* (2nd ed.). Silver Spring, MD: ANA.

American Nurses Association. (2017). ANA CAUTI Prevention Tool. https://www.nursingworld.org/practice-policy/work-environment/health-safety/infection-prevention/ana-cauti-prevention-tool/.

American Nurses Credentialing Center (ANCC). (2020). Magnet model-creating a magnet culture. https://www.nursingworld.org/organizational-programs/magnet/magnet-model/.

American Organization for Nursing Leadership. (2015). Nurse manager competencies. https://www.aonl.org/system/files/media/file/2019/06/nurse-managercompetencies.pdf.

American Society for Quality. (n.d.). *What is Six Sigma?* https://asq.org/quality-resources/six-sigma.

Aron, D. C., Tseng, C. L, Soroka, O., & Pogach, L. M. (2019). Balancing measures: Identifying unintended consequences of diabetes quality performance measures in patients at high risk for hypoglycemia. *International Journal for Quality in Health Care, 31*(4), 246–251. https://doi.org/10.1093/intqhc/mzy151.

Belrhiti, Z., Giralt, A. N., & Marchal, B. (2018). Complex leadership in healthcare: A scoping review. *International Journal of Health Policy and Management, 7*(12), 1073–1084. https://doi.org/10.15171/ijhpm.2018.75.

Benner, P. (1984). *From novice to expert: Excellence and power in clinical practice*. Menlo Park, CA: Addison-Wesley.

Benner, P., Sutphen, M., Leonard, V., & Day, L. (2010). *Educating nurses: A call for radical transformation*. San Francisco, CA: Jossey-Bass.

Blondon, K. S., Maitre, F., Muller-Juge, W., Bochatay, N., Cullati, S., Hudelson, P., Vu, N. V., et al. (2017). Interprofessional collaborative reasoning by residents and nurses in internal medicine: Evidence from a simulation study. *Medical Teacher, 39*(4), 360–367. https://doi.org/10.1080/0142159X.2017.1286309.

Braaten, J. S. (2015). Hospital system barriers to rapid response team activation: A cognitive work analysis. *American Journal of Nursing, 115*(2), 22–32. https://doi.org/10.1097/01.NAJ.0000460673.82070.af.

Campbell, D., & Dontje, K. (2019). Implementing bedside handoff in the emergency department: A practice improvement project. *Journal of Emergency Nursing, 45*(2), 149–154. https://doi.org/10.1016/j.jen.2018.09.007.

Centers for Medicare & Medicaid Services (CMS). (2020). *CMS releases proposed notice of benefit and payment parameters rule for 2021*. https://www.cms.gov/newsroom/press-releases/cms-releases-proposed-notice-benefit-and-payment-parameters-rule-2021.

Chang, W., Liu, H. E., Goopy, S., Chen, L. C., & Han, C. Y. (2017). Using the Five-Level Taiwan Triage Acuity Scale computerized system: Factors in decision making by emergency department triage nurses. *Clinical Nursing Research, 26*(5), 651–666. https://doi.org/10.1177/1054773816636360.

Chisengantambu, C., Robinson, G. M., & Evans, N. (2018). Nurse managers and the sandwich support model. *Journal of Nursing Management, 26*(2), 192–199. https://doi.org/10.1111/jonm.12534.

Chisengantambu-Winters, C., Robinson, G. M., & Evans, N. (2020). Developing a decision-making dependency (DMD) model for nurse managers. *Heliyon, 6*(1), e03128. https://doi.org/10.1016/j.heliyon.2019.e03128.

Clark-Burg, K., & Allix, S. (2017). A study of styles: How do nurse managers make decisions? *Nursing Management, 48*(7), 44–49. https://doi.org/10.1097/01.NUMA.0000520721.78549.ad.

Clancy, T. (2020). Artificial intelligence and nursing: The future is now. *Journal of Nursing Administration, 50*(3), 125–127. https://doi.org/10.1097/NNA.0000000000000855.

Dans, M., & Lundmark, V. (2019). The effects of positive practice environments: Leadership must-knows. *Nursing Management, 50*(10), 7–10. https://doi.org/10.1097/01.NUMA.0000580624.53251.29.

Effken, J. A., Brewer, B. B., Logue, M. D., Gephart, S. M., & Verran, J. (2011). Using cognitive work analysis to fit decision support tools to nurse work flow. *International Journal of Medical Informatics, 80*, 698–707. https://doi.org/10.1016/j.ijmedinf.2011.07.003.

Esan, O. T., Akanbi, C. T., Esan, O., Fajobi, O., & Ikenenbomeh, P. I. (2016). Application of quantitative techniques in decision making by healthcare managers and administrators in Nigerian public tertiary health institutions. *Health Services Management Research, 29*(3), 50–61. https://doi.org/10.1177/0951484816662490.

Fallman, S. L., Jutengren, G., & Dellve, L. (2019). The impact of restricted decision-making autonomy on health care managers' health and work performance. *Journal of Nursing Management, 27*(4), 705–714. https://doi.org/10.1111/jonm.12741.

Fischer, S. A., Horak, D., & Kelly, L. A. (2018). Decisional involvement: Differences related to nurse characteristics, role, and shared leadership participation. *Journal of Nursing Care Quality, 33*(4), 354–360. https://doi.org/10.1097/NCQ.0000000000000312.

Ganz, F. D., Wagner, N., & Toren, O. (2015). Nurse middle manager ethical dilemmas and moral distress. *Nursing Ethics, 22*, 43–51. https://doi.org/10.1177/0969733013515490.

Garcia-Sierra, R., & Fernández-Castro, J. (2018). Relationships between leadership, structural empowerment, and engagement in nurses. *Journal of Advanced Nursing, 74*(12), 2809–2819. https://doi.org/10.1111/jan.13805.

Gray, J., & Kerfoot, K. (2016). Expanding the parameters for excellence in patient assignments: Is leveraging an evidence-data-based acuity methodology realistic. *Nursing Administration Quarterly, 40*(1), 7–13. https://doi.org/10.1097/NAQ.0000000000000138.

Gummesson, C., Sundén, A., & Fex, A. (2018). Clinical reasoning as a conceptual framework for interprofessional learning: A literature review and case study. *Physical Therapy Review, 23*(1), 29–34.

Guo, K. L. (2008). DECIDE: A decision-making model for more effective decision making by healthcare managers. *The Health Care Manager, 27*, 118–127.

Harvey, C. L., Thompson, S., Willis, E., Meyer, E., & Pearson, M. (2018). Understanding how nurses ration care. *Journal of Health Organization and Management, 32*(3), 494–510. https://doi.org/10.1108/JHOM-09-2017-0248.

Hasanpoor, E., Belete, Y. S., Janati, A., Hajebrahimi, S., & Haghgoshayie, E. (2019). Nursing managers' perspectives on the facilitators and barriers to implementation of evidence-based management. *Worldviews on Evidence-Based Nursing, 16*(4), 255–262. https://doi.org/10.1111/wvn.12372.

Improta, G., Cesarelli, M., Montouri, P., Santillo, L. C., & Triassi, M. (2018). Reducing the risk of healthcare-associated infections through Lean Six Sigma: The case of the medicine areas at the Federico II University Hospital in Naples (Italy). *Journal of Evaluation in Clinical Practice, 24*(2), 338–346. https://doi.org/10.1111/jep.12844.

Institute for Healthcare Improvement. (n.d.). QI essentials toolkit: PDSA worksheet. http://www.ihi.org/resources/Pages/Tools/Quality-Improvement-Essentials-Toolkit.aspx.

Institute of Medicine (IOM). (1999). *To err is human: Building a safer health system*. Washington, DC: National Academies Press.

Institute of Medicine (IOM). (2011). *The future of nursing: Leading change, advancing health*. Washington, DC: National Academies Press.

Interprofessional Education Collaborative. (2016). *Core competencies for interprofessional collaborative practice 2016 update*. https://nebula.wsimg.com/2f68a39520b03336b41038c370497473?AccessKeyId=DC06780E69ED19E2B3A5&disposition=0&alloworigin=1.

Jansson, I., & Forsberg, A. (2016). How do nurses and ward managers perceive that evidence-based sources are obtained to inform relevant nursing interventions? An exploratory study. *Journal of Clinical Nursing, 25*, 769–776. https://doi.org/10.1111/jocn.13095.

Johansen, M. L., & O'Brien, J. L. (2016). Decision making in nursing practice: A concept analysis. *Nursing Forum, 51*(1), 40–48. https://doi.org/10.1111/nuf.12119.

Junious, D. L. (2020). Collaborative simulation training strategies used to teach root cause analysis leadership competencies. *Nursing Education Perspectives, 41*(1), 57–58. https://doi.org/10.1097/01.NEP.0000000000000404.

Karlsson, A., Lindeborg, P., Gunningberg, L., & Jangland, E. (2019). Evidence-based-nursing: How is it understood by bedside nurses? A phenomenographic study in surgical settings. *Journal of Nursing Management, 27*(6), 1216–1223. https://doi.org/10.1111/jonm.12802.

Keers, R. N., Plácido, M., Bennett, K., Clayton, K., Brown, P., & Ashcroft, D. M. (2018). What causes medication administration errors in a mental health hospital? A qualitative study with nursing staff. *PLOS ONE, 13*(10), Article e0206233. https://doi.org/10.1371/journal.pone.0206233.

Kowalski, M. O., Basile, C., Bersick, E., Cole, D. A., McClure, D.E., & Weaver, S. H. (2020). What do nurses need to practice effectively in a hospital environment? An integrative review with implications for nurse leaders. https://doi.org/10.1111/wvn.12401.

Kramer, M., Maguire, P., Halfer, D., Budin, W. C., Hall, D. S., Goodloe, L., et al. (2012). The organizational transformative power of nurse residency programs. *Nursing Administration Quarterly, 36*, 155–168. https://doi.org/10.1097/naq.0b013e318249fdaa.

Krishnan, P. (2018). A philosophical analysis of clinical decision making in nursing. *Journal of Nursing Education, 57*(2), 73–78. https://doi.org/10.3928/01484834-20180123-03.

Loresto, F. L., Welton, J., Grim, St., Valdez, C., & Eron, K. (2019). Exploring inpatient medication patterns. A big data and multilevel approach. *Journal of Nursing Administration, 49*(6), 336–342. https://doi.org/10.1097/NNA.0000000000000762.

Makary, M. A., & Daniel, M. (2016). Medical error-the third leading cause of death in the US. *BMJ, 353*. https://doi.org/10:1136/bmj.i2139.

Martinez, K., Borycki, E., & Courtney, K. L. (2017). Bring your own device and nurse managers' decision making. *CIN: Computers, Informatics, Nursing, 35*(2), 69–76. https://doi.org/10.1097/CIN.0000000000000286.

Massarweh, L. J., Tidyman, T., & Luu, D. H. (2017). Starting the shift out right: The electronic eAssignment sheet using clinical decision support in a quality improvement project. *Nursing Economic$, 35*(4), 194–200.

Mazer, B. L., & Nabhan, C. (2019). Strengthening the medical error "meme" pool. *Journal General Internal Medicine, 34*(10), 2264–2267. https://doi.org/10.1007/s11606-019-05156-7.

Medeiros, M. (2018). Shared governance councils: 10 essential actions for nurse leaders. *Nursing management, 49*(7), 12–13. https://doi.org/10.1097/01.NUMA.0000538920.83653.9b.

Moon, S. E., Van Dam, P. J., & Kitsos, A. (2019). *Healthcare, 7*(4), 132. https://doi.org/10.3390/healthcare7040132.

Morrison, J. (2016). Nursing leadership in ACO payment reform. *Nursing Economic$, 34*(5), 230–235.

Murphy, L. S., Wilson, M. L., & Newhouse, R. P. (2013). Data analytics: Making the most of input with strategic output. *Journal of Nursing Administration, 43*, 367–370. https://doi.org/10.1097/NNA.0b013e31829d60c7.

National Council of State Boards of Nursing. (2019). The clinical judgment and task model. https://www.ncsbn.org/NGN_Spring19_Eng_04_Final.pdf.

Nibbelink, C. W., & Brewer, B. B. (2018). Decision-making in nursing practice: An integrative literature review. *Journal of Clinical Nursing, 27*(5-6), 917–928. https://doi.org/10.1111/jocn.14151.

Nurses on Boards Coalition. (2020). About. https://www.nursesonboardscoalition.org/about/.

Orique, S. B., & Phillips, L. J. (2018). The effectiveness of simulation on recognizing and managing clinical deterioration: Meta-analysis. *Western Journal of Nursing Research, 40*(4), 582–609. https://doi.org/10.1177/0193945917697224.

Patient Protection and Affordable Care Act 42 U.S.C. 300gg–11. (2010). https://www.hhs.gov/sites/default/files/ppacacon.pdf.

Peltonen, L. M., Junttila, K., & Salantera, S. (2018). Nursing leaders' satisfaction with information systems in the day-to-day operations management in hospital units. *Studies in Health Technology & Informatics, 250*, 203–207. https://doi.org/10.3233/978-1-61499-872-3-203.

Peltonen, L. M., Sirrala, E., Juntilla, K, Lundgrén-Laine, H., Vahlberg, T, Löyttyniemi, E., Aantaa, R., & Salantera, S. (2019). Information needs in a day-to-day operations management in hospital units: A cross-sectional national survey. *Journal of Nursing Management, 27*(2), 233–244. https://doi.org/10.1111/jonm.12700.

Polancich, S., Williamson, J., Selleck, C. S., Talley, M., Frank, J., White-Williams, C., & Shirey, M. (2017). *Journal for Healthcare Quality, 39*(6), 391–396. https://doi.org/10.1097/JHQ.0000000000000112.

Porter-O'Grady, T. (2015). Through the looking glass: Predictive and adaptive capacity in a time of great change. *Nursing Management, 46*(6), 22–29. https://doi.org/10.1097/01.NUMA.0000465397.67041.bc.

Quality and Safety Education for Nurses (QSEN). (2020). QSEN Competencies. https://qsen.org/competencies/pre-licensure-ksas/.

Razieh, S., Somayeh, G., & Fariba, H. (2018). Effects of reflection on clinical decision-making of intensive care unit nurses. *Nurse Education Today, 66*, 10–14. https://doi.org/10.1016/j.nedt.2018.03.009.

Reed, C. C., Minnick, A. F., & Dietrich, M. S. (2018). Nurses' responses to interruptions during medication tasks: A time and motion study. *International Journal of Nursing Studies, 82*, 113–120. https://doi.org/10.1016/j.ijnurstu.2018.03.017.

Roshanzadeh, M., Vanaki, Z., & Sadooghiasi, A. (2019). Sensitivity in ethical decision-making: The experiences of nurse managers. *Nursing Ethics, 27*(5), 1174–1186. https://doi.org/10.1177/0969733019864146.

Sherman, R. O. (2015). How to avoid biased thinking. *American Nurse Today, 10*(3), 12–14.

Shirey, M. R., Ebright, P. R., & McDaniel, A. M. (2013). Nurse manager cognitive decision-making amidst stress and work complexity. *Journal of Nursing Management, 21*, 17–30. https://doi.org/10.1111/j.1365-2834.2012.01380.x.

Spiers, J. A., Lo, E., Hofmeyer, A., & Cummings, G. G. (2016). Nurse leaders' perceptions of influence of organizational restructuring on evidence-informed decision-making. *Nursing Leadership, 29*(2), 64–81. https://doi.org/10.12927/cjnl.2016.24805.

Stewart, K. R., & Hand, K. A. (2017). SBAR, communication, and patient safety: An integrated literature review. *MedSurg Nursing, 26*(5), 297–305.

Sveinsdóttir, H., Ragnarsdóttir, E. D., & Blöndal, K. (2016). Praise matters: The influence of nurse unit managers' praise on nurses' practice, work environment and job satisfaction: A questionnaire study. *Journal of Advanced Nursing, 72*, 558–568. https://doi.org/10.1111/jan.12849.

Tanner, C. A. (2006). Thinking like a nurse: A research-based model of clinical judgment in nursing. *Journal of Nursing Education, 45*, 204–211.

Thew, J. (2019, March). The Future of Nursing report: Where are we now?. *Health Leaders*. https://www.healthleadersmedia.com/nursing/future-nursing-report-where-are-we-now.

Thomson, C. L., Maskrey, N., & Vlaev, I. (2017). Making decisions better: An evaluation of an educational intervention. *Journal of Evaluation in Clinical Practice, 23*(2), 251–256. https://doi.org/10.1111/jep.12555.

Udon, S. A., Cummings, G., Care, W. D., & Jenkins, M. (2017). Impact of role stressors on the health of nurse managers. *Journal of Nursing Administration, 47*(3), 159–164. https://doi.org/10.1097/NNA.0000000000000459.

Weidema, F. C., Molewijk, A. C., Kamsteeg, F., & Widdershoven, G. A. M. (2015). Managers' views on and experiences with moral case deliberation in nursing teams. *Journal of Nursing Management, 23*(8), 1067–1075.

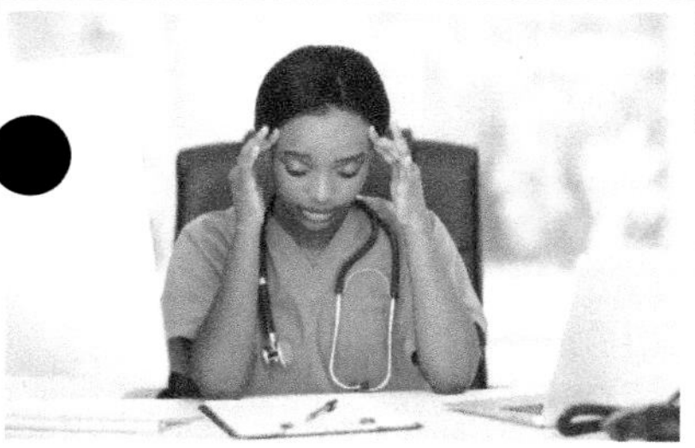

5

Managing Time and Stress

Susan R. Lacey, Debra V. Craighead

http://evolve.elsevier.com/Huber/leadership

The latest, most comprehensive study of workplace stress calculated that workplace stress, direct and indirect, costs organizations and businesses $300 billion per year in absenteeism, turnover, decreased productivity, and medical and legal fees (Rosch, 2001). Moreover, the Centers for Disease Control and Prevention (CDC, n.d.) estimated that stress is a leading workplace health problem surpassing physical inactivity and obesity. Clearly, workplace stress is a phenomenon that cannot be overlooked.

Stress can manifest as either negative or positive. There are physical, mental, and even professional benefits to good stress (eustress) (Nelson & Simmons, 2004). Good stress provides a feeling of accomplishment, but stressful experiences perceived as negative result in a variety of conscious or subconscious responses to regain stability or homeostasis (Seyle, 1950). The nature of these responses may be physical, mental, psychological, spiritual, or any combination of these. If these responses fail to achieve homeostasis, an individual's resources are depleted, which can threaten general well-being in an acute or chronic way. The warning signs of excessive workplace stress include feeling anxious; being irritable, depressed, or apathetic; or having sleeping problems, social isolation, and use of alcohol or drugs to cope (Segal et al., 2019). Long-term effects of stress may contribute to the development of chronic illnesses such as heart disease, high blood pressure, diabetes, depression, and anxiety (US Department of Health and Human Services National Institute of Mental Health [NIMH], n.d.).

The negative consequences of stress for individuals, organizations, society, and the economy are well documented (American Institute of Stress [AIS], n.d.). Work-related stress has been called the 21st Century Black Death (Lundberg & Cooper, 2011). In addition, work-related stress affects productivity and effectiveness at work, but it also may negatively affect personal lives and relationships (Rosch, 2001).

Joel Goh and colleagues reviewed more than 200 studies on workplace stress. They found that in some cases workplace stress raises the risk of illness and morbidity more than secondhand smoke (Goh et al., 2015). In addition, they calculated the cost of workplace stress as in excess of $190 billion, with 120,000 annual deaths.

COMPONENTS OF WORKPLACE STRESS

According to the World Health Organization (WHO), work-related stress has two key components: the content and context of work (WHO, 2010). Work content includes workload, work pace, and working hours. Context includes status and pay, role in the organization, and interpersonal work relationships. The content and context of work is perceived on the continuum of positive or negative. Central to this thesis is who is in control of these key components. The further away from control a person is from the context and content of work, the more problematic and stressful work can become. Thus, negative perceptions and lack of control translate into harmful job-related stress.

An article in *The Atlantic* provided a window into the impact and consequences of stress in relation to cost and personal health. The effects of stress are estimated to cost $180 billion or 5% to 8% of annual health care expenditures (White, 2015). Stress:

1. Increases the incidence of chronic and costly conditions, such as diabetes, Alzheimer's, and cardiovascular disease.
2. Increases addiction and mental health conditions associated with job insecurity, unjust dealings with employees, or poor leadership decisions that influence the working conditions of employees.
3. Is linked to over 120,000 deaths per year in the United States from physical and mental health conditions.

Governmental and organizational reports about work-related stress most often reference the work of Paul Rosch, MD, FACP, a leader in the field of occupational stress, specifically, his publication *The quandary of job stress compensation* (Rosch, 2001). Rosch calculated the combined direct and indirect cost of work-related stress to be a staggering $300 billion per year. Although the article is considered dated by academic standards, it remains the most widely referenced publication in support of national discourse, research, and large-scale planning in the area of work-related stress.

DEFINITIONS

Stress is defined as a negative emotional experience associated with biological changes that trigger the body to make adaptations (Rosenthal, 2002). This means stress can be a physical, mental, psychological, or spiritual response to a stressor experience that is evaluated by the individual as taxing or exceeding resources and threatening to one's sense of well-being. Furthermore, chronic stress can lead to acute and chronic health problems.

Job Stress

A seminal report by the National Institute of Occupational Safety and Health (NIOSH) defined job stress as the harmful physical and emotional responses that occur when the requirements of the job do not match the capabilities, resources, or needs of the worker. Job stress can lead to poor health and even injury (NIOSH, 1999).

Time Management

Time management is a deliberative process of identifying and focusing on the activities needed to accomplish tasks and goals in the time available. Since individuals cannot control time, they must learn to manage the available time more efficiently and effectively. This may be difficult, especially when behavior must be changed. At its core, time management is self-management.

BACKGROUND

The Relationship Between Time and Stress in the Health Care Setting

Situational stress and the need to respond in a timely manner are true for most types of work, and particularly in health care. Clinicians and leaders anticipate and even prepare for stressful situations. Time-sensitive care and decision-making may produce mild to severe stress. As if time sensitivity for single events were not stressful enough, it is typically compounded by multiple stressful events that occur at or near the same time. For example, there are specific times designated for medication administration, tests, and procedures, which may be interrupted by unplanned events with patients and/or families. Furthermore, if a clinician fails to complete the treatments or therapies within a defined window of time, a cascade of events may follow, from submitting an incident or variance report to patient harm. In life-threatening emergencies, response time is even more critical. Ineffective or inaccurate interventions may result in lasting consequences for patients—or even death.

The delivery of health care exists in an environment where time is finite and most often related to shift work. Nurses work shifts of time, such as 8- or 12-hour shifts. If time (a shift) is finite, the nurse must make accurate estimates of the amount of time each patient encounter will consume during that shift based on what needs to be done during each encounter.

During real or anticipated budgetary constraints, many organizations seek to reduce labor costs. Because labor expenditures are greatest within nursing, reducing the number of staff nurses on a unit is one strategy to improve the bottom line. However, there is also a need to increase reimbursement for good clinical outcomes and positive patient experiences, and this requires the presence of adequate numbers of nurses to deliver needed care.

The Centers for Medicare and Medicaid Services (CMS), the nation's largest payer, bases 30% of reimbursement on the patient experience and 70% on clinical outcomes (CMS, 2014). If the number of nurses is reduced on a given unit or shift, good outcomes may be compromised, and therefore reimbursement may be compromised. For instance, if normal nurse-to-patient ratios are modified from 1:5 to 1:7 without additional unlicensed assistive support, the time spent on patient encounters will naturally have to be decreased and the availability of nurses will be diminished. Chronic cycles of suboptimal staffing create stress and fatigue.

Evidence has linked lower patient-to-nurse ratios with better outcomes (Aiken et al., 2002). Many believe current staffing models are incongruent with professional practice standards, patient needs, and the organization's ability to maximize reimbursement. This perpetual grind makes it difficult for staff nurses to feel good about nursing or encourage others to join the profession. Many nurses have buyer's remorse for choosing nursing as their career, even more so compared with nurse practitioners and physicians (Peckham, 2015).

Lifecycle: Timing and Stress

"They say timing is everything. But then they say, there is never a perfect time for anything."

Anthony Liccioni (n.d.), poet, author

In life, we all routinely experience change. For generations, the timing of life events has created stress, both anticipated and unexpected. Plans for the work shift or for the future may change abruptly. Acknowledging that these changes are inevitable, and preparing for their occurrence, may make the difference between thriving and struggling to survive.

Timing affects our willingness to seek career advancement. This is often due to the time involved in developing a new work-related skillset. Nurses can prepare for career advancement by knowing about the task expectations involved when moving into new career roles. Sherman and Cohn (2019) examined the role timing plays in life and at work, and noted that demanding careers, coupled with a stressful life event such as caregiving, are common among nurses. Female nurses often feel unrelenting pressure to manage work and caregiving roles effortlessly. Recommended strategies to embrace in order to thrive during hectic life events include balancing life and career ambitions, self-advocacy, leveraging personal strengths, and co-creating work schedules (Sherman & Cohn, 2019).

We all work in a rhythm set by our unique biological clock. In his book *When: The secret to perfect timing*, author Daniel Pink (2018) asserted that timing is a science that can be studied and used to our benefit. He shared that productivity enhancement occurs when we recognize that 80% of us navigate each day in three predictable stages: peak, trough, and recovery. In the peak stage, we can concentrate deeply; in trough stage, we can accomplish routine tasks; and during the recovery stage we relax and therefore gain insight into the problems we face. Night owls move through these stages in the opposite order (recovery, trough, peak). Since our work tasks can be categorized as requiring either an insightful (awareness or creativity) or analytical (deliberate, attention to detail) type of focus, the time of the day chosen to complete a task can affect performance by up to 20% (Pink, 2018).

TIME MANAGEMENT STRATEGIES FOR NURSE LEADERS

Nurse leaders are expected to manage time effectively. The following time management strategies are useful and applicable in any work setting (Chutna & Boothby, 2017). Perform a time audit self-assessment to discover how you are spending your time and how to use small time increments effectively. Do tasks that prepare you in advance of the next workday. Engage in projects that require attention to detail while at your peak and save routine tasks (like answering e-mail) for a trough period. Convene meetings only when necessary, share the agenda in advance, and provide pre-meeting assignments. Moreover, nurse leaders need to model self-care because this augments time management and allows for recovery and rejuvenation (Chutna & Boothby, 2017).

Nurses are required to use time wisely due to facing new challenges hourly. We race to deliver patient-centered care and then chart care completion. Nurses often view time as an unforgiving foe; however, we can learn strategies to get the job done efficiently and effectively (Templeman, 2018). These strategies include cognitive stacking, prioritizing tasks, routinization, and time audits. Box 5.1 contains suggested time-saving strategies for nurses and nurse leaders.

BOX 5.1 Time-Saving Strategies for Nurses and Nurse Leaders

Strategy	Methods
Cognitive stacking	Mental list E-list
Prioritization	CURE: Critical, Urgent, Routine, and Extra Maslow's Hierarchy of Needs ABCs: airway, breathing, circulation
Routinization	Sequence activities and establish a time-frame expectation for routine task
Time audit	Track your time for 24 hours over 1–2 weeks; identify small time gaps (5–10 minutes) where small tasks may be completed

Cognitive stacking (creating mental, electronic, physical lists) is useful to plan the day before starting work. A list of what you need to accomplish should include what routinely needs to be completed on your shift. Prioritize tasks as appropriate using the CURE acronym, which stands for Critical, Urgent, Routine, and Extras. Other nursing prioritization frameworks include ABCs (airway, breathing, and circulation), Maslow's Hierarchy of Needs, and time-sensitive/safety indicators relevant to the care setting (Jesse, 2019). Establish a routine or routinization of work tasks and repeat what works best. Consistency in work routine aids time management (Templeman, 2018). Discover what works for you and use it to configure your daily work routine.

RESILIENCE

Countering the negative aspects of workplace stress is the concept of resilience. Resilience is defined as an ability to bounce back. Resilient people exhibit personal characteristics of an internal locus of control, prosocial behavior, empathy, positive self-image, a sense of optimism, and an ability to organize daily responsibilities (Pines et al., 2012). Several additional factors are associated with resilience, including:

- The capacity to make realistic plans and take steps to carry them out.
- A positive view of yourself and confidence in your strengths and abilities.
- Skills in communication and problem solving.
- The capacity to manage strong feelings and impulses. Empowered people are thought to be more resilient, and for nurses there is an association between stress resiliency and psychological empowerment. Because the behavioral skills needed to manage interpersonal conflict and its feelings of powerlessness and psychological distress can be taught, nurses can learn to resist stressors, manage conflict, and boost resilience (Pines et al., 2012).

Resilience is not a trait that people either have or do not have. It involves behaviors, thoughts, and actions that can be learned and developed by anyone. Today's nurse leader is required to be resilience competent in order to model and assist employees with developing this skill (Bernard, 2019). Nurse leaders model and support resilience development when they promote quality sleep, decompression from work, and assist staff with navigating ethically challenging situations (Bernard, 2019). The *Resilience and professional joy: A toolkit for nurse leaders* contains numerous evidence-based approaches useful for building resilient teams, leaders, organizations, and student nurses (Bernard, 2019).

LEADERSHIP AND MANAGEMENT IMPLICATIONS

Creating an Environment to Prevent and Address Work-Related Stress

To prevent and address work-related stress, creation and innovation are needed. A creation is something new that did not previously exist in that form and occurs in a multitude of fields, not just the arts (Merriam-Webster, n.d.a). Experts who study creativity may differ on the requisite attributes of creative individuals and exact steps in the creative process. However, most agree that intention is the critical first step (Ditkoff, 2010). Without intention, no action is ever taken.

Innovation and innovators in the health care industry are highly sought after, but to innovate is to alter, change, or transform something that exists in a stable system (Marshall, 2013). On the other hand, creativity is less frequently discussed in the industry, and in some cases, is maligned. For example, the term creative accounting is used to describe illegal or unethical activities and does not convey the positive aspect of creativity, which is to produce something needed or valued. Industry leaders prefer to predict the future based on the past and innovate within the current system as opposed to envisioning the future based on what is desired and creating it (Scott, 2003). The former is thought to use hard data, and the latter, subjective or unknown information, inspiration, and feelings. Creativity does not require one to suspend all intellect. Indeed, creative individuals use all of the senses, as well as abstract and concrete thought. Without concrete and abstract thought, it would have been impossible for Salvador Dalí to have painted *The persistence of memory*, or for British scientist Sir Tim Berners-Lee to have written code for the first web browser, which became the genesis of the world wide web (World Wide Web Foundation, 2015).

Getting Started

It is challenging to envision creating a health care organization focused not only on addressing work-related stress when it occurs but also on having structures and processes in place to prevent them from happening in the first place. This is particularly hard while in the midst of persistent demands from payers, consumers, regulators, and even the overarching uncertainty of the Affordable Care Act of 2010 (ACA) mandates. It has always been challenging to secure the necessary resources for prevention, even for patient care. However, failure to do so puts employees at risk, which in turn can jeopardize the lives of patients. It is no longer possible to wait for more evidence about the human and financial costs of work-related stress. Waiting for more stability in the industry, which may never come, wastes precious time. Once that is embraced and there is genuine intention, then design and creation can begin in earnest. This intention and corresponding action will call for bold leaders who reject reactionary quick fixes. Based on the evidence, this can lead to the interconnected outcomes of employees with greater resilience and performance, improved patient outcomes, and measurable and sustained financial benefits.

Strategies

Stress management. Stress management is important for nurses as they cope with stress at work. This is also true for nursing students and new nurses. Among the many stressors are needing to meet professional and academic demands, fear of failure, the workload of taking care of patients, and insecurity about clinical competence or lack of knowledge. Stress and anxiety are often high during times of education and training when the nurse or student is developing clinical skills. Two low-cost and easily implemented stress-management techniques are mindful meditation and biofeedback. Both were found to decrease anxiety, and mindfulness also significantly lowered stress levels in nursing students (Nowrouzi et al., 2015; Ratanasiripong et al., 2015).

Workplace intervention strategies for stress can be either individual-level stress management and burnout interventions or organizational-level workplace health-promotion programs. For the individual nurse, mindfulness-based stress reduction has evidence of effectiveness; for mental health, psychosocial interventions decrease burnout (Nowrouzi et al., 2015). The Research Note and Box 5.2 also provide some guidance on stress management for individuals suggested by the American Psychological Association (2018) and the CDC (n.d.).

Organization-directed prevention measures can be directed to management style, incentives and career structures, educational opportunities, salaries, and recruitment and retention practices (Nowrouzi et al., 2015). Research on conflict management styles found that nurses who worked in supportive work environments and who avoided conflict (avoidant style of managing conflict) experienced less work stress (Johansen & Cadmus, 2016). In addition, conflict and communicative stress feed off each other in a cycle that contributes to destructive working conditions. Nurses manage conflict and stress through respectful and caring communication and mismanage it through disrespectful communication. Building relationships can be fostered in organizations by formal and informal social gatherings, mentoring, social media, and deliberate culture creation (Moreland & Apker, 2016). Perceived supportive work environments are characterized by perceptions that supervisors are supportive, there is fairness, and there is open communication. Stress is reduced when nurses feel that win–win solutions occur in the work environment (Johansen & Cadmus, 2016).

One example is the implementation of new nurse residency programs. In response to the stress and anxiety ("transition shock") that new nurses feel in the transition from nursing education to nursing practice, organizations are instituting nurse residency programs.

BOX 5.2 Individual Strategies to Manage Stress

American Psychological Association (2018)	Centers for Disease Control and Prevention (n.d.)
• Journaling to track your stressors: record your thoughts and feelings and your reaction to stressful events.	• Reflect on positive experiences and express gratitude.
• Develop healthy responses to stress such as exercise, hobbies, pleasurable activities, adequate sleep.	• Participate in employer-sponsored programs/activities that target healthy lifestyle behaviors.
• Set boundaries by maintaining periods when you are not working or thinking about work (unplug from work e-mail in the evening and on days off).	• Adopt behaviors that promote stress management such as yoga, meditation, mindfulness.
• Take time away to recharge.	• Eat healthy meals, exercise, and get enough sleep.
• Learn relaxation techniques such as meditation, deep breathing, mindfulness (psychological state of moment-to-moment awareness of your current state without feeling inward judgement about your situation.	• Look for satisfaction and meaning in your work.
• Cultivate a social support system including family, friends, co-workers.	• Serve as wellness champion and participate in trainings.

They may be up to a year long. New nurses are mentored and guided during this residency in order to support their coping, reduce their stress, and augment their time-management capabilities. This is a major recruitment and retention strategy. In addition, it is a visible component of a supportive work environment (Rosenfeld & Glassman, 2016; Rush et al., 2013).

Informal nurse leaders can employ a combination of person-directed stress management techniques (for themselves) and organization-directed stress management techniques (for the sake of the work group). Clearly, a supportive work environment is critical, so any interventions that improve nurses' perceptions of the work environment are helpful. Role modeling and setting a tone of respectful and caring communication aids conflict resolution and stress reduction. Informal leaders can take the initiative to address workplace issues in a proactive and evidence-based manner so that nurses see that their issues are being evaluated fully and fairly for problem resolution.

Wellness programs in the larger context. There are a variety of strategies that individuals and organizations need to employ to prevent and address work-related stress. There is no shortage of research, workshops, websites, and blogs about how to reduce stress. Although sources may emphasize the benefits of one strategy over another, most include similar recommendations. Using these strategies can serve as the inspiration for creating this new, vital environment. Instead of employees trying to find their own way through the maze of strategies, the newly created health care environment would provide on-site (or reimbursement for) work-related stress prevention workshops and retreats. Just as the traditional employee health staff conduct new and ongoing physical health screening for risky behaviors such as smoking or substance use, additional screening for resiliency, coping strategies, and support networks needs to be a part of the work structure. Once screened and a profile developed, the employee can use the information to select from wellness options beyond smoking cessation, hypertension, and diabetes management programs in consultation with a wellness professional.

It is common practice to compensate employees who take advantage of preventive health care services. There are some organizations that pay for alternative health care, such as gym memberships, massage, and acupuncture, but that is not the norm. Given the costs of work-related stress, the health care environment of the future will provide full or partial compensation for a much wider array of prevention services that fit the needs of the individual employee. As personalized medicine forges a pathway to realize the potential of matching therapies to an individual's DNA for disease states, wellness offerings should match the employee's needs for work–life balance and prevention of work-related stress. Examples of wellness initiatives and programs might be offered in multiple formats, but could include self-care, setting boundaries, relaxation, and journaling.

Self-care. One of the most important strategies to mitigate individual stress is self-care. Though everyone needs to spend time on themselves, clinicians often put the needs of others ahead of their own. It is difficult to effectively care for patients and their families or be productive at work if clinicians and leaders do not care for themselves. Self-care is unique to each person, but the following are generally accepted as important self-care activities (Fischer & Keenan, 2010): taking personal time each day, getting enough sleep (7–8 hours), nutritious intake and adequate hydration, some form of exercise, and a strong support network, which includes friends, family, and counseling, if necessary. Box 5.2 displays personal strategies for decreasing stress at the workplace.

Setting boundaries. Setting boundaries is one way of engaging in self-care (Gionta, 2009). Family members and even friends faced with a health care question, concern, or crisis call on nurses and other clinicians to provide advice, and in some cases, direct care. To respond and be helpful, clinicians may overextend themselves, sacrificing their own needs or those of their direct family members. In some ways, it is flattering. It validates one's knowledge, skills, and expertise. However, when requests exceed a person's capabilities, it is reasonable to refer them to other experts and services.

Boundaries need not be exceedingly rigid and may change over time. For instance, someone who does not have a husband, wife, partner, or children may seem to have the capacity to take on extra work and may need to set more boundaries than those who have these commitments to others. Clearly, boundaries should be set based on individual needs, not gender, stereotypes, or even where someone is on the lifespan. The most important thing is that setting them should not induce more stress on the individual than not having them at all.

Relaxation. Finding ways to relax can also help one avoid and reduce stress. Because stress can produce both emotional and physical responses, it is important to learn to relax the body and mind, even for short periods. There are numerous relaxation techniques and even apps to download to help a person relax. It is not necessary to devote long periods or find a special environment to achieve a state of relaxation. One can relax anywhere and for any amount of time (Seaward, 2013). By calming the mind, physiological responses to stress are also reversed, which allows the individual to think more clearly.

Journaling. Keeping a diary or journal was a part of many individuals' lives when they were younger, but most do not continue the practice into adulthood. There are many benefits in keeping a journal. For those who recognize they are experiencing stress but are not fully cognizant of the specific triggers, experts suggest keeping a journal to identify situations that cause stress, the response or action to the stressor, and whether these actions lowered their stress or not (Ullrich & Lutgendorf, 2002).

The work of clinicians and leaders in health care is time sensitive, and time management is, for all intents and purposes, personal management. Journaling about situations that challenge personal time management will provide clarity. This clarity may shed light on learned behaviors that may be sabotaging one's quest for effective time management. Saunders (2013), an international expert and coach in the area of time management, outlined and described secrets to effective time investment. They are priorities, expectations, and routines. Fully understanding these three things can unlock the potential to manage even the most chaotic situation, regardless of the context, at work or home.

Organizational Recommendations

Clearly, organizations are experiencing financial pressures, which make adding the necessary work required to create a new environment that prevents and addresses work-related stress a challenge. However, either way, employees will experience work-related stress, which will negatively affect the organization in one way or another. Therefore, it is a matter of which approach (proactive or reactive) an organization wants to take, either being up front with prevention and early intervention or after the fact with employee loss of productivity, increased sick days, and/or turnover. If an organization chooses the proactive approach, beginning the work to create this environment does not seem as daunting and is a prudent business decision. Box 5.3 displays a list of institutional strategies to decrease stress in the workplace, suggested by Segal et al. (2019). This is not an exhaustive list, nor is it intended to be prescriptive. Instead, it is meant to

BOX 5.3 Institutional Strategies to Decrease Stress at the Workplace

- Assess stress levels and stress-management strategies of employees.
- Institute the AACN Standards for Establishing and Sustaining Healthy Work Environments.
- Ensure that management and leadership education include vital behaviors and competencies.
- Structure evaluations of managers, directors, supervisors, and senior-level management to evaluate leadership and management actions to provide stress management strategies.
- Ensure transparency of information and set effective communication patterns.
- Implement a top-down approach to sharing and owning quality improvement and outcomes.

generate discussions while this new environment is planned. Related evidence-based management strategies to address work-related stress include healthy work environment standards and empowerment strategies.

Healthy Work Environments Standards. A healthy work environment (HWE) is one that is safe, empowering, and satisfying. HWE standards are further discussed in Chapter 3. The American Association of Critical-Care Nurses (AACN) has established six standards that support healthy work environments (AACN, 2005). Although developed for nurses, they are applicable for all types of employees. Emerging research supports the positive effect of these standards to enhance critical-care nurses' work environments (Ulrich et al., 2019). These standards and supporting statements are displayed in Table 5.1.

Empowerment. Employees who are empowered in their jobs are also more engaged and satisfied. Research indicates that structural empowerment leads to higher productivity and satisfaction for the employee, which translates to more satisfied customers. Customer satisfaction stems from the empowered employee's ability to correct a problem at the time it occurs. This leads to better fiscal health for the organization in both direct and indirect labor and benefit costs (Woods, 2005). Empowerment for nurses is manifested in shared governance structures where nurses are engaged and participate in solving clinical practice issues. Shared governance structures are a hallmark of the Magnet Recognition Program®. There is a growing body of evidence that links Magnet hospitals to better clinical and patient level outcomes, as well as to better nursing outcomes (e.g., lower turnover and higher satisfaction), compared with non-Magnet hospitals (Aiken et al., 2008). Improved clinical and organizational outcomes translate to improved financial health.

Clinicians are also empowered by gaining new knowledge and skills beyond required clinical competence. In addition, if these new skills also allow them to be a part of developing solutions to clinical and organizational problems, this can lead to even greater engagement and satisfaction. For example, the Clinical Scene Investigator Academy is currently administered by

TABLE 5.1 AACN Standards for Establishing and Sustaining Healthy Work Environments

Standard	Statement
Skilled communication	Nurses must be as proficient in communication skills as they are in clinical skills.
True collaboration	Nurses must be relentless in pursuing and fostering true collaboration.
Effective decision-making	Nurses must be valued and committed partners in making policy, directing and evaluating clinical care, and leading organizational operations.
Appropriate staffing	Staffing must ensure the effective match between patient needs and nurse competencies.
Meaningful recognition	Nurses must be recognized and must recognize others for the value each brings to the work of the organization.
Authentic leadership	Nurse leaders must fully embrace the imperative of a healthy work environment, authentically live it, and engage others in its achievement.

American Association of Critical-Care Nurses (AACN). (2005). *AACN standards for establishing and sustaining healthy work environments: A journey to excellence.* Aliso Viejo, CA: AACN.

AACN (Lacey et al., 2012, 2017). This program teaches staff nurse teams skills in advanced leadership, quality improvement methods, project management, accurate data management, and how to translate nursing care into fiscal terms. To date, the national program has significantly improved nurse-sensitive outcomes, such as pressure ulcers, catheter-associated infections, ventilator-associated pneumonia, and patient satisfaction (Lacey et al., 2017).

Special Considerations for Nurse Managers

With any unit or department, workflow modifications creep into the manager's routines, creating chaos in a well-planned day. The unit manager has one of the most difficult jobs in meeting the challenges of managing and leading employees, as well as meeting priorities that flow from higher management. The challenge of meeting the expectations of the multiple roles of the nurse manager can produce stress that reveals itself as role strain, which is an unpleasant feeling of frustration and an intense labile emotional state (Richmond et al., 2009). This may lead to communication breakdowns, the sense of failing, and intense anxiety about job performance.

There is a scarcity of evidence about how stress affects the nurse manager role. However, Shirey et al. (2010) have provided a rich source of qualitative evidence about sources and factors related to stress, outcomes of this stress, and coping strategies used to decrease stress. In their study, nurse manager participants reported key sources of stress to include dealing with people (specifically related to people with negative attitudes or employees with subpar work performance); patient and family complaints; physician interactions; and working within the political nature of the hospital with a lack of transparency and collaboration. Staffing was noted as the most stressful part of their role. High stress is experienced by nurse managers and stems from the challenges of a multifaceted job with myriad sources of stress (Kath et al., 2012). Although there is a relationship between job satisfaction and intent to quit, when stress is high for nurse managers, other factors show strong relationships with stress (Kath et al., 2012). Having support from others (e.g., supervisors, co-managers, and co-workers) is a factor that decreases stress (Kath et al., 2012; Shirey et al., 2010). The amount of autonomy and predictability in the job mitigates the negative effects of stress as well (Kath et al., 2012).

There is nothing stopping us from creating this new environment that addresses work-related stress, except for the limits (real and imagined) placed on ourselves and organizations. It takes leadership and vision to see the business case for being proactive. Some of the most brilliant minds work in health care. Together nurses can build a preferred future state that results in managed stress and promotion of healthy work environments where all employees flourish.

CURRENT ISSUES AND TRENDS

Health care delivery environments are characterized by chaos, complexity, high risk, and high stress. This is not likely to change. Clinicians and leaders function in environments with increasing unknowns while trying to take appropriate daily actions as well as predict and plan for the future. This is a highly stressful situation. Individuals respond to unknowns in a fairly predictable pattern, which happens rapidly and primarily in one's subconscious. The process includes mentally triaging proven strategies used in similar situations, selecting and modifying the strategy, and evaluating the strategy in real time or as needed.

There is long-standing evidence that fear of the unknown is a normal part of human nature (Öhman, 2000). It is also known that fear is linked to the feeling of danger. A recently published study found that subjects presented with certain danger had significantly lower stress than subjects presented with potential danger (de Berker et al., 2016). In this study one group of participants, the certain danger group, was told when they picked up a rock a snake would be under it. The other group, the potential danger group, was told a snake may or may not be there. The researchers concluded that when participants knew something would occur ahead of time, they were able to mentally and physically prepare. In addition, physiological responses such as heart rate and breathing were significantly higher for participants in the potential danger group than those in the certain danger group.

Scientists in the field of psychology have studied a person's ability to predict or envision the future in normal and uncertain times. Noted psychologist Daniel Gilbert (2007) outlined his thesis in *Stumbling on happiness*, using scientific evidence coupled with analogies and real-world examples. What he and other social scientists found is that the need to control and predict the future is central to the human condition. It is part of what distinguishes us from other species. In addition, he offers compelling evidence that even those with a great deal of experience, expertise, and cultural wisdom find it difficult to accurately predict the future and make good choices when presented with new and uncertain situations. Specifically, prior experiences coupled with current realities do little to help accurately predict or envision the future, especially when the stakes are high. He extends the logic with additional evidence that in a person's struggle to gain control, make better predictions, and thus make effective plans and choices, individuals fill in details of missing information even if these details are inaccurate. As the brain is filling in inaccurate details from memories, perceptions, and emotions, it allows people to reweave the narrative to one they believe or want to be true.

The research supporting Gilbert's logic is applicable to the current health care industry. Clinicians and leaders make efforts to predict the future and make decisions based on their predictions. Unfortunately, just as Gilbert's work has proven, historical evidence supports the reweaving of narratives and undesirable outcomes. Organizations introduce new initiatives or cut services in response to expert predictions, only to realize when the future becomes the present that it looks nothing like the prediction, rendering the initiatives and related expenditures relatively useless.

An example of significant scale occurred in the 1980s. In response to payer demands, specifically the introduction of diagnosis-related groups (DRGs), reimbursements declined significantly (Fetter et al., 1980). Hospital leaders and external experts predicted vastly reduced margins, and experts recommended reducing expenditures as the best way to address the negative financial impact of DRGs. On face value, that was prudent, and a common business practice given the anticipated loss of revenue. They recommended consolidating organizations, reducing or eliminating services, and closing facilities, primarily within a defined geographical region. Nurse layoffs occurred. These recommendations led to a frenzy of mergers, acquisitions, and closings (Federal Antitrust Policy in the Health Care Marketplace, 1997). Some mergers created complicated partnerships. Many were ill conceived with little or no input from staff, referring physicians, or the communities served. Faith-based and secular hospitals merged, buildings were shuttered, and hybrid names and slogans emerged. Stark philosophical differences, disruption or elimination of services, and disgruntled staff and physicians made sustaining such mergers difficult. To make matters worse, loyal consumers of one hospital or another felt betrayed. It did not take long for many of these hospitals and systems to unmerge, costing even more money, all because experts inaccurately predicted the long-term consequences of this strategy. Some mergers did survive but rebuilding trust with providers and consumers took many years.

The current example is the odyssey surrounding the fate of the ACA, which has added formidable uncertainties not only for clinicians, leaders, organizations, and systems, but also for the industry's key drivers: payers, consumers, and regulators. The ACA passed along party lines and was signed into law on March 23, 2010 (US Department of Health and Human Services, 2014). Legal challenges were swift and aggressive. The Supreme Court upheld the constitutionality of the law, specifically the individual mandate, on June 28, 2012, after hearing arguments in the National Federation of Independent Business v. Sebelius case (Barnes, 2015). Nevertheless, challenges continue. These continued challenges create speculation regarding how decisions about the ACA will influence current external health care drivers and compound stress in the environment.

Even with the compelling evidence that we lack the ability to accurately predict the future, there is no evidence suggesting we cannot create our desired future. In fact, this advice is often suggested to nurses.

Predictions and Risk

A prediction is a statement or thought about a future event based on past experiences and knowledge (Merriam-Webster, n.d.b). Everyone makes predictions or forecasts about the future many times a day, most of which are made subconsciously. Some predictions involve low risk. Thus, an inaccurate prediction may cause a temporary inconvenience, but not stress. For example, a person driving to work who failed to listen to the current traffic report takes the regular route but is soon stuck for an hour behind an overturned vehicle.

Nurses make predictions in clinical practice based on assessment and clinical judgment. For example, a nurse may predict that following a standardized protocol will result in desired outcomes such as avoidance of catheter-associated urinary tract infections. If the protocol is evidence based, then prediction is low risk.

Other predictions would be considered high risk. If high-risk predictions are inaccurate, the consequences may cause intense stress, anxiety, depression, and even financial loss. Examples of personal situations that require high-risk predictions include choosing or leaving a job, selecting a partner, and buying or selling a large amount of company stock. Nurses are often faced with high-risk predictions in practice, and this is a source of work stress. For example, unstable patients, code situations, or rapid decompensation may result in the need for instant reactions and/or high-risk predictions about treatment.

One additional important aspect of making predictions is that predictions may affect others in positive or negative ways. When clinicians and leaders in health care initiate actions based on predictions, the actions often affect others in small and large ways. Clinicians make predictions every day based on tacit and empirical knowledge. Most would prefer using the term prognosis, not prediction, but they are similar. For example, a nurse predicts that if the patient has difficulty swallowing when provided a sip of water, then he may have difficulty eating solid food; recommendations and interventions occur based on this prediction. Likewise, when leaders make predictions and take subsequent actions about real or anticipated changes in demand from key drivers (e.g., payers, consumers, regulations, and the fate of the ACA), many people may be positive or negatively affected.

RESEARCH NOTE

Source

Chesak, S., Cutshall, S., Bowe, C., Montanari, K., & Bhagra, A. (2019). Stress management for nurses: Critical research review. *Journal of Holistic Nursing 17*(3), 288–295. https://doi.org/10.1177/0898010119842693.

Purpose

This systematic review examined current evidence on stress management interventions for nurses. The authors presented levels of evidence, findings, and instruments used to measure nurse stress.

Discussion

Evidence reviewed (n = 90) identified a wide variety of holistic interventions for nurse stress management. However, psychological skill training (coping, stress resilience, and cognitive behavioral therapy; n = 21) and mindfulness and meditation training (n = 24) were prevalent. Most interventions focused on handing individual stress, not workplace environmental stress. The authors identified a gap in the literature regarding system-level interventions. Randomized controlled trials are needed at the individual and system-level to add to the body of knowledge to support efficacious and cost-effective interventions.

Application to practice

This systematic review highlighted findings from evidence regarding stress management interventions for nurses. Holistic specialty nurses and the American Nurses Association have called for nurses to adopt self-care activities to promote personal health and well-being. Nurse leaders need to advocate for system-level interventions by demonstrating the significant return-on-investment to the organization.

NEXT-GENERATION NCLEX® EXAMINATION-STYLE CASE STUDY

Caitlin has been working on 2 North for 6 months since graduation from nursing school. Every day seems stressful, and every new situation makes her feel like she does not have what it takes to be a nurse. She often feels overwhelmed. There are very few senior experienced nurses on the unit, and they are burned out from constantly orienting new nurses. Productivity and effectiveness are low. Caitlin is concerned about her own coping yet also wants to build a higher functioning and more resilient team. There are lots of recommended stress reduction techniques. Key to success is choosing techniques that are practical and able to be accomplished by a busy nurse daily.

Choose the most likely options for the information missing from the question below by selecting from the list of options provided.

NEXT-GENERATION NCLEX® EXAMINATION-STYLE CASE STUDY—cont'd

Question

Caitlin spent two days observing the employees on the unit and noticed that they were always busy, skipped breaks and lunch, drank lots of coffee, and never had down time, confirming her personal perceptions. The top 3 strategies an employee may use while at work to relieve stress are:

1) ____________

2) ____________

3) ____________.

Options for Strategies

Getting a massage at the massage parlor 10 mts from work

Eat French fries

Drink 8 glasses of water a day

Taking scheduled lunches

Taking a long walk in nature

Taking yoga classes in your neighborhood

Eat at your desk

Use your getaway place

CRITICAL THINKING EXERCISE

Cindy and the unit council decide to explore strategies for stress reduction and resiliency in the document, *Resilience and professional joy: A toolkit for nurse leaders* (https://www.nurseleader.com/article/S1541-4612(18)30283-0/fulltext). They decide to select two interventions from Leading Self Individuals and Leading Teams for staff nurses and two strategies from Leader Leaders for the charge nurses.

1. What barriers should Cindy anticipate?
2. How should she address these barriers?
3. What should Cindy do first?
4. How should Cindy implement the interventions with the least impact on her unit budget?
5. Should Cindy engage staff and charge nurse champions to promote these interventions?
6. What factors should she continue to assess and analyze throughout the intervention phase?
7. How might Cindy use the $8000 for these efforts?

REFERENCES

Aiken, L. H., Clarke, S. P., Sloane, D. M., Lake, E. T., & Cheney, T. (2008). Effects of hospital care environment on patient mortality and nurse outcomes. *Journal of Nursing Administration, 38*(5), 223–229. https://doi.org/10.1097/01.NNA.0000312773.42352.d7.

Aiken, L. H., Clarke, S. P., Sloane, D. M., Sochalski, J., & Silber, J. H. (2002). Hospital nurse staffing and patient mortality, nurse burnout, and job dissatisfaction. *The Journal of the American Medical Association (JAMA), 288*(16), 1987–1993. https://doi.org/10.1001/jama.288.16.1987.

American Association of Critical-Care Nurses (AACN). (2005). *AACN standards for establishing and sustaining healthy work environments: A journey to excellence.* Aliso Viejo, CA: AACN.

American Institute of Stress (AIS). (n.d.). *Workplace stress.* http://www.stress.org/workplace-stress/.

American Psychological Association. (2018). *Coping with stress at work.* https://www.apa.org/helpcenter/work-stress.

Barnes, R. (2015, June 25). Affordable Care Act survives Supreme Court challenge. *Washington Post.* https://www.washingtonpost.com/politics/courts_law/obamacare-survives-supreme-court-challenge/2015/06/25/af87608e-188a-11e5-93b7-5eddc056ad8a_story.html.

Bernard, N. (2019). Resilience and professional joy: A toolkit for nurse leaders. *Nurse Leader, 17*(1), 43–48. https://doi.org/10.1016/j.mnl.2018.09.007.

Centers for Disease Control and Prevention (CDC). (n.d.). *Mental health in the workplace. Workplace health promotion.* https://www.cdc.gov/workplacehealthpromotion/tools-resources/pdfs/WHRC-Mental-Health-and-Stress-in-the-Workplac-Issue-Brief-H.pdf.

Centers for Medicare & Medicaid Services. (CMS). (2014). *HCAHPS: Patients' perspectives of care survey.* https://www.cms.gov/Medicare/Quality-Initiatives-Patient-Assessment-instruments/HospitalQualityInits/HospitalHCAHPS.html.

Chesak, S., Cutshall, S., Bowe, C., Montanari, K., & Bhagra, A. (2019). Stress management for nurses: Critical research review. *Journal of Holistic Nursing, 17*(3), 288–295. https://doi.org/10.1177/0898010119842693.

Chutna, K., & Boothby, J. (2017). Time management strategies for nurse leaders. *American Nurse Today, 12*(11), 10–11.

de Berker, A. O., Rutledge, R. B., Mathys, C., Marshall L., Cross G. F., Dolan R. J., et al. (2016). Computations of uncertainty mediate acute stress responses in humans. *Communications, 7*, 10996. https://doi.org/10.1038/ncomms10996.

Ditkoff, M. (2010). Intention: The root of creativity. *Innovation Excellence.* http://www.innovationexcellence.com/blog/2010/07/12/intention-the-root-of-creativity/.

Federal antitrust policy in the health care marketplace: Hearing before the committee on judiciary, senate, 105th Congress. 84. (1997). (Prepared statement of John C. McMeekin on behalf of the American Hospital Association). https://books.google.com/books?id=uwm1sG4a2_4C&dq=Federal+Antitrust+Policy+in+the+Health+Care+Marketplace:+Hearing+before+the+Committee+on+Judiciary,+Senate,+105th+Congress&source=gbs_navlinks_s.

Fetter, R. B., Shin, Y., Freeman, J. L., Averill, R. F., & Thompson, J. D. (1980). Case mix definition by diagnosis related groups. *Medical Care, 18*(2), 1–53.

Fischer, J., & Keenan, N. (2010). *Prioritizing self-care: The key to stress management.* http://ezinearticles.com/?Prioritizing-Self-Care:-The-Key-to-Stress-Management&id=5499316.

Gilbert, D. (2007). *Stumbling on happiness.* New York, NY: Vintage Books.

Gionta, D. (2009). Setting boundaries at work: Steps to making them a reality. *Psychology Today.* https://www.psychologytoday.com/us/blog/occupational-hazards/200901/setting-boundaries-work-steps-making-them-reality.

Goh, J., Pfeffer, J., Zenios, S. A., & Rajpal, S. (2015). Workplace stressors & health outcomes: Health policy for the workplace. *Behavioral Science and Policy, 1*(1), 43–52.

Jesse, M. (2019). Teaching prioritization: "Who, what, and why." *Journal of Nursing Education, 58*(5), 302–305.

Johansen, M. L., & Cadmus, E. (2016). Conflict management style, supportive work environments and the experience of work stress in emergency nurses. *Journal of Nursing Management, 24*(2), 211–218.

Kath, L. M., Stichler, J. F., & Ehrhart, M. G. (2012). Moderators of the negative outcomes of nurse manager stress. *Journal of Nursing Management, 42*(4), 215–221. https://doi.org/10.1097/NNA.0b013e31824ccd25.

Lacey, S. R., Goodyear-Bruch, C., Olney, A., Hanson, D., Altman, M. S., Varn-Davis, et al. (2017). Driving organizational change from the bedside: The AACN Clinical Scene Investigator Academy. *Critical Care Nurse, 37*(4), e12–e25. https://doi.org/10.4037/ccn2017749.

Lacey, S. R., Olney, A., & Cox, K. (2012). The Clinical Scene Investigator Academy: The power of staff nurses improving patient and organizational outcomes. *Journal of Nursing Care Quality, 27*(1), 56–62.

Liccioni, A. (n.d.) Goodreads. https://www.goodreads.com/quotes/7167475-they-say-timing-is-everything-but-then-they-say-there.

Lundberg, U., & Cooper, C. L. (2011). *The science of occupational health: Stress, psychobiology and the new world of work.* Chichester, UK: Wiley-Blackwell.

Marshall, D. (2013). There's a critical difference between creativity and innovation. *Business Insider Australia.* http://www.businessinsider.com.au/difference-between-creativity-and-innovation-2013-4.

Merriam-Webster. (n.d.a.). Creation. *Merriam-Webster's online dictionary.* http://www.merriam-webster.com/dictionary/creation.

Merriam-Webster. (n.d.b.). Prediction. *Merriam-Webster's online dictionary.* http://www.merriam-webster.com/dictionary/prediction.

Moreland, J. J., & Apker, J. (2016). Conflict and stress in hospital nursing: Improving communicative responses to enduring professional challenges. *Health Communication, 31*(7), 815–823.

National Institute for Occupational Safety and Health (NIOSH). (1999). *Stress…at work.* https://www.cdc.gov/niosh/docs/99-101/default.html.

Nelson, D. L., & Simmons, B. L. (2004). Eustress: An elusive construct, an engaging pursuit. In P. L. Perrewé, & D. C. Ganster (Eds.). *Research in occupational stress and well-being* (3, (pp. 265–322). Oxford, UK: Elsevier.

Nowrouzi, B., Lightfoot, N., Lariviere, M., Carter, L., Rukholm, E., Schinke, R., et al. (2015). Occupational stress management and burnout interventions in nursing and their implications for healthy work environments. *Workplace Health & Safety, 63*(7), 308–315.

Öhman, A. (2000). Fear and anxiety: Evolutionary, cognitive, and clinical perspectives. In M. Lewis, & J. M. Haviland-Jones (Eds.), *Workplace health & safety, handbook of emotions* (pp. 573–593). New York, NY: The Guilford Press.

Peckham, C. (2015). Nurses tell all! Salaries, benefits, and whether they'd do it again. *Medscape*. http://www.medscape.com/viewarticle/854372.

Pines, E. W., Rauschhuber, M. L., Norgan, G. H., Cook, J. D., Canchola, L., Richardson, C., et al. (2012). Stress resiliency, psychological empowerment and conflict management styles among baccalaureate nursing students. *Journal of Advanced Nursing, 68*(7), 1482–1493. https://doi.org/10.1111/j.1365-2648.2011.05875.x.

Pink, D. H. (2018). *When: The scientific secrets of perfect timing*. New York: Riverhead Books.

Ratanasiripong, P., Park, J. F., Ratanasiripong, N., & Kathalae, D. (2015). Stress and anxiety management in nursing students: Biofeedback and mindfulness mediation. *Journal of Nursing Education, 54*(9), 520–524.

Richmond, P. A., Book, K., Hicks, M., Pimpinella, A., & Jenner, P. A. (2009). C.O.M.E. be a nurse manager. *Nursing Management, 40*(2), 52–54. https://doi.org/10.1097/01.NUMA.0000345875.99318.82.

Rosch, P. J. (2001). The quandary of job stress compensation. *Health and Stress, 3*, 1–4.

Rosenfeld, P., & Glassman, K. (2016). The long-term effect of a nurse residency program, 2005–2012: Analysis of former nurse residents. *Journal of Nursing Administration, 46*(6), 336–344.

Rosenthal, M. S. (2002). *50 ways to prevent and manage stress*. New York, NY: McGraw-Hill.

Rush, K. L., Adamack, M., Gordon, J., Lilly, M., & Janke, R. (2013). Best practices of formal new graduate nurse transition programs: An integrative review. *International Journal of Nursing Studies, 50*(3), 345–356. https://doi.org/10.1016/j.ijnurstu.2012.06.009.

Saunders, E. G. (2013). *The 3 secrets to effective time investment: Achieve more success with less stress*. New York, NY: McGraw-Hill.

Scott, D. L. (2003). *Wall Street words: An A to Z guide to investment terms for today's investor*. Boston, MA: Houghton Mifflin.

Seaward, B. L. (2013). *Essentials of managing stress* (3rd ed.). Burlington, MA: Jones & Bartlett Learning.

Segal, J., Smith, M., Robinson, L., & Segal, R. (2019). *Stress in the workplace*. HelpGuide.org. https://www.helpguide.org/articles/stress/stress-in-the-workplace.htm.

Seyle, H. (1950). Stress and general adaption syndrome. *British Medical Journal, 1*(4667), 1383–1392.

Sherman, R., & Cohn, T. (2019). Leadership challenge: The role of timing in work and life. *American Nurse Today, 14*(10), 15–17.

Shirey, M. R., McDaniel, A. M., Ebright, P. R., Fisher, M. L., & Doebbeling, B. N. (2010). Understanding nurse manager stress and work complexity. *Journal of Nursing Administration, 40*(2), 82–91. https://doi.org/10.1097/NNA.0b013e3181cb9f88.

Templeman, J. (2018). Time: A nurse's friend or foe. *American Nurse Today, 13*(6), 54–55.

Ullrich, P. M., & Lutgendorf, S. K. (2002). Journaling about stressful events: Effects of cognitive processing and emotional expression. *Annals of Behavioral Medicine, 24*(3), 244–250.

Ulrich, B., Barden, C., Cassidy, L., & Varn-Davis, N. (2019). Critical care nurse work environments 2018: Findings and implications. *Critical Care Nurse, 39*(2), 67–84. https://doi.org/10.4037/ccn2019605.

US Department of Health and Human Services. (2014). *Key features of the Affordable Care Act*. http://www.hhs.gov/healthcare/facts-and-features/key-features-of-aca/index.html.

US Department of Health and Human Service National Institute of Mental Health. (n.d.). *Five things you should know about stress*. Mental Health Information. NIH Publication No. 19-MH-8109. https://www.nimh.nih.gov/health/publications/stress/index.shtml#pub3.

White, G. B. (2015). The alarming, long-term consequences of workplace stress. *The Atlantic*. http://www.theatlantic.com/business/archive/2015/02/the-alarming-long-term-consequences-of-workplace-stress/385397/.

Woods, E. (2005). *Employee development at the workplace: Achieving empowerment in a continuous learning environment* (2nd ed.). Dubuque, IA: Kendall Hunt.

World Health Organization (WHO). (2010). *Stress at the workplace*. https://www.who.int/occupational_health/topics/stressatwp/en/.

World Wide Web Foundation. (2015). *Sir Tim Berners-Lee*. http://webfoundation.org/about/sir-tim-berners-lee.

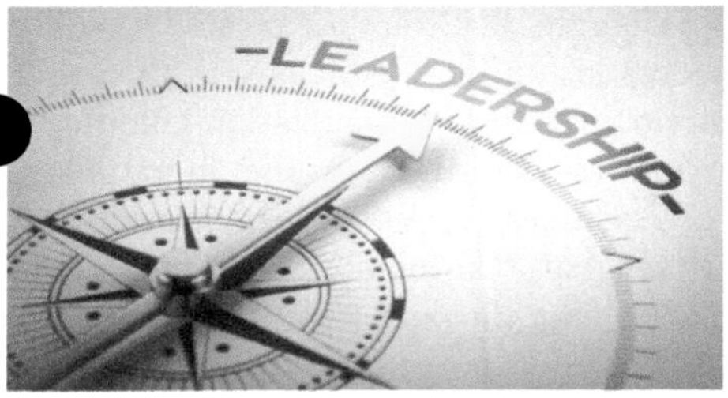

6

Role Management

Veronica Rankin

http://evolve.elsevier.com/Huber/leadership

Health care organizations in the United States continue to experience persistent nursing shortages with increasing demand for complex, low-cost health care services for a higher acuity patient population. Nurse leaders of today need to serve as change agents to innovatively approach practice in a way that will recruit, develop, and retain the nurses of tomorrow through role management. With the impending exodus of the baby boomer population from the health care workforce, leaders must also begin preparing nurse leaders of tomorrow who do not have as many years of nursing experience as those leaving the workforce.

According to the Institute of Medicine (2010) and other sources, these significant nurse staffing deficits are expected to worsen within the next decade as more nurses, belonging to the baby boomer generation, prepare for retirement (Beck & Boulton, 2016; Yeager et al., 2016). These factors, coupled with the highly competitive nurse recruitment environment, require nurse leaders to approach practice differently than ever before. Chism (2016) described nursing as dynamic, noting that nursing continues to evolve to meet the needs of society by caring for its people and maintaining health and well-being. With this in mind, nurse leaders need to be transformational and effectively manage the various roles of nursing in a way that promotes engagement, empowers innovation, builds long-lasting relationships, and supports continued growth and development of nurses. This chapter will explore the nurse staffing issues plaguing health care and provide insight into how nurse leaders can successfully overcome these challenges, while adapting to the ever-changing world of health care. Strategies are presented to help nurse leaders achieve success and combat challenging factors such as nurse leader vacancies and the reality of an expected influx of less experienced nurse leaders to guide frontline nursing staff. Nurse leaders cannot successfully manage the many roles within nursing without exploring ways in which to address the challenges of health care.

Although a definition of role management was not found in the literature, the definition to be used in this work refers to the activities necessary for leaders to successfully develop and maintain role definitions over time. In order to effectively manage roles, one must define the role, educate others, select the right person to implement the role, provide adequate support, master role development, and continuously evaluate the role for needed changes and sustainment purposes.

DEFINITIONS

Effective leadership, regardless of the discipline type, requires mutual understanding of the meaning and context of concepts used. Role management, and any other leadership function, cannot be accomplished if professionals lack the ability to speak and understand the same language. The following are definitions used in this chapter.

Change agent: an individual who effects change within themselves and builds the capacity for change in others to transform organizational systems (Stefancyk et al., 2013).

Change coach: an individual who alters human capabilities while supporting and influencing others towards change (Stefancyk et al., 2013).

Health care innovation: the process of rethinking and re-creating health care methods of practice and care delivery that extends farther than creating an electronic medical record (Porter-O'Grady & Malloch, 2018).

Innovation: the incessant adaptation to an ever-changing environment and available resources, which requires the creation of new business models and strategies to ensure that the organization survives and thrives in the future (Porter-O'Grady & Malloch, 2018).

Leadership: the science and skill of influencing or guiding a group of individuals towards the achievement of set goals (Carmen, 2002; McArthur, 2006). Leadership denotes accompaniment, whereas management denotes control and supervision.

Management: a guiding influence on an organization and its unit's market, production, and/or resource operations that may address human and non-human problems and is exerted by many individuals through either anticipatory norm-setting or situational intervention with a goal of achieving set objectives (Kaehler & Grundei, 2019).

Nursing: a dynamic practice that continues to evolve to meet the needs of society by caring for its people and maintaining health and well-being within various stages of health and illness (Chism, 2016).

Nursing practice: the independent, yet collaborative care of diverse populations through the use of health promotion, illness prevention, and care of the sick, disabled, and/or dying (International Council of Nurses, 2014).

Role management: the activities necessary for leaders to successfully develop and maintain role definitions over time, based on standardized expectations within an organization.

Transformational coaching: a method of activities used to transport individuals through the process of accepting change and accomplishing desired outcomes (Porter-O'Grady & Malloch, 2018).

BACKGROUND

Role Management

As the complexities of health care continue to evolve, the role of nurse leader must also continue to evolve to meet the needs of the patient population and the staff. Nursing literature lacks a definition of role management; therefore, a concept analysis was conducted to create a definition for the purpose of this chapter. Classic role theory suggests that roles are created based on standard expectations and are associated with distinguishable positions within an organization (Biddle, 1986). Management, as described in the literature, implies control of resources through supervision and training to achieve set goals (Carmen, 2002; Garrison & McBryde-Foster, 2004). For the purpose of this chapter, role management is defined as the activities necessary for leaders to successfully develop and maintain role definitions over time, based on standardized expectations within an organization. Leaders must think proactively, exceeding the basic definition of management by taking a more creative approach in effective role management. In order to function in this capacity, leaders must fully understand and practice the following activities:

- defining the role
- educating others
- selecting the right personnel
- providing adequate support
- mastering role development
- constantly evaluating the role to ensure maintenance

Defining the Role

There are many roles within nursing that can be categorized in many different ways. Regarding practice, the categories could include administration, clinical, and educational. Within education categories, nurses can be grouped by such education levels as diploma, associates, bachelor's, master's, or doctorate. Regarding specialty training, the opportunities are endless. Furthermore, each category previously mentioned contains its own subcategories and variations posing the potential for what Stanley (2006) refers to as role confusion due to the lack of clarity to delineate one nursing role from another. This confusion further intensifies chaos between nursing staff within a workplace and hampers collaboration and productivity.

Identity plays a critical role in the realm of individual engagement because it serves as the fundamental way in which people define, label, and find themselves within an environment (Armstrong et al., 2018). Role theory postulates that teammates within an organization take on different responsibilities and roles within the organization (Biddle, 1986). Matta et al. (2015) argued that according to role theory, an individual's acted-out behavior is centered on the definition and evolution of their role. Consequently, when clear definitions of duties and role expectations are not provided, the individual may experience ambiguity that increases dissatisfaction, hesitation to practice, confusion, and ineffective performance (Biddle, 1986; Kahn et al., 1964). It is therefore very important for the nurse leader to define the nurse's role and scope of practice prior to implementation, setting expectations, or attempting to educate others about the role. Nelson (2017, p. 407) supported this premise by strongly advising leaders to define and ensure that definitions are created, kept clear, and thoroughly communicated repetitively to avoid "a blurring of the boundaries."

Furthermore, although defining the role is important, equally important is the need to identify the team to which the role will belong. Foster (2017) supported this premise by noting that team identification is critical because the nature of the new role is ultimately determined by the skills and competencies that are required from the clinical team to which the role belongs. Through completely defining a role, all parties involved enter the partnership with a clear understanding of group dynamics to enhance collaboration and teamwork.

Educating Others

The natural progression after defining a role is to educate others regarding the findings. This act is important for not only those partaking in the education, but also to build confidence and personal understanding for the individual. It is also important while educating to explain the role's impact or fit within the team. Armstrong et al. (2018) noted that the interpretation of new information is grossly affected by the way in which individuals align themselves with the responsibilities and purpose of their group. This means that the individual filling the role and the team should be clearly educated on each entity's purpose, goals, objectives, and collaborative expectations (Foster, 2017). Since defining the role was already completed prior to this step, this information should be readily accessible. Education to the team must be provided frequently, as new members join the team, responsibilities or duties of the team change, or group dynamics evolve over time.

Chism (2016) noted the importance of effective education in role management based on findings from the literature that the perceptions of patients, nurses, and other professionals are significantly influenced by previous experiences. A study by Gooden and Jackson (2004) revealed that nurses' attitudes about other nurses in the health care environment could affect the patient's attitudes and impact health care outcomes. Richmond and Becker (2005) recommended that although attitudes about nurses were positive, these attitudes needed to be cultivated by nurses for sustainment. These authors recommended that nurses take on characteristics that are helpful in promoting credibility and trust that lead to understanding of the role and building of mutual relationships. Important characteristics include clarity in role and vision, commitment to practice, effective communication, collaboration, credibility through credentialing, contributions to patient outcomes, self-confidence, and solution-oriented practice (Richmond & Becker, 2005).

Role modeling is an effective way to educate through demonstration, which can be more impactful than verbal explanation. Chism (2016) noted that effective education depends on consistent demonstration of the value and expertise the nurse brings to health care delivery. The author explained that through role modeling, the nurse develops leadership abilities and interprofessional collaboration skills that enhance success in practice. Furthermore, other health care providers will be more receptive to the role and education offered about the role when evidence in the form of demonstrated outcomes is actualized.

Selecting the Right Personnel

A critical component of role management begins with selecting the right individual for the role. This may require leadership training and coaching for new leaders because an individual's clinical knowledge base or performance at the bedside does not predicate automatic selection for all nursing roles. Contrary to popular belief, the habit of hiring the highest performing nurse who is the most experienced on the unit into a nurse leader role may result in confusion, personal struggles, and poor leadership that ultimately potentiates poor care quality and patient outcomes (Stanley, 2006). It is critical for leaders to learn how to recruit, transition, and retain upcoming leaders more effectively for not only the organization but also for the future of nursing (Sherman & Saifman, 2018).

Koehn (2017) described the lives of five influential leaders in history. This author noted that all of the leaders discussed in the work were made into leaders, meaning they were not born leaders. Koehn postulated that although each leader was gifted in various skills, they each lacked something that was cultivated or had to be learned to become the successful leader that they were. Koehn (2017) listed the following attributes that successful leaders must possess:

1. Be accountable and willing to self-improve.
2. Be able to reflect on their actions and encounters to seek learning.
3. Be able to take instruction.
4. Take inventory of their strengths and weaknesses and maximize their own capabilities.
5. Excel in emotional intelligence, empathy, and intentionality.
6. Develop resilience.
7. Become comfortable with solitude and detachment.
8. Envision the big picture and potential impact.

The recruitment process also needs to include a thorough assessment of the individual's goals, expectations, and essential retention factors as related to the role. Yeager and Wisniewski (2017) conducted a cross-sectional study that examined recruitment and retention perspectives of more than 3000 nurses and non-nurses who worked in public health arenas. Of the 12 organizational factors included in the survey, results revealed that the top five retention factors the nurses reported were autonomy/employee empowerment, flexibility of work schedule, specific duties and responsibilities, opportunities for training/continuing education, and ability to innovate. Understanding the factors that matter to potential employees is critical to successful recruitment and retention efforts (Beck & Boulton, 2016). Present day leaders expecting to master role management need to be cognizant of their employees' driving forces upfront to combat the nursing shortage issues resulting from excessive turnover that are expected to worsen in the future.

Providing Adequate Support

According to Press Ganey (2018), nurse leader support is a key driver in positively impacting novice nurse intent to stay. The same holds true for experienced nurses whether the interest lies in staying at the bedside in a clinical position or aspiring to the executive board room. Bradley and Moore (2019) noted that nurse leaders are often inadequately prepared, developed, and supported in their roles. This undoubtedly perpetuates turnover and poor interest in nursing leadership positions. As leaders prepare to approach practice differently, multiple methods of support should be explored and implemented within the work setting.

Support can be achieved in various ways. One major method strongly supported in the literature is mentoring or coaching. Mentors are absolutely vital to the success of a new leader (Martin & Warshawsky, 2017). Evidence from the literature validates the positive effects of mentored onboarding for leadership success. Coaching is a commonly used technique implemented to help develop the skills of upcoming inquisitive leaders capable of instigating organizational impact. Roussel et al. (2020) noted that there is growing evidence supporting the use of developmental coaching for all new leaders as it has emerged as a cornerstone of learning organizations. Furthermore, in addition to employee retention and patient outcomes, evidence substantiates the fact that coaching promotes engagement among leaders and staff members, enriches communication skills, and advances motivation and decision-making skills (Blackman et al., 2016).

Through coaching, professionalism can be fostered seamlessly. Blackman et al. (2016) noted that the demonstration of personal excellence, genuineness, and credibility of coaches facilitates sustainable progress and continued learning for those who are coached. Now is the time for coaches to role-model to upcoming leaders the power of open communication, self-reflection, responsibility, respect for humankind, and each nurse's responsibility to advocate for professionalism (Roussel et al., 2020).

The concept of a change coach is introduced in the literature by Stefancyk et al. (2013) as a leader who uses behaviors such as guiding, facilitating, and inspiring followers to elicit change. A change coach is described as someone who can alter human capabilities through support and influence. Although both roles of change agent and change coach result in change, the change coach accomplishes change through influence and inspiration more so than hands-on action as with a change agent. A successful leader is described as being one who can easily move between the roles of change agent and change coach as required by the situation.

Competencies such as those provided by the American Organization of Nurse Executives (AONE, 2015), now the American Organization for Nursing Leadership, can serve as a helpful tool in developing a plan for role development and training. By studying these and other competency and role development tools, one can approach mentorship with a certain level of expectancy by being better prepared with the ability to voice needs to the mentor (Moyo, 2019).

Another way in which support can be provided to nurse leaders to effectively manage the various roles of nursing is relationship building or the formation of alliances. According to Siren and Gehrs (2018), nurse leaders are the connecting link between executive leaders and nursing staff at the bedside. They are also expected to foster relationships with interdisciplinary teammates as well as promote physician engagement and collaborative partnerships with nursing (Nelson, 2017). Alliances are automatically built as health care providers collectively share in meeting the needs of patients, communities, and organizations (Harris et al., 2018). By creating alliances, leaders can leverage differences within the team to achieve goals.

Mastering Role Development

Historically, clinical nurses from the frontline are "cut and pasted" into their new leadership role with little to no prior leadership development or mentoring (Sherman & Saifman, 2018). It sounds contradictory that although nursing leadership is well supported in the literature as being one of the most demanding roles in health care (Goodyear & Goodyear, 2018), more guidance and training is oftentimes devoted to new graduate nurses than new nurse leaders who are held accountable to retain them (Sherman & Saifman, 2018). Strategic planning and succession planning need to be devoted to rectifying this finding.

The literature recommends beginning succession planning with role development activities now to train and prepare the nurses of tomorrow. Although Moyo (2019) provided seven key strategies to help millennial nurse leaders achieve success, the literature shows that these strategies are applicable to all leaders, regardless of their generational category (Roussel et al., 2020). These strategies include:

1. Seek out opportunities to learn.
2. Remain confident and optimistic.
3. Show respect and be unbiased.
4. Work on getting to know and understand your staff early.
5. Be firm, yet fair, and always consistent.
6. Be helpful and supportive to your staff.
7. Reflect on your learning and progress.

Saifman and Sherman (2019) conducted a qualitative study on a national sample of 25 millennial nurse managers to explore their experiences as nurse managers. The purpose of this study was to better understand the organization's influential factors on the nurse manager's job satisfaction, development, intent to stay, and their perspectives regarding their role expectations and support as leaders. Findings revealed seven common themes from the participants: "coming into the role, learning as I go, having the support of my director, making an impact, helping staff succeed, and managing change" (Saifman & Sherman, 2019, p. 367). The findings of this study reveal pertinent opportunities leaders should prepare for in order to develop and retain millennial leaders. This study supports the importance of succession planning and formal standardized leadership development processes. Lastly, findings also suggest innovative approaches to modifying the design of the nurse leader role to enhance the desirability of the role for millennials.

Nurse leader training and preparation needs to be strategically planned to ensure that new leaders are trained, equipped, and empowered to achieve success. Simmers (2019) noted that this process begins with a review of the literature to identify best practices, evidence regarding the role, and barriers and challenges to role development and implementation. Once this process has been completed, role development needs to include adequate training, a needs assessment, relationship building, education, and support groups for sustainment.

A study by Warshawsky et al. (2013) led to the creation of a Nurse Manager Practice Environment Scale that assessed factors affecting nurse manager job performance. This study found that the success of a nurse manager is predicated on the manager's ability to create an innovative work culture, foster relationships, facilitate patient safety, and provide adequate resources and staffing. This tool is one of many that can be used to not only assess nurse leader satisfaction or burnout, but it can also be used to assist in developing action plans or strategies for improvement.

Fischer-Cartlidge et al. (2019) conducted a successful multiphase journey to rebuild a Clinical Nurse Specialist team after years of open vacancies and role confusion. The approach included innovative recruitment strategies, development of a talent pipeline through enhancement of student clinical placements, team and individual development activities, and value identification. As a result of the role development activities, the authors achieved role standardization and optimization, increased representation on hospital-wide committees and councils, and were able to quantify their work.

Yeager and Wisniewski (2017) stressed the importance of clearly defined duties and responsibilities that align within the organization's strategic plan, mission and vision statement, and values to enhance role management. Additional recommendations include detailed job descriptions emphasizing activities that the employee will participate in, benefits from organizations that offer training and continuing education, and partnering with local colleges and universities. Offering opportunities for employees to gain new skills and training on the job not only helps to identify future leaders, but it also helps to strengthen engagement by creating a community of invested partnership (Yeager & Wisniewski, 2017).

Role Evaluation/Maintenance

Adequate leadership is critical to role development and nurse positioning to achieve quality improvement and efficient health care delivery (Kraaij et al., 2020). Long-term maintenance of role management depends on the leader's ability to continue to develop and support the role as well as serve as an influential leader on all levels of nursing. Harris and Roussel (2010) noted that professional values, including such concepts as altruism, accountability, responsibility, human dignity, integrity, and other ethical principles, facilitate successful role implementation and management. These values and principles are essential to nursing practice because they govern how professionals communicate, form relationships, manage conflicts, deliver compassionate care, enculturate diversity, evaluate failures and successes, and handle stress (Harris & Roussel, 2010).

An important component of role management maintenance is reward and recognition along the journey. Stefancyk et al. (2013) advised leaders to celebrate successes and view innovations that may not have been seen initially as successful, as learning opportunities. Leaders need to consistently express confidence in the staff, in the role, and in the organization to encourage continued work and engagement. This action will also motivate followers to seek out bigger issues on the unit that can impact quality care.

In role management, maintenance depends upon direct focus on progress and on challenges and barriers to achieving progress. Porter O'Grady and Malloch (2018) advised leaders to address problems directly by approaching barriers proactively. The importance of proactive approaches to problem solving was stressed to avoid the "firefighting" phenomenon that can easily consume nurse leader's workday. Real-time problem-solving helps to develop leaders and strengthens the transformational impact one can have on a work setting. The recommendation is to avoid the error of finding quick fixes, but to instead drill down to the root of the problem to prevent recurrence.

Many evaluation frameworks exist to assess the success of implementations. These frameworks can be used to understand the phases, stages, and circumstantial factors that may be positively or negatively affecting a role or process. Roussel et al. (2020) provided examples of commonly used frameworks such as Reach X Efficacy-Adoption, Implementation, Maintenance (RE-AIM) and Precede-Proceed framework with the explanation that leaders need to be aware of the differences of such tools to ensure that the correct framework is chosen to meet the assessment needs of the leader. Additional assessment methodologies such as theories and process models can also be used to determine aspects of success with role management. Some of the more common quality and performance improvement strategies used to assess progress include Six Sigma, LEAN, Plan-Do-Study-Act, and standardization in practice (Roussel et al., 2020). Regardless of the strategy used, nurse leaders need to know what measures or metrics the role is expected to impact in order to assess progress. With having some method in which to assess progress of the implemented work, the leader can continuously perform pulse checks of the work to ensure that expectations are being met, adequate support is provided, and that the employee understands their role and what is expected of them.

LEADERSHIP AND MANAGEMENT IMPLICATIONS

Role management is defined as the activities necessary for leaders to successfully develop and maintain role definitions over time, based on standardized expectations within an organization. In order to tackle the nursing shortages as well as all of the other demanding challenges of health care, nurse leaders need to approach practice differently than ever before. Nurse leaders need to serve as change agents, change coaches, mentors, and transformational leaders at the bedside to attract clinical nurses into the worsening nurse leader vacancies expected in the near future. In order to successfully serve as role managers, nurse leaders need to define the role, educate others, select the right personnel, provide adequate support, champion role development, and continuously evaluate the role for maintenance. Succession planning for the nurse leaders of tomorrow need to start now to advance care quality because it is an immediate imperative. In addition to innovative practice approaches, leaders and nursing professionals at all levels need to thoroughly understand and practice delegation and ethical decision making to function effectively within their roles. These foundational components of nursing practice are essential to practice. They provide the capacity for nursing professionals to work within a collaborative team construct, impact health outcomes, and demonstrate compassionate, person-centered care.

Change Agents

Through basic nursing education, nurses are aware of the common change theories used in quality improvement work such as Lewin's 3-step Change Theory, Lippitt's Phases of Change Theory, and Prochaska and DiClemente's Transtheoretical Change Model (Kritsonis, 2005). The literature supports the fact that nurse leaders need to exceed change awareness. They need to understand the theories and be skilled at applying and coaching staff through change (Stefancyk et al., 2013). Stefancyk et al. (2013) noted that regardless of the model or method used, effective change penetrates far beyond the processes and structure of an organization to impact the organization's culture.

Leadership is the science and skill of influencing or guiding a group of individuals towards the achievement of set goals (Carmen, 2002; McArthur, 2006). Nurse leaders inhabit a critical position in creating a culture that is accepting of change. As transformational coaches, leaders are responsible for creating a culture of change and the structure in which change is to be actualized, thereby fostering adaptation and employee engagement (Porter-O'Grady & Malloch, 2018). Leadership, not to be confused with management, denotes accompaniment, whereas management denotes control and supervision. Through role modeling nurse leaders serve an important part in leading change at the front line of care delivery and therefore can be the most influential change agents in an organization.

Stefancyk et al. (2013) defined a change agent as an individual who transforms themselves and influences the capacity for change within individuals around them for the sake of an organization. Rogers (2003) defined a change agent as an individual who influences another person's innovative decisions towards the desirable wishes of an organization. Both definitions imply alignment with some party or institution's goals or action plan. Rogers (2003) also provides stages in the role of change agent which include:

1. Developing a need for change
2. Disseminating information
3. Identifying the problem
4. Developing the client's intent to change
5. Translating intent into action
6. Hardwiring adoption and preventing noncompliance
7. Achieving termination/adjournment

In order to serve as an effective change agent, nurse leaders must understand and put these steps into practice. Couros (2014) expands this work by defining five characteristics that change agents need to employ to be truly effective: having a clear vision, being patient yet tenacious, exploring tough uncertainties, being knowledgeable and role modeling, and building trusting relationships. Stefancyk et al. (2013) supported this information by noting that successful nurse leaders promote and hardwire a culture of change by strategically homing in on the leadership elements of human resource management, foundational thinking, relationship building, and the power of influence.

Transformational Leadership

Transformational leaders create an environment that allows individuals to contribute their fullest potential to achieve the best outcomes possible (Porter-O'Grady & Malloch, 2018). Leaders of today are responsible for inspiring and motivating staff despite the chaos of an unstable and extremely fast-paced environment. Consequently, it is because of the high demand for health care services to be provided at a faster pace to a sicker population, using fewer resources, that transformational leaders are critical to the success of the nursing profession. Tuuk (2012) noted that transformational leaders obligate individuals to take action, transform followers into leaders, and then change leaders into change agents. The author also noted that these types of leaders do not use power to repress and control, but instead empower individuals to create a vision and then trust them to work towards achieving that vision. The most effective way to tackle the challenges of health care is to enlist transformational leaders who are dedicated to serving as change agents.

Delegation

Effective leadership and role management in health care necessitates delegation in order to complete tasks in an efficient manner and to promote continued development (Bake, 2020). In fact, according to the National Council of State Boards of Nursing (NCSBN, 2019), delegation is a critical competency for nurses in all areas of practice, especially nurse leaders. Hewertson (2015) defined delegation as the planned learning of new skills and opportunities for an individual that transfers duties or tasks to that individual for a purpose that is mutually beneficial for the individual and delegator. As a critical competency, all licensed nurses must fully understand the laws and rules of their specific state or jurisdiction, since they can differ from location to location.

When tasks require delegation, the delegation process and the nurse practice act of that jurisdiction must be thoroughly understood to ensure that the process is handled in a safe and ethically sound manner (NCSBN, 2019). The licensed nurse must make the decision regarding the patient's condition, the competence of the delegatee, and the degree of supervision required and available to guarantee safe practice. Delegation goes beyond the delegatee's basic educational training, permitting the performance of tasks that are not routinely performed by the delegate, and may extend beyond their customary role or basic responsibilities. The delegating nurse is still ultimately responsible for making sure that the task is performed correctly. The national guidelines of the NCSBN (2019) outlined five rights of delegation that include: (1) delegation of the right task, (2) delegation under the right conditions, (3) delegation to the right individual, (4) delegation by providing the right instructions and effective communication, and (5) delegation with the right supervision and assessment. In order to comply with these five important steps, the following criteria by the NCSBN (2019) must be met:

- The delegate must have been trained and validated as competent to perform the task or responsibility.
- The nurse cannot delegate a task that requires nursing judgment or critical thinking.
- Delegation can only occur by an individual that owns delegating authority.
- The delegated task must be within the scope of practice of the delegator and the delegate according to the nurse practice act.

Although the licensed nurse is ultimately responsible for the overall well-being of the patient, once the task has been appropriately delegated and accepted by the delegate, the delegatee is responsible for the delegated task or duty (NCSBN, 2019). The delegation process is multidimensional within every health care setting, beginning at the administrative level. Administrators are responsible for setting the criteria and creating the policies and procedures regarding the delegation of nursing responsibilities. Administrators are also responsible for periodically assessing the delegation process and promoting a healthy working environment. Delegation is infused throughout all aspects of nursing; therefore, all nurses should become well versed in the process.

Nurse leaders need to role-model proper and effective delegation through role management. Effective role management requires skills and knowledge in delegation. The principles of delegation as noted by Hewertson (2015) include:

1. Select the right individual.
2. Demonstrate and teach considering various learning styles.
3. Assign and delegate new work that is challenging, yet rewarding and exciting.
4. Provide adequate time for training and development.
5. Delegate gradually while monitoring progress continuously.
6. Align responsibility and authority to manage delegated tasks.
7. Avoid splitting one job if possible, by delegating a job as a whole unit.
8. Share the expected results and outcomes of the job.
9. Avoid holes and overlaps due to incomplete planning.
10. Trust the delegate and allow autonomy within established boundaries.

These principles align with the activities of role management, which include role definition, education, personnel selection, support provision, role development, and evaluation/assessment. It is especially important to transcribe the plan in writing for future reference and to ensure complete understanding. Hewertson (2015) noted that the delegation plan should be a signed and dated document that includes such details as the names of the delegate and delegator, the delegated job duty, the details of the authority, time frame including time allotted for training and practice, agreed milestones, the plan for communication, performance criteria, risk factors, and needed resources.

Ethical Issues

Effective nurse leadership hinges on a thorough understanding of ethics due to the frequency of ethical dilemmas requiring sound decision-making that nurses find themselves in within the role. A definition provided by Butts and Rich (2008, p. 4) described ethics as "the study of ideal human behavior and ideal ways of being." Roussel et al. (2020) explained the meaning of ethics as an individual's conformity to the standards of a professional group. The premise of these definitions center on personal beliefs and moral philosophy that delineates right actions from wrong actions and an individual's adaptability to change behavior based on perceived good and bad intent.

A code of ethics as described by Pozgar (2010), defined the criteria of behavior and specific principles as they apply to the duties of professionals. The Code of Ethics for Nurses, created by the American Nurses Association (ANA, 2015), is considered to be the standard for ethical nurse behavior, regardless of the nursing position or role (Chism, 2016). This code needs to be role modeled by leaders within the workplace to ensure that nursing practice upholds the four responsibilities of nurses, which are "to promote health, to prevent illness, to restore health, and alleviate suffering" (International Council of Nurses [ICN], 2006, p. 1).

Leaders oftentimes find themselves in situations known as ethical dilemmas in which difficult decisions must be made between equally unfavorable options in clinical practice. These dilemmas develop as a result of conflict between principles and rules regarding socially approved human behavior, professional code of ethics standards, public policies of government agencies, business related ethics of an organization, and personal values held by each individual provider. Chism (2016) pinpointed four ethical principles that serve as the cornerstone of biology and medicine to include autonomy, beneficence, nonmaleficience, and justice. When ethical dilemmas arise, these principles are raised to help examine the situation and find resolution. Many authors have provided definitions of these principles for health care providers (Beauchamp & Childress, 2009; Butts & Rich, 2008; Cooper, 2014; Pozgar, 2010) that include:

- Autonomy is an individual's right for self-governance, free from controlling interference by others.
- Beneficence means doing good by helping others with compassionate care.
- Nonmaleficence means to avoid causing harm to others.
- Justice is the provision of fair and equal treatment, consistent with equal distribution of benefits and burden.

Leaders need to become champions of ethics and ensure that resources are available to help guide staff and themselves through ethical decision-making. Chism (2016) advised leaders to be ethically conscious and competent while being committed to consistently doing that which is right. Leaders are also advised to be courageous enough to abide by their own competence despite uneasiness or what is popular. Leaders are further advised to remain open and straightforward to directly address the ethical issue or dilemma. By accomplishing these recommendations in practice, a culture strong in autonomy, beneficence, nonmaleficence, and justice will be actualized.

CURRENT ISSUES & TRENDS

One concern found in the literature relates to the baby boomer exodus expected to worsen within the next decade, which will weaken the supply of seasoned, well-experienced nurse leaders (Beck & Boulton, 2016; Moyo, 2019; Yeager et al., 2016). This vacancy will require millennial nurses to fill in nurse leader vacancies. In fact, it has been estimated that 50% of the entire nursing workforce will soon be filled by millennials (Holland, 2015). This issue is of further concern because nurse leader recruitment has become extremely difficult over the years as manifested by increasing turnover rates (McCright et al., 2018). A way in which nurse leaders of today can ensure that care quality does not suffer from this unavoidable shift is to serve as change agents and approach leadership practice in an innovative, more strategic way. Porter-O'Grady and Malloch (2018) defined innovation as a continuous adaptation to an ever-changing environment and the availability of resources that require the creation of new business models and strategies to ensure that the organization survives and thrives in the future. The authors further defined health care innovation as the process of rethinking and re-creating health care methods of practice and care delivery extending beyond the electronic medical record (Porter-O'Grady & Malloch, 2018). This requires new leadership mindsets that are skilled in delegation and ethical decision-making to manage the seemingly contradictory expectations of stability and uncertainty within which health care exists today.

RESEARCH NOTE

Source

Siren, A., & Gehrs, M. (2019). Engaging nurses in future management careers: Perspectives on leadership and management competency development through an internship initiative. *Nursing Leadership, 31*(4), 36–49.

Purpose

The purpose of the article is to describe the process of creating a nurse management internship program and also explore the experience of an intern who completed the program. The article explores the intern's perspective regarding the program's competency development and the impact of mentorship support on personal resilience.

Discussion

Nurse managers have an important part in leading change at the front lines of care delivery. They need to manage and empower their team, support healthy and collaborative work environments, maintain patient safety, and address satisfaction concerns of patients and their families. As one of the most challenging roles in health care that continues to evolve over time, the nurse manager is the indispensable connector between senior leadership and staff at the point of care. For this purpose, new nurses preparing for nursing management benefit from a structured approach to preparation. The current state of the economy has caused many nurse leaders of the baby boomer generation to delay their retirement. As these leaders exit the workforce, new less-experienced nurses will need to fill the open leadership positions. The challenge with this situation is the fact that many younger generation nurses do not find nursing leadership roles desirable. They perceive the nurse manager role as requiring too much work and being both time consuming and inadequately compensated for the workload. In order to overcome these challenges and draw younger nurses into this role, organizations need to mentor and begin succession planning for the nurse managers of tomorrow. Orientation plans, support networks, and ongoing educational training need to be appropriately structured and adequately provided to nurse manager candidates.

In this article, a 10-year investment was arranged to create an advanced practice nursing scholarship initiative for 23 individuals employed at the addiction and mental health center. The purpose was to help the center "attract, develop, and retain skilled nurses for management, advanced practice and other relevant leadership roles" (Siren & Gehrs, 2018, p. 39). In addition to these scholarships, two 6-month paid internships were made available for 18 individuals over the 10-year period. The purpose was to "offer a period of enhanced professional nursing leadership development by applying knowledge and skills that foster confidence, critical thinking and leadership competency development..." (Siren & Gehrs, 2018, p. 39). A heterogeneous committee made up of senior nursing leaders and other interprofessional leaders monitored both the scholarship and internship processes over the course of the initiative.

The article provides the following steps of creating a successful nurse manager internship that includes selecting the right individual, selecting the right competency context, operationalizing the intern's development plan, identifying a mentorship network, and transitioning into the role. One lesson learned from the process was that novice-level leadership development content is lacking in the literature. Although this internship was especially designed for a novice leader, most of the evidence found related only to senior-level leadership. Another lesson learned from feedback provided by interns was the need for the intern to be within close proximity of their primary mentor for real-time learning. Other lessons included the benefit of a mentorship network, innovative approaches that inspire young nurses to consider management, and formal networking opportunities between novice nurses and senior leaders. The authors recommended further exploration regarding innovative methods to enhance work–life balance of nurse managers, which is extremely important for younger nurses.

Application to Practice

This article provided steps to consider when seeking to attract, recruit, and retain nurse leaders of tomorrow. Through providing the scholarships and internships, this addiction and mental health center was able to create an effective novice-level nurse management development program. The authors presented feedback from an intern

RESEARCH NOTE—cont'd

who completed the program to help others considering replication of similar processes. The application to practice centers on the need to combat the challenges of nurse leader vacancy, turnover, and ill-prepared leaders to handle the growing demands of health care. By applying evidence found in the future, nurse executives have a better chance of recruiting and retaining competent, satisfied, and effective leaders to manage front line care delivery.

CASE STUDY

You are an Assistant Vice President of the neuroscience division at a Level 1 Trauma Center. You have been informed that the Chief Nurse Executive wishes to discuss a new nursing role with you. In preparation for the meeting, you quickly research new nursing roles but are unable to find anything substantial. In the meeting, your Chief Nurse describes a new nursing role called the Clinical Nurse Leader (CNL). She explains that this role is the newest master's prepared role added to the profession of nursing in more than 30 years. The title and initials of the role are the exclusive property of the American Association of Colleges of Nursing, in that only individuals who have completed the program and passed the certification exam may use them. Within her high-level overview, she describes the advanced clinician role as an "attending nurse." She shares that this role was designed to provide the resource and clinical expertise of nurses at the bedside with advanced education who can coach and mentor nurses in order to improve patient outcomes and maintain patient safety. As a fellow nurse leader of the institution, she reminds you of the current state of opportunities on the medical units outside of the intensive care units. She explains the high influx of inexperienced nurses, the climbing acuity levels of patients serviced by the hospital, and constant pressure from administration to do more with less. She further explains her intent to implement the role at your hospital. She knows that the need for this role is much greater in the medical surgical areas as evidence by internal data and nationwide evidence from the literature. The Chief Nurse explains her plan to apply for grant funding, create a partnership with a local university to provide the CNL track, and recruit a certified CNL to serve as CNL Program Coordinator prior to implementing the role. She has not ironed out the rest of the details, but she would like to assess how you feel about the idea altogether. She would like to assess your ideas regarding role implementation and role management. What are first steps to consider in the process? What are critical components that should go into the planning of this initiative? What are pitfalls you can plan to avoid ensuring success of this role?

CRITICAL THINKING EXERCISE

Situation: You've been asked to implement a new role at your facility that you know very little about. Your executive leader has provided the finances needed to implement the role effectively, but, due to pressing matters, cannot lead the implementation of the role and has therefore delegated the task to you to lead. The leader has provided the return on investment expectations that he expects from the role but has left all other details to you to arrange. What are your first steps? What interdisciplinary teammates must be involved in planning this initiative? Follow the steps provided in this chapter to outline an approach that you can present to your executive leader.

REFERENCES

American Nurses Association (ANA). (2015). *Code of ethics for nurses with interpretive statements.* Silver Spring, MD: Nursebooks.org.

American Organization of Nurse Executives (AONE). (2015). *Nurse manager competencies.* http://www.aone.org/resources/nurse-manager-competencies.pdf.

Armstrong, A. K., Krasny, M. E., & Schuldt, J. P. (2018). Identity. In A. K. Armstrong, M. E. Krasny, & J. P. Schuldt (Eds.), *Communicating climate change: A guide for educators* (pp. 43–48). Ithaca, NY: Cornell University Press.

Bake, M. (2020). Health care management. *Radiologic Technology, 91*(3), 297–299.

Beauchamp, T. L., & Childress, J. F. (2009). *Principles of biomedical ethics* (6th ed.). New York: Oxford University Press.

Beck, A. J., & Boulton, M. L. (2016). The public health nurse workforce in U.S. state and local health departments, 2012. *Public Health Reports, 131*(1), 145–152.

Biddle, B. J. (1986). Recent developments in role theory. *Annual Review of Sociology, 12*, 67–92. https://doi.org/10.1146/annurev.so.12.080186.000435.

Blackman, A., Marscado, G., & Gray, D. (2016). Challenges for the theory and practice of business coaching: A systematic review of empirical evidence. *Human Resource Development Review, 15*(4), 459–486.

Bradley, J., & Moore, L. (2019). The perceptions of professional leadership coaches regarding the roles and challenges of nurse managers. *Journal of Nursing Administration, 49*(2), 105–109.

Butts, J. B., & Rich, K. L. (2008). *Nursing ethics: Across the curriculum and into practice* (2nd ed.). Sudbury, MA: Jones & Bartlett.

Carmen, T. (2002). *Love em' and lead 'em: Leadership strategies that work for reluctant leaders*. Lanham, MD: Scarecrow Press.

Chism, L. (2016). *The doctor of nursing practice: A guidebook for role development and professional issues*. Burlington, MA: Jones & Bartlett.

Cooper, R. W. (2014). Legal and ethical issues. In D. L. Huber (Ed.), *Leadership and nursing care management* (5th ed., pp. 94–110). St. Louis, MO: Elsevier.

Couros, G. (2014). *5 characteristics of a change agent*. http://georgecouros.ca/blog/archives/3615.

Fischer-Cartlidge, E., Houlihan, N., & Browne, K. (2019). Recruitment, role development, and value identification. *Clinical Nurse Specialist: The Journal for Advanced Nursing Practice, 33*(6), 266–272.

Foster, C. (November, 2017). Aiming high is the key to role development. *Imaging & Therapy Practice*, 6–10. ISSN: 2052-0727

Garrison, D. R., & McBryde-Foster, M. J. (2004). The baccalaureate nurse as a leader in health care delivery. In L. C. Haynes, H. K. Butcher, & T. A. Boese (Eds.), *Nursing in contemporary society: Issues, trends, and transition to practice* (pp. 504–525). Upper Saddle River, NJ: Pearson/Prentice Hall.

Gooden, J., & Jackson, E. (2004). Attitudes of registered nurses toward nurse practitioners. *Journal of American Academy of Nurse Practitioners, 16*(8), 360–364.

Goodyear, C., & Goodyear, M. (2018). Career development for nurse managers. *Nursing Management, 49*(3), 49–53.

Harris, J., & Roussel, L. (2010). *Initiating and sustaining the clinical nurse leader role: A practical guide*. Sudbury, MA: Jones and Bartlett Publishers.

Harris, J., Roussel, L., & Thomas, P. (2018). *Initiating and sustaining the clinical nurse leader role: A practical guide* (3rd ed.). Sudbury MA: Jones and Bartlett Publishers.

Hewertson, R. (2015). *Lead like it matters, because it does matter*. New York: McGraw-Hill Education.

Holland, C. (2015). Practice and education: Partnering to create a pipeline of nurse leaders. *Nursing Management, 46*(1), 8–10.

Institute of Medicine. (2010). *The future of nursing: Leading change, advancing health*. Washington, DC: National Academics Press.

International Council of Nurses [ICN]. (2006). *Code of ethics for nurses*. http://www.icn.ch/images/stories/documents/about/icncode_english.pdf.

International Council of Nurses [ICN]. (2014). *Definition of nursing*. http://www.icn.ch/about-icn/icn-definition-of-nursing.

Kaehler, B., & Grundei, J. (2019). The concept of management: In search of a new definition. *HR governance: A theoretical introduction*. (pp. 3-23). Cham: Springer. https://doi.org/10.1007/978-3-319-94526-2.

Kahn, R. L., Wolfe, D., Quinn, R., Snoek, J., & Rosenthal, R. (1964). *Organizational stress: Studies in role conflict and ambiguity*. New York: Wiley.

Koehn, N. (2017). *Forged in crisis: The power of courageous leadership in turbulent times*. New York: Simon & Schuster.

Kraaij, J., Oostveen, C., Vermeulen, H., Heinen, M., Huis, A., Adriaansen, M., & Peters, J. (2020). Nurse practitioners' perceptions of their ability to enact leadership in hospital care. *Journal of Clinical Nursing, 29*(3/4), 447–458. https://doi.org/10.1111/jocn.15105.

Kritsonis, A. (2005). Comparison of change theories. *International Journal of Scholarly Academic Intellectual Diversity, 8*(1), 1–7. http://www.nationalforum.com/Electronic%20Journal%20Volumes/Kritsonis,%20Alicia%20Comparison%20of%20Change%20Theories%20IJMBA%20V8%20N1%202005.pdf.

Martin, E., & Warshawsky, N. (2017). Guiding principles for creating value and meaning for the next generation of nurse leaders. *Journal of Nursing Administration, 47*(9), 418–420.

Matta, F. K., Scott, B. A., Koopman, J., & Conlon, D. E. (2015). Does seeing "eye to eye" affect work engagement and organizational citizenship behavior? A role theory perspective on LMX agreement. *Academic Management Journal, 58*, 1686–1708. https://doi.org/10.5465/amj.2014.0106.

McArthur, D. (2006). The nurse practitioner as leader. *Journal of the American Academy of Nurse Practitioners, 18*(1), 8–10.

McCright, M., Pabico, C., & Roux, N. (2018). Addressing manager retention with the pathway to excellence framework. *Nursing Management, 49*(8), 6–8.

Moyo, M. (2019). Millennial nurse manager: Leading staff nurses more experienced than you. *Nurse Leader, 17*(3), 253–256. https://doi.org/10.1016/j.mnl.2018.09.005.

National Council of State Boards of Nursing – American Nurses Association. (2019). *National guidelines for nursing delegation*. https://www.ncsbn.org/NGND-PosPaper_06.pdf.

Nelson, K. (2017). Nurse manager perceptions of work overload and strategies to address it. *Nurse Leader, 15*(6), 406–408.

Porter O'Grady, T., & Malloch, K. (2018). *Quantum leadership: Creating sustainable value in health care.* Burlington, MA: Jones & Bartlett.

Pozgar, G. D. (2010). *Legal and ethical issues for health professional* (2nd ed.). Sudbury, MA: Jones & Bartlett Learning.

Press Ganey Nursing Special Report. (2018). *Optimizing the nursing workforce: Key drivers to intent to stay for newly licensed and experienced nurses*. http://healthcare.pressganey.com/2018-Nursing-Special-Report?s=White_Paper-PR.

Richmond, T., & Becker, D. (2005). Creating an advanced practice nurse-friendly culture: A marathon not a sprint. *AACN Clinical Issues, 16*(1), 58–66.

Rogers, E. M. (2003). *Diffusion of innovations* (5th ed.). New York: Free Press.

Roussel, L., Thomas, P., & Harris, J. (2020). *Management and leadership for nurse administrators*. (8th ed.). Burlington, MA: Jones & Bartlett Learning.

Saifman, H., & Sherman, R. (2019). The experience of being a millennial nurse manager. *The Journal of Nursing Administration, 49*(7/8), 366–371.

Sherman, R., & Saifman, H. (2018). Transitioning emerging leaders into nurse leader roles. *Journal of Nursing Administration, 48*(7/8), 355–357.

Simmers, P. (2019). Development of a new nurse navigator program. *JONS-online, 10*(11), 474.

Siren, A., & Gehrs, M. (2018). Engaging nurses in future management careers: Perspectives on leadership and management competency development through an internship initiative. *Nursing Leadership, 31*(4), 36–49.

Stanley, D. (2006). Role conflict: Leaders and managers. *Nursing Management, 13*(5), 31–37.

Stefancyk, A., Hancock, B., & Meadows, M. (2013). The nurse manager change agent, change coach? *Nursing Administration Quarterly, 37*(1), 13–17.

Tuuk, E. (2012). *Transformational leadership in the coming decade: A response to three major workplace trends*. http://www.cornellhrreview.org/transformational-leadership-in-the-coming-decade-a-response-to-three-major-workplace-trends/.

Warshawsky, N. E., Rayens, M. K., Lake, S. W., & Havens, D. S. (2013). The nurse manager practice environment scale: Development and psychometric testing. *Journal of Nursing Administration, 43*(5), 250–257.

Yeager, V. A., Beitsch, L. M., & Hasbrouck, L. (2016). A mismatch between the educational pipeline and the public health workforce: Can it be reconciled? *Public Health Reports, 131*(3), 507–509.

Yeager, V. A., & Wisniewski, J. M. (2017). Factors that influence the recruitment and retention of nurses in public health agencies. *Public Health Reports, 132*(5), 556–562.

7

Legal and Ethical Issues

(Carol) Susan Johnson

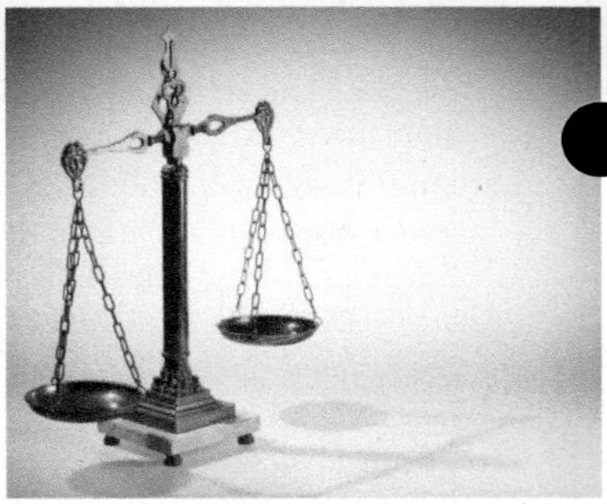

http://evolve.elsevier.com/Huber/leadership

"In civilized life, law floats in a sea of ethics."
Earl Warren, Chief Justice of the United States (1891–1974)
(Pozgar, 2019)

It takes a special person to consider a career in nursing. Not only is a nurse smart and technically savvy, but there is an essence of caring that simply cannot be taught. Because nursing is known as the profession of caring, society grants nursing autonomy or control over its own practice. The American Nurses Association's (ANA) *Nursing's Social Policy Statement: The Essence of the Profession* (2010, p. 25) indicates "competence is foundational to autonomy: the public has a right to expect nurses to demonstrate professional competence." The profession ensures nursing competence through professional regulation of nursing practice via standards and ethical codes of practice, legal regulation of nursing practice via state licensure requirements and law pertaining to criminal and civil wrongdoing, and self-regulation in which all nurses retain personal accountability for their own practice (American Nurses Association, 2015a).

The practice of nursing is constrained by both legal and ethical boundaries. Law and ethics are two sides of the same coin. Whether a legal mandate or an ethical obligation, the results are the same. Ethics "informs every aspect of the nurse's life" (ANA, 2015b, p. Preface vii). It is fitting to begin this chapter by addressing how ethics is essential as nurses confront and handle legal issues.

DEFINITIONS

Ethical concepts contain a variety of specific terms requiring definition.

Ethical Terms

The four principles that form the cornerstone of biomedical ethical decision-making are the following: (1) autonomy, (2) beneficence, (3) nonmaleficence, and (4) justice.

Autonomy: The client's right of self-determination and freedom of decision-making.

Beneficence: Doing good for clients and providing benefit balanced against risk.

Nonmaleficence: Doing no harm to clients.

Justice: The norm of being fair to all and giving equal treatment, including distributing benefits, risks, and costs equally (ANA, 2015b).

Biomedical ethics also recognizes a number of rules that are related to the four fundamental ethical principles and, likewise, provide guidance in dealing with ethical dilemmas. Examples of commonly applied rules are fidelity, veracity, confidentiality, and privacy. *Fidelity* means being loyal and faithful to commitments and accountable for responsibilities. *Veracity* is the norm of

Photo used with permission from Photos.com.

Disclaimer: The information contained in this chapter is for educational purposes only. It is not legal advice, which can be given only by an attorney admitted to practice in the jurisdiction/state(s) in which you practice.

telling the truth and not intentionally deceiving or misleading clients. Falsification of records is an example of violating veracity in the patient record. *Confidentiality* prohibits some disclosures of some information gained in certain relationships to some third parties without the consent of the original source of the information. *Privacy* is a right of limited physical or informational inaccessibility (ANA, 2015b).

ETHICAL COMPONENTS

Nurses and nurse managers are often faced with ethical dilemmas in connection with decision-making. Ethical dilemmas require that decisions be made about what is right and wrong in situations in which an individual has to make a choice between equally unfavorable alternatives. Like other health care professionals, nurses traditionally have faced ethical dilemmas arising primarily out of clinical practice. These dilemmas have involved conflicts among principles and/or rules attributable to common morality (socially approved norms of human conduct), standards articulated in professional codes of ethics, public policies promulgated by government agencies, and the personal values of the health care professionals themselves. Ethical dilemmas faced by nurses and nurse managers also arise as clashes between the principles, rules, values, and standards of clinical/professional ethics and those of organizational/business ethics.

Although the domain of clinical ethics is the care of clients, the domain of organizational ethics is a facility's business-related activities, including, among others, marketing, admissions, transfer, discharge, billing, and the relationship of the facility and its staff members to other health care providers, educational institutions, and payers. These are activities that also directly affect the care of patients. Organizational ethics reflect a health care facility's basic values that serve as guides for proper and acceptable behavior in decision-making. Together, clinical and organizational ethics reflect a health care facility's concern that, whether related to the continuum of care or the continuum of services related to that care, ethical dilemmas should be resolved based on values-centered principles that focus on doing the right thing and taking the right action.

Professional responsibility is something each nurse must deal with every day in their practice. If an error occurs, but no one knows, is it any less an error? This is the point where ethics and legal mandates come together. If the nurse accesses a client's record without a valid reason, but does not use the information, it is considered a Health Insurance Portability and Accountability Act (HIPAA) violation. The question is, is it wrong? Or is it wrong only if I get caught? In this author's opinion, it is fundamentally wrong, and accepting responsibility for such errors in judgment and practice are the duty of each and every nurse. "Nurses bear primary responsibility for the nursing care that their patients and clients receive and are accountable for their own practice" (ANA, 2015b, p. 15). Whether nurses are discussing distance practice, medication errors, HIPAA violations, or any other deviation from acceptable nursing practice, it is that accountability that sets nurses apart as the most trusted profession.

Code of Ethics

In addition to these basic moral principles and rules of biomedical ethics, nurses are also provided standards of conduct by professional codes of ethics. For example, the ANA's *Code of Ethics for Nurses with Interpretive Statements* (2015b) provides nonnegotiable standards as to the ethical obligations and duties of those who enter the nursing profession. The ANA indicated that the Code was developed as a guide for carrying out nursing responsibilities to be consistent with quality in nursing care and the ethical obligations of the profession. The focus is not on giving precise answers to specific ethical problems, but rather on providing general guidance as to how to act when faced with ethical dilemmas.

Ethical Decisions

Many of the decisions nurses and nurse managers make on a daily basis have an ethical component and may involve conflicts among ethical responsibilities. These conflicts may involve clashes between the following:

- Two ethical duties to the client (e.g., duty to respect autonomy and duty to benefit the client);
- The client's rights and benefits (e.g., withholding or withdrawing treatment in respect for a client's right to die by forgoing treatment at any time, and treating or continuing treatment that is expected to produce better results for the client);
- Duties to self and duties to the client (e.g., a nurse's desire to remain on the same shift because of parental responsibilities, and the need to advocate for better treatment of the clients by some health care practitioners on that shift);

- Professional ethical provisions and religious ones (e.g., a professional code requiring the recognition of the client's right to self-determination and a nurse's religious beliefs prohibiting abortion).

When ethical dilemmas are encountered in dealing with clinical matters, health care professionals commonly refer to various principles, rules, and standards for guidance in making moral decisions. Principles and rules are normative generalizations that provide guidance in ethical decision-making. Although rules are more specific in content and restricted in scope than principles, neither can fully guide action but instead must be complemented by judgment for a decision to be made (ANA, 2015b, p. 15). Many organizations employ an ethicist and have ethics committees that operate to provide a source of support and guidance for ethical dilemmas faced by nurses in organizations.

All nurses, regardless of position, must apply ethics in their daily practice using the Provisions of the *ANA Code of Ethics for Nurses with Interpretive Statements* (2015b). These Provisions include:

1. Practicing with compassion and respect for every person's worth, dignity, and unique attributes;
2. Demonstrating a primary commitment to the patient;
3. Protecting the patient's rights, health and safety;
4. Making decisions and acting to promote health and provide optimal care;
5. Maintaining own health and safety, integrity, competence, and personal and professional growth;
6. Improving the ethical environment at work and employment conditions conducive to safe, quality health care;
7. Advancing the profession through scholarly inquiry, development of professional standards, and creating nursing and health policy;
8. Collaborating with others to reduce health disparities, protect human rights, and promote health globally;
9. Engaging in professional organizations to communicate nursing values and ethics that promote health and social justice (ANA, 2015b).

Another issue with ethical, as well as legal, implications is bullying within the nursing profession. Incivility and bullying are common in workplace settings. According to the American Nurses Association, incivility is "one or more rude, discourteous, or disrespectful actions that may or may not have a negative intent behind them," whereas bullying is defined as "repeated, unwanted, harmful actions intended to humiliate, offend, and cause distress in the recipient" (American Nurses Association, 2019). Either of these actions are unacceptable and adversely impact the ability of the nurse to care for patients and self. Such actions violate the fifth Provision of the *ANA Code of Ethics for Nurses with Interpretive Statements* (2015b) and result in moral distress and threats to personal integrity. It is essential that such behavior be promptly and thoroughly addressed. Incivility and bullying have no place in any health care facility, and everyone is responsible for ensuring a safe work environment.

LEGAL PERSPECTIVES

Unlike scientific facts, with black and white boundaries, the law provides guidance, mandates, and parameters for lawful practice, and the facts are ever-changing. For example, when nurses see a blood culture result, the result can be placed on a finite range of acceptable norms. However, when examining legal requirements, there may be shades of gray.

No one can practice as a nurse without meeting the legal requirements of the state(s) of licensure. When embarking on a nursing career—or if the nurse has been licensed for some number of years—it is critical that the state board of nursing websites be checked regularly for practice alerts and new laws, as well as legal and regulatory changes for all state(s) in which the nurse practices. A complete list of all state boards of nursing can be found at https://www.allnursingschools.com/how-to-become-a-nurse/state-boards/. Although foundational nursing theory is time honored, it is critical in today's fast-moving digital world that nurses take responsibility for their own knowledge and stay current. The nursing license is a privilege, not a right, which the nurse is given by meeting the licensing requirements throughout their career.

Some laws are designed to protect the nurse, and other laws are there to protect the public from errors or wrong practices done by the nurse. As health professionals, nurses have a duty to perform their practice consistent with all relevant laws, scopes of practice, standards of practice, and codes of ethics consistent with the nurse's education and experience. The concept of title protection, which pertains to who can call themselves "nurse," is designed to provide the public with safe, effective nurses who can be relied on to practice to the current standard of care. By establishing minimum mandatory standards, complemented by specialty certifications and mandatory continuing education, the public can depend on nurses regardless of location or facility where practice occurs. It is imperative that nurses acquire and maintain nursing practice skills and competencies. Patient outcomes rely on competent professional practice.

LEGAL DEFINITIONS

Legal concepts contain a variety of specific terms requiring definition.

Legal Terms

Cross-examination: The opportunity for the attorney to ask questions in court of a witness who has testified in a trial on behalf of the opposing party. The questions on cross-examination are limited to the subjects covered in the direct examination of the witness, but it is important to note that the attorney may ask leading questions, in which he or she is allowed to suggest answers or put words in the witness's mouth (Hill & Hill, 2019). These questions are usually answered with "yes" or "no."

Damages: The amount of money that a plaintiff (the person suing) may be awarded in a lawsuit. There are many types of damages. Special damages are those that were actually caused by the injury and include medical and hospital bills, ambulance charges, loss of wages, property repair or replacement costs, or loss of money due on a contract. The second basic area of damages is general damages, which are presumed to be a result of the other party's actions, but are subjective both in nature and determination of the value of the damages. These include pain and suffering, future problems and crippling effect of an injury, loss of ability to perform various acts, shortening of lifespan, mental anguish, and loss of companionship.

Deposition: The taking and recording of the testimony of a witness under oath before a court reporter in a place away from the courtroom before trial. A deposition is part of permitted pretrial discovery (investigation) set up by an attorney for one of the parties to a lawsuit demanding the sworn testimony of the opposing party (defendant or plaintiff), a witness to an event, or an expert intended to be called at trial by the opposition.

Direct examination: The first questioning of a witness during a trial or deposition (testimony out of court), as distinguished from cross-examination by opposing attorneys, and redirect examination when the witness is again questioned by the original attorney. Questions on direct examination cannot be answered with "yes" or "no."

Expert testimony: Opinions stated during trial or deposition (testimony under oath before trial) by a specialist qualified as an expert on a subject relevant to a lawsuit or a criminal case.

Expert witness: A person who is a specialist in a subject, often technical, who may present their expert opinion without having been a witness to any occurrence relating to the lawsuit or criminal case. This is an exception to the rule against giving an opinion in trial, provided that the expert is qualified by evidence of their expertise, training, and special knowledge. If the expertise is challenged, then the attorney for the party calling the expert must make a showing of the necessary background through questions in court, and the trial judge has discretion to qualify the witness or rule that they are not an expert or are an expert on limited subjects.

Fact witness: A lay witness who has firsthand knowledge of certain facts, having made observations, and can testify to material facts.

Lay witness: A witness who is not an expert witness.

Liable: Responsible or obligated. Thus, a person or entity may be liable for damages due to negligence.

Material fact: A fact upon which all or part of the outcome of a lawsuit depends.

Malpractice: See *professional negligence.*

Negligence: Failure to exercise the care toward others that a reasonable or prudent person would do in the circumstances, or taking action that such a reasonable person would not.

Profession: "Any type of work that needs special training or a particular skill, often one that is respected because it involves a high level of education" (Cambridge Dictionary, 2020a).

Professional judgment: "The application of professional knowledge and experience in defining objectives, solving problems, establishing guidelines, reviewing the work of others, interpreting results and providing and assessing advice or recommendations and other matters which have an element of latitude or decision-making" (Law Insider, 2019).

Professional negligence: An act or continuing conduct of a professional that does not meet the standard of professional competence and results in provable damages to their client or patient. Such an error or omission

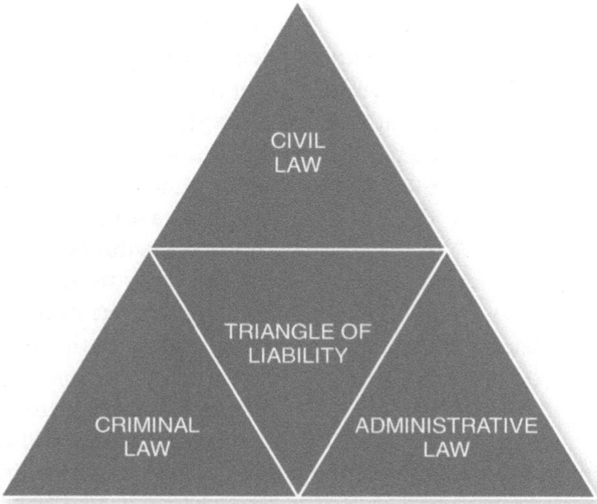

Fig. 7.1 Triangle of liability. From DePietro, S. C. (2016). *Legal and ethical issues in nursing professional development.* In C. M. Smith, & M. G. Harper (Eds.), Leadership in nursing professional development: An organizational & system focus (pp. 78–109). Chicago, IL: Association for Nursing Professional Development (ANPD).

may be through negligence, ignorance (when the professional should have known), or intentional wrongdoing. However, malpractice does not include the exercise of professional judgment even when the results are detrimental to the client or patient.

Types of Law

Administrative and Regulatory Law: These are **regulations** and rules that are created and enforced by federal and state agencies. Regulations about the workplace environment by the Occupational Safety and Health Administration (OSHA) and rules promulgated by the state board of nursing are examples.

Case Law: These are established by courts. **Case** law includes common law and the interpretation of statutes, including civil and criminal laws.

Statutory Law: These are laws passed by **legislative** bodies.

- **Civil:** Private law dealing with lawsuits between private individuals or parties.
- **Criminal:** Public law based on **statute** (enacted by federal or state legislatures) or **common law** (results from rules decided by the judiciary in court cases and referred to as a precedent set by a court), which consists of federal or state laws that make specific behaviors illegal (De Pietro, 2016).

Fig. 7.1 depicts the triangle of legal liability that displays the junctions of responsibility and accountability for health care professionals.

BACKGROUND

State Law and Nursing: Education and Licensure

Part of the way that a profession improves itself is to review its educational requirements and update as appropriate. More than ever, today's nurse is well-educated, because many states and territories are moving toward a minimum educational level of a bachelor's degree in nursing (BSN) for new nurses entering into the profession (NursingLicensure.org, 2019). This trend has been accelerated by *The Future of Nursing*, a report of the Institute of Medicine (IOM, now called the National Academies of Sciences, Engineering, and Medicine, Health and Medicine Division) (IOM, 2011) and its 80% BSN by 2020 challenge. New York was one of the first states to propose "BSN in 10," a concept that would require all nurses with an associate degree in applied sciences/nursing (AAS) or 3-year diploma from a hospital nursing program to obtain a BSN by their 10th year of licensure. Many hospitals, particularly those with the Magnet Recognition Program (R) designation, have established policies that reflect this model, even though states have not yet enacted such laws. Although the National Council of State Boards of Nursing's Licensure Examination (NCLEX) is a national standard, it is also a minimum national standard and may be only one element of the legal requirements for licensure in a state or territory. In addition, advanced practice is another area where state law defines the requirements, both educationally and clinically, for who may practice with a state-issued certification and/or supplemental license (laws and regulations vary by state), especially for nurse practitioners (Advanced Practice Registered Nurses [APRNs]).

> *"APRNs include certified registered nurse anesthetists, certified nurse-midwives, clinical nurse specialists and certified nurse practitioners. Each has a unique history and context but shares the commonality of being APRNs. While education, accreditation, and certification are necessary components of an overall approach to preparing an APRN for practice, the licensing boards—governed by state regulations and statutes—are the final arbiters of whom is recognized to practice within a given state. Currently, there is no uniform model of regulation of APRNs across the states. Each state independently determines the APRN legal scope of practice, the roles that are recognized, the criteria for entry into advanced practice, and the certification examinations accepted for entry-level competence assessment. This has created a significant barrier for APRNs to easily move from state to state and has decreased access to care for patients"*
>
> ***(APRN Joint Dialogue Group Report, 2008, p. 5).***

In each state the nurse practice act, administered by the state board of nursing, is the singular authoritative source to identify the educational, clinical, continuing education, fees, and all other requirements to satisfy the state's licensure requirements.

Administrative Law and State Boards of Nursing

The most well-known administrative laws are regulations that set the minimum standards for a licensed practitioner. These regulations are enforced by the state licensing board for that profession. The scope of practice for nurses is defined by the state and enforced by the state board of nursing. APRNs may be regulated by a separate practice act, or their scope of practice may be included in the state nurse practice act for registered nurses (RNs). Although regulations and state boards of nursing vary by state, the board of nursing can initiate disciplinary actions against nurses in any level of practice for the following:

1. Incompetence or failure to use knowledge, care, skill, and experience of a competent nurse;
2. Gross negligence or departure from standard of care;
3. Unprofessional conduct involving felony conviction, practicing medicine without a license, or possessing or using controlled or illegal drugs; and
4. Crimes such as theft, assault, abuse, fraud, or sexual offenses (De Pietro, 2016).

Disciplinary actions may include probation, suspension, or revocation of the nurse's license.

THE LEGAL SYSTEM AND SOURCES OF LAW

Nurses, nurse managers, and health care facilities are all subject to being found **legally liable** (i.e., legally responsible) for harm caused to others by civil wrongs. More specifically, liability is created when the law imposes a civil obligation on a wrongdoer to compensate an injured party for the consequences of a wrongful act. As shown in Fig. 7.2, there are two sources of legal liability: torts and contracts (Pozgar, 2019).

The most common source of legal liability for nurses and nurse managers is a *tort*. A tort is a wrongful act (other than breach of contract) committed against another person or organization or their property that causes harm and can be remedied by a civil (rather than criminal) lawsuit. Intentional torts are common civil lawsuits and include assault, battery, false imprisonment, property conversion, trespassing, and intentional infliction of emotional distress. In a health care setting, examples of an intentional tort are fear or apprehension of being touched in an offensive manner (assault) or the actual touching of someone without their consent (battery). Nurses should obtain consent before

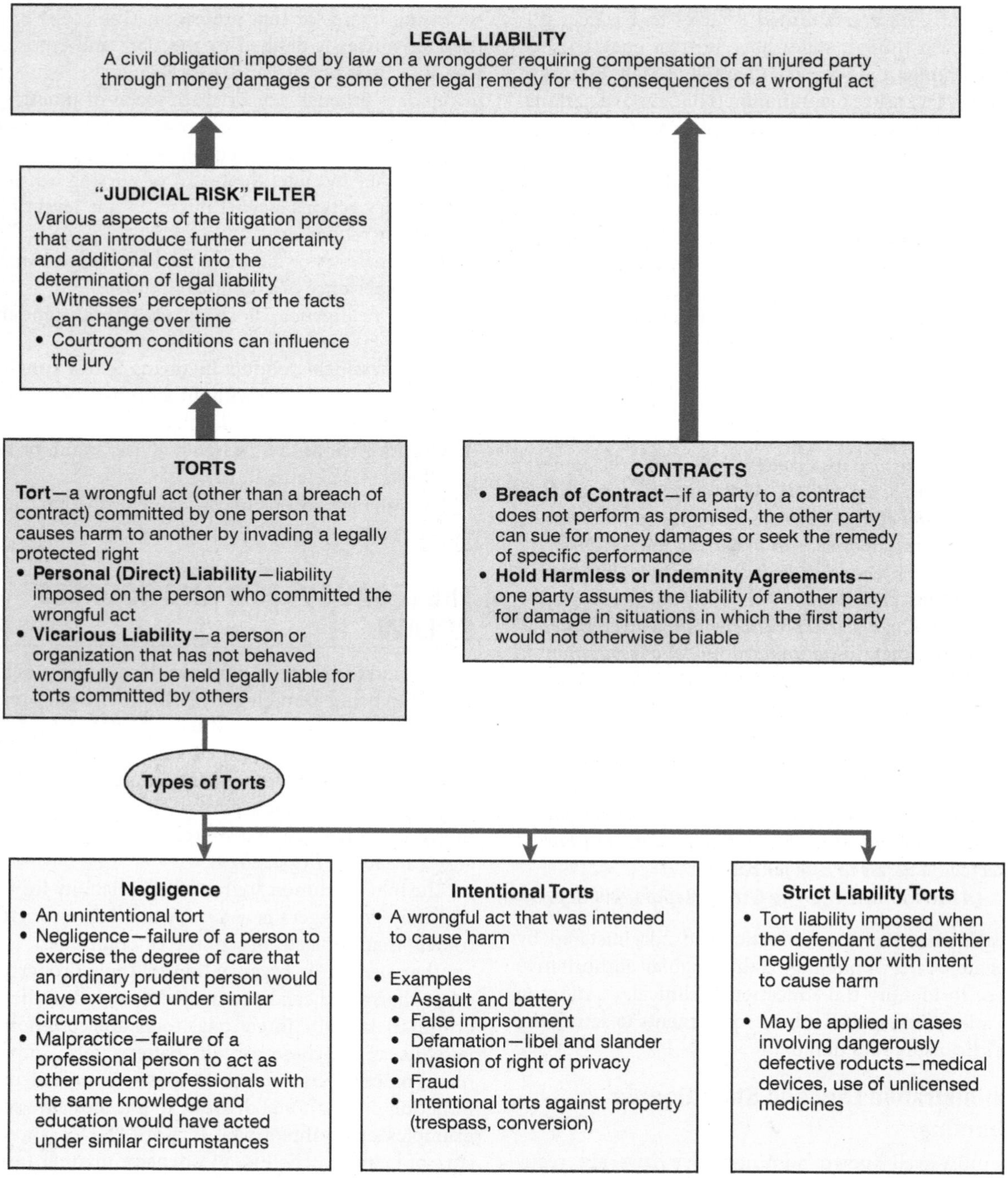
LEGAL LIABILITY
A civil obligation imposed by law on a wrongdoer requiring compensation of an injured party through money damages or some other legal remedy for the consequences of a wrongful act
"JUDICIAL RISK" FILTER
Various aspects of the litigation process that can introduce further uncertainty and additional cost into the determination of legal liability
• Witnesses' perceptions of the facts can change over time
• Courtroom conditions can influence the jury
TORTS
Tort—a wrongful act (other than a breach of contract) committed by one person that causes harm to another by invading a legally protected right
• Personal (Direct) Liability—liability imposed on the person who committed the wrongful act
• Vicarious Liability—a person or organization that has not behaved wrongfully can be held legally liable for torts committed by others
CONTRACTS
• Breach of Contract—if a party to a contract does not perform as promised, the other party can sue for money damages or seek the remedy of specific performance
• Hold Harmless or Indemnity Agreements—one party assumes the liability of another party for damage in situations in which the first party would not otherwise be liable
Types of Torts
Negligence
• An unintentional tort
• Negligence—failure of a person to exercise the degree of care that an ordinary prudent person would have exercised under similar circumstances
• Malpractice—failure of a professional person to act as other prudent professionals with the same knowledge and education would have acted under similar circumstances
Intentional Torts
• A wrongful act that was intended to cause harm
• Examples
• Assault and battery
• False imprisonment
• Defamation—libel and slander
• Invasion of right of privacy
• Fraud
• Intentional torts against property (trespass, conversion)
Strict Liability Torts
• Tort liability imposed when the defendant acted neither negligently nor with intent to cause harm
• May be applied in cases involving dangerously defective roducts—medical devices, use of unlicensed medicines

Fig. 7.2 Sources of legal liability.

initiating physical contact with clients (De Pietro, 2016). False imprisonment is seen when clients want to leave against medical advice or when they are restrained. An adult who has the capacity to make health care decisions and wants to leave the premises cannot be required to remain. The client must be informed about the consequences of this action, and organizational policies must be followed to address this issue. Nurses must also understand and follow their state's laws regarding clients restrained for psychiatric reasons (prevention of self-harm or harm to others) as these laws vary from state to state (De Pietro, 2016). Although torts most commonly give rise to *personal* (or *direct*) liability for the person committing the wrongful act, in some cases another person or organization may also be held *vicariously* liable for the same wrongful act they did not commit. For example, when a nurse commits a tort, the nurse may be found to be directly liable and the nurse's employer also may be found to be vicariously liable for the nurse's wrongful action (Pozgar, 2019).

As indicated in Fig. 7.2, determination of legal liability as a result of a tort depends on more than just the various technical elements of the tort that must be proved by the injured party (plaintiff), the presentation of various available defenses by the defendant, and the formal rules of the judicial system regarding the litigation process. In the case of torts, the legal outcomes are often influenced also by what may be termed *judicial risk*. This refers to various aspects of the litigation process that can introduce further uncertainty and additional cost into the determination of legal liability. Judicial risk can result in findings with respect to legal liability that are not based solely on the merits of the case nor on the rules of law applicable to the case (Pozgar, 2019).

What we refer to as the legal system is a multifaceted structure of federal, state, and local laws. In addition, there are regulations, which are rules that have full force and effect of law. In other words, in addition to statutes, there is a whole structure of rules created through an enabling statute. Such statutes give authority to an agency, such as the state board of nursing. There are two major divisions in the structure of the law: civil law and criminal law.

Civil Law

There are different standards by which defendants are judged in civil litigation: simple or regular negligence and professional negligence or *malpractice*.

Tort

A tort is a civil or personal wrong, compared with a crime, which is a public wrong. The purpose of tort law is to adjust losses by compensating one person because of the actions of another. Therefore the only remedy available in a civil lawsuit based on tort is monetary damages (i.e., money). Each intentional tort represents a direct interference with a person's physical integrity or right to property. Personal freedom is a fundamental right. One does not waive a fundamental right, such as personal integrity, automatically. On the contrary, a person must be aware that they possess a particular right and can intentionally relinquish it. This is the basis for the concept of informed consent.

Informed consent is a good example of a knowing and voluntary waiver of rights in the medical setting. In the absence of such a waiver of rights, a person touching or keeping another in a clinic, hospital, or any place they choose not to be, may be liable for assault, battery, or false imprisonment. Informed consent is a statutorily created right given to potential recipients of medical treatment. Most state statutes express that it is the duty of the physician to fully inform the patient as to the risks and benefits of a proposed procedure. The physician must also advise the patient of alternative treatments, if any, as well as the option to refuse any treatment. For the patient to be fully informed, the physician must advise the patient of all the potential risks and benefits of each option, including refusing the proposed treatment. Unless there is a specific statute, such as in the case of some APRNs, the physician's duty of informed consent is never transferred or delegated to a nurse.

Intentional torts are deliberate invasions of a person's legal rights and include assault, battery, false imprisonment, and trespassing. Unintentional torts result from negligence. These terms are often confused because they also exist within criminal law. Examples of an intentional tort in health care are forcing unwanted medical care on a patient or holding someone against their will.

Negligence. For a civil lawsuit to be successful in negligence, there are four required elements. These elements are commonly referred to as duty, breach, cause, and harm. All four of the elements must be proven, and the burden of proof is on the plaintiff (the one who brings the complaint). The plaintiff must prove that there was a well-established duty and an obvious breach of such duty. These proofs are not sufficient without also establishing the causal connection to the harm claimed. Proof of damages (harm) is an essential element to a negligence case. Negligence is sometimes referred to as simple negligence, compared with malpractice or professional negligence. This standard is used in cases such as motor vehicle accidents, personal injury (outside the medical setting), and property damage. The *standard of proof* for a simple or regular negligence case is that of a reasonably prudent person.

The concept of negligence is based on the idea that there can be a generally uniform standard of human behavior. The simplest example of this is that when one drives a car, there is a generally accepted expectation that each person will operate the vehicle in a reasonably prudent and careful manner. Each time there is a motor vehicle accident, it is likely that one or more persons deviated from the reasonably prudent person's standard, and liability may attach. However, state statutes may limit or expand a person's ability to bring a cause of action via a lawsuit (De Pietro, 2016).

Professional Negligence (Malpractice). The standard by which a licensed professional nurse (RN) will be judged comes from a governmental standard. The nurse's licensure and scope of practice are derived from the state's nurse practice act. All states and also US territories (Puerto Rico and Guam), have a nurse practice act. Links to all state boards of nursing and those states' nurse practice acts, can be found on individual state board of nursing websites or through the National Council of State Boards of Nursing (NCSBN, 2020a). Nurse practice acts provide broad statements defining nursing practice, delineating the educational and other requirements for licensure and renewal, giving notice to the public of the sort of behavior that can be expected from a nurse, and identifying what unacceptable practices might subject a nurse to disciplinary review or sanctions.

Professions develop a standard for themselves through a complex process of discussion and interaction within the profession and with other professions; knowledge dissemination such as peer reviewed professional journals; meetings; development of standards, guidelines, and statements; networking with colleagues; and the development and refining of academic programs both at the undergraduate and graduate levels for the profession. In addition, each profession has an obligation to monitor its members and self-police the behavior of its own.

For more than 17 years, nursing has been recognized by the general public in a Gallup poll as a highly esteemed profession for ethics and honesty (Brenan, 2018). Nurses have the respect and admiration of the American people and were acknowledged as the most trusted profession. Nurses should take great pride in this recognition. However, it also reminds nurses that they are always being watched by the public and are expected to conduct themselves in a professional, ethical, and truthful manner. Such accolades could easily be lost.

Professional Safeguards

Civil law controls those circumstances when an individual, the plaintiff, feels that he or she has been harmed by another. If the other person, known as the defendant, is a professional, the law provides for *professional liability,* also known as *malpractice*. Professionals are provided with many safeguards to avoid them being wrongfully accused of malpractice. Some of these safeguards include:

Statute of Limitations. A statutory time limit (most commonly 2 years) by which a plaintiff must file a lawsuit against a professional or lose that opportunity forever. In many states, there are exceptions to the time limitation for infants (children under a prescribed statutory age at the time of the alleged event) and an extension of time if the plaintiff was unaware of the injury at the time. One example is if a surgical count was incorrect at the completion of a procedure, an instrument or other substance was left in the patient's abdominal cavity in error, and the nurses "signed off" on the count. The patient is discharged, goes home, and does not have any symptoms or problems for 30 months, at which time it is discovered that the item has encapsulated, become infected, and the patient now requires additional surgery and/or suffers some other harm, even death. It is possible that a lawsuit could be filed as late as 2 years after the discovery of the indwelling item. The standard basis to file a professional liability/malpractice lawsuit is the time when the patient knew or should have known.

Affidavit of Merit. Another safeguard to protect the professional is the requirement of an affidavit of merit. An affidavit of merit is a sworn document by a like kind of professional (a doctor for a doctor defendant and a nurse for a nurse defendant) who reviews the injured patient's chart, and based upon the reviewer's education and experience, makes a statement that the case has merit and should be permitted to go to trial. Their opinion will also include that there is a likelihood of the plaintiff's success at trial. The person who reviews the record and provides the affidavit may never testify or have any other contact with the case.

Sources of Law. Laws are found in case books and online in official reports and legal research services. A reported case is one that can be found in an official reporter. There are state and also federal reporters. When entered into a reporter, the case is printed and becomes part of the ever-growing body of case law. It is important to remember that what is heard on the news, no matter the source, is simply news (maybe entertainment) and is not admissible as evidence at trial (De Pietro, 2016). Official sources of law need to be consulted and used when drawing conclusions.

Under both federal and state rules of evidence, the only way to prove professional negligence is through the use of expert witnesses. Expert witnesses need to be knowledgeable and up to date in their fields and familiar with texts, journals, and the relevant accepted standards of practice. These individuals are often published authors, leaders in the field, or academics.

The Nurse as Witness

There are times when a nurse is called on to testify at a deposition or appear to testify in court. The nurse may have been present in the hospital, clinic, or office setting where they made certain observations. This does not mean necessarily that the nurse is a party to the case; the nurse may not be a defendant. There are two general categories of witnesses who testify at trial: the fact witness and the expert witness.

A **fact witness** is someone who can testify from their own observations. In other words, the nurse can apply their senses to a fact or set of circumstances (e.g., I saw…, I heard…, I smelled…). For example, the nurse might have observed a patient fall in a hospital hallway, but it was not their patient; the person was with another staff member, but the nurse saw the fall. That nurse could testify as a fact witness (sometimes referred to as an eyewitness) to those events that were seen, heard, or felt. A fact witness may not offer an opinion, but must testify only as to personal knowledge.

An **expert witness** is a person with specialized knowledge who aids the judge and jury (in the case of a jury trial) to understand something that is beyond the scope of the average individual. There are multiple standards in determining whether one can be considered an expert witness. Experts base their opinions and their testimony on their knowledge, education, and experience. State and federal rules of evidence require that a patient claiming that a professional is responsible for their injuries and damages use a "like-kind" expert witness to prove their case (Federal Rules of Evidence 703,704; Legal Information Institute, 2020).

A professional liability case cannot be proven without an expert witness who can testify as to actions or inactions of the professional defendant. Simply put, only a nurse can testify as to the standard of care and scope of practice of another nurse. If the nurse works in a specialty area such as professional case management, the operating room, or the emergency department (ED), a like-kind nurse should be the one to testify as an expert for that particular nurse defendant.

There are typically two experts: one for the plaintiff and one for the defendant nurse. An expert witness is only as good as their education and experience in two critical ways: first by establishing and maintaining credibility by having expertise in the required field, and second by withstanding cross-examination by the plaintiff's attorney. The fastest way to be excluded as an expert witness is to "step outside your sandbox." Any document, text, or other material that an expert refers to in their written report and/or testimony must be available, and in most cases, is admissible into evidence.

It is important to note that if the expert refers to such a document, they must be fully familiar with the entire document. It would be appropriate cross-examination for the nurse to be asked about something in the text or other reference that has nothing to do with the present case and that the expert made no reference to; it goes to the expert's credibility. In other words, did the expert simply "cherry pick" a small portion of a reference that related to the facts, or is that expert fully familiar with the foundational materials? In recent years, some states have permitted professionals whose practice area overlaps with the defendants to testify, although other states interpret the "like-kind" expert strictly. The attorney who seeks a nurse's assistance as an expert should be fully familiar with the criteria in the jurisdiction. However, even those experts who are experienced in courtroom testimony can be enticed to step outside their area of expertise. The next thing that happens is that there is an objection to the witness and their testimony in whole or in part, the expert's credibility is ruined, and an otherwise solid case begins to crumble (De Pietro, 2016).

Criminal Law

Criminal law is based on statutes. Statutes are laws created by the legislature and signed into law by the executive, the governor for state laws, and the president of the United States for federal laws.

Crimes are prohibitions against behaviors that are so egregious that they offend society, not just the individual victim. Crimes are punishable with fines and/or jail, depending on the level of the offense and other factors, and these consequences are delineated in the criminal statute. Nurses can be subject to criminal law for such behaviors as stealing or misusing narcotics, practicing without a license, or intentionally causing physical harm to a person in their care. These criminal offenses violate the public trust and safety and carry serious consequences.

LICENSURE, MULTI-STATE, AND DISTANCE PRACTICE

There is no doubt that the world in which nurses' practice today has been dramatically and forever affected by advances in technology. Gone are the days when the only interaction between nurse and patient was at arm's length. Today, with the advent of electronic health records (EHR), telephonic, e-mail, text, and video connections, nurses and patients can interact from across town or across the country. Distance communications need to be considered with great caution: just because we can, does not mean we should. The law is slow to catch up with technical advances. Although there has been much talk about cost-effective interventions through electronic means, the nurse must adhere to the law. As it stands today, nurses must be licensed in each and every state/jurisdiction in which they practice.

> *"Uniform Licensure Requirements (ULRs) are the essential prerequisites for initial, endorsement, renewal and reinstatement licensure needed across every NCSBN jurisdiction to ensure the safe and competent practice of nursing. ULRs protect the public by setting consistent standards and promoting a health care system that is fluid and accessible by removing barriers to care and maximizing portability for nurses. They also assure the consumer that a nurse in one state has met the requirements of the nurses in every other state. ULRs support the fact that the expectations for the education of a nurse and the responsibilities of a nurse are the same throughout every NCSBN member board jurisdiction in the United States."*
>
> ***(NCSBN, 2019)***

The Nurse Licensure Compact (NLC) allows nurses to have one multistate license, with the ability to practice in both their home state and other compact states. There are currently 34 states in the NLC (NCSBN, 2020b). In 2015 significant revisions were made to the NLC Model Act, requiring all legislatures to revisit the issue. Revisions were made, in part, in response to objections from some states, and it is hoped that the NLC will grow significantly in the coming years to make it easier for nurses to work across state lines. If a nurse lives or works near another state's border, it is often tempting, and may be requested, that the nurse speak telephonically or go in person to deliver care to persons in the neighboring state. Thus it is imperative that nurses be licensed in each state in which they deliver care; otherwise care can only be legally delivered to patients in the state in which the nurse is licensed.

Distance practice is nothing new, but the tools and technologies available today make distance practice far easier and are predicted to become more common. Telehealth, telemedicine, and case management practice are examples where distance practice occurs. There is a two-pronged test to determine if a distance communication is permitted, whether by telephonic, e-mail, or another electronic device. The first test is that the nurse must examine the content of the communication, and the second test is whether that communication constitutes the practice of nursing.

Example #1: Nursing process begins with assessment. Assessment is a "systematic, dynamic way to collect and analyze data about a client, the first step in delivering nursing care. Assessment includes not only physiological data, but also psychological, sociocultural, spiritual, economic, and life-style factors as well" (ANA, 2020). Assessment can start with a simple telephone call, "Good morning. How are you?" If the nurse asks that simple question, "How are you?" and the patient responds with symptoms, then the nurse, based on their knowledge and experience, uses critical thinking, makes professional judgments, and takes action. That is the practice of nursing. To conduct such a dialogue across state lines, the nurse must be licensed in the state where the patient is located. Therefore in this example the nursing process has been established, and licensure is necessary.

Example #2: The caller contacts the patient and says, "Good morning, I'm calling to follow up and remind you of your appointment with Dr. Smith. I've arranged for transportation; the car will pick you up tomorrow morning. Is that ok? Is there anything else I can do for you?" No assessment occurred, no nursing process was initiated, and no nursing skill, based on education and training, was required to conduct this communication. Anyone with minimal training (such as a high school graduate) could perform this task. Review of Chapter 6 on role management will be helpful and provide parameters for appropriate task delegation.

LEGAL DOCUMENTS AND THE NURSE

It is important for the nurse to have a working knowledge of certain legal documents that affect practice. It is not uncommon for the nurse to encounter powers of attorney or advance directives for health care (also referred to as living wills or powers of attorney for health care, depending on the jurisdiction). Patients are asked before admission whether they have a living will or similar document, but what happens to that document varies greatly from facility to facility, even in the same state. The most important thing that the nurse must take away from a discussion of legal documents is that the nurse must actually see the document. It is not enough for an individual to say, "I am the health care representative/proxy" or "I'm the power of attorney," which is simply a misuse of the term.

Power of attorney is the document used for the appointment of another person, referred to as the principal, and empowers that person (the attorney-in-fact or agent) to act on behalf of the principal. In other words, by way of a legal document, one person gives authority to another to act and perform certain functions on behalf of that person. The power of attorney is a document, a writing, prescribed by state law, which can grant very limited or very broad powers to the attorney-in-fact (the agent). It is common to hear people say, "I have power of attorney." That may be a true statement if there is a document that assigns such a power, but it is actually incorrect to say, "I am the power of attorney." Misusing these terms overextends or improperly limits the authority of the attorney-in-fact.

Confusion regarding these terms often stems from those states that permit the use of the term "power of attorney" to extend to health care proxies and directives, commonly called living wills. New York, Michigan, and California are among the states that use a durable power of attorney for health care as the legal document for use as a living will. Other states, like New Jersey, use an advanced directive for health care (*The New Jersey Advance Directives for Health Care Act*, NJ. Stat. §. 26:2H-53–78). No matter what "power" an individual is asserting, without actually seeing the document (or a facsimile thereof where permitted), the nurse may risk a Health Information Portability and *Accountability Act of 1996* (HIPAA) violation or other liability exposure by disclosing information to one who is not entitled to such access (De Pietro, 2016; Pozgar, 2019).

Guardianship

Parents are the guardians of their children until the child reaches the age of majority in the particular state. Typically, this is at 18 years of age, but there are exceptions. Certain states have greatly reduced the age of consent, particularly in the medical setting. It is important to understand the purpose of the rule of law and the requirements in the state(s) in which the nurse practices.

A *guardian* is a person appointed by a court via a judge. In the normal course of events, a parent is the guardian of their child, but all that changes on the child's eighteenth birthday. There are many types of guardians. *A general guardian* is appointed if the court finds that an individual is incapacitated, according to that state's legal definition of incapacity, to govern or manage their affairs. The general guardian exercises all rights and powers of the incapacitated person concerning both the rights of the person and their financial assets, income, and responsibilities (NJ. Stat. §3B:12—24.1). The nurse must pause when any person represents to the nurse, the hospital, or the agency that they are the guardian of a person or custodian of that person's affairs. They *must* provide you with a copy of the specific court order naming them as the guardian over a named person, with any limitations to that guardianship.

Guardian ad litem is a temporary appointment of a person by a court to act on behalf of another for a specific purpose. Typically it is an adult who will take legal action on behalf of a minor child or an adult who is unable to handle their own affairs, even when represented by an attorney. For example, the *guardian ad litem* may file a lawsuit for a child who is injured in an automobile accident or by some other means. *Guardian ad litem* may also be appointed following the death of a person in order to file claim against an estate on behalf of a child or incompetent adult (Phillips & Walsh, 2018).

The Problem of the Adult Child

When a child reaches the age of majority—18 years in most jurisdictions—the parent no longer has access to medical records, nor do parents have the right to make medical decisions for their children. It is difficult for a devoted loving parent to simply stop, when yesterday the privilege and burden of making medical decisions for their child(ren) fell to them, and then the next day, on the eighteenth birthday, this stopped. The problem is further magnified when the child has a disability and special needs. The nurse is in a unique position to have insight and understanding into the child's (now a young adult) needs. In cases where the young adult is not competent to make their own medical decisions, guardianship may be a viable option. In most states, this is a complex procedure requiring an attorney's advice and at least one court appearance.

For a child who is unable to communicate but has the mental capacity to make their own choices, the legal documents described in this chapter are useful tools. It is the nurse's legal and ethical duty to protect the adult "child's" autonomy and not simply accept a parent's intervention, without lawful authority, just because it may seem easier at the moment. Along with incredible advances in prosthetics, electronic aids, and assistive devices, children and adults who were once unable to function in schools, universities, and the workforce are now able to. Thus the limits are being tested with regard to individual autonomy.

Confidentiality and Access to Medical Information

Patient confidentiality has been a central theme to medical and nursing practice for generations, but the rules governing access and release of medical records were solidified about 25 years ago with the advent of HIPAA (Public Law 104–191). Even though HIPAA is federal law and preempts state law, there is great variation from state to state. HIPAA is a minimum mandatory standard. States are permitted to provide additional protections to their residents, but no law can limit or reduce a right provided under federal law. An interactive map is available at: https://medcitynews.com/2017/06/need-interactive-map-understand-disparity-healthcare-data-sharing-u-s/ and provides a state-by-state comparison. Iowa, Alabama, and New Hampshire are examples of states whose law was preempted by HIPAA and provides no additional access or rights. California, Colorado, New York, and Nevada provide greater access and protection; they require release of medical records to those who properly make requests in a specific number of days, even though providers are permitted to charge reasonable fees for accessing and copying records (Zaleski, 2017). One of the goals of EHRs was to make provision of medical records to patients who request them easier to access, faster and less expensive to copy, and more accessible to patients (Pozgar, 2019). See the Research Note (Ben-Assuli, 2015) and De Simone (2019) for a discussion of electronic records as important legal documents.

Demonstrating Compliance

Legal compliance is demonstrated by holding and maintaining a professional license in each and every jurisdiction in which the nurse practices, whether in person, telephonically, or through other means of electronic communication. The nurse must maintain up-to-date knowledge through continuing education as mandated by the state(s) of licensure and adhere to all applicable laws and regulations.

Adhering to all applicable federal, state, and local laws and employer policies, is the general principle of necessary compliance, but there is a hierarchy to these duties. Federal law *preempts* state law. Law will always supersede hospital or other employer policies and procedures. Legal compliance is broader than simply following the rules for correct drug dosage, route, and observations of the patient; it starts with patient assessment and goes through full discharge of duties at the standard of care of a reasonable and prudent nurse.

Regulatory Compliance

Regulations are rules that have the same effect as laws. They are created based on a statute, giving authority to an agency or the director of an agency, to create regulations to further the purpose of the enabling statute. HIPAA has now been a part of health care and health care practice for about 25 years. Protecting health information is the core of the law and all the regulations that followed. Nurses need to be familiar with who the privacy officer is in whatever entity they work and use resources to educate and reeducate themselves with the requirements in their state.

The HIPAA Privacy Rule was published on December 28, 2000, with the goal of providing consumers with greater rights for protection of individually identifiable health information, sometimes referred to as personal health information (PHI). In the spring of 2003, there were further modifications to the Final Privacy Rule. The key to HIPAA, and all the changes and improvements over time, is meeting the educational requirement (at minimum, a yearly update) and demonstrating genuine compliance. The Privacy Rule is only part of HIPAA compliance requirements. There are complex regulations controlling the use of electronic communications, including telephone, fax, e-mail, and text messaging, as well as, billing and reporting requirements (Pozgar, 2019).

HIPAA responsibilities come to us as building blocks. The patient privacy rules and access to medical records do not go away when a new responsibility is added. Each new aspect, addition or modification of the law requires that each practitioner have not only a basic understanding of HIPAA (1996), but an ever-enlarging knowledge base regarding HIPAA, the *Health Information Technology for Economic and Clinical Health (HITECH) Act*, which is a portion of the *American Recovery and Reinvestment Act of 2009 (ARRA) 26 USC 1* and the Final Omnibus Rule (2013), and subtle changes that continue to be made. In January 2016, the HIPAA restriction on the disclosure of PHI was modified by agency amendment. "The Department of Health and Human Services issued a final rule expressly permitting certain HIPAA covered entities to provide to the [National Instant Criminal Background Check System] NICS limited demographic and other necessary information about these individuals" (Obama, 2016, p. 1). It is important to obtain and update knowledge of all HIPAA and state privacy and confidentiality mandates.

The Personal Representative

The Department of Health and Human Services (HHS, 2020, p. 1) "recognizes that there may be times when individuals are legally or otherwise incapable of exercising their rights, or simply choose to designate another to act on their behalf with respect to these rights. Under the Rule, a person authorized (under State or other applicable law, e.g., tribal or military law) to act on behalf of the individual in making health care related decisions is the individual's 'personal representative.' Section 164.502(g) provides when, and to what extent, the personal representative must be treated as the individual for purposes of the Rule. In addition to these formal designations of a personal representative, the Rule at 45 CFR 164.510(b) addresses situations in which family members or other persons who are involved in the individual's health care or payment for care may receive protected health information about the individual even if they are not expressly authorized to act on the individual's behalf."

Incident Reports

Incident-reporting systems are set up as a way to report errors, especially safety errors. They are used to gather data and information about patient safety occurrences for organizational learning. There are three types of incidents: a harmful incident, a no-harm incident, and a near miss. Incident-reporting systems are part of risk-management efforts and are voluntary but set an expectation for reporting. Barriers to reporting include personal reasons such as fear, accountability, and nurse characteristics, in addition to organizational factors such as culture, the reporting system, and management behavior (Vrbnjak et al., 2016; Wang et al., 2019). One study found that hospital personnel frequently encounter safety problems that they themselves can resolve on the spot. Fixing and forgetting, instead of fixing and reporting, was the main choice when handling near misses (seen as unworthy of reporting), solving a patient's safety problem (seen as unique or a one-time event), or encountering recurring problems (seen as inevitable, routine events). Although common, fixing and forgetting does not serve as the best organizational handling of patient safety or its risk-management efforts because it does not make patient safety more preventive. This leads to workarounds that may be a set-up for recurring problems (Huber et al., 2019). Nurses may incur liability and risk, with possible ethical implications, if incidents are not properly reported so that investigation and organizational intervention can occur.

LEADERSHIP AND MANAGEMENT IMPLICATIONS

By the very nature of their work, nurses and nurse managers are decision makers who are constantly faced with making choices in personal, clinical, and organizational situations. These decision-making situations are commonly fraught with legal and ethical issues that often become entwined. As members of a profession, nurses and nurse managers are guided by both legal and ethical considerations in making decisions. The legal aspects of nursing management center on decision-making and supervision. Because all nurses retain personal accountability for their own acts and the use of knowledge and skills in the provision of care, personal accountability cannot be assumed by another. Nurse managers keep their own personal accountability for their own specific acts, but they are accountable also for their acts of delegation and supervision (Pozgar, 2019).

Nurse managers carry the major responsibility for developing and upholding the standards of care for the staff. Nurses and nurse managers carry the accountability for the supervision of others, who are often unlicensed assistive personnel. Supervision includes monitoring the tasks performed, ensuring that functions are performed in an appropriate fashion, and ensuring that assigned tasks and functions do not exceed competency or require a license to perform. Nurse managers use their autonomy to make decisions about practice situations. They are accountable for carrying out supervisory responsibilities; proper notification; assessing the competency of staff; training, orientation, and evaluation of staff; reasonable staffing decisions; and monitoring and maintenance of professional treatment relationships with clients, called *non-abandonment* (Pozgar, 2019).

The managers of any health care organization are responsible to the policy-making body of the organization and hold an obligation to comply with the laws of society at local, state, and national levels. Managers are responsible for ensuring that laws are adhered to in the actions of management itself and also in the actions of those employees who assist the managers in carrying out the mission of the organization. Concern for the law involves three general areas: personal negligence in clinical practice, liability for delegation and supervision, and liability of health care organizations (Pozgar, 2019).

Personal Negligence in Clinical Practice

Activities of clinical client care involve corresponding legal accountability and risk. Errors do happen, and some lead to injury to a client. At minimum, nurses have an ethical obligation to nonmaleficence, or to do no harm to clients. This duty is discharged in part by remaining competent in knowledge and skills and the standards of practice. Nursing negligence/malpractice occurs when the nurse's actions are unreasonable given the circumstances, fail to meet the standard of care, or when the nurse fails to act and causes harm. In nursing, harm related to clinical practice commonly arises from negligent acts or omissions (unintentional torts) and a variety of intentional acts (intentional torts), such as invasion of privacy or assault and battery. To establish legal liability on the grounds of malpractice (professional negligence), the injured client (plaintiff) must prove these four elements:

1. A duty of care was owed to the injured party.
2. There was a breach of that duty.
3. The breach of the duty caused the injury (causation).
4. Actual harm or damages were suffered by the plaintiff.

When errors occur, nurses are advised to work with organizational risk management and establish a strategy for disclosure and apology (Russell, 2018).

Common clinical practice areas that give rise to allegations of malpractice include the general areas of treatment, communication, medication, and the broad category of monitoring/observing/supervising/surveillance. Examples of common negligence allegations in nursing malpractice suits include patient falls, use of restraints, medication errors, burns, equipment injuries, retained foreign objects, failure to monitor, failure to ensure safety, failure to take appropriate nursing action, failure to confirm accuracy of physicians' orders, improper technique or performance of treatments, failure to respond to a patient, failure to follow hospital procedure, and failure to supervise treatment (Pozgar, 2019). Although there is little research into cases where a nurse lost a license or was sued by a patient, there are some case studies recounting specific situations. For example, Wilson (2018) described a long-term care case where the facility was sued for inaccurate recordkeeping and failing to document and report changes in condition. Accurate documentation and prompt reporting by nurses were major issues.

Both nurses and nurse managers have a duty to follow organizational policies and procedures when reasonable. Nurse managers are advised to review policies and procedures carefully, including the language used, in order to adhere to legal and ethical parameters more closely. Clearly management in nursing practice means that nurses must fulfill obligations and duties both to clients and to the organization. This means using knowledge, skill, and decision-making abilities to reduce the incidence of negligence and malpractice by employees as a way to reduce harm to clients and legal risk to the organization. As the primary coordinators of care, nurses need to manage the environment of care delivery. Ensuring staff competence and reporting incompetent practice are key activities. For example, in nursing, legal and ethical issues arise when a nurse is impaired by substance abuse. The overall consideration is protecting the client from harm. Confronting suspected abuse must be done carefully, but when an incident occurs, the nurse manager has a responsibility to intervene (Pozgar, 2019).

Liability of Health Care Organizations

Health care facilities face extensive exposure to legal liability from several sources, in addition to the liability faced by nurses and nurse managers arising out of malpractice in clinical practice, and negligence in the process of delegating and supervising. These sources include negligence of their employees, negligence of independent contractors, corporate negligence arising out of the facility's responsibilities to hire qualified employees and monitor and supervise their activities, and failure to comply with numerous laws and regulations, especially those related to employment issues. Nurse managers have important roles to play in helping their organizations control facility liability arising from each of these sources (Pozgar, 2019).

Nurse managers can help the facility avoid corporate liability by, among other things, ensuring that those who report to them remain competent and qualified and have current licensure. Nurse managers should also report dangerously low staffing levels, incorrect mixes of staff for effectively meeting the health care needs of clients, and report incompetent, illegal, or unethical practices to appropriate authorities. Nurse managers have an important role to play in compliance with human resources (HR) areas of hiring, performance appraisal, management of employees with problems, and termination (Pozgar, 2019).

HR management is a major area for organizational liability. Nursing is a labor-intensive occupation. Some organizations are unionized. Labor and employment law include various laws and regulations that deal with issues related to hiring, firing, employee benefits, compensation, overtime, workplace safety, privacy, drug testing, and preventing discrimination, harassment, and violence. Because of the volume, variety, and complexity of local, state, and federal HR-related laws and regulations, organizations have HR departments whose function is to implement strategies and policies related to employee management.

Mandatory Reporting

Among the many duties under one's professional license to practice nursing is the duty to report. This duty sits firmly on the fence between legal and ethical responsibilities and is a good example of those times when a legal obligation is affected by ethics. This duty to report includes observations of children, elders, disabled, developmentally compromised, and anyone who is at risk or in a vulnerable situation. Licensed professionals have had an affirmative "duty to warn" ever since the 1976 decision of the Supreme Court of California in the case of *Tarasoff v. Regents of the University of California*, 551 P.2d 334 (1976). Since that time, nurses and other health professionals have struggled to identify the triggering point in a patient relationship that rises to the statutory "duty to warn" (Muller & Fink-Samnick, 2015). Initially, the case stood for the concept that if there was a specific threat against an individual, the therapist (in that case) was legally obligated to warn that individual and enable him/her to take steps to protect themselves. In other words, the threat had to be specific to an identifiable individual. Citing previous cases, the court said, "We recognize the difficulty that a therapist encounters in attempting to forecast whether a patient presents a serious danger of violence. Obviously, we do not require that the therapist, in making that determination, render a perfect performance; the therapist need only exercise 'that reasonable degree of skill, knowledge, and care ordinarily possessed and exercised by members of [that professional specialty] under similar circumstances'" (Tarasoff v. Regents of the University of California, 1976, p. 8).

In 2007 the California legislature codified Tarasoff, along with subsequent cases. The then-new law increased the duty to one that is twofold: (1) the duty to inform the potential victim of the risk, and (2) the duty to inform appropriate law enforcement. In the passage of time, states have adopted varying duties for nurses, therapists, social workers, physicians, and other practitioners. It is critical that nurses make inquiry and be fully familiar as to the requirement(s) of the state(s) in which they practice. The National Conference of State Legislatures (NCSL, 2019) lists those states that have laws in place. There are three types of laws: mandatory reporting, permissive reporting, and no reporting requirement at all.

CURRENT ISSUES AND TRENDS

Legal Issues and the Changing Family Dynamic

The ideal American family is no longer a mother, father and 2.6 children (Gao, 2015), and even if the number of children remains constant, the makeup of the family has changed. According to one definition, a family is "a social group of parents, children, and sometimes grandparents, uncles, aunts, and others who are related" (Cambridge Dictionary, 2020b). On June 26, 2015, the US Supreme Court issued its decision in *Obergefell et al. v. Hodges, Director, Ohio Department of Health, et al.* The court held that, "The Fourteenth Amendment requires a State to license a marriage between two people of the same sex and to recognize a marriage between two people of the same sex when their marriage was lawfully licensed and performed out-of-State" (Obergefell v. Hodges, 2015, pp. 3–28).

The traditional US concept of a family is clearly undergoing change. Nurses are confronted with families who may be structured in ways that are completely different from their own life experience and beliefs. Although nurses are entitled to their personal beliefs, those beliefs must remain outside the nurse–patient relationship. The duty as a nurse is to obey the law and act toward all patients, their families, and/or family caregiver with respect, providing them with the care and education that the circumstance requires. This issue is also directly related to the issue of consent and who may give consent for treatment on behalf of the patient. Questions in the practice setting should be referred to supervision, administration, or legal counsel within the facility or practice setting.

Staffing

In view of the significant degrees of change and uncertainty associated with the legal and ethical aspects affecting decision-making in nursing care management, there are important current issues and trends in this area. A major current and continuing issue is the nurse shortage, which for a number of reasons is expected to continue in the foreseeable future. This issue gives rise to a number of legal and ethical challenges for nurse managers and staff nurses. The nurse shortage has resulted in a major problem called short staffing caused largely by increases in cost-cutting measures and other financial constraints, and also from deterioration of working conditions. Short staffing refers to the use of an insufficient nursing staff on a unit or in a facility for the number of patients requiring care at various acuity levels. Consequences commonly associated with short staffing include:

- Deterioration of patient outcomes in terms of increased mortality and failure-to-rescue rates (Needleman et al., 2020; Walker, 2018);
- A general decline in the quality of patient care (Bridges et al., 2019; Carthon et al., 2019);
- Deterioration of nurse outcomes resulting from increased burnout and greater job dissatisfaction (Van Bogaert et al., 2017);
- Increases in organizational costs resulting from increased turnover (NSI Nursing Solutions, Inc., 2019);
- Legal liability.

In an effort to deal with short staffing, nurse managers are often required to do the following: float nurses to areas in which they are not cross-trained, an action that also increases the client-to-nurse ratio closer to staffing requirements; use agency (temporary) personnel; and use unlicensed personnel. Staff nurses, nurse managers, and health care facilities all face numerous possibilities of legal liability—as well as dilemmas involving conflicts between clinical and organizational ethics—as a result of short staffing and actions taken in an effort to temporarily solve this problem (Broadway, 2019).

Nurses need to focus on their use of expert judgment in practicing the highest legal and ethical standards in the quest for high-quality care and services. In some instances, they may also be called on to demonstrate moral courage, which is the courage to honor ethical core values in the face of personal risk. Strategies that are available to the nurse leader chiefly focus on the use of multidisciplinary teams because they can provide an expert group approach to addressing moral and ethical issues. Although not providing definitive answers, the use of a group approach increases the knowledge and ideas that can be brought to bear on the situation and increases analysis that helps to shape the best possible decision under difficult circumstances.

RESEARCH NOTE

Source

Ben-Assuli, O. (2015). Electronic health records, adoption, quality of care, legal and privacy issues, and their implementation in emergency departments. *Health Policy, 119*(3) 287–297.

Purpose

The purpose of this article was to review and analyze proposed and actual uses of electronic health records (EHR) and health information exchanges (HIE) in the emergency department (ED) and the implications and impact of use of these technologies from the clinical and legal standpoint. The focus was on the current body of evidence regarding the status of care quality as Health Information Technology (HIT) implementation becomes more common.

Discussion

The study reviewed use of EHR around the world and found varying degrees of success. One large and successful study was that of the veterans' health system in the United States. This particular study included over 1000 hospitals. Overall, the study found a greater degree of success in non-profit public (government run) hospitals. Training and readiness had a direct impact on the success and compliance with the newly adopted programs. Regulations requiring EHR have a direct impact on compliance and Medicare and Medicaid use, which—although lower at the time of the study—has increased due to regulatory mandates for phased-in implementation. In the ED, ease of use and accessibility of the system may well be a barrier to adoption if the system design does not take into account physicians' busy workflow.

Legal and privacy concerns are significant due to the rapid advancement of technology. Portable devices and security of patient information are paramount in analysis of the costs and benefits of EHR. One concern was that convenience may lead to carelessness, such a "cut and paste." The issue of accidents or mistakes while using these new systems (due to information technology [IT] glitches and bugs) raises new and unanswered questions about potential liability as it relates to professional liability (malpractice). In addition, there is concern that interaction with the IT system may negatively affect the quality of care, thus again exposing medical professionals to liability. Protecting and maintaining patient privacy has always been a nursing responsibility, but with the advent of uploading and sharing of medical information through an electronic system, these burdens take on new concerns.

Application to Practice

Particular concerns were raised with regard to certain practice areas, such as maternity, contraception, and sexual and mental health. Logic would also indicate that other sensitive areas such as drug and alcohol use, HIV/AIDS, sexual orientation, and transgender issues would generate privacy issues. Would patients resist being forthcoming with sensitive information, knowing that their information would be put into "the system"? Nurses need to be sensitive to patient concerns and use interviewing and observational skills to overcome potential gaps in necessary information.

Policies and procedures are critical to framing how nursing will use electronic access, information, and reporting. Safeguards must be established in cooperation with the IT department. Nurses must always be mindful of HIPAA implications and participate whenever possible in the creation and modification of polices affecting patient privacy. Segregating personal information from patient information and protecting patient privacy must never become lax. Compliance with HIPAA and state privacy laws must be at the forefront of practice.

CASE STUDY

Falsification of records is an ethical as well as legal issue. Mary Smith is a registered nurse in a Transitional Care Nursery and one of her responsibilities is to perform heel stick blood glucose determinations for all newborn infants within 1 hour of admission from Labor and Delivery. The patient care assistant assigned to the unit notices that some neonates have no heel stick marks. All documentation in the electronic medical record shows acceptable glucose readings. The patient care assistant reports her concerns to the nursing supervisor who checks the heels of several infants with charted glucose readings by the registered nurse. There is no evidence that the heel sticks have been performed.

1. What actions does the nursing supervisor take and why?
2. What ethical principle has been violated?
3. What ethical rule has been violated?
4. How has ANA's *Code of Ethics for Nurses with Interpretive Statements* (2015) been violated?

CRITICAL THINKING EXERCISE

Michael Jones is the nursing professional development coordinator who is orienting eight newly employed nurses. Five are new graduates and three are experienced nurses who are transitioning to positions in the hospital. This is the third day of orientation. Michael notices that one of the experienced nurses (Amy) constantly corrects one of the new graduates and the graduate nurse (Beth) is no longer asking questions or offering comments. At the end of the day, Michael is in his office preparing for tomorrow's class. Beth asks to speak to him. It is obvious that she has been crying. Michael asks what he can help her with, and she says she overheard Amy tell her experienced colleagues that Beth would never succeed as a nurse. Beth's self-confidence is clearly shaken, and she doesn't know what to do.

1. What action should Michael take?
   a. Tell Beth that she will have to deal with negative people and not take what she hears personally.
   b. Talk with Beth about approaches she can use to diffuse negative comments.
   c. Ensure that Beth is safe to go home and plan to talk with Amy privately before the next class.
2. How can Michael address bullying behavior?
   a. Ask Amy to explain why she is picking on Beth.
   b. Discuss with Amy why such bullying behavior cannot be tolerated in the organization and explore approaches with her to resolve this issue.
   c. Tell Amy that you don't want to hear any more complaints during orientation.
3. What is Michael's responsibility when bullying or incivility occurs?
   a. Maintain a safe positive learning environment.
   b. Avoid calling attention to negative behavior.
   c. Tell both parties to deal with the issue outside class.

REFERENCES

American Nurses Association. (2010). *Nursing's social policy statement: The essence of the profession* (3rd ed.). Silver Spring, MD: American Nurses Association.

American Nurses Association. (2015a). *Nursing: Scope and standards of practice* (3rd ed.). Silver Spring, MD: American Nurses Association.

American Nurses Association. (2015b). *Code of ethics for nurses with interpretive statements* (2nd ed.). Silver Spring, MD: American Nurses Association.

American Nurses Association. (2019). *Violence, incivility, & bullying*. https://www.nursingworld.org/practice-policy/work-environment/violence-incivility-bullying/.

American Nurses Association (ANA). (2020). *The nursing process*. Silver Spring, MD: American Nurses Association. https://www.nursingworld.org/practice-policy/workforce/what-is-nursing/the-nursing-process/.

APRN Joint Dialogue Group Report. (2008,July 7). *Consensus model for APRN regulation: Licensure, accreditation, certification & education*. http://www.nursingworld.org/ConsensusModelforAPRN.

Ben-Assuli, O. (2015). Electronic health records, adoption, quality of care, legal and privacy issues, and their implementation in emergency departments. *Health Policy, 119*(3), 287–297.

Brenan, M. (2018). Nurses again outpace other professions for honesty, ethics. https://news.gallup.com/poll/245597/nurses-again-outpace-professions-honesty-ethics.aspx.

Bridges, J., Griffiths, P., Oliver, E., & Pickering, R. M. (2019). Hospital nurse staffing and staff-patient interactions: An observational study. *BMJ Quality & Safety, 28*(9), 706–713. https://doi.org/10.1136/bmjqs-2018-008948.

Broadway, M. A. (2019). Legal and ethical issues. In P. Yoder-Wise (Ed.), *Leading and managing in nursing* (7th ed.) (pp. 32–61). St. Louis, MO: Elsevier.

Cambridge Dictionary. (2020a). *Profession*. https://dictionary.cambridge.org/us/dictionary/english/profession.

Cambridge Dictionary. (2020b). *Family*. https://dictionary.cambridge.org/us/dictionary/english/family.

Carthon, J. M., Hatfield, L., Dierkes, A., Davis, L., Hedgeland, T., Sanders, A. M., et al. (2019). Association of nurse engagement and nurse staffing on patient safety. *Journal of Nursing Care Quality, 34*(1), 40–46.

Department of Health and Human Services (HHS). (2020). *Personal representatives*. http://www.hhs.gov/hipaa/for-professionals/privacy/guidance/personal-representatives/.

De Pietro, S. C. (2016). Legal and ethical issues in nursing professional development. In C. M. Smith, & M. G. Harper (Eds.), *Leadership in nursing professional development: An organizational & system focus* (pp. 78–109). Chicago, IL: Association for Nursing Professional Development (ANPD).

De Simone, D. M. (2019). Data breaches are not just information technology worries! *Pediatric Nursing, 45*(2), 59–62.

Gao, G. (2015, May 8). *Americans' ideal family size is smaller than it used to be*. https://www.pewresearch.org/fact-tank/2015/05/08/ideal-size-of-the-american-family/.

Hill, G., & Hill, K. (2019). Cross examination. *LAW.COM*. https://dictionary.law.com/Default.aspx?selected=408.

Huber, D. L., Bair, H., & Joseph, M. L. (2019). Roadmap to drive innovativeness in health care. *Nurse Leader, 17*(6), 505–508.

Institute of Medicine (IOM). (2011). *The future of nursing: Leading change, advancing health*. Washington, DC: National Academies Press.

Law Insider. (2019). Definition of professional judgement. https://www.lawinsider.com/dictionary/professional-judgement.

Legal Information Institute. (2020). *Federal rules of evidence*. https://www.law.cornell.edu/rules/fre.

Muller, L. S., & Fink-Samnick, E. (2015). Mandatory reporting: Let's clear up the confusion. *Professional Case Management, 20*(4), 199–203.

National Council of State Boards of Nursing (NCSBN). (2019). *Uniform licensure requirements*. https://www.ncsbn.org/3884.htm.

National Council of State Boards of Nursing. (2020a). *Contact a U.S. member*. https://www.ncsbn.org/contact-bon.htm.

National Council of State Boards of Nursing. (2020b). Nursing licensure compact. https://nursinglicensemap.com/resources/nursing-licensure-compact/.

National Conference of State Legislatures (NCSL). (2019). *State legislative websites directory*. www.ncsl.org/aboutus/ncslservice/state-legislative-websites-directory.aspx.

Needleman, J., Liu, J., Shang, J., Larson, E., & Stone, P. W. (2020). Association of registered nurse and nursing support staffing with inpatient hospital mortality. *BMJ Quality & Safety, 29*(1), 10–18. https://doi.org/10.1136/bmjqs-2018-009219.

NSI Nursing Solutions, Inc. (2019). *2019 National health care retention & RN staffing report*. www.nsinursingsolutions.com.

NursingLicensure.org. (2019). *LPN/LVN and registered nurse license requirements by state*. NursingLicensure.org: https://www.nursinglicensure.org/.

Obama, B. H. (2016, January 6). *New executive actions to reduce gun violence and make our communities safer*. https://www.whitehouse.gov/the-press-office/2016/01/04/fact-sheet-new-executive-actions-reduce-gun-violence-and-make-our.

Obergefell v. Hodges, 576 U.S. __ (2015) (U>S> Supreme Court, 2015). https://supreme.justia.com/cases/federal/us/576/14-556/

Phillips, J., & Walsh, M. A. (2018). Teaming up in child welfare: The perspective of guardians ad litem on the components of interprofessional collaboration. *Children and Youth Services Review, 96*(2019), 17–26.

Pozgar, G. D. (2019). *Legal Aspects of Health Care Administration* (13th ed.). Burlington, MA: Jones & Bartlett Learning, LLC.

Russell, D. (2018). Disclosure and apology: Nursing and risk management working together. *Nursing Management, 49*(6), 17–19.

Tarasoff v. Regents of the University of California, 17 Cal.3d 425, 131 Cal. Rptr. 14 (California Supreme Court 1976).

Van Bogaert, P., Peremans, L., Van Heusden, D., Verspuy, M., Kureckova, V., Van de Cruys, et al. (2017). Predictors of burnout, work engagement and nurse reported job outcomes and quality of care: A mixed method study. *BMC Nursing, 16*(5), 1–14. https://doi.org/10.1186/s12912-016-0200-4.

Vrbnjak, D., Denieffe, S., O'Gorman, C., & Pajnkihar, M. (2016). Barriers to reporting medication errors and near misses among nurses: A systematic review. *International Journal of Nursing Studies, 63*, 162–178.

Walker, A. (2018, March 2). *Nursing satisfaction impacts patient outcomes, mortality*. Nurse.org: https://nurse.org/articles/nursing-satisfaction-patient-results/.

Wang, Y., Coiera, E., & Magrabi, F. (2019). Using convolutional neural networks to identify patient safety incident reports by type and severity. *Journal of the American Medical Informatics Association, 26*(12), 1600–1608.

Wilson, W. C. (2018). Inadequate nurse's notes lead to lawsuit. *Caring for the Ages, 19*(3), 14–15.

Zaleski, A. (2017). *You need a (interactive) map to understand the disparity of healthcare data sharing in the U.S.* https://medcitynews.com/2017/06/need-interactive-map-understand-disparity-healthcare-data-sharing-u-s/.

8

Communication Leadership

Bob Dent

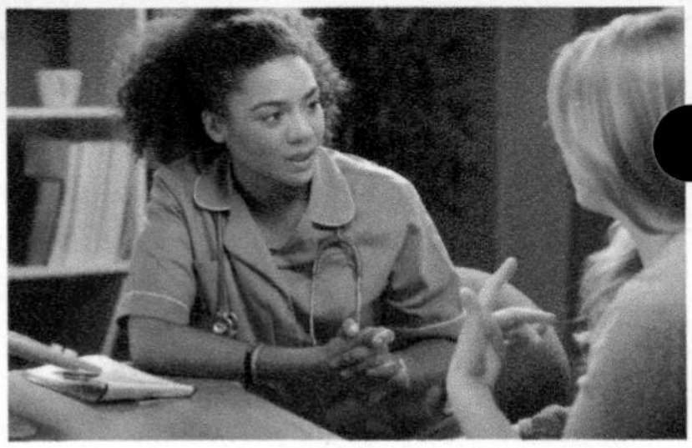

http://evolve.elsevier.com/Huber/leadership

Communication is a process by which meaning is assigned to the needs, feelings, perceptions, and interpretation of what is brought to our awareness. There are several variables that influence how we assign meaning to our experience and thus affect how we communicate. Successful health care outcomes are dependent on clear communication; therefore all nurses need proficiency in interpersonal skills. Nurse leaders and managers need to be mentors, coaches, and role models for effective interpersonal and team communication in order to ensure safe patient outcomes, effective teamwork, and staff satisfaction.

The purpose of this chapter is to enhance nurse leaders' understanding of the pivotal role that communication plays in health care by elucidating the complexities present in human communication, by addressing current key communication issues in health care, and by offering pragmatic strategies using communication models that can be applied to a variety of health care settings.

DEFINITIONS

Communication is based on mutual understanding. Clarity of meaning is derived from a clear definition of terms related to communication. Relevant definitions are as follows:

- **Interpersonal communication:** Communication between two or more individuals involving face-to-face interaction while all parties are aware of the others on an ongoing basis. Each person sends and receives information while continually adapting to the other actors.
- **Interprofessional communication:** Communication between two or more members of the interdisciplinary care team.
- **Intercultural communication:** Communication across cultural contexts. It applies equally to domestic cultural differences such as ethnicity and gender and to international differences such as those associated with nationality or world region (Bennet, 2013).
- **Non-verbal communication:** Unspoken, this communication is composed of affective or expressive behavior.
- **Persuasion, negotiation, and bargaining:** Persuasion is the conscious intent by one individual to modify the thoughts or behaviors of others. Negotiation is a dialogical discussion between two or more parties to arrive at an agreement about some issue. To bargain is to make a series of offers and counteroffers about what each party will do, give, receive, etc., until an agreement is reached to the satisfaction of all. All three of these involve communication. Persuasion uses argumentation and appeals to logic, whereas negotiation and bargaining may involve some sense of compensation and perhaps coercion, such as bullying or condescending behaviors.
- **Verbal communication:** Includes both written and spoken communication.

BACKGROUND

The literature supports the importance of effective team and interpersonal communication at all levels of an organization. Not only is this key in preventing medical errors, but effective communication and team functioning have also been shown to contribute to patient and staff satisfaction (Nicotera et al., 2014). Over 20 years ago, the Institute of Medicine (IOM, 2001) reported that 98,000 patient deaths per year stemmed from preventable medical errors. Not much has changed in the past 20 years. Health care still has a prevalent culture of silence. Frontline workers worried about litigation or job loss cover up mistakes, and leaders fail to address medical errors even in a preemptive fashion, almost as if not to jinx their luck (Aguilar, 2019).

Furthermore, individual, team, and interprofessional communication is influenced by organizational climate and culture (see Chapter 3). An organization with a rigid bureaucratic one-way communication network or lack of transparency will impede effective communication among all levels of the organization. A less rigid, more open, transparent structure will encourage creative problem-solving and healthy conflict resolution, elements that are needed for healthy organizations. Open communication practices are important because this builds trust. Trust, respect, and empathy are three ingredients that foster positive communication outcomes. The Joint Commission (2015) recognized that the leading causes of sentinel events—a patient safety event that reaches a patient and results in death, permanent harm, or results in severe temporary harm and interventions required to sustain life—relate to poor communication and leadership (The Joint Commission Online, 2015).

Stephen R. Covey (2004), the author of *The 8th Habit: From effectiveness to greatness*, discussed the emotional bank account derived from relationships built with each other. He explained the concept with the metaphor: "It is like a financial bank account into which you make deposits and withdrawals—only in this case, you make emotional deposits and withdrawals in your relationships that either build or destroy them" (p. 165). If a nurse leader breaches the trust of their staff, other leaders, or the medical staff, they may not ever be able to make enough deposits to get out of debt.

Proficiency in verbal, non-verbal, and written communication is a core leadership competency. Leaders need to possess the skills necessary to inspire a shared vision, ensure the mission, and establish a culture where this can be achieved. Leaders also need special communication skills in order to implement change.

Interpersonal relationship skills—including the ability to communicate—are as essential to a leader's personal set of leadership skills as psychomotor skills are for a clinical nurse. Leadership ability is predicated on a facility for communication. Human interaction issues are an area where leaders can spend a considerable amount of time. Power and conflict become important focal points of human interaction in organizations that may need managerial intervention or resolution through persuasion or negotiation. Because nurses may frequently be in situations in which they need to persuade others to cooperate, proficiency in managing conflict, bargaining, negotiating, and the art of "crucial conversations" is essential for nurses and nurse leaders. The foregoing skills require practice, experience, assertiveness, and confidence, which are necessary elements in the nurse leader's armamentarium.

Nurses need to be able to feel safe enough to articulate needs, viewpoints, and ideas for improvement of health care and the work environment. Feeling that one has not been heard can be a source of true frustration, anger, and conflict.

Nurse leaders play a crucial role in the management of information and communication for the purpose of effective care coordination and to prevent unsafe and error-prone care situations. Providers need high-quality information and access to health care information systems and effective communication models. Nurse leaders are responsible for developing care delivery systems with adequate structure and an effective communication system that enhances care coordination. These systems of communication need to enable patient rescue and safety by coordinating care, preventing information loss, and improving methods of surveillance. For example, there is a distinction between interprofessional collaboration and merely working on the same task together. This occurs when multiple health care providers are taking care of the same patient, but in a mode where multiple providers are simultaneously doing different jobs rather than there being collaborative efforts.

Successful nurse leaders are effective communicators establishing trust and respect. Nurse leaders need to model behavior and language that sets the tone for a positive and supportive work environment. Equally critical is the development and fostering of similarly effective communication skills in all nurses for peer-to-peer, interprofessional, intercultural, and followership interactions.

COMMUNICATION THEORIES AND MODELS

Communication is a process in which information, perception, and understanding are transmitted from person to person. It is important to nurses and is an integral part of any relationship. Nurse leaders and managers can view communication as a tool to accomplish work and meet goals. The significance of communication revolves around its effectiveness and the climate in which communication occurs. Effective communication is enhanced by clear, direct, straightforward, and frequent message transmission. Trust, respect, and empathy are the three ingredients needed to create and foster effective communication.

Much of what was written in the past with respect to communication in health care was about teaching techniques and skills such as interviewing and how to elicit information from patients. These works also included explanations regarding how to reflect, clarify, summarize, provide feedback, use silence, and actively listen. Learning communication techniques is not enough. Communication is more than messages, and human beings are more than senders and receivers. Further, communication models specifically written for nursing are limited, and rigorous studies using randomized controlled trials or systematic reviews to determine the effectiveness of models applicable to nursing practice are not well documented.

Communication is a process that is affected by several internal and external variables, takes place on multiple levels of complexity, is difficult to measure, and for which standardized instruments are lacking (Foronda et al., 2015).

COMMUNICATION TO FACILITATE CHANGE: KOTTER

In alignment with the goals of the Institute of Medicine's (IOM, 2011) report on *The Future of Nursing*, nurses are called upon to "lead change to advance health," yet the report acknowledges that several barriers exist that prevent nurses from responding to this call and participating fully in the rapidly changing health care environment. In a classic work, Kotter (1996) proposed a model in business for making change in organizations. This framework underscores that all change is made by communication, and the effectiveness and sustainability of the change is based on the skilled communication of the leadership and stakeholders endorsing the change process.

BOX 8.1 Kotter's Eight-Stage Process of Creating Major Change

1. Establishing a sense of urgency
2. Creating the guiding coalition
3. Developing a vision and a strategy
4. Communicating the change vision
5. Empowering broad-based action
6. Generating short-term wins
7. Consolidating gains and producing more change
8. Anchoring new approaches in the culture

From Kotter, J. (1996). *Leading change* (p. 21). Boston, MA: Harvard Business School Press.

Kotter (1996) suggested the following are needed to empower people to make change: communicate the vision to employees, make structures compatible with the vision, provide the training employees need, align information and personnel systems, and confront supervisors who undercut needed change. Further, he suggested that structures, skills, systems, and supervisors are generally the four barriers to any transformational process. Before implementing change, the nurse leader is well advised to first analyze the communication pattern currently in place at the macro and micro level and to be cognizant of the organization's general culture, climate, and politics. Box 8.1 outlines the points of Kotter's change process.

Leadership needs to be part of the guiding coalition in all of these stages to be supportive and communicate needed change. Kotter stated that the barriers that can interfere with change are as follows: "inwardly focused cultures, paralyzing bureaucracy, parochial politics, a low level of trust, lack of teamwork, arrogant attitudes, a lack of leadership in middle management, and general human fear of the unknown" (p. 20). He also stated that organizations that are more manager versus leader oriented will not produce needed change that is sustainable, because managers "plan, organize and control," whereas leaders "establish direction, align people, and motivate and inspire," qualities that are needed to "produce extremely useful change" (p. 26).

Intrapersonal and Interpersonal Communication

Decades ago, Abraham Maslow developed a model for understanding human needs. He identified that how we respond, react, and behave is based on our needs and whether they are being met. Thus this model is still relevant and is a useful framework for understanding human communication. At the bottom of Maslow's pyramid of human needs are our most basic needs for survival, followed by safety and security, love and belonging, esteem and appreciation, and finally altruistic needs, like fulfillment by helping others and reaching psychological maturity.

Our most basic needs will not be met if we are not able to communicate. Babies cry when they are hungry, tired, uncomfortable, and in need of safety and security. They do not usually speak until about age 1 year, and then they start to form words, yet their caregivers know what they want and provide for them in their preverbal state. This happens because we use body language, facial expressions, and other sounds to communicate. Thus, as a species, we would not survive without communication between and among us, and unmet needs can be a source of conflict, misunderstanding, and anger. There are several factors that can influence how we respond.

Words and language are powerful tools that can be used to harm or heal (Sears, 2010). Non-verbal communication, such as use of the body and face, can also convey a strong message. To be most direct and straightforward, verbal and non-verbal communication should be congruent, meaning that our verbal and non-verbal are consistent. Communication problems in interpersonal relationships, whether personal or occupational, can be a source of conflict due to misinterpretation of what was said or meant. Conflict is natural, inherent, and inevitable in hospitals, and can arise in the work environment with heavy workloads, limited resources, unclear policies, organizational changes, poor communication, and differences in employees' abilities, skills, and personalities (Mosadeghrad & Mojbafan, 2019). However, there is an optimum conflict level necessary and beneficial for individual growth and organizational productivity.

Unresolved conflict can lead to resentment, backbiting, bullying, and other dysfunctional behaviors. A supportive work environment, positive communication between staff nurses and leadership, and frequent feedback on job performance, facilitate nurse job satisfaction. Setting a positive and cooperative tone within a work group is each member's responsibility. Moreover, it is incumbent upon nursing leadership to set the tone of the work environment (such as promoting a healthy work environment) and model impeccable interpersonal communication for the staff.

Tools for Improved Communication

Many times individuals get caught in a situation and are just at a loss for words or cannot come up with the response that feels just right at the time. Effective communication tools can help.

Tools for effective communication and speaking up. Poor communication has consequences for patient safety and can be deadly. Medical errors can be avoided, and work environments can become healthier if health care professionals acquire the ability to speak up and discuss emotionally or politically risky topics. Communication breakdowns can be either honest mistakes or undiscussables. Honest mistakes are accidental or unintentional slips and errors such as confusing labels, competing tasks, language barriers, distractions, or gaps during handoffs. Undiscussables occur when someone knows of risks or something being wrong, but does not speak up or chooses to ignore or avoid it. A person may back down from the conversation (Maxfield et al., n.d.).

VitalSmarts, the Association of periOperative Registered Nurses, and the American Association of Critical-Care Nurses worked on research to address communication failures and avoidable medical errors. Their 2005 study called Silence Kills was followed by the 2010 study The Silent Treatment, which confirmed that poor communication is harmful and that despite encountering resistance, nurses need to be enabled to speak up about dangerous shortcuts, incompetence, and disrespect. A safety culture where people speak up when there is a strong suspicion of risk needs to be developed using the communication skills of exceptional nurses and organizational strategies (Maxfield et al., 2010).

There are useful tools developed by the Agency for Healthcare Research and Quality's TeamSTEPPS program (AHRQ, 2020) (discussed later in this chapter). With scripting, these tools help nurses and interprofessional teams to communicate fully and clearly as well as speaking up when appropriate. For example, AHRQ has developed a pocket guide (https://www.ahrq.gov/teamstepps/instructor/essentials/pocketguide.html#passbaton) that presents CUS assertive statements. The CUS model is a tool to help nurses speak up/speak out in uncomfortable situations. A script is presented, using "I am concerned," "I am uncomfortable," or "This is a safety issue." "Stop the line" is one script used. A constructive approach for managing and resolving conflict is the DESC script: *D*escribe the situation, *E*xpress how the situation makes you feel,

Suggest other alternatives, and state Consequences in terms of impact on team goals.

Another helpful tool for effective communication and speaking up is called crucial conversations, which gives guidance on providing constructive feedback. Based on a book by Patterson et al. (2011), a crucial conversation is defined as a discussion between two or more people where the stakes are high, opinions vary, and emotions run strong. Billed as tools for talking when the stakes are high, the focus is on alleviating failure to communicate. The choices when facing crucial conversations are to avoid them, face them but handle them poorly, or face them and handle them well. Examples of crucial conversations range from ending a relationship, to talking to a team member who is not keeping commitments or has a personal hygiene problem, to giving an unfavorable peer or performance review. Dialogue skills are learnable. The book and training courses help people learn how to create conditions that make dialogue the path of least resistance; how to use key skills related to talking, listening, and acting together; and how to master tools for talking when the stakes are high. For nurses, this training promotes a culture of safety because team members can then talk about issues and concerns openly even when they touch on areas of silence in health care—such as incompetence, poor teamwork, and disrespect—or are difficult, risky, or emotionally charged. Some organizations have crucial-conversations training for staff to build skills in how to speak and be heard.

Evidence-Based Practice and Communication

Evidence-based practice (EBP) was developed following several reports by the Institute of Medicine (IOM), now called the National Academies of Sciences, Engineering, and Medicine, that cited staggering numbers of poor patient outcomes related to preventable medical errors. EBP is the preferred model of nursing care now and for the future. EBP encompasses clinical knowledge coupled with research evidence and patient preference to develop best practices, and it is supported by a number of regulatory organizations. However, despite growing evidence for support of EBP, incorporation of this model into daily clinical practice "remains inconsistent and presents complex challenges" (Pryse et al., 2014, p. 244). For EBP to work in an organization, nurse leaders and those in the work environment must be well informed and supportive of individual nurses who wish to incorporate EBP principles into their nursing care. Pryse et al. (2014) developed and tested two psychometric instruments, the EBP Nursing Leadership Scale and the EBP Work Environment Scale that can be used by nurse leaders to determine support for EBP within their organization.

One example of EBP that can be readily learned and implemented by nurses is moving shift report to the bedside. McAllen et al. (2018) completed a literature review finding numerous studies supporting the positive impact of bedside shift report (BSR) on nurse-sensitive outcomes including patient falls, and patient and nurse satisfaction. The results of the quality improvement project were positive. Patient falls decreased by 24%. Patient satisfaction showed statistically significant improvements ($P = .03$) in their general surgery unit after BSR implementation. Implementation of BSR did not increase the average total time required for change of shift report. Earlier identification and correction of potential errors during BSR may have improved the quality of patient care.

Recent research highlighted the complexity of providing quality nursing care with regard to fulfilling patients' expectations (Sharifabad et al., 2019). Effective communication impacts how care is provided to patients and impacts patients' expectations and the perceptions of the quality of nurses' services. Their five service quality of care factors were (1) tangibles: the appearance of the physical environment, equipment, and nurses; (2) reliability: nurses'/organization's ability to provide the right services in a timely fashion; (3) responsiveness: nurses' willingness and urgency in helping patients; (4) assurance: nurses' ability to earn patients' trust with task competence and humility; and (5) empathy: nurses' ability to demonstrate an interest in patients and their care. How care is provided communicates to patients other messages that impact their perceptions and ultimate well-being.

Transformational Leadership and Communication Style

Transformational leadership is a leadership style of communicating that relates to systematic variants such as job satisfaction, change commitment, leadership trust, cooperative conflict management, and market orientation (Yang, 2012). The basic goal of transformational leadership is to empower staff to take ownership of their own development (see Chapter 1).

The American Nurses Credentialing Center's (ANCC) Magnet Model (ANCC, 2020) recognized transformational leadership as one of the five core model components of a Magnet organization. ANCC describes the following to describe transformational leadership:

> *It is relatively easy to lead people where they want to go; the transformational leader must lead people to where they need to be in order to meet the demands of the future. This requires vision, influence, clinical knowledge, and a strong expertise relating to professional nursing practice. It also acknowledges that transformation may create turbulence and involve atypical approaches to solutions.*
>
> *The organization's senior leadership team creates the vision for the future, and the systems and environment necessary to achieve that vision. They must enlighten the organization as to why change is necessary, and communicate each department's part in achieving that change. They must listen, transformational way of thinking should take root in the organization and become even stronger as other leaders adapt to this way of thinking.*
>
> *The intent of this Model Component is no longer just to solve problems, fix broken systems, and empower staff, but to actually transform the organizations to meet the future. Magnet-recognized organizations today strive for stabilization; however, healthcare reformation calls for a type of controlled destabilization that births new ideas and innovations (ANCC, 2020).*

Kouzes and Posner (2017) identified the Five Practices of Exemplary Leadership model. This model continues to prove its effectiveness as a clear, evidence-based path to achieving the extraordinary for individuals, teams, organizations, and communities. These leaders:

- **Model the way**. Leaders establish principles concerning the way people should be treated and the way goals should be pursued.
- **Inspire a shared vision**. Leaders passionately believe they can make a difference and enlist others in their dreams.
- **Challenge the process**. Leaders search for opportunities to change the status quo.
- **Enable others to act**. Leaders foster collaboration and build spirited teams.
- **Encourage the heart**. Leaders recognize the contributions of individuals and teams.

ORGANIZATIONAL CULTURE AND CLIMATE

Health care organizations are complex, and role expectations and responsibilities of leadership can change from facility to facility. Some health care organizations are moving away from bureaucratic and hierarchical organizational structures to more facilitative professional governance models. Some have even adopted the model of servant leadership.

Because nurses make up the bulk of the health care workforce, having nurse leaders strategically positioned within the organization to effectively influence other executive stakeholders, including the board of directors or board of trustees, is imperative to achieve the level of influence required to lead others.

Dent and Tye (2018, p. xi) stated, "The first responsibility of the nurse leader is to be clear about his or her own values, and to make a concerted daily effort to assure that these values are reflected in the attitudes they bring to work, the way they treat people, their approach to dealing with conflict, the criteria they use for making decisions, and how they deal with obstacles and setbacks. The second responsibility – the one that more than any other single quality defines the heart of a nurse leader—is to help the people whom they lead do the same thing."

According to workplace specialists, job satisfaction has been found to include much more than salary increases, decreased overtime, and tangible rewards. Appreciation, trust, and respect are not quantifiable but are extremely valuable. These, as well as support for individual growth and a sense of purpose, have been identified as important factors in job satisfaction. Job satisfaction means having a leader who is fair and honest, listens to concerns, and helps the team to develop knowledge, attitudes, and skills to advance their careers. Some have suggested that nurses probably do not leave agencies; they leave dehumanizing nursing leaders. Nurse leaders need to be in touch with the degree to which nursing staff are satisfied. Job satisfaction remains an important issue in the workplace environment, given nurse shortages and high reported levels of burnout.

Nurse leaders set the tone and expectations with every interaction. Much has been written about the effectiveness of informal power and that often, those without official title and position have more influence among leaders and peers than those with formal title and position. Therefore any nurse can exert influence on the cultural norms and climate of the organization, and nurse leaders should model this empowerment approach for all nurses.

Registered nurses (RN) form the backbone of health care in the United States, providing critical health care to the public wherever it is needed, and recognized as the key to the health of our nation. There are over 4 million RNs in the United States today. That means that one in 100 people is an RN. It is forecasted that there will be a shortage of RNs across the country between 2009 and 2030 (American Nurses Association [ANA], 2020). It is imperative then for nurse leaders to establish positive and healthy workplace environments to attract and retain nurses.

Communication in Patient and Family Engaged Care

Patients and their families are the reasons nurses exist in health care. Nurses and nurse leaders need to create an environment with structures and processes to improve patients' care and experiences. Patient and family engaged care (PFEC) is care planned, delivered, managed, and continuously improved in active partnership with patients and their families (or care partners as defined by the patient) to ensure integration of their health and health goals, preferences, and values. It includes explicit and partnered determination of goals and care options, and it requires ongoing assessment of the care match with patient goals (Frampton et al., 2017). Fig. 8.1 depicts the framework of PFEC with

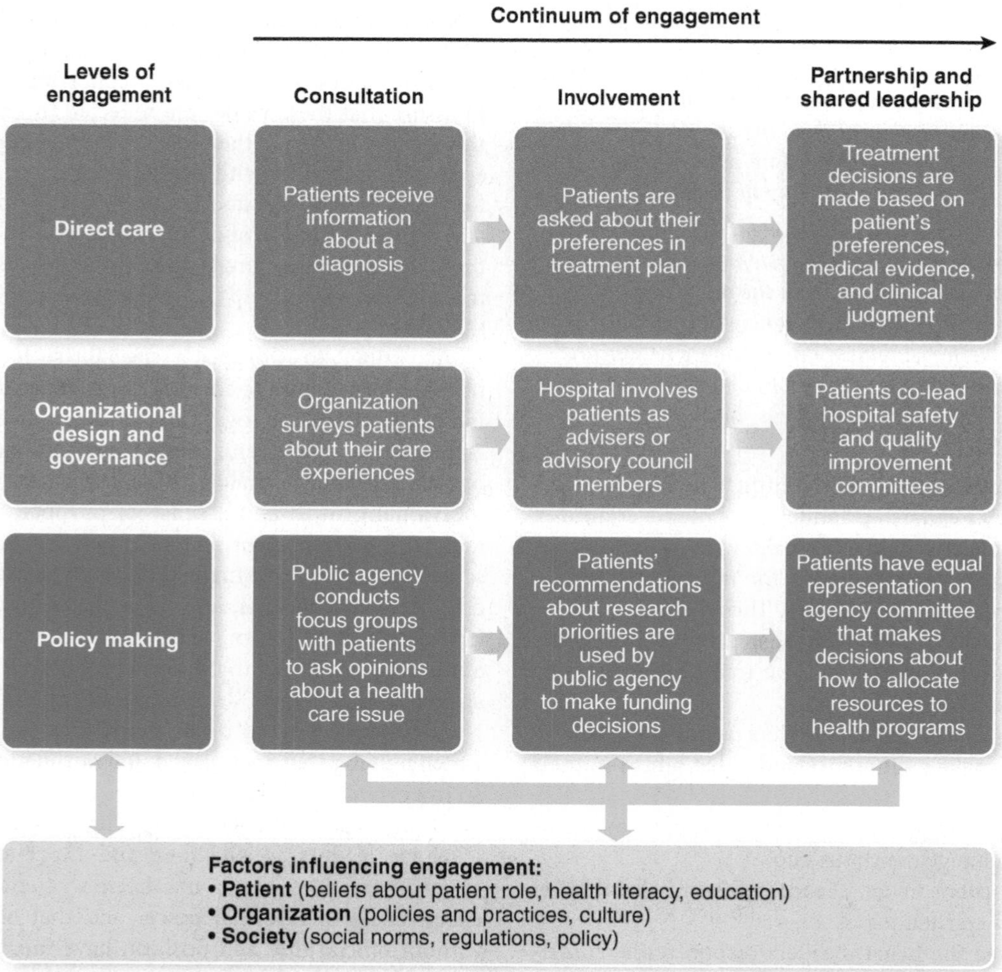

Fig. 8.1 Patient and family engaged care: a guiding framework (Frampton et al., 2017).

many of the key elements identified for improved engagement outcomes such as better culture, better care, better health, and lower costs.

The IOM defined patient-centered care as "providing care that is respectful of and responsive to individual patient preferences, needs and values, and ensuring that patient values guide all clinical decisions" (IOM, 2001, p. 40). Berwick (2009, p. 560) defined patient-centered care as "the experience (to the extent the informed, individual patient desires it) of transparency, individualization, recognition, respect, dignity and choice in all matters, without exception, related to one's person, circumstances, and relationships in health care."

Fooks et al. (2015) described three concepts that represent the principles of good patient relationships (see Box 8.2). Recognizing partnerships, equality, communication, trust, and respect are crucial levers for change. Carman et al. (2013) provided a multidimensional framework for patient and family engagement in health and health care as depicted in Fig. 8.2. The Joint Commission (R^3 Report, 2011) has patient-centered communication standards for hospitals. The standards assure hospitals lead by example every day, as hospitals and health care providers demonstrate what it means to honor people's needs and their differences, providing health equity. Effective communication is critical to the successful delivery of health care services. The Joint Commission requires hospitals to effectively communicate with patients when providing care, treatment, and services by (1) identifying the patient's oral and written communication needs, including the patient's preferred language for discussing health care, and (2) communicating with the patient during provision of care, treatment, and services in a manner that meets the patient's oral and written communication needs (R^3 Report, 2011).

BOX 8.2 Principles of Good Patient Relationships

1. ***Patient-centered care*** is an overall philosophy and approach that ensures that everything individual providers or health care organizations do clinically or administratively is based on patient needs and preferences.
2. ***Patient engagement*** is the way in which individual providers or health care organizations solicit patient needs and preferences to ensure they are delivering patient-centered care.
3. ***Patient experience*** is how patients perceive and experience their care. This involves the ability to hear what is being said, measure the experience, and develop the capacity to use the information to change practice, policies, and rules.

From Fooks, C., Obarski, G., Hale, L., & Hylmar, S. (2015). The patient experience in Ontario 2020: What is possible? *Healthcare Papers, 14*(4): 8–18.

LEADERSHIP AND MANAGEMENT IMPLICATIONS

Spears (2019, p. 1) stated, "[A]lmost all successful leaders understand that effective leadership really comes down to influence: influencing outcomes, influencing direction, influencing decisions, influencing atmosphere, and influencing people. The degree to which a leader can successfully influence people and teams becomes the 'lid' in his or her role. The only reliable tool we have to influence others is communication."

Effective leadership starts with communication, and progressive leaders need to understand how to ensure that their interventions lead to positive outcomes (Spears, 2019). Box 8.3 displays four conversations for the leader to get right. Strong communication is critical to supporting, guiding, and influencing; a leader's connections with others heighten the ability to influence, as well as the quantity and quality of work performance (Pater, 2016). The leader's communication has implications for success in achieving the organization's mission, vision, and strategic objectives. It is important for nurse leaders to be self-aware of their communication styles and know how to leverage their own and those of their teams. There are many valid and reliable tools to assess their own personality type and the personality types of their teams. These include Meyers-Briggs Type Indicator (MBTI) (https://www.myersbriggs.org/my-mbti-personality-type/mbti-basics/home.htm?bhcp=1), StrengthsFinder (https://www.gallup.com/cliftonstrengths/en/strengthsfinder.aspx), DISC (https://www.discprofile.com/what-is-disc/overview/), HBDI (http://www.hbdi.com/WholeBrainProductsAndServices/programs/thehbdi.php), and others.

For example, one's top five strengths are learned from taking the Strengths Finder survey. Experienced nurse leaders recognize that in all groups there is at least one person who has the positivity strength. When delivering bad news (e.g., outcomes, changes), the leader has to add in something positive to avoid demoralizing the

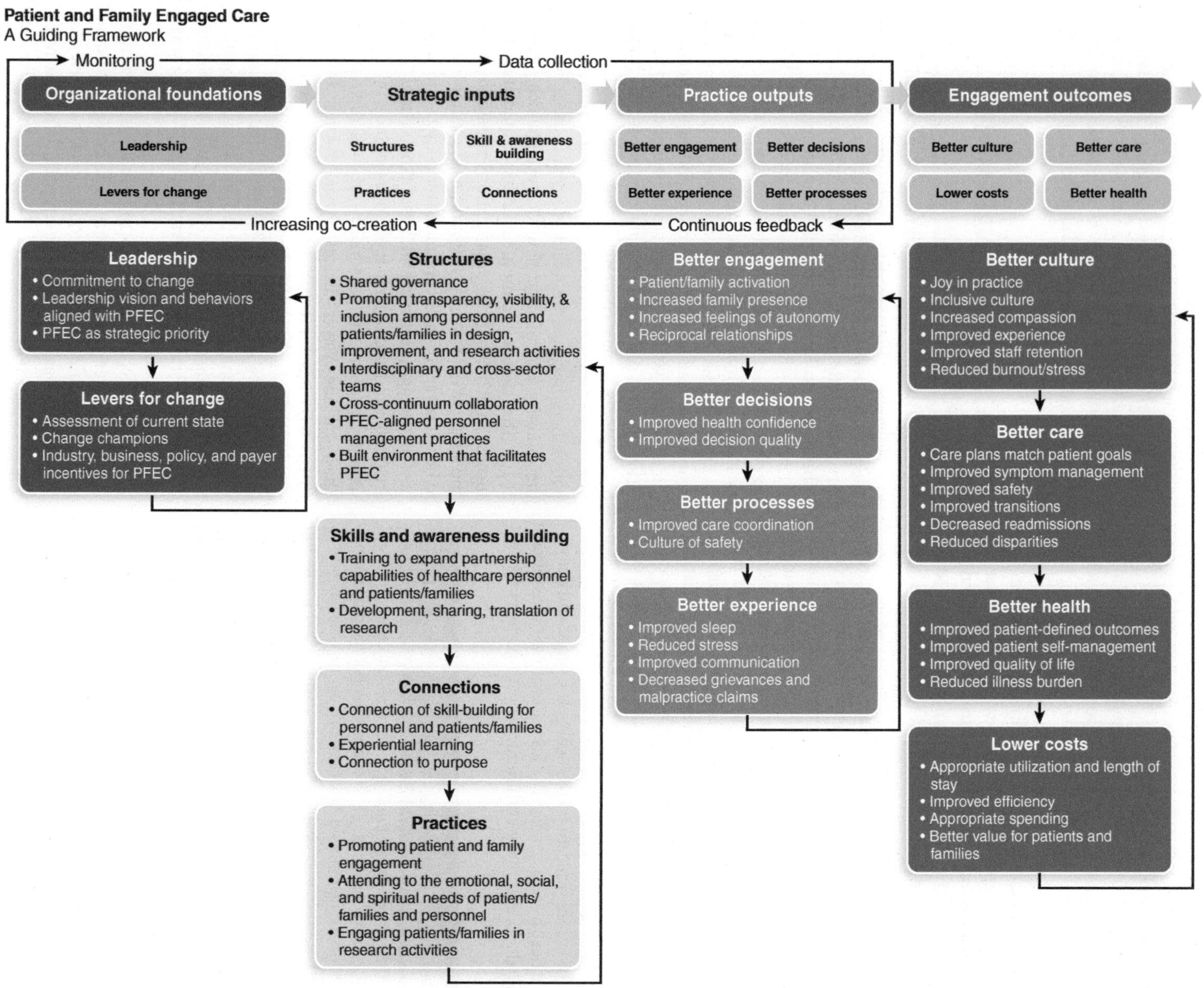

Fig. 8.2 Framework for patient and family engagement in health and health care (Carman et al., 2013). Note: movement to the right on the continuum of engagement denotes increasing patient participation and collaboration.

BOX 8.3 Spears Four Conversations You Must Get Right as a Leader

1. **The Timely Talk**. A must-have conversation for specific situations.
2. **The Rock Star Reminder**. An opportunity to influence growth and development and ultimate success with someone who has amazing potential.
3. **The Now or Never Conversation**. This conversation should always follow a failed Timely Talk (#1). The person knows that the performance or behavior or other issue cannot continue and has had some time to make changes. This person is now at risk.
4. **The Stay Interview**. A conversation with a proven and valued team member whom you very much want to stay. Add these to your calendar quarterly.

From Spears,T.L. (2019). *The four conversations you must get right as a leader.* American Association for Physician Leadership. https://www.physicianleaders.org/news/the-four-conversations-leader

person. Often the person with a positivity strength will chime in with something positive.

HBDI helps identify how the leader and the team would respond under normal circumstances and under pressure. On any given day, it helps to know how teammates are responding. Noting the responses reveals they are under pressure.

Understanding the different needs and expectations of others in communication requires leaders to customize their approach to communication, including listening and speaking (Fitzgerald & Kirby, 1997). Plonien (2015) discussed how to approach the MBTI in a perioperative setting to improve communication. For the nurse leader, knowledge of personality type provides an opportunity to enhance communication and improve team dynamics. Personality indicators such as the MBTI provide insight into the type of communication needed to connect with personnel, as well as within the interdisciplinary team.

It is imperative for nurse leaders to assess the workplace environment including observing the interactions of their teams regularly, recognizing top performers and addressing negative interactions quickly. No one is exempt from communicating effectively and working as a team. Leaders need to set realistic goals and model appropriate communication practice in establishing a more positive and healthier workplace environment. The next section discusses models that can be employed by nurse leaders to address issues in the health care environment resulting from ineffective communication.

Promoting Healthy, Inclusive Work Environments

In September 2017, the Tri-Council for Nursing (American Association of Colleges of Nursing [AACN]; American Nurses Association [ANA]; American Organization of Nurse Executives [AONE]; and the National League for Nursing [NLN]) issued a press release on the Proclamation on Nursing Civility. To emphasize how critical civil behavior is to excellence in nursing practice and to outstanding congruent care for all patients, the Tri-Council for Nursing issued a bold call to advance civility in nursing. The resolution called upon "all nurses to recognize nursing civility and take steps to systematically eliminate all acts of incivility in their professional practice, workplace environments, and in our communities" (Tri-Council for Nursing, 2017, para. 2). The Tri-Council urged that nursing civility be practiced throughout the United States "to establish healthy work environments that embrace and value cultural diversity, inclusivity, and equality" (Tri-Council for Nursing, 2017, para. 2). It noted that people of all racial, religious, ethnic, sexual orientation, socio-economic, political, geographic, and other differences are to be treated respectfully. "It's no secret that acts of disrespect, and other overt or subtle negative emotional behavior create a toxic work environment which contributes to burnout, fatigue, depression and other psychological stresses. Eliminating assaults to anyone's self-esteem is essential to providing a healthy work and learning environment," noted Alexander (Tri-Council for Nursing, 2017, para. 3). "The Tri-Council recognizes that instilling an ethic of civility from the very beginning of a nurse's education and throughout the profession will begin to eliminate the dangers that inevitably arise when it is lacking." "Manifesting civility is key to enhancing the patient care experience and ensuring quality team-based care," said Sebastian (Tri-Council for Nursing, 2017, para. 4). "As the most trusted healthcare provider, registered nurses understand the connection between treating patients with respect, establishing open lines of communication, and realizing positive care outcomes" (Tri-Council for Nursing, 2017, para. 4).

"AONE (AONL) is committed to providing nurse leaders with the tools and resources to prevent workplace violence and ensuring the safety of all health care workers and patients. Through its work with the American Hospital Association, AONL is partnering to increase awareness of the issue and support AHA's

Hospitals against Violence initiative," stated Clark (Tri-Council for Nursing, 2017, para. 5). "Civility forms the foundation of a culture of respect for one another and is non-negotiable for a healthy, safe and ethical work environment" (Tri-Council for Nursing, 2017, para. 6). "The ANA has zero-tolerance for any form of incivility, violence, or bullying in the workplace in order to safeguard patients, nurses, and other healthcare team members" (Tri-Council for Nursing, 2017, para. 6). The Tri-Council identified other potential measurable hazards to health care of incivility, intolerance, and disregard for emotional health: difficulty in nurse recruitment and retention, aggravating the persistent shortage of nurses, and poor communication and teamwork giving rise to preventable errors that risk patient safety. Noting that nurses currently enjoy a reputation as the most ethical and honest profession in the country, the council's statement articulates a nurse's ethical obligation to care for others and themselves (Tri-Council for Nursing, 2017, para. 7).

There is support on a national level to promote effective communication and collaboration. It is important that positive interdisciplinary relationships are established and are active in the organizational culture. The workplace does not have to be hostile. Nurse leaders have a responsibility to communicate zero tolerance for bullying and a hostile environment. The ANA (2015) developed a position statement on incivility, bullying, and workplace violence: "ANA's Code of Ethics for Nurses with Interpretive Statements states that nurses are required to 'create an ethical environment and culture of civility and kindness, treating colleagues, co-workers, employees, students, and others with dignity and respect.'" Similarly, nurses must be afforded the same level of respect and dignity as others (ANA, 2015). Thus the nursing profession will no longer tolerate violence of any kind from any source. All registered nurses and employers in all settings, including practice, academia, and research, need to collaborate to create a culture of respect, free of incivility, bullying, and workplace violence. Best practice strategies based on evidence need to be implemented to prevent and mitigate incivility, bullying, and workplace violence; to promote the health, safety, and wellness of registered nurses; and to ensure optimal outcomes across the health care continuum. This position statement, although written specifically for registered nurses and employers, is also relevant to other health care professionals and stakeholders who collaborate to create and sustain a safe and healthy interprofessional work environment. Stakeholders who have a relationship with the worksite have a responsibility to address incivility, bullying, and workplace violence.

According to the Workplace Bullying Institute (2019), although many good nurses have been driven out by toxic environments, many other nurses have just accepted those environments. Decoster, a cultural anthropologist in Cusco, Peru, described culture as a people's adaptation to an environment (Dent, B., A personal interview of Dr. Jean-Jacques Decoster in Cusco, Peru, October, 2018). It is imperative for nurse leaders to establish more positive and healthier workplace environments where nurses can be and perform at their best.

Tye and Dent (2017) described toxic emotional negativity as the name for the whole collection of behaviors that include gossiping, eye-rolling, bullying, and work-shirking. Toxic emotional negativity is so ubiquitous that often it is hardly even noticed it unless making a concerted effort to do so. The emotional climate of the workplace is defined by expected behaviors and tolerated behaviors; over time, the tolerated behaviors will dominate the expected behaviors. Thus it is imperative for nurses and nurse leaders to establish more positive and healthy workplace environments rid of toxic behaviors that erode teamwork and communication resulting in poor outcomes.

Nonviolent Communication

Expanding on nonviolent communication (NVC) concepts developed by Rosenberg (2004) and Sears (2010) critiqued the health care system. In a nutshell, NVC is predicated on the notion that our language, which is based on our culture and experience, is replete with judgment, criticisms, labels, and phraseology that is bound to create defensive reactions in others and is considered violent. Further, and more importantly, "the labels, analyses and judgments of others are tragic expressions of your own unmet needs" (Sears, 2010, p. 56).

Recalling the earlier discussion of Maslow's hierarchy of needs, this makes perfect sense. Unmet needs in the area of belonging—a basic need—can create issues of safety or feelings of insecurity or of feeling threatened. Anger or helplessness are two responses that may be seen in people trying to protect themselves. No one is safe in a hostile work environment. Therefore when someone feels threatened or unsafe, they may regress to an earlier stage of development to when they felt safe and thus respond in a childlike manner. This may account for behavior that we may consider to be immature.

Sears proposed a four-part nonviolent communication process grounded in compassion, empathy, and honesty. She stated, "Empathy is one of the simplest yet most potent technologies on the planet. It is a low-cost, high yield solution that everyone can use" (Sears, 2010, p. 88). The four parts include making an observation, expressing a feeling, expressing a need, and making a request without demanding. Table 8.1 is an adaptation of these four parts of NVC developed by Rosenberg (2004).

Nurses are by and large caretakers of others and thus may be great at making observations. But they may lack the ability to express their own feelings and needs and lack the ability to make a straightforward request. By becoming proficient at expressing their own feelings and needs and communicating requests in a clear, direct manner, nurses are providing for their own self-care. Only in this way can nurses truly care for others.

Team/Group Communication: TeamSTEPPS and SBAR

Nurse leaders need to be familiar with group theory because little is accomplished in a health care facility without individual participation in a team, group, or meeting. Participation in groups is a necessary part of the functioning of the larger organization. In principle, the degree to which individual need satisfaction is achieved differentiates effective from ineffective groups; the greater the individual's satisfaction, the higher the probability of group effectiveness (Hersey et al., 2013).

Group theorists have articulated different stages of group development. One of the most popular theories, first postulated by Tuckman in 1965, contains four stages as follows: forming, storming, norming, and performing. In the forming stage the group needs direction in defining tasks, goals, and objectives. Members are unclear regarding their respective roles in the group. This initial period can be chaotic and confusing. The next stage is storming. As the name connotes, there can be conflict, and indeed there must be conflict for the group to sort through issues such as leadership, power, and roles. Usually there is some willingness to accept the group goals and objectives, but there are still differences of opinion, competition for recognition, and attempts to influence the group. During the norming period, there is greater agreement on the task goals as the group develops cohesiveness and adjusts to the group and task. Finally, during the performing period, the members are thinking as one and willingly performing the task. There is camaraderie and team spirit as the group becomes self-managing (Hersey et al., 2013).

Members assume a variety of roles within the process of a group. Most are constructive in nature, contributing to the discussion, solving the problem, and achieving the group goals. These roles may be questioning, suggesting possibilities, taking notes, and summarizing the group's progress. However, some roles are not helpful. The most disruptive periods in group process are with intergroup dissonance and competition. It is at these levels that members may behave in roles that hinder group effectiveness, such as criticizing, attacking, or name-calling. The leader needs to intervene as appropriate with discussions of goals, standards, and feedback on behavior and progress for individuals or the group, depending on the situation. The degree to which roles are not helpful probably influences member satisfaction, and certainly interferes with communication and collaboration (Hersey et al., 2013). For example, using a generic team-based communication

TABLE 8.1 Four Parts of Nonviolent Communication (NVC)

Clearly Expressing (Without Blaming or Criticizing)	Empathetically Receiving (Without Hearing Blame or Criticism)
1. Making an observation	1. What you observe
2. Expressing a feeling	2. How you feel based on your observation
3. Stating what you need	3. How you feel based on what you are hearing
4. Making a request (without demanding)	4. Hearing the request for an action to be taken

From Rosenberg, M.B. (2004). *We can work it out: Resolving conflicts peacefully and powerfully.* Encinitas, CA: Puddledancer Press.

model, Matzke et al. (2014) analyzed conversations between nurses and physicians. Their findings indicated that although about half of the conversations were considered collegial, communication was status-based rather than team-based. Status-based communications were described as patterns that allow an individual with more perceived power to be more forceful and directive in their communication toward other team members. Unfortunately, this autocratic style of communication does not support team building or promote good working relationships, and this can lead to preventable medical errors.

Research in small task group process has also revealed movement from an initial organization through a period of disorganization or chaos to reorganization at a level that achieves a goal. A group is defined as two or more people, and it exists to meet the needs of everyone in the group so that each will be satisfied. The leader's four major styles of communication used with task groups are similar to those for individuals (telling, selling, participating, and delegating). The process includes moving from defining, clarifying, and involving to empowering according to the leader's assessment of the readiness of the group (Hersey et al., 2013). The relationship styles of defining, clarifying, involving, and empowering suggest the highest probability of success for the manner in which the leader relates to the group.

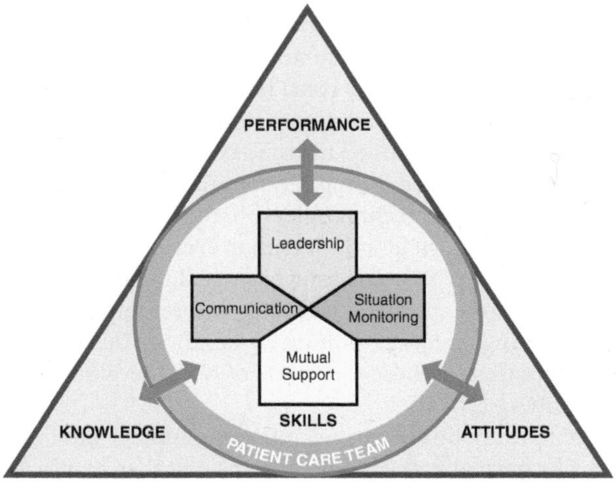

Fig. 8.3 Team competency outcomes. (From Agency for Healthcare Research and Quality. [2020]. *Pocket guide: TeamSTEPPS 2.0: Team Strategies & tools to enhance performance and patient safety.* Rockville, MD: AHRQ. https://www.ahrq.gov/sites/default/files/wysiwyg/professionals/education/curriculum-tools/teamstepps/instructor/essentials/pocketguide.pdf).

TeamSTEPPS

The Agency for Healthcare Research and Quality (AHRQ) has collected data regarding patient safety over many years. They continue to show that communication problems are found to be the most common root causes of medical errors. After discovering the staggering number of preventable medical errors and recognizing that communication problems were cited as the number one contributor, the AHRQ partnered with the Department of Defense (DOD) and developed the Team STEPPS program (AHRQ, 2020).

TeamSTEPPS is an evidence-based, comprehensive education and training program designed to improve patient safety by eliminating preventable medical errors related to ineffective team communication. TeamSTEPPS stands for Team Strategies and Tools to Enhance Performance and Patient Safety. TeamSTEPPS has been adapted and implemented effectively in several health care settings and across numerous specialty areas. Much support exists in the literature documenting the utility and effectiveness of TeamSTEPPS. The program consists of five key principles: team structure, leadership, situation monitoring, mutual support, and communication. Fig. 8.3 is a visual depiction of the five key principles of the TeamSTEPPS program. Extensive education and training programs are available on the AHRQ website.

SBAR and Handoff Communication

To address the "communication arm" of the TeamSTEPPS model pictured at the left side of Fig. 8.3, strategies such as SBAR have been created to enhance teamwork communication. One of the strategies that has been well documented and is familiar to nurses is SBAR, which stands for: Situation, Background, Assessment, and Recommendation. Fig. 8.4 demonstrates the four steps involved in SBAR. The SBAR tool provides members of the interprofessional team a great template to enhance communication such as framing conversations on a leadership agenda; framing email communication addressing specific concerns; or for more efficient communication with policymakers (Jurns, 2019).

Tiered daily huddles are becoming the norm in many hospitals and health systems. Hurle (2019),

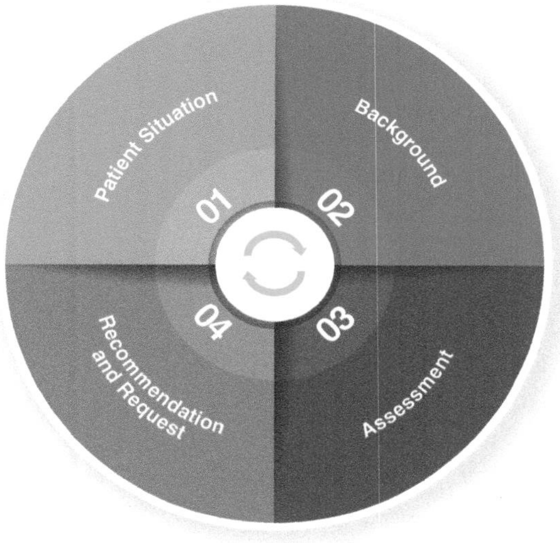

Fig. 8.4 Four steps in the SBAR process.

senior director of enterprise continuous improvement at Cleveland Clinic, built their tiered huddles upon existing practices focusing on patient safety and quality issues, caregiver safety issues, and providing access to care for their patients. They discovered that huddles needed to be smaller, connected, and standardized.

Midland (TX) Memorial Hospital holds daily leadership huddles in the hospital's lobby. These huddles helped drastically increase patient satisfaction, patient safety, and transformed a culture (Thrall, 2020). The huddle lasts no more than about 14 minutes, with information cascading to leaders shortly thereafter to share with employees in departments throughout the hospital.

Emory Healthcare in Georgia also has created leader standard work with tiered readiness huddles performing SMESS checks. SMESS communicates needs associated with Safety, Methods, Equipment, Supplies, and Staffing. Tier 1 Huddles are performed at the unit or department level engaging frontline employees. Unresolved issues or relevant information are escalated to Tier 2 Huddles, which are service line or division-based leaders. Unresolved issues or relevant information from Tier 2 are escalated using the same SMESS process in Tier 3 Huddles, which are organization-wide and include leaders from administration. As Emory Healthcare is a large health care system, unresolved issues or relevant information is then escalated to Tier 5 Huddles, where senior members of Emory Healthcare lead these huddles to guide resolution for systems-related issues. Huddles improve communication and teamwork resulting in improved outcomes.

CURRENT COMMUNICATION ISSUES AND TRENDS

Teaching Communication

The Research Note at the end of the chapter highlights how important it is to teach team communication strategies. These may be such things as TeamSTEPPS, SBAR, NVC model, and others. There is a need to determine a theoretical and evidence-based approach to teaching communication. It is important that this approach be most effective in developing interpersonal, interprofessional, and intercultural communication skills to ensure that nurses have the highest probability of responding in an empathetic manner with patients in critical life situations. More of this teaching can be done in simulated environments with interprofessional teams. Clearly, communication content builds. Nurses work first on therapeutic communication and then progress to mastering communication as a leader (see Table 8.2).

Patient Privacy

A related concern for the management of information and communication is how to prevent breaches of patient confidentiality. *The Health Insurance Portability and Accountability Act* (HIPAA) provisions have heightened awareness about and presented strategies to protect patients' privacy and data security in health care transactions. For example, fax transmissions need to be secure, and security measures need to be taken to protect computerized databases and electronic transmissions. End-user encryption is commonly used for data security. Health care providers' actions that disseminate confidential information can harm patients. For example, some nurses are uncomfortable performing handover reporting at the patient's bedside because of the risks of sharing patient information where other persons may be within earshot. Discretion and sensitivity are best used in these situations. Systems, processes, and structures can be altered to protect patient privacy.

TABLE 8.2 Practical Applications to Improve Communication and Build Relationships

Application	Frequency
1. Safety huddles	Every shift
2. Leadership rounds	Daily
3. Gemba walks	Daily
4. Newsletters (print or electronic)	Weekly/monthly
5. New employee experience (orientation) to receive foundational training and set expectations	Each orientation
6. Performance check-ins	Monthly
7. Professional governance (formal)	Monthly
8. CNO Advisory Councils (frontline staff and frontline nurse leaders)	Monthly
9. Mentoring/coaching	Monthly or as needed
10. CNO town hall meetings (live and virtual using technology)	Quarterly
11. Social media (e.g., Facebook, Yammer, LinkedIn, Twitter, Instagram)	Regularly

Adapted from Dent, B. (Fall 2019) Commentary: Communications. *Frontiers of Health Services Management, 36*(1), 2.

Communication in Emergencies

Communication effectiveness becomes crucial in times of emergency or disaster. In fact, often one of the key outcomes of disaster drills is to identify breaks in the communication system so they can be fixed before a real-time event occurs. TeamSTEPPS was developed to address communication issues between nurses and providers during critical patient events. Communication at these times must be impeccable. The AHRQ offers a plethora of team communication tools on their website for teams to practice and role-play so that they can be prepared to address issues efficiently during emergency situations.

Written Communication

The entire health care system relies on reliable, efficient tools and methods to produce timely and accurate patient documentation. The nursing profession, at the hub of the health care system, is called upon to produce the lion's share of the day-in, day-out documentation that exists in health care facilities. Proficiency and professionalism are imperative in all written documentation. Nurses need to have a command of the English language in order to produce written information that is useful and readable. Patient documentation is only one form of written communication needed by nursing staff. Promotions and awards in the profession are usually based on written documentation of performance and outcomes endorsing an individual staff member. Grants and funds for projects are based upon extensive written proposals that address specific criteria. Quality improvement initiatives within a hospital can be awarded based on both written proposals and oral presentations, such as those making a business case for a clinically based initiative. Sharing information with colleagues is nurses' professional responsibility, such as by authoring textbooks and journals and providing expertise as peer reviewers and subject matter experts.

Electronic Communication and Social Media

With the advent of e-mail and explosion of social media and cell phones, the avenues of communication have changed. Health care systems have kept pace by developing extensive internal information technology (IT) departments that have engineered electronic medical records, secured e-mail servers for communication between patients and their providers, and developed numerous health care "apps." Electronic communication has assisted nurses in being better informed regarding patients. However, within the professional health care realm, there is a tendency to rely on these modes of communication when other methods would be preferable and more appropriate. For instance, there are definite times when a face-to-face conversation is preferred to an e-mail. Warrell (2012) noted that there are four times you should never use e-mail: (1) when you are angry, (2) when rebuking or criticizing, (3) if there is any chance your words could be misunderstood, or (4) when you are canceling or apologizing. In our busy professional lives, it is easier to send off a quick e-mail than to pick up the phone or walk down the hall; however, e-mail distances us from others and is really only the preferred means of communication when information is simply being conveyed. It is not appropriate for a back-and-forth dialogue where feelings need to be expressed and opinions heard.

Similarly, there is an appropriate use of texting, social media, Facebook, Twitter, and hashtags (#). However, this form of communication can be overused, making face-to-face conversations a thing of the past. Video chatting provides a nice way to have a conversation and actually see the person. There are several very good health care apps that have been produced for downloading on smartphones for free or at a fairly minimal cost. Some of these apps are very useful; some are a waste of time and money. The important thing to remember is to maintain professionalism and appropriate boundaries when using social media and to be judicious in what information is shared about yourself and others publicly. Many organizations have formal social media policies to help nurses navigate around what is appropriate for sharing on social media. Patient privacy, potential HIPAA violations, perceived bullying, and damage to reputations are major concerns.

RESEARCH NOTE

Source

Raley, J., Meenakshi, R., Dent, D., Willis, R., Lawson, K., & Duzinski, S. (2016). The role of communication during trauma activations: Investigating the need for team and leader communication training. *Journal of Surgical Education, 74*(1), 173–177.

Purpose

Fatal errors due to miscommunication among members of trauma teams are two to four times more likely to occur than in other medical teams, yet most trauma team members do not receive communication effectiveness training. The purpose of this study is to demonstrate that communication training is necessary and highlight specific team communication competencies that trauma teams should learn to improve communication during activations.

Study Design

Data were collected in two phases. Phase 1 required participants to complete a series of surveys. Phase 2 included live observations and assessments of pediatric trauma activations using the assessment of pediatric resuscitation team assessments (APRC-TA) and assessment of pediatric resuscitation leader assessments (APRC-LA). Data were collected at a southwestern pediatric hospital. Trauma team members and leaders completed surveys at a meeting and were observed while conducting activations in the trauma bay. Trained research scientists and clinical staff used the APRC-TA and APRC-LA to measure trauma teams' performance and communication effectiveness. The sample included 29 health care providers who regularly participate in trauma activations. Additionally, 12 live trauma activations were assessed.

Discussion

Findings from the study suggest that the medical performance and communication effectiveness of trauma teams seem to be linked. Accordingly, health care providers working in trauma settings have begun to verbalize their concerns about miscommunication between team members. Trauma team members who participated in the study believe communication training is important and necessary, and if given the chance, they would attend this type of training. Team communication training is associated with increases in group cohesion and decreases in communication errors. Nurses and providers believe that communication training may improve patient safety and reduce the number of errors made in emergency settings.

Application to Practice

Although this study focused on communication in a pediatric hospital during trauma activations, communication mishaps in health care settings continue to be a leading cause of patient safety events. Communication training for all teams may help build team cohesion, relationships built on trust, and improve outcomes associated with patient safety.

NEXT-GENERATION NCLEX® EXAMINATION-STYLE CASE STUDY

Nurse Manager Tyler has been in his job for 9 months in a busy academic medical center and is just beginning to settle in. He has noticed a spike in medication errors on the unit. It is difficult to manage health care providers' incoming orders as well as the confusion and complexity of multiple provider teams (e.g., neuro, cardiovascular, oncology) rounding independently and making medication and treatment changes that sometimes conflict. Tyler just got the latest data on his unit's quality and safety measures. The medication error rate has increased. He calls the Chair of the unit's Shared Governance Council (SGC) to help evaluate ideas to address communication breakdowns.

Which communication strategies will Tyler, the nurse manager, use to support effective communication interventions? **Select all that apply.**

_____ **A.** Confrontive communication style
_____ **B.** AHRQ's CUS assertive statements.
_____ **C.** Incident reporting
_____ **D.** Crucial Conversations
_____ **E.** Formal referral to immediate supervisor
_____ **F.** TeamSTEPPS SBAR

CRITICAL THINKING EXERCISE

You are the new nurse leader of a heart and vascular service line. You note the outcomes for this area are poor (e.g., patient experience, quality of care, labor expenses). Interprofessional relationships are strained. The equipment in the area needs to be updated. More than 75% of nurses are contract labor. The team has been unsuccessful in recruiting, leaving some RN requisitions open for up to 2 years. However, you are asked by the senior leaders to accommodate adding additional cardiovascular providers and position your team for growth.

1. What are your priorities for this area as the new nurse leader?
2. What communication strategies would you use with your team?
3. Using the SBAR tool, describe how you would communicate requests to the CNO and other members of the senior leadership team, as needed.

REFERENCES

Agency for Healthcare Research and Quality (AHRQ). (2020). *TeamSTEPPS*. Rockville, MD: AHRQ. https://www.ahrq.gov/teamstepps/index.html.

Aguilar, A. (2019). Culture of silence contributes to lack of progress on patient safety. *Modern Healthcare, 49*(44), 34.

American Nurses Association (ANA). (2015). *Incivility, bullying, and workplace violence. ANA Position Statement.* https://www.nursingworld.org/practice-policy/nursing-excellence/official-position-statements/id/incivility-bullying-and-workplace-violence/.

American Nurses Association (ANA). (2020). *What is nursing?* https://www.nursingworld.org/practice-policy/workforce/what-is-nursing/.

American Nurses Credentialing Center (ANCC). (2020). *Magnet model.* https://www.nursingworld.org/organizational-programs/magnet/magnet-model/.

Bennet, M. J. (2013). *Intercultural communication.* https://www.idrinstitute.org/resources/intercultural-communication/.

Berwick, D. M. (2009). What 'patient-centered' should mean: Confessions of an extremist. *Health Affairs – Web Exclusive.* https://www.healthaffairs.org/doi/pdf/10.1377/hlthaff.28.4.w555.

Carman, K., Dardess, P., Maurer, M., Sofaer, S., Adams, K., Bechtel, C., et al. (2013). Patient and family engagement: A framework for understanding the elements and developing interventions and policies. *Health Affairs, 32*(2), 223–231.

Covey, S. R. (2004). *The 8th habit: From effectiveness to greatness.* New York: Free Press.

Dent, B., & Tye, J. (2018). *The heart of a nurse leader: Values-based leadership for healthcare organizations.* Monee, IL: Joe Tye and Bob Dent.

Dent, B. (Fall 2019). Commentary: Communications. *Frontiers of Health Services Management, 36*(1), 2.

Fitzgerald, C., & Kirby, L. K. (1997). *Developing leaders: Research and applications in psychological type and leadership development*. Palo Alto, CA: Davies-Black Publishing.

Fooks, C., Obarski, G., Hale, L., & Hylmar, S. (2015). The patient experience in Ontario 2020: What is possible? *Healthcare Papers, 14*(4), 8–18.

Foronda C. L., Alhusen J., Budhathoki C., Lamb M., Tinsley K., MacWilliams B., et al. (2015). A mixed-methods, international, multisite study to develop and validate a measure of nurse-to-physician communication in simulation. *Nursing Education Perspectives, 36*(6), 383–388.

Frampton, S. B., Guastello, S., Hoy, L., Naylor, M., Sheridan, S., & Johnston-Fleece, M. (2017). Harnessing evidence and experience to change culture: A guiding framework for patient and family engaged care. *National Academy of Medicine Perspectives, 7*. https://doi.org/10.31478/201701f.

Hersey, P., Blanchard, K., & Johnson, D. (2013). *Management of organizational behavior: Leading human resources* (10th ed.). Upper Saddle River, NJ: Pearson Education.

Hurle, N. (2019). How we improved our tiered daily huddles. *The Lean Post*. https://www.lean.org/LeanPost/Posting.cfm?LeanPostId=1095.

Institute of Medicine (IOM). (2001). *To err is human: Building a safer health system*. Washington, DC: National Academies Press (pp. 40).

Institute of Medicine (IOM). (2011). *The future of nursing: Leading change, advancing health*. Washington, DC: National Academies Press.

Jurns, C. (2019). Using SBAR to communicate with policymakers. *The Online Journal of Issues in Nursing, 24*(1). https://doi.org/10.3912/OJIN.Vol24No01PPT47.

Kotter, J. (1996). *Leading change*. Boston, MA: Harvard Business School Press.

Kouzes, J. M., & Posner, B. Z. (2017). *The leadership challenge: How to make extraordinary things happen in organizations* (6th ed.). Hoboken, NJ: John Wiley & Sons, Inc.

Matzke, B., Houston, S., Fischer, U., & Bradshaw, M. J. (2014). Using a team-centered approach to evaluate effectiveness of nurse-physician communications. *JOGNN: Journal of Obstetric, Gynecologic & Neonatal Nursing, 43*(6), 684–694. https://doi.org/10.1111/1552-6909.12486.

Maxfield, D., Grenny, J., Lavandero, R., & Groah, L. (n.d.). *The silent treatment: Why safety tools and checklists aren't enough to save lives*. http://www.silenttreatmentstudy.com/silencekills/.

Maxfield, D., Harmon, H., & McDonald, C. (2010). Crucial conversations for motivating colleagues and patients. *American Nurse Today, 5*(5), 16–18.

McAllen, E. R., Stephens, K., Swanson-Biearman, B., Kerr, K., & Whiteman, K. (2018). Moving shift report to the bedside: An evidence-based quality improvement project. *The Online Journal of Issues in Nursing, 23*(2). https://doi.org/10.3912/OJIN.Vol23No02PPT22.

Mosadeghrad, A. M., & Mojbafan, A. (2019). Conflict and conflict management in hospitals. *International Journal of Health Care Quality Assurance, 32*(3), 550–561.

Nicotera, A., Mahon, M., & Wright, K. (2014). Communication that builds teams: Assessing a nursing conflict intervention. *Nursing Administration Quarterly, 38*(3), 248–260.

Pater, R. (2016). Preventing strained communications. *Occupational Health & Safety, 85*(8), 50.

Patterson, K., Grenny, J., McMillan, R., & Switzler, A. (2011). *Crucial conversations: Tools for talking when stakes are high* (2nd ed.). New York, NY: McGraw-Hill Education.

Plonien, C. (2015). Using personality indicators to enhance nurse leader communication. *AORN Journal, 102*(1), 74–80.

Pryse, Y., McDaniel, A., & Schafer, J. (2014). Psychometric analysis of two new scales: The Evidence-Based Practice Nursing Leadership and Work Environment Scales. *Worldviews on Evidence-Based Nursing, 11*(4), 240–247.

R^3 Report. (2011). *Requirement, rationale, reference*. The Joint Commission (pp. 2). February 9, 2011. https://www.jointcommission.org/-/media/tjc/documents/standards/r3-reports/r3-report-issue-1-20111.pdf on March 9, 2020.

Raley, J., Meenakshi, R., Dent, D., Willis, R., Lawson, K., & Duzinski, S. (2016). The role of communication during trauma activations: Investigating the need for team and leader communication training. *Journal of Surgical Education, 74*(1), 173–177.

Rosenberg, M. B. (2004). *We can work it out: Resolving conflicts peacefully and powerfully*. Encinitas, CA: Puddledancer Press.

Sharifabad, M. A. M., Ardakani, M. F., Bahrami, M. A., & Fallahzadeh, H. (2019). Nurses' communication skills and the quality of inpatient services from patients' viewpoints. *Medical Science, 23*(96), 163–167.

Sears, M. (2010). *Humanizing health care: Creating cultures of compassion with nonviolent communication*. Encinitas, CA: Puddledancer Press.

Spears, T. L. (2019). *The four conversations you must get right as a leader*. American Association for Physician Leadership. https://www.physicianleaders.org/news/the-four-conversations-leader.

The Joint Commission. (2015). *Sentinel event statistics released for 2014*. Joint Commission Online. April 29, 2015. https://www.jointcommission.org/-/media/deprecated-unorganized/imported-assets/tjc/system-folders/joint-commission-online/jconline_april_29_15pdf.pdf?db=web&hash=DEFFBC41623A360F1C1428A5E9602773.

Thrall, T. H. (2020). How a 14-minute meeting transformed this hospital. *Hospitals & Health Networks*: Advisory Board Daily Briefing. March 15, 2016, republished on January 10, 2020. https://www.advisory.com/daily-briefing/2016/03/15/14-minutes.

Tri-Council for Nursing. (2017). *Tri-Council for nursing issues proclamation on nursing civility*. http://www.nln.org/docs/default-source/newsroom/tri-council-civility-proclamation-draft-2-krk-bm-tri-092617.pdf?sfvrsn=2.

Tuckman, B. W. (1965). Developmental sequence in small groups. *Psychological Bulletin, 63*(6), 384–399. https://doi.org/10.1037/h0022100.

Tye, J., & Dent, B. (2017). *Building a culture of ownership in healthcare: The invisible architecture of core values, attitude, and self-empowerment*. Indianapolis, IN: Sigma Theta Tau International.

Warrell, M. (2012, August 27). Hiding behind email? Four times you should never use email. *Forbes*. http://www.forbes.com/sites/margiewarrell/2012/08/27/do-you-hide-behind-email/#dc8f0e97bf00.

Workplace Bullying Institute (WBI). (2019). *WBI—the Workplace Bullying Institute*. https://www.workplacebullying.org/.

Yang, Y. (2012). Studies of transformational leadership in consumer service: Leadership trust and the mediating-moderating role of cooperative conflict management. *Psychological Reports, 110*(1), 315–337.

9

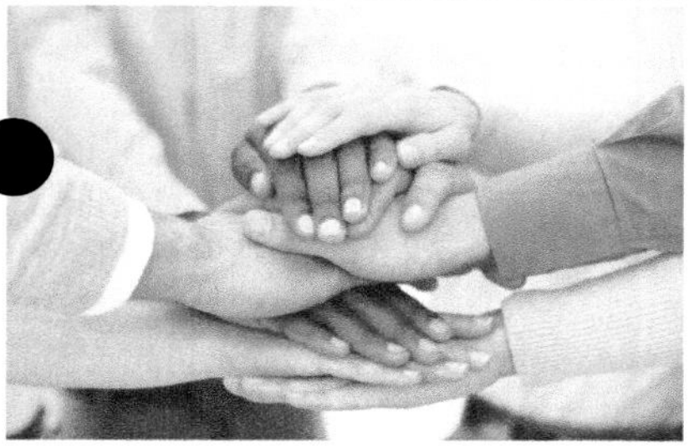

Team Building and Working With Effective Groups

Sandra Lynne Swearingen

http://evolve.elsevier.com/Huber/leadership

Nurse leaders in today's health care organizations must be skilled communicators, collaborators, and facilitators with an exquisite ability to lead the collective work of individuals. At times they will serve as a leader for a team or group, and at other times they will serve as a member. Being capable of both leading and following are essential skills for nurses. A significant percentage of work completed in organizations today is done through the collaborative efforts of different types of teams or work groups. There is an even greater emphasis on shared leadership in nursing, as well as in working with other health care professionals as part of an interdisciplinary or multidisciplinary team. Understanding the characteristics of teams, groups, and the basic principles for attaining successful outcomes increases the leader's effectiveness.

Health care leaders recognize that an interdisciplinary, team-based approach is essential for high-quality, patient-centered, coordinated, and effective health care. Teamwork allows for greater exchange of information, ideas, and problem-solving to address the complex issues of health care. Engaging teams in this process allows for diverse points of view, creativity, innovation, and an enhanced ability to adapt to continuous or sudden change. The health care environment continues to evolve at an unprecedented rate with new specialized knowledge, scientific and technological advances, and redesign of care processes. A high degree of specialization exists, even within a profession. The nursing profession, for example, includes individuals with a variety of different roles, including direct care registered nurses, clinical nurse leaders, licensed practical nurses, nurse practitioners, clinical nurse specialists, nurse educators, nurse midwives, and nurse anesthetists. Establishing effective teamwork across various specialties within and across professions is key to interdisciplinary collaboration to address and adapt to the constant state of change in health care.

The ability to collaborate is essential for optimal patient outcomes. The focus of health care organizations today is to achieve the Institute of Health Care Improvement's (IHI, 2016) Triple Aim. The goal is "simultaneously improving the health of the population, enhancing the experience and outcomes of the patient, and reducing per capita cost of care for the benefit of communities." This Triple Aim has been expanded to a fourth "Quadruple Aim" workforce element of improving the experience of providing care (Sikka et al., 2015). The shift in payment methodologies from fee-for-service to value-based purchasing and accountable care has created incentives and penalties for organizations to improve quality, efficiency, and the overall value of health care. The expectation for health care leaders is to continuously improve while delivering safe, high-quality patient care. Changing reimbursement methodologies, increasing governmental regulation, and managing care across the continuum require a high level of engagement between clinical disciplines, non-clinical staff, and senior management. Just as in other industries, rapid information dissemination and the shift to a knowledge worker–based service society are some of the social and economic forces operative in health care. These forces converge to create the tumultuous change currently underway in health care delivery. Teamwork is the solution.

Employees who work in a collaborative manner with others and who can work effectively within a team context can provide the strength, structure, and resiliency to deal with work complexities and changes. Today's health care organizations are considered *learning organizations*, and there is a renewed emphasis on the role of teams. Just as interdisciplinary teams play an important role in delivering mental health, home care, rehabilitation, hospice, and other community-based services, hospitals and large health care systems engage teams as an essential element of their core processes and structure. This is the general way now that business gets done in all health care settings. The Institute of Medicine (IOM, now called the National Academies of Sciences, Engineering, and Medicine, Health and Medicine Division) suggested that working as part of an interdisciplinary team is an essential core competency of health care professionals and that professionals cooperate, collaborate, communicate, and integrate care in teams to be sure that care is continuous and reliable (Altman et al., 2016).

Because health care professionals are specialists, it is incumbent on leaders to bring people together in groups and teams to build on their knowledge and strengths and ultimately to ensure safe, effective care. Leaders have an ever-increasing role to ensure that teams are effective, efficient, and productive. In their book *The wisdom of teams: Creating the high-performance organization*, Katzenbach and Smith (2015) claimed that teams should be the basic unit of organization for most businesses as a way to reach the highest levels of performance.

Team building is a strategy for designing, implementing, developing, and nurturing work teams in organizations. These work teams are a specialized subset of the many types of groups that form or are formed in organizations.

In nursing, group process theory relates to both how to be therapeutic with clients and how to work as an employee within an organization, which is often large and complex. Nursing has an integral role as a member of the health care team. As a caregiver, the nurse serves a key role as a patient advocate and frequently serves as the coordinator of care with other members of the team. The nurse tracks whether different interventions have been effective or whether alternative strategies might be needed. As a care provider spending significant time with the patient, often a nurse will see fine, distinct changes in a patient's condition before other members of the health care team. Nurses oversee the plan of care and are involved more intimately and more proximately than any of the other health care providers in managing the total health care of the patient. Therefore understanding and developing skills in group process and group dynamics is essential within the context of leadership and management in nursing because of the group functioning and coordinative aspects of nursing practice. Equally important is the nurse's role in coordinating multidisciplinary and interdisciplinary teams. Because care is complex and involves the expertise of many disciplines, nurses need strong group process and interaction skills to communicate clearly and collaborate effectively with a variety of colleagues.

DEFINITIONS

A **group** is defined as any collection of interconnected individuals working together for some purpose. Groups are important in organizations, not only because of informal network dynamics, but also because of the multitude of formal committees, task forces, councils, and teams in the contemporary organization. A **committee** is a relatively stable and formally composed group. Committees are a specific type of group in that they are stable, meet periodically, and have an identified purpose that is part of the organizational structure. There is a mechanism for maintaining and selecting members. Typically, committees have official status and sanction within an organization. For example, there are policy and procedure committees, quality and patient safety committees, and ethics committees.

A **task force** is a temporary group of individuals formed to carry out a specific mission or project. Task forces may solve a problem that requires a multidisciplinary approach. A **council** is an advisory group of individuals who may be elected or appointed and that has a defined charter or purpose and meets regularly. In a nursing professional shared governance model, the councilor structure is commonplace. Councils promote collegiality and engagement. Nursing may have unit practice councils, a hospital practice council, and a leadership council, as well as specific areas of focus, such as a nursing research council or education council.

Collaboration is defined as people undertaking harmonizing roles and jointly working to share responsibility for problem-solving and decision-making to formulate and carry out plans (Baggs & Schmitt, 1998; Christensen & Larson, 1993). It is a complex phenomenon that brings together two or more individuals, often from different professional disciplines, who work to achieve shared aims and objectives such as working together toward a common goal for the patient.

Communication is a process by which information is exchanged between individuals through a common system of symbols, signs, or behavior (Merriam-Webster, 2019). It includes the style and extent of interactions both among members and between members and those outside the team. It also refers to the way flows of conflict, decision-making, and day-to-day interactions occur.

Team building is defined as the process of deliberately creating and unifying a group into a functioning team. A **team** is made up of persons working on individual tasks that impact the overall objectives of the group. Team members need to collaborate with each other to combine individual tasks into a cohesive product that meets the goals of the team (Turner et al., 2018). Genuine communication is also a requirement of information exchanges within the team (Kayser, 2011). Finally, if a team is to remain effective in an ever-evolving, complex environment, it also needs to be adaptable (Kozlowski & Ilgen, 2006). Teams are interdependent, with shared responsibility to achieve their goals and for their successes or failures. Teams have the authority to coordinate activities and tasks; team members may have defined roles, duties, or responsibilities.

In today's workplace culture, working in a team is imperative to the success of many health care organizations. Teams tend to demonstrate synergy and therefore make better decisions as a group than as singular individuals. In addition, due to increasing technology, one individual cannot be an expert in all work processes. Health care workers are made up of many experts from many fields and occupations. Each of these team members may have expertise that is beyond the scope of one manager (Belker et al., 2019).

The distinction between a work group and a true team is crucial. Health care leaders may mistakenly assume that simply calling a group a *team* actually makes it a team. As Katzenbach and Smith (2015) emphasized, the group becomes a true team only by doing its collective work. The team goes through a developmental process that takes time and the investment of energy to materialize. Many collective entities in today's organizations are called *teams* yet clearly function more as work groups than true teams.

A **work group** is a collection of individuals who are charged with completing a specific activity or mission. Work groups come together to share information and ideas, and they may make some decisions mutually. However, the members of the work group have individual work products for which they are responsible, and these consume their major focus and effort. For example, in a patient care unit, the unit clerk has certain responsibilities, as do the charge nurse, direct care nurse, and nurse manager. The boundaries remain clearly separated when the collective entity is a work group. Each person may view their role as being individually accountable, but there is little to no collective accountability.

This is in contrast with a true team, which is a collective entity where leadership rotates and is shared by various members of the team, depending on appropriateness and fit of skills and abilities. In a true team, there are collective work products, for example, the provision of quality patient care to all patients housed in the department or seen in the clinic. There is group as well as individual accountability. If one member of the team is having a problem, it is not just that individual's problem; instead it becomes a team problem for all members of the team to pull together to resolve. An example of team thinking is "No one sits down until we can all sit down" or "No one goes home until we all go home." If quality outcomes are difficult for one team member, all team members are affected by this and become engaged in helping the affected team member meet expectations. In the management book *The goal* (Goldratt & Cox, 2016), the author tells a parable about taking a Boy Scout troop on a hike. When it was discovered that Scout Herbie was slowing the whole group down, the weight in his backpack was redistributed, and the troop sped up. This is how a high-performing team works.

BACKGROUND

Group interactions are a pervasive element of the health care environment in which nurses work. A basic understanding of groups helps nurses function more effectively. These principles apply to any group, whether an actual team, a committee, task force, council, or an informal group effort. Team effectiveness has nine core processes composed of the following elements (Turner et al., 2018):

- *Coaching:* The establishment of goals and behaviors in order to accomplish the team's work. This includes any activity performed individually and collaboratively for team effectiveness. It also includes person-to-person interactions that assist in the synchronization and utilization of resources in accomplishing the work of the team.

- *Cognition:* The ability of team members to mutually understand the task of the team. This includes the ability to make appropriate judgments, solve problems, incorporate information, forecast, and acquire information.
- *Cohesiveness:* The degree to which members of the team desire to remain in the team and meet the goals of the team. Feeling that they fit in the team and identify with the group are important to cohesiveness in the group.
- *Collective efficacy:* The team is capable, competent, and empowered to meet the team's goals successfully.
- *Collective identity:* A person's sense of being an individual is replaced by being a team member.
- *Communication:* The process by which people share information within the team. Communication should allow for the mutual exchange of information.
- *Conflict:* Any perceived incompatibility of opinions, benefits, or principles held by team members that are perceived threatening to other members of the team.
- *Cooperation:* Involves the group members working together towards a common goal. It is a structure where the success of one person improves the chances of success of the group.
- *Coordination:* Includes the progressive composition of codependent actions that impact the team's goals. Coordination also references the team's ability to use assets and turn tasks into desired outcomes of the team.

Marks et al. (2001) presented a taxonomy of team processes categorized into three different phases: the transition phase, the action phase, and the interpersonal phase.

- *Transition phase:* This is the phase when team members distribute duties, schedule actions, and allocate assets needed to meet the goals of the team. Three identified processes take place during this phase: mission analysis, goal specification, and strategy formation.
- *Action phase:* This phase pertains to activities relating to the attainment of established goals. There are four processes that take place in the action phase: monitoring goal progress, monitoring systems, monitoring the team itself, and activities that coordinate the work of the team.
- *Interpersonal phase:* This phase is about relationships between team members and other stakeholders. This is a phase that is typically present throughout the duration of the team and includes three processes: controlling conflict within the group, building the confidence and drive of the team members, and facilitation of emotive equilibrium between team members.

WHY GROUPS ARE FORMED

In nursing, the formation of groups occurs primarily for one of two reasons: (1) to provide a personal or professional socialization and exchange forum, or (2) to provide a mechanism for interdependent work accomplishment. Groups can be social, professional, or organizational in purpose. The following are some reasons why groups would be established in organizations:

- Group activities can create a sense of status and esteem, allowing an individual to be part of something bigger themselves.
- Groups allow an individual to test and establish reality.
- Groups allow engagement of individuals with leaders to share responsibility, decision-making, and accountability for outcomes.
- Groups function as a mechanism for individuals to work collectively and cooperatively to get a job done.
- Groups address complex problems or tasks by a diverse group of individuals with specialized knowledge and/or skill.
- Groups can maximize leaders' strengths and minimize their weaknesses.

A major part of the working environment of nurses is accomplishment of work through group activity. The work group provides an institutional and professional identity for an individual nurse, and work groups become a focus for interpersonal relationships, support, and social integration. Job satisfaction, positive relational leadership, and positive quality outcomes are linked (Wong et al., 2013). Factors related to job satisfaction include working conditions, job stress, role conflict and ambiguity, role perception, role content, and organizational and professional commitment (Lu et al., 2012). In addition, being part of a healthy group or team is related to the level of organizational commitment by the team member. Cultural issues that become barriers to effective teamwork and communication include workplace discrimination, bullying, fear of discipline, lack of feedback, and strong hierarchical models (Teunissen et al., 2020). Individuals with an emotional connection to their work group have lower levels of turnover and higher levels of engagement (Manion, 2009).

Work groups can be disrupted by factors such as downsizing, reorganization, absenteeism, loss of leadership, bullying, and turnover. Work group disruption has been linked to negative outcomes (Kalisch & Lee, 2010). In a study of four hospitals, interpersonal relations were found to be an important part of nurses' job satisfaction. Interpersonal relationships are integral to work group functioning. Things get done because of relationships among people. Nurses need to build successful collaborative relationships among multiple levels of intra- and interdisciplinary colleagues, other members of the organization, and patients. The level of nursing teamwork has been found to be directly linked to missed nursing care (Kalisch & Lee, 2010).

One vulnerable group of nurses are new graduates. There has been extensive research suggesting that workplace bullying occurs particularly with new graduates. Read and Laschinger (2013) found the sense of community and similarity between the ideals and beliefs of the nurses within a work unit affected the perception of bullying. Some of the job characteristics related to workplace bullying include workload, job control, reward, and recognition. Budin et al. (2013) found that support from their leader or a mentor had an impact on the likelihood of a new graduate being a victim of bullying. Bullying may affect trust, communication, and cohesiveness in a group. Furthermore, informal work group norms exert a strong influence on nurses' behavior and functioning within a group. Nurse residency programs for new graduate nurses are an antidote.

Work group relationships can reinforce behaviors and rationalization, thus leading to deviant behaviors such as workarounds that become passively or actively accepted. Debono et al. (2013) conducted an extensive literature search of studies concerning nurse workaround behaviors. There were several themes related to teamwork. First, workarounds may be individual or supported by a group who share the belief that rules are "flexible." When that is the case, there is also an understanding of who will and will not perform a workaround. Second, nurses may justify working around policies and procedures as necessary to benefit the patient. Finally, acceptance or proliferation of workarounds can be affected by a variety of factors, including group norms, leadership, professional structures, personal relationships, and organizational culture. A culture of innovativeness can be fostered as a fixing and reporting method for broken processes or systems failures so that there are more permanent and precise solutions to workarounds (Huber et al., 2019).

Clearly, there is a strong relationship between work groups, interpersonal relationships, leadership, and outcomes such as nurses' behaviors and perceptions. Work group relationships are a powerful mechanism influencing both good and bad outcomes in nursing practice.

ADVANTAGES OF GROUPS

Groups have the potential for being a driving force for change in an organization. Ronco (2005) identified positive impacts groups can have on an organization:

1. *Synergy:* Groups have potential to perform at higher levels than an individual would on their own.
2. *Positive individual impacts:* Groups have potential to improve every member of the group or at least help each one reach their highest potential.
3. *Motivation:* Groups have potential to motivate their individual members and provide encouragement, constructive criticism, and praise.
4. *Diverse thinking:* Groups have potential to engage in diverse thinking, thereby identifying problems that might otherwise go unnoticed or ignored and exploring solutions.
5. *Linkage to the larger organization:* Groups have potential to make individuals feel more connected to the larger organization.

Working as a team has advantages over working alone relative to solving problems. The main benefit of teamwork is it allows organizations to achieve goals that individuals working alone cannot. This is due to inherent advantages built into teamwork such as (Lumen Learning, 2020):

1. *Increased efficiency.* By combining the skills of individuals, the work effort is increased, allowing the team to accomplish more than an individual can.
2. *Speed.* Since there are many contributors in a team effort, tasks and activities are completed more rapidly.
3. *Reflection in ideas.* Different people have different ideas and perceptions of an issue. Combining such differences can achieve previously unidentified solutions.

4. *Superior effectiveness.* Teams work together and divide the work at hand. Through harmonization of tasks and efforts the work is shared out to better address issues.
5. *Social aspects.* Teamwork improves the work experience for individual team members because they receive support and assistance when they work on mutual tasks. This type of support helps people achieve normally unattainable goals. This also leads to team members having a greater sense of achievement.

Groups are one vehicle for creative problem-solving, stimulating innovation, and building consensus. To be successful, the leader must be skilled at facilitation, ensuring meetings have a clear purpose and are organized, focused, and productive, with balanced participation by team members. An effective meeting will start and finish on time and result in a balanced discussion of pros and cons on a topic or issue, with required next steps, actions, follow-up, and specific member assignments and accountabilities. These practices demonstrate the leader's organizational skills and respect for contributions by all team members and their time. It is imperative that there is a clearly defined purpose for a group, particularly when the group is part of a larger organization. Ideally this is an early discussion by the group and is determined with input from all members. The purpose and value of the group needs to be evaluated periodically in addition to evaluating whether the team is meeting its goals. Is it functional? Is it accomplishing the task to which it was assigned or committed? If not, should the group be disbanded or reorganized?

When the work output of any group is analyzed, meetings can be costly endeavors. For example, when the number of hours spent by all committee members is multiplied by their individual hourly salary along with fringe benefit costs, the sum of costs for the group may be astounding. This is one reason for paying attention to how well the group is functioning. Just as important is assessing whether the group adds value to the organization and the individuals involved. If team members are not actively contributing to the group's charge, their role and time on the team may be wasted energy, resulting in a drain on enthusiasm and effectiveness in the group. The cost of group work can be balanced by calculating benefits such as increased productivity or risk/cost avoidance.

A highly functioning group may have a profound impact on an organization. Such groups often identify and solve complex problems. Participation and involvement in a group decision typically results in individuals being more engaged and committed to a decision, even if there is disagreement. Disagreement and conflict are important elements for the leader to guide teams through and are often productive factors in solving problems. In this way, leaders of teams can demonstrate effective means of resolving differences, which are commonplace in health care.

DISADVANTAGES OF GROUPS

Ronco (2005) identified six potential negative impacts groups can have on an organization, including negativity, passivity, individual focus, groupthink, vocal minority, and the ethical dark side. A seventh is disruptive conflicts.

1. *Negativity:* Research suggests that people working in groups tend to be more negative than if they work individually.
2. *Passivity:* People may become passive participants in a group versus being active participants. Unbalanced participation may lead to feelings of resentment, jealousy, and disillusionment. Some may "slide by" on the work effort of others.
3. *Individual focus and individual domination:* Individuals may have difficulty thinking globally and objectively. They may focus on how a discussion affects them as an individual instead of as a group. Some individuals may also dominate the group, compromising group process. Strong opinions of group members may stifle discussion, creativity, and innovation. As a result, the group or leader may need to divert its energy and productivity into working out interpersonal dynamics rather than moving forward on the group's task.
4. *Groupthink:* Groups may reach quick agreement and be unwilling to challenge or debate. Sometimes decisions result from pressure—by the group, leader, or external deadlines—to complete the work. Groups may influence individual members when most of the group feels a certain way about an issue or task. Minority group members, who may disagree, experience an element of pressure due to psychological dynamics related to subtle pressure for group acceptance and conformity. Creative and innovate ideas may be lost if a group reaches decisions too quickly.

5. *Vocal minority:* Groups tend to allow the most vocal members of a group to represent overall group views even when they are the minority of members. It may be difficult to be a devil's advocate or to adopt the role of bringing alternative critique points to the group for consideration due to a concern about not being socially accepted or fear of conflict. For example, derision and humiliation can occur if members react negatively.
6. *Ethical dark side:* Groups have potential, based on power in the group, to not support ethical choices.
7. *Disruptive conflicts:* If people perceive an adverse effect on a group member or if they feel threatened, conflict emerges. Conflicts can accelerate in a competitive environment when members vest in their own position and are not willing to consider a different point of view. Conflicts about substantive issues actually help the group become more effective in decision-making. However, when conflicts occur over differences in personality, opinions, or values, conflicts can become destructive. Interdisciplinary teams may experience conflict due to team instability or differences in personal and professional priorities (Teunissen et al., 2020). Although it may seem contradictory, conflicts can serve as a control mechanism in a group and may result in far superior outcomes. When group members are comfortable respectfully disagreeing with each other, a premature acceptance of decisions can be avoided since opposing viewpoints are considered.

GROUP DECISION-MAKING

Group work can be—and typically is—a slow process. It takes more time for a group to arrive at a decision than for one person to make the decision.

In addition, a continuum of decision-making power may be vested in a group (Fig. 9.1). A group or committee has certain powers, tasks, and functions, and also certain parameters or latitude in terms of how far to go in deciding. Decision power is a matter of degree, with four distinct points on the continuum of authority for decision-making: authoritative, consultative, joint, and delegated.

On one end of the continuum is *authoritative decision-making*, where the leader makes the decision. In this process there is input, perhaps, but not necessarily a vote. One example of this is in some medical emergencies, such as cardiac arrest: there is no time for discussion, and the leader needs to take control and direct the team. Authoritative style is generally ineffective in non-emergencies because it can generate increased cynicism and employee disengagement.

Consultative decision-making occurs when decisions involve employee participation, but the leader still makes the final decision. Group members may make certain recommendations, to the leader, chairperson, or head of the group, who will make the final decision. There is increased participation in this type of procedure, but the ultimate decision is not under the control of group members. Consultative decision-making is used in nursing with task forces, quality committees, and shared governance councils.

Some decision procedures result in *joint decision-making*. In this approach, the entire group makes a decision by a two-thirds vote, simple majority, consensus, or some other process. In a joint decision procedure, team members have as much influence as the leader. The leader has one voice, one vote. The leader can use persuasion, but when it comes to the final vote, the leader's vote is equivalent to that of any other group member. This is fundamentally different from the leader making the decision with group input. This type of decision-making is used in a high functioning multidisciplinary team. Every team member is heard and valued equally. In nursing, individual unit and hospital councils may

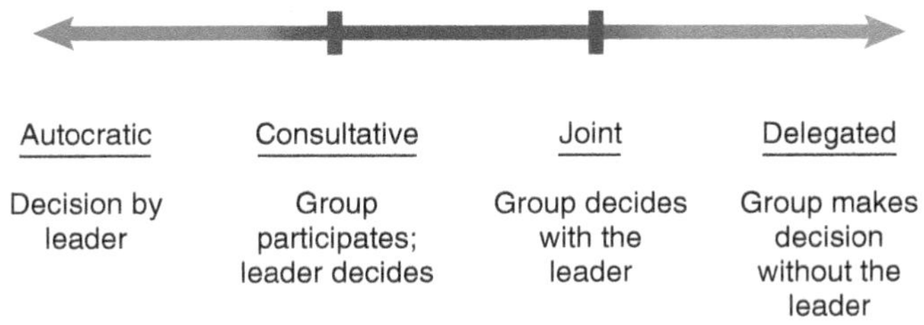

Fig. 9.1 Range of decision powers.

have authority to implement certain decisions related to clinical practice.

At the other end of the decision-making continuum is a *delegated decision procedure*. This occurs when the committee chair or leader allows participants to make the final decision. For example, establishment of a self-directed work team for the purpose of self-scheduling involves decision delegation. The leader may set up basic parameters to follow, such as ensuring an appropriate number of staff by role and experience for a shift or for the entire schedule before it is released. In nursing, many leaders use self-scheduling to engage the team and allow for flexibility in scheduling. The true test of delegation decision-making is whether the leader overrides the followers' decision. Technically, the leader would not have authority to veto or override unless he or she determined the decision made would compromise safety or organizational well-being. For example, new legal mandates supersede group decision-making. If it is truly a delegation situation, the leader would go forward with the approach that the decision is the group's choice. The group then becomes accountable for outcomes and is responsible for resolving any issues. Hersey et al. (2013) labeled these same four procedures as *authoritative, consultative, facilitative*, and *delegative* decision-making styles.

It is advisable for followers in any group to determine who has authority to make decisions. Knowledge about the type of group and the delegation or decision-making to be anticipated is critical to participation. A leadership or conflict moment may occur when a group assumes that they have the authority to make decisions, but the leader disagrees. Clarity before beginning work on an issue prevents unnecessary conflict and augments productivity. However, group members and leaders need to become skilled and comfortable in handling interpersonal dynamics.

Group decision-making may be time consuming. The leader needs to be skilled at allowing appropriate amounts of discussion to occur, ensuring that varying opinions are presented before a decision is made. A decision can be derailed if the leader is not skilled at facilitation, does not have a clear purpose for meeting, or is disorganized, unfocused, or allows unbalanced participation or discussion. Meetings that do not start and finish on time show a lack of respect for participants. When there is limited discussion of pros and cons of a topic or issue, members of the group may feel disenfranchised and limit their attendance or participation. Leaders need to be skilled at ensuring there is equal participation and ideas and suggestions by all group members are considered. Group members and leaders need to become skilled and comfortable in handling interpersonal dynamics, including conflict.

TEAM BUILDING

There are five stages of team development as defined by Newell and Kirkwood (2020): (1) Forming: This is where ground rules are assessed, set, and discussed by the group. The team begins to gather information about goals in this stage. (2) Storming: This is a period of conflict with and between team members as they work to understand their positions in the team. This stage ends when the team members can agree about issues and resolve conflict. (3) Norming: The team comes together and begins building cohesion between members. The team also agrees about established norms for the group. (4) Performing: The team begins to produce work. This is where the generation and application of problem-solving skills to problems identified in earlier stages is completed. (5) Adjournment is when the team completes their goals and disengages/breaks up the team.

Teams use processes to function. There are different views of ways to study the processes of a team. Einola and Alvesson (2019) discussed three processes often used in the study of teams:

1. *Entity-based process view.* In this view, the team process is seen as the logic applied to explain the relationships or actions of individuals or organizations. The concepts of this process are things such as verbal interactions, alliance building, dispute management, and the sorting of inputs and outputs. Team process is seen as a linear, input-process-outcome framework. This process view also coincides with the form, storm, norm, and perform model.
2. *Dynamic entity-based process view.* In this model, the process is focused on a flow in which entities (team members) travel. The focus is still on input-process-outcome, but the frameworks are more robust and profound. Team processes are categorized as transition, action, or interpersonal processes; these groups are further split into subprocesses. It is felt that this view focuses on structure, function, and how stages follow each other in the team process. Outcomes from one stage are often seen as inputs for successive stages.

3. *Fluid process view.* This view is one where the interest focuses on how teams came to be, are reproduced, how they adapt to the environment, and how stable they are. Under fluid process view a team is not a given entity, but just a possibility. Teams under fluid process view are partial, fragile, shifting, inconsistent, or stable (stable in this view is a temporary state and not a fixed state or definitive outcome). This view is about situational sensemaking (turning complex and confusing situations into something understandable) and relationships in the team. Process refers more to the process of being the team based on team interactions that shift experiences and meanings.

WORKING WITH TEAMS

In health care, multidisciplinary and interdisciplinary care teams are necessary for survival. Teamwork affects clinical performance, and team training is an effective strategy for improving patient safety. Implementation strategies and organizational conditions matter (Salas & Rosen, 2013). Organizational design principles and management approaches that strive to prevent patient injury and improve quality include use of high-reliability theory. High-reliability health care organizations are characterized by an organizational commitment to safety, redundancy of processes, safety measures, and an organizational culture for continuous learning (Riley et al., 2010). These organizations provide safe care and use deliberate design to minimize errors. Applied to nursing, the concept is *high-reliability teams*. Using reliability principles, multidisciplinary and interdisciplinary teams can focus on reducing flaws in care processes, increase the consistency of appropriateness of care delivery, and improve patient outcomes. Team training and system design are the key hallmarks of high-reliability patient care units. Members of high-reliability teams have four key behaviors: situational awareness, use of standardized communication, closed-loop communication, and a shared mental model, which can be enhanced with interdisciplinary team training (Riley et al., 2010). High-performance teams are essential to an organization's efficiency and effectiveness. High-quality work outcomes and cost control suffer without communication, collaboration, and teamwork. Interdisciplinary team members rely on each other's skills in a highly dynamic work environment (Teunissen et al., 2020).

Nurse leaders need to learn how to create, lead, and manage teams; all nurses also need to know how to be effective team players. Skilled leaders listen, invite, and encourage participation by team members. They understand the individual strengths and weakness of each member. Formation of a well-functioning group or team is never the work of just the leader. Members, as followers, give input, participate in decision-making, share responsibility, and hold themselves and each other accountable for group outcomes. A highly skilled and effective professional is not necessarily a highly skilled and effective group member. Distinct skill sets are required and are beneficial for nurses. Leaders and staff members alike should be able to function both independently and interdependently with others. They need to have the judgment to know when and which form of functioning is more appropriate. Regardless of the role as leader or group member, vision, and goals of the group need to be effectively embraced.

Types of Teams

Three types of teams found in health care are: (1) primary work teams, (2) leadership teams, and (3) ad hoc teams (Manion, 2011). Primary work teams include all forms of operational teams, including patient care teams such as a medical intensive care team and teams organized by a focused area, such as the rapid response team or a quality improvement team. In the operating room, teams are often based on the specialty (e.g., a cardiovascular or orthopedic team). The senior executive team is an example of an executive or management leadership team. At the hospital department level there may be a leadership team composed of the nurse manager, charge nurses, and perhaps an educator. Project teams and problem-solving teams are examples of ad hoc teams found across settings and sites. Specific problem-solving teams in departments are other examples of ad hoc teams, frequently referred to as task forces. The chief characteristic of these teams is that they are created to perform a specific piece of work. When work is completed, the team dissolves. Designing, building, and implementing effective work teams requires a specific methodology and process. A primary work team fails if it behaves like a collection of individuals operating from narrowly defined jobs; if it is composed of the wrong mix of members, size, structure, responsibility, or expertise, or if it cannot fluidly shift activities and adapt to changes. Teams need to be designed based on work responsibilities, skills, and competencies required by the work of the team. After the team design is determined, the next step is to build the team by incorporating essential elements needed to function. These include a common purpose, agreed-on performance goals or results-driven structure, competent members, a common approach for the work, complementary skills, collaborative relationships, mutual accountability, standards of excellence, external support, and principled leadership (Manion, 2011). The complementary skills needed in the right mix to do the team's task fall into at least three categories: technical or functional expertise, problem-solving and decision-making skills, and interpersonal skills. These are defined characteristics of *highly effective teams* (Wynia, 2012, pp. 1327–1328) (Table 9.1).

Managing this development process is a key leadership function. The leader guides the team in development of its purpose. Team members are more likely to coalesce into a strong team if they have been given time and opportunity to carefully reflect on their purpose and agree on what they do and for whom they do it. This leads to a unified commitment. A team becomes a true team by doing its work. Specific performance goals give it direction and provide evaluative criteria to measure success. Unnecessary conflict can occur if the leader and team members have not established key processes. Agreement is needed about how things are going to be done and by whom. This ranges from establishment of team behavioral norms to agreement on procedural issues. This step usually requires a significant amount of time and will continue to be addressed throughout the lifetime of the team. When foundations are laid carefully, effective teams can emerge (Manion, 2011).

Team Dynamics

The dynamics of interdisciplinary teams create some unique challenges. When teams are composed of professionals who have been educated, socialized, and are used to a unique vocabulary, professional values, and standards and practices, then it may become challenging for them to work across disciplines. Regrouping people into multidisciplinary groups increases team diversity

TABLE 9.1 Values and Principles of High-Functioning Health Care Teams

Share Values Among Team Members	Principles to Guide Team-Based Care
Honesty Put a high value on open communication within the team, including transparency about aims, decisions, uncertainty, and mistakes.	Clear roles Have clear expectations for each member's functions, responsibilities, and accountabilities.
Discipline Carry out roles and responsibilities even when inconvenient and seek out and share information to improve even when it is uncomfortable.	Mutual trust Earn each other's trust, creating strong norms for reciprocity and greater opportunities for shared achievement.
Creativity Be excited by the possibility of tackling new or emerging problems, seeing errors and unanticipated bad outcomes as potential opportunities to learn and improve.	Effective communication Prioritize and continuously refine communication skills using consistent channels for candid and complete communication.
Humility Recognize differences in training but do not believe that one type of training perspective is uniformly superior; recognize that team members are human and will make mistakes.	Shared goals Work to establish shared goals that reflect patient and family priorities and that can be clearly articulated, understood, and supported by all members.
Curiosity Delight in seeking out and reflecting on lessons learned and using those insights for continuous improvement.	Measurable processes and outcomes Agree on and implement reliable and timely feedback on successes and failures in both the overall functioning of the team and achievement of specific goals.

Data from Wynia, M.K., Von Kohorn, I., & Mitchell, P.H. (2012). Challenges at the intersection of team-based and patient-centered health care: Insights from an IOM working group. *Journal of the American Medical Association, 308*(13), 1327–1328.

and is essential to ensure high-quality, coordinated, reliable care.

Challenges occur when:

- There is confusion about the team's work.
- The team lacks real authority.
- Structural team building is not done.
- Dysfunctional behavior occurs, and team members do not know how to constructively deal with it.
- Team-based outcome measures and coaching are lacking.

Trust and communication are critical elements of building effective work teams. It is not enough to simply structure the team. Team members need to learn to work collaboratively and interdependently. Team performance and effectiveness are important managerial concerns.

Teams form, grow, and mature in stages. Team dynamics change throughout this process. Teams benefit from team building and developmental training. Articulating and negotiating expectations for healthy interpersonal behavior benefits team development. A key characteristic of an emotionally intelligent team is establishment of norms to guide team member behaviors (Cherniss & Goleman, 2001).

Team norms are best established when the team initially forms. They are continually revisited, modified, and expanded throughout the team's life. The process for developing norms is usually leader initiated and begins with a team conversation about how team members behave and contribute. Norms are usually developed during a group meeting in which ideas are shared, refined, and finally negotiated with all team members. Appropriate topics for behavioral norms include, but are not limited to, expectations around communication, both at individual and group levels; how team members treat each other; how support is to be demonstrated; decision-making processes; and how conflict is to be handled. For example, one team developed the following expectations of each other.

I expect you to:

- Communicate in an open, honest, and direct manner with me;
- Give me feedback when my behavior creates a difficult or uncomfortable situation for you;
- Persist and work with me on difficult issues until we reach a mutually agreeable resolution;
- Pitch in gladly, provide help when asked, and look for ways to help each other out;
- Respect confidences and not share sensitive information we discuss with others without my knowledge or permission;
- Be trustworthy as evidenced by honoring and meeting commitments made, including being on time and staying engaged (being present) throughout the meeting;
- Refrain from using technology and "multitasking" during meetings;
- Be loyal to absent team members, and present them in the best light to others.

Often these norms are referred to as the *team operating agreement*, the *code of conduct*, ground rules, or *articulated expectations*. Once the norms are identified, team members sign them, indicating agreement, and the norms often are posted in the workplace. These norms are more than just a paper exercise. They signify that team members agree to live by established expectations and address other team members who do not. As new members join the team, it is important to share team members' expectations. It is also beneficial to revisit defined expectations on a regular basis.

Team effectiveness is dependent not only on how individual team members perform and adhere to norms, but also on the degree of communication, cooperation, and emotional intelligence of individual members and the team's leader. The ability to manage conflict and have self-awareness is essential for a team to reach peak performance. The greater the performance of a team, the greater is the advantage to group members, patients, and the organization.

COMMITTEES

An essential part of any nurse's role is to be involved in committee and group work. Work is accomplished through people, and quality of care is furthered through committee actions. It positively impacts nurses' job satisfaction and autonomy to have an avenue of involvement and participation to actively solve problems and retain autonomy over nursing care. Professional shared governance models incorporate staff nurse participation in groups and committees as a core element of how work gets accomplished.

Some people prefer not to participate in committees because they dislike the time involved or because they are frustrated with psychodynamics of group process and decision-making. However, committees are a mainstay of organizations and can be an important way to make changes in clinical practice. Understanding committee workings facilitates the process of being a more effective nurse.

Committee structures are preferable in two kinds of situations:

1. *Situations in which each member's input is needed to attain a certain goal.* For example, a committee may be set up to review patient safety issues in a department, such as patient falls. If the work cannot be done alone or if there is a need to have everyone's agreement or support, then a committee is probably appropriate.
2. *Situations in which diverse representation facilitates implementation of proposed activities.* To have a diverse group of people provide input in order to get the job done, a committee should be created. For example, a multidisciplinary product committee could be established to develop a process in which existing and new products would be reviewed before large purchases are made. This approach allows nurses to evaluate new products and look at value to patient care, safety, efficacy, and cost. It also provides a disciplined approach to product review, with an aim of preventing duplication of products and promoting good financial stewardship.

Types of Committees

Several types of committees are found in organizations. One kind is the *standing* committee, that is a constant, ongoing part of the organizational mission, performing critical and essential functions. For example, policy committees are standing committees because there always are policies to write and review. The same is true for a patient safety committee because these functions and activities are ongoing and continuous.

Contrasted with a standing committee is the task force, also called a *project team* or *ad hoc committee.* This committee is developed in response to some emergent or immediate need. A task force is not part of the organizational core mission. It is formed in response to a specific circumstance that arises or to study a specific problem. The committee is expected to disband when the issue is resolved. Examples are a search committee to replace an advanced practice nurse or a problem-solving group dealing with emergency department patient throughput and hospital bed availability.

Some groups or committees are structured to gather members *based on organizational position or job position.* For example, all the nurse managers may belong to a group of nurse managers, or staff nurses may belong to a staff nurse council. By holding a position of nurse manager, a person belongs to that committee. Committee involvement provides an opportunity for peer interaction, support, and problem-solving.

There are multidisciplinary interdivisional committees. A *multidisciplinary* committee includes participants from several divisions, locations, or specialties. Participants may be from within the institution or from both inside and outside the organization. These committees are often used to coordinate and eliminate boundary conflicts. Some examples are a product committee, risk management committee, or patient safety committee in which nurses, physicians, and allied health colleagues work together to improve patient care and reduce interprofessional conflicts. In some cases, multidisciplinary teams are formed using a committee structure (e.g., to develop a critical pathway such as sepsis screening). Other committees may be cross-functional (e.g., nurses meeting with members from information technology or facilities management department to discuss and resolve issues).

Within organizations, committees perform a central role in the implementation of the strategic plan. A committee is a group that can assume responsibility and be held accountable for planning, implementing, and evaluating outcomes of a strategic goal translated to the operational level. Committees accomplish some departmental activities and provide a mechanism for increasing staff participation in decision-making. In an environment characterized by complex work, committees become a major vehicle for resolving issues related to the organization's mission. Two elements promote efficient and effective committee decision-making: appropriate representation (by including people affected by changes) and delegation of an appropriate level of authority to the committee (Manion, 2011).

Committees evolve over time. To remain vital, committees need to be evaluated regularly for congruence with organizational mission and contribution to outcomes. The committee's goals and outcomes need to be reviewed annually, with membership reevaluated and changed as necessary. If asked to be on a committee as a department representative, it is advisable for the nurse to explore the nature and characteristics of the committee.

The nurse needs to determine the authority level delegated to this committee, remembering that delegation may be formal or informal. Another factor involves assessing the personal level of interest in the work of the committee. Other factors include whether people on the committee are highly motivated, whether they are task- or relationship-oriented people, and what committee politics exist. Feedback mechanisms and the committee's productivity are key characteristics. The track record of the committee is reflected in its output. These characteristics are important for the nurse to understand before deciding whether to participate. Preparation for followership enhances both personal and committee productivity. It is also helpful to clarify any expectations for the committee role being considered. For example, is the nurse there to share individual opinions or to represent others in the department? The latter role requires more active solicitation of colleagues' opinions and ideas.

EFFECTIVE MEETINGS

Meetings are common occurrences in health care organizations. Whether a meeting involves a group, committee, or team, the leader's role is to maximize the benefits of the meeting. Structuring a meeting for effectiveness requires preparation and effort. To manage effective meetings, the leader needs to consider the meeting's purpose. Some of the most common reasons meetings are ineffective relate to a lack of clarity of purpose, or too many competing issues on the agenda for a single meeting. For example, a brief team huddle would become ineffective if it turned into a decision-making group about a key department issue.

Probably the most common type of meeting is held for *information dissemination or sharing*. For example, the designated leadership person calls the group together to let members review the organization's performance scorecard. That may include organization and individual department performance in financial management, patient experience scores, quality scores, and employee measures such as turnover. A meeting is called to disseminate information about what is happening and to provide time for questions and answers. This also occurs when there has been an organizational change, such as the decision that one unit is going to be consolidating with another unit or that a new building, department relocation, or new service is being planned or implemented.

One familiar form of information sharing is the end-of-shift report. Pertinent, important information about patients is reviewed and discussed by staff members from the outgoing and incoming shift. The shift handoff report is a very common form of this type of meeting. This is a very short meeting at the beginning of shift with all team members to review the upcoming shift or any emergent topics that need to be communicated. These meetings may be called huddles.

Second, there are meetings held for *opinion seeking*. The goal of these meetings is open dialogue to solicit group and individual opinions and ideas on specific topics or issues. This purpose does not imply that decision-making is the prerogative of the group. Seeking opinions is an input strategy and may be used for gathering data or testing group reactions. For example, an opinion-seeking meeting may be called to invite input on equipment purchases for budget requests.

The third type of meeting is held for *problem-solving and/or decision-making*. The meeting is structured to solicit help in clarifying, analyzing, and solving a specific problem. This type of meeting is action oriented. Group participation in decision-making is encouraged. For example, group problem-solving or unit meetings may be called to discuss ways to solve problems related to patient safety issues, or complex and challenging patients or family members. Meetings for problem-solving need to follow a methodical structure, otherwise they are likely either to deteriorate into a complaint session or to result in ineffective or unacceptable recommendations. Effectively leading these groups requires strong facilitation skills and knowledge in problem-solving techniques. It is helpful to focus on common agreed-on goals such as patient safety.

Yet another type of meeting is a *strategy* meeting. These meetings are less frequent—perhaps quarterly or annually—and focus on reviewing the organization's vision and strategic goals, developing future goals and strategies for the department or work group, or tackling one issue in great depth, such as implementing a professional shared governance model or a new model of care delivery. This may be called by executive nursing leaders as a "summit," a "retreat," or "town hall meeting."

Preparing for Meetings

In the most effective groups, all members are clear about the purpose of the meeting they are attending, are prepared, and help the group to stay focused. When the group becomes distracted by other issues (for example, getting side-tracked by operational issues during a strategy meeting), focus is lost, and meeting time is wasted. This is a sign that the meeting structure may need to be evaluated.

In preparing for a meeting, a leader should make certain that the committee's process stays true to the purpose of the meeting. There is a caution about having a mix of items in the same meeting. For example, basic information dissemination is best addressed at a quarterly strategic meeting. This does not mean that any of these items are less important, but introducing them in the wrong venue or with the wrong timing will reduce the effectiveness of the meeting.

A timed agenda may be a helpful way to facilitate the group's process. This involves identifying on the agenda, next to each item, the anticipated amount of time allotted for discussion. It might be beneficial to review proposed time allotments with committee members before meeting to ensure realistic estimates. Time estimates should serve as a guideline rather than a rigid parameter. It is important not to cut off discussion prematurely or force a decision when a discussion is productive but taking longer than anticipated. One effective strategy is to do a time check with members and adjust accordingly. This may require an adjustment in the agenda. Many leaders organize agenda items according to priority topics. Some leaders have a brief agenda and add to it to cover any pressing issues or topics based on the team's input. This can be done at the beginning of the meeting or after planned agenda items are covered. Meetings can rapidly become disorganized without an agenda or a carefully facilitated discussion. The leader must be mindful of the time allotted for the meeting.

Leader Duties

The leader of the group can facilitate meeting effectiveness by preparing and dealing with both the task and people involved. The leader should listen carefully, process interactions, control flow, and keep the meeting directed toward accomplishing objectives. The ideal size of a group depends on work to be accomplished. If group interaction and getting everyone's input is important, then the size of the ideal group needs to be small, ideally 4 to 7 people, with 12 being the upper limit. Members should be carefully selected for providing best input, being representative, and having potential contribution to the work.

The leader needs to start on time and be alert to seating positions. Some leaders assign seating to maximize group participation and prevent disruption. The leader can facilitate effectiveness ensuring that all members of the team have an ability to actively participate. The leader may need to control compulsive talkers, draw out silent members, protect junior members, encourage the respectful clash of ideas, discourage the clash of personalities, prevent squashing of creative ideas, and close on a note of achievement (Jay, 1982). The leader also needs to attend to careful meeting wrap-up. Summarizing the group's accomplishments after the meeting and verifying task assignments are important leader responsibilities. Box 9.1 presents a checklist for leading effective meetings.

Without thought and preparation, people may go into a meeting focused on their own issues, biases, and perspectives; they may not be focused on being productive

BOX 9.1 Effective Meetings Checklist for Leaders

- Identify the purpose of the meeting. Is it for:
  - Information dissemination
  - Opinion seeking
  - Problem-solving
- Prepare an agenda and related materials
- Identify time needed for each item on the agenda
- Identify the category of each agenda item. Is it:
  - For information
  - For development
  - For implementation
  - For change in the system
- Identify the number and type of members needed
- Carefully select members (based on skill and expertise)
- Distribute agenda and related materials such as previous minutes well in advance of meeting with instructions for assignments due and materials to be reviewed before the meeting
- Listen carefully and summarize discussion and assignments at the end of the meeting
- Process group interactions to ensure balanced dialogue by all members
- Control the flow of interactions
- Keep the meeting directed toward accomplishing objectives
- Start on time and finish on time

Data modified from Jay, A. (1982). How to run a meeting. *Journal of Nursing Administration, 12*(1), 22–28.

within the meeting. However, even in a negative situation, individuals may choose to participate in a way that assists or enhances the process by making constructive suggestions about how things could be done better. This is an ideal situation, one to be encouraged, structured, and facilitated by the leader.

The duties of the chairperson include preparing the physical environment. Comfort and convenience engineering are part of the leader's responsibility in terms of preparing an environment that is conducive to people being satisfied, productive, positive, and working together. The worst-case situation occurs if the meeting room is uncomfortable, including being too cold, too hot, too noisy, too small, or too large. Another challenge is when technology does not work. The chairperson needs to ensure the meeting room, including technology, is set up appropriately. Consider how to facilitate group work through hosting functions related to breaks, food, and beverages. It is human nature for members to be more relaxed and productive in comfortable surroundings. With the reliance on technology versus the need for people to "be present" during a meeting, many leaders have added mechanisms to foster group interactions.

As all nurses are pressured to do more with less under severe time and travel constraints, conducting meetings assisted by technology has become a major strategy. The prevalence and ease of technology, such as video conference calls, webinars, Internet-based meeting technology, real-time (synchronous) discussion boards, and related audio or video technology strategies are commonly employed. These become useful ways to save time by eliminating travel to a remote site. However, specific problems may occur, such as technology incompatibility, speed of transmission, connection failures, or other delays in transmission that result in inconsistent communication, a lack of interpersonal modulation due to absence of body language, or a tendency to forget about people who are not actually in the room. Ensuring that the agenda, minutes, assignments, and presentations are sent in advance will mitigate some technology difficulties. Despite these known issues, nurses will increasingly experience meetings assisted by technology.

Positive meeting dynamics are a shared responsibility between the leader and group members. A leader has a responsibility to prepare in advance for meetings and provide participants support in preparation. The participants' responsibility is to read and be prepared, show up on time, participate openly and positively, share responsibility for managing the group's dynamics, and attend to the task at hand. Depending on the meeting, the leader needs to prepare an agenda with handouts and background materials and distribute them to the members to give them time to review. A leader who does not distribute materials in advance may limit effectiveness of the meeting because members will not be prepared. Most materials can be sent electronically to members. The better prepared members are, the more they can participate, positively affect the quality of decisions, and feel gratified by their participation.

If the leader's preparation activities include generating an agenda or reviewing the status of agenda topics, questions to ask when organizing and preparing include the following:

- Where are we/what is the current status?
- What else needs to be done?
- What supporting materials might help the committee members?
- Who should be invited?
- Are there other experts or people from other departments that can contribute to this committee's process?
- What do we hope to accomplish?

CONSTRUCTIVE GROUP ROLES AND BEHAVIORS

Savvy group leaders and members understand that people in groups assume a variety of roles. In a now-classic work, Lancaster (1981) identified both group building roles and group maintenance roles as being a part of group interactions. Group building roles include *initiator, encourager, opinion giver, clarifier, listener,* and *summarizer.* Group maintenance roles include *tension reliever, compromiser, gatekeeper,* and *harmonizer.* The group building roles concentrate more on relationship functions than on task functions; the group maintenance roles focus more on task functions than on relationship functions. Effective groups need a balance of members and roles.

Beyond the more general group, roles are specific, structured roles that can help increase the effectiveness of the group. For example, one positive way to handle meetings is to identify a facilitator. This is often the formal group leader or individual in a position of authority, but it does not have to be. If this is a true team, the role of facilitator may rotate among team members. In a committee, the facilitator is probably the committee chairperson. A facilitator conducts the meeting, ensuring that everyone can speak, maintains the focus of the meeting, and ensures group dynamics remain positive.

A group recorder is also needed. The task of taking minutes or summarizing discussion and decisions may need to be delegated to a clerical support person (if possible) if group members are averse to taking on the task of recording outcomes. However, a recorder who is a group member technically can do far more than just take minutes. This person should be in tune with group processing and with inputs and roles of group members. In addition, they can help keep the group on time. The recorder can provide feedback to the facilitator in terms of how to improve the process. One key tip is to construct a standardized meeting agenda and a record (or minutes) to facilitate group process. It is helpful to decide in advance the level of detail required in the minutes to avoid lengthy minutes and potentially unnecessary effort.

One useful way to expedite group work is to use a laptop computer to directly enter draft minutes. It is also valuable to summarize actions and assignments at the end of the meeting. Some leaders choose to allow the recorder to summarize discussion on a topic versus composing detailed minutes on each topic. Sending out minutes and talking points or a summary of items discussed, and decisions made shortly after the meeting can support continued engagement and communication of the group.

Finally, group members who believe they can be active participants—with equal status in the meeting—are generally more engaged and feel empowered. The three components of facilitator, recorder, and group members contribute to the design of a positive working group. All can share in the basic group role functions. As with teams, leaders should establish ground rules for members of the group to facilitate maximum engagement. Some common rules may include:

- Meetings begin and end on time
- Members need to be on time, prepared, and stay for the entire meeting
- No cell phone or computer use during the meeting except on scheduled breaks
- One person speaks at a time
- No sidebar conversations.

DISRUPTIVE ROLES AND BEHAVIORS

Another role that the group leader assumes is that of process facilitator. The leader needs to observe group members' actions and be prepared to control or redirect disruptive behaviors. It is important to focus on behavior that needs to be adjusted and not label an individual in a group. Although the leader has a responsibility to deal with nonproductive behaviors, in a mature team or highly effective group, monitoring of behaviors is also a responsibility of other group members. If the issue is not addressed by a fellow group member, then the leader needs to be prepared to address it. However, it is hierarchical thinking to leave this responsibility solely to the leader and doing so reinforces formal hierarchy in the group. It is also important that the leader, facilitator, or group member avoids embarrassing a member of a group publicly, because the impact on the group will be equally disruptive. Many times, individuals do not have insight concerning their own behavior or its impact on the group. It can be a "teachable moment" to enhance an individual professionally by diplomatically redirecting to positive behavior. The following section delineates types of disruptive group members that are encountered (Jacobs & Rosenthal, 1984), with strategies for the leader to use in managing the behavior of the group member.

Compulsive Talkers

A common disruptive behavior is seen in individuals who are compulsive talkers. Often their behavior can be modified. One suggestion is to thank them for their input and then ask to hear from others on that same topic before they are given the opportunity to speak again. This will serve as a way of guiding and opening up the meeting to be more effective. If this behavior continues to affect the group negatively and the individual is not receptive to subtle feedback, meeting with the person after group work and giving direct, constructive feedback about the negative impact of the behavior may be necessary. There are techniques that can be shared to assist them in future meetings, such as asking them to keep track of the number of times they have spoken on a subject. In a mature team, it would be expected that this issue could be brought up and dealt with by any team member.

Nontalkers

The nontalkers are the quiet ones. They may not be comfortable speaking in front of a group or may process information more slowly than other members of the group. It is important to create a safe environment where their ideas are considered. Some approaches include offering the option of submitting their ideas in writing or directly asking them to share their thoughts on the matter at hand. Anyone in the group can specifically ask them questions to draw them out, thereby encouraging a broader range of group input. Preparing members in advance by distributing the agenda or letting them know where their input will be crucial is also a way to include nontalkers. Sometimes these individuals need time to think through their thoughts before they engage in a conversation, unlike more spontaneous and verbal peers. It is important to understand their communication style and not embarrass them in front of a group if they are not engaged in discussion.

Interrupters

The facilitator must address the interrupter because this person demonstrates a lack of awareness or self-control. The interrupter can be a problem in groups because they can stifle group conversation. Individuals who are interrupted may feel violated and wonder why they are not given the courtesy of finishing a thought and having their full input considered. Anyone in the group can halt the interruption, control, and redirect the interrupter. This can be accomplished by saying, "Let's allow Joan to finish what she was saying." If the group does not intervene, it is the responsibility of the facilitator. One consideration when developing ground rules for the group is to list no interruptions as an expectation. Interrupters may be individuals who process information quickly. It might be beneficial to meet with them privately to give them some examples. They might not have insight concerning their behavior and actions needed to support communication within the group.

Squashers

Squashers try to squash an idea before it is even developed. Suggestions about processes or procedures that have not been proven or even tried are much easier to criticize than are facts or opinions. Persons who are averse to change may have a litany of reasons why a potential solution would never work or why this proposed project simply cannot or should not happen. Often these are people who do not want to take a personal risk or undergo the personal effort of making a change, so it is easier to squash everything and maintain the status quo. Especially during brainstorming sessions, the leader needs to be alert to and have a method for containing the squasher. An easy way to influence this is to set the expectation at the beginning of the session by saying, for example, "For this exercise, please do not engage in analyzing or saying anything negative about the ideas thrown out until we have them all identified." There will be time later that allows dissecting and critiquing a new idea. Negative remarks adversely affect the level of creativity in any group, but the individual may have a wealth of experience and knowledge such that they discern pitfalls and barriers more quickly than others. Careful team discussion guidance is needed.

Distracted or Unreliable Members

Unreliable members really may not be committed to the group's work. They may be distracted, which they exhibit in a variety of ways including arriving late, leaving early, answering phone calls, texting, or reading e-mails during the meeting. They may not be prepared for the meeting. Ultimately, they are not contributing to the ongoing group work or the task at hand nor are they invested in the group's goals. The leader needs to address this issue with them. One possible solution is to meet with them privately and discuss whether they are interested and able to be part of the group. There are times when individuals overcommit, and as a result do not fulfill their obligations to the group. Sharing observed group behaviors and explaining expectations is essential if they wish to be part of the group. If they do, it might be beneficial to give them a specific assignment with accountability. If this does not work, they may need to be released from the group or placed in an advisory role.

MANAGING DISRUPTIVE BEHAVIOR IN GROUPS

The most useful way to have an impact on negative behaviors is to lead the group through clarification of working expectations. When group members have clearly identified what is needed to productively work together in a group setting, they have established norms for acceptable and unacceptable behavior.

The nurse leader can take an active role in structuring group work for positive processing and effective outcomes. It is important to control communication flow to modulate disruptive group members without enhancing conflict. Another way is to structure positive and constructive group roles among members. Peer pressure is a powerful group behavior modification tactic, especially for group members for whom approval of the rest of the group is important. The leader's vision, enthusiasm, interpersonal relationship skills, and empowerment of followers all facilitate group effectiveness.

LEADERSHIP AND MANAGEMENT IMPLICATIONS

Leaders play a significant role in the success of an organization and, specifically, patient safety, quality, and joy at work. The ability to work with a committed collaborative group, team, or committee is essential for an organization to continue to grow and improve, and also retain top talent. It is well documented in the literature that nursing job satisfaction and burnout correlate with the degree of teamwork, work environment, professional practice, and degree of professional and collaborative working relationships with both the nursing team and medical staff. For example, new nurses in nurse residency programs report difficulty in working on project and patient care teams if they have not had prior exposure or background. Because of the growing use of interdisciplinary teams, leaders and managers can structure in mentored experiences so new nurses specifically can grow in knowledge and skill in teamwork. Health care organizations that have managers with an effective management style that allows a degree of autonomy, promotes interdisciplinary relationships, and promotes professional development have a lower turnover among the nursing staff.

The leadership and management roles are essential in ensuring groups, teams, and committees are effective. With limited resources the leader should consider the work to be accomplished, determine the structure most suited to do the work, put the structure in place, and facilitate work processes. This requires a leader who understands basic differences among work groups and teams, committees, and informal groups. A leader also needs to be able to think carefully about the work to be accomplished and determine whether it is primarily collective or individual work.

A leader's role includes selecting the right members, inspiring participation, preparing critical questions, developing agendas and background materials, summarizing minutes and developing talking points, continually coaching the group for effective functioning, and guiding long-range strategy. This is the planning, coordinative, and tracking function. Leaders and managers address questions such as:

- What is the task?
- What is the best way for this task to be accomplished?
- Is collective work involved?
- Do we need a team, or will a good work group or committee suffice?
- How many meetings will it take?
- How much effort is required?
- How can the tasks be divided?
- How can they be delegated?
- What measures will demonstrate success?

In planning for meetings, a good leader puts in time and effort needed to provide preliminary information and documents so that all members are prepared when they come to the meeting, know what the issues are, and are familiar with the background of the task to be accomplished. The leader facilitates the group in agreeing about norms for decision-making, length of discussion, when to vote or use consensus, and processes through which the task is completed efficiently and effectively. This is done as a deliberate agenda item that the leader initiates, opens for discussion, and brings to closure. Sometimes an off-site retreat is used to employ high-relationship and group-forming strategies. Nurses may find the group leader role challenges them to plan, organize, coordinate, and evaluate the work of the group.

An effective leader understands a process is involved in creating effective, engaged work teams, highly functioning groups, and committees. The process requires facilitation and significant amounts of coaching from the leader. The leader's style needs to fit the group development stage. The leader will need to supply more extensive structure and direction in early stages and minimal structure and direction in later stages. The leader needs to support the work and at times coach the team or group. Group skill, capability, and readiness need to be assessed. Ensuring appropriate resources is imperative. Finally, celebrating successes of the group, team, or committee is essential, with the understanding that recognition is related to personal preferences. Although some individuals enjoy public recognition, others prefer private recognition such as a note or private comment about a job well done.

CURRENT ISSUES AND TRENDS

Creating Healthy Workplaces

Creation of a positive and healthy work environment is a key issue in health care. Organizations continue to struggle with attracting and retaining highly qualified nurses and other members of the health care team. They also struggle with motivating employees who are highly engaged and experience joy in work. There is much evidence that confirms that an unhealthy work environment contributes to unsafe conditions that result in medical errors, poorly coordinated and ineffective care, and conflict and stress among members of the health care team (Roth et al., 2015). In 2005 the American Association of Critical-Care Nurses (AACN, 2005) released *AACN Standards for Establishing and Sustaining Healthy Work Environments: A Journey to Excellence*. The six standards are as follows: skilled communication, true collaboration, effective decision-making, appropriate staffing, meaningful recognition, and authentic leadership. These are recognized in nursing as the gold standard for health care organizations.

A healthy work environment assumes relationships a person has with colleagues and co-workers are positive and respectful. Leadership plays an important role in supporting the nursing team. Ensuring adequate staff, an appropriate workload, and mutual respect among the nursing team and other disciplines is critical to creating and sustaining a healthy work environment. A positive work environment for nurses demonstrates problem-solving and resolution of issues resulting in workplace conditions improving. Effective problem-solving groups are a crucial aspect of making this happen.

TeamSTEPPS

In the early 2000s, the Agency for Healthcare Research and Quality (AHRQ), in partnership with the Department of Defense, began working on a patient safety initiative that was directed at improving teamwork in health care settings. TeamSTEPPS was the result (AHRQ, 2016). The acronym stands for Team Strategies and Tools to Enhance Performance and Patient Safety. The premise is quite simple. Anyone who touches a patient (nurse, physician, pharmacist, technician) must work together to ensure the delivery of safe and high-quality care. It is aimed at helping health care professionals work together more effectively as a team. TeamSTEPPS teaches professionals to understand each other's roles and collaborate to improve the quality of care delivered. The aim is to foster a culture where any member of the team has freedom to respectfully question authority when an error may be occurring. It teaches the team that questioning authority need not be threatening. In the airline industry, there is similar training known as crew resource management.

One example is a structured process for communication to ensure information is clearly exchanged between team members. There is a specific training curriculum used to integrate teamwork principles. This program is like a boot camp in teamwork and interdependent relationships. It offers a host of innovations such as team huddles, patient handoff briefings, time-outs before commencement of a surgical procedure, and the SBAR (situation, background, assessment, and recommendation) technique for communicating information in a concise manner. The website http://www.ahrq.gov/teamstepps/index.html offers an impressive number of resources.

Innovation Centers

Fostering innovation is essential as health care continues to transform with targeted focus on continuous improvement and breakthrough novel ideas and approaches to patient care (see Chapter 2). Health care organizations today are being measured on quality results, the patient experience, and cost of care. Innovation groups and committees are engaged in total quality management (TQM) initiatives, continuous quality improvement (CQI) methods using techniques such as Lean, Six Sigma, and rapid response teams.

A common response to problems is to look for an individual to blame. The result of systems thinking is to capture the energy of teams to resolve systems problems. An overall focus on quality has led to adoption of business management concepts such as Lean and Six Sigma. These are customer-focused and data-driven approaches to deriving best practices. The focus is on reducing process variation and improving process capability. Lean focuses on process speed and reduction of waste and inefficiencies; Six Sigma focuses on process quality with the aim of fewer defects.

A current innovation in health care is the MakerNurse project from the Robert Wood Johnson Foundation (https://www.rwjf.org/en/how-we-work/grants-explorer/featured-programs/maker-nurse.html). Nurses are adept at problem-solving, creating work-arounds, and suggesting care innovations. MakerNurse is an initiative that listens to and gathers stories to detail the natural abilities of nurses to solve problems in an inventive, creative, innovated manner. From these stories a database of information has been built to support nurses with tools and resources that enable nurses to continue innovation at the patient's bedside.

Many organizations have created innovation centers to discover new ways to address health care challenges. New health care products and services are being tested—and in some cases commercialized—through collaboration with clinicians, scientists, entrepreneurs, and business partners. Innovation centers are focused on disruptive innovation to expedite change. This may involve developing new techniques and approaches to operational efficiency including testing new workflows, patient care redesign, standardization, and teamwork through simulation and hands-on experiential learning.

Leaders are cautioned that creativity and innovation at a team level require diversity in membership and perspective. Diverse teams have freedom to challenge the status quo and engage in creative problem-solving. Nursing leaders play a crucial role integrating with other disciplines in making a commitment to ensure teams feel supported and have freedom to creatively identify new ways to address clinical processes and care redesign. Leaders who understand and use these techniques and processes of innovation can be effective in disseminating and implementing novel approaches to patient care.

Multidisciplinary Quality Improvement Teams

Whether using CQI, TQM, Lean, Six Sigma, or some related quality improvement program, direct care nurses are expected to participate more actively in multidisciplinary quality improvement teams. In an organization that identifies problems as systems problems, the next step is to acknowledge that anyone involved in the system needs to be engaged in solving problems. Therefore coordinating patient care and solving problems through interdisciplinary committees and groups with people of equal status is the strategy best suited to solving systems problems.

The strategy behind systems-based approaches is to bring together interdisciplinary, collaborative groups. This means that if there is a problem in patient care, physicians, nurses, ancillary staff, and other direct caregivers work together to identify issues and possible solutions. Solutions identified can be tested and evaluated through collaboration. The facilitator does not have to be a content expert or have the most expertise in that problem area. In fact, having the most expertise in a problem area can be problematic when functioning as a facilitator because it becomes too tempting to take over the process. The individual's facilitation skills are crucially important.

Establishing equality among peers regardless of status and using expertise and responsibility result in a different way of looking at work. This has implications in terms of how nursing practice may change. It also means nurses are going to continue to be substantially involved in groups, committees, and teams. Multidisciplinary teams are not just for problem-solving and process improvement. The current pace and complexity of the world today also demands that new approaches to care delivery be considered by teams.

RESEARCH NOTE

Source

Miller, C.J., Kim, B., Silverman, A, & Bauer, M.S. (2018). A systematic review of team-building interventions in non-acute healthcare settings. *BMC Health Services Research, 18*:146, 1–21. https://doi.org/10.1186/s12913-018-2961-9.

Purpose

A systematic review was done to identify team-building interventions. The process identified 14 team-building interventions that pertained to nonacute care settings along with 25 documents describing observed studies of the interventions.

Discussion

The authors developed a Team Effectiveness Pyramid as a conceptual model of nonacute health care. The authors proposed that the pyramid was in four levels: (1) Foundational Resources such as leadership support, staffing, space, civility, and respect, (2) Team Building Interventions such as knowledge of team work principles and attitudes towards teamwork, (3) Enhanced Team Functioning demonstrated by shared purpose and goals, coordination and communication, role clarity, increased civility and respect, and capacity to improve process, and (4) Patient Impact including patient outcomes and patient satisfaction. Three authors independently rated a subset

RESEARCH NOTE—cont'd

of 10 manuscripts using a descriptive approach to report the characteristics of team-building interventions/empirical studies and to catalogue support for each intervention.

Results

Evaluations of team building strategies were mostly positive with mixed results in relation to team functioning and patient impact. Only one study demonstrated statistically significant improvement in teamwork attitudes and knowledge.

Application to Practice

This systematic review found that the evidence base for health care team-building interventions for nonacute settings demonstrated a paucity of information when compared to short-term team function in acute care settings. One intervention was found to be tested in multiple nonacute settings. The positive findings in relation to team-building interventions were moderated by variables such as few control conditions, inconsistent measures of outcomes, and bias. The results of this study determined a great need for further research in the area of nonacute team building.

CASE STUDY

Developing Leadership Teams to Improve Clinical Metrics

A new C-Suite team was formed to lead a midsized community hospital. Members included the Hospital Chief Executive officer (CEO), Chief of Nursing (CNO), Chief of Finance (CFO), Medical Chief of Staff (COS), various directors of nursing services, directors of ancillary services, and the associate chiefs of staff for various medical/surgical services. The team was established to improve clinical metrics throughout the hospital. Clinical metrics were chosen, thresholds were set to demonstrate needed improvement, and subcommittees were established by the C-Suite to address individual metrics.

Due to the numerous metrics, it was felt that subcommittees would need to be established in order to tackle the enormous amount of data that needed to be reviewed. Nursing was tasked with establishing subcommittees working on metrics that were directly related to nursing; physicians were tasked to established subcommittees to work on metrics directly related to clinical outcomes demonstrated as a result of physician interventions. The Director was tasked to address patient and staff satisfaction indicators. All subcommittees would routinely report the status of their metrics to the C-Suite members composed of the CNO, CFO, COS, and the CEO.

Subcommittee chairs and subchairs were established with the understanding that it was imperative that subject matter experts and stakeholders be on the team and to ensure those chosen would be able to work as a team in improving metrics. Within a month of forming the teams, it was noted that many of the teams were not functioning as well as it was hoped they would be. An outside team-building group was commissioned to evaluate and remediate issues affecting team functioning. Issues identified by the team building group included:

- Lack of accountability in some teams leading to some of the team members doing most of the work of the group
- Domination of the group and its processes by one or two people with strong personalities or of higher status
- An overall lack of trust within the group that was undermining group efforts
- Constant conflict between some members who were negatively influencing team performance
- Lack of teaming skills causing an inability to work with others
- Lack of understanding of group goals, roles, tasks, and priorities
- Teams too large to easily come to consensus
- Groupthink was present in some groups causing a limitation of creativity.

The team-building group met with the C-Suite members to discuss their findings and to provide them assistance in forming efficient, effective teams. The first task undertaken was to solidify group goals, roles, tasks, and priorities by clearly delineating them in writing and reviewing them with each low performing team. During this process it was noted that people had been placed on committees who had no concept of the metrics they were supposed to fix, or teams were missing vital specialists on their teams. For example, housekeepers were placed on HEIDIS teams but did have any concept about what they were being asked to do. The Sepsis team was miss-

continued

CASE STUDY—cont'd

ing an all-important clinical pharmacist on their team, and the team working on patient infections did not have an infection disease doctor as a member.

The team building group, with the assistance of the C-Suite, assisted the teams in realigning personnel assigned to each team, sometimes changing chairpersons to those who better understood the issues at hand. Once the teams were reselected, all teams went through formal training to be an effective, efficient team. Team sizes were reduced and conflicts among members were addressed as part of the team building training. Chairpersons and co-chairs were given special training in how to lead a team, improve team communication, deal with difficult team members, and decrease conflict. Each team was reviewed to assure that the appropriate subject matter experts were part of the individual teams.

After 6 months of monitoring and revising teams as needed, the facility stabilized their metrics and, in many cases, exceeded the thresholds that had been established.

CRITICAL THINKING EXERCISE

Organize into a small group, then select a leader. Take a few minutes to do this, and then select or appoint a process recorder. Here is your assignment:

The leader is a nursing director for hospital services at Deering Hospital. He has been asked to lead a task force to establish the safety of toxic therapeutic drug handling at the staff level. The task force is to create a methodology to identify toxic therapeutic drugs used in the hospital, proper methods to be employed to protect the staff, proper methodologies for disposal of toxic medications, and proper education of staff in relation to the handling and disposal of toxic medications. The leader must select the team members, lead them while preserving teamwork, and produce a viable product that will protect staff from harm. A process recorder is part of the team and will record and report as requested.

1. Observe the process the group uses to select its own leader. Did anyone try to avoid selection? Was someone an enthusiastic volunteer? How long did the process take? Were the selection criteria discussed? What were the selection criteria?
2. What method was used to select/appoint a process recorder? What power strategy was used to make this decision?
3. What is the problem identified in the task?
4. What did the group leader do to handle the situation?
5. What should the group leader do to handle the situation?
6. How did group members respond to the task?
7. What leadership and management strategies might be effective?
8. What could the leader and followers consider changing in the situation?
9. How did group members feel about what happened?

Follow up this exercise with one that tackles a similar problem: this time the leader has just been informed of patient complaints about staff watching TV at night on their phones, ignoring call lights, and keeping patients awake through loud laughing and talking on night shift. There are only a few nurses partaking in this behavior, but they are very intimidating, and most of the staff do not want to get involved in the issue. Evidently this issue has been going on for years, reported continually but never addressed. The staff now exhibits a sense of hopelessness in relation to resolving the issue.

REFERENCES

Agency for Healthcare Research and Quality (AHRQ). (2016). *TeamSTEPPS strategies and tools to enhance performance and patient safety*. http://www.ahrq.gov/professionals/education/curriculum-tools/teamstepps/index.html.

Altman, S., Butler, A., & Shein, L. (Eds.). (2016). *Assessing progress on the Institute of Medicine Report – The Future of Nursing*. Washington, DC: National Academies Press. www.nap.edu.

American Association of Critical-Care Nurses (AACN). (2005). *AACN standards for establishing and sustaining healthy work environments: A journey to excellence*. http://www.aacn.org/wd/hwe/docs/hwestandards.pdf.

Baggs J., & Schmitt, M. (1998). Collaboration between nurses and physicians. *Journal of Nursing Scholarship, 20*, 145–149.

Belker, L., McCormick, L., & Topchik, G. (2019). *Team dynamics*. https://www.amanet.org/articles/team-dynamics/.

Budin, W. C., Brewer, C. S., Chao, Y. Y., & Kovner, C. (2013). Verbal abuse from nurse colleagues and work environment of early registered nurses. *Journal of Nursing Scholarship, 45*(3), 308–316.

Cherniss, C., & Goleman, D. (2001). *The emotionally intelligent workplace: How to select for, measure, and improve emotional intelligence in individuals, groups, and organizations*. San Francisco, CA: Jossey-Bass.

Christensen, C., & Larson, J. (1993). Collaborative medical decision making. *Medical Decision Making, 13*, 339–349.

Debono, D. S., Greenfield, D., Travaglia, J. F., Long, J. C., Black, D., Johnson, J., et al. (2013). Nurses' workarounds in acute healthcare settings: A scoping review. *BMC Health Services Research, 13*(1), 175. https://doi.org/10.1186/1472-6963-13-175.

Einola, K., & Alvesson, M. (2019). The making and unmaking of teams. *Human Relations, 72*(12), 1891–1919.

Goldratt, E. M., & Cox, J. (2016). *The goal: A process of ongoing improvement* (3rd ed.). Abingdon, UK: Routledge.

Hersey, P., Blanchard, K. H., & Johnson, D. E. (2013). *Management of organizational behavior: Leading human resources* (10th ed.). Upper Saddle River, NJ: Pearson Education.

Huber, D. L., Bair, H., & Joseph, M. L. (2019). Roadmap to drive innovativeness in health care. *Nurse Leader, 17*(6), 505–508.

Institute for Healthcare Improvement (IHI). (2016). *Triple aim initiative*. http://www.ihi.org/engage/initiatives/tripleaim/pages/default.aspx.

Jacobs, B., & Rosenthal, T. (1984). Managing effective meetings. *Nursing Economic$, 2*(2), 137–141.

Jay, A. (1982). How to run a meeting. *Journal of Nursing Administration, 12*(1), 22–28.

Kalisch, B., & Lee, K. H. (2010). The impact of teamwork on missed nursing care. *Nursing Outlook, 58*(5), 233–241.

Katzenbach, J. R., & Smith, D. K. (2015). *The wisdom of teams: Creating the high-performance organization* (reprint ed.). Boston, MA: Harvard Business Review Press.

Kayser, T. (2011). *Building team power: How to unleash the collaborative genius of teams for increased engagement, productivity, and results*. New York: McGraw Hill Professional.

Kozlowski, S., & Ilgen, D. (2006). Enhancing the effectiveness of work groups and teams. *Psychological Science of Work Groups and Teams, 7*(3), 77–124.

Lancaster, J. (1981). Making the most of meetings. *Journal of Nursing Administration, 11*(10), 15–19.

Lu, H., Barriball, K. L., Zhang, X., & While, A. E. (2012). Job satisfaction among hospital nurses revisited: A systematic review. *International Journal of Nursing Studies, 49*(8), 1017–1038.

Lumen Learning.com. (2020) *Boundless management. Defining a team*. https://courses.lumenlearning.com/boundless-management/chapter/defining-teams-and-teamwork/.

Manion, J. (2009). *The engaged workforce: Proven strategies to build a positive healthcare workplace*. Chicago, IL: AHA Press.

Manion, J. (2011). *From management to leadership: Strategies for transforming health care*. San Francisco, CA: Jossey-Bass.

Marks, M., Mathieu, J., & Zaccaro, S. (2001). A temporary based framework and taxonomy of team processes. *The Academy of Management Review, 26*(3), 356–376.

Merriam-Webster. (2019). Communication. *The Merriam-Webster.com Dictionary*, Merriam-Webster Inc. https://www.merriam-webster.com/dictionary/communication.

Miller, C., Kim, B., Silverman, A., & Bauer, M. (2018). A systematic review of team-building interventions in non-acute healthcare settings. *BMC Health Services Research, 18*(146), 1–21. https://doi.org/10.1186/s12913-018-2961-9.

Newell, S., & Kirkwood, H. P., Jr. (2020). Teams and teamwork. Adameg, Inc. https://www.referenceforbusiness.com/management/Str-Ti/Teams-and-Teamwork.html.

Read, E., & Laschinger, H. K. (2013). Correlates of new graduate nurses' experiences of workplace mistreatment. *Journal of Nursing Administration, 43*(4), 221–228.

Riley, W., Davis, S. E., Miller, K. K., & McCullough, M. (2010). A model for developing high-reliability teams. *Journal of Nursing Management, 18*, 556–563.

Ronco, W. (2005). *Partnering solutions*. Franklin Lakes, NJ: Career Press.

Roth, C., Wieck, K. L., Fountain, R., & Haas, B. K. (2015). Hospital nurses' perceptions of human factors contributing to nursing errors. *Journal of Nursing Administration, 45*(5), 263–269.

Salas, E., & Rosen, M. A. (2013). Building high reliability teams: Progress and some reflections on teamwork training. *BMJ Quality & Safety, 22*(5), 369–373.

Sikka, R., Morath, J., & Leape, L. (2015). The Quadruple Aim: Care, health, cost and meaning in work. *BMJ Quality & Safety, 24*(10), 608–610. https://doi.org/10.1136/bmjqs-2015-004160.

Teunissen, C., Burrell, B., & Maskill, V. (2020). Effective surgical teams: An integrative review. *Western Journal of Nursing Research, 42*(1), 61–75.

Turner, J. R., Baker, R., & Morris, M. (2018). Complex adaptive systems: Adapting and managing teams and team conflict. *IntechOpen, Chapter 5*, 65–94. https://doi.org/10.5772/intechopen.72344.

Wong, C. A., Cummings, G. G., & Ducharme, L. (2013). The relationship between nursing leadership and patient outcomes: A systematic review update. *Journal of Nursing Management, 21*(5), 709–724.

Wynia, M. K., Von Kohorn, I., & Mitchell, P. H. (2012). Challenges at the intersection of team based and patient-centered health care: Insights from the IOM working group. *Journal of the American Medical Association, 308*(13), 1327–1328.

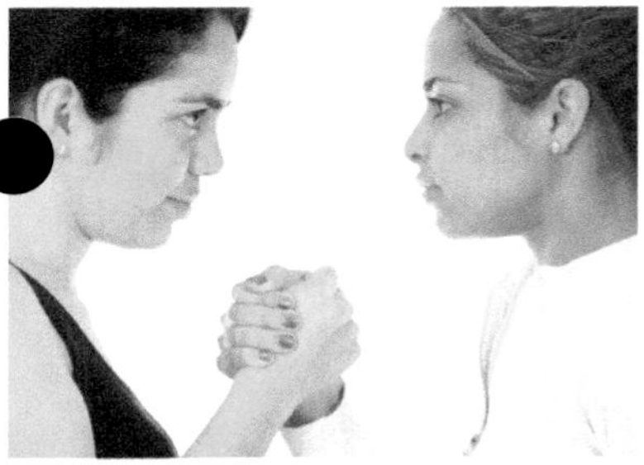

10

Power and Conflict

Mary Louanne Friend

http://evolve.elsevier.com/Huber/leadership

POWER

Nurses are increasingly recognized as leaders who can transform and influence health outcomes by becoming full partners with physicians and other health care professionals to redesign delivery of care in the United States. Several prestigious organizations have acknowledged that nurses are uniquely qualified to lead health care reform, but they must first significantly change their current roles, educational preparation, and responsibilities. The landmark report, *The Future of Nursing: Leading Change, Advancing Health* (Institute of Medicine [IOM], 2011), included recommendations for nurses to improve: (1) access to care, (2) interprofessional collaboration, (3) nursing leadership, (4) nursing education, (5) diversity in nursing, and (6) collection of workforce data. Likewise, in 2010 the Robert Wood Johnson Foundation, in conjunction with the American Association of Retired Persons (AARP) and AARP Foundation, developed the Future of Nursing (n.d.) Campaign to empower nursing to achieve the IOM's recommendations with a nationwide initiative designed to strengthen the power of nursing to help Americans lead longer, healthier lives.

In 2014 the Robert Wood Johnson Foundation requested that the IOM, now called the National Academies of Sciences, Engineering, and Medicine, Health and Medicine Division, assess advancements made since the recommendations of *The Future of Nursing* (IOM, 2011). This follow-up report, *Assessing Progress on the Institute of Medicine Report The Future of Nursing* (National Academies of Sciences, Engineering, and Medicine, 2016), described substantial improvements including increasing the number of: (1) baccalaureate prepared nurses, (2) nurses with doctoral degrees, (3) states where advanced practiced registered nurses (APRNs) can work to their full capacity, (4) interprofessional educational opportunities, (5) nurses who hold positions on corporate boards, and (6) states that collect nursing workforce data.

However, less progress has been noted in efforts to increase diversity in nursing. Of note, the lack of diversity in nursing has been associated with identified underrepresented groups preferring careers in medicine due in part to the perceived ability to overcome stereotypes, while rejecting nursing to avoid negatively stereotyped careers (Alexander & Diefenbeck, 2020). Additionally, men in nursing have been criticized for being competitive and for receiving preferential leadership opportunities with differential compensation (Brody et al., 2017). These findings are disappointing and suggest the profession has much work to do in terms of improving the image of nursing to increase diversity in both ethnicity and gender.

The authors of the 2016 follow-up report suggested that efforts to increase the numbers of APRNs who practice to the full extent of their education will require ongoing collaboration with other health professions and policy makers to remove scope of practice restrictions. Other recommendations included developing nursing leaders who can (1) lead ongoing reforms to the health care system, (2) direct research on evidence-based improvements to care, (3) translate research findings into practice, (4) be full partners on the health care team, and (5) advocate for policy change (National Academies of Sciences, Engineering, and Medicine, 2016). The accomplishments made thus far are the direct result of nursing leaders working together and collaborating with others to increase their influence. However, nurses also need to learn not only to embrace but also to *value* power if these accomplishments are to be maintained. The process of becoming powerful is not static and will continue to be influenced by societal expectations, emerging technologies, and regulation (Nancarrow & Borthwick, 2005). Both power and conflict have a long history of theoretical development and research primarily found within the business literature. Influential traditions of thought are reviewed in this chapter as they formed the foundation for power and conflict research within nursing.

DEFINITIONS

Power eludes definition but is easy to recognize by its consequences: "the ability of those who possess power to bring about the outcomes they desire" (Salancik & Pfeffer, 1977, p. 3). The general and nursing literature continue to lack a clear definition of power because the construct is often used interchangeably with terms including empowerment, status, leadership, and influence. Power is also defined differently based on the unit of analysis including the individual, groups and institutions. Broadly, **power** is defined as control over resources and is considered to be relational in nature (Fiske, 2010). Power is often described as being either positional (legitimate) or personal.

SOURCES OF POWER

A frequently cited reference related to power is French and Raven's (1959) classic work where power in leadership is defined as the ability of an agent to influence a target within a certain system or context. French and Raven identified five bases of power: (1) reward, (2) coercive, (3) legitimate, (4) expert, and (5) referent (Box 10.1). When reward power is used, people comply because doing so produces positive benefits. Coercive power depends on fear. An individual reacts to the fear of the negative consequences that might occur for failure to comply. Referent power is based on admiration for a person who has desirable resources or personal traits. Legitimate power represents the power a person receives

BOX 10.1 French and Raven's Five Sources of Power

1. ***Reward power*** is giving something of value. For example, in nursing, rewards may be a pay raise, praise, a promotion, or a job on the day shift. Reward power is based on the ability to deliver desired rewards.
2. ***Coercive power*** is force against the will. For example, in nursing, coercive power can be the threat of firing, of disciplinary action, or other negative consequences. Coercive power is the power derived from an ability to threaten punishment and deliver penalties. It is a source of power used to apply pressure so that others will meet what is demanded.
3. ***Expert power*** means the use of expertise. It is knowledge, competence, communication, and personal power all combined in a reservoir of knowledge and experience. Expert power is a source of power held by those with some special knowledge, skill, or competence in a particular area. For example, the nurse with the greatest expertise in wound dressings will be sought out by other people in the work environment for this expertise. Expertise is an artful combination of skill and knowledge. It may be founded on depth of knowledge and/or psychomotor skill. There is power in the use of knowledge and skill (i.e., because people need you or can benefit from your expertise, power exists). Therefore the use of expertise can be structured to accomplish or influence movement or action toward certain goals.
4. ***Referent power*** is a little more difficult to understand because it is subtle. It is the use of charisma to influence others. The followers of someone with referent power respond positively to the interpersonal communication and image of the charismatic person. In organizations, this translates into an informal leadership based on liking, charisma, or personal power. Referent power comes from the affinity other people have for someone. They admire the personal qualities, the problem-solving ability, the style, or the dedication the person brings to the work. Referent power can be viewed as an inspirational power because people's admiration for someone allows that person to influence without having to offer rewards or threaten punishments. For example, in the political arena, occasionally there are charismatic political figures or orators. Their influence comes from their followers' liking or identification with them. An example in nursing is Florence Nightingale, who became a symbol of professional nursing. An emotional upsweep is felt by associating with a charismatic person. Referent power is a personal liking and identification experienced by others. Followers attribute referent power to a leader based on the leader's personal characteristics and interpersonal appeal. Physical attractiveness may contribute to referent power.

BOX 10.1 French and Raven's Five Sources of Power—cont'd

5. ***Legitimate power*** means positional power. It is the right to command within the organizational structure based on the hierarchical position held. The president of the United States has power because of holding the position. Legitimate power is the most common source of power. It is what most often is called *authority*. The authority of position gives the person the right to act, order, and direct others. However, leadership and influence need not be confined to those with authority. Every person possesses the ability to tap different sources of power to use in a variety of situations.

Data from French, J., & Raven, B. (1959). The bases of social power. In D. Cartwright (Ed.), *Studies in social power* (pp. 150–167). Ann Arbor, MI: University of Michigan, Institute for Social Research.

as a result of his or her position in the formal organizational hierarchy. Expert power results from expertise, special skill, or knowledge. This typology is often considered negative because it implies legitimate authority to use positive and negative sanctions (Friend, 2013). Raven later added a sixth base of power, informational or persuasion. *Information power* can stem from any person in the organization and is based on another's perception that the influencer either possesses or has access to information that is valuable to another (Raven, 1965).

Personal power has been associated with social relationships and personal characteristics, including having expertise in knowledge and skills (Yukl, 2013). Yukl suggested that informal power includes referent, expert, or persuasive power. Referent power results from the desire of others to please an agent and is associated with someone who is friendly, charming, and trustworthy. For nurses, clinical competence (expert power) is a considerable source of power because peers will follow a nurse who is perceived to be clinically competent. This personal expertise power is one way that a nurse becomes an informal leader (Mannix et al., 2013). Referent and expert power have reportedly been widely utilized by nurses to implement patient care. *Persuasive power* refers to skill in making rational appeals and is an essential source of personal power (Yukl & Falbe, 1991). It has been suggested nurses' recurrent and direct access to patients increases their informal power in health care settings, yet they continue to lack formal power (Paynton, 2009).

The most recent source of power has been described as capital (Oakes et al., 1998; Ocasio, 2002). There are different types of capital, including economic, cultural, social, and symbolic, which can be used to access valued resources within relationships (Bourdieu, 1985). Bourdieu conceptualized economic capital as material resources that can be converted into money. Cultural capital included cultural and class distinctions acquired through socialization (embodied cultural capital), the possession and display of cultural artifacts that reflect class distinctions (objectified cultural capital), and the acquisition of formal degrees (Ocasio et al., 2020). Social capital is defined by Bourdieu (1985) as resources that can be acquired through access to social relationships and membership in social groups. Symbolic capital included sources such as family names, titles and ranks that provide status and collective recognition. Nahapiet and Goshal (1998) later described three dimensions of social capital including structural, relational, and cognitive social capital. Social capital has been associated with healthy work environments in primary care (DiCicco-Bloom et al., 2007). Social capital theory has also been identified as a framework to understand and measure nurses' contribution to rural health care (Lauder et al., 2006).

SOCIAL CAPITAL IN NURSING

A concept analysis of social capital identified nursing social capital as "nurses' shared assets and way of being and knowing that are evident in, and available through nurses' network of social relationships at work" (Read, 2014, p. 997). Read suggested that future research should include developing tools to measure social capital and that nurse leaders need to focus on strategies to enhance social capital, including improved communication, positive leadership practices, and cultivating a culture of trust among nurses. Laschinger et al. (2014) evaluated the impact of social capital and structural empowerment finding positive correlations between social capital on unit work effectiveness and individual nurses' perception of unit quality. They suggested nursing units that support strong social capital are a value-added investment in patient care quality.

In summary, although power remains an elusive concept, negative connotations of power as individuals imposing their will on another person are still included within nursing textbooks (Catalano, 2019), the constant in many students' lives in relation to literature

(Huntington & Gilmour, 2001). One could even argue that little has changed in nursing since Cohen (1992) wrote the "crises facing nursing today can be summarized under three headings: status and power; economics; and numbers" (p. 113). However, the portrayal of power being absolute or existing only when one agent is dependent upon another is changing, in part due to the scholarship of nursing theorists, who have expanded the characterizations of power as both positive and essential to nursing.

NURSING THEORY AND POWER

The significance of conceptual frameworks of nursing has been well documented (Alligood & Tomey, 2010; Butts et al., 2012; Fawcett, 1999). According to Fawcett, by definition, a profession has unique perspectives and subsequently, requires specific theoretical foundations in order to adequately examine their phenomena of interest. Nurse phenomena of interest are the human as a whole being, the environment, and health (Barrett, 2017). The significance of utilizing nursing knowledge has been increasingly highlighted in the literature because "without theory, nursing becomes a trade who are not professional but instead are ancillary and placed into the despised category of midrange practitioners" (Turkel et al., 2018, p. 186).

Barrett's (1989) Theory of Power as Knowing Participation in Change was developed from a perspective of Rogers' Science of Unitary Human Beings (1970; 1990), and power was identified as one way that human beings participate in patterning their potentials toward well-being. Barrett conceptualized power as a process that can be quantified using the Power as Knowing Participation in Change Tool Version II (PKPCT V II) (Barrett, 2010). Power is making choices, feeling free to act on intention, and creating change. According to Barrett, there are two types of power: power as control and power as freedom, and both are continuously available. Barrett (2017) recommended this framework to be utilized as a structure for strategic planning for the profession.

Sieloff's Theory of Work Team/Group Empowerment within Organizations© (1995) was developed using King's definition of power as a positive resource for nurses within health care organizations, defined as "the capacity to achieve goals" (King, 1981, p. 127). Sieloff's theory defined and measured power at the group level, essential to the work of nurses. The related instrument, The Sieloff-King Assessment of Group Outcome Attainment within Organizations (SKAGOAO) can be utilized to measure the level of nursing group power within organizations (Sieloff, 2003).

Likewise, Chinn's emancipatory theory of Peace and Power (Chinn & Falk-Raphael, 2015) posited that all human relationships involve power that can be used to "create harmony, collective strength, and individual well-being" (p. 62). Chinn rejected the patriarchal view of power as "power over" and instead theorized that power is an exercise to join with others to direct collective energies "toward a future you seek together" (Chinn & Kramer, 1995, p. 8). By incorporating these positive aspects of power, and expanding the concept of power to include groups, nurses have the discipline-specific theoretical foundation and instruments to advocate for and measure their power.

Without power the profession will be unable to challenge ongoing barriers that prohibit nurses' abilities to autonomously provide access to high-quality, patient-centered, affordable care to decrease health inequities. The capability of nursing to collectively embrace their political power at the institutional, community, and national levels is essential. Nursing has been consistently identified as being the highest rated profession in terms of honesty and ethics (Gallup, 2020), while Americans rate their congressman and legislators as having the least honesty and ethical standards. When it comes to public trust in various groups trying to improve the US health care system, Americans generally do not trust any interest major groups, except for nurses (The Commonwealth Fund, 2019). Those who support hierarchal relations are typically those with power (Sidanius & Pratto, 1999). If nurses are disadvantaged in terms of their political power, they need to assemble to collectively challenge the status quo.

POLITICAL POWER

Political power or capital has been defined as the variety of economic, social, and cultural resources available to individuals and groups to affect organizational decisions, actions, and outcomes (Ocasio, 2002). The nursing literature has scant mention of the importance of political power and instead discusses power at the individual, intrapersonal, or institutional levels. This is significant since there are more than three times as many RNs in the United States as physicians, with more than 3.8 million registered nurses (RNs) nationwide

(American Association of Colleges of Nursing [AACN], 2008; Rosseter, 2018). Medicine has historically been perceived as more powerful than nursing (Manojlovich, 2007), and their power has resulted from strategic planning and deliberate actions. These steps included moving into powerful positions in government and creating a strong political voice, while also concentrating on regulation and limiting licensure for other health professions (Nancarrow & Borthwick, 2005).

Nurses have a unique opportunity to unify in efforts to impact health care inequities and disparities that currently plague the American health care system; however, they must understand the political process and how they as individuals can participate. Nurses have historically been apolitical (Des Jardin, 2001) and oblivious to the power they possess (Pelc, 2009). The profession's ongoing values of altruism and caring are associated with nursing's lack of power (Baer, 2009; Bassett, 2002; Cook, & Cullen, 2003). In order to increase political activism, nurse educators need to prepare graduates with the skills required to lead others and develop policy.

Nursing Education and Political Power

The AACN Essentials documents (AACN, 2008, 2011) call for nurses to achieve 12 health policy competencies at the baccalaureate level. However, there are few faculty qualified to teach policy in many schools and some faculty reportedly do not appreciate the importance of policy as it relates to nursing practice and research (Boswell et al., 2005; Des Jardin, 2001; Heiman et al., 2016). This gap in nursing education has been addressed by researchers who incorporated political perspectives within a public health nursing curriculum. Student feedback suggested the course influenced students' values of the political process and increased their knowledge of public policy, the legislative process, teamwork, and organizational skills (Byrd et al., 2004). Service learning has also been utilized to teach baccalaureate students health policy. Course evaluations suggested the experiences were valuable in helping students learn social justice, determinants of health, and the policy process (O'Brien-Larivée, 2011). Recently, recommendations have been made to stage policy education within nursing by tailoring content in undergraduate and graduate courses to prepare students to participate in health policy development. At a bare minimum, future nurses need to be provided with an introduction to how health policy is drafted along with the opportunity to meet local political leaders to learn how to serve their communities on local school boards and city councils. Novice nurses would greatly benefit from learning how their colleagues have shaped important legislation influencing nursing practice, including mandatory patient/staff ratios (Spetz et al., 2008), mandatory nursing overtime, and mandated staffing committees (ANA, 2015).

Group/Team Power

The strategic contingencies theory of power (Hickson et al., 1971) hypothesized that organizations consisted of interdependent subunits, thus shifting the emphasis of power from individuals to groups (Friend & Sieloff, 2018). The concept of group power is essential to nurses who practice in teams regardless of their setting. Team power has been defined as the ability of teams to control resources to enable the influence of others (Greer et al., 2011). However, this definition is based upon providing or withholding resources or punishments (French & Raven, 1959). In contrast, Sieloff defined group power as the group's ability to achieve goals, rejecting the paternalistic view of power as depending upon either the environment or other individuals within that environment rather than on the efforts of the work team (Sieloff & Friend, 2015). Group power has profound impact on the social realities of nursing, which has repeatedly been referred to as oppressed.

Powerlessness/Oppression

Nursing has been described as powerless and unable to control its own destiny (D'Antonio et al., 2010). Powerless implies being unable to exercise your capacities to produce the goals you are capable of (Sieloff, 2004; Abood, 2007). The profession has often also been referred to as oppressed. According to Webster, oppression is "the unjust or cruel exercise of authority or power; or a sense of being weighed down in body or mind" (Merriam-Webster, n.d.). Frye (1983) described oppression as living one's life shaped by barriers that restrict or penalize motion. The nursing profession, historically restrained by the barriers of hospital bureaucracy, physicians, and senior nurse authority, may be compared to this analogy (Friend, 2013). Oppressed or powerless nurses were first described by Roberts (1983) who affirmed that submissive, passive-aggressive behaviors in nursing develop in response to domineering practices of physicians and hospital administrators.

The nursing literature is replete with manuscripts describing negative nursing interactions characterized as incivility, horizontal and lateral violence, and nurse bullying in academic and clinical environments (Baltimore, 2006; Clark, 2008; Roberts, 2015; Trossman, 2014). Regardless of the label for these behaviors, these actions are consistently associated with increased burnout and turnover intentions, and decreased job satisfaction and commitment (Smith et al., 2010; Laschinger et al., 2009). Of note, these toxic nursing behaviors are not limited to the United States but have also been reported worldwide (Flateau-Lux & Gravel, 2014; Losa Iglesias & Becerro de Bengoa Vellajo, 2012a; Nixon, 2014). A review of the literature proposes these nursing actions are the result of a cycle where behaviors are tolerated and repeated, suggesting that noxious nursing practices are learned from one generation and passed on to another (Hutchinson & Jackson, 2013). What is less clear is how to break the cycle of oppressed behaviors in order to support a unified, powerful profession that can impact individual, community and global health outcomes.

Empowerment

Empowerment, like power, is complex and has multiple perspectives, including structural, psychological, and group. Rappaport (1987) suggested that the ability to identify the absence of empowerment was easier than actually defining the concept. Historically, empowerment gained momentum during the civil right struggles and, unlike power, is consistently considered positive and is either an outcome or process (Friend & Sieloff, 2018). Empowerment has also been described at the individual, organizational, and community levels.

Empowerment was first described within the nursing literature at a time of hospital down-sizing, a nursing shortage, and initiation of quality improvement projects (Bartunek & Spreitzer, 2006). Nursing empowerment was initially described in terms of individual nurses empowering their patients until Rodwell (1996) reported that nurses cannot empower patients and only people can empower themselves. Rao (2012) later defined nurse empowerment as a state in which an individual nurse has assumed control over their practice, enabling them to successfully fulfill professional nursing responsibilities within an organization. Of note, much of the nursing research related to nursing empowerment has been conducted using theoretical frameworks other than nursing, including the social-structural and psychological theories of empowerment.

Empowerment Theories

The social-structural empowerment theory (Kanter, 1977; 1993) focused on how social, political, and organizational forces create powerlessness. Kanter (1977) defined power as the capacity to mobilize resources to accomplish work and believed that workers become empowered by their work environments, not as a result of their personal predisposition. According to Kanter, empowerment is influenced by the degree of formal and informal power an individual has within an organization. Kanter's perspective emphasizes changing organizational policies and practices that support top-down control systems, where power is held by few (Friend, 2013). The concept of psychological empowerment, first described by Conger and Kanungo (1988), suggested empowerment involves more than sharing power. Thomas and Velthouse (1990) expanded upon Conger and Kanungo (1988) by conceptualizing psychological empowerment as intrinsic task motivation consisting of four dimensions: meaning, competence, self-determination, and impact. Spreitzer (1996) built upon Thomas and Velthouse and confirmed that psychological empowerment consisted of four dimensions including meaning, competence, self-determination, and impact. An additional description of power espouses a poststructuralist approach based on the work of Foucault (1980) who believed power is not fixed but instead changes based on context and induces pleasure. Bradbury-Jones et al. (2008) suggested this poststructuralist perspective should be used by nurses to "consider hierarchical observation, normalizing judgment, the examination and knowledge/power relationships in order to illuminate taken-for-granted areas of nursing practice" (p. 264). However, they also asserted that this approach can be used by other disciplines other than nursing. Since nursing is a unique profession, nursing empowerment is best examined using discipline-specific theories and frameworks including Sieloff's nursing theory of group empowerment within organizations (Sieloff & Bularzik, 2011).

Nursing Theory and Empowerment

Sieloff utilized the strategic contingencies theory of power (Hickson et al., 1971) to provide conceptual guidance to understand nursing's lack of power within organizations (Sieloff, 2007). The strategic contingencies theory of power (Hickson et al., 1971) hypothesized that organizations consist of interdependent subunits and that there is a distribution of power in the division of labor, thus shifting the emphasis of power from persons to groups. Three concepts are included within the theory: (1) centrality, (2) coping with uncertainty, and (3) substitutability (Hickson et al., 1971). The centrality of a subunit is the degree to which its activities are interlinked into the system. Centrality refers to working in a central part of the organization giving one a critical role and bargaining power. Uncertainty is defined as "lack of information about future events so that alternatives and their outcomes are unpredictable" (Hickson et al., 1971, p. 5). Substitutability is defined as the ability of the organization to obtain alternative performance for the activities of a subunit. Power comes from the ability to cope with uncertainty, substitutability, and centrality.

Sieloff reconceptualized the concepts of organizational power to address the human context of nursing (Sieloff, 1995). Centrality, coping with uncertainty, and substitutability were relabeled as position, controlling the effects of environmental forces, and role, respectively. In addition, Sieloff (1995) added resources as a fourth source of power. According to Sieloff, these four variables contribute to a group's empowerment capacity. To explain why some groups are not empowered despite empowerment capacity, four variables associated with group empowerment were identified through observations and labeled based on the results of a factor analysis of instrument data (Sieloff, 1995). The variables were (1) communication competency, (2) goal/outcome competency, (3) nurse leaders' empowerment competency, and (4) empowerment perspective (Friend, 2013). The theory has been refined and an associated instrument developed, the Sieloff King Assessment of Work Team/Group Empowerment within Organizations (SKAWGEO) (Friend & Sieloff, 2018).

Gaps in knowledge. Past research has attempted to examine the relationship between work team/group empowerment and nursing-sensitive patient outcomes and safety (Sieloff, 2010). However, due to a lack of the availability of consistent data, this relationship has yet to be studied. It is critical to establish whether a relationship exists between work team/group empowerment and the achievement of safe and quality care as the identification of a relationship between work team/group empowerment and safe, quality nursing care may provide a foundation for future interventional research designed to identify processes to increase cost effective quality nursing care.

Furthermore, past research has identified that work team/group empowerment is a unique construct that exists within all nursing work settings. However, it is not known which factors have the most effect on improving a work team's/group's overall empowerment. If this knowledge could be identified, strategies could be selected using the most effective, yet least expensive, approaches. Rather than using non-nursing theories to develop knowledge to effect nursing work environments, the use of a nursing-theory based perspective and reliable and valid instrument may generate sufficient knowledge to change workplace practices both now and in the future. Regardless of the definition, power is an essential concept because power differentials in health care settings are universal.

The perspective that nurses wait for empowerment to occur as a result of something or someone else has supported the patriarchal view of empowerment and the perception that nurses are oppressed. There is a current need to focus on empowerment at the group or work team level as a strategy to transform nursing education, practice, and research. If, as the nursing literature suggests, factors associated with nursing's oppressed group behavior continue to include lack of empowerment, authoritative leadership, oppression, learned helplessness (Lewis, 2006), negative nursing unit culture and toxic work environment (Freshwater, 2000; Hamlin, 2000), suppressed anger and gender issues (Rowell, 2005), and low self-esteem (Longo & Sherman, 2007), empowered nursing teams are desperately needed.

AUTHORITY AND INFLUENCE

Definitions

Authority and influence are two major content dimensions of power identified in classic theory. Barnard (1938, p. 161) defined authority as "the character of a communication (order) in a formal organization by virtue of which it is accepted by a contributor to or 'member' of the organization as governing the action he contributes." Weber's (1968) work is considered the most influential related to authority. He defined three types of authority: traditional, rational-legal, and charismatic authority. Weber defined traditional authority as resulting from customs and traditions passed from one generation to the next. Rational-legal authority was born from laws, rules, and power with a legitimate office. Charismatic authority is the result of personal abilities to inspire. Authority generally refers to those who have expertise (theoretical authorities) or practical authorities who have particular positions in an organization or social system (Wendt, 2018).

Influence has been defined as the capacity to impact agendas and outcomes and to bring other people on board (Heath, 1988). Influence is associated with leadership as a way to request a behavior that encourages followers to act (Gardner & Avolio, 1998), and the ability to influence others has been described as the most important determinant of managerial effectiveness (Yukl, 1989). Influence then is the attempt to affect or control the behaviors of others (Bierstadt, 1950; Pfeffer, 1992). Beauchamp and Childress (1994) stated that persuasion is one of three categories of influence and includes convincing someone to believe in something through the merit of reasons by another person.

Typically, influence is considered as something that flows downhill from powerholders to subordinates (Oc et al., 2019). However, followers may also use influence tactics upwardly, impacting organizational effectiveness (Goldrick et al., 1994). There have been three conceptualizations of authority and influence: (1) some authors equate these terms, (2) others tend to equate power with influence and assert that authority is a special case of power, and (3) still others view authority and influence as distinctly different dimensions of power. Several points of contrast are summarized in Table 10.1.

TABLE 10.1 Authority and Influence Contrasted

Authority	Influence
Authority is the static, structural aspect of power in organizations.	Influence is the dynamic, tactical element.
Authority is the formal aspect of power.	Influence is the informal aspect.
Authority refers to the formally sanctioned right to make decisions.	Influence is not sanctioned by the organization and is therefore not a matter of organizational rights.
Authority implies involuntary submission by subordinates.	Influence implies voluntary submission and does not necessarily entail a superior–subordinate relationship.
Authority flows downward, and it is unidirectional.	Influence is multidirectional and can flow upward, downward, or horizontally.
The source of authority is solely structural.	The source of influence may be personal characteristics, expertise, or opportunity.
Authority is circumscribed.	The domain, scope, and legitimacy of influence are typically ambiguous.

Influence Tactics

Nurse Managers (NMs) confront multiple challenges as they are often charged with fiscal, quality, and human resource responsibilities (Bradley & Moore, 2019). Managers operate at the nexus between the nurse and central decision authority levels. Thus they influence the flow and implementation of resources and support. Most of the research on influence has been conducted within the psychology, business, and organizational frameworks. Kipnis et al. (1980) were among the first to investigate the influence behavior of managers. Content analysis led to the identification of 370 different forms of influence behavior, which were condensed into 14 categories. Subsequently, factor analysis brought about the following eight forms of influence behavior:

1. Assertiveness means expressing one's own position to another without inhibiting the rights of others.
2. Ingratiation means trying to make the other person feel important, giving praise or sympathizing. Ingratiation is attempting to advance oneself by trying to make another person feel important.
3. Rationality means using logical and rational arguments, providing pertinent information, presenting reasons, and laying out an idea in a logical, structured way.
4. Sanctions are threats. Positive sanctions, or rewards, are addressed within motivation mechanisms.
5. Exchange means that to persuade, an exchange is offered; this is sometimes called "scratching each other's back."
6. Upward appeal means going to a higher authority. It is the childhood threat of "if you don't play by my rules, I am going to go tell Mom." Upward appeal simply means taking the appeal to a higher authority to arbitrate.
7. Blocking means deliberately keeping others from getting their way, threatening to stop working with them, ignoring them, not being friendly, or simply

attempting to make sure others cannot accomplish their aims. This may take the form of bullying.

8. Coalitions are the result of a group of people getting together to speak or negotiate as one voice.

Influence behaviors translate into power strategies. In their three-nation study of managerial influence styles, Kipnis et al. (1984) identified the most to least popular strategies (Table 10.2). Yukl and Falbe (1991) continued the work of Kipnis et al. (1980). They developed the Influence Behavior Questionnaire (IBQ), an instrument to measure the influence behavior of managers. In later studies, the IBQ was developed further, and psychometric tests were performed (Yukl et al., 1992, 1993, 2008). The resulting 11 tactics cover a wide range of influence behavior relevant for managerial effectiveness or, in a broader sense, for getting things done in an organization. Influence tactics are identified in Table 10.3. Research

TABLE 10.2 Most to Least Managerial Influence Strategies Used in All Countries

Strategy Popularity	Managers Influencing Superiors	Managers Influencing Subordinates
Most popular	Reason	Reason
↑	Coalition	Assertiveness
	Friendliness	Friendliness
	Bargaining	Evaluation
	Assertiveness	Bargaining
↓	Higher authority	Higher authority
Least popular	Sanction	

Modified from Kipnis, D., Schmidt, S.M., Swaffin-Smith, C., & Wilkinson, I. (1984). Patterns of managerial influence: Shotgun managers, tacticians, and bystanders. *Organizational Dynamics, 12*(3), 58–67.

TABLE 10.3 Definitions of Influence Tactics

Tactic	Definition
Rational persuasion	The agent uses logical arguments and factual evidence to show that a proposal or request is feasible and relevant for important task objectives.
Inspiration appeals	The agent appeals to the target's values and ideals or seeks to arouse the target's emotions to gain commitment for a request or proposal.
Consultation	The agent asks the target to suggest improvements or help plan an activity or change for which the target's support is desired.
Ingratiation	The agent uses praise and flattery before or during an attempt to influence the target to carry out a request or support a proposal.
Personal appeals	The agent asks the target to carry out a request or support a proposal out of friendship or asks for a personal favor.
Exchange	The agent offers something the target person wants or offers to reciprocate at a later time if the target complies with the request.
Coalition tactics	The agent enlists the aid of, or uses the support of, others to influence the target to do something.
Legitimating tactics	The agent seeks to establish the legitimacy of a request or verify that he or she has the authority to make it.
Pressure	The agent uses demands, threats, frequent checking, or persistent reminders to influence the target to do something.
Collaboration	The agent offers to provide assistance or necessary resources if the target will carry out a request or approve a proposed change.
Apprising	The agent explains how carrying out a request or supporting a proposal will benefit the target personally or help to advance the target's career.

From Yukl, G., Seifert, C.F., & Chavez, C. (2008). Validation of the extended Influence Behavior Questionnaire. *The Leadership Quarterly, 19*(5), 609–621.

utilizing the IBQ suggests that university administrative employees most often used rational persuasion while influencing their superiors (Ghalazi et al., 2012). Nursing research utilizing a modified IBQ suggested that professional practice leaders most frequently used consultation (mean = 4.4, standard deviation [SD] = 0.71) and rational persuasion (mean = 4.3, SD = 0.67), followed by moderate use of inspirational appeal (mean = 3.8, SD = 0.89), legitimizing (mean = 3.8, SD = 0.82), and collaboration (mean = 3.9, SD = 0.72), whereas coalition (mean = 3.0, SD = 0.80) was described as being used occasionally with the manager group (Lankshear et al., 2013). The authors concluded their results were consistent with existing research in that rational persuasion and consultation were often used when trying to influence superiors (Yukl et al., 1993).

Nursing Influence

Historically, nursing influence has focused on how to promote change and outcomes as opposed to how it is acquired and best used (Shilliam et al., 2018). However, the nursing literature currently describes efforts to enhance and to quantify nursing influence. The Adams Influence Model (AIM), originally developed in 2003 to gain an understanding of nurse executive influence, describes the attributes, factors, and processes of influence relating specifically to nurse leaders (Adams & Natarajan, 2016). The original model was based upon French and Raven (1959) and Kipnis and Schmidt (1988) and has since been adapted using three nursing conceptual models, including Neuman's Theory of Health as Expanding Consciousness, Roy's Adaption Model and King's Interacting System Framework and Theory of Goal Attainment.

The current version of the AIM presents an open system model involving a two-person dyad of the influence agent and the influence target. Within the AIM Version V, "there are significant areas of overlap between Barrett's and Sieloff's definitions of power and concepts presented in the AIM, since all three emphasize the role of relationships and intentionality in nurse leaders' efforts to shape the care environment and effect change" (Adams & Natarajan, 2016, p. E 50) (Fig. 10.1). Iteration V of the AIM was evaluated using secondary data analysis resulting in a revised list of influence factors and attributes. The AIM addresses three issues for nursing as identified by King (1964), including the need to further define the nurse leader's practice domain, to identify a standardized, professional language for nurse leaders, and to articulate a theoretical basis for nurse leaders' practice (Adams & Natarajan, 2016). The AIM was recently used to develop an instrument, the Leadership Influence Self-Assessment (LISA©) to help nurse leaders assess and enhance their influence capacity. Factor analysis of the 145-item instrument supports validity and reliability of the tool (Shilliam et al., 2018).

LEADERSHIP AND MANAGEMENT IMPLICATIONS

According to Yukl, "leadership is the process of influencing others to understand and agree about what needs to be done and how it can be done effectively, and the process of facilitating individual and collective efforts to accomplish the shared objectives" (2010, p. 8). Nurses require expertise regarding politics, policy and power to become effective leaders. In order to do this, they must embrace influence and learn to deliver messages that appeal to a wide variety of stakeholders including politicians, policymakers, the media, and the public (Salvage et al., 2019). Dynamic, complex health care organizations require nurse leaders who have the competencies to collaborate across hierarchical boundaries and to influence others towards performance improvement (Dougall et al., 2018). By collaborating across boundaries, nurses can initiate and sustain change from within.

CONFLICT

There are many interpretations of conflict within the literature. **Conflict** is a process that begins when one party perceives that another party has negatively affected, or is about to negatively affect, something that the first party cares about (Robbins, 1998). Marquis and Huston (2012) defined conflict as the consequences of experienced or perceived variations in common goals, values, ideas, attitudes, beliefs, feelings, or actions.

The consequences of unresolved or dysfunctional conflict "hinder organizational performance" (Kreitner & Kinicki, 2010, p. 375). Estimates suggest that US employees spend 2.8 hours per week dealing with unnecessary conflict, corresponding to approximately $359 billion in paid hours and 385 million working days each year (CPP Global Human Capital Report, 2008; Dunford et al., 2020). Conflict between health

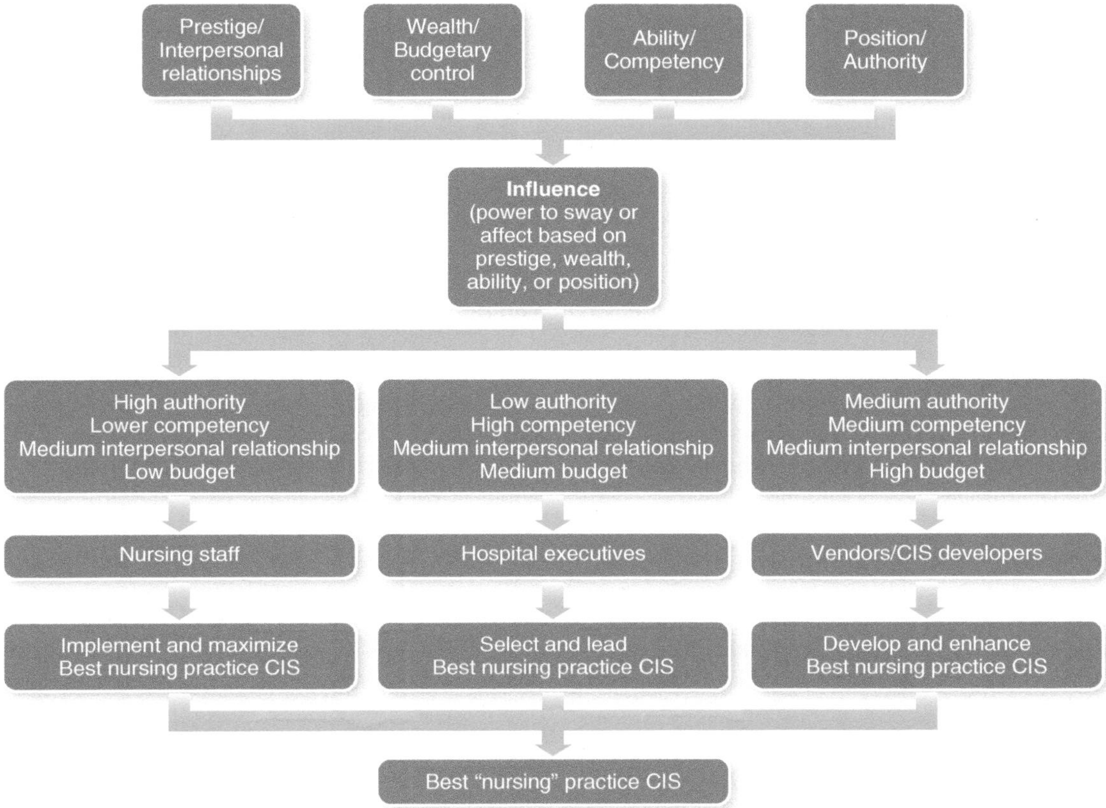

Fig. 10.1 Adams Influence Model, iteration 1. Note: CIS is clinical information systems. (From: Adams, J., & Natarajan, S. (2016). Understanding influence within the context of nursing: Development of the Adams influence model using practice, research, and theory. *Advances in Nursing Science*, 39(3):E40–E56, Figure 1).

care professionals has been associated with decreased providers' attention to patient care, employee satisfaction and morale, and increased turnover (Rosenstein & O'Daniel, 2005). The most damaging outcome of conflict is dysfunctional organizational culture, which stifles change, innovation, and organizational effectiveness. Sentinel events, defined as patient safety events that result in death, permanent harm, or severe temporary harm, have been associated with hospital leadership that fails to establish cultures of safety in hospitals (Smetzer et al., 2010). Conflict resulting in disruptive behaviors in hospitals prompted The Joint Commission (2017), the agency that provides hospital accreditation, to develop a new leadership standard that addressed intimidating behaviors in its elements of performance. Specifically, the standard mandates Chief Executive Officers (CEOs) to advance trust within the organization by adopting and modeling appropriate behaviors and championing efforts to eradicate intimidating behaviors.

Conflict in nursing has been associated with job dissatisfaction. Nurses have also reported that their managers and nursing colleagues are the most common source of conflict (Bishop, 2004; Lawrence & Callan, 2006; Warner, 2001). Conflict has been reported by 53% of nurses as common (Dewitty et al., 2009) and as contributing to practice errors (Rowe & Sherlock 2005). Unresolved conflict may have negative impacts on organizations, individuals, and patient outcomes (Johansen, 2012; McKibben, 2017). Interpersonal conflicts can lead to nurse attrition and thereby contribute to increasing nurse shortages (Almost et al., 2010; Brinkert, 2010).

Conflict is not inherently undesirable, and, in some situations, a certain amount of conflict is needed as it can improve the quality of decision-making, stimulate involvement in discussion, and build group cohesion (Henry, 2009). What is required is to make a distinction between poorly managed conflicts and properly managed ones. Ideally, conflicts are resolved at the lowest organizational level possible to avoid higher levels of management (Costantino & Merchant, 1996) suggesting nurses need to appreciate how to address conflict at the individual level. However, nurses receive very little training in conflict management but are extensively trained in therapeutic communication (Northam, 2009). Conflict management should be viewed less from a perspective that aims to solve conflict and more towards the idea to manage conflict in a constructive way to enhance group outcomes (Bagshaw & Lepp, 2005; Leksell et al., 2015; Rahim, 2002).

DEFINITIONS

There is no universally accepted definition of conflict (Patton, 2014), although the construct has been studied for a long time. Scholars view the lack of consensus as a major obstacle to progress within the field because research results cannot be generalized from one study to another (Mikkelsen & Clegg, 2018). **Conflict** is defined as a situation where the concerns of two people appear to be incompatible (Thomas & Kilmann, 1974). Conceptual analysis suggested that conflict is a multidimensional construct with both detrimental and beneficial effects (Almost, 2006). The source of conflicts in nursing can be categorized in terms of the degree to which individual characteristics, interpersonal factors, and organizational factors affect working relationships. (Almost, 2006).

Organizational conflict is defined as the struggle over scarce organizational resources. Values, goals, roles, money, or structural elements may be the specific locus of the struggle for scarce organizational resources. For example, two parties may be in opposition because of perceived differences in goals, a struggle over budget allocations, or interference in goal attainment. This opposition prevents cooperation (Deutsch, 1973). **Workplace conflict** emerges when one party—be it an individual or a group of individuals—perceives its goals, values, or opinions being thwarted by an interdependent counterpart (Pondy, 1967; Thomas, 1992; Wall & Callister, 1995). These conflicts may result from scarce resources, such as time, responsibilities, status, or budgets or they may involve different political preferences, or religious convictions or a combination of issues (De Dreu & Gelfand, 2007; Deutsch, 1973; Druckman, 1994; Kelley & Thibaut, 1969; Rapoport, 1960). **Task-related conflicts** are about the way the team is doing its job, including the pros and cons of certain task approaches (Jehn, 1994). Task conflict is often viewed as healthy because it stimulates discussions and prevents premature consensus, leading to enhanced work-team effectiveness and performance (De Dreu & Beersma, 2005). **Relationship conflicts** are about people, their values, political convictions, or religious preference (Jehn, 1994, 1995; Simons & Peterson, 2000). Relationship conflict leads to biased information-processing and rigid stances, which negatively affect decision-making (de Wit et al., 2013). **Process conflict** involves incompatibilities in views about how the work should be accomplished (e.g., distribution of workload, order of tasks to be completed) (Jehn, 1997).

CONFLICT MANAGEMENT

There has been a decrease in the negative connotation of conflict to include a more positive view where conflict is seen as an inevitable phenomenon that can have beneficial effects and lead to personal, as well as organizational, growth (Almost, 2006; Alper et al., 2000; Brinkert, 2010; Slabbert, 2004). Conflict is functional, or constructive, when it improves the quality of decisions, stimulates creativity and innovation, encourages interest and curiosity, provides a medium through which problems can be aired and tensions released, and fosters an environment of self-evaluation and change (Box 10.2). In contrast, dysfunctional or destructive outcomes

BOX 10.2 Effects of Conflict

Constructive Effects

- Improves decision quality
- Stimulates creativity
- Encourages interest
- Provides a forum to release tension
- Fosters change

Destructive Effects

- Constricts communication
- Decreases cohesiveness
- Explodes into fighting
- Hinders performance

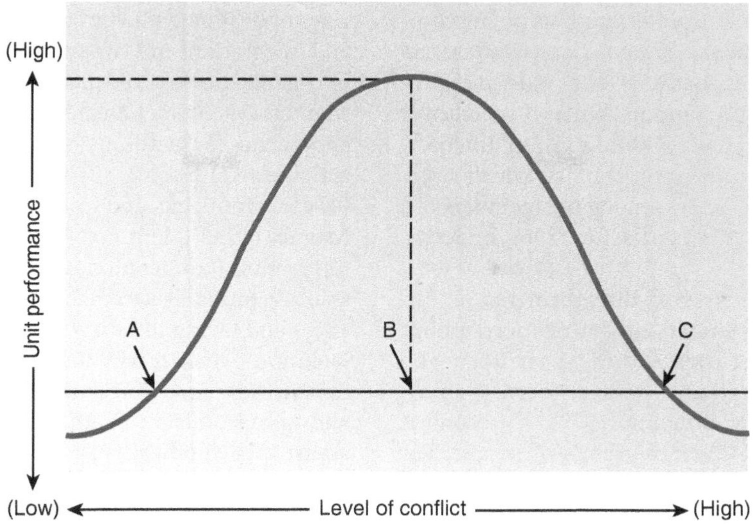

Fig. 10.2 Conflict and unit performance. (Modified from Brown, L.D. [1983]. *Managing conflict at organizational interfaces.* Reading, MA: Addison-Wesley Publishing.)

include a degrading of communication, reduction in group cohesiveness, and subordination of group goals to the primacy of infighting among members. Extremely high or low levels of conflict hinder performance. An optimal level is high enough to prevent stagnation and stimulates creativity, releases tension, and initiates change. However, it is not so high as to be disruptive or counterproductive (Brown, 1983) (Fig. 10.2).

LEVELS OF CONFLICT

Thomas (1992) identified two broad types of conflict. The first refers to incompatible response tendencies within an individual, which Rahim and Bonoma (1979) referred to as intrapersonal conflict (Fig. 10.3). Intrapersonal conflict means discord, tension, or stress inside—or internal to—an individual that results from unmet needs, expectations, or goals. Intrapersonal conflict is conflict that generates from within an individual (Rahim, 1983). It is often manifested as a conflict over two competing roles. For example, a parent with a sick child who has to go to work faces a conflict: the need to take care of the sick child against the need to make a living. A nursing example occurs when the nurse determines that a patient needs teaching or counseling, but the organization's assignment system is set up in a way that does not provide an adequate amount of time. When other priorities compete, an internal or intrapersonal conflict of roles exists.

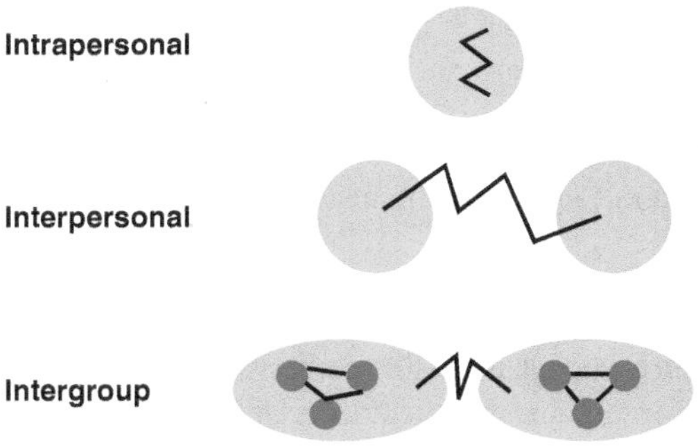

Fig. 10.3 Types of conflict.

The second use refers to conflicts that occur between different individuals, groups, organizations, or other social units. Rahim and Bonoma (1979) identified these as interpersonal conflict, a category that includes intragroup conflict, intergroup conflict, and interorganizational conflict. Interpersonal means conflict emerging between two or more people, such as between two nurses, a doctor and a nurse, or a nurse manager and a staff nurse. In this case, two people have a disagreement, conflict, or clash. Either their values or styles do not match or there is a misunderstanding or miscommunication between them. Interpersonal conflict can be viewed as happening between two individuals or among individuals within a group. When it specifically involves multiple individuals within a group, interpersonal conflict is called intragroup conflict, which refers to disagreements or differences among the members of a group or its subgroups about goals, functions, or activities of the group.

Intergroup conflict refers to disagreements or differences between the members of two or more groups or their representatives over authority, territory, and resources. Interorganizational conflict occurs across organizations (Rahim & Bonoma, 1979). It is conflict occurring between two distinct groups of people. For example, physicians and nurses may disagree about role functions and activities, or lay midwives may seek to perform home deliveries without being prepared as licensed nurse midwives. Intergroup conflict may also arise during decision-making about the use of postoperative life-sustaining treatment in the intensive care unit due to their perceptions of professional roles and responsibilities (Pecanac & Schwarze, 2018). Sometimes the conflict arises between departments or units as groups. For example, hospital nurses might find themselves in conflict with central purchasing if supplies are provided that do not meet nursing needs or are defective.

CONFLICT MANAGEMENT

Conflict management is used within the organization when facing disagreement or conflict to achieve organizational goals like effectiveness and efficiency. According to De Dreu et al. (2001), conflict management is the intention of a person's actions tailored with their conflict experiences. Follett (1940) identified three main ways of dealing with conflict: domination, compromise, and integration; and two other ways of handling conflict in organizations: avoidance and suppression. Blake and Mouton (1964) later created a framework for classifying approaches for handling interpersonal conflicts into five activities: (1) forcing, (2) withdrawing, (3) smoothing, (4) compromising, and (5) problem-solving. Rahim and Magner (1995) identified five ways of handling conflict: integrating (cooperation among the parties to reach a solution mutually acceptable), obliging (reducing differences and trying to satisfy the other party), dominating (solution-oriented win–lose or behavior forced to win the position), avoiding (behavioral withdraw or escape), and compromising (both parties give and accept or adjust to each other).

Thomas and Kilmann (1974) developed a model of conflict management based on assertive behavior (the desire to satisfy yourself) and cooperative behavior (the desire to satisfy the other party). They identified five strategies involved with conflict resolution including: competing, collaborating, avoiding, accommodating, and compromising. Competing strategy is characterized by the urge to maximize benefits to the individual, but it is a loss for others. Compromising includes not taking sides and involves making concessions towards the resolution of the conflict. Avoiding involves escape from the conflict. Accommodating behaviors involve sacrificing self-interest for satisfying the needs of others. Models including five management strategies have been most widely utilized in the literature (Kristanto, 2017).

Pondy (1967), Filley (1975), and Thomas and Schmidt (1976) described conflict dynamics across a temporal sequence of stages or phases. These models provide significant insight into understanding the nature of conflict phenomena (Table 10.4). These models are similar in that all indicate that conflict follows a

TABLE 10.4 Comparison of Four Process Models of Conflict

Pondy (1967)	Filley (1975)	Thomas (1976)	Robbins & Judge (2016)
1. Latent (antecedent conditions)	1. Antecedent conditions	1. Frustration	1. Potential opposition
2. Perception and feeling	2. Perceived conflict	2. Conceptualization	2. Cognition and personalization
3. Behavior manifestation (manifest)	3. Felt conflict	3. Behavior	3. Intentions
4. Aftermath	4. Manifest behavior	4. Others' reactions (interaction)	4. Behavior
	5. Resolution or suppression	5. Outcome	5. Functional or dysfunctional outcomes
	6. Conflict aftermath		

predictable course. However, they differ in the number of identifiable stages or elements in a particular pattern. The following elements exist in all the models:

- Causes, identified as conditions, that occur before the conflict
- Core processes, including the perception that conflict exists, followed by some kind of affective state or emotional response
- Conflict behaviors, including a variety of behaviors from very subtle to violent
- Effect that includes outcomes such as resolution or aftermath consequences

Cause, Core Process, Effect

Wall and Callister (1995) described a generic model of conflict. As with any social process, there are causes and a core process that have effects. These effects in turn have an impact on the original cause. This conflict cycle takes place within a context (environment), and the cycle flows through numerous iterations. Wall and Callister (1995) indicated that the model is a general one that displays how the major pieces in the conflict puzzle fit together. The value of this model is that concepts from all other models may be subsumed under the major concepts of this generic model. In addition, the simplicity of the model facilitates the discussion of conflict according to cause, core process, and effect. Fig. 10.4 uses Wall and Callister's model as a beginning and incorporates the work of Boynton (2012), Patton (2014), and Robbins and Judge (2016). A recent meta-analysis of the literature to identify and synthesize key triggers and impact of healthcare conflicts identified three gaps in the research literature including: (1) lack of holistic approaches to understanding the multilayered factors involving healthcare conflicts, (2) few studies associating resource depletion and low psychological capital with conflict triggers, and (3) the need to understand the role of psychological safety in healthcare power hierarchy (Kim, 2017, p. 3).

Causes of Conflict

According to Wall and Callister (1995), conditions that occur before conflict is identified are causes. Patton (2014) identified some causes of conflict as personality differences, value differences, blurred job boundaries, battle for limited resources, constraints on the decision-making process, communication, departmental competition, unmet expectations for co-workers, and the complexity of organizations. Additional causes of conflict include lack of clarity with expectations or

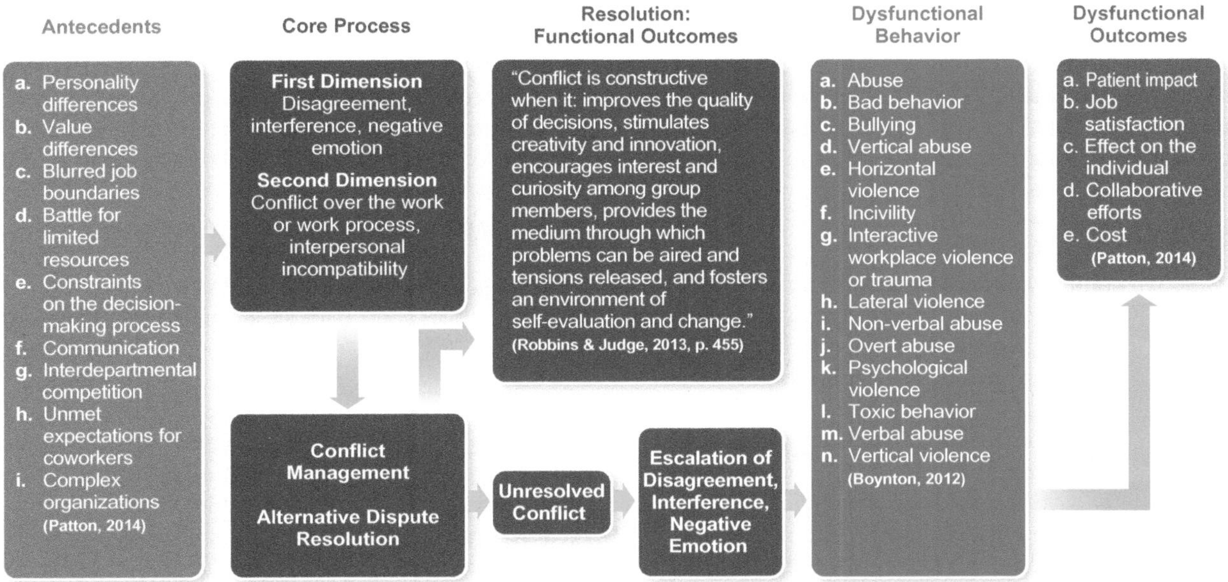

Fig. 10.4 Conceptual framework: antecedents, core process, and functional and dysfunctional outcomes of intragroup conflict.

guidelines, poor communication, lack of clear jurisdiction, personality differences, conflicts of interest, and changes within the organization (Umiker, 1999).

A recent longitudinal study to explore health care professionals' experiences of conflicts and their characteristics identified six sources of conflict: relationships, patient-related tasks, other tasks, team processes, structural processes, and social representations (Bochatay et al., 2017). The authors suggested that disagreements on patient care tended to be the primary trigger of conflict, whereas sources related to communication contributed to conflict escalation without directly triggering conflict.

Moore's Circle of Conflict Model (Moore & Kordick, 2006) included five sources of conflict: (1) data based, (2) interest based, (3) structural based, (4) relationship based, and (5) value based. Data-based conflict occurs when important information is withheld, late, error ridden, irrelevant, or poorly interpreted to the patient or family. Interest-based conflicts occur when a health facility's protocols, processes, or policies frustrate patients' or their loved ones' goals or objectives. Relationship conflicts may not involve important interests, yet they evoke strong reactions. An example of relationship conflict includes poor bedside manner. Structural conflicts arise from the health care system's essential makeup and culture. At the organizational level, structural conflicts involve resource allocations, status differences, role assignments, spatial and organizational relationships, and rules and regulations. Values-based conflicts involve most deeply held beliefs and moral systems that fuel conflicts which are often edgy, "angry," emotional, unforgiving, and disruptive to good care; they are also strongly linked to staff burnout and turnover (Nelson, 2012).

The Core Process of Conflict

Although conflict has been defined in many ways, disagreement, interference, and negative emotion are thought to underlie conflict situations (Barki & Hartwick, 2001). Disagreement, interference, and negative emotion can be viewed as reflecting cognitive, behavioral, and affective manifestations of interpersonal conflict. Disagreement is the most commonly discussed and assessed cognition in the literature. Although a number of different behaviors have been associated with and may be typical of conflict, they do not always indicate the existence of conflict. Conflict exists when the behavior of one party interferes with or opposes another party's attainment of its own interests, objectives, or goals. Several affective states have been associated with conflict. However, it is the negative emotions such as fear, anger, anxiety, and frustration that have been used to characterize conflict. Barki and Hartwick (2001) proposed that interpersonal conflict exists only when disagreement, interference, and negative emotion are present in the situation.

In Barki and Hartwick 2004, conducted a comprehensive review of the literature, and two dimensions of conflict were identified. The first dimension identifies disagreement, interference, and negative emotion as three properties generally associated with a conflict situation. The second dimension identifies relationship and task content or task process as two targets of interpersonal conflict encountered in organizational settings. Conflict management and alternative dispute resolution (ADR) are also components of the core process of conflict.

Effects of Conflict

Patton (2014) noted that conflict has an impact on job satisfaction, individuals, collaborative efforts, and organizational costs. However, the most serious effect is the negative impact on patients. Positive functional outcomes of conflict include increased group performance, improved quality of decisions, stimulation of creativity and innovation, encouragement of interest and curiosity, provision of a medium for problem-solving, and creation of an environment for self-evaluation and changes. In contrast, dysfunctional outcomes include development of discontent, reduced group effectiveness, disrupted communication, reduced group cohesiveness, and infighting among group members, which then overrides the focus on group goals (Robbins & Judge, 2016).

BULLYING AND DISRUPTIVE BEHAVIOR

Interestingly, many authors addressed the negative impact of unresolved conflict, but few have addressed the escalation of conflict to dysfunctional behavior. Disruptive behavior is defined differently but includes behavior that can negatively impact labor relations, effectiveness of communication, information transfer, and the care process and its outcomes (Rosenstein et al., 2002). Disruptive Behavior in Healthcare Work is a theoretical construct made from the combination of several attributes that represent a spectrum of behaviors ranging from incivility to physical and/or sexual violence (Oliveira et al., 2016, p. 695). After a meta-analysis,

Oliveira and colleagues promulgated the following definition: "any inappropriate behavior, confrontation or conflict—ranging from verbal abuse (abusive, intimidating, disrespectful, or threatening behavior) to physical or sexual harassment—which can negatively impact labor relations, effectiveness of communication, information transfer, and the care process and its outcomes." Disruptive behaviors have been classified as including primarily psychological violence, followed by incivility, and physical or sexual violence. There are an increasing number of professionals in hospital organizations whose behavior includes intimidation and hostility, reflected in poor communication and reduced information transfer endangering patient safety (Walrath et al., 2013).

Precursors of disruptive behavior include intrapersonal, organizational, and interpersonal antecedents. Consequences of disruptive behavior primarily affect the worker/health team followed by the patient and the health care organization (Oliveira et al., 2016). Disruptive behavior in the workplace is shown to have significant negative effects on individuals and on patient care and safety, and it can undermine the organization itself (Small et al., 2015). Consequences for workers and the health care team were most often cited, including burnout and decreased morale. Disruptive behaviors were also associated with decreased job satisfaction of nurses and their decisions to leave the profession (Rosenstein & O'Daniel, 2005). Of note, many nurses who reported disruptive behaviors often did not report or comment about them to their peer or manager (Oliveira et al., 2016). The authors also identified three themes of disruptive behavior: incivility, psychological aggression, and violence (Walrath et al., 2010). Given that disruptive behaviors can result in compromised patient safety and costs to the organization and physical violence, nurses need to understand how to address the antecedents of these behaviors and have the difficult conversations to address them head on. Likewise, hospital leaders must strive to decrease the organizational antecedents of disruptive behaviors, including high workload pressure, volume, and number of patients, in addition to unsolved systemic problems (Oliveira et al., 2016.)

Prevention of conflict would be ideal; however, the multiple antecedents and diverse nature of hospital environments preclude preventing conflict. The use of Conflict Management Interviews (CMIs) has gained popularity in health care settings. CMIs are private in-person meetings between two individuals to confront and resolve emerging conflict (Cummings & Worley, 2015). In CMIs, communication and feedback are exchanged in both directions between the supervisor and subordinate as opposed to the top-down method with traditional performance appraisal-related meetings (Dunford et al., 2020). A recent study evaluated a major preventive conflict management initiative in a US health care system in the eastern United States over an 8-year period. The initiative consisted of training and enabling employees and supervisors to conduct CMIs (Boss 1983; Whetten & Cameron, 2016) with one another throughout the health system. The authors used a combination of survey and administrative data and analyzed using ordinary least squares (OLS) and fixed effects panel regression models to test how line managers' participation in CMIs with their employees affected formal grievances, their employees' perceptions of department culture, and actual retention. Study findings suggested that high quality CMIs are associated with a lower likelihood of formal grievances, significantly more perceptions of participative department culture, and lower turnover rates (Dunford et al., 2020).

CONFLICT SCALES

Three conflict inventories are available to measure conflict. The Rahim Organizational Conflict Inventory-I (Rahim, 1983) is designed to measure three dimensions of conflict: intrapersonal, intragroup, and intergroup. The Perceived Conflict Scale (Gardner, 1992) contains four subscales of conflict: intrapersonal, interpersonal, intergroup/other departments, and intergroup/support services. This scale is designed to measure conflict in nursing. Cox (2014) developed a new intragroup conflict scale based on Barki and Hartwick's two dimensions. The scale consists of six subscales: (1) interference over the task, (2) negative emotion over the task, (3) negative emotion and interference related to interpersonal incompatibilities, (4) disagreement over the task process, (5) disagreement over the task, and (6) disagreement related to interpersonal incompatibilities.

CONFLICT MANAGEMENT AND ALTERNATIVE DISPUTE RESOLUTION

Although conflict management and conflict resolution are often used interchangeably, there are differences in the terms (Rahim, 2010). Conflict management involves the control, but not resolution, of a long-term or deep-rooted conflict. In contrast, conflict resolution involves eliminating all forms of conflict. Negotiation, mediation, and arbitration are often referred to in discussions of conflict resolution. These terms are also included under the umbrella of ADR. ADR consists of several forms of conflict resolution that are used to avoid going to court (Brubaker et al., 2014).

Conflict Management Styles

Although other labels have been used for conflict management styles, those identified by Thomas and Schmidt in 1976 are the most frequently cited. The author labeled the five conflict management styles as accommodating, avoiding, collaborating, competing, and compromising.

- **Accommodating** results when one party seeks to appease an opponent; that party is willing to be self-sacrificing.
- **Avoiding** emerges when a person recognizes that a conflict exists and wants to withdraw from it or suppress it.
- **Collaborating** ensues when the parties to conflict each desire to fully satisfy the concerns of all parties. The intention is to solve the problem by clarifying differences rather than by accommodating.
- **Competing** occurs when one person seeks to satisfy his or her own interests regardless of the impact on the other parties to the conflict.
- **Compromising** may develop when each party to the conflict seeks to give up something and sharing occurs, with the result of a compromised outcome. There is no clear winner or loser, and the solution provides incomplete satisfaction of both parties' concerns (Robbins & Judge, 2016).

Shargh et al. (2013) indicated that each of the conflict management styles can be used for different situations. The challenge is for nurses to know when to use each style. Thomas (1976) identified situations for the appropriate use of each conflict management style (see Table 10.5).

Conflict Competence

Conflict competence is the ability to develop and use cognitive, emotional, and behavioral skills that enhance productive outcomes of conflict while reducing the likelihood of escalation or harm (Runde & Flanagan, 2010). An essential skill associated with this competency includes being able to have difficult or crucial conversations. A crucial conversation is defined as "a discussion between two or more people where (1) the stakes are high, (2) opinions vary, and (3) emotions run strong (Patterson et al., 2005). In addition to the ability to hold crucial conversations, one must also be able to confront someone about their behavior face to face (Patterson et al., 2005).

Carefronting

Sometimes conflict between two individuals can be managed by carefronting, which is defined as "a method of communication that entails caring enough about one's self, one's goals, and others to confront courageously in a self-asserting, responsible manner" (Kuperschmidt, 2008, p. 12). Issues are the focus of the interaction. Individuals speak for themselves but in a way that decreases defensiveness and allows another person to hear the message. "I" messages are used; "you" messages are avoided.

Studies of Conflict Management in Nursing

Historically, nursing experienced intrapersonal conflict because of role confusion (Benne & Bennis, 1959). They identified four sources of role confusion for nursing, including institutional expectations, expectations from other nurses including peers and supervisors, professional associations, and the nurse's own self expectations. They summarized role conflicts as involving (1) frustration between their image of "real" nursing and the functions they assume in actual work situations, (2) the nurse–doctor relationship as often a tension area, and (3) promotion for the nurse all too frequently being a conflict between a desire for higher status and a psychological need to give bedside care. Of note, they identified that many of these role conflicts were related to continuing and accelerated change in the health field, stating that change has become the law of contemporary organizational life. Through their research they identified three patterns that nurses use to address conflict: (1) the nurse may lose interest in the job or forsake the effort to find satisfaction in it, (2) the nurse rationalizes away the conflicting demands by calling the schools of nursing and the professional associations "impractical," "theoretical," and "disoriented to the realities of nursing" (Benne & Bennis, 1959, p. 383), and (3) the nurse may formally or informally organize with others to resist the demands of the institution where they work, including a slowdown of efforts and watering down of orders in the execution of them.

TABLE 10.5 Use of Conflict Management Styles According to Situation

Conflict Management Style	Situation
Collaborating	When both sets of concerns are too important to be compromised When objective is to learn To merge insights from people with different perspectives To gain commitment by incorporating concerns into a consensus To work through feelings that have interfered with a relationship
Accommodating	To allow a better position to be heard and to show reasonableness When issues are more important to others than yourself To build social credit for later issues To minimize loss when you are outmatched and losing When harmony and stability are especially important To allow subordinates to develop by learning from mistakes
Competing	When quick, decisive action is vital On important issues where unpopular actions need implementing On issues vital to organization and when you know you are right Against people who take advantage of non-competitive behavior
Avoiding	When an issue is trivial, or more important issues are pressing When you see no chance of satisfying your concerns To let people "cool down" and regain perspective Gathering information supersedes the immediate decision When others can resolve the conflict more effectively
Compromising	When goals are important but not worth potential disruption of more assertive modes When equal power opponents are committed to mutually exclusive goals To find temporary settlements of complex issues To arrive at expedient solutions under time pressure

Adapted from Thomas, K.W. (1977). Toward multidimensional values in teaching: The example of conflict behaviors. *Academy of Management Review, 2*(3), p. 487.

Nursing conflict has been examined widely since then, with older studies finding that avoiding and compromising were the most frequently used conflict handling intentions in nursing. For example, Sportsman and Hamilton (2007) conducted a study to determine prevalent conflict management styles chosen by students in nursing and to contrast these styles with those chosen by students in allied health professions. The associations among the level of professional health care education and the style chosen were also determined. A convenience sample of 126 university students completed the Thomas-Kilmann Conflict Mode Instrument (TKI). The difference was not significant between the prevalent conflict management styles chosen by graduate and undergraduate nursing students and those in allied health. Some of the students were already licensed in their discipline; others had not yet taken a licensing examination. Licensure and educational level were not associated with choice of styles. Women and men had similar preferences. The prevalent style for nursing students was compromise, followed by avoidance. The prevalent style for allied health students was avoidance, followed by compromise and accommodation. Compared with the TKI norms, slightly more than one-half of all participants chose two or more conflict management styles—commonly avoidance and accommodation—at the 75th percentile or above. Only 9.8% of the participants chose collaboration at that level.

Professional nurses in Madrid, Spain, who worked in either a university setting, or a clinical care setting were surveyed to identify conflict resolution styles based on TKI (Thomas & Kilmann, 1974). The styles most frequently used by nurses overall were compromising (27.7%) and competing (26.2%), followed by avoiding

(23.1%) and accommodating (18.5%). Very few participants (4.6%) were assessed as using a collaborating approach (Losa Iglesias & Becerro de Bengoa Vallejo, 2012b). The authors suggested that these results confirm previous findings (Shell, 2001; Valentine, 1995). They concluded that the inclination toward compromise may reflect the powerlessness associated with some nursing positions.

CONFLICT RESOLUTION

Conflict resolution involves eliminating all forms of conflict. Negotiation, mediation, and arbitration are often referred to in discussions of conflict resolution. These terms are also included under the umbrella of ADR. According to Knickle et al. (2012) the resolution continuum includes negotiation, mediation, arbitration, and litigation as a spectrum of third-party dispute resolution.

Negotiation: Negotiation can be used by individuals to come to an agreement or in third-party negotiations such as ADR. Negotiation is the major process used in any ADR technique. It is the process whereby two or more parties come to an agreement. There are no official rules for the negotiation process. Robbins and Judge (2016) described negotiation as a five-step process: (1) preparation and planning, (2) definition of ground rules, (3) clarification and justification, (4) bargaining and problem-solving, and (5) closure and implementation.

Principled negotiation: Principled negotiation is an approach proposed by Fisher et al. (1991), who urged negotiators to use the following five fundamental principles to negotiate effectively with each other instead of against each other:

1. Separate the people from the problem.
2. Focus on interests, not positions.
3. Invent options for mutual gain.
4. Insist on using objective criteria.
5. Know your BATNA (Best Alternative to Negotiated Agreement).

The authors were also the first to coin the acronym BATNA. This term essentially describes the need to conceive of creating and developing backup plans when all else fails. Invariably, not even the best intentions to find agreement will necessarily come to fruition.

Conciliation: A conciliator is like a third friend who might attempt to intercede in an argument between two other friends. Conciliators attempt to diffuse the negative emotions that are often involved in the conflict, and they strive to establish more effective communications between the parties. They attempt to understand each party's point of view as a basis for common ground. The conciliator might also meet with managers and co-workers who are involved in order to have greater insight into the conflict situation (Brubaker et al., 2014).

Mediation: Mediation is often used when the parties have tried to negotiate on their own, but the negotiation has not been successful. The mediator is a process expert and acts as a neutral third party. Although the mediator controls the process, the parties control the outcome. The mediator's job is to listen to the evidence, assist the parties to understand each other's viewpoint regarding the controversy, and then facilitate the negotiation of a voluntary resolution to the conflict situation (Brubaker et al., 2014).

Arbitration: Arbitration also involves the use of a neutral third party, which may be an individual or panel. The arbitrator(s) make the decision for the parties in conflict. Arbitration may be binding or non-binding (Brubaker et al., 2014).

There are several advantages of ADR. It is usually faster and less costly than litigation. Everyone in the conflict situation has the opportunity to explain their perceptions of the situation. ADR is more flexible and responsive to the individual needs of the people involved, and it is less formal than litigation. Because of the parties' involvement in the process, greater commitment results, and the parties may be more compliant. Confidentiality is maintained as well as the relationship, which is especially important if the relationship will continue.

Face Negotiation Theory

Face negotiation is the focus of a theory developed by Ting-Toomey to describe and explain differences in responses to conflict based on cultural backgrounds (Ting-Toomey, 1988; Ting-Toomey & Kurogi, 1998). This theory draws on the idea that face is a metaphor for our public identity, or self-image, and is an important element of social situations throughout the world. The theory suggested that face influences conflict behavior because in any conflict individual parties have to consider protecting self-interest and/or honoring or attacking another person's conflict goals (Ting-Toomey & Kurogi, 1998). Specifically, face refers to a claimed sense of favorable social self-worth that people want others to have of them (Ting-Toomey & Kurogi, 1998). In the theory, facework refers to a set of communicative behaviors that people use to regulate their social dignity. All individuals want others to see them in a certain way, even though they may not be consciously aware of this desire.

Ting-Toomey (1988) originally considered face negotiation theory as a way to explain differences in conflict communication styles stemming from cultural preferences for individualism versus collectivism. She proposed that those in cultures best described as collectivistic would be more likely to seek to uphold "other-face," whereas those in individualistic cultures would more likely seek to uphold "self-face."

Face negotiation theory builds on the five-style dual-concern framework developed by Rahim (1983, 2002) and is based on the degree to which a person is concerned with self-interest, as well as with the interests of others. The five styles are problem-solving (also called integrating, collaborating, or cooperating), forcing (also called competing or dominating), avoiding (also called suppressing or withdrawing), yielding (also called obliging, accommodating, or smoothing), and compromising (Putnam & Poole, 1987; Rahim, 2010). The theory posits that collectivistic cultures favor the avoiding, yielding, and compromising styles; in contrast, individualistic cultures reputedly favor forcing and problem-solving styles (Ting-Toomey, 1988).

In 1998, the face negotiation theory was revised, and the dimension of self-construal (self-image) was discussed in terms of the independent and interdependent self, or the degree to which people conceive of themselves as relatively autonomous from or connected to others (Ting-Toomey & Kurogi, 1998). The revised theory posits that the degree to which people see themselves as autonomous (independent; self-face) or connected to others (interdependent; other face) is a better predictor of conflict interaction than their cultural or ethnic background. Ting-Toomey and Kurogi (1998) also added the concept of power to the theory to explain communicative differences based on the cultural dimension of power distance. In low power-distance cultures, differences in treatment based on status are less accepted. On the other hand, in high power-distance cultures, differences in treatment based on status are more accepted. The authors proposed that individuals of different status levels in low power-distance cultures are more likely to use the forcing style to resolve conflict, whereas in high power-distance cultures, those in lower status roles may use styles such as yielding.

Two cross-cultural empirical tests of the revised face negotiation theory supported much of the theory (Oetzel & Ting-Toomey, 2003; Oetzel et al., 2001). The 2001 study involved a cross-cultural comparison of four national cultures (Oetzel et al., 2001). In the 2003 study of face negotiation theory, Oetzel and Ting-Toomey tested the underlying assumption that face mediates the relationship between cultural or individual-level variables and conflict styles. The findings provide supportive evidence of the face negotiation theory, especially that face concerns provide a mediating link between cultural values and conflict behavior. The authors also suggested that these findings are particularly significant given the relatively large sample size across four national cultures.

Results of the studies indicated that nursing administrators need to be more attuned to face issues in the conflict dialogue process. The findings of Oetzel and Ting-Toomey (2003) demonstrated that display of other-face concern, which is maintaining the poise or pride of the other person and being sensitive to the other person's self-worth, can lead to a collaborative, win–win integrative approach or an avoiding approach. In contrast, individuals who are more concerned with maintaining self-pride or self-image during a conflict episode would devote effort to defending their conflict position to the neglect of other-face validation issue. Face negotiation theory has been applied to physician communication in the operating room (Kirschbaum, 2012). Study findings suggested (1) the theory and instrument can be utilized for health communication research, (2) face-negotiation theory can be expanded beyond traditional intercultural communication boundaries, and (3) theoretically-based communication structures applied in a medical context could help explain physician miscommunication in the operating room to assist future design of communication training programs for operating-room physicians (p. 292).

Conflict Resolution Outcomes

Whatever conflict resolution style is used, the individual needs to be aware of the outcome that results from the strategy selected. The outcomes of conflict are what actually happens as a result of the conflict management process. The three ways in which conflicts resolve are (1) win–lose, (2) lose–lose, and (3) win–win (Filley, 1975) (Box 10.3). Filley (1975) described the win–win resolution as the optimum conflict management. Win–lose and lose–lose resolutions also occur, but effective managers should seek win–win resolutions. Win–win strategies focus on problem-solving.

BOX 10.3 Conflict Resolution Outcomes

Win–Lose
One party exerts dominance.

Lose–Lose
Neither side wins.

Win–Win
An attempt is made to meet the needs of both parties simultaneously.

Data from Filley, A.C. (1975). *Interpersonal conflict resolution.* Glenview, IL: Scott, Foresman; Filley, A., House, R., & Kerr, S. (1976). *Managerial process and organizational behavior.* Glenview, IL: Scott, Foresman.

Conflict Resolution Inventories

Several instruments have been developed to measure conflict-handling styles. In the Organizational Conflict Inventory-II, Rahim (1983) divided the handling of interpersonal conflict into the two dimensions of concern for self and concern for others—both in high and low degrees—to form a grid. Rahim then adapted Blake and Mouton's (1964) five types of handling interpersonal conflict (forcing, withdrawing, smoothing, compromising, and problem-solving) into five styles of handling interpersonal conflict (avoiding, obliging, compromising, integrating, and dominating). The inventory measures the five identified styles.

Thomas and Kilmann (1974) also developed a style assessment and diagnosis inventory, called the TKI. Their grid uses dimensions of assertiveness and cooperativeness on high to low degrees. The five styles are avoiding, accommodating, compromising, competing, and collaborating. This model blends a description of an individual's behavior on assertiveness and cooperativeness dimensions in situations in which the concerns of two people appear to be incompatible. The behaviors of individuals are thought to be a function of both personal predispositions and situational contingencies. Avoiding is low on both assertiveness and cooperativeness; collaborating is high on both aspects. Competing is high on assertiveness and low on cooperativeness; accommodating is low on assertiveness and high on cooperativeness. Compromising is in the middle.

LEADERSHIP AND MANAGEMENT IMPLICATIONS

Organizational Conflict

Thomas and Schmidt (1976) identified a "big picture" structural model of conflict that examines four factors that seem to influence the way conflict is handled in organizations: behavioral predispositions of individuals, social pressure in the environment, the organization's incentive structure, and rules and procedures. Different levels of power exist as a result of bureaucratic hierarchy and the resultant position power.

Organizational conflict is a form of interpersonal conflict that is generated from aspects of the institution, such as the style of management, rules, procedures, and communication channels. Conflicts that arise when an individual's needs and goals cannot be met within the system are generally organizational. Conflict may be necessary to groups and organizations. Conflict serves to unify and bind together a group by setting boundaries and strengthening a group's identity. Conflict may help stabilize a group by serving as a test of opposing interests within the group. Conflict may help integrate a group by distributing power. Thus conflict may be necessary for the growth of a group and its members and serves to stimulate creativity, innovation, and change.

Organizational leadership sets a tone for conflict and conflict management. This occurs because leaders and managers model behaviors of positive or negative conflict management and choose when and how to intervene in conflict situations. Choice of intervention style and timing of conflict management are functions of the individuals' behavioral predispositions and environmental pressure coupled with the organization's reward structure and coordination and control methods.

Specifically related to organizational conflict and the focus on groups in organizations, Pondy (1967) identified three strategies to use when attempting to resolve organizational conflicts by using bargaining; rules, procedures, and administrative control; and a systems integrator. Bargaining might be useful when a conflict exists over scarce monetary resources. The administrative control approach might be helpful when clarification of role boundaries is needed, such as disagreements over delegation by RNs. The systems integrator approach might be appropriate in a matrix structure or where there is a need to coordinate personnel in vertical and horizontal organizational structures.

Ellis and Abbott (2011) recommended avoiding the seven Cs as ground rules before approaching conflict:

Commanding by way of telling people how to behave

Comparing the person or situation to other people and situations

Condemning individuals

Challenging behavior and condescension

Contradictory or Confusing actions may lead to uncertainty and frustration

Johansen (2012) identified strategies for NMs to use to resolve conflict. The strategies are also useful for all nurses:

- Recognize conflict early. Recognizing the early warning signs of conflict is the first step toward resolution. Pay attention to body language and be cognizant of the moods of the staff.
- Be proactive. Address the issue of concern at an early stage. Avoiding the conflict may cause frustration and escalate the problem.
- Actively listen. Focus attention on the speaker. Try to understand, interpret, and evaluate what is being said. The ability to listen actively can improve interpersonal relationships, reduce conflicts, foster understanding, and improve cooperation.
- Remain calm. Keep responses under control and emotions in check. Do not react to volatile comments. Calmness will help set the tone for the parties involved.
- Define the problem. Clearly identify and define the problem. A clear understanding of the issues will help minimize miscommunication and facilitate resolution.
- Seek a solution. Manage the conflict in a way that successfully meets the goal of reaching an acceptable solution for both parties.

The goal of conflict resolution is to create a win–win situation for all. Although it is not realistic to think that every conflict can be resolved in such an ideal fashion, a win–win solution is a worthy goal requiring hard work, creativity, and sound strategy.

CURRENT ISSUES AND TRENDS

There are numerous trends and issues in the continually changing health care environment that have an impact on nursing and health care organizations related to power and conflict. The availability of nursing theories that conceptualize power and group power as a positive resource are essential to advancing discipline-specific knowledge to help nurses identify how to obtain and use power to achieve goals. Nursing theorists strove to understand nursing as a practice from theoretical points of view that moved beyond a task orientation and served to demarcate distinctive boundaries for nursing as a practice and a realm of knowledge (Meleis, 2018; Walker & Avant, 2019). Walker suggested that the "gifts" of nursing theorists including Orlando, Johnson, Roy, and Orem, are as relevant today as they were in the 60s and 70s and are "are worthy of rediscovery and reformulation as nursing navigates present-day challenges" (Walker, 2020, p. 2).

The one constant in health care is change and by using nursing theory and adopting instruments developed using conceptual frameworks of nursing, the profession will be able to address these changes in discipline specific ways. Issues with health care access, quality, and costs of care will continue to be addressed by nursing leaders who must develop conflict competency, in addition to core competencies including knowledge of health systems, health technology, and policy development. Nurses have been and will continue to be essential to reducing medication errors, reducing infection rates, and ensuring safe transitions of care from hospital to home.

Perhaps the most important reason for nurses to stay at the forefront of technological advances is that medical errors are the third leading cause of death in the United States (Makary & Daniel, 2016). Medical errors are defined by the IOM (1999) as the failure of a planned action to be completed as intended or the use of a wrong plan to achieve an aim. James (2013) referred to medical errors as preventable adverse events and separated the errors into these categories: (1) errors of commission, (2) errors of omission, (3) errors of communication, (4) errors of context, and (5) diagnostic errors. Ehteshami et al. (2013) indicated that a variety of technologies reduce medical errors, especially medication errors, and prevent them in the health care system. Nurses are at the forefront of implementing information technology and use their expertise power throughout the process.

Healthcare information technology (HIT) has been widely adopted with four goals including to (1) inform clinical practice, (2) interconnect clinicians, (3) personalize care, and (4) improve population health (Thompson, & Brailer, 2004). Electronic health records

(EHRs) are an example of technology that increases the effectiveness of health care and reduces medical errors through reminders, alerts, and internal intelligent capabilities. EHRs directly or indirectly improved patient safety by minimizing medicals errors, improving documentation of data, enhancing the completeness of data, and improving the sustainability of data (Tubaishat, 2017). By improving interpersonal communication and collaboration, EHRs may also help decrease intragroup and intergroup conflict and litigation.

Participation in High-Level Decision-Making

Nurses need to participate in high-level decision-making in order to influence patient care and the nursing profession. Power needs to be leveraged and conflict managed. The Robert Wood Johnson Foundation's (RWJF, 2018) Future of Nursing Campaign for Action advocated for a nurse in every boardroom. Thew (2016) suggested that if nurses are interested in entering the boardroom, they need to (1) find an organization in which they are interested, (2) know their own strengths, (3) express interest, and (4) not allow time constraints to interfere with participation in the boardroom.

Stalter and Arms (2016) described six competencies needed by nurses who are serving on boards and/or policy committees so that they can contribute in a productive manner. These competencies include a professional commitment to serving on a governing board; knowledge about board types, bylaws, and job descriptions; an understanding of standard business protocols, board member roles, and voting processes; a willingness to use principles for managing and leading effective and efficient board meetings; an appreciation for the ethical and legal processes for conducting meetings; and the ability to employ strategies for maintaining control during intense/uncivil situations.

Building a Personal Power Base

Huston (2008) emphasized the importance of building a personal power base and proposed 11 strategies that can be used by both NMs and staff to establish a personal power base. These are demonstrating expertise possibly through certification, identifying positive role models and seeking mentoring relationships, networking and coalition building, maintaining freedom of maneuverability, being aware of self, staying focused on goals, choosing battles carefully, demonstrating willingness to take risks, giving up some ego, working hard and being a team player, and finally, taking care of oneself. The author concluded that building a personal power base will take time, but the outcome is the ability to achieve personal and professional goals and is therefore well worth the effort.

Political Action

With 3.8 million RNs in the nation, the nursing profession should be a tremendous force in political and public policy debates. This is an area for nurses to unite and use their power to improve patient care. Nurses have great potential to contribute to the development of health policy through political action, and their involvement in health policy development ensures that health care is safe, of a high quality, accessible and affordable. Knowledge, skills, and abilities in understanding, using, and managing power and conflict are crucial to nursing in both personal and professional arenas.

RESEARCH NOTE

Source

Kang, S. W., Lee, S., & Choi, S. B. (2017). The impact of nursing leader's behavioral integrity and intragroup relationship conflict on staff nurses' intention to remain. *JONA: The Journal of Nursing Administration, 47*(5), 294–300.

Purpose

This study tested a multilevel model examining the effect of nursing leaders' (NL) behavioral integrity and intragroup relationship conflict on staff nurses' intent to remain.

Discussion

This study was the first to examine the impact of the NL behavioral integrity on hospital nurses' intention to remain. In addition, the effect of unit-level intragroup relationship conflict on hospital nurses was examined. The study was framed methodologically using the Social Exchange perspective, which proposed both leaders and followers enter into reciprocal relationships to maximize their benefits. The theory suggests that a NL's behavior integrity causes staff nurses to perceive them as trustworthy and believe that they have the best interests of

RESEARCH NOTE—cont'd

staff nurses in mind, because of the congruence between their words and actions. In contrast, when a nursing unit is subjected to a high level of intragroup relationship conflict, the quality of social exchange between staff nurses is often poor, and it is important that they maintain good social exchange with the NL. Therefore, in nursing units with a high level of intragroup relationship conflict, the impact of the NLs' behavioral integrity on staff nurses' intention to remain is stronger relative to that in units without this conflict.

Sample and design. The survey participants were RNs working at a large public hospital in South Korea. Surveys were distributed to RNs from 34 nursing units, and English survey items were translated into Korean. Of 552 RNs, 480 returned completed questionnaires (response rate, 87%). Measures of the NLs' behavioral integrity and staff nurses' intention to remain were used as individual-level variables, and intragroup relationship conflicts were aggregated to a unit level as specified in a hypothesized research model.

Data analysis. The model was tested using a multilevel technique (i.e., hierarchical linear modelling) to examine the relationships between individual- and unit-level variables simultaneously. The program 28 STATA Data Analysis and Statistical Software 12.1 (StataCorp, College Station, TX) was used in the analysis.

Results. Nursing leaders' behavioral integrity was positively related to nurses' intention to remain (b = 0.34, $P < .001$). In addition, job stress and individual perceptions of intragroup relationship conflict exerted a negatively significant effect on staff nurses' intention to remain ($b = -0.22$ [$P < .001$] and $b = -0.12$ [$P < .05$], respectively). The simple slope analysis indicated that the coefficient for the relationship between the NLs' behavioral integrity and staff nurses intention to remain differed significantly from zero when the level of intragroup relationship conflict was either low (b = 0.23, $P < .01$) or high (b = 0.48, $P < .001$).

Discussion. The main implication of the study is that it presented a specific means of enhancing staff nurses' intention to remain. Another implication of the study was that NLs should care about intragroup relationship conflict in the workplace. The experience of relationship conflict with other nurses could intensify staff nurses' intention to resign. Specifically, workplace bullying or nurse–nurse interpersonal conflict can cause problems, and NLs need to disseminate the anti-bullying message through nursing units and provide group activities to foster teamwork to decrease interpersonal conflict between staff nurses.

Application to Practice

This study presents a practical solution to this issue in that the impact of the NLs' behavioral integrity on staff nurses' intention to remain is stronger in units where levels of intragroup relationship conflict are high relative to those where levels are low. Staff nurses working in an unfriendly workplace often engage in social exchanges with the NL they trust, instead of their co-workers, and try hard to maintain high-quality social exchange with the NL. In this circumstance, the impact of the NL on staff nurses can be intensified. Therefore NLs assigned to nursing units with a high level of intragroup relationship conflict should endeavor to maintain their behavioral integrity to promote staff nurses' intention to remain.

CASE STUDY

A new nurse manager, 2 years post-graduation from a large baccalaureate program, is experiencing increased unit conflict among her staff, presumably due to ongoing increased patient acuity and the recent resignations of two senior nurses. The unit had previously enjoyed a healthy work environment with a stable team, but morale is low and unit nurses are considering transferring to another unit or choosing to work at the larger local hospital with Magnet status. The nurse manager has never received conflict management training, has limited experience dealing with conflict, and tends to utilize avoidance when confronted. She has promised her nurses that she is working to improve morale and has worked many additional shifts to help the staff. However, when staff come to the manager for help and to discuss their issues with one another, the nurse manager has little feedback and tells them "to work it out among themselves." The nurse manager has asked hospital leadership to provide formal staff development to help nurse mangers deal with staff conflict and believes that the training would be beneficial not only for new nurse mangers, but also for experienced managers who may have never thought about nor analyzed their conflict management or leadership styles. When she reaches out to several of the more senior nurse managers, they report that their units are doing well and they do not feel additional training would be

Continued

CASE STUDY—cont'd

helpful, but instead would simply add additional workload to their overburdened schedules. The Chief Nursing Officer (CNO) has stated she is reluctant to offer the training due to financial constraints and has requested that the nurse mangers collectively identify evidenced-based support for the additional education with documentation that the associated expense would benefit the organization. The CNO has been with the organization for 20 years and is widely respected for her clinical expertise.

1. What is the relationship between intragroup conflict and nursing intent to leave?
2. What examples of behavioral integrity are demonstrated by the nurse manager? What is she doing well and how could she improve?
3. If the nurse manager is unable to resolve the unit conflict, what are the possible consequences to patient care?
4. How can the nurse manager convince the other managers that this training would be helpful to the organization?
5. What resources could the nurse manager use to convince the CNO that this training would be helpful?
6. In lieu of the additional staff development, what could the nurse managers do to ensure a healthy work environment within their hospital?

CRITICAL THINKING EXERCISE

Mary is a registered nurse who graduated 2 years ago from a Bachelor of Science in Nursing (BSN) program. She has worked on a very busy unit and in a short period of time has established herself as a natural leader. She loves the unit that she works on and intends to stay with the organization. She has been invited by her chief nursing executive to become the nurse manager for a unit with an ongoing history of nurse turnover and intragroup conflict. Mary has never served in a management position but would like to accept the offer. She has aspirations to become a nursing manager and during her undergraduate education was required to attend interprofessional conflict management training during senior year. Mary also participated in a capstone project where she facilitated an anti-bullying campaign with her preceptor on a busy medical surgical unit. While deliberating about whether to accept the position, she met with the Chief Nursing Officer (CNO) and asked her impressions about issues with the previous nurse manager for recommendations to help turn the unit around. She asked the CNO about the unit. They suggested the previous manger had become burned out and typically avoided staff when they demonstrated bullying behaviors or approached her for advice about how to deal with conflict. She increasingly refused to help her staff to provide direct patient care and instead stayed in her office most of the day except to attend mandatory meetings. The CNO also indicated that when first hired, the nurse manger had been outstanding, but as the conflict within her unit grew, she became distant.

1. What is significant about Mary's undergraduate training in relation to the nurse manager opportunity?
2. What information did the CNO share with Mary about the previous nurse manger that may be helpful?
3. If Mary accepts the new position, what should she do *first* to demonstrate behavioral integrity to her staff?
4. What could the CNO have done to prevent burnout of the previous nurse manager and to assist with improving morale on the unit?
5. What should CNOs understand about the relationship between intragroup conflict and nurse turnover?
6. Why is behavioral integrity important for NMs to demonstrate as related to staff turnover and patient outcomes?

REFERENCES

Abood, S. (2007). Influencing health care in the legislative arena. *OJIN: The Online Journal of Issues in Nursing, 12*(1), 2.

Adams, J. M., & Natarajan, S. (2016). Understanding influence within the context of nursing. *Advances in Nursing Science, 39*(3), E40–E56.

Alexander, R. K., & Diefenbeck, C. (2020). Challenging stereotypes: A glimpse into nursing's difficulty recruiting African Americans. *Journal of Professional Nursing, 36*(1), 15–22.

Alligood, M. R., & Tomey, A. M. (2010). *Nursing theorists and their work* (7th ed.). Maryland Heights, MO: Mosby.

Almost, J. (2006). Conflict within nursing work environments: concept analysis. *Journal of Advanced Nursing, 53*(4), 444–453.

Almost, J., Doran, D. M., McGillis Hall, L., & Spence Laschinger, H. K. (2010). Antecedents and consequences of intra-group conflict among nurses. *Journal of Nursing Management, 18*(8), 981–992.

Alper, S., Tjosvold, D., & Law, K. S. (2000). Conflict management, efficacy, and performance in self-managing work teams. *Personnel Psychology, 53*(3), 625–642.

American Association of Colleges of Nursing (AACN). (2008). *The essentials of baccalaureate education for professional nursing practice*. Washington, DC: AACN. http://www.aacn.nche.edu/education-resources/BaccEssentials08.pdf.

American Association of Colleges of Nursing (AACN). (2011). *The essentials of master's education in nursing*. http://www.aacn.nche.edu/education-resources/MastersEssentials11.pdf.

American Nurses Association (ANA). (2015). Optimal nurse staffing to improve quality of care and patient outcomes: Executive summary [White paper]. https://cdn.ymaws.com/www.anamass.org/resource/resmgr/docs/NurseStaffingWhitePaper.pdf.

Baer, E. D. (2009). "Do trained nurses… work for love, or do they work for money?" nursing and altruism in the twenty-first century. *Nursing History Review, 17*, 28–46.

Bagshaw, D., & Lepp, M. (2005). Ethical considerations in drama and conflict resolution research in Swedish and Australian schools. *Conflict Resolution Quarterly, 22*(3), 381–396.

Baltimore, J. J. (2006). *Nurse collegiality: Fact or fiction? Nursing Management, 37*(5), 28–36.

Barki, H., & Hartwick, J. (2001). Interpersonal conflict and its management in information system development. *MIS Quarterly, 25*(2), 195–228.

Barki, H., & Hartwick, J. (2004). Conceptualizing the construct of interpersonal conflict. *International Journal of Conflict Management, 15*(3), 216–244.

Barnard, C. I. (1938). *The functions of the executive*. 7th printing. Cambridge, MA: Harvard University Press.

Barrett, E. A. M. (1989). A nursing theory of power for nursing practice: Derivation from Rogers' paradigm. In J. Riehl (Ed.). *Conceptual models for nursing practice* (3rd ed.) (pp. 207–217). Norwalk, CT: Appleton & Lange.

Barrett, E. A. M. (2010). Power as knowing participation in change: What's new and what's next. *Nursing Science Quarterly, 23*(1), 47–54.

Barrett, E. A. M. (2017). Again, what is nursing science? *Nursing Science Quarterly, 30*(2), 129–133.

Bartunek, J. M., & Spreitzer, G. M. (2006). The interdisciplinary career of a popular construct used in management: Empowerment in the late 20th century. *Journal of Management Inquiry, 15*(3), 255–273.

Bassett, C. (2002). Nurses' perceptions of care and caring. *International Journal of Nursing Practice, 8*(1), 8–15.

Beauchamp, T. L., & Childress, J. F. (1994). Principles of biomedical ethics (4th ed.). New York: Oxford University Press.

Benne, K. D., & Bennis, W. (1959). Role confusion and conflict in nursing: The role of the professional nurse. *The American Journal of Nursing, 59*(2), 196–198.

Bierstadt, R. (1950). An analysis of social power. *American Sociological Review, 15*, 730–738.

Bishop, S. R. (2004). *Nurses and conflict: Workplace experiences*. Dissertation, University of Victoria (Canada).

Blake, R. R., & Mouton, J. S. (1964). *The managerial grid*. Gulf Publishing.

Bochatay, N., Bajwa, N. M., Cullati, S., Muller-Juge, V., Blondon, K. S., Perron, N. J., et al. (2017). A multilevel analysis of professional conflicts in health care teams: Insight for future training. *Academic Medicine, 92*(11S), S84–S92.

Boss, R. W. (1983). Team building and the problem of regression: The personal management interview as an intervention. *Journal of Applied Behavioral Science, 19*(1), 67–83.

Boswell, C., Cannon, S., & Miller, J. (2005). Nurses' political involvement: responsibility versus privilege. *Journal of Professional Nursing, 21*(1), 5–8.

Bourdieu, P. (1985). The social space and the genesis of groups. *Information (International Social Science Council), 24*(2), 195–220.

Boynton, B. (2012). *Disruptive behavior, bullying, & incivility: A glossary of violence in healthcare workplaces*. https://www.confidentvoices.com/2012/04/04/disruptive-behavior-bullying-incivility-workplace-abuse-a-glossary-of-violence/.

Bradbury-Jones, C., Sambrook, S., & Irvine, F. (2008). Power and empowerment in nursing: a fourth theoretical approach. *Journal of Advanced Nursing, 62*(2), 258–266.

Bradley, J. M., & Moore, L. W. (2019). The perceptions of professional leadership coaches regarding the roles and challenges of nurse managers. *The Journal of Nursing Administration, 49*(2), 105–109.

Brinkert, R. (2010). A literature review of conflict communication causes, costs, benefits and interventions in nursing. *Journal of Nursing Management, 18*(2), 145–156.

Brody, A. A., Farley, J. E., Gillespie, G. L., Hickman, R., Hodges, E. A., Lyder, C., et al. (2017). Diversity dynamics: The experience of male Robert Wood Johnson Foundation nurse faculty scholars. *Nursing Outlook, 65*(3), 278–288.

Brown, L. D. (1983). *Managing conflict at organizational interfaces*. Reading, MA: Addison Wesley Publishing Company.

Brubaker, D., Noble, C., Fincher, R., Park, S. K. Y., & Press, S. (2014). Conflict resolution in the workplace: What will the future bring? *Conflict Resolution Quarterly, 31*(4), 357–386.

Butts, J. B., Rich, K. L., & Fawcett, J. (2012). The future of nursing: How important is discipline-specific knowledge? A conversation with Jacqueline Fawcett. *Nursing Science Quarterly, 25*(2), 151–154.

Byrd, M. E., Costello, J., Shelton, C. R., Thomas, P. A., & Petrarca, D. (2004). An active learning experience in health policy for baccalaureate nursing students. *Public Health Nursing, 21*(5), 501–506.

Catalano, J. T. (2019). *Nursing now: Today's issues, tomorrows trends*. F.A. Davis.

Chinn, P. L., & Falk-Rafael, A. (2015). Peace and power: A theory of emancipatory group process. *Journal of Nursing Scholarship, 47*(1), 62–69.

Chinn, P. L., & Kramer, M. K. (1995). *Theory and nursing a systematic approach*. Mosby.

Clark, C. M. (2008). Faculty and student assessment of and experience with incivility in nursing education. *Journal of Nursing Education, 47*(10), 458–465.

Cohen, L. B. (1992). Power and change in health care: Challenge for nursing. *Journal of Nursing Education, 31*(3), 113–116.

Conger, J. A., & Kanungo, R. N. (1988). The empowerment process: Integrating theory and practice. *Academy of Management Review, 13*(3), 471–482.

Cook, P. R., & Cullen, J. A. (2003). CARING as an imperative for nursing education. *Nursing Education Perspectives, 24*(4), 192–197.

Costantino, C. A., & Merchant, C. S. (1996). *Designing conflict management systems: A guide to creating productive and healthy organizations*. San Francisco: Jossey-Bass.

Cox, K. B. (2014). The new Intragroup Conflict Scale: Testing and psychometric properties. *Journal of Nursing Measurement, 22*(1), 59–76.

Cummings, T. G., & Worley, C. G. (2015). *Organization development and change* (10th ed.). Stamford, CT: Cengage.

D'Antonio, P., Connolly, C., Wall, B. M., Whelan, J. C., & Fairman, J. (2010). Histories of nursing: The power and the possibilities. *Nursing Outlook, 58*(4), 207–213.

De Dreu, C. K., Evers, A., Beersma, B., Kluwer, E. S., & Nauta, A. (2001). A theory-based measure of conflict management strategies in the workplace. *Journal of Organizational Behavior: The International Journal of Industrial, Occupational and Organizational Psychology and Behavior, 22*(6), 645–668.

De Dreu, C. K., & Beersma, B. (2005). Conflict in organizations: Beyond effectiveness and performance. *European Journal of Work and Organizational Psychology, 14*(2), 105–117.

De Dreu, C. K. W., & Gelfand, M. J. (2007). Conflict in the workplace: Sources, dynamics, and functions across multiple levels of analysis. In C. K. W. De Dreu, & M. J. Gelfand (Eds.), *The psychology of conflict and conflict management in organizations*. New York: Lawrence Erlbaum.

Des Jardin, K. E. (2001). Political involvement in nursing—Education and empowerment. *AORN Journal, 74*(4), 467–475.

de Wit, F. R., Jehn, K. A., & Scheepers, D. (2013). Task conflict, information processing, and decision-making: The damaging effect of relationship conflict. *Organizational Behavior and Human Decision Processes, 122*(2), 177–189.

Deutsch, M. (1973). *The resolution of conflict: Constructive and destructive processes*. New Haven: Yale University Press.

Dewitty, V. P., Osborne, J. W., Friesen, M. A., & Rosenkranz, A. (2009). Workforce conflict: What's the problem? *Nursing Management, 40*(5), 31–33, 37.

DiCicco-Bloom, B., Frederickson, K., O'Malley, D., Shaw, E. Crossan, J.C. & Looney, J. A. (2007). Developing a model of social capital: Relationships in primary care. *Advances in Nursing Science, 30*(3), E13–E24.

Dougall, D., Lewis, M., & Ross, S. (2018). *Transformational change in health and care. Reports from the field*. London: The King's Fund.

Druckman, D. (1994). Determinants of compromising behaviour in negotiation: A meta-analysis. *Journal of Conflict Resolution, 38*(3), 507–556.

Dunford, B. B., Mumford, K. J., Boss, R. W., Boss, A. D., & Boss, D. S. (2020). Integrated conflict management systems pay off with lower levels of formal grievances and lower turnover rates. *ILR Review, 73*(2), 528–551.

Ehteshami, A., Rezaeil, P., Tavakoli, N., & Kasaei, M. (2013). The role of health information technology in reducing preventable medical errors and improving patient safety. *International Journal of Health System and Disaster Management, 1*(4), 195–199.

Ellis, P., & Abbott, J. (2011). Strategies for managing conflict within the team. *British Journal of Cardiac Nursing, 7*(3), 138–140.

Fawcett, J. (1999). The state of nursing science: hallmarks of the 20th and 21st centuries. *Nursing Science Quarterly, 12*(4), 311–315.

Filley, A. C. (1975). *Interpersonal conflict resolution*. Glenview, IL: Scott, Foresman.

Filley, A., House, R., & Kerr, S. (1976). *Managerial process and organizational behavior*. Glenview, IL: Scott, Foresman.

Fisher, R., Ury, W., & Patton, B. (1991). *Getting to yes: Negotiating agreement without giving* (2nd ed.). New York: Penguin Group.
Fiske, S. T. (2010). Interpersonal stratification: Status, power, and subordination. In S. T. Fiske, D. T. Gilbert, & G. Lindzey (Eds.) (5th ed.), *Handbook of social psychology* (pp. 941–982). Hoboken, NJ: John Wiley & Sons Inc.
Flateau-Lux, L. R., & Gravel, T. (2014). Put a stop to bullying new nurses. *Home Healthcare Now, 32*(4), 225–229.
Follett, M. P. (1940). Constructive conflict. In H. C. Metcalf & L. Urwick (Eds.), *Dynamic administration: The collected papers of Mary Parker Follett* (pp. 30–49). New York and London: Harper.
Foucault, M. (1980). *Power/knowledge: Selected interviews and other writings*, 1972–1977). New York: Vintage.
French, J., & Raven, B. (1959). The bases of social power. In D. Cartwright (Ed.), *Studies in social power* (pp. 150–167). Ann Arbor, MI: University of Michigan, Institute for Social Research.
Freshwater, D. (2000). Crosscurrents: Against cultural narration in nursing. *Journal of Advanced Nursing, 32*(2), 481–484.
Friend, M. L. (2013). *Group empowerment capacity and capability in schools of nursing* (Doctoral dissertation). Retrieved from ProQuest Dissertations & Theses. (Order No. 3577616).
Friend, M. L., & Sieloff, C. L. (2018). Empowerment in nursing literature: An update and look to the future. *Nursing Science Quarterly, 31*(4), 355–361.
Frye, M. (1983). *The politics of reality: Essays in feminist theory*. Trumansburg, NY: Crossing Press.
Future of Nursing. (n.d.). *Campaign for action: Campaign progress—dashboard indicators*. Center to Champion Nursing in America. http://campaignforaction.org/dashboard.
Gallup. (2020). *Nurses continue to rate highest in honesty, ethics*. Gallup. https://news.gallup.com/poll/274673/nurses-continue-rate-highest-honesty-ethics.aspx.
Gardner, D. L. (1992). Conflict and retention of new graduate nurses. *Western Journal of Nursing Research, 14*(1), 76–85.
Gardner, W. L., & Avolio, B. J. (1998). The charismatic relationship: A dramaturgical perspective. *Academy of Management Review, 23*(1), 32–58.
Ghazali, M., Hashim, R., & Ismail, N. M. (2012, April). Gender and influence tactics among university administrative employees. In *2012 IEEE Business, Engineering & Industrial Applications Colloquium (BEIAC)* (pp. 237–240), IEEE.
Goldrick, B., Leclair, J., & Larson, E. (1994). Intraorganizational influence in the health care setting: A study of strategies preferred by head nurses and infection control practitioners. *American Journal of Infection Control, 22*(1), 6–11.
Greer, L. L., Caruso, H. M., & Jehn, K. A. (2011). The bigger they are, the harder they fall: Linking team power, team conflict, and performance. *Organizational Behavior and Human Decision Processes, 116*(1), 116–128.
Hamlin, L. (2000). Horizontal violence in the operating room. *British Journal of Perioperative Nursing (United Kingdom), 10*(1), 34–42.
Heath, R. L. (Ed.). (1988). *Strategic issues management: How organizations influence and respond to public interests and policies*. Thousand Oaks, CA: Jossey-Bass.
Heiman, H. J., Smith, L. L., McKool, M., Mitchell, D. N., & Roth, C. (2016). Health policy training: A review of the literature. *International Journal of Environmental Research and Public Health, 13*(1), ijerph13010020.
Henry, O. (2009). Organizational conflict and its effects on organizational performance. *Research Journal of Business Management, 2*(1), 16–24.
Hickson, D. J., Hinings, C. R., Lee, C. A., Schneck, R. E., & Pennings, J. M. (1971). A strategic contingencies theory of intraorganizational power. *Administrative Science Quarterly, 16*(2), 216–229.
Huntington, A. D., & Gilmour, J. A. (2001). Re-thinking representations, re-writing nursing texts: possibilities through feminist and Foucauldian thought. *Journal of Advanced Nursing, 35*(6), 902–908.
Huston, C. (2008). Preparing nurse leaders for 2020. *Journal of Nursing Management, 16*(8), 905–911.
Hutchinson, M., & Jackson, D. (2013). Hostile clinician behaviours in the nursing work environment and implications for patient care: A mixed-methods systematic review. *BMC Nursing, 12*(1), 25.
Institute of Medicine (IOM). (1999). *To err is human: Building a safer health system*. Washington, DC: National Academies Press.
Institute of Medicine (IOM). (2011). *The future of nursing:* Leading change, advancing health. Committee on the Robert Wood Johnson Foundation Initiative on the Future of Nursing. Washington, DC: National Academies Press. https://www.nap.edu/read/12956/chapter/1#v.
James, J. T. (2013). A new, evidence-based estimate of patient harms associated with hospital care. *Journal of Patient Safety, 9*(3), 122–128.
Jehn, K. (1994). Enhancing effectiveness: An investigation of advantages and disadvantages of value-based intragroup conflict. *International Journal of Conflict Management, 5*, 223–238.
Jehn, K. A. (1995). A multi-method examination of the benefits and detriments of intragroup conflict. *Administrative Science Quarterly, 40*, 256–282.
Jehn, K. A. (1997). A qualitative analysis of conflict types and dimensions in organizational groups. *Administrative Science Quarterly, 42*(3), 530–557.

Johansen, M. L. (2012). Keeping the peace: Conflict management strategies for nurse managers. *Nursing Management, 43*(2), 50–54.

Kang, S. W., Lee, S., & Choi, S. B. (2017). The impact of nursing leader's behavioral integrity and intragroup relationship conflict on staff nurses' intention to remain. *JONA: The Journal of Nursing Administration, 47*(5), 294–300.

Kanter, R. M. (1977). *Men and women of the corporation*. New York: Basic Books.

Kanter, R. M. (1993). *Men and women of the corporation* (2nd ed.). New York: Basic Books.

Kelley, H. H., & Thibaut, J. (1969). Group problem solving. In G. Lindzey & E. Aronson (Eds.), *The handbook of social psychology* (2nd ed.). Reading, MA: Addison-Wesley.

Kim, S. (2017). A new focus in healthcare conflict research. *Journal of Community and Public Health Nursing, 3*(4), 1–2.

King, I. M. (1964). Nursing theory—Problems and prospect. *Nursing Science, 2*(5), 394–403.

King, I. M. (1981). *A theory for nursing: systems, concepts, process*. New York: Wiley & Sons.

King, I. M. (1992). King's theory of goal attainment. *Nursing Science Quarterly, 5*(1), 19–26.

Kipnis, D., & Schmidt, S. M. (1988). Upward-influence styles: Relationship with performance evaluations, salary, and stress. *Administrative Science Quarterly, 33*, 528–542.

Kipnis, D., Schmidt, S. M., Swaffin-Smith, C., & Wilkinson, I. (1984). Patterns of managerial influence: Shotgun managers, tacticians, and bystanders. *Organizational Dynamics, 12*(3), 58–67.

Kipnis, D., Schmidt, S. M., & Wilkinson, I. F. (1980). Intraorganizational influence tactics: Explorations in getting one's way. *Journal of Applied Psychology, 65*(4), 440–452.

Kirschbaum, K. (2012). Physician communication in the operating room: Expanding application of face-negotiation theory to the health communication context. *Health Communication, 27*(3), 292–301.

Knickle, K., McNaughton, N., & Downar, J. (2012). Beyond winning: Mediation, conflict resolution, and non-rational sources of conflict in the ICU. *Critical Care, 16*, 308. https://doi.org/10.1186/cc11141.

Kreitner, R., & Kinicki, A. (2010). *Organizational behavior* (9th ed.). Boston: McGraw-Hill Higher Education.

Kristanto, H. (2017). Demographic characteristics and conflict management strategies. *International Journal of Economic Perspectives, 11*(4), 566–580.

Kupperschmidt, B. R. (2008). Conflicts at work? Try care fronting. *Journal of Christian Nursing, 25*(1), 10–17.

Lankshear, S., Kerr, M. S., Laschinger, H. K. S., & Wong, C. A. (2013). Professional practice leadership roles: the role of organizational power and personal influence in creating a professional practice environment for nurses. *Health Care Management Review, 38*(4), 349–360.

Laschinger, H. K. S., Read, E., Wilk, P., & Finegan, J. (2014). The influence of nursing unit empowerment and social capital on unit effectiveness and nurse perceptions of patient care quality. *JONA: The Journal of Nursing Administration, 44*(6), 347–352.

Lauder, W., Reel, S., Farmer, J., & Griggs, H. (2006). Social capital, rural nursing and rural nursing theory. *Nursing Inquiry, 13*(1), 73–79.

Lawrence, S., & Callan, V. J. (2006). *Interpersonal conflict and support mobilization: Nurses' experience of coping in the workplace*. Paper at Annual Meeting of the Academy of Management. Glassboro, NJ: June 2006. https://www.researchgate.net/publication/29462063_Interpersonal_conflict_and_support_mobilisation_Nurses'_experience_of_coping_in_the_workplace.

Leksell, J., Gardulf, A., Nilsson, J., & Lepp, M. (2015). Self-reported conflict management competence among nursing students on the point of graduating and registered nurses with professional experience. *Journal of Nursing Education and Practice, 5*(8), 82–89.

Lewis, M. A. (2006). Nurse bullying: organizational considerations in the maintenance and perpetration of health care bullying cultures. *Journal of Nursing Management, 14*(1), 52–58.

Longo, J., & Sherman, R. (2007). Leveling horizontal violence. *Nursing Management, 38*(3), 34–37.

Losa Iglesias, M. E., & Becerro de Bengoa Vallejo, R. (2012a). Prevalence of bullying at work and its association with self-esteem scores in a Spanish nurse sample. *Contemporary Nurse, 42*(1), 2–10.

Losa Iglesias, M. E., & Becerro de Bengoa Vallejo, R. (2012b). Conflict resolution styles in the nursing profession. *Contemporary Nurse, 43*(1), 73–80.

Makary, M. A., & Daniel, M. (2016). Medical error—the third leading cause of death in the US. *British Medical Journal, 353*, i2139.

Mannix, J., Wilkes, L., & Daly, J. (2013). Attributes of clinical leadership in contemporary nursing: An integrative review. *Contemporary Nurse, 45*(1), 10–21.

Manojlovich, M. (2007). Power and empowerment in nursing: Looking backward to inform the future. *Online Journal of Issues in Nursing, 12*(1), 2.

Marquis, B. L., & Huston, C. J. (2012). *Leadership and management tools for the new nurse: A case study approach*. Philadelphia: Lippincott Williams & Wilkins.

McKibben, L. (2017). Conflict management: Importance and implications. *British Journal of Nursing, 26*(2), 100–103.

Meleis, A. I. (2018). *Theoretical nursing: Development and progress* (6th ed.). Philadelphia, PA: Wolters Kluwer.

Merriam-Webster. (n.d.). *Oppression*. https://www.merriam-webster.com/dictionary/oppression.

Mikkelsen, E. N., & Clegg, S. (2018). Unpacking the meaning of conflict in organizational conflict research. *Negotiation and Conflict Management Research, 11*(3), 185–203.

Moore, J. B., & Kordick, M. F. (2006). Sources of conflict between families and health care professionals. *Journal of Pediatric Oncology Nursing, 23*(2), 82–91.

Nahapiet, J., & Ghoshal, S. (1998). Social capital, intellectual capital, and the organizational advantage. *Academy of Management Review, 23*(2), 242–266.

Nancarrow, S. A., & Borthwick, A. M. (2005). Dynamic professional boundaries in the healthcare workforce. *Sociology of Health & Illness, 27*, 897–919. https://doi.org/10.1111/j.1467-9566.2005.00463.x.

National Academies of Sciences, Engineering, and Medicine (was the IOM). (2016). *Assessing progress on the Institute of Medicine Report The Future of Nursing*. Washington, DC: National Academies Press.

Nelson, H. W. (2012). Dysfunctional health service conflict: Causes and accelerants. *The Health Care Manager, 31*(2), 178–191.

Nixon, J. (2014). Looking at the culture of nursing through fresh eyes. *Kai Tiaki: Nursing New Zealand, 20*(1), 26–27.

Northam, S. (2009). Conflict in the workplace: Part 1. *AJN The American Journal of Nursing, 109*(6), 70–73.

Oakes, L. S., Townley, B., & Cooper, D. J. (1998). Business planning as pedagogy: Language and control in a changing institutional field. *Administrative Science Quarterly, 42*(3), 257–292.

O'Brien-Larivée, C. (2011). A service-learning experience to teach baccalaureate nursing students about health policy. *Journal of Nursing Education, 50*(6), 332–336.

Oc, B., Bashshur, M. R., & Moore, C. (2019). Head above the parapet: How minority subordinates influence group outcomes and the consequences they face for doing so. *Journal of Applied Psychology, 104*(7), 929.

Ocasio, W. (2002). Organizational power and dependence. In J. Baum (Ed.), *Companion to organizations* (pp. 363–385). Malden, MA: Blackwell.

Ocasio, W., Pozner, J. E., & Milner, D. (2020). Varieties of political capital and power in organizations: A review and integrative framework. *Academy of Management Annals, 14*(1), 303–338.

Oetzel, J. G., & Ting-Toomey, S. (2003). Face concerns in interpersonal conflict: A cross-cultural empirical test of the face negotiation theory. *Communication Research, 30*(6), 599–624.

Oetzel, J., Ting-Toomey, S., Masumoto, T., Yokochi, Y., Pan, X., Takai, J., et al. (2001). Face and facework in conflict: A cross-cultural comparison of China, Germany, Japan, and the United States. *Communication Monographs, 68*(3), 235–258.

Oliveira, R. M., Silva, L. M. S. D., Guedes, M. V. C., Oliveira, A. C. D. S., Sánchez, R. G., & Torres, R. A. M. (2016). Analyzing the concept of disruptive behavior in healthcare work: An integrative review. *Revista da Escola de Enfermagem da USP, 50*(4), 695–704.

Patterson, K., Grenny, J., McMillan, R., & Switzler, A. (2005). *Crucial confrontations: Tools for resolving broken promises, violated expectations, and bad behavior*. New York: McGraw-Hill.

Patton, C. M. (2014). Conflict in health care: A literature review. *The Internet Journal of Healthcare Administration, 9*(1), 1–11.

Paynton, S. T. (2009). The informal power of nurses for promoting patient care. *OJIN: The Online Journal of Issues in Nursing, 14*(1). http://ojin.nursingworld.org/MainMenuCategories/ANAMarketplace/ANAPeriodicals/OJIN/TableofContents/Vol142009/No1Jan09/ArticlePreviousTopic/InformalPowerofNurses.html.

Pecanac, K. E., & Schwarze, M. L. (2018). Conflict in the intensive care unit: Nursing advocacy and surgical agency. *Nursing Ethics, 25*(1), 69–79.

Pelc, K. (2009). The political power of nurses: power to influence, power to change. *AAACN Viewpoint, 31*(6), 1.

Pfeffer, J. (1992). Understanding power in organizations. *California Management Review, 34*(2), 29–50.

Pondy, L. R. (1967). Organizational conflict: Concepts and models. *Administrative Science Quarterly, 12*(2), 296–320.

Putnam, L. L., & Poole, M. S. (1987). Conflict and negotiation. In F. M. Jablin, L. L. Putnam, K. Roberts, & L. W. Porter (Eds.), *Handbook of organizational communication* (pp. 549–599). Newbury Park, CA: Sage.

Rahim, M. A. (1983). *Rahim organizational conflict inventories: Experimental edition: Professional manual.* Palo Alto, CA: Consulting Psychologists Press.

Rahim, M. A. (2002). Toward a theory of managing organizational conflict. *International Journal of Conflict Management, 13*(3), 206–235.

Rahim, M. A. (2010). *Managing conflict in organizations* (4th ed.). Piscataway, NJ: Transaction Publishers.

Rahim, M. A., & Bonoma, T. V. (1979). Managing organizational conflict: A model for diagnosis and intervention. *Psychological Reports, 44*(3), 1323–1344.

Rahim, M. A., & Magner, N. R. (1995). Confirmatory factor analysis of the styles of handling interpersonal conflict: First-order factor model and its invariance across groups. *Journal of Applied Psychology, 80*(1), 122.

Rao, A. (2012). The contemporary construction of nurse empowerment. *Journal of Nursing Scholarship, 44*(4), 396–402.

Rapoport, A. (1960). *Fights, games, and debates*. Ann Arbor: University of Michigan Press.

Rappaport, J. (1987). Terms of empowerment/exemplars of prevention: Toward a theory for community psychology. *American Journal of Community Psychology, 15*(2), 121–148.

Raven, B. H. (1965). Social influence and power. In I. D. Steiner, & M. Fishbein (Eds.), *Current studies in social psychology* (pp. 371–382). New York: Holt, Rinehart, Winston.

Read, E. A. (2014). Workplace social capital in nursing: an evolutionary concept analysis. *Journal of Advanced Nursing, 70*(5), 997–1007.

Robbins, S. P. (1998). *Organizational behaviour.* (8th ed.). Englewood Cliffs, NJ: Prentice Hall.

Robbins, S. P., & Judge, T. A. (2016). *Organizational behavior* (17th ed.). Upper Saddle River, NJ: Prentice Hall Publishing.

Robert Wood Johnson Foundation (RWJF). (2018). *Nurses and nursing. Future of nursing: Campaign for action.* https://www.rwjf.org/en/our-focus-areas/topics/nurses-and-nursing.html.

Roberts, S. J. (1983). Oppressed group behavior: Implications for nursing. *Advances in Nursing Science, 5*(4), 21–30.

Roberts, S. J. (2015). Lateral violence in nursing: A review of the past three decades. *Nursing Science Quarterly, 28*(1), 36–41.

Rodwell, C. M. (1996). An analysis of the concept of empowerment. *Journal of Advanced Nursing, 23*(2), 305–313.

Rogers, M. E. (1970). *An introduction to the theoretical basis of nursing.* Philadelphia: F. A. Davis.

Rogers, M. E. (1990). Nursing: Science of unitary, irreducible, human beings: Update 1990. In E. A. M. Barrett (Ed.), *Visions of Rogers' science-based nursing* (pp. 5–11). New York: National League for Nursing.

Rosenstein, A. H., & O'Daniel, M. (2005). Disruptive behavior & clinical outcomes: Perceptions of nurses & physicians: Nurses, physicians, and administrators say that clinicians' disruptive behavior has negative effects on clinical outcomes. *Nursing Management, 36*(1), 18–28.

Rosenstein, A. H., Russell, H., & Lauve, R. (2002). Disruptive physician behavior contributes to nursing shortage: Study links bad behavior by doctors to nurses leaving the profession. *Physician Executive, 28*(6), 8–11.

Rosseter, R. (2018). *Nursing faculty shortage fact sheet.* American Association of Colleges of Nursing. https://www.aacnnursing.org/News-Information/Fact-Sheets/Nursing-Fact-Sheet.

Rowe, M. M., & Sherlock, H. (2005). Stress and verbal abuse in nursing: Do burned out nurses eat their young? *Journal of Nursing Management, 13*(3), 242–248.

Rowell, P. A. (2005). Being a "target" at work: Or William Tell and how the apple felt. *JONA: The Journal of Nursing Administration, 35*(9), 377–379.

Runde, C., & Flanagan, T. (2010). *Developing your conflict competence: A hands-on guide for leaders, managers, facilitators and teams.* San Francisco, CA: Jossey-Bass.

Salancik, G. R., & Pfeffer, J. (1977). Who gets power—and how they hold on to it: A strategic-contingency model of power. *Organizational Dynamics, 5*(3), 3–21.

Salvage, J., Montayre, J., & Gunn, M. (2019). Being effective at the top table: developing nurses' policy leadership competencies. *International Nursing Review, 4*, 449. https://doi.org/10.1111/inr.12567.

Shargh, F. S., Soufi, M., & Dadashi, M. A. (2013). Conflict management and negotiation. *International Research Journal of Applied and Basic Sciences, 5*(5), 538–543.

Shell, R. (2001). Perceived barriers to teaching for critical thinking by BSN nursing faculty. *Nursing Education Perspectives, 22*(6), 286–291.

Shillam, C. R., Adams, J. M., Bryant, D. C., Deupree, J. P., Miyamoto, S., & Gregas, M. (2018). Development of the leadership influence self-assessment (LISA©) instrument. *Nursing Outlook, 66*(2), 130–137.

Sidanius, J., & Pratto, F. (1999). *Social dominance: An intergroup theory of social hierarchy and oppression.* New York: Cambridge University Press.

Sieloff, C. L. (1995). Development of a theory of departmental power. In M. Frey & C. L. Sieloff (Eds.), *Advancing King's systems framework and theory of goal attainment* (pp. 46–65). SAGE Publications.

Sieloff, C. L. (2003). Measuring nursing power within organizations. *Journal of Nursing Scholarship 35*(2), 183–187.

Sieloff, C. L. (2004). Leadership behaviors that foster nursing group power. *Journal of Nursing Management, 12*(4), 246–251.

Sieloff, C. L. (2007). The theory of group power within organizations—Evolving conceptualization within King's conceptual system. In C. L. Sieloff & M. A. Frey (Eds.), *Middle range theory development: Using King's conceptual system* (pp. 196–214). New York: Springer Publishing Company.

Sieloff, C. L. (2010). Improving the work environment through the use of research instruments: An example. *Nursing Administration Quarterly, 34*(1), 56–60.

Sieloff, C. L. (2012). *Theory of group empowerment within organizations.* https://sites.google.com/site/theoryofnursinggrouppower.

Sieloff, C. L., & Bularzik, A. M. (2011). Group power through the lens of the 21st century and beyond: Further validation of the Sieloff-King Assessment of Group Power within Organizations. *Journal of Nursing Management, 19*(8), 1020–1027.

Sieloff, C. L., & Friend, M. L. (2015, November 9–10). *A global resource for Nurses: Work team empowerment.* Poster session presented at Sigma Theta Tau International Conference. Las Vegas, NV.

Simons, T. L., & Peterson, R. S. (2000). Task conflict and relationship conflict in top management teams: The pivotal role of intragroup trust. *Journal of Applied Psychology, 85*, 102–111.

Slabbert, A. D. (2004). Conflict management styles in traditional organisations. *The Social Science Journal, 41*(1), 83–92.

Small, C. R., Porterfield, S., & Gordon, G. (2015). Disruptive behavior within the workplace. *Applied Nursing Research, 28*(2), 67–71.

Smetzer, J., Baker, C., Byrne, F. D., & Cohen, M. R. (2010). Shaping systems for better behavioural choices: lessons learned from a fatal medication error. *The Joint Commission Journal on Quality and Patient Safety, 36*(4), 152–AP2.

Smith, L. M., Andrusyszyn, M. A., & Spence Laschinger, H. K. (2010). Effects of workplace incivility and empowerment on newly-graduated nurses' organizational commitment. *Journal of Nursing Management, 18*(8), 1004–1015.

Spence Laschinger, H. K., Leiter, M., Day, A., & Gilin, D. (2009). Workplace empowerment, incivility, and burnout: Impact on staff nurse recruitment and retention outcomes. *Journal of Nursing Management, 17*(3), 302–311.

Spetz, J., Donaldson, N., Aydin, C., & Brown, D. S. (2008). How many nurses per patient? Measurements of nurse staffing in health services research. *Health Services Research, 43*(5p1), 1674–1692.

Sportsman, S., & Hamilton, P. (2007). Conflict management styles in the health professions. *Journal of Professional Nursing, 23*(3), 157–166.

Spreitzer, G. M. (1996). Social structural characteristics of psychological empowerment. *Academy of Management Journal, 39*, 483–504.

Stalter, A. M., & Arms, D. (2016). Serving on organizational boards: What nurses need to know. *Online Journal of Issues in Nursing, 21*(2). https://ojin.nursingworld.org/MainMenuCategories/ANAMarketplace/ANAPeriodicals/OJIN/TableofContents/Vol-21-2016/No2-May-2016/Articles-Previous-Topics/Serving-on-Organizational-Boards.html.

The Commonwealth Fund/The New York Times/Harvard T.H Chan School of Public Health. (2019). *Americans' values and beliefs about national health insurance reform.* https://cdn1.sph.harvard.edu/wp-content/uploads/sites/94/2019/10/CMWF-NYT-Harvard_Final-Report_Oct2019.pdf.

The Joint Commission. (2017). Sentinel Event Alert 57. *Leadership committed to safety.* The Joint Commission. https://www.jointcommission.org/-/media/tjc/documents/resources/patient-safety-topics/sentinel-event/sea_57_safety_culture_leadership_0317pdf.pdf.

Thew, J. (2016). *4 strategies for nurses who want to enter the boardroom.* HealthLeadersMedia. https://www.healthleadersmedia.com/nursing/4-strategies-nurses-who-want-enter-boardroom.

Thomas, K. W. (1976). Conflict and conflict management. In M. D. Dunnette (Ed.), *The handbook of industrial and organizational psychology* (pp. 889–935). Chicago, IL: Rand McNally.

Thomas, K. W. (1977). Toward multidimensional values in teaching: The example of conflict behaviors. *Academy of Management Review, 2*(3), 487.

Thomas, K. W. (1992). Conflict and negotiation processes in organizations. In M. D. Dunnette, & L. M. Hough (Eds.), *The handbook of industrial and organizational psychology* (2nd ed., Vol. 3. pp. 651–717). Palo Alto, CA: Consulting Psychologists Press.

Thomas, K. W., & Kilmann, R. H. (1974). *Thomas-Kilmann conflict mode instrument.* Tuxedo, NY: Xicom.

Thomas, K. W., & Schmidt, W. H. (1976). A survey of managerial interests with respect to conflict. *Academy of Management Journal, 19*(2), 315–318.

Thomas, K. W., & Velthouse, B. A. (1990). Cognitive elements of empowerment: An "interpretive" model of intrinsic task motivation. *Academy of Management Review, 15*(4), 666–681.

Thompson, T. G., & Brailer, D. J. (2004). *The decade of health information technology: delivering consumer-centric and information-rich health care.* Washington, DC: US Department of Health and Human Services.

Ting-Toomey, S. (1988). Intercultural conflict styles: A face negotiation theory. In Y. Y. Kim & W. Gudykunst (Eds.), *Theories in intercultural communication* (pp. 213–235). Newbury Park, CA: Sage.

Ting-Toomey, S., & Kurogi, A. (1998). Facework competence in intercultural conflict: An updated face-negotiation theory. *International Journal of Intercultural Relations, 22*(2), 187–225.

Trossman, S. (2014). Healthy work environment toward civility. ANA, nurses promote strategies to prevent disruptive behaviors. *The Oklahoma Nurse, 59*(2), 6.

Tubaishat, A. (2017). Evaluation of electronic health record implementation in hospitals. *CIN: Computers, Informatics, Nursing, 35*(7), 364–372.

Turkel, M. C., Fawcett, J., Amankwaa, L., Clarke, P. N., Dee, V., Eustace, R., et al. (2018). Thoughts about nursing curricula: Dark clouds and bright lights. *Nursing Science Quarterly, 31*(2), 185–189.

Umiker, W. (1999). Principles of workforce stability. *Health Care Manager, 18*(2), 58–64.

Valentine, P. E. (1995). Management of conflict: Do nurses/women handle it differently? *Journal of Advanced Nursing, 22*(1), 142–149.

Walker, L. O. (2020). Gifts of wise women: A reflection on enduring ideas in nursing that transcend time. *Nursing Outlook.* https://doi-org.libdata.lib.ua.edu/10.1016/j.outlook.2020.01.004.

Walker, L. O., & Avant, K. C. (2019). *Strategies for theory construction in nursing* (6th ed.). New York: Pearson.

Wall, J. A., & Callister, R. R. (1995). Conflict and its management. *Journal of Management, 21*(3), 515–558.

Walrath, J. M., Dang, D., & Nyberg, D. (2010). Hospital RNs' experiences with disruptive behavior: A qualitative study. *Journal of Nursing Care Quality, 25*(2), 105–116.

Walrath, J. M., Dang, D., & Nyberg, D. (2013). An organizational assessment of disruptive clinician behavior: Findings and implications. *Journal of Nursing Care Quality, 28*(2), 110–121.

Warner, I. J. (2001). Nurses' perceptions of workplace conflict: Implications for retention and recruitment. MA dissertation, Royal Roads University, Canada. Retrieved from Dissertations & Theses: Full Text. (Publication No. AAT MQ62041).

Weber, M. (1968). *Economy and society: An outline of interpretive sociology* (Vol 3). New York: Bedminster Press.

Wendt, F. (2018). *Authority*. Hoboken, NJ: John Wiley & Sons.

Whetten, D. A., & Cameron, K. S. (2016). *Developing management skills* (9th ed.). Boston: Prentice Hall.

Yukl, G. (1989). Managerial leadership: A review of theory and research. *Journal of Management, 15*(2), 251–289.

Yukl, G. (2010). *Leadership in organizations* (7th ed.). Upper Saddle River, NJ: Prentice Hall.

Yukl, G. (2013). *Leadership in Organizations* (9th ed.). Harlow, UK: Pearson Education Limited.

Yukl, G., & Falbe, C. M. (1991). Importance of different power sources in downward and lateral relations. *Journal of Applied Psychology, 76*(3), 416–423.

Yukl, G., Falbe, C. M., & Youn, J. Y. (1993). Patterns of influence behavior for managers. *Group & Organization Management, 18*(1), 5–28.

Yukl, G., Lepsinger, R., & Lucia, T. (1992). Preliminary report on development and validation of the Influence Behavior Questionnaire. In K. E. Clar, M. B. Cla, & D. P. Campbell (Eds.), *The impact of leadership* (pp. 417–427). Greensboro, NC: Center for Creative Leadership.

Yukl, G., Seifert, C. F., & Chavez, C. (2008). Validation of the extended Influence Behavior Questionnaire. *The Leadership Quarterly, 19*(5), 609–621.

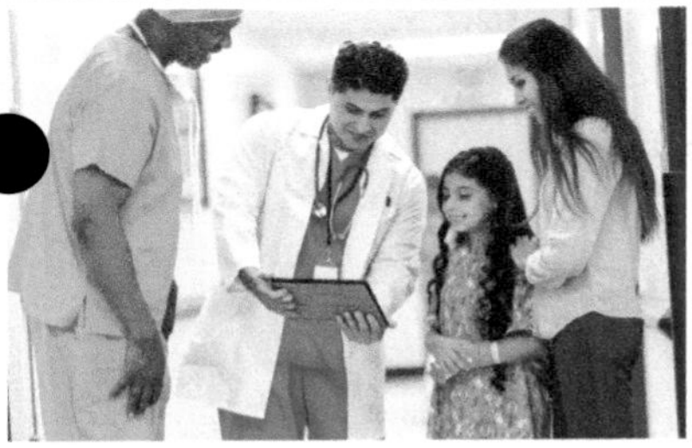

11

Workplace Diversity and Inclusion

Kupiri Piri Ackerman-Barger

http://evolve.elsevier.com/Huber/leadership

Health care values include service to others, quality care, and justice. However, a paradox in health care occurs when values fall short of outcomes. In response to this, nursing organizations are prioritizing workforce diversity as an essential approach to promoting health equity (American Association of Colleges of Nursing [AACN], 2019; Campaign for Action, 2019; National League for Nursing [NLN], 2016). This chapter guides nurses through definitions needed to understand the value of workplace diversity as well as strategies for creating and maintaining workplace diversity and inclusion.

DEFINITIONS

A long existing and pernicious issue in health care is health disparities. **Health disparities** can be defined as "a particular type of health difference that is closely linked with social, economic, and/or environmental disadvantage. Health disparities adversely affect groups of people who have systematically experienced greater obstacles to health based on their racial or ethnic group; religion; socioeconomic status; gender; age; mental health; cognitive, sensory, or physical disability; sexual orientation or gender identity; geographic location; or other characteristics historically linked to discrimination or exclusion" (Healthy People 2020, 2020). Health equity "means that everyone has a fair and just opportunity to be as healthy as possible. This requires removing obstacles to health such as poverty, discrimination, and their consequences, including powerlessness and lack of access to good jobs with fair pay, quality education and housing, safe environments, and health care" (Braveman et al., 2017, p. 2). The term **health equity** encompasses health disparities data, but also includes a purposeful focus on actions and solutions to mitigate health disparities.

Diversity in its broadest sense refers to the condition of having or being composed of different elements (Merriam-Webster, 2020). In terms of racial/ethnic diversity a student or patient cannot be diverse as an individual but may add diversity to an otherwise homogeneous group of people. A group of people who are all black or all Hispanic are not necessarily a diverse group of people. A racially/ethnically diverse group of people would have representation from multiple groups. Nursing has historically and continues to be comprised of primarily white females: a homogeneous group of people who create policies and procedures, define nursing theories, create nursing school curricula, and decide what and how topics will be researched. This creates a problem on several levels. One is that perspectives of white women are overrepresented while perspectives of other groups are underrepresented. Another issue is the lack of **cognitive diversity**, which refers to differences in information, knowledge, representations, mental models, and heuristics to better outcomes on specific tasks such as problem-solving, predicting, and innovating (Page, 2017). In other words, when groups of health care providers who think differently, who have different perspectives, and who hold varied world views come together, there is an increased likelihood that some of the complex health issues such as health disparities can be solved. It is imperative that nurses do not oversimplify the value of workforce diversity by reducing it to **compositional diversity (identity diversity)** or by looking at demographics as the sole indicator for diversity. Neither one should be a proxy for the other, rather to truly leverage the value of diversity, representation, and inclusion of the many social identities that exist such as race/ethnicity, gender identity and sexual orientation, political viewpoints, socio-economic status, diversability as well as the many ways these identities can intersect are needed.

Inclusion is the binding force for diversity and the foundation for the kind of teamwork and collaboration that is necessary for health care providers to provide quality care. It is the process by which individuals view themselves as active members of the workplace, where their background, insights, and contributions are valued as part of the creativity and productivity of the organization (Ackerman-Barger et al., 2016).

Intersectionality: Crenshaw (1989) developed a framework called "intersectionality" designed explore how the overlapping and interdependent forms of social stratification (such as race/ethnicity, gender, gender identity, sexual orientation, socio-economic status, and diversability) shape the experiences of individuals. Intersectionality is an important framework to help nurses provide patient-centered care and avoid stereotyping and anchoring biases. The concept of intersectionality also suggests that it is difficult to assess someone's "culture" based on assumptions, stereotypes, or generalizations about culture. It is important to engage with patients, families, and communities authentically and with **cultural humility** (see discussion below).

Representation refers to the degree to which the nursing workforce accurately reflects the patient demographic. This can be analyzed from a national, state or regional perspective. There are several groups that are underrepresented in nursing. The percentage of black/African American patients was 22.16% and Hispanic/Latino was 36.27 in 2018 (Health Resources and Service Administration, 2018). However, according to Smiley et al. (2018) only 6.2% of the nursing workforce is black/African American, and 5.3% is Hispanic/Latino. Men compose nearly half the patient population but only 9.1% of the nursing workforce. Each of these groups are *underrepresented in nursing.*

Cultural competence: Leininger is one of the first nurse scholars to advocate the importance of culture in the profession of nursing. Leininger (2006) stated that culture was one of the broadest, most comprehensive, holistic, and universal features of humans and that it must be understood in order to provide care to clients. Leininger emphasized the interdependence of the concepts of culture and care, and developed The Culture Care Theory. Leininger's work set the stage for the concept of cultural competence.

A widely used definition of cultural competence describes a set of congruent behaviors, attitudes, and policies that come together in a system, agency, or among professionals and enables that system, agency, or those professionals to work effectively in cross-cultural situations (Cross et al., 1989; Isaacs & Benjamin, 1991). AACN (2008) defined cultural competence as "the attitudes, knowledge and skills necessary for providing quality care to diverse populations" (p. 1). Campinha-Bacote (2007) created a conceptual framework for cultural competence that included the following components: cultural desire, cultural awareness, cultural knowledge, cultural skill, and cultural encounters. **Cultural desire** is when the health care provider is motivated to become engaged in becoming culturally competent because they want to not because they have to. She stated the concepts of love and caring, the capacity to sacrifice biases, a commitment to social justice, and humility are central to cultural desire. **Cultural awareness** "is the deliberate self-examination and in-depth exploration of our personal biases, stereotypes, prejudices and assumptions that we hold about individuals who are different from us" (p. 27). Cultural awareness helps the health care provider avoid cultural imposition. Cultural imposition was defined by Purnell and Paulenka (2003) as the intrusive application of the majority group's cultural view upon others. **Cultural knowledge** is the process of actively seeking knowledge about culturally diverse groups. **Cultural skill** refers to the ability of the health care provider to collect culturally relevant data about patients and to conduct culturally based physical assessments. **Cultural encounter** is the process of engaging in direct contact with culturally diverse groups to understand more about those groups. Campinha-Bacote (2007) warned that interacting with three or four people from a particular group does not make the health care provider an expert on that group.

The term cultural competence has been controversial. The criticism about this term is the implication that an individual can take a class or classes and become competent. Competence suggests a state of arrival that allows us to relinquish accountability for actively engaging in lifelong learning about others. If individuals view themselves as competent in understanding the myriad of cultures and intersections of cultures, identities, or roles that an individual inhabits, they are prone to stereotyping and likely to miss critical nuances. Fundamentally, the idea of cultural competence is not a set of functions or skills that are applied in certain situations but a way of being in the world. Cultural competence comes from recognizing one's own biases and taking the time to understand others in the context of their worldview. Davidhizar et al. (1998) warned against using a "cookbook" approach for assessing cultural and ethnic differences. Cultural knowledge should serve as a framework for inquiry rather than a strategy to generalize ethnic groups, which can lead to stereotyping.

Cultural humility is a term that first appeared in the health professions literature in 1998 in an article written by Tervalon and Murray-Garcia (1998). It provides a lens for how to learn about other people and other cultures. Cultural humility is rooted in the idea that one can never be competent in a culture other than one's own, but that we continue to grow and learn about others throughout our lives. Cultural humility has three tenets: (1) a lifelong commitment to self-evaluation, self-critique and growth; (2) a recognition of the existence of power differentials, to understand how they shift and to level them during interactions; and (3) a partnership with communities and groups who advocate for others by having them serving as experts on their own respective communities (Tervalon & Murray-Garcia, 1998).

Structural and institutional inequities are those factors that are largely responsible for historical inequities and perpetuate them into current inequities. The weight of structures and institutions is far more powerful than individual intent. This means that unless there are intentional and active efforts to reverse inequities, the status quo will remain unchanged. A health professions workforce armed with structural competencies has the potential to move the dial toward health equity. Hansen and Metzel (2016) stated that the notion of structural competency suggests that many health disparities are the consequence of downstream decisions about larger structural contexts, including health care and food delivery systems, zoning laws, local politics, urban and rural infrastructures, structural racisms, or even the very definitions of illness and health. **Structural competencies** are therefore necessary to identify upstream causes of health inequities. They "direct clinical training and healthcare systems to intervene at the level of social structures, institutions and policies that must be altered to improve population health and promote health equity" (Hansen & Metzel, 2016, p. 180).

BACKGROUND

Statistics show that the racial/ethnic profile of nurses, who are predominantly white and female, does not reflect the general patient population. Nurses from non-white backgrounds represent 19.2% of the nursing population, whereas 80.8% of the nursing population is white/Caucasian (Smiley et al., 2018). In contrast, according to the National Health Center Data, the total number of non-white patients based on race/ethnicity in 2019 was 62.99% (Health Resources and Services Administration, 2019), indicating a wide gap in racial/ethnic representation of the patient population compared with nursing (Table 11.1).

There are many benefits to having a nursing workforce that reflects the patient population. First is the concept of racial concordance (also known as racial match), which indicates that patients are more comfortable and satisfied with nurses (and other health care providers) who speak their language and understand their culture. This care symmetry can increase the likelihood that patients and families will seek medical care and follow through with treatments. Second, diverse perspectives can provide a greater number of innovations and solutions to health care challenges because differing

TABLE 11.1 Racial Ethnicity of Nurses Compared With Patients

	% Nurses by Race Ethnicity	% Patients by Race Ethnicity
White	**80.8**	**40.99**
Black/African American	6.2	21.69
Asian	7.5	4.22
Hispanic	5.3	36.84
American Indian/Native Alaskan	0.4	1.45
Two or more races	2.6	3.45
Non-white totals	**19.2**	**62.99**

Source: Health Resources and Services Administration (HRSA). (2019). *Total patients by age and race/ethnicity from 2016 to 2018.* US Department of Health and Human Services, National Health Center Data. https://bphc.hrsa.gov/uds/datacenter.aspx; Smiley et al., 2018).

experiences, ideas, and ways of thinking lead to better problem-solving. Third, increasing workforce diversity can make it much easier to recruit and retain minority nurses.

CREATING DIVERSITY AND INCLUSION IN THE WORKPLACE

Effective leaders will seek a diversity of people and ideas knowing that they will then have a wide selection of options from which to choose in order to solve problems. However, when teams represent a diversity of backgrounds, communication and interaction can be more challenging than when individuals are from the same culture. We tend to be attracted to people who are more like us than different from us (a concept known as *homophily*). In fact, those who are different from us can make us feel uncomfortable or even anxious. Yet fostering comfort with the unfamiliar and promoting inclusion must be a standard that is upheld consistently for an organization to benefit from diversity. Nurse managers who supervise diverse teams need to be aware of how cultural difference and backgrounds can affect interactions and communications between the health care team and with patients. To reduce miscommunications across diverse groups and to improve patient satisfaction, health care practitioners need to have skills. Communicating across cultures can take effort and is a skill that needs to be developed and nurtured over time because in the health care field, miscommunications can be fatal.

Another important concept that nurse managers need to be aware of when leading teams is that each of us carry biases, whether unconscious or not, that have the potential to hamper communication, negatively impact interactions and relationships, and ultimately impede quality patient care. Unconscious (or implicit) bias refers to beliefs and prejudices that reside outside of our awareness. There are many ways that these can manifest. Ross (2014) outlined multiple types of unconscious bias.

Selection attention (intentional blindness) is a mental process through which we selectively see some things but not others. We select what information to retain and what to discard. We tend to discard information that complicates our individual views of the world (Ross 2014). The notion of the existence of racism in current times is difficult for many white people to acknowledge. Dovidio et al. (2017) discussed the concept of aversive racism, which describes individuals who hold egalitarian values but maintain racial implicit bias. Because of the cognitive dissonance related to having one's values and beliefs in conflict, selection attention can be a helpful tool in avoiding painful realities. For example, an individual may say, "I don't think racism exists anymore. I have never seen it." Closely related to selection bias is **confirmation bias,** which is a tendency to gather information or respond to a circumstance in a way that confirms an already established belief or idea. **Commitment confirmation** supports selection attention and confirmation bias. It is when our minds become attached to particular points of view, even when they are wrong, and can lead to a form of confidence bias or self-motivated reasoning. This is an over attachment to being right rather than a genuine seeking of the truth.

Diagnosis bias is the propensity to label people, ideas, or things based on our initial opinions or first impressions (Ross, 2014). For example, if you believe that women and black people are prone to exaggerating their pain or discomfort, as a provider, you might be less likely to believe women or black people or black women, in particular, about their pain. This may account for the chronic disparities in pain management that exist for people of color. Another example is the account of an otherwise healthy black woman who died shortly after giving birth. In 2018 Charles Johnson shared the story of his wife, who had many signs of hemorrhaging after the delivery of their baby, but whose care was delayed because, as her husband described, she was not considered a priority. When asked whether he thought this incident was related to her being black, he responded, "The very fact that we have to ask that question is a problem." (This video can be found on YouTube in the video titled, "Charles Johnson shares the tragic story of his wife Kira's death hours after giving birth.")

Pattern recognition is the tendency to sort and identify information based on prior experience or habit. Stereotyping is an example of pattern recognition (Ross, 2014). This shortcut is common among health care providers. "If you have seen one drug-seeker, you have seen them all" is typical pattern recognition bias. We remember the patient who complained of back pain and was treated generously with opioids only to discover that he did not really have back pain, but rather was addicted to pain killers. Now, every time someone complains of back pain, we think we recognize a pattern and are determined not to be tricked again. However, we are not always correct in pattern recognition. And when we are wrong, we risk undertreating patients who are indeed experiencing excruciating pain.

Value attribution is the inclination to imbue a person or thing with certain qualities based on initial perceived value (Ross, 2014). Although nurses are highly educated and skilled health care providers, many nurses have experienced a time when they explained a procedure or condition to a patient or family only to have them respond with doubt or skepticism. However, when the physician explained the exact same information, the patient and family believed the physician. This is related to a perception that the information provided by the physician is more credible and therefore more valuable. Nurses internalize value attribution in favor of a physician's decision-making at the cost of their own. An example of this is when nurses do not question or clarify physician's orders and simply follow them because "the doctor said." This is disempowering at best and can have catastrophic consequences for patients.

Anchoring bias is a tendency to rely too heavily on one trait or piece of information when making decisions (Ross, 2014). Members of the transgender community often experience anchoring bias when health care providers are too focused on their gender identity rather than their reason for entering the health care system. For example, a common story from transgender patients is that they have endured a genital exam even when they have come in for a cough or respiratory issue. In other words, they receive an exam for a respiratory issue although cisgender people rarely have this exam when they present with the same symptoms.

Group think is a function of accepted patterns of bias that have become part of the organizational culture. When people respond to questions with "This is how we have always done it," they exemplify group think. When health care providers prioritize group membership over independent thought, they tend to conform to unit norms rather than think differently or question the status quo. Ross (2014) stated that this kind of bias is one of the greatest deterrents to true diversity of thought.

LEADERSHIP AND MANAGEMENT IMPLICATIONS

Valuing and Leveraging Diversity

Health care services in the United States are arguably unnecessarily complex and inefficient, with often disappointing outcomes. Further, the state of health care leaves many consumers of health and health care providers frustrated and powerless. How, then, can we change health care and health care organizations to meet the health care needs of the United States? The answer is certainly not simple, but there are ways to begin. Ross (2011) stated, "Organizations across every part of the economic spectrum—hospitals, corporations, schools, religious institutions, banks, utility companies, law offices, architectural firms, government agencies, and nonprofits and charities—all share a common link. They are bound together in the acknowledgement that the way to a new future cannot be found by using the old models of limited leadership and participation. It can only be discovered by constructing a new way of *being with each other* in organizations" (p. 15). Page (2017), who used logic models to explain the value of diversity, stated, "Complexity increases in a problem's dimensionality and interdependencies. On complex tasks, no single person's repertoire will be sufficient, so teams will be needed, and those teams need to be diverse" (p. 68). Page argued that it is cognitive diversity that increases problem-solving and innovation and that identity diversity is the source of cognitive diversity. The following outlines some aspects of diversity and how they can be beneficial to health care. This is not intended to be an exhaustive list, rather an illustrative list.

Racial and Ethnic Minority Employees

The concept of race is often understood as a biological or genetic difference between groups of people. Our historical medical knowledge has often sought to differentiate individuals based on a construct of race and to even ascertain from a scientific perspective the inferiority and superiority of groups of people. However, science has not been able to make this association. The National Human Genome Research Institute (n.d.) stated, "Race is a fluid concept used to group people according to various factors including, ancestral background and social identity. Race is also used to group people that share a set of visible characteristics, such as skin color and facial features. Though these visible traits are influenced by genes, the vast majority of genetic variation exists within racial groups and not between them. Race is an ideology and for this reason, many scientists believe that race should be more accurately described as a social construct and not a biological one." Yudell et al. (2016, p. 564) stated, "In the wake of the sequencing of the human genome in the early 2000s, genome pioneer and social scientists alike called for an end to the use of race as a variable in genetic research." The concept of race is a social construct rather than a biological construct. Racism therefore describes something that we do to each other, not what we are. Disparities based on race that exist across institutions indicate that racism still exists and influences the access to resources and availability to opportunities for individuals in the United States.

One of the ways to ameliorate racial disparities in health care is to diversify the health care workforce by hiring, retaining, and promoting more individuals of color. In the hiring process, nurse leaders must be attentive to mitigating bias in individuals on hiring committees and bias that might be embedded into hiring processes. In order to retain nurses of color, nurse leaders need to acknowledge that nurses of color are often dealing with burdens that their white counterparts are not, such as discrimination and racial microaggressions. Acts of discrimination can be a patient stating they do not want a nurse of color caring for them. Racial microaggressions describes interactions, whether intentional or not, that convey negative messages about specific groups of people, in subtle but powerful ways (Sue, 2007; Sue et al., 2019). Examples of microaggressions are, "You were only hired to increase diversity in our department" (this implies that the individual of color was somehow less qualified for the job and should not have been hired). These interactions can be extremely taxing and tend to wear on nurses of color. Nurses of color are also notably absent in leadership positions, often overlooked and passed up for promotion. To foster diversity and representation in nursing there will need to be active steps taken to move the dial forward. This means that acknowledging the problem and stating values will not be enough. Neither will good intentions. It means that organizations need to take active steps to set the tone for valuing diversity and requiring inclusion excellence, creating and adhering to policies that protect from workplace discrimination, and establishing transparent career ladders that provide equal opportunities for professional growth.

LGBT (Lesbian, Gay, Bisexual, and Transgender) Employees

Minority stress, a concept coined by Meyer (2003), describes the excess stress individuals from stigmatized social groups experience as a result of their social position and often as a member of a minority group. This term highlights how stigma, prejudice, and discrimination create a hostile and stressful social environment that causes mental health problems. The model describes stress processes, including the experience of prejudice events, expectations of rejection, hiding and concealing, internalized homophobia, and ameliorative coping processes. Some health disparities that exist for LGBT individuals that may be the result of minority stress include higher rates of depression and anxiety, higher rates of smoking and substance abuse, higher rates of obesity (Institute of Medicine [IOM], 2011; Medley et al., 2016; Meyer, 2003; National LGBT Health Education Center 2016). Some of the most staggering suicide attempt rates are among transgender individuals. McNeil et al. (2017) conducted a systematic literature review to summarize the evidence concerning factors that correlate with suicide ideation and attempts in transgender populations. They found suicide attempt rates that ranged from 37% to 83% in the general transgender population. Toomey et al. (2018) found that suicide rates for transgender youth were as high as 50.8%. Additional health factors are higher rates of HIV (human immunodeficiency virus) and STI (sexually transmitted infection) transmission for men, and lower rates of mammography and Pap smear screening for women (National LGBT Health Education Center, 2016). One way to mitigate these health disparities in LGBT populations is care given by openly LGBT health care providers and staff.

National LGBT Health Education Center (2015) recommended several strategies for recruiting and retaining LGBT employees, such as commitment statements to LGBT employees from boards and senior management, sponsoring LGBT employee resource groups, attending LGBT job fairs, advertising positions in LGBT publications, ensuring that health benefits plans include same-sex partners, and having health benefits cover the health needs of transgender employees, including transition-related expenses. They further recommended that all employees receive training on culturally affirming care for LGBT people and have policies that reflect the needs of LGBT people. Individuals can promote inclusive workplace environments for LGBT co-workers by recognizing the tendency to make gender-binary assumptions about others. Respect for LGBT individuals can be shown by asking for their preferred pronouns. Many organizations recommend that when you introduce yourself, you state your name and your preferred gender pronouns, which opens the door for the person you are speaking with to reciprocate. For example, "Hello, my name is XXX and my preferred gender pronouns are she/her. What is your name and what are your preferred gender pronouns?" Leveraging allyship means that you use your social privilege to advocate for LBGT inclusive work environments, policies, and training.

Divers-ability

Workplace diversity focuses on inclusiveness beyond race and LGBT. It also applies to being inclusive of persons with hearing, vision, mobility, and other challenges. There are many differing abilities that have often been called "disabilities." The term divers-ability reframes how we think about abilities and provides an opportunity to value the perspectives that people with divers-abilities bring to the workplace. For example, consider an employee who is hard of hearing and reminds speakers to use the microphone during a forum. A co-worker states "my voice is loud, I don't need to use a microphone." The employee who is hard of hearing explains that although using a raised voice may work for people who have normal hearing, for those who are hard of hearing the pitch of raised voice is often difficult to hear. She also explains that many people who are hard of hearing feel uncomfortable having to request a microphone. That department then adopted a custom of using a microphone when speaking to large groups as a standard practice. It is also served as a reminder that shouting to communicate with patients who are hard of hearing is not effective.

Under the ADA, employment discrimination is prohibited regarding qualified individuals with disabilities. This 180 PART III Communication and Relationship Building applies to persons who have impairments; these must substantially limit major life activities such as seeing, hearing, speaking, walking, breathing, performing manual tasks, learning, caring for oneself, and working. An individual with epilepsy, paralysis, HIV infection, AIDS, a substantial hearing or visual impairment, mental retardation, cancer, mental illness, or a specific learning disability is covered (US Equal Employment Opportunity Commission, n.d.).

Politics

Navigating political differences at work can be challenging and doing so poorly can quickly lead to conflict. However, when viewed through a lens of cognitive diversity, political differences, whether Democratic/Republican, liberal/conservative, or even rural/urban, can be a way of deepening the collective understanding of topic areas and problem-solving in such a way to meet health needs for the broadest possible groups of people. Although it may not be wise to debate politics at work, it is important to listen to and value differing viewpoints.

Language Diversity

Culturally and linguistically appropriate health care and services are broadly defined as care and services that are respectful of and responsive to the cultural and linguistic needs of all individuals. These are increasingly seen as essential to reducing disparities and improving health care quality. The National Standards for Culturally and Linguistically Appropriate Services in Health and Health Care (the National CLAS Standards) were originally developed in 2000 by the US Department of Health and Human Services Office of Minority Health (OMH) (2013) and then enhanced in 2010. They were intended to advance health equity, improve quality, and help eliminate health care disparities by providing a blueprint for individuals and health and health care organizations to implement culturally and linguistically appropriate services. The original National CLAS Standards provided guidance on cultural and linguistic competency, with the ultimate goal of reducing racial and ethnic health care disparities. The HHS Office of Minority Health undertook the National CLAS Standards Enhancement Initiative from 2010 to 2012 to recognize the nation's increasing diversity, reflect the tremendous growth in the fields of cultural and linguistic competency over the past decade, and ensure relevance with new national policies and legislation, such as the Affordable Care Act. A compendium titled *National Standards for Culturally and Linguistically Appropriate Services in Health and Health Care* (US Department of Health and Human Services, 2016) is a comprehensive view of the 15 standards and recommendations for implementing and maintaining culturally and linguistically appropriate services.

Nurses encounter patients who do not speak or understand the English language well. Patients who are limited English proficient (LEP) are likely to require the services of an interpreter. This person should be a neutral outsider instead of a family member, especially in the case of a bilingual child of the patient, except in extreme emergencies. Robust and readily available policies and procedures are needed to guide health care personnel in the use of interpreter services. Knowledge about the major ethnic and cultural groups in the patient population is a key aspect of success. Health care interpreters can be trained bilingual staff, on-staff interpreters, contract interpreters, telephone interpreters, and trained volunteers. Some people, however, should **not** serve as health care interpreters: patients' family and friends, children under 18 years old, health care personnel not involved in direct care, other patients or visitors, and untrained volunteers.

Communication style

reflects social, cultural, and family structures and varies among groups of people. Anthropologists Hall and Hall (1990) introduced the concept of 'low-context' and 'high-context' communication styles. Low-context people tend to communicate with the purpose of exchanging information directly and clearly, separating personal and professional relationships, and one situation from another. Low-context individuals feel less need to be subtle and worry less about how their communication will be received by others (Ward et al., 2016). Although a low-context style can be efficient and direct it can also be reductionist, narrow, and lacking in sensitivity. High-context communicators tend to focus more on relationship building and connecting ideas or situations, giving meaning to a broader or more contextual whole. High-context communicators tend to be more conflict avoidant and deferential to those perceived as having a higher position in the social hierarchy. Low-context communicators are more likely to speak up and share their views in work settings than high-context communicators (Ward et al., 2016). In terms of culture, Western societies like the United States tend to be low context and Eastern cultures like Japan tend to be high context (Hall & Hall, 1990; Ward et al., 2016). In health care, physicians might be considered largely low context and nurses high context.

Neither communication style should be considered more valuable than the other. Rather, both are essential to any team and exemplify how cognitive diversity can enhance problem-solving. Physicians specialize in specific systems and are trained in minute detail about the inner workings of that system. This knowledge is essential for diagnosing and providing medical interventions. Consider, however, nurses who are trained to understand how individuals, families, and communities experience illness and to create care plans that ensure patients can and will follow through with medical interventions. These approaches represent interdependent ways of thinking and addressing illness that, viewed as a whole, can produce better outcomes.

Generational Diversity

A growing challenge in nursing leadership for both nurses in practice and for nurse managers is the management of generational workforce diversity. Sociologists categorize generational groups into cohorts, called *generational markers*. These cohorts are members of a generation who are linked through shared life experiences in their formative years. Phillips (2016) stated that it is important to appreciate and embrace these differences and outlined some of the general descriptions of each generation.

Baby boomer nurses (1946–1964). Baby boomers, the second largest generational group, currently occupy many of the leadership positions, including those in health care organizations. Having been influenced by the Vietnam War, Watergate, and the Civil Rights movement they have questioned traditional authority structures, blurred gender roles, and made vigorous attempts to push systems toward their ideas of perfection. They grew up thinking they could ignore or break rules and still be successful. Consequently, financial security is a central issue for this generation, and many boomers will work past the age of retirement. In the workplace they tend to be loyal, team-oriented, and appreciative of promotions and monetary gains. Their preference is for a more participative and less authoritarian workplace (Hendricks & Cope, 2013; Phillips, 2016). The impending retirement of large numbers of baby boomer nurses is predicted to create further nurse and nurse faculty shortages.

Generation X nurses (1965–1980). People from Generation X (Gen X) grew up in a time of rapid social, economic, and technological change. Many were latchkey children who watched their parents work long hours (Phillips, 2016). Although they tend be averse to authority like baby boomers, they tend to seek work–life balance. Gen X nurses learned to set limits and manage their own time. They are self-directed, do not feel obligated to work in teams, and practice very comfortably by themselves. Gen X nurses desire facts rather than emotions. They believe quality of life is important, and they are self-reliant and resourceful (Phillips, 2016).

Millennial nurses (1981–1996). As the largest group in US history, millennial workers are the most demographically diverse generation. The common marker of their developmental years is technology. These workers have astonishing multitasking skills. They also tend to have a positive outlook and a desire to improve the world. People from older generations tend to believe that millennials are shallow on basic skills; but because they grew up with computers, they can create solutions that other generations could not have imagined. Technology guides their every move. They are problem-solvers who grew up in a flourishing economy. Millennials matured in a world in which shortcuts, manipulation of rules, and situational ethics seem to have reigned. They got the message somehow that the final word is not the final word. They do not live to work; they work to live. Thus they have a different set of expectations about the world of work. Phillips (2016) noted that millennial nurses, like Gen X nurses, strive for work–life balance, and prefer flexible work shifts and job portability. Millennial nurses also tend to have a great sense of morality and civic duty.

Generation Z nurses (1997–2012). The newest cohort just entering the workforce is called Generation Z (Gen Z). Projections about the overarching influences for Gen Z are speculative. They are the most racially and ethnically diverse adult generation. Most members of Gen Z have no memory of the 9/11 terrorist attack. Donald Trump would be the first US president most Gen Z's know as they turn 18. The political environment in 2020 may influence the attitudes and engagement of Gen Z. Technology and the internet explosion are generation-shaping elements, with the rapid way people communicate and interact, including social media and an "always-on" technology environment that has produced dramatic shifts in behaviors, attitudes, and youth lifestyles (Dimock, 2019).

Like any demographic group, people from different generations have their own cultural perspectives and social expectations. These can cause workplace conflict. However, there is great potential for cross-generational growth and support as each generation has experienced its own set difficulties and has developed its own strengths. Barry (2014) suggested that by acknowledging the strengths of each generation there is the potential for effective mentoring, reducing work-place conflict, and diversification of the nursing workforce.

It is acceptable to take a sincere interest in a co-worker's or patient's background or culture. However, many Americans are afraid to ask people about their culture or background because they worry, "I don't want to offend anyone." The challenge with this thinking is that if nurses do not ask about people's differences, then the only option is to make assumptions. It is far more likely that others will be offended by people making assumptions than asking them directly about differences in their behavior or beliefs. In fact, asking other people directly about their culture can often help build rapport and a much deeper working relationship than simply talking about the weather or current events. Exploring and assessing the individual's preferences can bring to light the impact of culture on health care needs. Their culture could have an impact on their views about health issues such as health care, diet, and lifestyle. When people do not ask others about their cultural differences, those unasked questions can create a kind of "cultural static" that can keep the nurse from hearing a co-worker or patient clearly. This is a part of patient assessment and is also important for fostering co-worker relationships. Nurses can miss important facts that would enlighten care delivery and healthy work environments. However, it is important to note that is not an obligation for individuals to teach you about their culture.

Generational differences can be seen as both a challenge and an opportunity (Douglas & Gray, 2020). This is because of the acceleration of change and radical shifts in technology and information processing. There can be more than four generations working together in the workplace. Part of the complexity is whether or not the individuals grew up immersed in technology. Despite all of this, a highly qualified nurse workforce is desperately needed. A holistic perspective that considers generational differences along with universal human characteristics will aid in creating a foundation that sustains nursing through the path ahead (Douglas & Gray, 2020).

CURRENT ISSUES AND TRENDS

Strategies for Creating and Maintaining Workplace Diversity

The Pipeline

An important step in increasing nursing workforce diversity is looking at the long-term pipeline. The American Association of Colleges of Nursing (2019) and National League for Nursing (2016) outlined steps they are taking to increase nursing workforce diversity, including recruiting and retaining students from diverse backgrounds. A significant portion of nursing student education occurs in the practice setting. This means that hospitals, clinics, nursing homes, and other practice settings can contribute to workforce diversity by ensuring that students from underrepresented backgrounds feel welcomed, included, and valued during their clinical experiences. Ackerman-Barger et al. (2020) found that students of color experienced racial microaggressions from preceptors during their clinical rotations. Organizations can take steps to promote inclusion by having strong mission and vision statements related to diversity, inclusion and health equity; staff who exemplify and uphold the mission statement; and by having staff nurses and nursing leaders who reflect the characteristics of the general population.

Outreach and Recruitment

Advertisements for positions need to include inclusive language, organizational diversity, and inclusion statements. Increased recruiting efforts from historically black colleges and universities, Hispanic serving institutions, and Native American communities can help. Targeting the networks of underrepresented groups like minority nursing organizations and LGBT groups like Gay and the Lesbian Medical Association (GLMA), which has a nursing branch, can increase diversity. Using connections to personally reach out to potential candidates is also a helpful strategy.

Hiring

Organizations need to develop hiring committees with diverse compositions. Individuals who serve on hiring committees should undergo unconscious bias training. This training can include how to account for bias that may be present in letters of recommendation. Further, prior to reviewing applications the committee needs to discuss the qualification criteria for candidates and processes that will be followed during the hiring process. A discussion about the value that diversity brings to the organization and to patient care should be central in conversations about hiring. Be flexible in reviewing resumes and tend toward inclusion versus exclusion when deciding upon which applicants to invite for interview. Recognize that some applicants, often women and individuals from collectivist cultures, may not include or may minimize their accomplishments as opposed to those from individualist cultures who may be more comfortable with self-promotion. Include diversity, inclusion, and health equity themed questions to ask candidates during the interview. An iterative appraisal process of hiring procedures should occur periodically to ensure that biased processes have not become embedded into hiring procedures. Things to ask during periodic appraisals are: how does the pool of people hired compare with the list of who to interview and who applied for the position? Are applicants from underrepresented groups held to different standards than well-represented groups? If there was a high percentage of underrepresented groups who did not make it to the interview or hiring pool, why did this occur?

Retention and Promotion

Organizations are better served when they invest in long-term employees. There are cost savings and valuable institutional memory that is retained when turnover rates are reduced. Women and employees of color have historically and are currently paid less and are promoted less compared with their male and white counterparts. This is true in nursing as well. A first step is to consistently offer competitive and transparent hiring packages. Note that not all individuals have the same comfort with, or knowledge about, how to negotiate. For example, men and women tend to negotiate differently, in ways that leave women at a disadvantage. There are cross-cultural differences as well. In the United States, Canada, Western Europe, and a few other countries, people only negotiate the most expensive purchases like cars and houses, whereas they will pay exactly what is asked on almost everything else. In countries and regions such as Mexico, Asia, India, South America, and the Philippines, negotiation is a daily expectation (Lewis, 2017). Suggestions for equitable negotiations are as follows:

- Provide education to business office staff, individuals serving on hiring committees, and managers about how negotiating styles can vary based on gender, culture, and individual background.
- Create a fair, transparent hiring process. Organizations who 'low-ball' their new employees on hiring may pay a much bigger price later in turnover when disgruntled employees leave the organization.

RESEARCH NOTE

Source

O'Connor, M.R., Barrington, W.E., Buchanan, D.T., Bustillos, D., Eagen-Torkko, M., Kalkbrenner, A., et al. (2019). Short-term outcomes of a diversity, equity, and inclusion institute for nursing faculty. *Journal of Nursing Education, 58*(11), 633–640.

Purpose

The purpose of this study was to develop faculty knowledge and effectiveness in addressing diversity, equity, and inclusion (DEI) topics in teaching. Specific objectives were to provide school of nursing faculty with the knowledge and skills they need to create truly inclusive learning environments, facilitate crucial conversations on racism and other-ism, and incorporate DEI topics through all curricula. To this end, the researchers offered a 3-day DEI Institute that included content experts, exercises on how to facilitate conversations on racism and other-isms led by social justice facilitators, and active learning opportunities such as individual self-reflection and small and large group discussions.

Discussion

This study found that the DEI Institute resulted in overwhelmingly positive increases in satisfaction and impact and statistically significant increases in DEI-related teaching self-efficacy post institute. These results suggest that workshops such as these show promise as interventions to create more inclusive learning environments. The researchers noted that significant institutional support from both the university and school of nursing were needed for the success of their DEI Institute. They discussed the importance of allowing participants to self-select into the workshop because of the evidence showing that mandatory DEI workshops may have the opposite effect than intended. Finally, they highlighted that a singular event or approach is not adequate to create inclusive learning environments, rather institutions need multiple resources and activities and ongoing trainings and discussions to make an impact.

Application to Practice

Training and skills are needed to achieve diversity, equity, and inclusion. An important place to start this process is in schools of nursing where future nurses can have DEI modeled for them and bring these skills to clinical practice. Although this study focused on nursing academic settings, it highlights the value and impact DEI training can have on participants, which could be applicable in multiple workplace settings.

CASE STUDY

Carol, a black nurse, has been assigned to care for a patient. When she walks into the patient's room and introduces herself, the patient responds, "I don't want you to be my nurse. I need a nurse who is not a (insert racial epithet)." A co-worker observed this interaction and called the nurse manager. The nurse manager comes to the floor.

1. Describe the impact this interaction could have had on Carol.
2. What would support for her look like?
3. Describe the impact this interaction could have had on other members of the unit who belong to marginalized groups.
4. What would support for them look like?
5. Describe the impact that not addressing this issue could have on unit as a whole.
6. What response should be made to the patient?
7. Imagine this same scenario but the nurse is a white male instead of a black female. What would be similar and/or different about the response?

CRITICAL THINKING EXERCISE

With the ever-increasing use of social media in our society, health care is grappling with new issues. Platforms like LinkedIn, Facebook, and Instagram have been helpful in recruiting nurses and can be a mechanism for providing news and education. However, there have also been challenges related to social media in the form of posts made with images of patients in clinical environments and complaints about co-workers and/or hospitals. A nurse manager is preparing a staff development workshop about the positive and negative aspects of social media platforms currently in health care.

1. What differing generational perspectives should the nurse manager anticipate when developing this training? In what ways might millennial nurses view social media differently than baby boomers?
2. What facilitation strategies could the nurse manager use to ensure all participants feel included and valued during the social media workshop?
3. Describe some activities the nurse manager can use to build community and create meaningful and productive dialogue among participants during the social media workshop.

REFERENCES

Ackerman-Barger, K., Boatright, D., Gonzalez-Colaso, R., Orozco, R., & Latimore, D. (2020). Seeking inclusion excellence: Understanding microaggressions experienced by underrepresented medical and nursing students. *Academic Medicine, 95*(5), 758–763. https://doi.org/10.1097/ACM.0000000000003077.

Ackerman-Barger, K., Valderama-Wallace, C., Latimore, D., & Drake, C. (2016). Understanding health professions students' self-perceptions of stereotype threat Susceptibility. *Journal of Best Practices in Health Professions Diversity, 9*(2), 1232–1246.

American Association of Colleges of Nursing (AACN). (2008). *Cultural competency in baccalaureate nursing education*. https://www.aacnnursing.org/Portals/42/AcademicNursing/CurriculumGuidelines/Cultural-Competency-Bacc-Edu.pdf.

American Association of Colleges of Nursing (AACN). (2019). *Enhancing diversity in the nursing workforce*. https://www.aacnnursing.org/Portals/42/News/Factsheets/Enhancing-Diversity-Factsheet.pdf.

Barry, M. (2014). Creating a practice environment that supports multigenerational workforce collaboration. *American Nurse, 46*(1), 13.

Braveman, P., Arkin, E., Orleans, T., Proctor, D., & Plough, A. (2017). *What is health equity? and what difference does a definition make?* Princeton, NJ: The Robert Wood Johnson Foundation: National Collaborating Centre for Determinants of Health.

Campaign for Action: Center to Champion Nursing in America. (2019). *The importance of diversity in nursing*. https://campaignforaction.org/the-importance-of-diversity-in-nursing/.

Campinha-Bacote, J. (2007). *The process of cultural competence in the delivery of healthcare services: The journey continues*. Cincinnati, OH: Transcultural C.A.R.E. Associates.

Crenshaw, K. (1989). Demarginalizing the intersection of race and sex: A Black feminist critique of antidiscrimination doctrine, feminist theory and antiracist politics. *The University of Chicago Legal Forum, 140*(1989), 139-167.

Cross, T., Bazron, B., Dennis, K., & Isaacs, M. (1989). *Towards a culturally competent system of care: A monograph on effective services for minority children who are severely emotionally disturbed (volume I)*. Washington, DC: Georgetown University Child Development Center.

Davidhizar, R., Dowd, S. B., & Giger, J. N. (1998). Educating the culturally diverse nursing student. *Nurse Educator, 23*(2), 38–42.

Dimock, M. (2019). *Defining generations: Where Millennials end and Generation Z begins*. Pew Research Center. January 17. https://www.pewresearch.org/fact-tank/2019/01/17/where-millennials-end-and-generation-z-begins/.

Douglas, K., & Gray, S. (2020). Generational complexities present new challenges for nurse leaders. *Nurse Leader, 18*(2), 126–129.

Dovidio, J. F., Gaertner, S. L., & Pearson, A. R. (2017). Aversive racism and contemporary bias. In C. G. Sibley & F. K. Barlow (Eds.), *The Cambridge handbook of the psychology of prejudice* (pp. 267–294). Cambridge, UK: Cambridge University Press.

Hall, E. T., & Hall, M. R. (1990). *Understanding cultural differences*. Boston: Intercultural Press.

Hansen, H., & Metzl, J. M. (2016). Structural competency in the U.S. healthcare crisis: Putting social and policy interventions into clinical practice. *Bioethical Inquiry, 13*, 179–183.

Health Resources and Services Administration (HRSA). (2018). *Total patients by age and race/ethnicity from 2016 to 2018*. US Department of Health and Human Services, 2018 National Health Center Data. https://bphc.hrsa.gov/uds/datacenter.aspx.

Healthy People 2020. (2020). *Disparities*. https://www.healthypeople.gov/2020/about/foundation-health-measures/Disparities.

Hendricks, J. M., & Cope, V. C. (2013). Generational diversity: What nurse managers need to know. *Journal of Advanced Nursing, 69*(3), 717–725.

Isaacs, M., & Benjamin, M. (1991). *Towards a culturally competent system of care. Programs which utilize culturally competent principles (volume II)*. Washington, DC: Georgetown University Child Development Center.

Institute of Medicine (IOM). (2011). *The health of Lesbian, Gay, Bisexual, and Transgender people: Building a foundation for better understanding*. Washington, DC: National Academies Press.

Leininger, M. M. (2006). Culture care diversity and universality theory and evolution of the ethnonursing method. In M. M. Leininger & M. R. McFarland (Eds.), *Culture care diversity and universality: A worldwide nursing theory* (2nd ed) (pp. 1–41): Sudbury, MA: Jones and Bartlett.

Lewis, B. (2017). *Negotiation tactics: How to haggle like your life depends on it*. https://www.fluentin3months.com/negotiation-tactics/.

McNeil, J., Ellis, S. J., & Eccles, F. J. R. (2017). Suicide in trans populations: A systematic review of prevalence and correlates. *Psychology of Sexual Orientation and Gender Diversity, 4*(3), 341–353. https://doi.org/10.1037/sgd0000235.

Medley, G., Lipari, R. N., Bose, J., Cribb, D. S., Kroutil, L. A., & McHenry, G. (2016). *Sexual orientation and estimates of adult substance use and mental health: Results from the 2015 National Survey on Drug Use and Health*. Substance Abuse and Mental Health Services Administration. https://www.samhsa.gov/data/sites/default/files/NSDUH-SexualOrientation-2015/NSDUH-SexualOrientation-2015/NSDUH-SexualOrientation-2015.pdf.

Merriam-Webster. (2020). *Diversity*. https://www.merriam-webster.com/dictionary/diversity.

Meyer, I. H. (2003). Prejudice, social stress, and mental health in Lesbian, Gay, and Bisexual populations: Conceptual issues and research evidence. *Psychological Bulletin, 129*(5), 674–697.

National Human Genome Research Institute. (n.d.). *Race*. https://www.genome.gov/genetics-glossary/Race.

National League for Nursing (NLN). (2016). *Achieving diversity and meaningful inclusion in nursing education: A living document from the National League for Nursing*. http://www.nln.org/docs/default-source/about/vision-statement-achieving-diversity.pdf?sfvrsn=2.

National LGBT Health Education Center. (2015). *10 things: Creating inclusive health care environments for LGBT people*. https://www.lgbthealtheducation.org/wp-content/uploads/Ten-Things-Brief-Final-WEB.pdf.

National LGBT Health Education Center. (2016). *Understanding the health needs of LGBT people*. https://www.lgbthealtheducation.org/publication/understanding-health-needs-lgbt-people/.

Page, S. (2017). *The Diversity bonus: How great teams pay in the knowledge economy*. Princeton, NJ: Princeton University Press.

Phillips, M. (2016). Embracing the multigenerational nursing team. *MEDSURG Nursing, 25*(3), 197–200.

Purnell, L. D., & Paulenka, B. J. (2003). *Transcultural health care: A culturally competent approach* (2nd ed). Philadelphia, PA: F.A. Davis.

Ross, H. (2011). *Reinventing diversity: Transforming organizational community to strengthen people, purpose, and performance*. Lanham, MD: Rowman & Littlefield.

Ross, H. (2014). *Everyday bias: Identifying and navigating unconscious judgments in our daily lives*. Lanham, MD: Rowman & Littlefield.

Smiley, R. A., Lauer, P., Bienemy, C., Berg, J. G., Shireman, E., Reneau, K. A., et al. (2018). The 2017 national nursing workforce survey. *Journal of Nursing Regulation, 9*(3), S1–S88.

Sue, D. W., Capodilupo, C. M., Torino, G. C., et al. (2007). Racial microaggressions in everyday life: Implications for clinical practice. *American Psychologist, 62*(4), 271–286. https://doi.org/10.1037/0003-066X.62.4.271.

Sue, D. W., Alsaidi, S., Awad, M. N., Glaeser, E., Calle, C. Z., & Mendez, N. (2019). Disarming racial microaggressions: Microintervention strategies for targets, white allies, and bystanders. *American Psychologist, 74*(1), 128–142.

Tervalon, M., & Murray-Garcia, J. (1998). Cultural humility versus cultural competence: A critical distinction in defining physician training outcomes in multicultural education. *Journal of the Healthcare Poor and Underserved, 9*(2), 117–123.

Toomey, R. B., Syvertsen, A. K., & Shramko, M. (2018). Transgender adolescent suicide behavior. *Pediatrics, 142*(4), 1–8.

US Department of Health and Human Services, Office of Minority Health (OMH). (2013). *National standards for CLAS in health and health care: A blueprint for advancing and sustaining CLAS policy and practice*. https://thinkculturalhealth.hhs.gov/pdfs/EnhancedCLASStandardsBlueprint.pdf.

US Department of Health and Human Services, Office of Minority Health (OMH). (2016). *National standards for culturally and linguistically appropriate services in health and health care: Compendium of state-sponsored national CLAS standards implementation activities*. U.S. Department of Health and Human Services. https://thinkculturalhealth.hhs.gov/pdfs/CLASCompendium.pdf.

US Equal Employment Opportunity Commission. (n.d.). *Americans with Disabilities Act: Questions and answers*. https://search.ada.gov/search?query=Americans+with+Disabilities+Act%3A+Questions+and+ans&search=go&sort=date%3AD%3AL%3Ad1&output=xml_no_dtd&ie=iso-8859-1&oe=UTF-8&client=default_frontend&proxystylesheet=default_frontend&affiliate=justice-ada.

Ward, A.-K., Ravlin, E. C., Klaas, B. S., Ployhart, R. E., & Buchan, N. R. (2016). When do high-context communicators speak up? Exploring contextual communication orientation and employee voice. *Journal of Applied Psychology, 101*(10), 1498–1511.

Yudell, M., Roberts, D., DeSalle, R., & Tishkoff, S. (2016). Taking race out of human genetics. *Science, 351*(6273), 564–565.

12

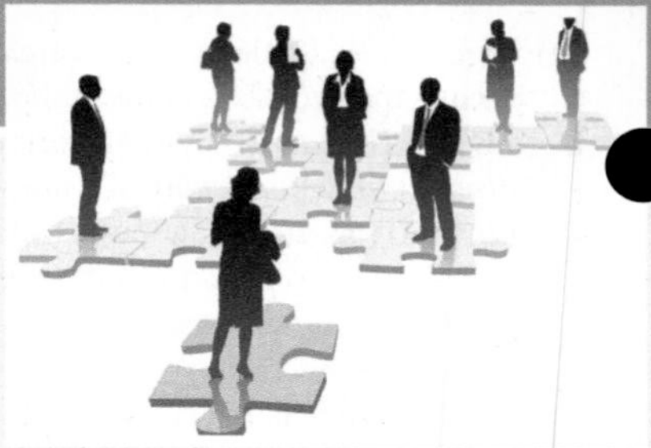

Organizational Structure

Christopher J. Louis

http://evolve.elsevier.com/Huber/leadership

Organizations are essentially social structures that rely on human activity. An organization meaningfully coordinates group activity toward a shared goal because collective efforts are often necessary to manage large-scale work processes and outcomes efficiently and effectively. Many types of organizations are necessary in order to deliver nursing and health care services to diverse populations across sectors and geography. In health care, obvious organizational goals might be safety and quality of care, cost reduction, and increased efficiency. Yet the challenges and consequences of system fragmentation and care coordination continue to plague the US health care system (Louis et al., 2019). Understanding organizational structure helps nurses be more effective and efficient in their work lives.

Whether as employees or as independent practitioners, nurses work for or interact with organizations. How nurses' roles interface with the structure of the organization influences the accomplishment of organizational goals. Research examples throughout this chapter highlight associations between the organizational structures in which nurses work and clinical, nurse, and organizational outcomes.

DEFINITIONS

Structure refers to the arrangement of the parts within a larger whole. In Donabedian's (1980) classic quality framework of structure, process, and outcomes, structure affects process, which affects outcomes. **Organizations** are entities that contain groupings that consolidate smaller elements into a larger, systematized whole. **Organizational social structure** is defined as the ways in which work is divided and coordinated among members and the resulting network of relationships, roles, and work groups (e.g., units, departments). The social structure of an organization influences the flow of information, resources, and power among its members.

BACKGROUND

Organizational Theory

Organizations are complex and dynamic. Yet for nurses to function as effective health care workers, an understanding of organizations is essential. There are many ways to understand organizations, and each understanding reflects different assumptions and tensions regarding the nature and dynamics of organizations. The history of organizational theory has been shaped by multiple disciplines, including management, engineering, psychology, sociology, and anthropology, and by study over a long period of time. Although this has created a rich and varied understanding of organizations, the field of organization theory contains a variety of approaches to and assumptions about the phenomenon of "organization." Objectivism, subjectivism, and postmodernism reflect three broad perspectives regarding the nature of reality and the nature of knowledge with respect to the concept of "organization" (Hatch & Cunliffe, 2013). These perspectives are reviewed briefly with attention to the meanings of social structure, management, and power.

Objective Perspective

The objective (also called modern) perspective centers interest on causal explanation that entails describing the antecedents and results of a particular phenomenon (Hatch & Cunliffe, 2013). When approached as an objective entity, an organization exists as an external reality, independent of its social actors. Organizations are viewed as logical and predictable objects with identifiable and scientifically measurable characteristics (e.g., size) that can be predicted, observed, or manipulated (Hatch & Cunliffe, 2013). The purpose is to uncover laws that enhance the generalizability of knowledge. Organizational structure is a consequence of both the division of and the coordination of labor, which results in a formal set of interrelated and interdependent roles and work groups. Management determines the formal relationships and standardizes the behaviors of individuals and groups in order to align organizational functioning with internal demands (e.g., technology) and external demands (e.g., market conditions, regulatory standards) (Reed, 1992). Typically, power is conceptualized as a resource to be allocated among roles and groups. Modernist theories related to bureaucracy and systems—as well as the schools of scientific management and human relations—have focused on improvements to efficiency, motivation, and performance in the achievement of collective goals (Reed, 1992). These theoretical approaches, which focus on the *formal* aspects of organizations, are examined in detail in this chapter.

Subjective Perspective

In contrast to objectivism, a symbolic or subjective approach to the phenomenon of organization asserts that an organization cannot exist independent of its social actors. The organization is a social reality that can be known only through human experience, relationships, and shared meanings and symbols (Hatch & Cunliffe, 2013). Because knowledge is considered to be relative, open to interpretation, and context dependent, the purpose of inquiries is to uncover collective meanings and understandings that resonate with the experiences of those involved (Hatch & Cunliffe, 2013). Social structure therefore arises from and is continuously transformed through social interaction, which is played out against a backdrop of formal rules and material resources directed by management (Reed, 1992). Power is reflected in the struggle between social actors who proactively and self-consciously shape organizational arrangements and secure scarce resources to serve their interests (Hatch & Cunliffe, 2013; Reed, 1992).

The subjective perspective focuses on the *informal* aspects of organization and on the freedom of individuals to make choices and to influence organizational life. Symbolic–interpretive theorists are interested in "how the everyday practices of organizational members construct the very patterns of organizing that guide their actions" (Hatch & Cunliffe, 2013, p. 113). Examples of daily social practices include routines (e.g., clinical protocols), interactions, and communities of practice. For example, instead of viewing routines as mechanisms to standardize the behavior of individuals (i.e., an objective approach), a subjective approach might examine the changing nature or pattern of routines as members selectively modify, adapt, and retain practices in response to varying conditions and evidence-based practice. In a community of practice, learning occurs through voluntary social interaction whereby clinicians who are committed to a common interest self-organize informally to build ongoing relationships, partake in joint activities, and share resources (Wenger, 2008). An example in nursing would be an informal group of staff nurses who routinely have lunch together and who come to rely on this activity as a source of knowledge related to patient care in terms of problem-solving, information exchange, and networking.

Postmodern Perspective

Departing from the polarization between objectivism (or modernism) and subjectivism (symbolism), the postmodern view offers critique and appreciation by challenging the meanings and interpretations associated with the concept of organization. The basic premise is that the world is known through language. Because language is continually reconstructed and context dependent, knowledge is essentially a power play (Hatch & Cunliffe, 2013). Notions of order and structure are the subject of scrutiny, and organizations may be thought of as chaotic entities characterized by conflicts and misunderstandings (Reed, 1992). Managerial practices and structures within organizations are seen to legitimize the interests of those in power. Even classic organization theorists such as Weber (1978) cautioned that bureaucracies were essentially domination structures that shape the form and purpose of social action through a system of rational rules and norms. Those who control bureaucracies therefore exert significant power over social action. For example, occurrences of sexual harassment can be either ignored or aggressively sanctioned as consistent with organizational values and norms. Thus the postmodern organization is understood both as an arena in which power struggles between dominant and subordinate groups play out and as a text to be rewritten to free its members from exploitative and controlling influences (Hatch & Cunliffe, 2013; Reed, 1992).

Postmodernists challenge the assumption that social structure results from the division and coordination of work among roles and groups. Clegg (1990) suggested that excessive fragmentation of work results in a disjointed and confusing experience for workers who become dependent on more powerful members in the hierarchy to make sense of workflow and goals. To counter this excess control over member actions, he proposed the idea of **differentiation**, whereby people self-manage and coordinate their own activities. Other examples of postmodern approaches to organization include feminist critiques of bureaucracies (e.g., Eisenstein, 1995) and anti-administration theory (Farmer, 1997). Each perspective contributes to stretching the thinking about how organizations are structured and function.

KEY THEORIES OF ORGANIZATIONS AS SOCIAL SYSTEMS

In the field of organizational design, the organization is most commonly approached as a social system from the objective perspective. Different theories within this tradition have contributed to understanding organizational social structure over an extensive period of study. However, these theories have also been critiqued for rationalizing social action, for favoring efficiency and productivity over other values (e.g., equity, justice), and for adopting an elitist view of management (e.g., O'Connor, 1999).

Bureaucratic Theory

Although often criticized for its oppressive qualities and administrative burden, the concept of bureaucracy may be better understood when placed within a historical context. Theorist Max Weber (1864–1920) was a German lawyer, professor, and political activist who noted the push of industrialism toward mass production and technical efficiency (Prins, 2000). Weber sought to explain from a historical perspective how the bureaucratic structure of large organizations differed from and improved on other forms of societal functioning (e.g., feudalism). He viewed bureaucracy as a social leveling mechanism founded on impartial and merit-based selection (i.e., legal authority), rather than a social ordering determined by kinship (i.e., traditional authority) or personality (i.e., charismatic authority) (Weber, 1978). However, Weber warned of the potential dehumanizing effects of bureaucracies that emphasized purely economic results (i.e., formal rationality) at the expense of other important social values such as social justice and equality (i.e., substantive rationality) (Weber, 1978). Weber's descriptions of authority and rationality are foundational concepts in the study of organizations. His interpretation of hierarchy and its relevance to health care organizations are explored later in the chapter.

Scientific Management School

Arising from the experiences and ideas of business leaders and engineers in manufacturing industries, the scientific management school sought to determine the single best way to structure an organization. A well-known theorist in this field is Frederick W. Taylor (1856–1915), an engineer who authored *The Principles of Scientific Management* in 1914 (Prins, 2000). Along with colleagues, Taylor's vision was to improve labor relations and the low industrial standards that plagued the American manufacturing industry by the application of technical solutions (e.g., time and motion studies) (Prins, 2000). The goal was to enhance organizational performance in a milieu of improved cooperation between management and labor by matching the work performed with the worker's skills and with economic incentives. However, the experiments and engineering techniques associated with this approach were ultimately criticized for reducing the worker to a mere input in the production process (Prins, 2000). The application of scientific principles to improve the task performance and productivity of workers reflected a bottom-up approach to organizational design (Scott, 1992). In nursing, efforts to redesign nursing jobs, such as by using nurse practitioners or to measure nursing workload, often rely on this tradition.

Classical Management Theory

In contrast, classical theorists such as Fayol, Urwick, and Gulick evolved a top-down approach to organizational design. Based on experience as company executives, they identified principles of administration and management functions that could be applied in the design of organizations. Key concepts such as differentiation, coordination, the scalar principle, centralization, formalization, specialization, and span of control became central to the study of organizational structure. These concepts, which describe the *formal* aspects of an organization's social structure and their application to health care organizations, are examined in relation to nursing later in the chapter.

Human Relations School

Theorists in the human relations school emphasized the *informal*, rather than *formal*, aspects of organization social structure. The disciplines of industrial psychology and industrial relations founded this approach, which now persists as the field of organizational behavior (O'Connor, 1999). The social and psychological needs and relationships of workers and groups were thought to be important to work productivity. Improved cooperation between management and workers was proposed to enhance performance and reduce industrial strife (O'Connor, 1999). The famous Hawthorne experiments were influential in this school of thought. Initial interpretations of the Hawthorne experiments suggested that psychological factors influenced worker motivation because improved worker productivity was observed when researchers gave special attention to workers, regardless of changes to physical surroundings (Scott, 1992). Concepts such as job enlargement and job rotation were promoted to offset the alienation workers experienced because of excessive **formalization** and division of work processes (Scott, 1992). Formalization is the extent to which the organization uses explicit rules, procedures, job descriptions, and communications to prescribe roles and role interactions, govern activities, and standardize behaviors (Hatch & Cunliffe, 2013).

Streams of study included leadership behavior, small group dynamics, participative decision-making, morale, motivation, and other worker characteristics and behaviors (Scott, 1992). In nursing, this school of thought is reflected in efforts to meet the professional development needs of nurses, enhance nurse autonomy and empowerment, and involve nurses in decision-making processes to improve organizational functioning.

Open System Theory

Open system theory emphasizes the dynamic interaction and interdependence of the organization with its external environment and its internal subsystems. Meyer and O'Brien-Pallas (2010) conceptualized the health care organization as an open system characterized by energy transformation, a dynamic steady state, negative entropy, event cycles, negative feedback, differentiation, integration and coordination, and equifinality. *Inputs* (i.e., characteristics of care recipients, nurses, resources), *throughputs* (the delivery of nursing services arising from the nature of the work, structures, and work conditions), and *outputs* (i.e., clinical, human resource, and organizational outcomes) were theorized to interact dynamically to influence the global work demands placed on nursing work groups at the point of care in production subsystems.

Contingency theory is a subset of open system theory positing that there is no single right way to structure an organization. Effective organizational performance depends on the fit between the structure and multiple contingency factors such as technology, size, and strategy. Mark et al. (1996) applied contingency theory to the evaluation of nursing care delivery system outcomes. The basic premise was that to perform effectively and produce quality outcomes, an organization must structure and adapt its nursing units to complement the environment and technology.

Technology is a core concept in contingency theory and refers to the work performed. Technology can be examined in terms of task uncertainty (i.e., repetitive nature of the task), diversity (i.e., number of different components), and interdependence (i.e., degree to which work processes are interrelated) (Scott, 1992). Highly repetitive and distinct tasks are amenable to mass production technologies (e.g., manufacturing industry). In contrast, highly uncertain and interdependent tasks require discretion, improvisation, and more intense coordination structures across team-driven networks. The work performed by health care professionals such as nurses is often considered to be highly uncertain, diverse, interdependent, and reliant on group coordination. For example, in a study of hospital care for persons with joint replacements, the use of teams with high levels of shared knowledge and goals and mutual respect positively influenced patient-assessed quality of care despite shortened lengths of stay (Gittell, 2004). In this study, task uncertainty was intensified by time constraints (i.e., shorter lengths of stay), task diversity was reflected by the multidisciplinary roles, task interdependence resulted as multidisciplinary work was performed concurrently, and the coordination device was teamwork.

Newer Organizational Theories

In this section, two newer organizational theories that have been applied in health care—including **complexity theory** (see Chapter 1), which suggests that organizations are complex adaptive systems, and **network theory**—are briefly reviewed. Complexity science arose out of the field of physical sciences in the latter half of the twentieth century. It has also provided new perspectives to reconsider both natural and human systems. The theory carries specific assumptions about systems characterized by nonlinearity and feedback loops (Hatch & Cunliffe, 2013; McDaniel et al., 2013). Complexity science is concerned with complex systems and problems that are constantly changing, multidimensional, and unpredictable, comprising interconnected diverse elements and relationships. Concepts such as chaos, self-organization, and complex adaptive systems (CAS) have been used to understand both irregular aspects of nature and provide frameworks to explore regularities that arise in complex systems. A hallmark of these ideas is the existence of nonlinearities in systems, which means that the behavior of the system is more than the sum of the behaviors of individual components (McDaniel et al., 2013).

The notion that organizations, and specifically health care systems, can be viewed as CAS has been proposed by organizational researchers (Hatch & Cunliffe, 2013; McDaniel et al., 2013). This perspective has been applied to current issues in today's health care organizations with the goal of finding new ways to understand the roles of individuals and groups (*agents*) and their effects on health care delivery processes. For example, CAS are *nonlinear and dynamic* and do not essentially reach stable equilibrium states. As a result, system behaviors may appear to be unplanned or chaotic (Rouse, 2008). As agents operate in the system, gain experience, or learn and change their behaviors, the overall system behavior naturally changes over time. This change or adaptation and learning tend to result in *self-organization* and these organizational behavior patterns can be viewed as evolving rather than being planned or constructed into the system. However, these emergent behaviors may range from valuable advances to unfortunate errors. In CAS, there is *no single point(s) of control*, and, as a result, the behaviors of CAS can usually be more easily influenced than controlled. That is, hierarchy plays a less significant role as knowledge, expertise, and decision-making are more distributed across organizational members than invested in authorities at the top of the organization. Leaders using the principles of complexity theory engage in influencing, collaborating, and relational activities rather than aiming for control of others and the future (McDaniel et al., 2013).

Theories of networks are also applied to organizational structure. Social network analysis, which builds on a system view of organizations, examines and interprets the structures and patterns of the formal and informal relationships among members of the organization (Tichy et al., 1979). A recent review of the literature by Bae et al. (2015) focused on health care provider social network analysis found that relationships among care providers were primarily built upon personal characteristics, practice settings and patient type (e.g., disease-oriented). This study also found that social networks affected some patient outcomes, care coordination approaches, and the utilization of health information systems (Bae et al., 2015). **Social capital** is another concept that has been identified in studies using social network theory and refers to resources produced by and rooted in social relationships. The concept is founded on the idea that the relationships among people in the workplace are resources that in turn can provide access to other resources through social exchange (Hatch & Cunliffe, 2013). The concept has been identified by health care leaders as an important resource that is instrumental to the success of health care organizations (Read, 2014) and that leadership in health care organizations was associated with increasing attention to social capital over time (Strömgren et al., 2017). It is receiving current attention in nursing research because greater knowledge about nurses' relationships at work may provide new insights into the creation of healthier work environments that promote positive outcomes for nurses, patients, and health care organizations.

KEY ORGANIZATIONAL DESIGN CONCEPTS

The structure of an organization can be described as the overall way work is divided into tasks and roles, grouped into subunits, and coordinated across an organization. Leaders need to address key elements when they design an organizational structure: division of labor (specialization), departmentalization, differentiation, hierarchy (chain of command), span of control, coordination (integration), centralization and decentralization, standardization, and formalization. In Table 12.1 each of

TABLE 12.1 Dimensions of Organizational Design

Dimension	Definition or Measure	Examples in Health Care and Nursing
Centralization and decentralization	The degree to which decision-making is concentrated at a single point in the organization versus the degree to which decisions are made by lower-level employees	Centralized or tall organization with several layers of management above the direct care unit level (e.g., unit coordinator, manager, director, vice president, chief executive officer [CEO]) versus flat organization with one layer (vice president) between unit manager and CEO
Coordination or integration	The coordination of activities through accountability, rules, and procedures, liaison roles, committees, task forces, cross-functional teams, or direct communication	Bed management specialist role who links across hospital units to manage access and efficient use of available beds, or a quality improvement team that works across patient care programs to improve a particular aspect of patient care such as infection rates, or inter-professional rounds on patient care units
Departmentalization	The basis by which jobs are grouped	Jobs may be grouped by function (e.g., the human resources department), or by product or service/ program (e.g., cardiac surgery, palliative care)
Differentiation	The process of dividing the work in an organization. *Vertical* differentiation is shown in the number of levels in the hierarchy, and *horizontal* differentiation is shown in the number of departments or divisions across an entire organization	*Vertical* includes several levels from care units to departments or programs/service lines to divisions, and *horizontal* refers to number of units or departments at the same level across the organization
Division of labor (or specialization)	The degree to which work activities/ tasks in an organization are divided into separate jobs	Large acute care hospitals with several levels of nursing care roles, such as patient care assistants, registered nurses, specialty nurses, advanced practice nurses, etc.
Formalization	The degree to which jobs within the organization are standardized and employee behavior is guided by rules and procedures	Formal job descriptions, certification and educational requirements for each role, standards of practice, clinical protocols, care guidelines, written procedures for various treatments, union contractual agreements
Hierarchy (or chain of command)	The structure of authority in an organization The chain of command is an unbroken line of authority that extends from the top of the organization to the lowest level and clarifies who reports to whom	CEO at the top has several vice presidents (e.g., patient care divisions, human resources, finance, etc.) who in turn have directors who in turn have unit managers who may have staff nurses and other professionals reporting to them
Size	Number of employees in the organization	Health system of multiple organizations with 2000 employees versus small rural hospital with 100 employees
Span of control	The number of subordinates a manager can efficiently and effectively direct	A nurse manager of an intensive care unit with 100 direct reports of nurses and charge nurses versus a manager of a small outpatient clinic with 20 direct reports of nurses plus support personnel
Standardization	The extent to which standard procedures govern the organization's functions and activities rather than using individual judgment	Mission and vision statements, organizational policies and procedures, clearly defined communication channels, or supervisory roles and functions

Adapted from: Hatch, M.J., & Cunliffe, A.L. (2013). *Organization theory: Modern, symbolic, and postmodern perspectives* (3rd ed.), p. 95. Oxford, UK: Oxford University Press.

these elements is presented, with definitions and examples, and the following sections describe them.

Division and Coordination of Labor

A formal organization that employs people to achieve predetermined goals divides the work among its members by assigning tasks and delegating responsibilities to positions and work units. Structure is a byproduct of the basic need to divide the labor into the specific tasks to be performed and a consequent need to coordinate these tasks to accomplish the activity or goal. The division (or differentiation) of work by occupation or by function is a form of **specialization**. As occupations and functions multiply in number, an organization increases in complexity and **size**. Size is a quantitative measure of personnel, physical capacity, volume of inputs or outputs, or discretionary resources of an organization.

The advantages of specialization include improved work performance and a critical mass of experts (Charnes & Tewksbury, 1993). In health care, specialist roles have emerged to address the increasing complexities of care and technology. Within nursing, specialist roles have also evolved to address particular areas of nursing practice and include advanced practice roles such as clinical nurse educators, nurse practitioners, and nurse anesthetists.

Organizations may also **differentiate** work units by function (also called **departmentalization**) to serve distinct client populations. For instance, rather than a single, general intensive care unit, an organization may establish several intensive care units by medical specialty (e.g., cardiovascular, neurosurgical, neonatal) or grouped into a "service line," such as palliative care or cardiac care programs. At the work group level, nursing care delivery models (e.g., team, primary, or total nursing care models) reflect different ways of dividing and coordinating the work among a team of nurses caring for clients.

Subdividing work may create breaks or fragmentation in work flow, which can be addressed in organizations by integrating work processes across roles and subunits using coordination devices (Hatch & Cunliffe, 2013). At the work group level, coordination may involve specific roles, standardization (programming), groups, or feedback devices. For example, handoff communication and techniques such as Situation, Background, Assessment, and Recommendation (SBAR) are used to coordinate between units or providers in the delivery of care.

In health care, common programming devices used to control work processes are the following:

- Standardization of worker skills coordinates work indirectly by stipulating the kind of training or education required to perform the work. In nursing, the standardization of worker skills might occur if specific degrees or certifications are required for certain roles such as nurse practitioners or critical care nurses.
- Standardization of work processes coordinates work by prespecifying or programming content before the work is undertaken, such as nurses being required to use clinical protocols or evidence-based best practice guidelines in practice.
- Standardization of work outputs coordinates work through the specification of the results, product, or performance desired or expected and includes the specification of outcome targets such as reduction of nosocomial infection rates.
- Standardization of communication methods coordinates work by providing a uniform structure for information delivery and flow in order to facilitate exchange among those involved in common work processes. In nursing, this might be achieved through electronic health records and relational databases with alerts that allow nurses and other care providers to have direct and simultaneous access to client information in a consistent format.

In addition, feedback mechanisms are used in the transfer of information in an adaptive and reciprocal manner to foster the exchange of information (Gittell, 2002):

- Mutual adjustment coordinates work by using simple informal communication and may occur when one nurse consults another nurse about practice issues, such as how to interpret a policy, or when nurses, physicians, and allied health professionals participate in clinical rounds.
- Direct supervision coordinates work through the use of a supervisor taking responsibility for the instruction and monitoring of the work of others, such as when a nurse supervises the work of assistive personnel.
- Boundary spanning roles coordinate work by managing relationships as well as the bidirectional flow of information and materials across functional divisions. For example, case managers exemplify boundary spanning because these roles manage relationships, exchange information, and negotiate resources with internal and external parties to facilitate care across occupations, services, sectors, funding agencies, and locations.

The types of **coordination** that are used may depend on the degree of stability and predictability of the work situation and the size of the work unit. For instance, acute health care settings are typically characterized as highly uncertain and interdependent work situations in which patient health needs, acuity, and care trajectories are often highly variable and unpredictable. To ensure comprehensive care, nurses coordinate patient care activities with the work of others in a reciprocal manner because the work performed is highly interdependent. As conditions become increasingly uncertain and variable, as in health care, coordination by feedback or specific liaison roles may be used. Improved health care team performance has been associated with both programming and feedback devices because standardized routines may enhance, rather than replace, the interactions among health care providers, particularly in situations of increasing uncertainty (Gittell, 2002). Recent research has shown that improved provider ratings of coordination in inpatient medicine units were linked with an organization's alignment and commitment to high-quality patient care, adequate staffing, resources that support health care professionals to do their jobs, and approaches that promote interactions and communication between nurses and physicians, such as regular multidisciplinary rounding (McIntosh et al., 2014).

At the organizational level, the coordination and division of labor influence the size and degree of organizational centralization and formalization. As organizations grow in size, work units are increasingly subdivided to ensure tasks are accomplished. However, this process slows as organizations become very large, because the gains achieved by subdividing work occur at the expense of the coordination mechanisms necessary to unify system functioning across subunits. In centralized structures, top leaders make all the decisions, and lower-level managers and staff have little decision-making discretion. In a highly formalized job, the individual has minimal discretion over what to do and when and how to do it. Organizational coordination is often measured by the degree of centralization and formalization. Health care organizations tend toward being decentralized and less formalized because professionals are employed to manage highly uncertain work. However, as organizations grow and the work becomes increasingly complex, specialized, and interdependent, there is a pull toward greater centralization and formalization (Hatch & Cunliffe, 2013).

Hierarchy

Hierarchy is the structure of authority in an organization. Authority is equated with the enforcement of regulations, which creates a governing order among the formal social relationships of organizational members (Weber, 1978). Authority is vested in positions, rather than in persons, and creates an impartial mechanism whereby the supraordinate position directs the actions and the norms expected of subordinate positions. Centralization is a multidimensional concept frequently associated with authority and hierarchy and describes the extent to which decision-making authority is concentrated in the top level of the hierarchy (i.e., centralized) versus spread down through the hierarchy (i.e., decentralized). In nursing, shared governance structures signify decentralization. **Hierarchical centralization** can vary according to the decision type.

Corporate strategy is likely to be decided by top executives, whereas procedural work decisions may be decentralized to work units or employees. For instance, a nurse executive could be required to centralize some budgetary decisions, whereas others could be decided at lower levels in the hierarchy. A specific example would be the need to centralize a component of professional development expenditures required by union contracts (e.g., organization-wide funding for nursing certification) in contrast to decisions at the work unit level to possibly fund nurses to attend their specialty conferences (some units do, some do not). Participation is an alternate dimension of centralization that refers to the scope of involvement and influence of organizational members in decision-making. Findings from a study of Belgian hospitals showed that nurses who perceived that their work decisions were tightly controlled by a supervisor (i.e., high hierarchical centralization) and they had little influence on program decisions (i.e., low participative centralization) reported lower job satisfaction (Willem et al., 2007).

In addition, hierarchy creates a reporting structure whereby formal lines of communication, in conjunction with role descriptions, delineate the responsibilities and accountability of each position for work processes and outcomes. Organizational positions are traditionally described in terms of staff and line positions (Hatch & Cunliffe, 2013). Staff positions are outside the direct hierarchical authority chain. These positions provide expertise and knowledge to support the line positions in meeting the organization's goals. The clinical nurse specialist (CNS) who is hired for knowledge development and expert consultation for selected patient groups is an example of a staff position. Line positions are in the direct line of hierarchical authority from top to bottom in an organization and are central to controlling or generating the product or service of the organization. Line positions include vice presidents, directors, managers, and frontline nurses because these positions are authorized either to supervise production processes or to produce the organization's output. In nursing, although frontline nurses are commonly referred to as "staff" nurses, these nurses hold line positions that deliver services to care recipients.

Hierarchy also enables organizations to assign responsibilities based on the complexity and skill requirements of the work and to ensure individual accountability. Responsibility is the obligation to take on and accomplish work and to secure the desired results. A manager assigns or delegates responsibility to a subordinate, and thus responsibility flows down the organizational chain. In accepting the obligation of an assigned task, the staff person is accepting responsibility to accomplish the task, whereas accountability is the liability for task performance and is determined in a retrospective analysis of what occurred. The assignment of responsibility and the granting of authority create accountability. Accountability flows upward or outward, from staff to manager or from provider to client. Reporting relationships are important for creating channels of appeal (Weber, 1978), to ensure employees are held accountable for the work assigned, and to invest managers with the necessary authority to ensure the completion of work. The manager represents the organization at the point of contact with staff, and thus the reporting relationship is also a mechanism by which staff can access organizational resources to identify and solve complex problems. Ideally, managers also apply their leadership skills to reporting relationships to release the energy and talents of people in ways that add value to the work performed. Examples of "value-added" outcomes include improved employee productivity, organizational commitment, and organizational citizenship behaviors.

Organizational Forms

The division and coordination of labor lead to varied organizational forms. As illustrated by the sloping triangles in Fig. 12.1, organizational forms reflect a trade-off between differentiation by function and integration by program. **Differentiation by function** refers to the division of work by occupation. **Integration by program** means the coordination of work around the delivery of particular products or services. Five basic organizational forms can be situated along a differentiation–integration continuum (Charnes & Tewksbury, 1993). Functional and program forms represent extreme examples of differentiation and integration. The matrix form represents the most balanced form. In reality, organizations are not usually found in these pure forms but instead reflect hybrids of the forms described next.

Functional Form

At the extreme left end of the continuum, dividing the work by occupation leads to a functional organization

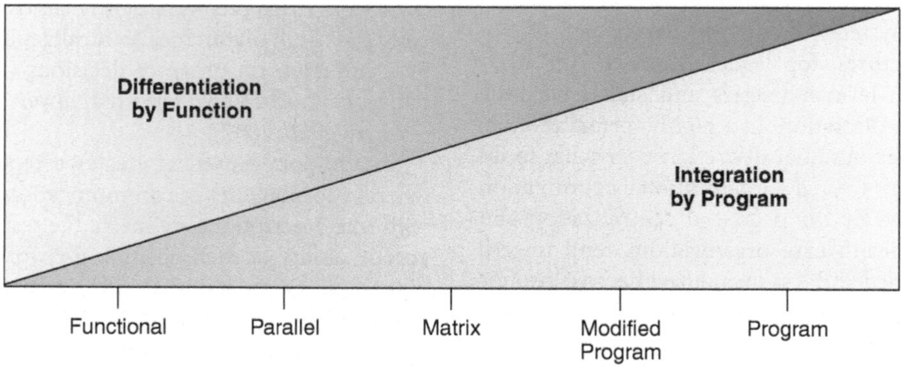

Fig. 12.1 Continuum of organizational configurations. (Adapted from Charnes, M., & Tewksbury, L. [1993]. *Collaborative management in health care: Implementing the integrative organization* [p. 28, Fig. 2.1]. San Francisco, CA: Jossey-Bass. This material is used by permission of John Wiley & Sons.)

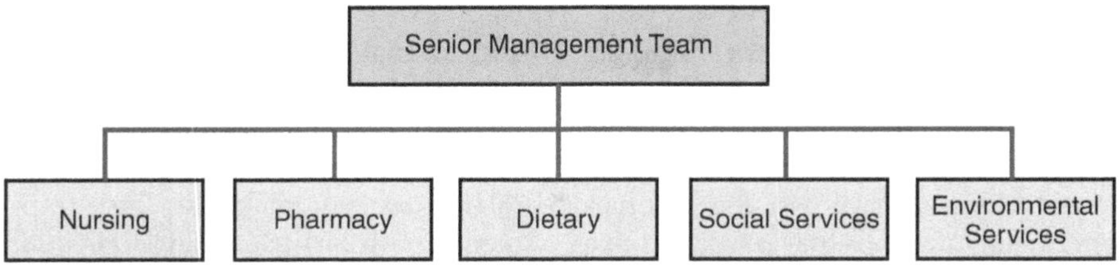

Fig. 12.2 Simplified functional form.

whereby health professions and nonprofessional services are arranged according to the type of work performed. The emphasis is on the human resources inputs to the organization (Fig. 12.2). Examples are nursing, respiratory therapy, admitting, and environmental services. Within each functional department, management develops specific structures, policies, procedures, and human resource practices. In this type of organizational form, professionals report directly to a discipline-specific supervisor (e.g., nurses would report to a nurse manager). Members of a functional group (e.g., nursing) are likely to interact more frequently, develop social relationships, receive supervision and evaluations from within the group, and conform to professional standards (Charnes & Tewksbury, 1993).

By dividing personnel according to the type of work performed, organizations can capitalize on the expertise, experience, efficiency, and professional standards that each discipline offers (Charnes & Tewksbury, 1993). Other benefits include cost reduction through shared resources; enhanced monitoring of cost, performance, and quality; and promotion of professional development, identity, autonomy, advocacy, and career advancement. Disadvantages of the functional form are its potential to overemphasize professional silos, discourage informal relationships across disciplines, and fragment care delivery (Charnes & Tewksbury, 1993). Coordination of activities becomes challenging because group members have functionally based differences in work goals, cognitive patterns, and status (Gittell, 2004). Because the work of nursing is highly interdependent with other professional and nonprofessional work, nurse leaders in functional forms may use coordination mechanisms and leadership behaviors to span the boundaries between disciplines and facilitate the flow and exchange of information, resources, and work activities. Although prevalent in health care in the 1980s, functional forms have gradually been replaced by program or matrix forms to enhance patient centeredness.

Program Form

At the extreme right end of the continuum, program organizations emphasize integration of the work by consumer, service, or geography (Charnes & Tewksbury, 1993). The emphasis is on the outputs of the organization (Fig. 12.3). In health care, programs may be managed according to consumer health needs (e.g., diabetes, cancer), consumer age (e.g., elderly, neonates, women),

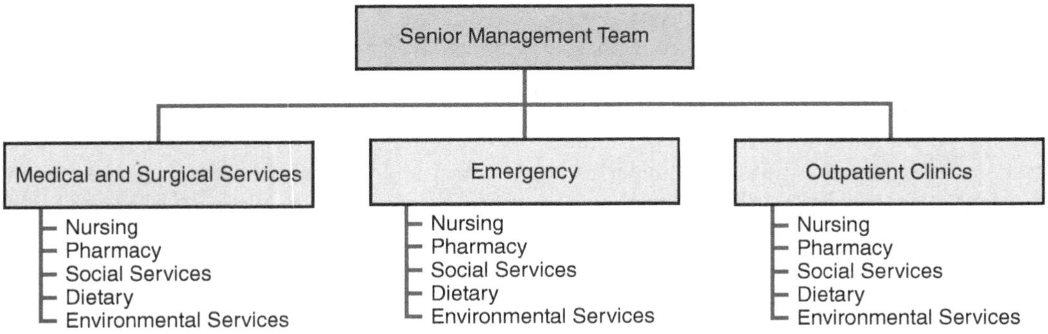

Fig. 12.3 Simplified program form.

services (e.g., addictions, rehabilitation), medical specialty (e.g., neurosciences, endocrinology), or geography (e.g., catchment areas). Although the corporate structure is shared, each program tends to operate as a semiautonomous unit with its own management team composed of medical, administrative, and nursing representatives (Charnes & Tewksbury, 1993). Professionals who work in program organizations may not report to a discipline-specific supervisor.

Program designs can optimize service delivery because local experts with accountability for costs, outcomes, and staffing control resources and can make timely operational decisions (Leatt et al., 1994). Patients can access integrated services from an array of health professionals with specific clinical expertise. With the program form, there is a push toward a multidisciplinary team approach. However, clients who require access to more than one program may find it difficult to coordinate services among different programs. Integration by program occurs at the expense of decreased coordination among programs (Charnes & Tewksbury, 1993). Although organizational relationships with medical staff are enhanced when programs are grouped by medical specialty, health care professionals may be isolated from their colleagues in other programs, and this has been associated with job dissatisfaction and lack of professional development opportunities (Young et al., 2004). For nursing, the concern is that no organization-wide mechanisms would exist to systematically handle professional nursing issues in terms of standards, resources, or professional advocacy. Because each program operates independently, processes and procedures are likely to be duplicated, and programs may compete for resources or develop goals that diverge from the corporate mission (Leatt et al., 1994).

Parallel Form

To address the challenges of purely functional forms, mechanisms in the parallel form assist in coordinating across functional departments (Charnes & Tewksbury, 1993). These mechanisms can include teams, specialists, task forces, liaison roles, and standing committees. For example, rather than each functional department separately establishing procedures to hire staff, a specialized human resource department may be created to deal with recruitment and employment issues across the organization. Another example is a rapid response team in a hospital that is composed of intensive care physicians and nurses and respiratory therapists. This team assists staff throughout the hospital in detecting and managing imminent patient deterioration and in resuscitating compromised patients. Likewise, in home care, nurses with specialized expertise such as wound care or palliative care might be responsible for referrals across multiple areas. Task forces bring together members from various divisions in an organization to address a concern. For example, developing and implementing critical pathways, evidence-based practices, disease management initiatives, case management projects, or outcomes management efforts generally require an interdisciplinary team of specialists. These types of mechanisms foster collaboration and cross-fertilization of knowledge across divisions and can reinforce consistency in clinical and management practices by standardizing procedures.

Modified Program Form

To offset the fragmentation and isolation of functions in pure program structures, organizations maintain the program structure and develop integrative mechanisms to unify functions and occupations across programs (Charnes & Tewksbury, 1993). For example, a nurse executive could address professional nursing issues related to standards, educational resources, and research activities across the organization. Unlike their counterpart in a functional nursing department who has line authority, a nurse executive in a modified program would not directly control operations, finances, or personnel issues (known as *staff authority*). A nurse executive with staff authority need to use personal influence and leadership skills to effect change.

Matrix Form

In a pure matrix form, people and work are organized along both functional and program dimensions (Charnes & Tewksbury, 1993). Essentially, the program form overlays the functional form (Fig. 12.4). Although some employees may have dual reporting relationships, staff members are evaluated by both supervisors. The budget and decision-making are shared between functional and program divisions. A matrix configuration has the flexibility to adapt to change and to deliver services innovatively and efficiently by drawing on a varied talent pool (Hatch & Cunliffe, 2013). In contrast, innovation in program forms is costly because additional cross-coordination may be required across functional

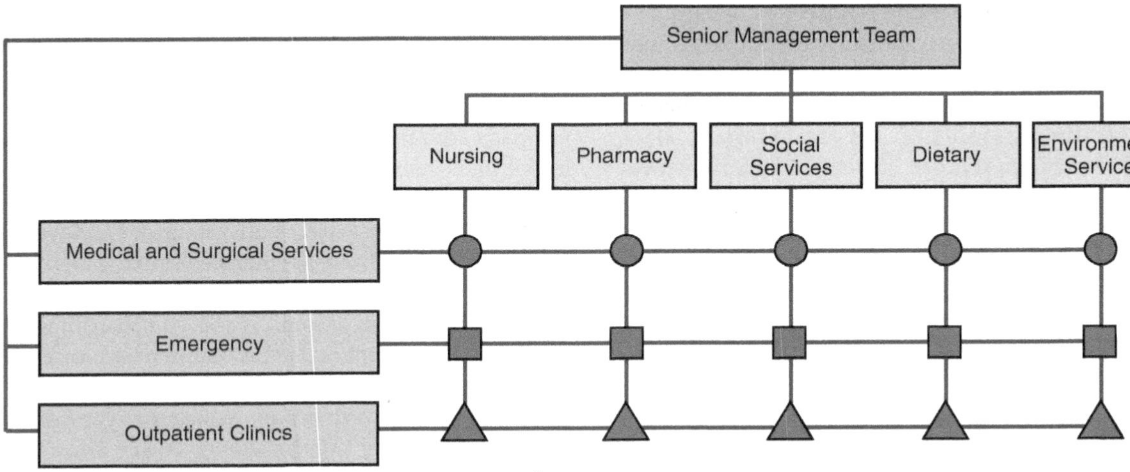

For example, team members for Outpatient Clinics (▲) are drawn from different functions.

Fig. 12.4 Simplified matrix form.

divisions, or specialists may need to be hired for each program. However, true matrix forms are rarely seen and are difficult to maintain because the additional management infrastructure is costly and dual reporting relationships may be ambiguous and lead to conflict (Charnes & Tewksbury, 1993). Success requires well-educated workers who can handle a multifaceted communication and authority web. Nurses in matrix organizations need strong interpersonal and teamwork skills to negotiate these complex environments.

ORGANIZATIONAL CHARTS

Hierarchy reflects the *formal* structure of the organization, which can be identified on an organizational chart. An organizational chart is a visual display of the organization's positions and the intentional relationships among positions. The organizational chart reflects the various positions and the formal relationships between and among the positions and, by extension, the people who are a part of the organization. The organizational chart generally presents the line positions, linked together by solid lines to show the flow of authority. Administrative roles are generally shown in vertical and horizontal dimensions. Staff positions or advisory bodies may be depicted on the chart with dotted lines to show consultative relationships. Organizational charts help with administrative control, policy making and planning, and the evaluation of the organization's strengths and weaknesses. They clearly depict who reports to whom. Charts are used to orient personnel because relationships and expected patterns of interaction within the formal organization are made clear. For example, an organizational chart of a matrix structure may show dotted lines for the project or interdisciplinary team relationships. Dotted lines mean that a relationship to the position or the group would form for a project. In the process of applying for a job, obtaining the employer's organizational chart will help understand the relative positioning of individuals within the organization and how the organization is structured—or at least how decision makers believe it is structured.

In addition to a *formal* structure, organizations are characterized by an *informal* structure. The *informal* structure is simply the network or pattern of social relationships and friendship circles that are outside the formal structure. It is an interconnected web of relationships that operate in and around the formally designated lines of communication. The *informal* structure does not appear on the *formal* organizational chart.

ORGANIZATIONAL SHAPES

The shape of an organization structure can be described as relatively tall or flat. Several structural factors influence the shape of an organization. The formal reporting relationships among positions ensure the assignment of responsibility, authority, and accountability and result in hierarchical levels. The **span of control** of managers—the number of employees reporting directly to a management position—also influences organizational shape (Meyer, 2008). For instance, when managers on average have fewer direct-report staff, the organizational shape is relatively taller. Another structural factor involves decisions about the number of management layers in the hierarchy (i.e., the **scalar principle**). Increased layers of management help the organization cope with increasing work complexity and extended timelines (Jaques, 1990). A tall organization structure assumes a pyramidal shape with multiple management layers (Fig. 12.5). In contrast, a flat organization structure has minimal management layers (Fig. 12.6). Advantages and disadvantages associated with tall and flat organizational shapes are summarized in Table 12.2. However, a narrow focus on the hierarchical structure of an organization without attention to the people and processes within the organization or the outcomes achieved can be misleading. For instance, factors that can potentially offset the effects of tall organizations include the competence and leadership of members, the use of merit-based rewards, the effectiveness of reporting relationships, and the sharing of information and authority (Jaques, 1990).

Span of management refers to the number and ordering of management positions and resources relative to other personnel and can be measured at organizational, departmental, managerial, work group, or employee levels (Meyer, 2008). There are many competing arguments about factors influencing the span of management, and decisions about the amount, type, and distribution of nursing management resources within health care organizations are influenced by a multitude of factors at the consumer, nurse, work group, manager, organizational, and regional levels (Meyer, 2008). A key controversy about the span of control of nurse managers relates to supervisory responsibilities. On the one hand, wider spans of control for managers are proposed because nurses and other health care professionals are experts committed to professional codes of ethics and regulated

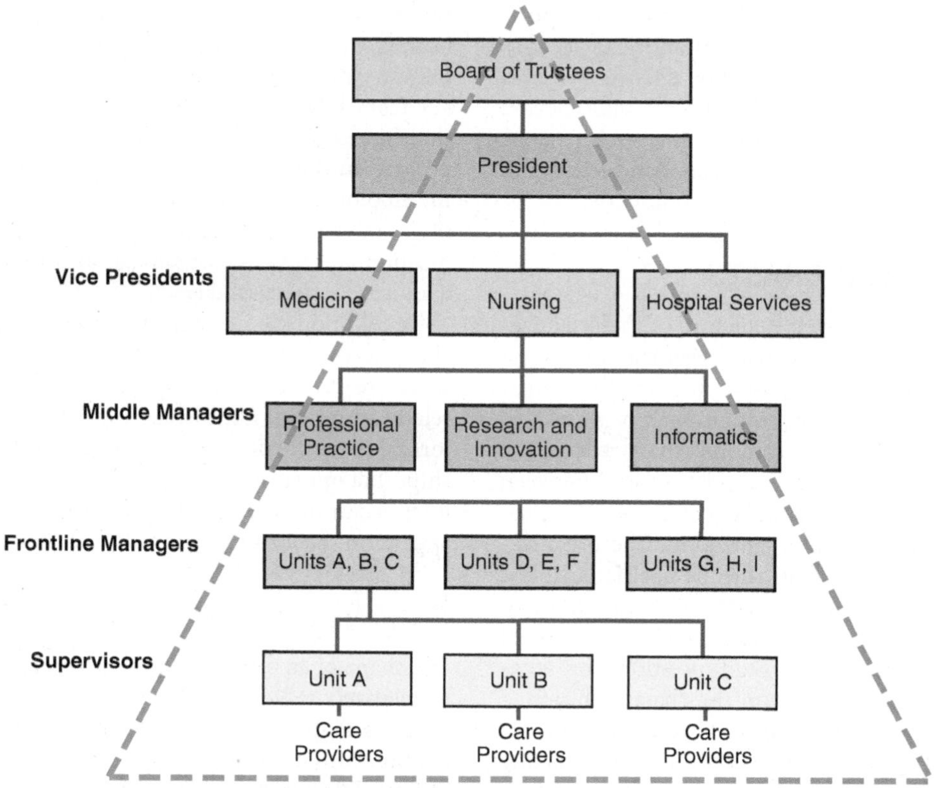

Fig. 12.5 Simplified tall organizational structure.

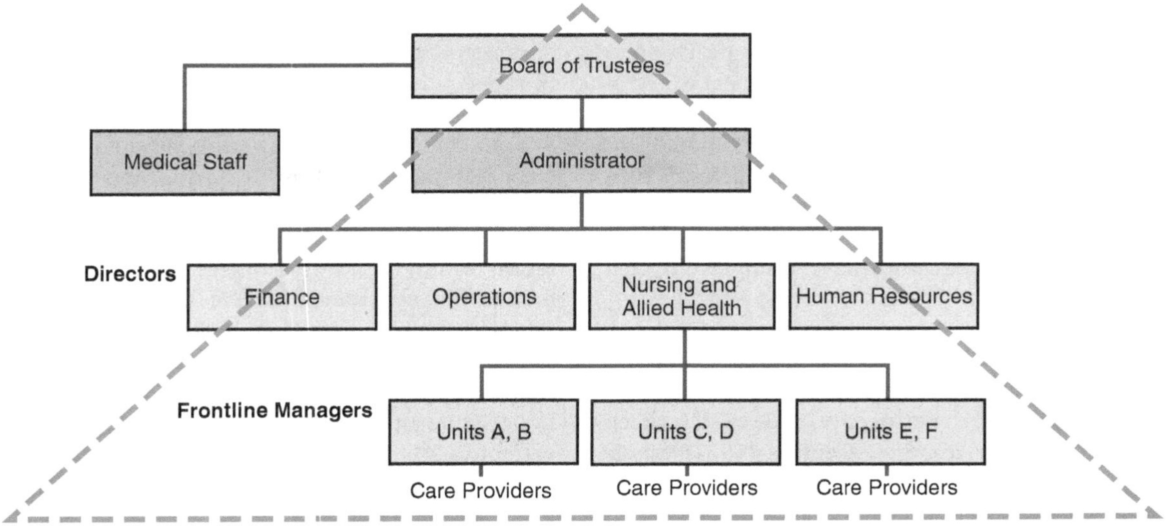

Fig. 12.6 Simplified flat organizational structure.

TABLE 12.2 Comparison of Flat and Tall Organization Structures

	Tall Organization	Flat Organization
Advantages	• Increased access to managers and organizational resources • Greater supervisory capability • Layers of skill to deal with varying degrees of work complexity • Layers of accountability for work completion • Layers of responsibility to address short, medium, and long-term issues and planning	• Fewer divisions facilitate streamlining of goals, problem-solving, and resource use • Greater hierarchical decentralization; potential for greater staff autonomy through increased delegation • Greater innovation • Enhanced responsiveness to consumers at point of service • Less cross-coordination required • Less costly management infrastructure
Disadvantages	• More hierarchical centralization; potential to micromanage staff activities • Slowed vertical decision-making and distorted communication • Less innovation • Difficult way-finding for consumers • Greater cross coordination required • Costly management infrastructure	• Decreased access to managers and organizational resources • Decreased supervisory capability • Overextension of managers • Vertical communication delays

 Table based on: Alidina & Funke-Furber, 1988; Jaques, 1990; Pabst, 1993.

standards, therefore requiring less direct supervision (Meier & Bohte, 2003). On the other hand, narrow spans of control are deemed necessary because (1) nurses require managerial support and access to organizational resources and information to coordinate complex work processes to achieve positive outcomes, and (2) the introduction of unlicensed workers into health care settings has required more direct, hands-on supervision to ensure that care standards and organizational expectations are met. This counterargument suggests that the span of control of frontline nurse managers should factor in the needs of staff nurses for their manager's support and supervision. In nursing, relationships between the span of control of frontline managers and manager, nurse, and clinical outcomes have been investigated (Wong et al., 2015).

STRUCTURAL POWER

Within the objective perspective, power has been conceptualized as a resource. Kanter's (1977) classic theory of the structural determinants of behavior in organizations has been investigated in nursing systems (Laschinger, 1996). For Kanter (1977, p. 166), power refers to "the ability to get things done, to mobilize resources." It is not the power to control or dominate others. When power is shared, rather than monopolized, employees are empowered, and the organization is more likely to benefit. More activity can be accomplished by organizational members, and the capacity for effective action is increased. Kanter (1977) described three work empowerment structures: opportunity, power, and proportion. The structure of *opportunity* refers to expectations and future prospects (e.g., opportunities for growth, mobility, job enrichment). The structure of *power* stems from access to information, support, and resources. The structure of *proportion* denotes the social composition of the organization's workforce (e.g., gender, minorities). Empowered work environments are those in which all employees have access to opportunities to learn and grow and to information, support, and resources necessary for the job. Indeed, frontline nurses' job-related or structural empowerment has been linked to positive nurse outcomes, including greater nurse job satisfaction (Cicolini et al., 2014; Wong & Laschinger, 2013), increased organizational commitment (Smith et al., 2010; Yang et al., 2013), feelings of trust and respect in the workplace (Laschinger et al., 2014), lower job and career turnover intentions (Choi et al., 2014; Laschinger & Fida, 2014), and lower burnout and workplace incivility (Laschinger et al., 2013). Nurses who occupy positions at higher levels in the nursing hierarchy reported increasingly greater degrees of empowerment (Laschinger et al., 2012), which may mean that nurses in management positions are likely to perceive greater access to opportunity and power structures than frontline nurses.

In Kanter's (1977) study, effective leaders were seen as both competent and powerful. Sensitivity with subordinates was secondary to having upward credibility within the organization; leaders to whom others listened, who accessed resources, and who produced results within the broader organization were perceived to be effective. Kanter (1977) proposed that effective leadership evolves from both *formal* and *informal* sources of power in the organization. *Formal* power is derived from work that is relevant to pressing organizational issues and that provides opportunities to perform extraordinary and highly visible activities; *informal* power comes from relationships and alliances with people in the organization.

Kanter (1977, p. 168) also theorized that "power begets power." Research indicates that nurses who are managed by empowered leaders are also empowered (Laschinger, 1996). For example, frontline nurses in organizations where chief nurse executives had line authority reported significantly greater global empowerment with respect to resources than their counterparts in organizations where chief nurse executives had staff authority (Matthews et al., 2006). The authors suggested that the *formal* power accessible to nurse executives with line authority enabled them to secure the staffing resources necessary for frontline nurses to provide high quality of care. Magnet hospitals typically consist of flat organizational structures with nursing councils that empower nurses through decentralized decision-making. This structure engages staff nurses in decisions affecting their work, for example, when inter-professional staff work together to redesign workflow. Considered overall, the research suggests that empowerment structures have a positive impact on both nurses and managers and can inform the design of the organizational structures in which nurses work.

LEADERSHIP AND MANAGEMENT IMPLICATIONS

The global and local challenges for nursing within organizations and across systems are numerous. Leaders and managers can influence the structure in which goals are accomplished. In fact, determining the structure is a key responsibility of leaders and managers in planning an organization that is conducive to high-quality nursing care. As environments and technologies evolve, the leadership and management team may need to rethink and redesign the organization and work group structures to better match the changing conditions and achieve the desired outcomes. In nursing, determining the structure is a planning and organizing aspect of the management process that can be informed by evidence and theory from the management field.

Leaders and managers may be involved in revising or changing organizational structures. *Restructuring* means revising or modifying the structure to reshape it or switch to another structural form. Restructuring efforts have typically been geared toward fixing existing operational processes. Lean, decentralized, self-governing organizations that empower first-line caregivers are the preferred structures. To begin anew, processes are analyzed from the point of view of the consumer (patient and family) as well as the requirement to achieve greater cost containment, quality, service, and speed. User-friendly processes, efficiency, and economy are key ideas. Job redesign focuses on who does what tasks and on maximizing flexibility, cross-training, and productivity.

Changes to organization structure afford opportunities to empower nurses. Strategies include maximizing nurses' scope of practice, creating autonomous and visible nursing roles relevant to organizational priorities, and providing more leadership opportunities for nurses at all levels. Fiscal and material resources can also be deployed to empower nurses by facilitating access to knowledge-development opportunities (e.g., courses, conferences) and by providing adequate resources for job completion (e.g., staffing). A decentralized, participative structure can be promoted through coordination mechanisms that involve nurses in shared governance councils and task forces (e.g., related to clinical practice or nurse retention) and in information exchange (e.g., newsletters, open forums, web technologies).

A transparent and participative approach to the development of programming devices to standardize work processes (e.g., clinical protocols, electronic health records) can be used to build shared goals for interdisciplinary teams. Organizations can also deliberately foster informal coordination mechanisms to enhance the relational and functional networks in which work is accomplished (Hatch & Cunliffe, 2013). For example, physical colocation, communal space, communities of practice, rotational job assignments, electronic chat groups, and interdisciplinary training programs can foster spontaneous interactions and relationships across functional, professional, and geographical silos, resulting in knowledge sharing, problem-solving, and innovation.

Hierarchical reporting relationships can be greatly enhanced by transformational leaders who establish trust with nurses by communicating role and behavior expectations, giving constructive performance feedback, and recognizing and rewarding successes (Wong & Laschinger, 2013). When workers fall outside organizational lines of authority (e.g., outsourced services, nursing agencies such as travelers), managers and leaders need skills in negotiating standards and performance outcomes, in resolving problems across organizational boundaries, and in building relationships and shared goals to overcome differing alliances (Porter-O'Grady & Malloch, 2014).

In more highly matrixed organizations, nurse managers and leaders need to network with interdisciplinary stakeholders within and across programs and support services. Success for leaders with line authority requires strong relational skills, credibility, an ability to link resource use to outcomes using a business model, and an in-depth understanding of the needs of clients and staff (Lorenz, 2008). The trends toward increased outsourcing, decreased reliance on traditional inpatient services for revenues, and increased specialization of health services require an entrepreneurial skill set and innovative leadership roles to build business partnerships and alliances and to foster change at the point of service delivery (Porter-O'Grady, 2015). In the context of nurse and manager shortages, organizations need to recruit and deploy management resources in line with objectives by reevaluating the number of management layers and the span of control of individual positions, as well as by developing a nursing leadership succession plan. To be supportive of nursing staff, nurse managers need access to the support and information of senior management and peers, professional development and mentorship, an office that is easily accessible to staff, administrative support, and a strong and shared organizational culture.

Organizational Assessment

Nurse leaders can use organizational assessment to generate data needed for analysis that serves as the foundation for planning and change management as well as to identify the status of quality and safety efforts. Organizational assessments focus on assisting teams, departments, organizations, and systems to better understand the organization as it is and to continuously improve by indicating areas in need of further development. There are a variety of organizational assessments. Some are commercial or not in health care, like the Organizational Assessment (Lusthaus et al., 2002). Some are both in business and industry as well as health care, such as the Malcolm Baldrige National Quality Award (American Society for Quality [ASQ], n.d.), which recognizes US companies that have implemented successful quality management systems. Some focus specifically on the unit, such as the Dartmouth Institute for Health Policy & Clinical Practice's (2010) Microsystems at a Glance and the Institute for Healthcare Improvement's (IHI) (2016) Clinical Microsystem Assessment Tool. In nursing, the Magnet Recognition Program (American Nurses Credentialing Center, n.d.) only focuses on the quality of nursing services and resources for nurses.

CURRENT ISSUES AND TRENDS

During the 1990s, health care systems in many developed countries were subjected to restructuring, decentralization, specialization, and performance management, resulting in the de-layering of management structures in an effort to contain costs and achieve outcomes (Mahon & Young, 2006). Those managers remaining in the system faced expanded roles. Instead of a traditional head nurse position responsible for patient care on a single unit, the role of the nurse manager typically grew to encompass the management of finances, operations, and human resources across multiple clinical areas and services in program management structures with regulated and unregulated multidisciplinary staff.

The twenty-first century has ushered in significant concerns related to the global community and public safety. These issues are intensified by calls for transparency, accountability, and public reporting in the management of health care services, which in turn have increased demands on the internal structures and external boundaries of organizations. In addition, at a societal level, preparedness for disasters, bioterrorism, and pandemics has required health care organizations, communities, and jurisdictions to pool resources and coordinate activities along the external boundaries of organizational structures. Furthermore, large companies in the business world have been working to eliminate *vertical* and *horizontal* boundaries within and to break down *external* barriers between the company and its customers and suppliers. This **boundaryless** organization seeks to eliminate the hierarchical chain of command, replace departments with empowered teams, and promote learning in order to keep pace with rapid change (Hatch & Cunliffe, 2013). Although achieving a boundaryless state may never be completely actualized, especially in health care organizations, there is evidence of moves to create better integration of care delivery processes across care sectors and organizations within health systems (Edgren & Barnard, 2012).

Attempts to remove vertical boundaries, flatten the hierarchy and implement cross-functional and cross-organizational teams (which include senior executives, middle managers, supervisors, employees, and care recipients), participative decision-making practices, and boundary-spanning leadership practices are being implemented in health care to break down vertical and horizontal boundaries (Shirey & White-Williams, 2015). With wide-ranging changes introduced with the Affordable Care Act (ACA) of 2010 and the Institute for Healthcare Improvement's (IHI's) Triple Aim framework for optimizing health system performance, a focus for organizations is on improving individual patient and family care experiences, increasing the health of populations, reforming primary care, and reducing overall costs. All of these priorities require high levels of system integration and even transformation (Shirey & White-Williams, 2015). One solution has been a rise in the number of health care organizations (hospitals, ambulatory facilities, continuing care homes, and home health) merging not only to achieve economies of scale but as also as a way of better organizing the clinical functions across different sites and locations (Kerfoot & Luquire, 2012; Shirey & White-Williams, 2015). With the emergence of these larger health systems, the role of the system chief nurse executive has increased (Bradley, 2014).

At a global level, increasing shortages of nurses and other health care professionals has engendered a call for developed countries to create self-sufficient and sustainable nursing workforces by increasing domestic supply (Gantz et al., 2012). At the organizational level, employers need to attract and retain nurses through changes to work conditions and structures such as creating full-time positions, re-dividing work to continue to remove non-nursing tasks, supplying adequate staffing and material resources to accomplish the work, and improving work climates that support exemplary professional nursing practice (Gantz et al., 2012). These strategies are necessary to stabilize the nursing workforce within organizations and to ensure that the knowledge, skills, and competence that nurses possess are retained and appropriately deployed in the organization.

Increased awareness and disclosure about medical errors and preventable adverse events have encouraged organizations to address consumer safety through risk reduction and the development of cultures of safety (DiCuccio, 2015). To address safety, new coordination mechanisms and explicit safety standards are based on the science of human factors engineering, which takes a systems approach to understanding and preventing critical incidents (Carayon et al., 2014). A systems approach considers how adverse events occur in relation to management, organization, and regulatory factors such as policies and procedures, information technology, staffing practices, and physical structures. Recall that policies, procedures, and information systems are coordination devices. For instance, safety risks may be reduced when nurses standardize care through the use of evidence-based clinical protocols. Organizations are also compelled to collaborate in the development and sharing of safety innovations. The Center for Quality Improvement and Safety in the United States and the Canadian Patient Safety Institute in Canada are examples of how safety innovations can be widely shared and standardized across organizations.

RESEARCH NOTE

Source

Louis, C. J., Clark, J. R., Gray, B., Brannon, D., & Parker, V. (2019). Service line structure and decision-maker attention in three health systems: Implications for patient-centered care. *Health Care Management Review*, *44*(1), 41–56.

Purpose

The aim of this study was to understand the role of service line structure in producing coordinated, patient-centered care.

Description

Prior research has identified a disconnect between the level at which structure is typically examined (the organization level) and where coordination effort actually takes place (e.g., the delivery of services). However, we know little about the role that structure plays in care coordination. In this study, a comparative case study approach was used to understand the role structure played in care coordination efforts at three different health systems. The study specifically investigated the delivery of breast cancer care, the care providers involved, and services provided.

Results

This study found that the three health systems had substantial variation in service line structure. Corresponding variation was also found in terms of where each health system primarily focused in coordinating care. These results draw a clear connection between the organization's structural characteristics and the dominant focus of attention (operational tactics, provider roles and relationships, or patient needs and engagement) at the service line level.

Application to Practice

The structure and design of health care organizations and service lines influences how care providers function and can enable (or hinder) their propensity to collaborate. In each of the organizations in this study, a different dominant focus of attention was found and ultimately influenced the level at which the care providers could put the patient at the center of care processes. Achieving a patient-centered attention may require careful internal planning of service line structure such that inter-departmental barriers are removed and collaborative efforts across provider specialties are prioritized. The alternative is a less desirable, more fragmented orientation where staff and care providers are constantly focusing on operational process workarounds and overcoming barriers to timely, efficient care.

CASE STUDY

Consolidation of Inpatient Services at Two Community Hospitals

Hospital A is the flagship hospital in a two-hospital health system and is located in the suburbs of a major US city. Hospital A is comprised of 240 medical/surgical and telemetry beds and has eight units, each with the maximum capacity of 30 beds. Over the past 12 months the average daily census (ADC) in this hospital is 40% (96 patients), with a peak census of 70% (168 patients). Hospital A also has 20 Intensive Care Unit (ICU) beds and the ADC over the past 12 months was 40% (eight patients), with a peak census of 90% (18 patients).

Hospital B is located 7 miles away from Hospital A and is in a rural location. Hospital B is comprised of 100 medical/surgical and telemetry beds and has five units, each with the maximum capacity of 20 beds. The ADC over the past 12 months is 33% (33 patients), with a peak census of 75% (75 patients). Hospital B also has a six-bed ICU, and the ADC over the past 12 months is 33% (two patients), with a peak census of 100% (six patients).

Health system leadership has noticed a steady decline in inpatient admissions at their two hospitals over the past 3 years resulting in the current census numbers. The organization has been running at a loss ("in the red") for the past 2 years. Moreover, challenges with patient throughput, care coordination, and timely discharge have plagued the organization for years. The current average length of stay (ALOS) across both hospitals for medical/surgical patients is 5.9 days and ICU patients is 9.8 days. When compared to other local competitors, these ALOS data suggest that they are approximately 10%–20% higher on average.

The current situation is not sustainable. Alternatives for restructuring were reviewed and evaluated. What is the best way to improve the functioning of inpatient services?

CRITICAL THINKING EXERCISE

Nursing leadership been asked to assess the feasibility of consolidating inpatient services across the two hospitals. Hospital A and Hospital B have a long history of serving the communities for decades, so the decisions must be considered carefully. They need your help in understanding the operational, cultural, and political benefits and drawbacks of each option. Financial analysis will be performed by the Finance team at the completion of this operational exercise and is not your responsibility.

1. What elements of organization structure and design must be considered in determining whether consolidation of inpatient services is feasible?
2. Who are the key internal and external stakeholders that would be impacted by a decision to consolidate inpatient units at the two hospitals? Why must their perspectives be considered?
3. What are the key operational challenges with consolidating the medical/surgical and telemetry units at both hospitals? What about with the intensive care units (ICUs)?
4. What role might improve care coordination, reduced average length of stay (ALOS), or more timely discharge play in your decision to consolidate units? Would consolidation prompt a culture change within the health system?
5. You are the Chief Nursing Officer. What is your recommendation to other health system leadership—do you recommend consolidating the inpatient units or not? Why or why not?

REFERENCES

Alidina, S., & Funke-Furber, J. (1988). First line nurse managers: Optimizing the span of control. *Journal of Nursing Administration, 18*(5), 34–39.

American Nurses Credentialing Center. (n.d.). *Magnet model–Creating a Magnet culture.* https://www.nursingworld.org/organizational-programs/magnet/magnet-model/.

American Society for Quality (ASQ). (n.d.). *Malcolm Baldrige National Quality Award (MBNQA).* http://asq.org/learn-about-quality/malcolm-baldrige-award/overview/overview.html.

Bae, S., Nikolaev, A., Seo, J., & Castner, J. (2015). Health care provider social network analysis: A systematic review. *Nursing Outlook, 63*(5), 566–584.

Bradley, C. (2014). Leading nursing through influence and structure: The system nurse executive role. *Journal of Nursing Administration, 44*(12), 619–621.

Carayon, P., Xie, A., & Kianfar, S. (2014). Human factors and ergonomics as a patient safety practice. *BMJ Quality & Safety, 23*(3), 196–205.

Charnes, M., & Tewksbury, L. (1993). The continuum of organization structures. In *Collaborative management in health care: Implementing the integrative organization*. (pp. 20–43). San Francisco, CA: Jossey-Bass.

Choi, S., Jang, I., Park, S., & Lee, H. (2014). Effects of organizational culture, self-leadership and empowerment on job satisfaction and turnover intention in general hospital nurses. *Journal of Korean Academy of Nursing Administration, 20*(2), 206–214.

Cicolini, G., Comparcini, D., & Simonetti, V. (2014). Workplace empowerment and nurses' job satisfaction: A systematic literature review. *Journal of Nursing Management, 22*(7), 855–871.

Clegg, S. R. (1990). *Modern organizations: Organization studies in the postmodern world*. Sage Publications.

Dartmouth Institute for Health Policy & Clinical Practice. (2010). *Microsystems at a glance*. https://studylib.net/doc/8879258/microsystems-at-a-glance—the-dartmouth-institute—micr...

DiCuccio, M. H. (2015). The relationship between patient safety culture and patient outcomes: A systematic review. *Journal of Patient Safety, 11*(3), 135–142.

Donabedian, A. (1980). *Explorations in quality assessment and monitoring: The definition of quality and approaches to its assessment* (Vol. 1). Ann Arbor, MI: Health Administration Press.

Edgren, L., & Barnard, K. (2012). Complex adaptive systems for management of integrated care. *Leadership in Health Services, 25*(1), 39–51.

Eisenstein, H. (1995). The Australian femocratic experiment: A feminist case for bureaucracy. In M. M. Ferree, & P. Y. Martin (Eds.), *Feminist organizations: Harvest of the new women's movement* (pp. 69–83). Philadelphia, PA: Temple University Press.

Farmer, D. J. (1997). The postmodern turn and the Socratic gadfly. In H. T. Miller, & C. J. Fox (Eds.), *Postmodernism "reality" and public administration* (pp. 105–117). Burke, VA: Chatelaine Press.

Gantz, N. R., Sherman, R., Jasper, M., Choo, C. G., Herrin-Griffith, D., & Harris, K. (2012). Global nurse leader perspectives on health systems and workforce challenges. *Journal of Nursing Management, 20*(4), 433–443.

Gittell, J. H. (2002). Coordinating mechanisms in care provider groups: Relational coordination as a mediator and input uncertainty as a moderator of performance effects. *Management Science, 48*(11), 1408–1426.

Gittell, J. H. (2004). Achieving focus in hospital care: The role of relational coordination. In R. E. Herzlinger (Ed.), *Consumer-driven health care: Implications for providers, payers, and policymakers* (pp. 683–695). San Francisco, CA: Jossey-Bass.

Hatch, M. J., & Cunliffe, A. L. (2013). *Organization theory: Modern, symbolic, and postmodern perspectives* (3rd ed.). Oxford, UK: Oxford University Press.

Institute for Healthcare Improvement (IHI). (2016). *Clinical microsystem assessment tool*. http://www.ihi.org/resources/pages/tools/clinicalmicrosystemassessmenttool.aspx.

Jaques, E. (1990). In praise of hierarchy. *Harvard Business Review, 68*(1), 127–133.

Kanter, R. M. (1977). *Men and women of the corporation*. New York, NY: Basic Books.

Kerfoot, K. M., & Luquire, R. (2012). Alignment of the system's chief nursing officer: Staff or direct line structure? *Nursing Administration Quarterly, 36*(4), 325–331.

Laschinger, H. K. S. (1996). A theoretical approach to studying work empowerment in nursing: A review of studies testing Kanter's theory of structural power in organizations. *Nursing Administration Quarterly, 20*(2), 25–41.

Laschinger, H. K. S., & Fida, R. (2014). A time-lagged analysis of the effect of authentic leadership on workplace bullying, burnout, and occupational turnover intentions. *European Journal of Work and Organizational Psychology, 23*(5), 739–753.

Laschinger, H. K., Wong, C. A., Cummings, G. G., & Grau, A. (2014). Resonant leadership and workplace empowerment: The value of positive organizational cultures in reducing workplace incivility. *Nursing Economics, 32*(1), 5–15, 44.

Laschinger, H. K., Wong, C. A., & Grau, A. (2013). Authentic leadership, empowerment and burnout: A comparison in new graduates and experienced nurses. *Journal of Nursing Management, 21*(3), 541–552.

Laschinger, H. K., Wong, C. A., Grau, A. L., Read, E. A., & Pineau Stam, L. M. (2012). The influence of leadership practices and empowerment on Canadian nurse manager outcomes. *Journal of Nursing Management, 20*(7), 877–888.

Leatt, P., Lemieux-Charles, L., & Aird, C. (1994). Program management: Introduction and overview. In L. Lemieux-Charles, P. Leatt, & C. Aird (Eds.), *Program management and beyond: Management innovations in Ontario hospitals* (pp. 1–10): Ottawa, ON, Canada: Canadian College of Health Service Executives.

Lorenz, H. L. (2008). Service line leadership. *Nurse Leader, 6*(1), 42–43.

Louis, C. J., Clark, J. R., Gray, B., Brannon, D., & Parker, V. (2019). Service line structure and decision-maker attention in three health systems: Implications for patient-centered care. *Health Care Management Review, 44*(1), 41–56.

Lusthaus, C., Adrien, M., Anderson, G., Carden, F., & Montalvan, G. P. (2002). *Organizational assessment: A framework for improving performance*. Inter-American Development Bank/International Development Research Centre. https://www.idrc.ca/sites/default/files/openebooks/998-4/index.html.

Mahon, A., & Young, R. (2006). Health care managers as a critical component of the health care workforce. In C. Dubois, M. McKee, & E. Nolte (Eds.), *Human resources for health in Europe* (pp. 116–139). Berkshire, UK: Open University Press.

Mark, B. A., Sayler, J., & Smith, C. S. (1996). A theoretical model for nursing systems outcomes research. *Nursing Administration Quarterly, 20*(4), 12–27.

Matthews, S., Laschinger, H. K. S., & Johnstone, L. (2006). Staff nurse empowerment in line and staff organizational structures for chief nurse executives. *Journal of Nursing Administration, 6*(11), 526–533.

McDaniel, R. R., Driebe, D., & Lanham, H. J. (2013). Health care organizations as complex systems: New perspectives on design and management. *Advances in Health Care Management, 15*, 3–26.

McIntosh N., Meterko M., Burgess J. F., Jr., Restuccia J. D., Kartha A., Kaboli P., et al. (2014). Organizational predictors of coordination in inpatient medicine. *Health Care Management Review, 39*(4), 279–292.

Meier, K. J., & Bohte, J. (2003). Span of control and public organizations: Implementing Luther Gulick's research design. *Public Administration Review, 63*(1), 61–70.

Meyer, R. M. (2008). Span of management: Concept analysis. *Journal of Advanced Nursing, 63*(1), 104–112.

Meyer, R. M., & O'Brien-Pallas, L. (2010). Nursing Services Delivery Theory: An open system approach. *Journal of Advanced Nursing, 66*(12), 2828–2838.

O'Connor, E. S. (1999). The politics of management thought: A case study of the Harvard Business School and the Human Relations School. *Academy of Management Review, 24*(1), 117–131.

Pabst, M. K. (1993). Span of control on nursing inpatient units. *Nursing Economic$, 11*(2), 87–90.

Porter-O'Grady, T. (2015). Confluence and convergence: Team effectiveness in complex systems. *Nursing Administration Quarterly, 39*(1), 78–83.

Porter-O'Grady, T., & Malloch, K. (2014). *Quantum leadership: Building better partnerships for sustainable health* (4th ed): Burlington, MA: Jones & Bartlett Learning.

Prins, G. (2000). *Testing theories on structure and strategy: An assessment of organizational knowledge.* Delft, The Netherlands: Eburon.

Read, E. A. (2014). Workplace social capital in nursing: An evolutionary concept analysis. *Journal of Advanced Nursing, 70*(5), 997–1007.

Reed, M. I. (1992). *The sociology of organizations: Themes, perspectives and prospects.* New York, NY: Harvester Wheatsheaf.

Rouse, W. B. (2008). Health care as a complex adaptive system: Implications for design and management. *Bridge-Washington-National Academy of Engineering, 38*(1), 17.

Scott, W. R. (1992). *Organizations: Rational, natural, and open systems* (3rd ed.). Englewood Cliffs, NJ: Prentice-Hall.

Shirey, M. R., & White-Williams, C. (2015). Boundary spanning leadership practices for population health. *Journal of Nursing Administration, 45*(9), 411–415.

Smith, L., Andrusyszyn, M. A., & Spence Laschinger, H. K. (2010). Effects of workplace incivility and empowerment on newly-graduated nurses' organizational commitment. *Journal of Nursing Management, 18*(8), 1004–1015.

Strömgren, M., Eriksson, A., Ahlstrom, L., Bergman, D., & Dellve, L. (2017). Leadership quality: A factor important for social capital in healthcare organizations. *Journal of Health Organization and Management, 31*(2), 175–191.

Tichy, N. M., Tushman, M. L., & Fombrun, C. (1979). Social network analysis for organizations. *Academy of Management Review, 4*(4), 507–519.

Weber, M. (1978). *Economy and society: An outline of interpretive sociology*. In E. Fischoff, H. Gerth, A. M. Henderson, F. Kolegar, C. W. Mills, T. Parsons, M. Rheinstein, G. Roth, E. Shils, & C. Wittich, (Eds.). Trans. (Vol. 2): Berkeley, CA: University of California Press.

Wenger, E. (2008). *Communities of practice: A brief introduction*. https://scholarsbank.uoregon.edu/xmlui/bitstream/handle/1794/11736/A%20brief%20introduction%20to%20CoP.pdf.

Willem, A., Buelens, M., & De Jonghe, I. (2007). Impact of organizational structure on nurses' job satisfaction: A questionnaire survey. *International Journal of Nursing Studies, 44*, 1011–1020.

Wong, C. A., & Laschinger, H. K. (2013). Authentic leadership, performance and job satisfaction: The mediating role of empowerment. *Journal of Advanced Nursing, 69*(4), 947–959.

Wong C. A., Elliot-Miller P., Laschinger H. K., Cuddihy M., Meyer R., Keatings M., et al. (2015). Examining the relationships between span of control and manager and unit work outcomes in Ontario academic hospitals. *Journal of Nursing Management, 23*(2), 156–168.

Yang, J., Liu, Y., Huang, C., & Zhu, L. (2013). Impact of empowerment on professional practice environments and organizational commitment among nurses: A structural equation approach. *International Journal of Nursing Practice, 19*(S1), 44–55.

Young, G. J., Charnes, M. P., & Heeren, T. C. (2004). Product line management in professional organizations: An empirical test of competing theoretical perspectives. *Academy of Management Journal, 47*(5), 723–734.

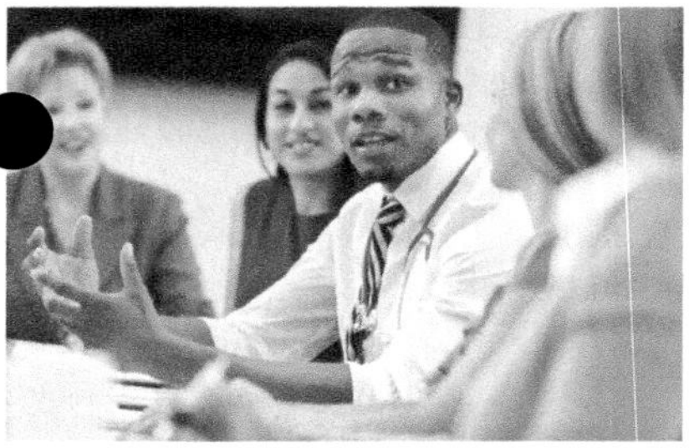

13

Decentralization and Governance

M. Lindell Joseph, Richard J. Bogue

http://evolve.elsevier.com/Huber/leadership

The US health care system is constantly adapting in the face of changes in governmental policies, payment mechanisms, population health priorities, local disasters, and to meet the daily challenges of patient care across the continuum of care. Among critical assets for adaptation in health care organizations are innovations that liberate the strengths of nurses, care teams, and the field of nursing. Such adaptations in health systems, hospitals, and clinics include ensuring that the right personnel, with the right training, the best situational understanding, and the authority and flexibility to act are free to meet any given challenge at the needed time. Promptly meeting these complex challenges requires teams composed of staff who feel encouraged to exercise their competencies to their full scope of practice in their respective part of the health system. This decentralization of authority is a core feature of shared governance: having authority for decision-making at the right level in the organization from the local work unit and up the levels of leadership, with ramifications for nursing participation at the level of the governing board.

Participation in shared governance, especially in unit-based councils, is an evidence-based practice that is integral to the Magnet Recognition Program® (https://www.nursingworld.org/organizational-programs/magnet). In a review of 20 articles, it was found that shared governance makes a meaningful difference for nurses. Shared governance promotes autonomy, higher job satisfaction, greater control over nursing practice, better quality and safety outcomes, greater engagement, and an improved work environment (Al-Marri & Kehyayan, 2018). In situations where nurses are dissatisfied and turnover is high, one significant remedy is to institute shared governance using unit-based councils to give nurses a venue for greater satisfaction and participation. This chapter reviews key definitions, approaches to operationalize decentralization and governance, implications for leadership, and current issues and trends.

DEFINITIONS

Board Governance

A **governing board** is a decision-making body with fiduciary and strategic accountability for an organization's mission and the assets for advancing that mission. Board members provide oversight for corporations, not-for-profits, agencies of government, and other entities by exercising four duties. These four duties are (1) Duty of Fiduciary, acting in the organization's best interests, ensuring that resources are used in a reasonable, appropriate, and legally accountable manner, (2) Duty of Care, making responsible decisions and providing appropriate oversight, (3) Duty of Loyalty, avoiding conflicts of interest or self-interest, and (4) Duty of Obedience, ensuring compliance with applicable laws, rules, and regulations, and to act within the scope of their authority under the organization's articles, bylaws, and applicable laws (American Hospital Association [AHA], 2009). The vision of the Nurses on Boards Coalition (NOBC), for example, is "to build healthier communities in America by increasing nurses' presence on corporate, health-related, and other boards, panels, and commissions" (2020).

Governance is how society or groups within it organize to make decisions or achieve collective action. It is defined as "Establishment of policies, and continuous monitoring of their proper implementation, by the members of the governing body of an organization. It includes the mechanisms required to balance the powers of the members (with the associated accountability), and their primary duty of enhancing the prosperity and viability of the organization" (Business Dictionary.com, 2020a).

Centralization and decentralization

Describe both the degree of hierarchical power distribution for decision-making authority in an organization *and* how power is manifested in the organizational structure, reflected in the locus of decision-making authority. In a highly centralized organization (BusinessDictionary.com, 2020b), the power of planning and decision-making are exclusively in the hands of top management. Decentralization (BusinessDictionary.com, 2020c) means that authority for planning and decision-making are widely distributed throughout the organization.

Structural Empowerment

Structural empowerment refers to organizational structures and procedures that help advance or maintain generally flat, flexible, and decentralized decision-making. In nursing, this means adopting shared governance and/or decentralized decision-making structures and processes that establish and reinforce standards of practice and opportunities for improvements that advance the performance of nurses and others up and down the organization's formal hierarchy (American Nurses Credentialing Center [ANCC], 2019).

Subsidiarity and Decentralization

The phrase "decentralization of authority" and the term subsidiarity both refer to one core feature of organizations aiming to be more effective and better democratized: engaging all members of the team in the journey toward excellence. **Subsidiarity** is the principle that "functions which are performed effectively by subordinate or local organizations belong more properly to them than to a dominant central organization" (Merriam-Webster, 2020); in other terms, decision-making power should be decentralized to the extent possible.

Tsagourias summarized the history of the principle of subsidiarity:

> "The origins of the principle of subsidiarity go back to Aristotle, but it is Catholic doctrine that popularized this concept. Subsidiarity was invoked in 1891 by the Catholic Church and has been reaffirmed since then in different contexts as a principle of social ordering of constituent parts in order to serve and attain the common good" (Tsagourias, 2011, p. 547).

The supranational European Union embedded subsidiarity in its constitution. From the Glossary of summaries in EUR-Lex we learn:

> "The principle of subsidiarity is defined in Article 5 of the Treaty on European Union. It aims to ensure that decisions are taken as closely as possible to the citizen and that constant checks are made to verify that action at EU level is justified in light of the possibilities available at national, regional or local level" (EUR-Lex, 2020).

The General Effective Multilevel Theory for Shared Governance (GEMS)

GEMS is a theory-based approach to nursing shared governance. It offers a precise, specific, and systematic approach to enacting, evaluating, and improving shared governance. GEMS guides the implementation of effective shared governance by using both the unit-level work team and the leadership team to improve outcomes at the individual level, unit level, department level, and organizational level (Bogue et al., 2009; Joseph & Bogue, 2016).

BACKGROUND

Approaches Used for Decentralization and Governance

Board Governance

The Institute of Medicine's (IOM, 2011) *The Future of Nursing: Leading Change, Advancing Health* report, challenged nurses to strive for board engagement. The recommendations encouraged nurses to participate in the redesign of care delivery, including by aspiring to board membership (IOM, 2011). Many nurses hold esteemed leadership roles throughout the health care field. However, they often cannot or do not participate at the highest level of organizational leadership—the governing board. An outcome of the report was a Campaign for Action. This campaign resulted in the development of NOBC. The primary mission of the NOBC is to get an additional 10,000 nurses on governing boards by 2020. According to the (NOBC, 2018), the positioning of nurses with diverse knowledge, expertise, and independence on boards has become essential to enable and capture diverse thoughts and contributions. The approaches of decentralization, governance, improvement methods, and innovations enable buy-in, collaborative decision-making, alignment, and sustainability for the reshaping of health care. As of April 11, 2020, there were 7309 nurses on boards (NOBC, 2020). The work of the NOBC will not end until the right nurses are serving on the right boards creating strategic value.

Regardless of nurses' level of education, background, or experience, there is a place on a board, commission, or other leadership entity for every nurse. Nurses are suited to impact board discussions and outcomes. Nurses are accustomed to using critical thinking skills, evidence-based approaches, good listening skills, and to formulate key questions that often result in new thinking, discussions, and outcomes. Each nurse who is appointed to a board brings America one step closer to the collective goal of healthier communities and a healthier nation. The following are strategies for an effective presence when on a board (Joseph & Benson, 2017 a,b,c; 2018; 2019):

1. Show attentiveness by using nonverbal cues that show understanding such as nodding, eye contact, and leaning forward
2. Be gracious by not using ungracious expressions such as "whatever" and reflect on your social skills
3. Use storytelling since it is an effective strategy that helps to build relationships, demonstrate effective communication, and engage others in the issues
4. Be confident by learning from setbacks, failures, and successes
5. Take an ethical stance by striving for the best possible outcomes for the benefit of all and express empathy

Nurses' Role in Health Care

Nursing has its own organizational structure within health care for extremely good reasons. Nurses, in teams, are expected to be persistently and readily at the call to care for patients, 24 hours a day, 7 days a week, all year around in hospitals. Each individual nurse is expected to apply their knowledge and skills of nursing to every moment that a patient needs them. In the performance of their duties, nurses are expected to represent the most flexible and persistently available health care professionals until a need arises that calls for a different configuration of the system. This is not true of physicians, let alone administrators or financial or IT managers, or any of the other roles that might be useful for other specific aspects of patients' needs within the system of health care. At least in inpatient settings, nursing is a unique role that demands effective, nurse-driven teamwork and problem-solving on a constant basis. Nursing, therefore, from top to bottom in the organization, requires its own organizational structure and can perform better using formal, organized, and effective methods for nursing shared governance.

As noted above, subsidiarity drives decision-making to the most local or personal level of a complex organization but also recognizes that certain decisions and actions may be more effective when addressed at the organizational level directly above the most local members. In the case of nursing, if the nursing team working together cannot effectively meet the demands of decision-making and action for a particular issue, that issue should be elevated to the nursing unit. If the unit cannot effectively handle an issue, that issue should be elevated to the department level or, if needed, higher in the organization.

Centralization Versus Decentralization on 4 East and 5 West

Organizations have an identifiable structure that affects decision-making authority and the power that nurses have to control and make improvements in their practice. The higher the degree of decentralization in an organization, the more decision-making is done at the point of activity or "the front line." Institutions organize and structure themselves by defining departmental function and authority to achieve a more coordinated effort. This drives plans and decisions about responsibilities and who reports to whom. The following two scenarios provide a contrast to illustrate the operationalization of centralization and decentralization in an institution:

- In scenario one, Abigail Hutton is the nurse manager in the primary care clinic, a medical nursing unit in General Medical Center. Once a candidate is screened for a position by the human resources department, Nurse Hutton interviews applicants to fill open nursing positions in the clinic. At the conclusion of the interviews, she decides whom to hire and notifies human resources. Although this is a somewhat simplistic example, of note is that the decision-making authority is vested solely in the nurse manager.

- In scenario two, Jordan Jones is the nurse manager of 4 East and 5 West, medical nursing units in City Hospital. With three staff nurse positions vacant, he posts the openings and asks the unit council—made up of nurses and other staff on the unit who have had human resources training on behavioral interviewing—to act as part of the selection committee. Based on the needs of the nursing unit and the availability of nursing applicants who match those criteria, human resource staff screen the files of the applicants. They pass on the applications of those nurses who meet the requirements for the positions to the selection committee, who then schedules interviews with the applicants. Once the selection committee has interviewed the candidates, they decide on the best candidate for each position. The committee's recommendations, along with the rationale for its choices, are relayed to the manager. The manager (1) meets with the candidates and takes into consideration the recommendations by the selection committee, (2) interviews them, and (3) makes the job offers.

In this second scenario, the staff nurses are involved in making a hiring decision that directly affects their work environment. This scenario clearly illustrates a more decentralized organizational philosophy. In such an organization, decision-making authority rests in levels closer to the point of service rather than in the executive levels. Decentralization encourages and facilitates greater innovation, more input, and faster response times because staff who are directly responsible for implementing changes and delivering care are a major part of decision-making at the point of implementation.

Nursing Shared Governance Effectiveness

The principle of subsidiarity—or decentralization—has been applied widely, including as a fundamental precept of models of nursing shared governance even if not worded in these terms. O'May and Buchan (1999) described types of nursing shared governance *based on the level at which councils operate*: the nursing unit, the department, the executive level (coordinating activities of lower-level councils), and system-wide (where representative staff participate through top-level cabinets). In any of these types, the target of shared governance is to guide and improve practice. In 2009, Bogue and colleagues argued for the importance of practice councils at the unit level, built on the concept of subsidiarity: where the action is. Subsidiarity works because it also illustrates the importance of pushing issues up the organization when that would be more effective. Effectiveness in nursing relies on "supportive nursing group power and the concomitant exercise of power by nursing work units—vertically aligned empowerment" (Bogue et al., 2009, p. 6).

There has been little research evidence available about best practices in establishing shared governance. GEMS theory represents an innovative and evidence-based approach to nursing shared governance that is based on the critical importance of the principle of subsidiarity. GEMS theory guides the implementation of shared governance using leadership strategies both within the unit work team and the leadership team, to improve outcomes for patients, nurses, and the overall organization. Such successes lead to increased understanding of challenges and improved performance in goal attainment (Bogue et al., 2009; Joseph & Bogue, 2016).

There are nine essential competencies required for unit-level work teams or nursing practice councils to become increasingly effective. These nine competencies are grouped into three major categories that reflect increasing levels of competence in goal achievement: team foundations, empowering, and aligning (Fig. 13.1). Team foundations for nursing practice council effectiveness include these competencies: (1) skillful group formation and group tasks, (2) creating group identity and norms, and (3) focusing on driving improvements in nursing practice. The empowering competencies include actively gaining the active support of management. The unit council must take responsibility for gaining the support of local management and do so while helping drive unit practices toward achieving outcomes and enabling excellence in patient safety initiatives. In the aligning competencies phase, the unit council leadership group is conducting highly efficient meetings that are oriented toward identifying, achieving, and regularly demonstrating an ability to identify, design, conduct, and promulgate evidence from their successes in a patient care improvement agenda; in the aligning phase, unit councils are practicing excellence and providing leadership in improving patient outcomes.

A local unit council may be fluid as to membership due to time, reassignments, family considerations, or other reasons. This means two things: (1) there may

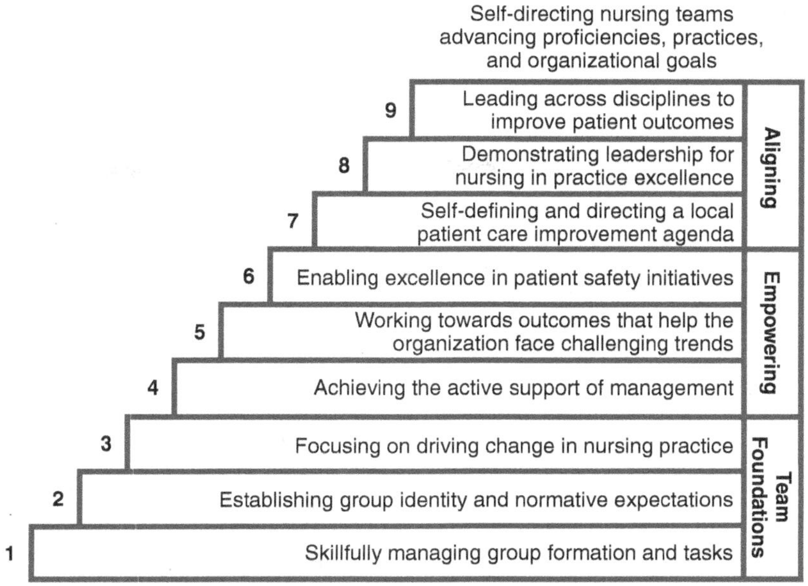

Fig 13.1 Competencies stair-stepping toward becoming self-directing nursing teams. From: Bogue, R. J. & Joseph, M. L. (2011, October 16–19). *A general theory for effective multilevel shared governance: A model for driving change in nursing practice.* International Conference on Communication in Healthcare, Chicago, IL.

be changes in the council membership, and (2) there must be ongoing, but not highly time-consuming, efforts to keep other nurses, nursing assistants, nurse practitioners, physicians, or others on the unit aware of and, ideally, engaged in the unit's progress. When a strong and mutually supportive relationship is developed between the unit manager(s), the nursing practice council, and other personnel who frequent the unit, this structure becomes more natural.

Nursing shared governance effectiveness can be reliably measured on GEMS' nine specific-nursing competencies using the Nursing Practice Council Effectiveness Scale (NPCes). Research has shown that higher NPCes scores were associated with improvements in various measures at the individual level, unit level, departmental level, and organizational level. These improvements included manager support, job satisfaction, self-efficacy, and pressure ulcer rates (Bogue et al., 2009; Joseph & Bogue, 2016).

It is inconceivable that an organization would implement a new shared governance process and expect it to flourish automatically. Ongoing improvement requires *kaizen*, a spirit of continuous improvement and a simple, clear, consistent process. GEMS theory describes and contains a developmental, iterative process that generates experience in reaching goals, as local councils and nursing units achieve higher levels of self-directed goal attainment. GEMS enables this through time-efficient methods, relying on goals inherent in the unit's aspirations but also an initial GEMS site visit, quick self-assessments twice per year for target setting, feedback reports at all levels, online or telephonic support as needed, and other assistance if desired.

Fig. 13.2 illustrates the overall framework of GEMS theory. The nursing unit work team, engaged by its local leadership and nursing practice council, accelerates progress toward goals by gaining and exercising the competencies shown in Fig. 13.1. The nursing leadership team provides clarity, effective communications, encouragement, and buffering from externalities that might otherwise disrupt progress. These two GEMS inputs from below and above interact in the process of GEMS effective shared governance to adopt and track target outcomes for improvement. These targets should respect the organization's goals and individual goals, as well as goals for the specific unit and for the nursing department.

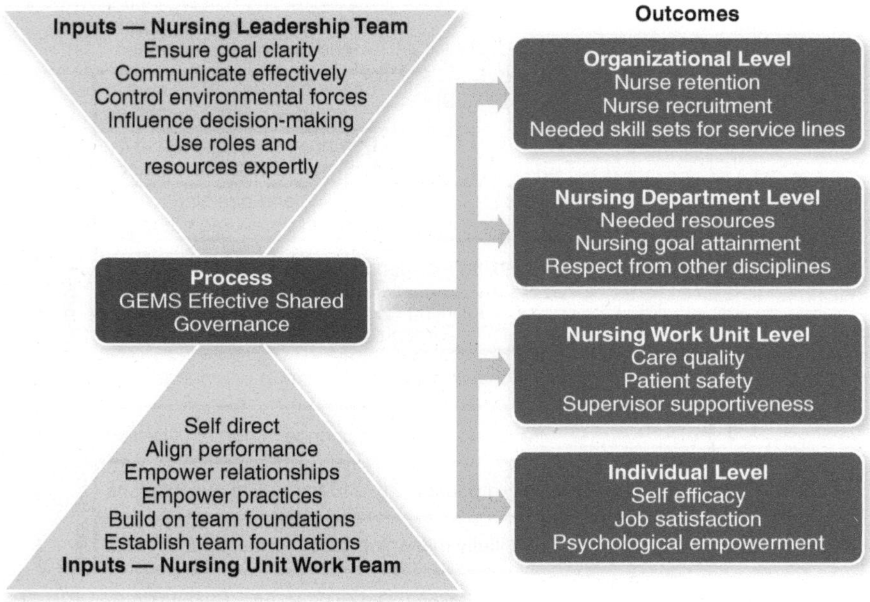

Fig. 13.2 GEMS, general theory for effective multilevel shared governance. From: Bogue, R. J. & Joseph, M. L. (2011, October 16–19). *A general theory for effective multilevel shared governance: A model for driving change in nursing practice.* International Conference on Communication in Healthcare, Chicago, IL.

Organizations Fostering Decentralization and Governance in Health Care

Magnet Hospitals

In the Magnet Recognition Program®, structural empowerment provides organizations with a framework for empowerment and governance (American Nurses Credentialing Center [ANCC], 2019). According to study findings (Spence Laschinger et al., 2003), empowering work conditions and Magnet Hospital characteristics were significantly predictive of nurses' satisfaction with their jobs. McHugh and et al. (2013) found that patients treated in Magnet hospitals had 14% lower odds of mortality and 12% lower odds of failure-to-rescue.

Structural empowerment (SE) is evaluated based on the following criteria (ANCC, 2019, pp. 26–27):

1. Clinical nurses are involved in interprofessional decision-making groups at the organizational level.
2. The health care organization supports nurses' participation in local, regional, national, or international professional organizations.
3. The organization supports nurses' continuous professional development.
4. Nurses participate in professional development activities designed to improve their knowledge, skills, and or practices in the workplace.
5. Professional development activities are designed to improve the professional practice of nursing or patient outcomes, or both.
6. Nursing education opportunities are provided for those interested in a nursing career.
7. The organization provides opportunities to improve nurses' expertise in effectively teaching a patient or family.
8. The organization facilitates the effective transition of registered nurses and advanced practice nurses (APRNs) into the work environment.
9. The organization provides educational activities to improve the nurse's expertise as a preceptor.
10. The organization supports nurses' participation in community health care outreach.
11. Nurses participate in the assessment and prioritization of the health care needs of the community.
12. Nurses are recognized for their contributions in addressing the strategic priorities of the organization.

The Lean Model

The Lean model is another illustration of the centrality of subsidiarity in more effective organizations. Lean has been widely used in health care and owes its existence to Toyota's kaizen quality improvement principles. The kaizen path refers to accelerating the implementation of kaizen (continuous incremental improvement) to processes within the organization (Black & Miller, 2008). Both kaizen and Lean rely upon the core importance of subsidiarity in fostering effective organizations. In both cases, the aim is to achieve continuous improvements that reduce waste and improve outputs. To do this, both models depend on workers at all levels in their various roles to notice problems and propose improvements, keeping in mind that the workers closest to production are also generally those who are furthest from the board, the CEO, and the management at division and department levels. The classic Toyota example is Toyota Principle #5: Build a culture of stopping to fix the problem, to get quality right the first time. This principle means that any worker on a production line can pull the cord to illuminate the location of a production problem and alert support personnel to immediately go to the location, identify, and resolve the problem (Gao & Low, 2014). In health care the same principle applies when workers at all levels, but starting where actual care processes occur, are empowered to ensure high-quality, defect-free health care (Black & Miller, 2008).

The Institute for Health Care Improvement (IHI)

The Institute for Health Care Improvement (IHI) was founded in 1991, but their work began in the late 1980s as part of the National Demonstration Project on Quality Improvement in Health Care. This group was created with the commitment to redesign health care into a system without errors, waste, delay, and unsustainable costs (IHI, 2019). IHI's structure and vision supports Follesdal's (1998) definition of subsidiarity, whereby powers or tasks should rest with the lower-level subunits of that order, and the higher-level central unit would ensure higher comparative efficiency or effectiveness in achieving health care improvement and health. IHI has been an influential force toward a journey of excellence in the United States and has had a rapidly growing influence in such countries as Canada, England, Scotland, Denmark, Sweden, Singapore, Latin America, New Zealand, Ghana, Malawi, South Africa, and the Middle East. IHI's governance structure is not an organization with walls but more of a movement for collaboration and change. IHI governance is organized around multiple stakeholders such as an Executive Team, Management Team, Board of Directors, Faculty, IHI Senior Fellows, IHI Alumni, IHI Scientific Advisory Group, and anyone who has a passion for improvement of patient care and who wants to profoundly change health and health care for the better. In addition to these groups, IHI uses a grassroots multiforum approach to enable engagement and participation (IHI, 2020). These include:

1. ihi.org
2. IHI Open School
3. Women's Health Initiative (WHI)
4. Conferences, seminars and direct consultations, such as:
    a. National Forum on Quality Improvement in Health Care
    b. International Forum on Quality and Safety in Healthcare
    c. Annual Summit on Improving Patient Care in the Office Practice and in the Community, Face-to-Face seminars and trainings
    d. Virtual Training Programs such as Virtual Expeditions
    e. IHI Open School
    f. the ability to bring IHI staff for consultation
5. Training in improvement skills such as the Breakthrough Series College and Patient safety Executive Development Program
6. Working strategically with IHI with programs such as IHI Leadership Alliance, and Cutting-Edge Innovation

LEADERSHIP AND MANAGEMENT IMPLICATIONS

Although shared governance shifts decision-making away from a health care organization's leader and into the hands of empowered staff, shared governance does not mean that leaders can ignore their responsibility in the decision-making process. Nor does it mean that all decisions are made by nurses. To be effective, leaders must be ready for and accepting of this shift. So too must leaders be prepared to empower staff.

"Staff who experience empowerment feel that they are respected and trusted to be active participants.

Staff who feel empowered also demonstrate a positive image to other healthcare team members, patients and their families, and the public. Nurses who do not feel empowered will not be effective in conveying a positive image, because they will not be able to communicate that nurses are professionals with much to offer. Empowerment that is not clear to staff is just as problematic as no staff empowerment. Empowered teams feel a responsibility for the team's performance and activities, which in turn can improve care and reduce errors" (Finkelman & Kenner, 2016, p. 457).

"An interprofessional approach to Shared Governance must be embedded throughout the organization adopting it, from the clinical decisions at points of service to the strategic priorities placed on interprofessional issues by senior leadership. A cornerstone of this approach to practice may be the inclusion of patients and families as full partners on both care teams and planning groups. Respecting and valuing the knowledge and service of all team members contributes to a trusting, openly communicative, learning environment and positive patient care and practice outcomes" (Swihart & Hess, 2014, p. 87).

An inter-professional approach:

"[O]ften engages patients and families as partners. Keys to successful implementation ... include active participation of all team members contributing to mutually respectful, trusting, collaborative, openly communicative, safe, and effective learning environments of care and practice across disciplines and departments. Interprofessional Shared Governance provides a unique structure for shared decision-making reflective of the current and devolving demands of an increasingly diverse and integrated care delivery system" (Swihart & Hess, 2014, p. 4).

CURRENT ISSUES AND TRENDS

There are four key issues and trends today. These include (1) whether to use the terms shared governance versus profession nursing governance, (2) types of councils, (3) whole system integration, (4) engagement, and (5) the appropriateness of selected measures.

Shared Governance Versus Professional Nursing Governance

A debate exists about using the terms shared governance versus professional nursing governance. Porter-O'Grady (2017) stated that in the early 1980s shared governance was an alternative term used for professional governance because the term professional was not considered as legitimate when applied to nurses. Because nursing has been a predominantly employed work group primarily composed of women, the usual requisites of ownership, control over practice, and membership were rarely applied to nurses.

However, in 1998 Hess published his seminal works on professional governance. Hess defined professional governance as a multidimensional organizational characteristic that encompasses the structure and processes by which professionals direct, control, and regulate goal-oriented efforts of one another. To measure these types of professional governance, he developed and tested the Index of Professional Nursing Governance and the Index of Professional Governance. The latter is a more generic version for nurses, physicians, pharmacists, and allied health professionals (Swihart & Hess, 2018).

Although both Hess and Porter-O'Grady have published on shared governance and professional governance extensively, the evidence-based knowledge for nursing shared governance and professional governance was sparse. In the early 2000s, there was a call for a stronger link between theory and practice so that evaluations can build nursing theory, science, and practice for shared governance (Anthony, 2004). And in 2011, the Institute of Medicine called for nurses to become active in building research knowledge. The seminal theory of GEMS has provided the most progressive evidence to advance nursing practice. GEMS is the only theory for shared governance in the field of nursing (Bogue et al., 2009; Joseph & Bogue, 2016).

Types of Councils

The decision to implement the most appropriate type of shared governance for an organization may be a challenging. In a blog by Lippincott (2019), the authors described three levels of councils. These include unit practice-level councils, hospital-level councils, and themed-level councils. In some institutions one, two, or all types may be implemented. The following core types are discussed. (1) **Unit practice councils are** organized and implemented by direct care nurses. This format offers direct care nurses the opportunity to share their opinions, suggest ways to improve the patient care experience, and make decisions regarding process improvements. (2) **Hospital councils are at the meso-system level.** Direct care nurses from many units gather to discuss issues affecting nursing practice and patient care throughout the entire organization. Members of nursing leadership should be present to support staff nurses in their decision-making and act as intermediaries between the staff and upper management. (3) **Themed councils are organized to address** broader issues such as quality and safety, professional development, or the healing environment.

The key in selecting the appropriate type of council is to ensure that councils are not too big so that they limit participant engagement and motivation. Williams noted, "I have observed hospital and themed councils with 60–100 participants but if you read the research on teams, the ideal group size should be based on your purpose. Are these shared governance councils convening to problem solve? How can 60–100 people engage? Secondly, alignment may be absent in many institutions. In many institutions nurses voice that they are usually delegated to by upper management and are sometimes working in a vacuum with minimal influence when alignment is absent" (J. Williams, personal communication, May 17, 2013).

Whole-System Integration

Practice leaders see the benefits of decentralization and the shared governance model extending beyond nurses and all care providers to all employees. "As for the future of Shared Governance, Susan Allen PhD, RN (assistant vice president, Cincinnati Children's Hospital) says it would be ideal to see whole-system integration involving all hospital staff. But will Shared Governance ever be the sole governing system or will there always be a traditional system to manage operations? Shared Governance would have to be highly integrated, says Allen" (Gray, 2013). Clearly, the next steps in this vision are to include patients and the community more deliberatively into the shared governance model. Allen says Cincinnati Children's Hospital has a family advisory council and a teen council that get involved in projects, including reviewing potential educational materials and designing a new learning center (Gray, 2013).

Engagement

Shared governance is the gold standard for engaging nurses in solving problems at the point of care. An ongoing challenge among US employers, including health care systems, is to keep employees engaged. A Gallup poll (2017) indicated that only 33% of employees in the United States report they are "engaged at work," meaning they are committed to their job and feel they are making positive contributions. Fifty-one percent reported they are "not engaged at work," meaning they are not likely to put effort into organizational goals. Sixteen percent are "actively disengaged," described as unhappy, unproductive and likely to spread negativity.

Perhaps improved technology can also make a difference. According to AHA (2016), "almost 30% of clinicians aren't satisfied with technology used by their organization." It will become more and more important for nurses to leverage the power of shared governance to improve practice and help deliver desired outcomes. Nurses need to both structure and participate in shared governance as a routine part of their work life.

Appropriateness of Selected Measures

Nursing Practice Council Effectiveness Scale (NPCes)

NPCes is a valid and reliable index of nursing practice council effectiveness. It measures nine competencies at the practice/unit council level. These competencies include skillfulness, usefulness, effectiveness, supported by management, empowering nurses and nursing, improves patient care, improves patient safety, leads with professional practice issues, and improves professional practice (Bogue et al., 2009). NPCes is used as a self-assessment tool for nursing practice councils, so they can identify their progress across the competencies and craft "lean" plans for improving their competencies as a group as they strive toward leadership.

The GEMS Self-Assessment

The GEMS self-assessment measures shared governance at the team level and leadership level to examine team effectiveness, alignment, and goal attainment. This measure consists of 21 items; initial uses indicate that the GEMS self-assessments are valid and reliable (Joseph & Bogue, 2016).

The Index of Professional Nursing Governance (IPNG)

IPNG is used to identify an organization's place on a continuum of traditional governance, shared governance, and self-governance. Two instruments currently exist: (1) the Index of Professional Nursing Governance, and (2) the Index of Professional Governance (this version evaluates the health care team). This is in multiple languages and may be perceived as lengthy (Swihart, & Hess, 2018).

The Structural Professional Governance Self-Assessment Survey (SPGS-A)

This is a new tool in development. It measures attributes of professional governance. These attributes include accountability, professional obligation, collateral relationships, and effective decision-making (Porter-O'Grady & Clavelle, 2019).

RESEARCH NOTE

Source

Al-Marri, A.H., & Kehyayan, V. (2018). Nurses' lived experience serving on unit-based councils: A literature review. *Journal of Nursing Education and Practice*, *8*(12), 21–28. https://doi.org/10.5430/jnep.v8n12p21.

Purpose

This literature review examined studies reporting results about nurses' lived experiences on unit-based councils (UBCs) within shared governance (SG) structures. The aims of the review were to describe whether and how UBCs affect decisions about nursing practice, standards of nursing care, nurse work environment, nurses' sense of empowerment, and any other findings.

Discussion

A literature review was designed to identify full texts of English-language empirical studies with results associated with shared governance that were published in peer-reviewed journals between January 2006 and January 2017. Search terms were "shared governance AND nurses' experience OR perspective OR view OR attitude," "shared governance AND healthcare," and "unit-based councils." This search strategy was employed in CINAHL, Academic Search Complete, and Academic Search Elite. Of 120 articles found, 15 were duplicates, 13 were excluded based on the title, 48 were excluded based on the abstract, and 35 were excluded based on full text review. The results are based on 20 articles, representing results from Belgium, Brazil, UK, Jordan, the Kingdom of Saudi Arabia, and the United States.

After extracting all the results associated with UBCs in SG, the study team reviewed general perceptions of UBCs and SG. General perceptions about UBCs in SG included (1) an increased desire for decisional involvement related to more experience in UBCs, and (2) participation in SG at the unit-level (UBCs) increases voice for nursing and for individual nurses, as well as greater voice in interdisciplinary contexts. Hospitals successfully achieving Magnet designation are "known for fostering positive work environments."

The researchers also identified four themes grouping results documented in one or another study. **Theme 1: Leadership and management** results demonstrated that UBCs in SG may promote autonomy among nurses, provide active support for engagement in SG, and increase the chance of offering patient care coverage and compensation for SG effort outside normal schedules, as well as mentoring staff nurses to improve performance and fostering a healthy work environment. **Theme 2: Increased job satisfaction** was composed of findings of higher job satisfaction from SG in UBC participation and greater control over nursing practice; job satisfaction was also positively associated with years of experience in one's current work Findings under **Theme 3: Improved patient care** demonstrated that nurses participating in decisions affecting nursing practice produced better quality and safety outcomes; moreover, quality and safety benefits appeared to increase as engagement in decision-making increased. **Theme 4: Improved work environment** suggests that SG facilities where UBCs enable greater engagement in SG, nurses are more empowered to have control over their own polices, thereby experiencing their work more as managing patient care, being bedside leaders. This demonstrates that nurses gain satisfaction when nurses enjoy greater active decision-making at the point of care. In general, older nurses and more experienced nurses both tend to be more satisfied and more active in shared governance.

Application to Practice

The findings from the studies in this review suggest that SG participation specifically in UBCs makes a meaningful difference. Where nurses cannot participate in SG at the level of UBCs, nurses are more likely to be confused about expectations for their roles in SG and/or perceive that SG does not make a difference. Participation in SG at the unit level tends to generate a different set of expectations that are associated with greater work satisfaction and more active engagement in improving performance

RESEARCH NOTE—cont'd

for patient experience and patient care quality. These findings offer a recommendation that hospitals and health systems can achieve greater performance and higher nurse satisfaction by investing in the establishment and maintenance of unit-level councils for nursing shared governance.

NEXT-GENERATION NCLEX® EXAMINATION-STYLE CASE STUDY

After one year of employment on 3 South, nurse Maria was invited to join the unit's Shared Governance Council Committee (SGCC). Maria has listened to her fellow nurses complain about not being listened to or valued, and the unit's nurse turnover rate is climbing. Morale is low. She is thrilled that this will be a venue to communicate ways to mitigate the increasing turnover and to communicate her peer's perceptions of being powerless and not having a voice. However, it is important that the SGCC operate as an effective structure. At the first meeting, Maria decided to observe and gain trust with the group versus voicing her concerns. After the meeting, Maria made an appointment with the chairperson (Elyssa) to discuss her observations about how the SGCC operates. Elyssa was open to her feedback.

Choose the most likely options to complete the question below.

Question

Which actions, observed while on the committee, indicate that the Shared Governance Council is demonstrating effectiveness? **Select all that apply.**

1. The council meetings are skillful
2. The council enables leadership
3. The information discussed is useful
4. The committee goals are supported by management
5. The council members are empowered to act
6. The council is improving patient safety
7. The council is improving nursing practice

CRITICAL THINKING EXERCISE

Kimani Joseph is a member of the unit-level SG council. A group of nurses approach him because the nurse manager has locked up all personal protective equipment (PPE) and is dolling them out sparingly. Nurses are afraid for personal safety; lately staff have been absent from work, and the unit's staff satisfaction scores are decreasing. Kimani is concerned about the complaints; he has observed them himself.

1. What are the areas of concern in this scenario?
2. Using the General Effective Multilevel Theory for Shared Governance, which competencies would be essential for the nursing team to execute?
3. With shared governance in mind, what should Kimani do? What would you do?

REFERENCES

Al-Marri, A. H., & Kehyayan, V. (2018). Nurses' lived experience serving on unit-based councils: A literature review. *Journal of Nursing Education and Practice, 8*(12), 21–28.

American Nurses Credentialing Center (ANCC). (2019). *Magnet recognition program: Application manual*. Silver Spring, MD: American Nurses Credentialing Center.

American Hospital Association (AHA). (2009). *The guide to good governance for hospital boards*. https://trustees.aha.org/sites/default/files/trustees/09-guide-to-good-governance.pdf.

American Hospital Association (AHA). (2016). *2016 American Hospital Association environmental scan*. http://www.hhnmag.com/articles/3199-american-hospital-association-environmental-scan.

Anthony, M. K. (2004). Shared governance models: the theory, practice, and evidence. *Online Journal of Issues in Nursing, 9*(1), 7.

Black, J., & Miller, D. (2008). *The Toyota way to healthcare excellence: increase efficiency and improve quality with Lean*: Chicago, IL: Health Administration Press. https://www.amazon.com/Toyota-Way-Healthcare-Excellence-Efficiency/dp/1567932932.

Bogue, R. J., Joseph, M. L., & Sieloff, C. L. (2009). Shared governance as vertical alignment of nursing group power and nurse practice council effectiveness. *Journal of Nursing Management, 17*(1), 4–14. https://doi.org/10.1111/j.1365-2834.2008.00954.x.

Bogue, R. J., & Joseph, M. L. (2011, October 16–19). *A general theory for effective multilevel shared governance: A model for driving change in nursing practice*, International Conference on Communication in Healthcare, Chicago, IL.

BusinessDictionary.com. (2020a). *Governance*. http://www.businessdictionary.com/definition/governance.html.

BusinessDictionary.com. (2020b). *Centralization*. http://www.businessdictionary.com/definition/centralization.html.

BusinessDictionary.com. (2020c). *Decentralization*. http://www.businessdictionary.com/definition/decentralization.html.

EUR-Lex. (2020). *EUR-Lex: Access to European Common Law*: Publications Office of the European Union. https://eur-lex.europa.eu/homepage.html.

Follesdal, A. (1998). Survey article: Subsidiarity. *The Journal of Political Philosophy, 6*(2), 190–218. https://philpapers.org/rec/ANDSAS.

Finkelman, A., & Kenner, C. (2016). *Professional nursing concepts*. Sudbury, MA: Jones & Bartlett Learning.

Gallup Inc. (2017). *State of the American workplace*. https://www.gallup.com/workplace/238085/state-american-workplace-report-2017.aspx.

Gao, S., & Low, S. P. (2014). The Toyota Way model: an alternative framework for lean construction. *Total Quality Management, 25*(6), 664–682. https://doi.org/10.1080/14783363.2013.820022.

Gray, B. B. (2013). *Taking control through shared governance*. https://www.nurse.com/blog/2013/02/18/taking-control-through-shared-governance-2/.

Hess, R. (1998). Measuring nursing governance. *Nursing Research, 47*(1), 35–42.

Institute for Healthcare Improvement (IHI). (2019). *Improving health and health care worldwide*. http://www.ihi.org/.

Institute for Healthcare Improvement (IHI). (2020). *About us*. http://www.ihi.org/about/Pages/History.aspx.

Institute of Medicine (IOM). (2011). *The future of nursing: Leading change, advancing health*. Washington, DC: The National Academies Press.

Joseph, M. L., & Benson, L. (2017a, May 30). Confidence and truthfulness. *Building a Healthier America Blog. https://www.nursingcenter.com/ncblog/may-2017/confidence-and-truthfulness.*

Joseph, M. L., & Benson, L. (2017b, September 18). Take an ethical stance! *Building a Healthier America Blog*. https://www.nursingcenter.com/ncblog/september-2017/take-an-ethical-stance.

Joseph, M. L., & Benson, L. (2017c, December 15). Influence and storytelling. *Building a Healthier America Blog*. https://www.nursingcenter.com/ncblog/december-2017/influence-with-storytelling.

Joseph, M. L., & Benson, L. (2018, June 12). The art of being gracious. *Building a Healthier America Blog*. http://lippincottsolutions.lww.com/blog.entry.html/2018/06/12/building_a_healthier-1F2z.html.

Joseph, M. L., & Benson, L. (2019, May 30). Nurses on Boards: 5 ways to show attentiveness while serving on a board. *Building a Healthier America Blog*. http://lippincottsolutions.lww.com/blog.entry.html/2019/05/30/nurses_on_boards5-8vKF.html.

Joseph, M. L., & Bogue, R. J. (2016). A theory-based approach to nursing shared governance. *Nursing Outlook, 64*(4), 339–351. PMID: 27005400. https://doi.org/10.1016/j.outlook.2016.01.004.

Lippincott. (2019, February 27). *How shared governance in nursing works*. http://lippincottsolutions.lww.com/blog.entry.html/2019/02/27/how_shared_governanc-oiGj.html.

McHugh, M. D., Kelly, L. A., Smith, H. L., Wu, E. S., Vanak, J. M., & Aiken, L. H. (2013). Lower mortality in Magnet hospitals. *Medical Care, 51*(5), 382–388. http://www.ncbi.nlm.nih.gov/pubmed/23047129.

Merriam-Webster. (2020). *Subsidiarity*. https://www.merriam-webster.com/dictionary/subsidiarity.

Nurses on Boards Coalition (NOBC). (2018). *Resources*. https://www.nursesonboardscoalition.org/resources/.

Nurses on Boards Coalition (NOBC). (2020). About. https://www.nursesonboardscoalition.org/about/.

O'May, F., & Buchan, J. (1999). Shared governance: a literature review. *International Journal of Nursing Studies, 36*(4), 281–300.

Porter-O'Grady, T. (2017). A response to the question of professional governance versus shared governance. *Journal of Nursing Administration, 47*(2), 67–71.

Porter-O'Grady, T., & Clavelle, J. (2019). The structural framework for nursing professional governance. *Nurse Leader, 18*(2), 181–189.

Laschinger, Spence, H. K., Almost, J., & Tuer-Hodes, D. (2003). Workplace empowerment and Magnet Hospital characteristics: Making the link. *Journal of Nursing Administration, 33*(7/8), 410–422.

Swihart, D., & Hess, R. (2014). *Shared governance. A practical approach to transforming interprofessional healthcare* (3rd ed): Danvers, MA: HCPro.

Swihart, D., & Hess, R. (2018). *Shared governance. A practical approach to transforming interprofessional healthcare* (4th ed): Danvers, MA: HCPro.

Tsagourias, N. (2011). Security Council Legislation, Article 2(7) of the UN Charter, and the principle of subsidiarity. *Leiden Journal of International Law, 24*(3), 539–559. https://www.cambridge.org/core/journals/leiden-journal-of-international-law/article/security-council-legislation-article-27-of-the-un-charter-and-the-principle-of-subsidiarity/B68B4E6DBDED98406FAA814DA80481FD.

14

Strategic Management

Cole Edmonson

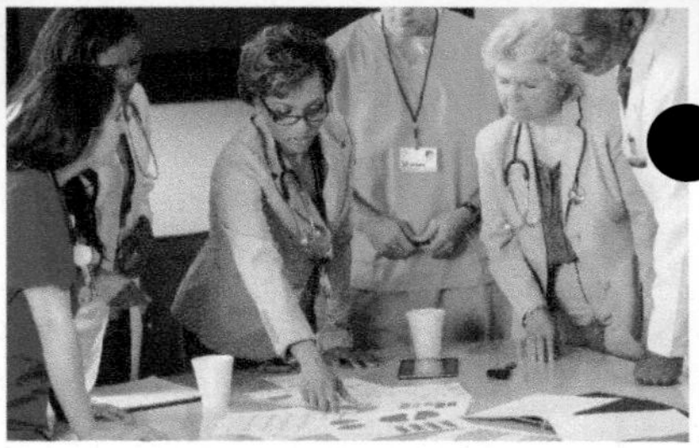

http://evolve.elsevier.com/Huber/leadership

Thinking and acting strategically are crucial for nurses to be proactive in a complex, fast-changing, rapid-cycle environment. Arising from the business field, strategic management has made its way into health care leadership, including nursing. The leadership role of nurses has become an area of increasing focus since the Institute of Medicine (IOM, now called the National Academies of Sciences, Engineering, and Medicine, Health and Medicine Division), in its 2010 *Future of Nursing* report, called for increased leadership development and participation in leadership among nurses. Evaluation of progress toward the *Future of Nursing* goals indicates that although leadership development opportunities have been created since the release of the IOM report, insufficient data exist to determine progress toward nurses serving on "executive management teams and other key leadership positions" (National Academies of Sciences, Engineering, and Medicine [NAM], 2015). Leadership development and participation continues to be an area of focus for nursing as the profession strives to fulfill the IOM goals.

In order to be effective leaders, nurses need to gain competence in a variety of areas. The American Organization for Nursing Leadership (AONL), formerly the American Organization of Nurse Executives (AONE), divided these competencies into five broad categories: communication and relationship management, knowledge of the health care environment, leadership, professionalism, and business skills and principles (AONL, 2015). One key area of business skills includes strategic management. Competencies that align with strategic management consist of several processes, including organizational assessment, planning, management of implementation, and evaluation. The American College of Healthcare Executives (ACHE) also provides a competency assessment tool that offers health care leaders an opportunity to conduct a self-evaluation of key competencies necessary for strategic leadership (ACHE, 2020).

In alignment with the competencies developed by AONL (2015), strategic management involves conducting an environmental scan, knowing the competition, establishing goals, setting targets, developing an action plan, implementing the plan, and evaluating success (Management Study Guide, 2020; Pearce & Robinson, 2012). This approach has long been used in business to ensure a competitive advantage over similar enterprises. Issues in the health care industry, including the Hospital Consumer Assessment of Healthcare Providers and Systems (HCAHPS) and the Hospital Value-Based Purchasing Program, among others, require health care organizations to function as businesses to obtain and maintain a competitive advantage. In the last 10 years, health systems are challenged with meeting the Institute for Healthcare Improvement's (IHI) Quadruple AIM (Sikka et al., 2015) that consists of improving care to the individual, optimizing health outcomes, and lowering overall cost while improving the work environment in health care. Bowles et al. (2018) described the importance of nurse leaders' roles and actions in accomplishing IHI's quadruple aims. The success of a health care enterprise depends on competitive advantages of how well it does something compared with similar efforts and how well it is able to continuously achieve superior performance. Those enterprises that do not do so fail to remain viable for long. Lasater et al. (2016) reported that hospitals known for their excellence in nursing also perform better on value-based purchasing outcomes.

Strategic management involves strategic planning and implementation. It provides a "blueprint" for operating a business, establishing a competitive position, ensuring customer satisfaction, and reaching strategic objectives or goals. Although most strategic planning occurs at the "macro" level (i.e., the executive levels of the health care institution), its implementation typically becomes the responsibility of the "micro" level, such as the nursing division, department, or unit and even the individual nurse. As a result, success depends on the engagement of the entire workforce (Jasper & Crossan, 2012). Fortunately, strategic management prepares nurses to adapt to the current health care environment and helps them achieve their goals, whether related to the workplace or to the profession.

DEFINITIONS

A review of literature by Jasper and Crossan (2012) determined that strategic management is a multifaceted concept that is difficult to define. These authors embraced the definition of strategic management offered by Nag et al. (2007, p. 944), which asserted that "strategic management deals with the major intended and emergent initiatives taken by general managers... involving utilization of resources, to enhance the performance of firms in their external environments." This definition encompasses the five characteristics of strategic management found by Jasper and Crossan (2012):

- Engagement of the entire workforce in organizational leadership
- Alignment with the external environment
- Future orientation
- Use of change management strategies to achieve performance goals
- Facilitation of decision-making with well-communicated decisions

The concept of strategic management includes strategic planning and strategy implementation (Management Study Guide, 2020). Additional terms associated with an organization's use of strategy include *organizational mission and vision, core values, core purpose, strategy, tactics, strategic plan, objectives,* and *stakeholders*. The **organizational mission and vision** collectively is a guiding framework that describes the organization's purpose and future direction (Society for Human Resource Management [SHRM], 2018). **Core values** define the characteristics or beliefs that underlie the organization's activities. The core purpose is the reason the organization is in business. **Strategy** is a competitive move or business approach designed to produce a successful outcome. **Tactics** are operational choices for action that are made to implement a strategy. A **strategic plan** is a document that specifies a plan for actualizing the mission. A strategic plan may also involve a *business plan* or an *action plan* (either as part of the strategic plan or as an adjunct to it) that consists of the who, what, by when, where, and in general terms, the costs involved in implementing the activities identified as objectives in the strategic plan. Weston (2020, p. 54) defined **strategic planning** as "a thoughtful, systematic process of determining a direction and course of actions for achieving a desirable envisioned future." **Objectives** are defined as the targets an organization wants to achieve. These can be financial or performance based with short-range or long-range targets. Finally, **stakeholders** are individuals, groups, or another institution with a financial interest in—or who are affected by—what happens with the organization (BusinessDictionary, 2020).

BACKGROUND

Strategic Planning Process

Strategic management generally begins with a strategic planning process, triggered by recognition of the need for an organization to establish its competitive position in the marketplace or to address some other perceived need (e.g., seeking Magnet Recognition from the American Nurses Credentialing Center's Magnet Recognition Program®, [2017], applying to become a Certified Comprehensive Stroke Center through The Joint Commission [2020], or simply establishing future directions). These are questions to be answered in the strategic planning process: Where are we currently? Where do we want to go? How will we get there? What differentiates us from other organizations?

The components of the nursing process—assessment, planning, implementation, and evaluation—are similar to those employed in strategic management. Although a variety of strategic planning frameworks

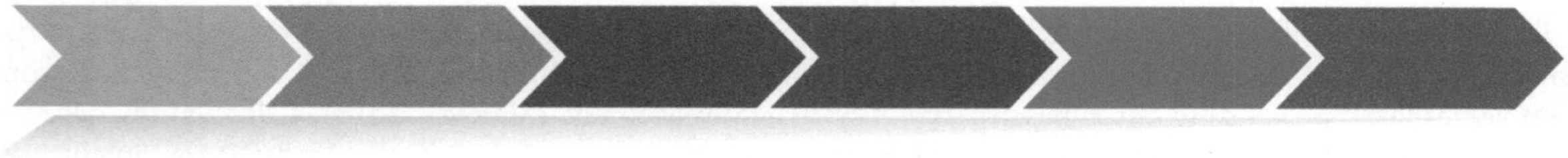

Fig. 14.1 Strategic planning process.

exist, they include the following six components, as shown in Fig. 14.1:

- Creating strategic mission and vision
- Assessing the environment
- Setting objectives
- Developing strategies to achieve the objectives
- Planning for implementation
- Planning for evaluation

The strategic plan provides a framework for strategic management, considering both external and internal environmental factors. Although the strategic planning process may appear to be sequential, it may be iterative as each stage illuminates new ideas for consideration.

Creating Mission and Vision Statements

The first step of the strategic planning process is to formulate or review and update as needed the organization's mission and vision in alignment with the organization's core purpose and values. The mission delineates what the organization does, while the vision articulates the preferred future state of the organization (SHRM, 2018). This step requires a determination of what the organization is, what business it is in and for whom, and where the business seeks to be in the future. The documentation of the mission and vision serves to communicate both purpose and direction to all stakeholders.

The mission and vision are informed by the core values of the organization. The core values held by an organization are those values that are held regardless of whether circumstances—either internal or external—change. They provide a standard for decision-making processes (SHRM, 2018). These core values are so embodied in the culture of the organization that even if they were seen as a liability, they would not be abandoned. Core values do not change even if the industry in which the organization operates changes. Thus, in health care, the organization that has as its core values quality care, patient safety, integrity, and social responsibility would retain those core values despite internal changes (e.g., changes in chief executive officers [CEOs]) or external changes (e.g., reimbursement, the nursing shortage).

The organization's core purpose is the reason the organization exists. The mission defines what the organization does, and the core purpose delineates why (Jones, 2018). The core purpose, like the core values, is relatively unchanging. It provides direction to the organization and contributes to the articulation and implementation of its mission.

In the strategic planning process, the following questions can help develop or revise vision and mission statements:

- What business are we in now?
- What business do we want to be in?
- What do our customers expect of us now?
- What will the customers' expectations be in the future?
- Who are our customers now?
- Who will our customers be in the future?
- Who are our current stakeholders (other than customers)?
- How will those stakeholders change in the future? What about their expectations?
- Who are our primary competitors currently?
- Who will our competitors be in the future?
- What about partners, now and in the future?
- What will the effect of technology be?
- What are the available and the needed resources, both human and financial?
- What is happening in the environment both internally and externally, now and in the future, that may affect us?

In many cases, the core values and the core purpose of the organization may have been defined previously, but if not, planners engaged in the strategic planning process should develop them using questions such as the following:

- What are the values on which we base our work?
- How central or essential are these to the organization?
- Would these values be supported if circumstances changed, or if the industry in which we currently operate changes?

The core purpose can be defined and refined by asking, "Why are we in business?" As a result, the initial response, "We are in the business of health care," may be further refined to "We want to contribute to the community in which we exist." Thus asking "why" may result in the core purpose of providing needed health care services to the community in which the organization is located. Sinek (2009) referred to the "why" in his book *Start with Why* as the core reason that individuals commit to a purpose, profession, or organization, which he later expounded on as an organization's "just cause" and, in his third book, *The Infinite Game* (2019), as the reason that individuals continue to engage in an organization and profession.

Responses to these questions by the principals involved in an organization (e.g., executive management, supervisory staff, department heads) shape an organization's mission, vision, strategic plan, and, as a result, its strategic management. However, involving individuals at all levels of the organization (e.g., staff nurses, clerical workers) in addition to those at the top of the hierarchy ensures a variety of perspectives and more buy-in to the final product. Such inclusion also engages all levels of staff in helping make the vision a reality. When everyone involved in an institution shares the same vision, individuals know where the organization is going and can be instrumental in helping it get there through their daily activities. As the old saying goes, "If you don't know where you're going, then any path will take you there." Conversely, if all of the individuals in the institution know the mission and vision, they are more likely to take the same path. Thus, although it is tempting to skip the mission, vision, and values review, sound strategic planning is premised on a firm linkage to them so that the plan then makes sense and flows out from this core.

Assessing the Environment

A key component of the strategic planning process is to assess the environment. This assessment, called environmental scanning, consists of analyzing both internal and external environmental factors. A SWOT analysis is often used in the environmental assessment and reviews four key areas: **s**trengths, **w**eaknesses, **o**pportunities, and **t**hreats (Centers for Disease Control & Prevention, 2015). A grid such as the one seen in Table 14.1 is often used for documenting the SWOT analysis. In this approach, strengths and weaknesses internal to the organization are identified. These strengths and weaknesses are generally related to resources, programs, and operations in key areas of the organization, examples of which are the following:

- *Operations:* efficiency, capacity, processes
- *Management:* systems, expertise, resources
- *Products:* quality, features, prices
- *Finances:* resources, performance

TABLE 14.1 SWOT Analysis Template

Internal factors	Strengths	Weaknesses
External factors	Opportunities	Threats

Once identified, these components are analyzed for the purpose of drafting a picture of the critical features of the organization, its achievements and failures, and its good points and bad points.

The external components are described as opportunities and threats, and they are identified in the same manner as the internal factors. Opportunities and threats may include changes in industry, marketplace, economy, political climate, technology, and competition.

Once identified, these strengths, weaknesses, opportunities, and threats must be analyzed for their impact on the organization. Next, priorities are established for the critical issues so that strategies are based on the priority issues. For example, a change in the market for the organization's services may be a threat but a low priority, so the organization determines it is not essential to target resources (e.g., human, financial) to deal with the threat when a higher priority is to take advantage of an opportunity involving technology. The SWOT analysis often leads to strategies in which the organization determines to build on **s**trengths, resolve or minimize **w**eaknesses, seize **o**pportunities, and avoid **t**hreats.

The strategies identified through the SWOT analysis help shape the strategic plan on which strategic management is based. The more carefully the analysis is conducted, the more reliable the strategic plan. A plan based on faulty assumptions or careless analysis does not serve the organization well and indeed may lead eventually to its demise.

There are a variety of methods used to analyze and craft a strategic plan. Besides the SWOT analysis, the SOAR (**s**trengths, **o**pportunities, **a**spirations, and **r**esults) planning model has been used in nursing to encourage innovation (Wadsworth et al., 2016). SOAR is a more positive alternative to the more traditional SWOT, places greater emphasis on the organization's future, and encourages employee involvement.

In addition to a SWOT or SOAR analysis of the current environment, individuals engaged in the strategic planning process must project the future. The assessment of future environmental impact takes the form of assumptions. These assumptions encompass the sociodemographic, political, economic, and technological aspects of the external environment. Of course, these assumptions are merely best guesses, because it is impossible to predict the future with certainty.

Setting Objectives

Once the organization's mission and vision have been established and the environmental assessment conducted, the next step in strategic planning is to develop the ways and means to achieve the vision. Strategic goals and objectives are crafted in this step. These objectives generally define the "who," "what," and "where" of the strategies to be implemented. Clearly defined objectives allow individuals to recognize where the organization wants to go and how much time it will take to get there. Absence of strategic objectives results in individuals trying to move in too many directions without a coordinated plan or not moving at all because of confusion about the organization's direction.

Strategic objectives provide a way of converting the rather abstract mission and vision of an organization into concrete terms. These are targets of performance that when taken together will achieve the mission and vision. Objectives also offer a way of measuring progress toward achieving the organization's mission and vision. These objectives generally are written to reflect not what *is* but what *should be*—activities that encourage the individuals implementing them to be creative, stretch beyond their current limits, and challenge themselves to improve their performance. These objectives must be achievable, however, lest individuals lose faith that they can accomplish them. If the strategic objectives are challenging but achievable, they prevent employees of an institution from becoming complacent or settling for the status quo.

Objectives may be written in terms of financial outcomes that relate to improvements in an organization's fiscal health and result in a stronger position for the institution in the industry. For example, a hospital may set a financial objective to decrease expenses by a specific percentage each year. This objective may be accomplished through tactics to decrease length of stay or prevent hospital-acquired conditions such as pressure ulcers (HAPU) or ventilator-associated pneumonia (VAP). In addition, the organization may have objectives to enhance their position as a health care provider or employer of choice. These objectives may relate to obtaining high scores on publicly reported data such as HCAHPS or achieving quality recognition such as Magnet designation.

Developing Implementation Strategies

Objectives are the targeted results and outcomes, and strategies are actions taken to achieve those outcomes. The strategies must be aligned with the organizational culture. In addition, they must be realistic, planned, and intentional, yet flexible enough to respond to unanticipated events.

In the strategic management process, tactics need to be developed with patient safety and quality care as the guiding force (Jasper & Crossan, 2012). Operational strategies need to be evidence based and engage employees at all levels of the organization. Because of this, individuals who develop implementation strategies need to be cognizant of the organizational culture and the impact of changes on those who are tasked with carrying out the plans. As Jasper and Crossan (2012, p. 843) stated, "[I]f we accept that part of the organization's culture is a sense of agreement among staff as to what constitutes the best way forward in any given situation then acknowledgment of those values and beliefs when formulating strategy will be key to successful implementation."

Plans that engage employees are realistic. The need for realistic yet flexible plans is emphasized by the American Nurses Association's (ANA, 2018) Leadership Institute Competency Model. This model identifies the leadership competency of strategic planning as the ability to "translates his or her vision into realistic business strategies" (ANA, 2018, p. 9). Behaviors that demonstrate this competency include:

- Adjusting plans as needed based on circumstances
- Developing plans with consideration for organization-wide needs
- Formulating realistic tactical plans that align with organizational strategies

- Creating contingency plans
- Balancing "long-term goals with immediate organizational needs" (ANA, 2018, p. 9)

This ability to rapidly adapt to changing environmental influences is referred to as *strategic agility* (Kotter, 2014; Shirey, 2015). Kotter maintains that organizations that are not able to shift their operational focus quickly are at risk in an environment of ever-increasing change. Strategic agility has become a key to organizational success. A flexible implementation plan helps an organization remain strong enough to withstand competition, overcome obstacles, and achieve peak performance. The organization's strategy needs to be flexible to respond appropriately to the following:

- Evolving needs and preferences of customers and stakeholders
- Advances in technology
- Changes in political climate and regulatory requirements
- New opportunities
- New entrants/disrupters in the market
- Economic variability
- Altered market conditions
- Disasters and crises

Planning for Implementation

Once the strategies have been delineated, the next step in the strategic planning process is planning for implementation. Implementation involves trying out the activities in a way that determines how best to close the gap between how things are done and what it takes to achieve the strategy. For example, given an objective related to improvement of the financial bottom line, the first step is to determine current cost and then compare it with desired cost to decide what needs to be changed to reach the desired lower cost.

If strategies are to be effective, they must be implemented proficiently, efficiently, and in a timely manner. For this to occur, the organization must attend to its capabilities, the reward structure, available support systems, and the organizational culture. For example, if employees are not rewarded in ways that are meaningful to them, they are unlikely to initiate or maintain efforts to implement the strategy. If the organizational culture does not support innovation or risk taking, or if the prevailing attitude is "if it's not broken, don't fix it," then efforts to improve performance or outcomes may be doomed. Support systems such as education, policies, and procedures must be developed to support the implementation plan.

Implementing strategy is closely linked to an organization's operations; it involves managing, budgeting, motivating, changing culture, supervising, and leading. Strategic planning and implementation are managerial processes that accomplish the following:

- Demonstrate leadership in implementation of the strategy
- Develop accountability structures
- Reward those who carry out the strategy successfully
- Allocate necessary resources to activities critical to the strategy
- Formulate policies and procedures that support the identified strategy
- Initiate continuous quality improvement activities
- Develop and reward best practices
- Maintain a culture that supports the strategy

Effective implementation is more likely when an action plan is developed with input from the individuals who are responsible for implementing the strategic plan. The action plan should include a priority order for achieving the strategic objectives or outcomes, the determination of who (individual or group) is responsible for achieving these objectives, an indication of available or necessary financial support, and a timetable outlining when achievement of the objectives can be expected. If the strategic objective is long term or complex, it may also be advisable to include interim activities and time frames so that progress can be evaluated.

Planning for Evaluation

The final step in the strategic planning process is developing the evaluation design. Planning for evaluation is imperative to ensure that systems and measurements are in place to determine whether the strategic plan has been achieved. During the strategic planning process, measures of success are delineated, responsible individuals are identified, and frequency of evaluation and reporting of these measures is determined. If these progress reports reveal that the measures of success are not being achieved, further evaluation—such as environmental scanning with additional SWOT analysis—may be indicated.

Strategic plan progress reports may appear in a variety of formats from a simple narrative to use of complex strategic management software. Whatever format is used, it should clearly indicate the organization's progress toward its strategic goals.

ELEMENTS OF A STRATEGIC PLAN

Strategic planning results in a written document called the strategic plan. This document may be written by the individuals involved in the strategic planning process or by the individual who facilitated the process (e.g., consultant). Strategic plan documents generally contain the following sections:

- **Executive summary:** A two- to three-page synopsis of the plan, written in language understandable by all potential readers.
- **Background**: A description of the institution, its history, and current state, including its accomplishments, as well as the situation that prompted the strategic planning process.
- **Mission, vision, and values:** A description of the philosophy of the organization.
- **Goals and strategies:** A list of the target objectives and the strategies identified to ensure achievement of the objectives.
- **Appendices:** All additional documentation related to the strategic planning process to provide the background information used by the strategic planners to arrive at the final plan.

Appendix materials may include the annual reports of the institution, SWOT analysis results, financial information, environmental scan results, staffing information, and current and projected programs and services. Other materials may be included as desired. Caution should be exercised, however, to not include confidential data that should not be viewed by individuals outside of the organization.

The strategic plan should be disseminated widely throughout the institution. However, the document does not need to be reproduced in its entirety for everyone in the institution. A decision needs to be made about which parts of the strategic plan are appropriate for the individuals who will receive them. Some may need the entire plan, others may need only the executive summary, and still others may need only the goals and strategies.

In any case, the strategic plan should be communicated to stakeholders: board members, management, and staff. Copies should be included in orientation programs for new employees. The institution's vision and mission—including the core values—should be displayed in public areas (e.g., waiting rooms, cafeteria), as well as in areas reserved for employees. The core values can be listed on employee identification badges and printed in all marketing materials for the organization. The strategic plan tenets should be incorporated into all of the institution's policies and procedures.

Copies of the plan may also be provided to trade or professional organizations with which the institution is associated. The public relations or community outreach department in the institution can use the strategic plan as the basis for a media campaign to educate the community and other stakeholders and audiences about the institution's vision and mission. Patients may be provided with a condensed summary of the strategic plan on admission, particularly those sections related to their care. Patients should be informed of the institution's core values as well.

IMPLEMENTATION OF THE STRATEGIC PLAN

At this point, strategic management often fails. Strategic plans are developed and then allowed to languish as the necessary commitment to implementation is not realized. Strategy projects are said to fail in the range of 50%–90% of the time (Weston, 2020). This may be due to lack of a well-executable plan or lack of follow-through. Often competing priorities impede implementation of the plan. Executives and staff in health care organizations have numerous responsibilities, and implementing strategic objectives adds another burden to an already overwhelming workload. To overcome this obstacle, the strategic plan needs to be integrated into the organization's daily activities. Everyone needs to be committed to implementing the strategic plan, from the leaders to the staff at all levels and in all departments. Focusing on the strategic plan and its meaning to the viability and future of the institution is imperative.

An operational plan is key to maintaining focus on implementation of the strategic plan. The operational plan breaks the strategic plan into manageable components with defined tactics, particularly for those individuals who were not directly involved in crafting the strategic plan. During implementation, the operational plan needs to become a living document that is constantly referenced, consulted, and discussed. The operational plan should be reviewed and updated at regular intervals. Actions that have been completed or those that do not move the organization toward achievement of its goals should be deleted, and new actions based on existing environmental conditions should be added. It may also be necessary to readjust the timeline for completion of some activities in response to external or internal factors that affect the ability to accomplish the desired activities.

Ensuring that the operational plan remains at the forefront of daily activities—whether in an institution as a whole, a department, or a unit—often requires a "champion." This champion is an individual who is passionate and committed to the implementation process and who can inspire others. Often a champion appears as the strategic planning process unfolds; generally, this individual contributes freely, is engaged in the work groups, and expresses interest in the process. Champions can be selected as well, but those who volunteer are usually more enthusiastic about the work than those who are "drafted." Leaders often consider not only formal champions, but also informal champions who have influence in the area of the operational plan in order to increase the chance for success.

LEADERSHIP AND MANAGEMENT IMPLICATIONS

Strategic management is useful for nursing leaders and managers because it can be used to analyze the environment for opportunities and threats; to set measurable, achievable goals and strategies; and to help determine the future of the nursing department or unit. There are two predominant schools of thought today related to strategic planning at the enterprise, facility, department, and unit level. First is the opportunity to develop strategic plans for each of the levels, to align them, and then deploy. Second is the idea that the only one strategic plan should be developed at the highest organizational level, meaning a health system would develop a strategic plan at the enterprise level and the remainder of the plans would then be operational plans to support the overarching strategic plan. Regardless of the approach, strategic plans need to cascade and align to link and relate to the organization's overall mission, vision, and values. Success in strategic planning and implementing the operational plan will position nursing well, and more importantly this is critical to the success of the organization. The process provides an opportunity for nursing to shine, because the similarities between the nursing process and the strategic planning process allow nurses to shortcut the learning curve and begin to move forward with the implementation phase while others may still be grappling with the planning process. Nursing skills and abilities make it relatively easy to plan strategically, and nurses, as 24-hour workers, can approach implementation as an ongoing, continuous, and seamless process. Nurses' involvement with continuous quality improvement and performance improvement systems provides a basis for participation in strategic planning that is systematic and thorough.

Implementation of the organization's strategic plan can be useful in unifying staff on a nursing unit or in a department. Collaboration and cooperation among staff generally are required to accomplish strategic objectives. Working together to accomplish a strategic objective keeps staff engaged. Involvement in decisions that ultimately will affect them is essential and often results in positive spin-offs; for example, staff members feel a sense of ownership in the process and pride in their accomplishments.

CURRENT ISSUES AND TRENDS

Many current issues and trends affect the strategic management process in health care organizations and nursing. These trends include a focus on the Institute for Health care Improvement's (IHI) Quadruple Aim, the effect of the Patient Protection and Affordable Care Act (ACA), and continued attention to the goals of the IOM's *Future of Nursing* report.

First proposed in 2008, the Triple Aim established by the IHI includes goals related to population health, improving the patient experience, and decreasing per capita cost (IHI, 2016; Whittington et al., 2015). The Triple Aim transformed to become the Quadruple Aim, with the fourth aim being that of improving work environments and the experience of health care workers (Sikka et al., 2015). The IHI posited that these goals can strengthen other health care reform measures such as accountable care organizations (ACOs), bundled payments, avoidance of penalties for preventable events such as hospital readmissions or hospital-acquired infections, and the conservation of human capital in health care. Strategic management in health care organizations requires attention to these goals in order to maintain optimal reimbursement and remain financially viable.

Tenets of the original Triple Aim were incorporated in the ACA, another trend that affects strategic management in health care organizations. Provisions of the ACA, which was implemented in 2010, continue to evolve (Rand Health Care, 2017). Overall, the ACA has resulted in fewer uninsured individuals but has also affected hospital and provider reimbursement. As the ACA's mandates continue to be phased into practice, health care organizations must strategically manage their impact on overall operations.

Finally, the continued focus on the IOM's (2010) *Future of Nursing* goals drives the strategic goals of health care organizations and nursing practice. Elimination of barriers to practicing at the full scope of practice, advancing educational preparation of nurses, creating diversity in the nursing workforce, leading change to promote health, and improving collection of nursing workforce data all require continued effort (NAM, 2015). However, the shifting health care environment requires more inter-professional collaboration and mandates that organizations and nursing professionals engage with a broad base of stakeholders to promote the Quadruple Aim targets of population health, patient satisfaction, and decreased costs of health care while also improving the care giver's experience.

CONCLUSION

Strategic planning is not reserved for activities such as seeking recognition through the ANCC Magnet Recognition Program® or for ameliorating workforce issues in a particular institution. Any business venture benefits from having a strategic plan. The plan provides for assessment of the environment, including current and future opportunities, and identification of specific, measurable, realistic ways of taking advantage of those opportunities. Most importantly, perhaps, the strategic plan answers the question, "What business are we in?" Clearly defining a mission and vision helps a nursing unit or department focus its efforts on its core business.

Strategic planning and strategic management are necessary components of business in today's competitive and highly unstable health care environment. Strategic planning is a process similar to the nursing process, with defined and specific steps to be taken to ensure that a comprehensive and thorough process occurs. Strategic management involves implementation of the strategic plan to ensure that the organization is responsive to changes in its environment as well as to internal events.

Strategic planning and strategic management are not reserved exclusively for organizations. Individuals such as nurses can use these techniques to determine their own direction and establish objectives to ensure that they meet the goals they have set for themselves. Nurses in all areas of practice and in all employment settings can use the principles of strategic planning to explore programs, projects, and services and to advance their careers. Nurses who are involved in any aspect of an institution's strategic planning efforts should incorporate those activities into a personal portfolio (Cope & Murray, 2018) and use those activities to reflect their competence and expertise as well as their own professional development.

RESEARCH NOTE

Source

Alvarez-Maldonado, P., Reding-Bernal, A., Hernandez-Solis, A., & Cicero-Sabido, R. (2019). Impact of strategic planning, organizational culture imprint and care bundles to reduce adverse events in the ICU. *International Journal for Quality in Health Care, 31*(6), 480–484.

Purpose

To evaluate the impact of a multi-faceted program on quality outcomes and adverse events in a respiratory intensive care unit (ICU) in a large tertiary care setting using a cross-sectional secondary analysis design.

Discussion

Adverse events in hospital settings contribute to significant morbidity and mortality and are responsible for approximately 400,000 deaths per year in hospitalized patients. The authors undertook the project with the primary goal of reducing the number of nosocomial infections related to mechanical ventilation and central venous catheters.

The team implemented a multi-pronged program based upon three "Es" from the Michigan Keystone organizational change model: Engage (strategic planning and organizational culture imprint), Educate (training and practice), and Execute (implementation of care bundles). The project leadership team then conducted strategic planning sessions and completed a SWOT analysis prior to implementing the project based on the three Es framework. Some of the threats identified included work overload, resistance to change and a lack of commitment to the organization's mission and vision. As part of the organizational

RESEARCH NOTE—cont'd

culture aspect of project implementation, key messages emphasized the importance of "belonging to the organization," also known as wearing the institution's t-shirt. The educational presentations centered on the organization's strong foundation and focus on the roles and value of all health care team members' contributions to care and implementation of specific care bundles aimed at reducing ventilator- and central venous catheter-associated infections.

As a result of the project, infections related to central venous catheters and mechanical ventilators were reduced by 40% per 1000 patient catheter or ventilator days. As a secondary finding in the analysis, the authors also monitored other adverse events and observed reductions in some of those patient outcomes as well, including accidental extubation, pneumothorax, endotracheal tube changes, and atelectasis. They observed an 18% reduction in ICU death rates.

Application to Practice

Current health care environments are filled with complexity. As organizations face ever-increasing demands to achieve quality clinical and financial outcomes, traditional linear approaches often no longer prove effective in solving problems or attaining desired goals and objectives. Interprofessional health care team members each bring unique knowledge, competencies and skill sets that bring value to care delivery and patient outcomes.

Strategic planning is the foundation of any organization, department, unit, and team initiative and involves bringing interprofessional teams together to conduct SWOT analyses, set goals, and plan, implement, and evaluate the project. Aligning processes with organization mission, vision, and values and engaging interprofessional team members and key stakeholders throughout the project is vital to success.

CASE STUDY

The Chief Nursing Officer (CNO) in a large urban health care facility approached the Chair of the organization's shared governance council (SGC) about engaging the council in a project to improve patient satisfaction scores. The senior leaders had implemented various strategies to improve the "patient experience" without successfully achieving health system targets. Senior executives and leaders were concerned about the impact of these patient outcomes on Centers for Medicare & Medicaid Services reimbursement and the organization's financial outcomes.

Since the SGC chair was working with council leadership to plan council activities and set goals for the coming year, she agreed that this initiative was certainly an important area of focus that impacted the majority of clinical areas represented by council members. The Chair also believed that council members' involvement and engagement in this work could have significant impact on patient, unit, and organization outcomes.

Once the CNO and SGC Chair set expectations and planned an approach, the CNO attended the January SGC meeting to present an overview of the organization's mission, vision, and values; a synopsis of strategies implemented and recent annual patient satisfaction outcome results. Following the formal presentation, the CNO hosted an open forum and question and answer session with council members regarding the patient experience.

Following the initial SGC meeting, the SGC Chair then worked with a task force of leaders and interprofessional team members to set goals, develop a timeline, and formalize the project overview and presented the information to the entire SGC membership at the next meeting. Following the task force presentation, the SGC Chair and task force members facilitated work group sessions with all SGC members present. Members were divided into small groups to complete their assigned tasks for the meeting.

CRITICAL THINKING EXERCISE

Pursuant to the Shared Governance Council's "patient experience" improvement project, the Chair charged the council members with homework assignments that included meeting with their managers and unit council leaders to present the project information and expectations. Each council member, in collaboration with their unit leaders, would identify and implement at least two interventions aimed at improving patients' experiences on their units.

As council members returned to their units and clinical areas to partner with their managers to complete their assignments and lead these efforts, each member engaged their interprofessional team members in finding the best evidence-based interventions that their disciplines could implement to improve patient satisfaction scores.

1. Which team members have the greatest impact on patients' satisfaction with their hospital experiences, and how can they be involved?
2. Once the team develops a plan for improving these patient experience outcomes, what elements of strategic planning, implementation, and evaluation will lead to accomplishing the best team, patient and unit outcomes?
3. What measures can team members use to periodically evaluate outcomes?

REFERENCES

Alvarez-Maldonado, P., Reding-Bernal, A., Hernandez-Solis, A., & Cicero-Sabido, R. (2019). Impact of strategic planning, organizational culture imprint and care bundles to reduce adverse events in the ICU. *International Journal for Quality in Health Care, 31*(6), 480–484.

American College of Healthcare Executives (ACHE). (2020). *ACHE healthcare executive 2020 competencies assessment tool.* https://www.ache.org/-/media/ache/career-resource-center/competencies_booklet.pdf.

American Nurses Association (ANA). (2018). *ANA leadership competency model.* https://www.nursingworld.org/~4a0a2e/globalassets/docs/ce/177626-ana-leadership-booklet-new-final.pdf.

American Nurses Credentialing Center (ANCC). (2017). *Magnet® application manual* 2019: Silver Spring, MD.: American Nurses Credentialing Center.

American Organization of Nurse Executives (AONE)/American Organization for Nursing Leadership (AONL). (2015). *AONE nurse executive competencies*: Chicago, IL: AONE. https://www.aonl.org/sites/default/files/aone/nec.pdf.

Bowles, J. R., Adams, J. M., Batcheller, J., Zimmermann, D., & Pappas, S. (2018). The role of the nurse leader in advancing the quadruple aim. *Nurse Leader, 16*(4), 244–248. https://doi.org/10.1016/j.mnl.2018.05.011.

BusinessDictionary. (2020). *Stakeholder.* http://www.businessdictionary.com/definition/stakeholder.html.

Centers for Disease Control & Prevention (CDC). (2015). Do a SWOT analysis. In *Communities of practice resource kit.* https://www.cdc.gov/phcommunities/resourcekit/evaluate/swot_analysis.html.

Cope, V., & Murray, M. (2018). Use of professional portfolios in nursing. *Nursing Standard, 32*(30), 55–63.

Institute for Healthcare Improvement (IHI). (2016). *IHI triple aim initiative: Better care for individuals, better care for populations, and lower per capita costs.* http://www.ihi.org/Engage/Initiatives/TripleAim/Pages/default.aspx.

Institute of Medicine (IOM. (2010). *The future of nursing: Leading change, advancing health.* https://www.nap.edu/read/12956/chapter/1.

Jasper, M., & Crossan, F. (2012). What is strategic management. *Journal of Nursing Management, 20*(7), 838–846.

Jones, B. (2018). Mission versus purpose: What's the difference? Talking point. *Disney Institute Blog.* https://www.disneyinstitute.com/blog/mission-versus-purpose-whats-the-difference/.

Kotter, J. P. (2014). *Building strategic agility for a faster moving world.* Cambridge, MA: Harvard Business Press Books.

Lasater, K. B., Germack, H. D., Small, D. S., & McHugh, M. D. (2016). Hospitals known for nursing excellence perform better on Value Based Purchasing measures. *Policy & Politics & Nursing Practice, 17*(4), 177–186.

Guide, Management Study (2020). *Strategic management—meaning and important concepts.* https://www.managementstudyguide.com/strategic-management.htm.

Nag, R., Hambrick, B. C., & Chen, M.-J. (2007). What is strategic management, really? Inductive derivation of a consensus definition of the field. *Strategic Management Journal, 28*, 935–955.

National Academies of Sciences, Engineering, and Medicine (NAM). (2015). *Assessing progress on the Institute of Medicine Report The Future of Nursing.* Washington, DC: The National Academies Press.

Pearce, J. A., & Robinson, R. (2012). *Strategic management* (13th ed.). New York, NY: McGraw-Hill/Irwin.

Rand Health Care. (2017). *The future of U.S. health care: Replace or revise the Affordable Care Act?* https://www.rand.org/health-care/key-topics/health-policy/in-depth.html.

Shirey, M. R. (2015). Strategic agility for nursing leadership. *Journal of Nursing Administration, 45*(6), 305–308.

Sikka, R., Morath, J. M., & Leape, L. (2015). The quadruple aim: Care, health, cost and meaning in work. *BMJ Quality & Safety, 24*(10), 608–610. https://doi.org/10.1136/bmjqs-2015-004160.

Sinek, S. (2009). *Start with why: How great leaders inspire everyone to take action.* New York: Portfolio.

Sinek, S. (2019). *The infinite game.* New York: Portfolio.

Society for Human Resource Management (SHRM). (2018). *Mission & vision statements: What is the difference between mission, vision and value statements?* https://www.shrm.org/resourcesandtools/tools-and-samples/hr-qa/pages/isthereadifferencebetweenacompany%E2%80%99smission,visionandvaluestatements.aspx.

The Joint Commission. (2020). *Stroke certification*. https://www.jointcommission.org/en/accreditation-and-certification/certification/certifications-by-setting/hospital-certifications/stroke-certification/.

Wadsworth, B., Felton, F., & Linus, R. (2016). SOARing into strategic planning: Engaging nurses to achieve significant outcomes. *Nursing Administration Quarterly, 40*(4), 299–306.

Weston, M. J. (2020). Strategic planning in an age of uncertainty: Creating clarity in uncertain times. *Nurse Leader, 18*(1), 54–58.

Whittington, J. W., Nolan, K., Lewis, N., & Torres, T. (2015). Pursuing the Triple Aim: The first 7 years. *Milbank Quarterly, 93*(2), 263–300. http://www.milbank.org/uploads/documents/featured-articles/pdf/Milbank_Quarterly_Vol-93_No-_2_Pursuing_the_Triple_Aim_The_First_7_Years.pdf.

15

Professional Practice Models

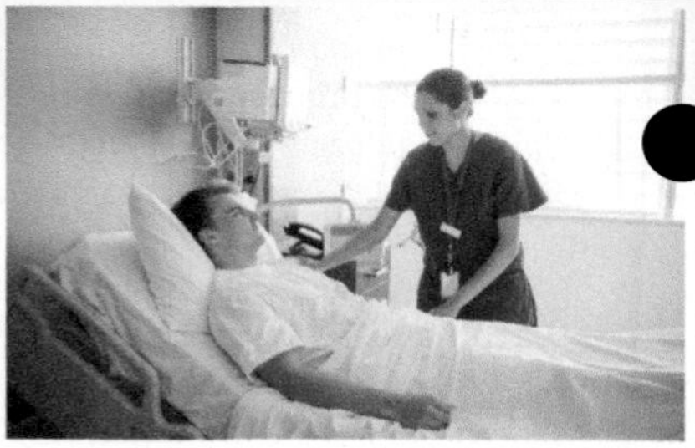

Joy Parchment

http://evolve.elsevier.com/Huber/leadership

Health care organizations continue to evolve with rapid speed to deliver safe, quality care that meets the needs of patients. Fueling this change is the adoption of the Centers for Medicare & Medicaid Services' (CMS) incentive programs that penalize or reward health care organizations for high quality value rather than the volume of services performed (CMS, 2019; Lasater et al., 2016). The achievement of patient outcomes that demonstrate the delivery of safe, high quality patient care requires organizations to match the caring side of the health care business with available and/or limited resources. The practice of nursing requires nurses to serve as patient advocates, to integrate the best evidence into the delivery of patient care, and to improve the health of individuals (American Nurses Association, 2015). Nurses, intricately linked to the delivery of patient care, are challenged to transform health care with innovative care models that result in positive, sustainable, valued-added benefits to patients, providers, and organizations.

Over 20 years ago, researchers identified nursing sensitive indicators (NSIs) or elements of patient care that nurses directly influence (Heslop & Lu, 2014). In addition to NSIs, the publicly reported patient's perception of care survey known as Hospital Consumer Assessment of Healthcare Providers and Systems (HCAHPS), is used by CMS and other accrediting bodies to determine clinical quality outcomes of patient care or high-quality value that is tied back to hospital reimbursements. Patient's perception of care or patient satisfaction, an outcome measure for all hospitals, includes the ability of nurses to identify and mitigate the inherent suffering that patients experience when receiving care (Dempsey et al., 2014) (Box 15.1). However, the ability to attain high quality outcomes depends on the organization's approach to matching human and material resources, patient characteristics, and health care needs to professional practice and care delivery models.

DEFINITIONS

The terms *professional practice model* and *care delivery model*, though used interchangeably in practice settings, are quite different. A **professional practice model (PPM** as defined by the American Nurses Credentialing Center (ANCC) is "a schematic depiction of a system, theory, or phenomenon that depicts how nurses practice, collaborate, communicate, and develop professionally to provide the highest-quality care for those served by the organization" (ANCC, 2017, p. 158). This visual representation serves as the foundational guide for how nurses' practice provides meaning for nurses and defines the structure and processes that enable nurses to achieve exemplary outcomes while practicing at top of license (Glassman, 2016; Stallings-Welden & Shirey, 2015).

Core elements of a PPM include a theoretical framework, nursing values or beliefs, leadership, care delivery model, collaborative relationships, autonomous decision-making, environment, research and innovation integration, and development and recognition (Duffy, 2016; Slayter et al., 2016). Organizations that utilize a PPM will typically include it on their website, in organizational documents, and in their nursing annual report.

BOX 15.1 Nursing Sensitive Indicators and Patient Satisfaction Outcomes

Nursing Sensitive Indicators

Structure

- Nursing hours per patient day
- Nursing turnover rate
- Registered nurse (RN) education/certification
- Staff or skill mix

Process

- Pediatric pain assessment and intervention, reassessment

Process and Outcome

- Patient falls
- Patient falls with injury
- Pressure injury (community, hospital, unit acquired)
- RN Survey (job satisfaction, practice environment)

Outcome

- Adverse outcomes of care: wrong site, side, patient, procedure, implant
- Antibiotic stewardship
- Delay in treatment
- Nosocomial infections (catheter-associated urinary tract infection [CAUTI]; central line-associated bloodstream infection [CLABSI]; clostridium difficile [CDIFF]; methicillin-resistant staphylococcus aureus [MRSA]; venous thromboembolism [VTE]
- Peripheral intravenous infiltration (PIV)
- Psychiatric physical/sexual assaults
- Pressure injuries, device related, hospital acquired

Patient Satisfaction

Outcome

- Patient engagement or patient-centered care
- Patient education
- Care coordination
- Safety
- Service recovery
- Courtesy and respect
- Responsiveness
- Pain
- Careful listening

(National Database for Nursing Quality Indicators, n.d.; Press Ganey, 2020; Centers for Medicare & Medicaid Services, 2020).

A **care delivery model (CDM** is integrated with the PPM and defines the operational mechanism for organizing care, the skill set needed to provide care, the setting for the care, and what the intended outcome could be for patients and families (ANCC, 2017). Inherent in all CDMs is the authority of the nurse to make informed clinical decisions, the accountability process for decision-making that maximizes quality and safety of nursing care, and the collaborative approach used with other members of the interdisciplinary team (ANCC, 2017). Several types of CDMs are noted in the literature. The two most prominent are total patient care and team nursing. In total patient care, one registered nurse (RN) is responsible for the total care of a patient or groups of patients. With team nursing, a team consisting of care providers with varying skill mix will care for groups of patients throughout their shift (Havaei et al., 2016).

BACKGROUND

Professional practice models were first described in the literature in the 1980s to articulate exemplary nursing practice, nurses' control over the delivery of care, and the practice environment; all core components of Magnet® organizations (ANCC, 2017). Nursing literature chronicles the influence of the work environment on nursing practice and identifies a strong correlation between work environments, safety, and the delivery of quality patient care (Olds et al., 2017). Executive leaders are responsible for designing strategies to create innovative work environments that support the practice of nurses. Given the complexity of nursing practice and the myriad of factors that influence patient, team, and organizational outcomes, nurse leaders need to actively collaborate with clinical nurses to determine the most effective models that can achieve quality outcomes (Wharton et al., 2016; Winslow et al., 2019). If these decisions are made only by executive nurse leaders, exemplary outcomes are less likely to occur.

The conceptual framework by Donabedian (1988) is frequently used to identify **s**tructures and **p**rocesses that promote positive **o**utcomes (S-P-O), and these concepts are causally linked. Structures support the care delivery process and focus on how the delivery of care is organized, the skill mix of the team, and the available number of care providers (ANCC, 2017).

Processes consist of two categories: clinical and interpersonal processes, such as collaborative teamwork, patient–provider communications, cultural sensitivity of care, and patient education. Outcomes answer the "so what" and are organized into three domains to include: patients, nurses, and the organization (ANCC, 2017; Donabedian, 1988).

PROFESSIONAL PRACTICE MODELS

An important predictor of RN job satisfaction is the presence of a PPM. Job satisfaction is directly associated with nurse turnover, which is a significant human resource challenge for nurse leaders (Sabei et al., 2020). Professional practice models consist of structures, processes, and values that support nurses' control over practice, enhance job satisfaction, and decision-making (Basol et al., 2015). Yet, the Magnet Recognition Program®, the highest recognition for nursing practice and known for being associated with organizations' success at attracting and retaining nurses, is credited with bringing to the forefront the PPM. Of the five components of the Magnet model, one component focuses on exemplary professional practice and the enculturation of the PPM into the practice environment (ANCC, 2017; Basol et al., 2015). Though many core elements of PPMs exist, seven major elements will be discussed: theoretical framework, leadership, autonomy and collaborative relationships, practice environment, development and recognition, research and innovation, and the CDM.

Theoretical Framework

PPMs are often grounded within a nursing or organizational theoretical framework, such as Kolcaba's comfort theory, Koloroutis' (2004) relationship-based care theory, systems theory; or PPMs are based on an established nursing concept like professional (shared) governance or Benner's novice to expert model (Cordo & Hill-Rodriguez, 2017; Kolcaba et al., 2006; Slayter et al., 2016). Nurse-driven PPMs prosper when nurse leaders at all levels support nursing professional practice. Evidence of professional practice support includes active professional (shared) governance councils and resources to engage and empower nurses in their practice (Cordo & Hill-Rodriguez, 2017; Glassman, 2016).

A strong link between the PPM, the vision, mission statements, and core values of the organization are vital to ensure adoption of the PPM. Also, alignment of nursing values with organizational values supports a culture of excellence throughout the organization (Slayter et al., 2016). Mission, vision, values, and philosophy also are fundamental to strategic planning. These foundational elements for PPMs will be briefly reviewed here.

Mission Statements

The purpose or goal of an organization is expressed by its *mission statement*. For health care organizations their sole existence is to deliver patient care. Publicly posted mission statements communicate to key stakeholders, the public, and employees the organization's purpose and identity. Mission statements provide information and support an organization's public relations. For management at all levels of an organization, the mission statement acts as a blueprint or foundational guide for developing specific measurable objectives and actions (Alegre et al., 2018).

Measurable *objectives and actions* associated with the mission statement explicitly represent what the organization is trying to do, and these initiatives keep an organization on track by providing guidelines and indicators for measuring present performance. Lack of goal alignment across an organization can trigger conflict and slow progress toward goal completion (Alegre et al., 2018). Nurse leaders are responsible for ensuring their unit, department, service line goals, and performance measures are in alignment with the organization's mission. A common source of conflict related to goal achievement within the complex health care environment is resource allocation, such as nurse staffing. However, an important leadership responsibility is to ensure that stakeholders agree with the mission statement and goals and support their enactment.

Vision Statements

Vision statements are often confused with mission statements. The difference is vision statements focus on the future direction of the organization and are crafted to describe the most desirable state at some future point in time. Vision statements are meant to be an inspirational tool for organizational leadership to reenergize and motivate stakeholders to ensure the fulfillment of the vision. Fully deployed vision statements have demonstrated a positive correlation with financial and growth performance metrics (Gulati et al., 2016).

Values Statements

Core *values* are strongly held beliefs and priorities that guide organizational decision-making. Values do not change but are anchors or fundamental beliefs that are constant and relate to the mission and vision of the organization. Values create the culture of the organization and drive the behaviors of team members. Furthermore, personally held values need to demonstrate congruency with organizational values because value congruency can predict compliance, autonomous practice, and conformity with organizational norms (Eva et al., 2017).

Philosophy

A statement of *philosophy* is defined as an explanation of the systems of beliefs, values, or ethics that determine how the mission and vision will be achieved. The philosophy is abstract; it describes an ideal state and gives direction to achieving the purpose. Philosophy statements typically begin with "we believe" and could be stated in any of the following ways:

- We believe everyone has a right to the highest quality of care.
- We believe we have an obligation to render quality care at a cost-effective price.
- We believe that any person who presents for care should receive care, regardless of his or her ability to pay.

The philosophy has implications for the role of the nurse. If an organization's stated mission includes patient care, education, and research utilization, then the expectation will be for nurses to embrace all aspects of the mission. Nurses develop new knowledge, integrate the best evidence into their practice to ensure exemplary patient outcomes, and participate in educating patients and nursing colleagues. For example, a correlation study of approximately 500 clinical nurses identified a positive significant relationship between the ethical climate of the organization, the level of support given to nurses, and turnover intentions (Abou Hashish, 2017). Nurse leaders, therefore, need to identify misaligned values, address possible sources of ethical conflict, and put strategies in place to decrease ethical conflicts before nurses take action and leave the organization.

Leadership

A key element identified in PPMs is the assumption that all nurses regardless of position are leaders. Leadership for organizational leaders includes setting the vision to ensure alignment with organizational values and strategies; ensuring that nurses have an equal voice at nursing and interprofessional decision-making groups, committees, forums, and councils; and empowering nurses to lead (Slayter et al., 2016). To ensure a professional practice environment of ownership, empowerment and engagement by nurses, some organizations have implemented professional (shared) governance structures at the unit, hospital, and or system levels. This structure has decreased the organizational bureaucratic layers found in most health care organizations and enabled relationship building leadership styles to flourish (Clavelle et al., 2016).

Autonomy and Collaborative Relationships

The practice of nursing is governed by nurses, and this grants nurses the authority to practice within identified scope and standards of practice to benefit patients, families, and communities. Nurses are given the self-governing right to define, credential, and evaluate nursing practice to promote health, protect patients/clients, and prevent illness and injury (Fowler, 2017). To accomplish these directives, nurses are granted the authority by their respective board of nursing to make autonomous decisions and/or to engage various collaborative health care providers to ensure the delivery of appropriate care to patients. Thus, collaborative relationships and/or partnerships built on trust involve effective communication techniques to not only engage patients with their care, but also to facilitate effective relationships between other interdisciplinary providers.

Practice Environment

The practice environment is a driver for nurse satisfaction, burnout, intent to leave, and patient mortality (Cicolini et al., 2014; Olds et al., 2017). Positive practice environments, also known as **healthy work environments,** are often found in Magnet designated organizations (Box 15.2). Magnet hospitals are known for their exemplary nursing care, transformative leadership,

BOX 15.2 Organizational Structures for Healthy Work Environment

- Effective leaders at all levels of the organization
- Professional development opportunities
- Staffing structures that consider nurse competencies, patient needs, and teamwork
- Interdisciplinary collaboration
- Empowered, shared decision-making
- Patient-centered culture/culture of safety
- Quality improvement infrastructure, evidence-based practice
- Visible acknowledgment of nursing's unique, valued contributions (e.g., professional practice model, vision/mission/philosophy statements)

(ANCC, 2017; AACN, 2005).

low turnover, and superior patient outcomes, such as higher patient care experiences and lower infection, mortality and morbidity rates over non-Magnet hospitals (Lasater et al., 2016; Park et al., 2016; Stimpfel et al., 2016). To achieve these outcomes, Magnet hospitals have structures and processes that support nursing professional practice (ANCC, 2017; Stimpfel et al., 2016). These structures and processes are differentiating factors for nurse satisfaction and quality patient outcomes. Most Magnet-like characteristics are easy to adapt to different work contexts. Characteristics such as involving nurses in practice decisions, providing resources for ongoing development, and utilizing a relationship building leadership style are demonstrated to have a dramatic impact on the environment where nurses practice.

Development and Recognition

Health care is constantly changing. What was current 2 years ago is perhaps now outdated. This never-ending evolution of health care practices and standards requires nurses to have a growth mindset, to pursue professional **development** activities to ensure the safety of patients, and to expand their professional knowledge and competence. Ulep (2018) suggested key strategies to retain millennial nurses included the availability of professional development resources, career advancement pathways or opportunities, and real-time coaching from their nurse leader. Strategies like intentional mentoring, the use of various conversations that help nurses understand that they make a difference in their practice, and the establishment of early accomplishments can build long-term loyalty with millennial nurses (Ulep, 2018).

Recognition of nurses is positively linked to job satisfaction and retention of nurses (Tang & Hudson, 2019; Ulep, 2018). To ensure a healthy practice environment, the American Association of Critical-Care Nurses (AACN, 2005) included meaningful recognition as an important strategy. Meaningful recognition consists of communicating the value that the nurse brings to the delivery of patient care, identifying exemplary nursing care, and celebrating their accomplishments and milestones. Though there are numerous ways that nurses can be recognized, many organizations utilize the DAISY Award™ (https://www.daisyfoundation.org/daisy-award), an international award program that has grown in notoriety and is described as continuing the legacy of thanks to ensure that nurses understand how critical their role is for the health of nations (Barnes et al., 2016).

Research and Innovation

The utilization of new knowledge and innovative strategies into the practice environment is critical to meet the evolving needs of patients and healthcare. **Research** is defined as "the systematic inquiry that uses disciplined methods to answer specific questions or solve problems. The goal of research is to develop, refine, and expand knowledge" (Polit & Beck, 2017, p. 3). Though the translation of research into the practice environment is slow, the improvement of patient outcomes cannot be undervalued. All completed research studies should be disseminated, but not all research can be adopted into practice because research needs to be evaluated for quality and relevancy to the population at hand (Curtis et al., 2017).

Innovation is described as the utilization of creative or problem-solving techniques that result in a widely adopted strategy, product, or service to fill a need in a way that is new, different, or was non-existent before. Innovations will typically consist of quality improvement or cost effective or efficiency measures that impact the practice environment (Kaya et al., 2016). When integrated together these two concepts of research and innovation focus on what is possible and what is needed. The innovation can be studied to prove a theory, assess feasibility across different populations, or to ensure generalizability. Innovations can also serve as solutions to issues in the current practice environment. Innovation can include new CDMs, new leadership styles, and or new processes that drive change and redefine the practice environment (Weberg, 2009).

STRUCTURES AND PROCESSES THAT SUPPORT CARE DELIVERY MODELS

The appropriate CDM is the one that maximizes existing resources while meeting organizational goals and objectives, specifically the mission of the organization. However, to ensure the effective delivery of patient care, structures and processes such as policies, procedures, and clinical protocols are part of the tools that allow nurses to practice accountably.

Policies and Procedures

Policies and procedures are two functional elements or written rules of an organization that are extensions of the mission statements. Together they determine the requirements of the unit, department, service line, or organization. Policies and procedures provide order and stability so that the unit functions in a coordinated manner within the larger structure of nursing and the health care organization. Standard *operating policies and procedures* integrate behaviors of team members to prevent random chaos and maintain order, function, structure, and most of all decision-making (Amadei, 2016).

Policies

A **policy** serves as a formal guideline that directs action for thinking about and solving recurring problems related to practice and or the objectives of the organization. Throughout the practice arena, specific instances exist when team members are not clear about who is supposed to do something, the circumstances that an action should occur, or what should be done about unusual circumstances (Amadei, 2016). Policies, therefore, clarify actions, direct decision-making, and serve as guides to increase the likelihood of consistency with decisions and actions. Though broad limits are available with policies, there could be some modifications made for unique circumstances.

Written policies are *formal* and general in nature to cover all team members. Unwritten policies are *informal* and are established by patterns of decisions and interpretation of observed behaviors. For instance, an unwritten policy of an organization is the expectation that all individuals will receive compassionate care. However, this expectation may not be written as a policy. Yet, by decisions and disciplinary actions that occur, a team member can infer there is a policy that will be enforced even though it is not written (Box 15.3).

BOX 15.3 Policies

- Serve as guides
- Help coordinate plans
- Control performance
- Increase consistency of action
- Should be written
- Usually are general in nature
- Refer to all employees

Some general nursing areas require the formulation of policies. These include areas where there is confusion about the locus of responsibility and where lack of guidance might result in the neglect, malpractice, or "malperformance" of an act necessary for the patient. Unambiguous policies are necessary for medication error reporting, the protection of patients' or families' rights, and matters of human resource management and personnel welfare. Conflicts arise when a lack of explicit criteria to inform decisions and actions exists (Amadei, 2016).

Procedures

Procedures are descriptions of step-by-step directions, methods for actions to take in common situations, and serve as a ready reference for all personnel. **Procedures** require the best evidence and should be written in enough detail to provide the information required by all persons engaging in the activity. This means procedures will have a statement of purpose, identify who is to perform the activity and include the steps necessary along with a list of supplies and equipment needed for the activity (Box 15.4).

BOX 15.4 Procedures

- Provide step-by-step methods
- Are written in detail
- Provide guidelines for commonly occurring events
- Provide a ready reference
- Guide performance of an activity
- Should include the following:
  - A statement of purpose
  - Identification of who performs activity
  - Steps in the procedure
  - A list of supplies and equipment needed

The similarities between policies and procedures are that both are a means for accomplishing objectives and are necessary for the smooth functioning of any work group, department, or organization. The difference between a policy and a procedure is that a policy is a directive that must be followed, for example, the use of restraints. A procedure provides direction, such as evidence-based steps to perform a urinary catheterization. There are legal implications to the application of policies and procedures. For instance, the nurse may be held liable for failing to follow written policies and procedures. Thus, it is important for nurses to be informed about policies and procedures governing practice in an organization. In addition, both policies and procedures need regular and periodic review (Amadei, 2016).

Clinical Protocols

Clinical protocols fall under the umbrella term of *structured care methodologies* (SCMs). SCMs are interdisciplinary tools that identify best practices, facilitate standardization of care, and provide a mechanism to track variances, quality, and outcomes (Cole & Houston, 1999). *Clinical or critical pathways, evidenced-based algorithms, clinical protocols, standards of care, order sets,* and *clinical practice guidelines* are all types of SCMs. However, the gold standard for clinical protocols is the use of best evidence to reduce practice variation in a patient outcome focused environment.

A *clinical pathway* is a written plan that identifies key, critical, or predictable incidents that must occur at set times to achieve patient outcomes within an appropriate length of stay in a hospital setting. As a pathway, it is a tracking system for the timing of treatments and interventions, health outcomes, complications, activity, and teaching/learning (Pound et al., 2017). Pathways are also considered a method of quality improvement to assist health care providers with clinical process innovation (Pound et al., 2017).

CARE DELIVERY MODELS

A variety of patient CDMs exist. The redesign of a CDM is influenced by fiscal responsibility, accountability to the consumer, available resources, and quality and safety considerations. Although all models have their advantages and disadvantages, there is no one right way to structure patient care. Quite often, aspects of older or traditional, models are incorporated into new delivery models. Therefore, it is important to understand the variety of models available. They may be old, traditional, new, evolving, and/or innovative. With the proliferation of numerous health care provider roles, expedited care processes, and increased patient acuity and needs, pure nursing models that flourished in less complex environments have yielded to collaborative practice and interdisciplinary approaches. Understanding the historical perspective helps nurses to better analyze options for current practice.

Traditional Nursing Care Delivery Models

Historians mark the emergence of modern nursing from the time of Florence Nightingale's work in the Crimea. Nightingale (1860) believed that nursing care of patients included spiritual well-being as well as their environment. Over the past century, the evolution of nursing models of care has resulted from the impact of economic, social, and political agendas. There are five traditional nursing models of care: (1) private duty, (2) functional, (3) team, (4) primary, and (5) case management. Of those, functional, team, primary, and case management were and are currently associated with hospital nursing practice. Private duty and case management were associated with public health, home health, and community health but have been adapted to the inpatient setting. Private duty, later called *case* or *case management*, was the original way nursing care was delivered; it later became the foundation for public health nursing and community service delivery (Muir, 2019; Whelan, 2012).

Private Duty Nursing

Private duty nursing is sometimes called *case nursing*, because it is based on the case method where each patient is a case. Another term for private duty nursing is total patient care. There are two ways of thinking about *total patient care*. One approach is holistic care of the total patient, including mind, body, and spirit. Another approach is functionally based, where a nurse assumes total care for one patient. Private duty nursing is the oldest care model in the United States. Between 1890 and 1929, graduate nurses in the United States served as private duty nurses, caring for patients in their homes (Muir, 2019; Whelan, 2012). Nurses did the cooking, cleaning, bathing of wounds, and organizing of the household functions, basically functioning as a home manager. A form of hospital case nursing evolved between 1900 and the 1930s. When the Great Depression hit, most families were too poor to afford private duty nurses and so nurses were without jobs. Hospitals then began to employ graduate nurses. As the graduate nurses who had been doing private duty moved into the hospital, the desire was to retain the type of care model to which they had become accustomed. Private duty was transplanted into hospital settings for as long as nurses were paid by patients. When nurses became employees of hospitals, the kind of care that private duty allowed was not possible within the organizational structure of hospital staff nursing (Muir, 2019; Whelan, 2012).

The advantages of private duty nursing were one-to-one care, the ability to foster close nurse–patient relationships, and attainment of a high degree of autonomy. The disadvantages were the high cost and low efficiency associated with this model. With the shift to hospital-based care, nurses' job security was questionable (Whelan, 2012).

Two main variations on the basic pattern of private duty nursing developed within hospitals: group nursing and total patient care.

Group nursing was a care model proposed in the 1930s by Geister, then the executive director of the American Nurses Association (ANA). Defined as nursing group practice, the idea of group nursing in hospitals was similar to divisional private duty in which several patients shared a private nurse. The plan was to reorganize private duty from individual to group practice both inside and outside the hospital. The intention was to link a group practice registry of private duty nurses to a community's public health nursing service, but after political pressure the plan died. Hospitals also experimented with a group nursing care modality, described as being halfway between a private duty arrangement and graduate nurse hospital staff nursing. Under this plan, patients were grouped together in a special unit where several patients shared a private nurse. Thus, three nurses could do 8-hour shifts for two patients instead of four nurses being needed for 12-hour shifts. The hospital paid the nurses' wages but charged the patients directly as a surcharge on the hospital bill. The advantages included shorter hours for nurses, order and regularity in hospital staffing, steady employment for nurses, slightly cheaper rates for patients, and responsibility for the total care of several patients for the nurse. Nurses had the autonomy and care delivery method of private duty without its isolation and uncertainty. Nurses were members of the hospital's staff, yet their time was specifically allocated only to a set number of patients who paid for this service directly. However, economic and political pressures for more efficiency, productivity, and service cut off the adoption of this system in hospitals (Baas, 1992; Muir, 2019; Reverby, 1987). There is a striking parallel between group nursing and how physicians are organized to practice medicine in today's health care environment.

Total patient care initially occurred in intensive care, hospice care, and home health care. The term total patient care has come to mean the assignment of each patient to a nurse who plans and delivers care during a work shift. With this model, continuity of care can be compromised as patients are allocated by shift, rather than allocated based on admission date to discharge (King et al., 2015).

Functional Nursing

Functional nursing emerged as a care model in the 1940s. With this model, the division of labor is assigned according to specific tasks and technical aspects of the job, such as medication administration and taking vital signs. Under functional nursing, the nurse identifies the tasks to be done for a shift. The work is divided and assigned to nursing and support personnel, such as care assistants.

From the late 1800s through the end of World War II, functional nursing was the norm in US hospitals. In the early 1900s, business and industry concepts of "scientific management" emphasized efficiency. The efficiency was gained by breaking down a work process into its component task steps and then analyzing and timing the steps, establishing standards, and determining the best way to perform each task. Thus, managerial control over the planning and execution of work could be established. Functional nursing was developed as a result of this concern for task analysis and proper division of the nursing workload. With this model, there could be a "temperature nurse," a "medication nurse," a nurse for the right side of the hall, and a nurse for the left side of the hall (Tiedeman, 2004). This model enabled hospitals to improve service efficiency and control labor costs by requiring fewer RNs. Another advantage of this model was clear division of labor. Over time, with the increased complexity of patient care needs, the functional model has become less favored due to the fragmentation of care and patient exposure to multiple care providers.

The focus on tasks diminishes nurses' critical thinking and the patient-centered approach of care delivery (Tiedeman, 2004).

Team Nursing

Team nursing is a care model that uses a group of care providers led by a knowledgeable nurse to achieve a common goal. This model utilizes a delivery approach that provides care to a group of patients by coordinating a team of RNs, licensed practical nurses, and care assistants under the supervision of one RN, called the *team leader*. Team nursing developed in the early 1950s in response to a shortage of RNs and in reaction to the dissatisfaction with functional nursing (Fairbrother et al., 2015; King et al., 2015).

Team nursing is designed to make use of each member's capabilities to meet the nursing needs of their group of patients. When making team assignments, the nurse leader considers the scope of practice, knowledge, and expertise of each team member and gives each team member their own patient assignments. This model requires effective team leadership, collaboration, frequent communication, and the expectation that team members will assist and support each other as needed. A benefit of an effective team is that team members provide extra surveillance for patients and give greater support for novice nurses (Dickerson & Latina, 2017). Blurring of the scope of practice along with educational preparation, critical thinking skills, and knowledge application are significant challenges for team nursing models (Martin & Weeres, 2016). Nursing literature suggests teams with a greater proportion of RNs or richer skill mix have better patient outcomes (Halm, 2019). A national study of nurses across 41 hospitals in the United States identified higher levels of collaboration between nurses, physicians, and their leaders had a strong impact on the quality of care given to patients and increased reports of the job satisfaction of nurses (Ma et al., 2015).

Primary Nursing

Primary nursing began in the 1960s by Manthey to overcome the discontent with functional and team nursing's emphasis on tasks and discrete functions that directed nurses' attention away from the holistic care of the patient. This matched a societal trend toward accountability, as well as nursing's rising level of professionalism. In this model, the primary nurse has 24-hour-per-day accountability for the patient's plan of care from admission to discharge. Associate nurses oversee patient care delivery when the primary nurse is not on shift and are expected to follow the primary nurse's plan of care. This model enhances continuity of care; maximizes RN utilization of professional competencies, such as critical thinking, collaboration, and teaching; and philosophically complements holistic, patient-centered care. Although this model is favored by RNs and patients due to its relational nature, it takes time and energy investment to have 24-hour accountability (Wessel & Manthey, 2015). However, Manthey (2002) believed that the implementation of primary nursing would be a vehicle to return nursing to its true professional role.

Fernandez et al. (2012) completed a systematic review of the literature to evaluate nursing models of care delivery, specifically team and primary nursing, on nurse and patient outcomes. This research team identified sparse differences with respect to quality of communication among staff, nurse job satisfaction, absenteeism rates, and role clarity, while the impact on patient outcomes was ambiguous. Team nursing was associated with significantly decreased medication errors, fewer adverse events involving intravenous management, and lower pain scores for patients, although there were no differences for patient fall rates. Overall, the researchers concluded that team nursing is often preferred when there are staff with less experience or skill level on a unit. In another systematic review, Mattila et al. (2014), revealed that the primary nursing model was less costly than a team nursing model and nurses on primary nursing units reported higher quality care delivery than nurses on team nursing units. Also, the Mattila team identified that primary nursing could have a higher impact in the maternity setting, as continuity of care was enhanced. Mothers reported less breast discomfort and engaged more effectively in breastfeeding. Dal Molin et al. (2018) assessed the relationship between nursing sensitive staff, and organizational outcomes and the effectiveness of primary nursing using a before and after research methodology. After the implementation of primary nursing, patient satisfaction with the care they received improved, and nursing sensitive outcomes such as urinary catheter infections, falls, and pressure injuries (ulcers) decreased.

Case Management

Case management as a nursing model of care evolved in the late 1980s, as both a process (a provider intervention), a CDM, and as a method to manage care. The Case Management Society of America (CMSA), a multidisciplinary organization is the professional organization representing the practice of case managers. The CMSA defined case management as "a collaborative process of assessment, planning, facilitation, care coordination, evaluation, and advocacy for options and services to meet an individual's and family's comprehensive health needs through communication and available resources to promote quality, cost-effective outcomes" (CMSA, 2017). **Care coordination,** an integral role of case managers, is the facilitation of resources, integration of providers to achieve the longitudinal plan for the best patient outcomes (Swan et al., 2019).

Case management and care coordination have been the CDMs used for years by public health and community health nurses, although case management can occur in any health sector (acute care, community), extend across the health care continuum, or be linked to a population focus, such as school nursing (Maughan et al., 2018). In the face of strong economic external forces, acute care hospitals turned to case management to help reduce provider practice variation and to ensure the appropriateness of care. The risk with case management models is that communication and coordination infrastructures, along with standardized practice guidelines, may not be available or integrated for effectiveness of care (Joo & Huber, 2018).

Case management has components of health services delivery, coordination, and monitoring, through which multiple service needs of patients are met. Hospital-based acute care nursing case management focuses on an entire episode of illness, crossing all settings in which the patient receives care. Care is directed by a case manager, who is not always a nurse, and can be unit or population focused (Joo & Huber, 2018). A longitudinal study to determine the effectiveness of a 12-month nursing case management intervention on the functioning of the family, stress of the mother, and outcomes of children with attention deficit hyperactivity disorder found improvement in the functioning of the family and behaviors of the child. Though there was not a statistically significant outcome with the mother's stress level between the intervention and the control group, this study determined that the nursing care management intervention promoted communication, empowered families to take ownership of their care, and strengthened the connection between providers (Churchill et al., 2018). Other research demonstrated that the use of RN case managers within the care delivery system can improve adherence to care treatments resulting in better patient outcomes (Mattei da Silva et al., 2020).

EVOLVING MODELS

Changes to the health care, economic, social, and political environments will continue to have a strong impact on the creation of **traditional and evolving** CDMs. Coupled with these transforming changes is the retirement of baby boomers, the delivery of care across the care continuum, and exploding technological advancements. The seminal and replicated work of Aiken and colleagues (Aiken et al., 2011, 2013, 2017) contributes a body of evidence that richer RN-specific skill mix reduces patient mortality. However, many of the resulting structures for patient care are skill mix models or mixed models that partner RNs with a variety of "extenders" or multi-skilled workers. Even though care teams consist of members with various skills, when redesigning the CDM, the professional practice standards of nursing and the Code of Ethics for Nurses are key drivers to frame any model.

Patient-and-Family-Centered Care

For more than 50 years, **patient-and-family-centered care (PFCC)** has been in the health care literature. However, during the 1980s the Institute for Patient-and-Family-Centered Care (IPFCC, n.d.) partnered with researchers to develop care principles, and they pushed these principles into the health care arena through the revolutionary book *Through the patient's eyes* (Gerteis et al., 1993). PFFC is care that is organized around the patient and family. Providers partner, support, connect, and communicate with patients and families to identify and satisfy their needs and cultural preferences (Institute for Patient-and-Family-Centered Care, n.d.) and to treat symptoms and prevent suffering (Press Ganey, 2014). When the Institute of Medicine (IOM, 2001), now called the National Academies of Sciences, Engineering, and Medicine, Health and Medicine Division, included PFCC as one of its major goals for twenty-first century

BOX 15.5 The Eight Dimensions of Patient-Family-Centered Care

1. Respect for patient preferences, values, needs
2. Information, education, communication
3. Coordination, integration of services
4. Emotional support
5. Physical comfort
6. Family/close other involvement
7. Continuity, safe transitions between care settings (e.g., hospital to home; hospital to long-term care)
8. Access to care and services

From Institute of Medicine (IOM). (2001) *Crossing the quality chasm: A new health system for the 21st century.* Washington, DC: National Academies Press.

health care improvement, many health care organizations utilized the framework for their CDM (Box 15.5). Foundational to PFCC is nurses' ability to connect with the patient, their determination of patient preferences, their provision of realistic care options, and their assistance with making care decisions based on patient values versus provider values (Ortiz, 2018). Organizing care around the patient is not a new practice for nurses as many nursing theorists did formulate their theories using the patient as a major focus, resulting in patient-centered care becoming a core component of nursing.

PFCC has been studied for its relationship to patient satisfaction. The framework of Compassionate Connected Care inherent in PFCC consists of domains that are linked to clinical excellence and other concepts that identify preventive measures to mitigate the suffering of patients and increase their overall perception of care. The use of this framework provides nurse leaders with the tools to evaluate their patient satisfaction data for the purpose of reducing patient suffering (Dempsey et al., 2014).

A randomized control trial to measure the effectiveness of patient-centered care on the patient's experience after a cardiac event supported the benefits of PFCC on the satisfaction of patients across the care continuum. Approximately 200 patients were randomized to either a standard cardiac care group or person-centered care group. Results demonstrated an increase in the communication between the care provider, the patient and family, increased involvement in decision-making, and improvement in documentation for those who were randomized to the patient care group (Wolf et al., 2019), suggesting a relationship between patient satisfaction with care and the use of a PFCC model of care.

Transitional Care Model

In the United States and other countries, many older citizens suffer from multiple chronic conditions that involve the interactions of physical, cognitive, and emotional health problems. Due to multiple comorbidities, these individuals have frequent care transitions (e.g., from home to hospital to assisted living) that involve many health care providers in different settings. To promote safe passage of senior patients between the various care continuum providers, the ***transitional care model* (TCM)** emerged as a nurse-led, team-based CDM for chronically ill older adults. The transitional care nurse (TCN) leader is typically an advanced practice, master's prepared nurse with population-specific clinical expertise. Three National Institute of Nursing Research funded randomized controlled trials using TCM have demonstrated improved quality of care outcomes and cost savings. Some notable outcomes are reduced numbers of unnecessary hospital readmissions and enhanced patient satisfaction (Naylor et al., 2018).

Patient-Centered Medical Home

A related CDM is the ***patient-centered medical home* (PCMH).** The PCMH was originally designed by the American Academy of Pediatrics to care for children with special needs with the goal of refocusing patient care from the hospital to the primary care setting. The current model has expanded to include care across the life span (Prokop et al., 2017). Approximately 25% of primary care patients have one or more chronic physical and psychiatric disorders, such as diabetes, heart disease, and psychological disorders, which can often impair the patients' capacity to manage their own care or the care of others. The use of the PCMH with this population is to decrease unnecessary primary care/specialty care visits and hospitalizations and to improve self-care management with diet, exercise, and medication adherence. The PCMH uses a nurse (i.e., care manager) to promote education and decision-making with treatment adjustments (e.g., medication management) and to track outcomes associated with the disorders. The nurse care manager connects weekly with a consultant and updates the PCMH primary care provider as needed. Nurse care managers are tasked with monitoring patients to ensure no one "falls through the cracks." After implementation of a PCMH, researchers identified improved care coordination and a reduction in hospital and emergency services admissions (Prokop et al., 2017).

INNOVATIVE MODELS

The complexity of health care delivery necessitates the use of dynamic and innovative models to ensure patient outcomes are met. The IOM's (2001) report *Crossing the quality chasm: a new health system for the 21st century* described the need for sweeping change and redesign of patient CDMs to foster innovation and improve the delivery of care. As defined by Asurakkody and Shin (2018) the term "innovative" describes an idea or product that has been reframed, something that is new and different from the original idea. Many of the innovative models have as their core component one of traditional CDMs that were previously discussed.

Virtual Nursing

In the 1870s with the invention of the telegraph, telehealth or telemedicine was first introduced into the health care environment. Since those early beginnings, the use of technology to integrate care continues to expand into urban and rural health care organizations to increase access for patients to health care services. The **virtual nursing CDM** is defined as the utilization of telecommunication technologies remotely to perform patient-centered surveillance evaluations, care interventions, and interpretation of data for the promotion of the patient's health and wellbeing. Virtual nursing is a care delivery mode that allows patients access to health care services in a financially responsible manner (American Academy of Ambulatory Care Nursing [AAACN], 2018). Over 19 years ago, the AAACN published the first telenursing scope and standards of practice for telehealth nursing. These standards outline six core roles for virtual nurses to embody: (1) patient education, (2) mentoring and education of teams, (3) surveillance of patient quality and safety using "real-time," (4) admission, (5) discharge activities, and (6) physician rounding (AAACN, 2018). The virtual nurse (VN) demonstrates competencies at the proficient and/or expert level for complex patients and has a strong acumen to lead teams, along with being technologically competent. Virtual nursing can occur in a variety of practice settings to include the home, clinics, long-term care, correctional facilities, hospitals, and essentially any setting where nursing care is needed (Cloyd & Thompson, 2020). Utilizing telephonic and video technology with high resolution, two-way audio and video communication to perform care, the VN serves as the clinical expert to support decision-making among all other members of the care delivery team (Schuelke et al., 2019).

One health care system implemented a virtually integrated care^{SM} (VIC) team model on two medical-surgical units at two separate hospitals. VN coverage was provided for only 12 hours per day, 5 days per week. Over a period of 2½ years after implementation of the new delivery model, both hospitals observed an increase in their patient satisfaction, teamwork between departments, emergency department throughput, length of stay, discharge times, and financial metrics. Education and mentoring of clinical nurses' efforts uncovered numerous anecdotal examples of conversations with nurses that resulted in the identification of care gaps and assistance with new procedures. This tailored mentoring became a recruitment tool for nurses coming into the unit (Denney & Evans, 2017; Schuelke et al., 2019).

Artificial Intelligence, Machine Learning, and Robotics

The use of artificial intelligence, machine learning, and robotics in the delivery of patient care are innovative technologies that are rapidly disrupting how nurses practice. Health care organizations are charged with achieving positive outcomes yet must attain these outcomes within financial margins that challenge their viability. Innovative technologies are poised to assist organizations to meet health care disruption by reducing the burden of less-value added tasks and increasing data processing, and medical information transfer for effective decision-making (American Hospital Association, 2019). Less value-added nursing activities, now completed by nurses, increases their workload and takes time away from patients; incorporating innovative technologies into the care delivery system could give time back to nurses.

Artificial intelligence (AI) is defined as a collection of technologies, that can learn, teach, perceive, and mimic the thought process of humans (Davenport & Kalakota, 2019; Robert, 2019). Many consumers have already embraced the use of various devices that recognize voice patterns to help achieve various mundane tasks in the home. In health care, the use of AI could be utilized to rank various types of data, provide applicable treatment options for care providers, and deploy a virtual assistant for nurses (Robert, 2019). **Machine learning (ML)** describes the practice of creating and utilizing algorithms to separate data, learn, and then make predictive decisions (Clipper et al., 2018). An example of ML is the use of a risk assessment tool to identify patients at risk for sepsis. Using prescribed algorithms, data are calculated in real time from medical record entries, such as nursing assessments and laboratory values. A predictive index score is then generated and based on the risk score, a prediction for patient safety risk is identified (Robert, 2019). **Robotics** describes the design, construction, and operation of robots through the integration of science and technology. As defined, robots are "re-programmable, physically embodied, intelligent and mobile systems, that can act autonomously or be teleoperated in an environment where the robot has the ability to sense" (Olaronke et al., 2017, p. 44).

A robotics company based in Austin, Texas, designed a robot to assist nurses with various mundane "hunting and gathering" tasks. The social intelligence features of the robot, Moxi, includes blinking eyes, soft curved edges, a neutral voice, and a moving head. Moxi has a robotic arm, can move through the hallways, and sense obstacles. Due to the AI integration, Moxi can learn various behavior patterns and has predictive abilities that allow for coordination of supplies with the patient's plan of care (Schwab, 2019; Stuart, 2019). During the successful beta trials of Moxi at several hospitals in Texas, team members and patients learned to appreciate the capabilities of this robot; essentially Moxi decreased the workload of nurses and other care providers (Schwab, 2019).

LEADERSHIP AND MANAGEMENT IMPLICATIONS

Fundamentally, a CDM is the way patients' needs are matched to health care resources to achieve positive clinical outcomes. Through many complex relationships, the CDM influences the quality of nursing care provided and its cost. Though multiple nursing CDMs have been developed, evidence suggests evolutionary changes are underway. Traditionally, care delivery was provided within a pure nursing framework. Over time, nursing care delivery methods were adapted to better fit external forces and the balance of the needs of patients and the needs of employing organizations. With these changes came variations in modes of delivery (e.g., team nursing, total patient care), skill mix, staffing levels, and nurse roles and accountabilities. The delivery of nursing care has become more complex as integration with other provider disciplines became essential to meet the patients' needs throughout the entire continuum of care. Future trends point to greater integration and inter-professional team collaboration models as health care reform drives changes within the health care industry.

Though the repeal, replace, or change of the Affordable Care Act (ACA) was not completed, the ACA mandates continue to alter the way health care is delivered (Vogenberg & Santilli, 2018). The Health and Medicine Division (HMD), formerly IOM, *Future of nursing report* (2010), is inclusive of the ACA's health care vision of accessible, equitable, and affordable care with a key feature being new CDMs. The themes of integration and coordination of care, addressing needs in a comprehensive manner with patients as key partners, and providing services efficiently continue to predominate and trigger a radical shift in the delivery of health care toward primary health care (Vogenberg & Santilli, 2018). Reimbursement structures and other incentives to health care providers are triggering new models and offering leadership opportunities for nurses (Porter-O'Grady, 2019).

Nursing leaders and managers need to have a broad vision to facilitate the design of CDMs that meet the objectives of cost containment, patient satisfaction, quality, and safety outcomes over the course of the care cycle. Nursing leaders are in the perfect position to lead the changes essential in care delivery redesign. Nursing, as a major percentage of the health care labor force, needs to be able to demonstrate its effectiveness in producing financial as well as clinical outcomes. The challenge to prove "value" will continue.

Mentoring staff to participate in the creation of new care delivery methods is an aspect of effective leadership. Many factors, including the environmental context, influence successful implementation of new models, and nurses need to be engaged in these quality improvement initiatives. Evidence demonstrates that professional practice models, particularly their valuing of nursing and their professional (shared) governance structures and processes, are critical to nurse satisfaction and retention. Furthermore, there is evidence that CDMs, a component of professional practice models, are associated with nurse, patient, and organizational outcomes. Nurses and nurse leaders, therefore, need to be visible and engaged when planning patient care delivery strategies at all levels of the organization. The challenge of nurse leaders is to balance risk taking and adoption of innovations with the practical necessity to be systematic, evaluative, and realistic. To assist nurse leaders with designing and adopting innovative CDMs, the American Organization for Nursing Leadership (AONL) developed a *Guiding principles for the role of the nurse in future patient care delivery* toolkit (2010). These principles outline five assumptions to guide nurse leaders: (1) use a systems approach with all disciplines involved in process and outcome models, (2) recognize that accountable care organizations will influence health care reform provisions to impact differing care delivery venues, (3) be mindful that an increasingly informed public will drive changes in care delivery based on safety concerns and outcomes, (4) remember that as health leaders gain knowledge of funding sources, they will strategically deploy funds to achieve desired outcomes, and (5) joint education of inter-professionals will become the norm to ensure shared knowledge and practice. Today these assumptions are still significant, with some assumptions emerging or peaking in health care environments.

CURRENT ISSUES AND TRENDS

The challenges for patient care in the future are massive. The work environment of the nurse is dramatically different. Cost containment and demands for quality and safety outcomes will continue to drive CDM redesign. The Donabedian S-P-O framework can be used to plan and test model structures and processes associated with safe quality care delivery outcomes.

Clearly, forces and pressures outside of professional nursing influence care models. What is not known is which model is the best CDM for each patient care setting, and there is limited research evidence to support specific inpatient and ambulatory nursing care models (Fernandez et al., 2012). Nurses are urged to examine their patient populations, understand and embrace the business aspects of health care, and remain vigilant in analyzing emerging economic and clinical trends in order to be active participants in the creation of future patient CDMs.

A final trend worth noting is the shift toward the integration of digital tools in the practice setting, big data management, and the use of evidence to make practice decisions. With this digital integration, practice changes will be time driven and fluid. Speed of implementation of new treatment processes into practice will become the new norm and a definer of value, quality, and effectiveness of care provided to patients (Porter-O'Grady, 2019). Nurses play a critical role in facilitating this transition by encouraging knowledge exchange, shared problem-solving, and the creation and reinforcement of patient-and-family-centered goals. Nurses are exceptionally skilled at building informal and formal relationships across levels, permitting more rapid coordination, practice integration, and more effective communication. The heightened awareness of the social determinants of health on communities will continue to propel nurses to improve access, identify, connect, and implement health care resources to ensure the sustainable health of individuals and communities. Nurse leaders, therefore, are important influencers for leading CDM redesign and developing innovations.

RESEARCH NOTE

Source

Havaei, F., MacPhee, M., & Dahinten, V. (2016). The effect of nursing care delivery models on quality and safety outcomes of care: A cross-sectional survey study of medical-surgical nurses. *Journal of Advanced Nursing, 75*(10), 2144–2155.

Purpose

Havaei et al. (2016) used an exploratory cross-sectional correlational methodology to study the effects of two delivery care modes (total patient care and team nursing), and skill mix on the quality of nursing care and adverse patient outcomes. Using secondary data from a larger study, this team examined four aspects: (1) the mode of delivery of nursing care on quality of nursing care and patient outcomes, (2) skill mix on quality of nursing care and patient outcomes, (3) the moderating effect of nursing delivery model of care between workload on quality nursing care and patient outcomes, and (4) the moderating effect of skill mix between workload on quality nursing care and patient outcomes.

Continued

RESEARCH NOTE—cont'd

Sample

The Havaei team surveyed 416 clinical nurses whose practice was in acute care medical and or surgical settings across hospitals in British Columbia, Canada. A power analysis identified a sample size of 226 individuals would garner a small effect size for the multiple regression analysis that would be used.

Study Variables

The *mode of delivery of nursing care* was measured using one item that asked nurses to describe how care was delivered on their unit during their shift. Clinical nurses were asked to select either total patient care (one nurse caring for the patient) or team nursing (different care providers caring for groups of patients at one time). *Skill mix* was measured by one item that asked clinical nurses to determine the number and type of nurse that gave nursing care to patients on their unit during their shift. Types of care providers included: registered nurses (RNs), registered practical nurses (RPNs), licensed practical nurse (LPNs), and unlicensed individuals (nursing assistants [NAs]). Based on these skill mix types, the research team further categorized skill mix into skill mix with all RNs and NAs and skill mix with RNs, LPNs, and NAs.

Workload factors included staffing levels inclusive of the number of nurses available to care for the specified number of patients on the unit, acuity level (not acute or very acute), and whether the patient was completely dependent or completely independent. *Work environment factors* were measured using the 28-item Practice Environment Scale-Nursing Work Index (PES-NWI), an instrument validated by Lake (2002).

Patient outcome variables focused on nurse reported quality of care, total number of nursing tasks left undone, and the frequency of adverse events of nurse sensitive measures that included medication errors, urinary tract infections, and patient falls with injuries.

Discussion

Key findings of the study were clinical nurses practicing in a team-based mode of care delivery reported a higher number of tasks left undone when compared with reports from clinical nurses practicing in a total patient care mode of delivery. Clinical nurses in a skill mix team model that included LPNs reported greater occurrences of patient adverse events when compared to a skill mix without LPNs. When the patient acuity level was very acute, clinical nurses in a team-based model reported increased numbers of adverse patient events when compared to clinical nurses in a total patient care model. Work environment factors, such as foundations of nursing care delivery and the availability of resources were linked to patient adverse events.

This study used a cross-sectional correlational design; therefore, findings only demonstrate a relationship between the study variables, rather than causation, and are not generalizable to other study populations. Though study findings are correlational, they are supported by other research where richer skill mix is associated with improved patient outcomes. Work environment factors, along with the mode of care delivery and skill mix impacted adverse patient outcomes. These findings are also supported by other research that documents the relationship between the work environment of nurses, patient outcomes, and staffing (Griffiths et al., 2019; Stalpers et al., 2015; Twigg et al., 2019). With the impetus for health care organizations to attain high quality metrics, all contributory factors that impact quality and safety must evaluated and embraced by all nurses.

Application to Practice

Nurse leaders need to utilize research evidence to deliberately structure and advocate for the adoption of innovative nursing care delivery models and practice environments that drive exemplary patient care.

CASE STUDY

Overview

Ceremony Medical Center (CMC), an 814-bed teaching hospital utilizes Kolcaba's theory of comfort as a framework for their nursing professional practice model (PPM). The values of the organization are quality, safety, teamwork, and service and though listed on CMC documents are not evident in the PPM nor do nurses "live" the organizational values. Total patient care is the care delivery model (CDM) for all areas. However, RNs of different experience levels have responsibilities for a group of seven to eight patients on four of the medical and surgical units, three to four patients on the four-step-down units, and one to two patients on the three-intensive care units. A nurse manager has 24/7 responsibility for two 36 bed units which serves a mixed population of patients with cardiac, renal, pulmonary, neurological, and

CASE STUDY—cont'd

gastrointestinal diagnoses. Assistant nurse managers are accountable for daily operations and, due to low staffing, must frequently have a patient assignment consisting of one to two patients. Novice nurses, those with less than 15 months of nursing experience, account for 48% of the team. The Registered nurse (RN) voluntary turnover rate for both units continues to climb above 25%. Certified nursing assistants (CNAs) are occasionally assigned to a nurse but are more likely given secretarial tasks to complete. Though responsibilities of the CNA include basic custodial care of patients, they also function as patient safety attendants and are assigned to serve as sitters for Baker Act patients or those patients at high risk for falls.

Complaints from patients and physicians are numerous and cite unsafe nursing care practices, poor transitions to and from various levels of care, and a general lack of responsiveness for the care needs of patients. Reporting of significant incidents and "near misses" have increased, with two incidents resulting in a nurse reporting the medical center to the accrediting agency for endangering the lives of patients. This prompted the accrediting agency to place the medical center on conditional accreditation. These findings trigger the service line nursing director to conduct a comprehensive assessment to ascertain the root cause.

Assessment and Findings

The assessment of the nursing director identified that the professional practice model that guides nursing practice is not fully embraced; this results in disjointed delivery of care. Timely and complete nursing assessments and reassessments, along with evidence of nursing care planning, were not identified in the electronic medical record. Consequently, nurses are unable to speak to the patient's diagnosis and medical plan of care. Novice nurses are challenged with critical thinking and effective decision-making yet can perform some care activities with limited knowledge. Though the policy of CMC requires nurses to begin discharge planning on admission to the unit, discharge education typically will not start until a discharge order is received from the physician; this frequently delays a timely discharge from CMC. Multiple caregivers perform patient care activities. However, communication of the plan of care at shift change is deficient due to a lack of continuity, numerous nurse callouts, poor problem identification, and incomplete coordination and prioritization of care activities. Inter-professional communication, specifically between physicians and nurses, is sporadic and inadequate. Nurses rarely use communication tools such as situation, background, assessment and recommendation (SBAR) and handoff reports to standardize and share critical information. Nurses are not comfortable with delegation of tasks to CNAs and frequently assume non-nursing functions rather than communicate the patient's care needs to their CNAs. Dedicated preceptors and learning professionals to support the knowledge, skills, and attitudes of novice nurses for the purpose of growing them into competent practitioners is inadequate.

Nursing quality data indicates high rates of catheter associated urinary tract infections (CAUTI), patient falls with injury, central-line associated bloodstream infections (CLABSI), physical assaults by patients on nurses, and delays in treatment. Patient satisfaction scores continue their downward trajectory and have never attained the intended 85th percentile benchmark in over 15 months. The most recent results of the NDNQI RN survey revealed poor teamwork across units, low marks for quality of care, and insufficient staffing and resources that support top of license practice.

Professional Practice Model Enculturation and Care Delivery Redesign

To meet the care needs of patients by "living" the organizational values of quality, safety, teamwork, and service, the nursing director and the vice president of nursing agreed that the PPM needed further enculturation, while a re-design of how care is delivered was also warranted. The nursing director initiated a redesign process by forming a team consisting of RNs, CNAs, and other inter-disciplinary care providers from the two 36 bed medicine units. Using the model for improvement framework, the team clarified the goal of the project, identified changes that can demonstrate improvement, and outlined specific success metrics. Provider focus groups, a focused literature review, discussions with patient representatives, and an assessment of CDMs from other hospitals rounded out the assessment process. Team meetings were used to align nursing practice to the components of the PPM, to brief everyone about planned changes, and to listen for consensus and any new ideas.

Given the spatial layout of the two medicine units, modular nursing was the best option. A form of team nursing, modular nursing allows the clustering of similar patients, grants exposure to, and increases learning about specific patient populations that are cared for within a structural module or pod. Complexity of needed services, patient acuity, and diagnosis are used to further group patients who are admitted to each pod. Based

Continued

CASE STUDY—cont'd

on preference, members of the care team are assigned permanently to a unit but understand that rotation to the sister unit is available after a trial period of 6 months. Each pod consists of 18 patients, an experienced nurse who is partnered with a novice or agency nurse, and one or two CNAs. Shift report is taken by all members of the modular care team. This practice facilitates communication and continuity of care if one team member is off the unit or is not scheduled the next day. Daily inter-disciplinary care planning rounds facilitated by nurses, are established for each pod. The evidence-based practices of bedside shift report, hourly rounding, and focused assessments are instituted to improve monitoring and surveillance of rapidly changing patient conditions.

To increase skills performance, a new CNA level is established, and competency assessments evaluated in the simulation lab. Members of the unit's professional (shared) governance council determined the most valued CNA skills to reduce the non-nursing tasks that nurses perform. Team-building workshops to facilitate understanding of delegation responsibilities and roles were given to both RNs and CNAs. Staffing levels were refined to ensure the assistant nurse manager is free of a patient assignment. This change facilitates communication between physicians, nurses, and other members of the care team, ensures the availability of resource, and establishes effective staffing levels.

Evaluation

Process and outcome indicators that measure quality, safety, patient satisfaction, RN satisfaction, and financial metrics were established and displayed in a dashboard. Clinical outcomes must follow successful implementation of processes. Therefore, the quality improvement project team made the decision to measure process indicators for 6 months, then quality indicators at 6 months, 1 year, 18 months, and 2 years post implementation.

Fast Forward: The End of the First Year

Nurses understand the components of the professional practice model and integrate the components into their practice. Nursing satisfaction, specifically intent to stay and perceptions of quality care delivery, improved. Nursing practice activities of assessment of psychosocial and clinical needs, evaluation of care treatments, documentation, delegation of non-nursing tasks, patient education, coordination of care, and safe transition to the next care setting are consistently identified in the electronic medical record. Agency usage is almost non-existent and novice nurse attrition is reduced by 10%. Patient satisfaction scores such as pain management, discharge preparation, and responsiveness to the care needs of patients demonstrated improvement by 24 percentage points. The number of patient falls with injury are significantly reduced, while patient assaults and delays in treatment are rare occurrences. Incidence of CAUTIs continues its downward trend, although metrics have not yet attained benchmark.

Conclusions

By using the model as an improvement framework, collaborative and deliberate planning with all stakeholders, and implementation and evaluation of adopted strategies, the enculturation of the PPM along with the redesign of the CDM was successfully achieved.

CRITICAL THINKING EXERCISE

After a 5-month search, your organization brought on a new chief nursing officer (CNO). Within 10 months of hire, all nurse leaders were part of a strategic alignment process with the CNO which resulted in clearly defined outcomes for each nurse leader. Though the PPM incorporates the theory of relationship-based care, the virtual CDM continues to interrupt workflow, exceed costs associated with the level of care, and hinder patient and family interactions. You are the nurse manager for a 72-bed orthopedic unit and your CNO has requested that you use the S-P-O Donabedian framework to determine what structures and processes need to be in place within your work environment to support exemplary VIC for your patients. To determine your outcomes or goals, you perform patient/family and team surveys to establish preferences and needs. Major care preferences for patients and families include real-time communication with the health care team, assistance with physical needs, and a clear understanding of the roles and responsibilities of the virtual care team. For the virtual care team, their desires centered around technical challenges, resistance to the new model, and interruption of their workflow.

1. What evidence-based structures are necessary to meet your VIC goals or outcomes?
2. What evidence-based processes are necessary to meet your VIC goals or outcomes?

3. Koloroutis' (2004) relationship-based care is a theoretical framework that some Magnet hospitals use for their nursing professional practice model. What Magnet-like characteristics can you use to change the culture of your work environment to become more relationship-based?

Hint: Consider using a matrix or table such as:

Structures	Processes	Desired Outcomes

REFERENCES

Abou Hashish, E. (2017). Relationship between ethical work climate and nurses' perception of organizational support, commitment, job satisfaction and turnover intent. *Nursing Ethics, 24*(2), 151–166.

Aiken, L., Cimiotti, J., Sloane, D., Smith, H., Flynn, L., & Neff, D. (2011). Effects of nurse staffing and nurse education on patient deaths in hospitals with different nurse work environments. *Medical Care, 49*(12), 1047–1053.

Aiken, L., Sloane, D., Bruyneel, L., Van den Heede, K., Sermeus, W., & Consortium, R. (2013). Nurses' reports of working conditions and hospital quality of care in 12 countries in Europe. *International Journal of Nursing Studies, 50*(2), 143–153.

Aiken L., Sloane D., Griffiths P., Rafferty A., Bruyneel L., McHugh M., et al. (2017). Nursing skill mix in European hospitals: Cross-sectional study of the association with mortality, patient ratings, and quality of care. *BMJ Quality & Safety, 26*(7), 559–568.

Alegre, I., Berbegal-Mirabent, J., Guerrero, A., & Mas-Machuca, M. (2018). The real mission of the mission statement: A systematic review of the literature. *Journal of Management & Organization, 24*(4), 456–473.

Sabei, Al, S. Labrague, L., Miner Ross, A., Albashayreh, A., Al Masroori, F., & Al Hashmi, N. (2020). Nursing work environment, turnover intention, job burnout, and quality of care: The moderating role of job satisfaction. *Journal of Nursing Scholarship, 52*(1), 95–104.

Amadei, L. (2016). Why policies and procedures matter. *Risk Management, 63*(9), 12–13.

American Academy of Ambulatory Care Nursing (AAACN). (2018). *Scope and standards of practice for professional telehealth nursing* (6th ed.). Pitman, NJ. AAACN.

American Association of Critical-Care Nurses, (AACN) (2005). AACN standards for establishing and sustaining healthy work environments: A journey to excellence. *American Journal of Critical Care*, (14(3), 187–197).

American Hospital Association (AHA). (2019. *AI and care delivery: Emerging opportunities for artificial intelligence to transform how care is delivered.* https://www.aha.org/system/files/media/file/2019/11/Market_Insights_AI_Care_Delivery.pdf.

American Nurses Association (ANA). (2015). *Nursing scope and standards of practice,* (3rd ed.). Silver Springs, MD. Nursebooks.

American Nurses Credentialing Center (ANCC). (2017). *2019 Magnet® application manual.* Silver Springs, MD. ANCC.

American Organization for Nursing Leadership (AONL). (2010). *Toolkit for patient care delivery*. https://www.aonl.org/toolkit-future-care-delivery.

Asurakkody, T., & Shin, S. (2018). Innovative behavior in nursing context: A concept analysis. *Asian Nursing Research, 12*(4), 237–244.

Baas, L. (1992). An analysis of the writings of Janet Geister and Mary Roberts regarding the problems of private duty nursing. *Journal of Professional Nursing, 8*(3), 176–183.

Barnes, B., Barnes, M., & Sweeney, C. (2016). Putting the "meaning" in meaningful recognition of nurses: The DAISY award. *Journal of Nursing Administration, 46*(10), 508–512.

Basol, R., Hilleren-Listerud, A., & Chmielewski, L. (2015). Developing, implementing, and evaluating a professional practice model. *Journal of Nursing Administration, 45*(1), 43–49.

Case Management Society of America (CSMA). (2017). Little Rock, AR. *What is a case manager?* https://www.cmsa.org/who-we-are/what-is-a-case-manager/.

Centers for Medicare and Medicaid Services (CMS). (2019). *Hospital CAHPS (HCAHPS). https://www.cms.gov/Research-Statistics-Data-and-Systems/Research/CAHPS/HCAHPS1.*

Centers for Medicare & Medicaid Services. (CMS). (2020). *CAHPS® Hospital Survey.* https://hcahpsonline.org/.

Churchill, S., Leo, M., Brennan, E., Sellmaier, C., Kendall, J., & Houck, G. (2018). Longitudinal impact of a randomized clinical trial to improve family function, reduce maternal stress and improve child outcomes in families of children with ADHD. *Maternal & Child Health Journal, 22*(8), 1172–1182.

Cicolini, G., Comparcini, D., & Simonetti, V. (2014). Workplace empowerment and nurses' job satisfaction: A systematic literature review. *Journal of Nursing Management, 22*(7), 855–871.

Clavelle, J., O'Grady, Porter, T. Weston, M., & Verran, J. (2016). Evolution of structural empowerment: Moving from shared to professional governance. *Journal of Nursing Administration, 46*(6), 308–312.

Clipper, B., Batcheller, J., Thomaz, A., & Rozga, A. (2018). Artificial intelligence and robotics: A nurse leader's primer. *Nurse Leader, 16*(6), 379–384.

Cloyd, B., & Thompson, J. (2020). Virtual care nursing: The wave of the future. *Nurse Leader, 18*(1), 1–4.

Cole, L., & Houston, S. (1999). Linking outcomes management and practice improvement. Structured care methodologies: Evolution and use in patient care delivery. Outcomes Management for Nursing Practice, 3(2), 53–60.

Cordo, J., & Hill-Rodriguez, D. (2017). The evolution of a nursing professional practice model through leadership support of clinical nurse engagement, empowerment, and shared decision making. *Nurse Leader, 15*(5), 325–330.

Curtis, K., Fry, M., Shaban, R., & Considine, J. (2017). Translating research findings to clinical nursing practice. *Journal of Clinical Nursing, 26*(5–6), 862–872.

Dal Molin, A., Gatta, C., Boggio Gilot, C., Ferrua, R., Cena, T., Manthey, M., & Croso, A. (2018). The impact of primary nursing care pattern: Results from a before–after study. *Journal of Clinical Nursing, 27*(5-6), 1094–1102.

Davenport, T., & Kalakota, R. (2019). The potential for artificial intelligence in healthcare. *Future Healthcare Journal, 6*(2), 94–98.

Dempsey, C., Wojciechowski, S., McConville, E., & Drain, M. (2014). Reducing patient suffering through compassionate connected care. *Journal of Nursing Administration, 44*(10), 517–524.

Denney, S., & Evans, E. (2017). Virtually integrated care: A new paradigm in patient care delivery. *Nursing Administration Quarterly, 41*(4), 288–296.

Dickerson, J., & Latina, A. (2017). Team nursing: A collaborative approach improves patient care. *Nursing,* 201947(10), 16–17 .

Donabedian, A. (1988). The quality of care. How it can be assessed. *Journal of the American Medical Association, 260*(12), 1743.

Duffy, J. (2016). *Professional Practice Models in Nursing: Successful Health System Implementation*. Springer Publishing Company.

Eva, N., Prajogo, D., & Cooper, B. (2017). The relationship between personal values, organizational formalization and employee work outcomes of compliance and innovation. *International Journal of Manpower, 38*(2), 274–287.

Fairbrother, G., Chiarella, M., & Braithwaite, J. (2015). Models of care choices in today's nursing workplace: Where does team nursing sit?. *Australian Health Review, 39*(5), 489–493.

Fernandez, R., Johnson, M., Tran, D. T., & Miranda, C. (2012). Models of care in nursing: A systematic review. *International Journal of Evidence-Based Healthcare, 10*(4), 324–337.

Fowler, M. (2017). *Guide to Nursing's Social Policy Statement: Understanding the profession from social contract to social covenant*. American Nurses Association.

Gerteis, M., Edgman-Levitan, S., Daley, J., & Delbanco, T. (1993). *Through the patient's eyes: Understanding and promoting patient-centered care*. John Wiley & Sons, Inc.

Glassman, K. (2016). Developing and implementing a professional practice model. *Nursing Science Quarterly, 29*(4), 336–339.

Griffiths P, Maruotti, A., Recio Saucedo, A., Redfern, O., Ball, J., Briggs, J., et al., Missed Care Study Group. (2019). Nurse staffing, nursing assistants and hospital mortality: Retrospective longitudinal cohort study. *BMJ Quality & Safety*, 28, 609–617.

Gulati, R., Mikhail, O., Morgan, R., & Sittig, D. (2016). Vision statement quality and organizational performance in U.S. hospitals. *Journal of Healthcare Management, 61*(5), 335–350.

Halm, M. (2019). The influence of appropriate staffing and healthy work environments on patient and nurse outcomes. *American Journal of Critical Care, 28*(2), 152–156.

Havaei, F., MacPhee, M., & Dahinten, V. (2016). The effect of nursing care delivery models on quality and safety outcomes of care: A cross-sectional survey study of medical-surgical nurses. *Journal of Advanced Nursing, 75*(10), 2144–2155.

Heslop, L., & Lu, S. (2014). Nursing-sensitive indicators: A concept analysis. *Journal of Advanced Nursing, 70*(11), 2469–2482.

Institute of Medicine (IOM). (2001). *Crossing the quality chasm: A new health system for the 21st century. Washington, DC*: National Academies Press.

Institute of Medicine (IOM). (2010). *The future of nursing: Leading change advancing health.* Washington, DC: National Academies Press.

Institute for Patient-and-Family-Centered Care (IPFCC). (n.d.). Patient-and-family-centered care. https://www.ipfcc.org/about/pfcc.html.

Joo, J., & Huber, D. (2018). Barriers in case managers' roles: A qualitative systematic review. *Western Journal of Nursing Research, 40*(10), 1522–1542.

Kaya, N., Turan, N., & Aydın, G.Ö (2016). Innovation in nursing: A concept analysis. *Journal of Community and Public Health Nursing, 2*(1), 108–112.

King, A., Long, L., & Lisy, K. (2015). Effectiveness of team nursing compared with total patient care on staff wellbeing when organizing nursing work in acute care wards: A systematic review. *JBI Database of Systematic Reviews and Implementation Reports, 13*(11), 128–168.

Kolcaba, K., Tilton, C., & Drouin, C. (2006). Comfort Theory: A unifying framework to enhance the practice environment. *Journal of Nursing Administration, 36*(11), 538–544.

Koloroutis, M. (2004). *Relationship-based care: A model for transforming practice.* Minneapolis: Creative Healthcare Management.

Lake, E. (2002). Development of the practice environment scale of the Nursing Work Index. *Research in Nursing & Health, 25*(3), 176–188.

Lasater, K., Germack, H., Small, D., & McHugh, M. (2016). Hospitals known for nursing excellence perform better on value-based purchasing measures. *Policy, Politics, & Nursing Practice, 17*(4), 177–186.

Ma, C., Shang, J., & Bott, M. (2015). Linking unit collaboration and nursing leadership to nurse outcomes and quality of Care. *Journal of Nursing Administration, 45*(9), 435–442.

Manthey, M. (2002). *The practice of primary nursing* (2nd ed.). Minneapolis, MN: Creative Health Care Management, Inc.

Martin, D., & Weeres, A. (2016). Building nursing role clarity on a foundation of knowledge and knowledge application. *Healthcare Management Forum, 29*(3), 107–110.

Mattei da Silva, Â. T., de Fátima Mantovani, M., Castanho Moreira, R., Perez Arthur, J., & Molina de Souza, R. (2020). Nursing case management for people with hypertension in primary health care: A randomized controlled trial. *Research in Nursing & Health, 43*(1), 68–78.

Mattila, E., Pitkänen, A., Alanen, S., Leino, K., Luojus, K., Rantanen, A., & Aalto, P. (2014). The effects of the primary nursing care model: A systematic review. *Journal of Nursing and Care, 3*(6), 1–12.

Maughan, E., Cowell, J., Engelke, M., McCarthy, A., Bergren, M., Murphy, M., & Vessey, J. (2018). The vital role of school nurses in ensuring the health of our nation's youth. *Nursing Outlook, 66*(1), 94–96.

Muir, K. (2019). Historical perspectives informing modern day nursing innovation and economics. *Nursing Economic, 37*(6), 284–293.

Naylor, M., Hirschman, K., Toles, M., Jarrín, O., Shaid, E., & Pauly, M. (2018). Adaptations of the evidence-based Transitional Care Model in the U.S. *Social Science & Medicine, 213*, 28–36.

Nightingale, F. (1860). *Notes on nursing: What it is, and what it is not.* New York. Appleton-Century.

Olds, D., Aiken, L., Cimiotti, J., & Lake, E. (2017). Association of nurse work environment and safety climate on patient mortality: A cross-sectional study. *International Journal of Nursing Studies, 74*, 155–161.

Olaronke, I., Oluwaseun, O., & Rhoda, I. (2017). State of the art: A study of human-robot interaction in healthcare. *International Journal of Information Engineering and Electronic Business, 9*(3), 43–55.

Ortiz, M. (2018). Patient-Centered Care: Nursing knowledge and policy. *Nursing Science Quarterly, 31*(3), 291–295.

Park, S., Gass, S., & Boyle, D. (2016). Comparison of reasons for nurse turnover in Magnet® and non-Magnet hospitals. *Journal of Nursing Administration, 46*(5), 284–290.

Polit, D., & Beck, C. (2017). *Nursing research: Generating and assessing evidence for nursing practice* (11th ed.). Philadelphia: Wolters Kluwer | Lippincott Williams & Wilkins.

Porter-O'Grady, T. (2019). Turning the page: Nursing in the digital age and beyond. *Nursing Management, 50*(9), 40–47.

Pound C., Gelt V., Akiki S., Eady K., Moreau K., Momoli F., et al. (2017). Nurse-driven clinical pathway for inpatient asthma: A randomized controlled trial. *Hospital Pediatrics, 7*(4), 204–213.

Press Ganey. (2014). *Reducing suffering: The path to patient-centered care.* https://www.pressganey.com/resources/white-papers/reducing-suffering-the-path-to-patient-centered-care.

Press Ganey. (2020). *Capture Nursing Specific Measures.* https://www.pressganey.com/solutions/clinical-excellence/capture-nursing-specific-measures.

Prokop, J., LaPres, M., Barron, B., & Villasurda, J. (2017). Implementing a health home: Michigan's experience. *Policy, Politics & Nursing Practice, 18*(3), 149–157.

Reverby, S. (1987). *Ordered to care: The dilemma of American nursing* 1850–1945. Cambridge, MA: Cambridge University Press.

Robert, N. (2019). How artificial intelligence is changing nursing. *Nursing Management, 50*(9), 30–39.

Schuelke, S., Aurit, S., Connot, N., & Denney, S. (2019). Virtual nursing: The new reality in quality care. *Nursing Administration Quarterly, 43*(4), 322–328.

Schwab, K. (2019). A hospital introduced a robot to help nurses. They didn't expect it to be so popular. https://www.fastcompany.com/90372204/a-hospital-introduced-a-robot-to-help-nurses-they-didnt-expect-it-to-be-so-popular.

Slayter, S., Coventry, L., Twigg, D, & Davis, S. (2016). Professional practice model for nursing: A review of the literature and synthesis of key components. *Journal of Nursing Management, 24*(2), 139–150.

Stallings-Welden, L., & Shirey, M. (2015). Predictability of a professional practice model to affect nurse and patient outcomes. *Nursing Administration Quarterly, 39*(3), 199–210.

Stalpers, D., de Brouwer, B., Kaljouw, M., & Schuurmans, M. (2015). Associations between characteristics of the nurse work environment and five nurse-sensitive patient outcomes in hospitals: A systematic review of literature. *International Journal of Nursing Studies, 52*(4), 817–835.

Stimpfel, A., Sloane, D., McHugh, M., & Aiken, L. (2016). Hospitals known for nursing excellence associated with better hospital experience for patients. *Health Services Research, 51*(3), 1120–1134.

Stuart, S. (2019). When nurses are busy, it's Moxi the robot to the rescue. https://www.pcmag.com/news/when-nurses-are-busy-its-moxi-the-robot-to-the-rescue.

Swan, B., Haas, S., & Jessie, A. (2019). Care coordination: Roles of registered nurses across the care continuum. *Nursing Economic, 37*(6), 317–323.

Tang, J., & Hudson, P. (2019). Evidence-based practice guideline: Nurse retention for nurse managers. *Journal of Gerontological Nursing, 45*(11), 11–19.

Tiedeman, M. (2004). Traditional models of care delivery: What have we learned?. *Journal of Nursing Administration, 34*(6), 291–297.

Twigg, D., Kutzer, Y., Jacob, E., & Seaman, K. (2019). A quantitative systematic review of the association between nurse skill mix and nursing-sensitive patient outcomes in the acute care setting. *Journal of Advanced Nursing, 75*(12), 3404–3423.

Ulep, K. (2018). The nurse leader's pivotal role in retaining millennial nurses. *Journal of Nursing Administration, 48*(12), 604–608.

Vogenberg, F., & Santilli, J. (2018). Healthcare trends for 2018. *American Health and Drug Benefits, 11*(1), 48–55.

Weberg, D. (2009). Innovation in healthcare: A concept analysis. *Nursing Administration Quarterly, 33*(3), 227–237.

Wessel, S., & Manthey, M. (2015). *Primary nursing: Person-centered care delivery system design*. Minneapolis, MN: Creative Health Care Management, Inc.

Wharton, G., Berger, J., & Williams, T. (2016). A tale of 2 units: Lessons in changing the care delivery model. *Journal of Nursing Administration, 46*(4), 176–180.

Whelan, J. C. (2012). When the business of nursing was the nursing business: The private duty registry system, 1900–1940. *Online Journal of Issues in Nursing, 17*(2), 1–1.

Winslow, S., Cook, C., Eisner, W., Hahn, D., Maduro, R., & Morgan, K. (2019). Care delivery models: Challenge to change. *Journal of Nursing Management, 27*(7), 1438–1444.

Wolf, A., Vella, R., & Fors, A. (2019). The impact of person-centered care on patients' care experiences in relation to educational level after acute coronary syndrome: Secondary outcome analysis of a randomised controlled trial. *European Journal of Cardiovascular Nursing, 18*(4), 299–308.

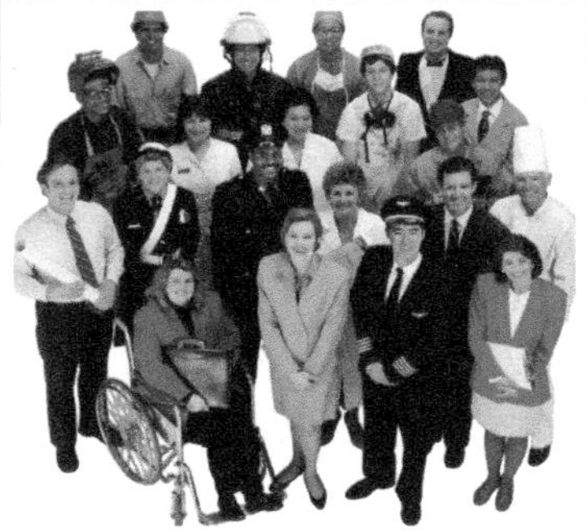

16

Case and Population Health Management

Ellen Fink-Samnick, Teresa M. Treiger

http://evolve.elsevier.com/Huber/leadership

Events of recent decades have thrown the health care system into a radical reformation. This revolution continues to unfold in ever-changing ways. Care delivery has shifted from acute institution-based interventional care to a patient-centered primary care model where quality-driven prevention and outpatient management are the preferred method of operating. Case and population health management (PHM) are multidisciplinary by nature. Nurses provide these services and work in these care delivery models, as do many other disciplines (see Chapter 15).

The modern era of case, disease, and PHM began in the early 1990s. The effectiveness of what was called case management (CM) in producing quality and cost containment outcomes began to be noticed anecdotally by providers in the field. More importantly, it was noticed by health insurance companies that came to believe it worked. However, CM services were rarely paid for outside of rehabilitation and some social services areas, which severely limited the widespread implementation of CM and inhibited care integration. Despite funding restrictions, the belief in the effectiveness of CM spurred research and the development of the knowledge base and evidence for practice. Major professional, certification, and trade associations have also grown in this time period.

The field split first into CM and disease management (DM) (Huber, 2005). With the criticism that not all health conditions, such as behavioral health, are "diseases," the term **DM** was dropped in favor of **PHM**. Rigorous research and federal government–funded demonstration grants continued to solidify the evidence base for practice.

When necessary services other than acute care are actually added to/provided for in the mix of health care, it is difficult to demonstrate cost savings. However, CM, DM, and PHM strategies all have shown positive clinical outcomes. What is clear is that **care coordination** is the core element common to all provider interventions in CM, DM, and PHM.

DEFINITIONS

Case management (CM): "A collaborative process of assessment, planning, facilitation, care coordination, evaluation, and advocacy for options and services to meet an individual's and family's comprehensive health needs through communication and available resources to promote patient safety, quality cost-effective outcomes" (Case Management Society of America, 2017a).

Disease management (DM): Chronic DM is an "integrated care approach to managing illness which includes screenings, check-ups, monitoring and coordinating treatment, and patient education. It can improve your quality of life while reducing your health care costs if you have a chronic disease by preventing or minimizing the effects of a disease" (HealthCare.gov, n.d.).

Population health management (PHM): "A population health management program strives to address health needs at all points along the continuum of health and well-being through participation of, engagement with and targeted interventions for the population. GOAL: Maintain or improve the physical and psychosocial well-being of individuals through cost-effective and tailored health solutions" (Population Health Alliance, n.d.). A more succinct definition is "the process of addressing population health needs and controlling problems at a population level" (Nash et al., 2016).

BACKGROUND

Distinguishing Components of the Health Care Management Continuum

This chapter primarily discusses CM and DM. Before launching into these individual areas, it is essential to frame the health care management continuum and provide perspective on where CM and DM reside within and relate to the whole of PHM.

The health care management continuum (or spectrum as it is sometimes referred) is not synonymous with the continuum of health care practice settings or continuum of care. Although health care management is practiced across the continuum of care, the depth and scope of these services are often driven by the primary purpose of the organization or department (e.g., acute care hospital, emergency department, managed care organization) and the organizational resources available to take on the challenge of these services.

The health care management continuum is better known as PHM. PHM is the overarching umbrella under which CM and DM exist, along with a number of other health management initiatives.

Generally speaking, CM programs serve a smaller percentage of the overall population. Enrollees are complex from a medical–behavioral, health–social vulnerability perspective. Health plans often target the top 5% to 10% high utilizers of their population for CM consideration. The case manager performs an initial screening followed by an in-depth individual assessment involving the client, family caregiver, and other care team members. From the information gathered a CM plan of care is developed. This plan includes highly individualized goals and desired outcomes. DM programs serve a larger percentage of patients whose main problem is one or more chronic condition(s). These individuals generally have similar primary needs regarding health condition education and accommodation strategies. Assessments focus on health condition-specific issues, and programs take a more standardized approach to education and resources. Table 16.1 contains definitions and additional distinguishing characteristics.

CASE MANAGEMENT

CM evolved from a chain of social developments and historical events that made apparent the health, social, and human service needs of disadvantaged, ill, and injured populations through the identification and provision of social services and coordination of care (Treiger and Fink-Samnick, 2013, 2016). Although initially not formally labeled as CM, this history provides a rich context for understanding how CM evolved into what it is today, intertwined with social and legislative events, trends, and changes.

Before government-sponsored interventions, government programs were not addressing the most basic human needs in an organized manner. The federal government had not yet expanded into areas of social support or health care realms, and so efforts to provide social assistance and supportive services for individuals in need were humanitarian and grassroots in nature. Charitable and community-based organizations with wealthy benefactors began to address and fill the local population's needs. The history of caring for the disadvantaged arose from the context of social–political–industrial changes, which piqued more liberal attitudes of social consciousness.

Landmark Legislation

A major influence on CM practice was the continuous stream of socially motivated legislation beginning with the 1935 Social Security Act and extending through to the Patient Protection and Affordable Care Act of (2010) (ACA). These laws put both federal and state governments—as well as newly created regulatory agencies—in a position of responsibility for support and care of the general population. Accompanying these major pieces of legislation was the demand for accountability, service quality, and consumer protection. The role of the case manager (also identified as a service or care coordinator), was first seen in the school setting with the Education for All Handicapped Children Act, (Library of Congress, 1975). Passage of federal and state law mandated CM services for elders (Older Americans Act, 1965), the mentally ill (the Community Mental Health Centers Act, 1963), and the developmentally disabled (the Developmentally Disabled Assistance and Bill of Rights Act, 1975), as noted in the classic resource by Weil and Karls (1985). The ACA further leveraged the concept of case management, envisioning roles within various programs, including the Patient Centered Medical Home (PCMH) and Accountable Care Organizations (ACOs).

CM is not merely the outcome of a single event, piece of legislation, company's risk reduction strategy, or a

TABLE 16.1 Case Management, Disease Management, and Population Health Management Side by Side

Case Management	Disease Management	Population Health Management
"...A collaborative process of assessment, planning, facilitation, care coordination, evaluation, and advocacy for options and services to meet an individual's and family's comprehensive health needs through communication and available resources to promote patient safety, quality cost-effective outcomes."*	Chronic disease management is an "integrated care approach to managing illness which includes screenings, check-ups, monitoring and coordinating treatment, and patient education. It can improve your quality of life while reducing your health care costs if you have a chronic disease by preventing or minimizing the effects of a disease" (HealthCare.gov, n.d.).	Population health management (PHM): "A population health management program strives to address health needs at all points along the continuum of health and well-being through participation of, engagement with and targeted interventions for the population. GOAL: Maintain or improve the physical and psychosocial well-being of individuals through cost-effective and tailored health solutions" (Population Health Alliance, n.d.).
• CMSA definition is used by URAC and NCQA although multiple CM definitions exist • Relies on client-centered assessment, planning, facilitation, care coordination, evaluation, and advocacy • Standards of practice • Individual certifications • Program accreditation and certification available	• Multiple DM definitions • DM program usually focuses on single condition • Relies on a structured system of interventions that focus on a specific condition • No standards of practice • Program content and interventions are evidence and guideline based • Program accreditation and certification available	• Multiple PHM definitions • PHM is a term that overarches the spectrum of health care management • Practice standards exist for components within PHM • Certification and accreditation programs exist for components within PHM

DM, Disease management; *NCQA*, National Committee for Quality Assurance; *PHM*, population health management; *URAC*, Utilization Review Accreditation Commission.

*Data from Case Management Society of America (CMSA). (2016). *Standards of practice for case management.* Little Rock, AR: Author; Disease management. HealthCare.gov. (n.d.). *Chronic disease management.* https://www.healthcare.gov/glossary/chronic-disease-management/; Population health management. Population Health Alliance. (n.d.). *PHM-defined.* https://populationhealthalliance.org/research/understanding-population-health/.

particular professional affiliation. CM is an organically developed practice specialty; it is an insightful response to the interplay of biology, psychology, sociology, health care system factors, and the influences exerted on individuals with complex illnesses and injuries.

Case Management Models

A single and universally accepted CM model does not exist. The diversity of practice models stems from there being multiple definitions of CM. Having infiltrated virtually every practice setting and area of specialization across the health care continuum, it seemed to be an unrealistic expectation that a single model could garner global agreement. However, this assumption hinged on the definition and characteristics of the practice models themselves. Among other influencers is the lack of title protection for case managers, resulting in the widespread misapplication of the case manager job title.

Contemporary approaches, defined on a foundation of practice competencies, have been introduced. One model sparked the notion that a universal practice paradigm is not only possible but is essential to the continued growth of professional CM practice. This section addresses the background and characteristics of CM models and highlights the current trend of practice models being general to practice settings and competency-based practice models.

Practice Models Background

There are a very large number of identifiable CM practice models. Some are nursing models, others are non-nursing models, and still others are team oriented.

The core elements of CM models center on a case manager who coordinates, and monitors care rendered to clients by multiple health care providers and services in an attempt to decrease service fragmentation and improve the quality of care.

By definition, CM is identified as a cycle. The CM process steps align with components of the nursing process. The CM process identifies needs, risks, and resources, and coordinates care and services while educating the client–caregiver to be better self-advocates for health care. CM is designed to support and foster an individual through the health care system using patient-focused care coordination strategies. "Case management should be considered a bridge, not a crutch" (Treiger, 2012). The CM process may be identified differently because of proprietary branding, and it is affected by legislation, regulation, organizational policy, and care setting. However, at its foundation is an approach that defines the various parts of the CM process. Voluntary practice standards provide a frame for qualifications and expectations in all health care practice settings.

Weil and Karls (1985) identified eight main service components common to all CM models:

1. Client identification and outreach
2. Individual assessment and diagnosis
3. Service planning and resource identification
4. Linking clients to needed services
5. Service implementation and coordination
6. Monitoring service delivery
7. Advocacy
8. Evaluation

These components remain a part of the basic CM process framework to the present day.

CM exists in many contexts, settings, and programs. This includes but is not limited to inpatient care, payer-based, ACOs, employer-based, workers' compensation, social services, independent practice, for-profit companies, non-profit organizations, PCMHs, nursing practice, public health nursing, home health care agencies, maternal–child care, and behavioral health settings.

CM programs incorporate a variety of key activities, some of which vary according to practice setting. These activities include (but are not limited to):

- Identification and screening of participants
- Assessment
- Needs identification
- Planning
- Service and product acquisition and implementation
- Coordination of care
- Ongoing monitoring

These and other activities focus on the achievement of client and organizational outcomes that should be accomplished within effective and appropriate time frames and through efficient utilization of available resources. The time span for CM engagement may be for an episode of care in a single care setting (e.g., acute hospital, rehabilitation) lasting a few days/weeks or may span across care settings (e.g., ACOs) over a number of years or for life. In the setting of patient-centered primary care, a client may engage with a case manager for multiple distinct episodes of care or for years of management due to the client's complexity of needs profile.

A model of CM may be designed for a large, rather generic target group or population (e.g., hospitalized, long-term care, chronic care, rehabilitation) or for a specified segment on the health care continuum (e.g., an episode in one setting, in one organization, or for the whole continuum). Historically, these CM models specify organizational policies and processes for care delivery, resource use, and job responsibilities based on general position descriptions. Depending on the organization's care process, the case manager may or may not be a direct care provider.

Many types of CM models and labels are found in literature. There are discipline-specific models as well as generally accepted overarching models. Two factors are common across all CM models: The core component is coordination of care, and the core principle is advocacy. There are fairly common process elements in CM models in addition to coordination of care, advocacy, brokering of services, and resource management. Models may be tailored to fit unique target groups (e.g., vulnerable populations, care setting) or discipline-specific factors.

Nursing and health care models tend to focus on the management of health/illness or disease, or the rehabilitation needs of an individual or population. These models are sometimes called medical models, medical–social models, acute care nursing CM models, or DM models. There has been some confusion in the nursing literature about whether CM is a care delivery model or an intervention that entails a process. In both nursing and social work, there is a differentiation between CM designed to deliver services and CM designed to coordinate the provision of services. This is a key distinction that impacts staffing and roles.

Several frameworks and other methods of classifying activities have been considered when discussing CM models. Because of the variability in how CM programs are designed and administered, classification into models helps describe—as well as compare and contrast—each type. Using distinctive classifications, CM models may be understood relative to perspective (e.g., organization, setting based), scope (e.g., services delivered within an organization, cross-continuum), and time (e.g., single or multiple episode of care). A methodology for consistent classification of CM practice models has neither been proposed nor accepted. The likelihood of universal acceptance is dim within the current health care context due to the issues associated with the variety of professions practicing CM, competing professional organizations, and the multitude of available individual certifications, among a number of other important influences. Unfortunately, there is no common understanding about what is meant by "doing case management."

Seminal Nursing Case Management Models

There are two historical nursing CM programs cited in nursing literature as forerunners of modern-day nursing CM. These programs are the *New England Medical Center (NEMC) model* and the *Carondelet St. Mary's model.* The NEMC model is considered to be acute care nursing CM, whereas the Carondelet model is a community-based model.

The NEMC model is an extension of primary nursing methodology referred to as nursing CM. It focuses on the acute care episode and is a hospital-based model of CM. It leverages principles of planning and management from engineering and other fields to extend primary nursing into outcomes management.

Carondelet St. Mary's Community Nursing Network, or the Arizona Model (Forbes, 1999), used professional nurse case managers (baccalaureate and master's level) organized as a nursing health maintenance organization (HMO) at the hub of a network to broker services. This model type is known as a beyond-the-walls, medical–social, across-the-continuum of care model. It is best known for its innovative work in moving beyond the inpatient episode of care and into across-the-continuum of care (Cline, 1990).

Social Work Models

CM has been integral to social work since the founding of the profession (Herman, 2013). From their roots in charitable efforts there has been considerable evolution in CM models across the social work profession. Originally known as "social casework," the intervention was used to track the growing needs, progress, and changes for each person. The emphasis has traditionally been on society's most vulnerable populations. These persons are at risk of poor physical, psychological, or social health. Examples include individuals with chronic physical and/or mental illness, intellectual and/or physical disability, and housing insufficiency. By the 1980s, use of the term caseworker was on the wane as use of the term case manager was on the rise (Summers, 2016).

The function of CM remains part of most social work jobs and constitutes a core function of—and specialty within—social work practice. In 2013, standards of practice were developed by the National Association of Social Workers (NASW) to further elaborate on the distinctions for CM from the lens of social work. The six guiding principles are (1) person-centered services, (2) primacy of the client–social worker (SW) relationship, (3) person-in-environment framework, (4) strengths perspective, (5) collaborative teamwork, and (6) intervention at the micro, mezzo, and macro levels of practice (NASW, 2013, pp. 17–18).

More than a dozen different models of contemporary social work CM have been identified in the literature (including medical, social advocacy, managed care, outreach, ecological, intensive, and clinical) (Berger, 2015; Herman, 2013; Summers, 2016). Those most commonly mentioned include: brokerage, primary therapist, interdisciplinary team, comprehensive, and strengths.

The **brokerage model** emphasizes the case manager's traditional linkage function. Clients are linked to a network of providers and service coverage using assessment and referral to ensure the availability of service activities. The case manager plans a comprehensive service package and negotiates through barriers that prevent clients from accessing needed services.

In the **primary therapist model**, the case manager's relationship to the client is primarily therapeutic, and CM functions are undertaken as a part or an extension of therapeutic intervention. The client has one person to relate to about treatment, service access, and case coordination. However, the therapist may feel that CM is a secondary activity to therapeutic work (Weil and Karls, 1985).

The **interdisciplinary team model** uses a specialized team of various professional disciplines in which each member has a specific responsibility for service activities in their area of expertise. Team structures vary considerably. In some, all case managers on the team are interchangeable and serve the total group of clients. Other programs consist of multidisciplinary teams of up to six different professions, often driven by client-specific issues and needs. One team member is identified as the lead, with the other members combining their knowledge to share information about the client.

The **comprehensive service center model** is used in agencies that provide comprehensive services and community-based programming that can include psychosocial support, vocational training, rehabilitation, and care coordination. Examples of settings include community health centers, community-focused programs, continuing care communities (e.g., nursing homes, assisted living facilities), and public housing programs. Case managers in these practice settings may engage in high levels of advocacy, often interacting with members of the client's health care team from other agencies and/or programs.

Interdisciplinary Models

A growing number of interdisciplinary models for CM collaboration exist across practice settings. These models blend the unique competencies and knowledge that underlie nursing and social work education, a full listing of which are shown in Box 16.1. The strength of the social work profession lies in its ability to assess human behavior of patient and families in the context of the social environment. Social work's lens encompasses a multidimensional perspective, which incorporates the biological, psychological, sociological, and spiritual domains (Ashford and LeCroy, 2017). Skilled in psychopathology, and the clinical minutia of behavioral health symptoms, SWs are able to evaluate the premorbid condition of a client's unique situation. In addition, they possess understanding of available community resources and how to access them. Nursing addresses understanding of the pathophysiology of illness with the core of practice to deliver holistic patient-focused care incorporating assessment, diagnosis, outcomes/planning, implementation, and evaluation.

The CM **dyad team model**—composed of a nurse case manager and SW—has been found in hospitals.

BOX 16.1 Professional Competencies of Nursing and Social Work

Nursing
- Clinical judgment
- Advocacy and moral agency
- Caring practices
- Collaboration
- Systems thinking
- Response to diversity
- Facilitation of learning
- Clinical inquiry

Social Work
- Demonstrate ethical and professional behavior
- Engage diversity and difference in practice
- Advance human rights and social, economic, and environmental justice
- Engage in practice-informed research and research-informed practice
- Engage in policy practice
- Engage with individuals, families, groups, organizations, and communities
- Assess individuals, families, groups, organizations, and communities
- Intervene with individuals, families, groups, organizations, and communities
- Evaluate practice with individuals, families, groups, organizations, and communities

Data from American Association of Critical-Care Nurses (AACN). (n.d.). *AACN Synergy Model for patient care.* https://www.aacn.org/nursing-excellence/aacn-standards/synergy-model; Council on Social Work Education. (2015). *Educational policy and accreditation standards for baccalaureate and master's social work programs.* Alexandria, VA: Council on Social Work Education Commission on Accreditation, Commission on Educational Policy.

The dyad structure presents an opportunity for nurses and SWs to integrate their strengths and expertise in a collaborative patient-centered effort (Carr, 2009). These two helping professions align the power of their respective clinical knowledge: social work's proficiency in psychopathology, psychosocial issues, and resource linkage with nursing's emphasis on pathophysiology and the disease process. Both disciplines share the innate value of expertise in empathic listening, advocacy, and critical thinking. This skill set is a forceful combination when used to collaborate with team members in their efforts to evaluate, manage, plan, treat, and coordinate important aspects of the patient's care (Carr, 2009). There is some variation in roles and functions assigned to each discipline, with the distinct scope of job responsibilities defined by each organization.

Through its unique structure, the nurse and social work dyad provides the implementation of collaborative interventions that focus on (1) minimization of inpatient transitions, (2) reduction of cost by decreasing the length of stay, (3) promotion of patient and family satisfaction through efforts of advocacy, and (4) enhanced discharge planning (Carr, 2009).

Hospitals are also increasingly motivated to address readmissions and safe care transitions. Both of these issues are greatly affected by *social determinants*. Social determinants of health (SDoH) are defined by the World Health Organization (2019) as "the conditions in which people are born, grow, live, work and age. These circumstances are shaped by the distribution of money, power, and resources at global, national and local levels. The social determinants of health are mostly responsible for health inequities—the unfair and avoidable differences in health status seen within and between countries." The five domains associated with these non-clinical social service needs, are among the costliest and most complex for health care organizations to care for:

1. Economic stability
2. Education
3. Health care access and quality
4. Neighborhood and built environment
5. Social and community content (HealthyPeople.gov, 2019a)

Current literature has identified that inclusion of these factors, and attention to the SDoH, can lead to a pronounced effect on calculated hospital readmission rates for patients across disease states (Fink-Samnick, 2019b; Gillespie, 2016; Hu et al., 2014; Nagasako et al., 2014; Rice, 2016). When barriers to access to care (e.g., poverty, housing insufficiency, health literacy, medication adherence) are clearly identified by the nurse and SW, specific goals can be established, system processes can be developed or changed, and initiatives can be set into motion to provide patients with safe transitions (Ellsworth, 2015).

Healthy People 2020

The government-sponsored program known as Healthy People "provides science-based, 10-year national objectives for improving the health of all Americans. For 3 decades, Healthy People has established benchmarks and monitored progress over time in order to:

- Encourage collaborations across communities and sectors.
- Empower individuals toward making informed health decisions.
- Measure the impact of prevention activities (HealthyPeople.gov, 2019b).

Healthy People 2020 is a 10-year agenda for improving the nation's health and is the result of local, state, and federal planning processes. A key feature is the engagement of local and state communities to reflect the input from diverse groups (HealthyPeople.gov, 2019b).

The Chronic Care Model

The one general, overarching interdisciplinary model that is becoming widely accepted as the generic CM model is Wagner's **Chronic Care Model** (Improving Chronic Illness Care, 2006–2019). The Chronic Care Model addresses concerns about how to manage chronic illnesses. The six elements of the health care system that encourage quality chronic illness care are the community, the health system, self-management support, delivery system design, decision support, and clinical information systems. The specific concepts related to the six elements are patient safety, cultural competency, care coordination, community policies, and CM. CM is an attractive strategy because it is aimed at care coordination and decreased system-related fragmentation.

A close relative of the Chronic Care Model is the **Collaborative Care Model**. The latter is actively being implemented in primary care practices to address the increased costs for and numbers of patients with co-occurring physical and mental health needs. Patients who have a co-occurring behavioral health condition receive intervention from the health care system significantly more frequently, with bills that are anywhere from 50% to 175% higher than similarly ill patients without a behavioral health condition (Gupta, 2015; Milliman, 2014). Collaborative models for mental and physical health use a team approach to deliver care. The general features of Collaborative Care models are (Bullock et al., 2017):

- Screening for mental health conditions
- Assessing and documenting baseline symptoms using valid instruments for mental health
- Provision of patient and family education to support self-management
- Provision of clinical support and supervision

In the Collaborative Care Model, dedicated team members address the needs of patients though a comprehensive and strategic care delivery process. Included in the team are a primary care provider, a case manager who is trained in behavioral health, and psychiatric consultants and/or behavioral health specialists (Unützer et al., 2013). This comprehensive approach to care serves as a proactive means to screen and track mental health conditions within the primary care setting.

Outcomes indicate that the Collaborative Care Model is clinically sound and cost effective in treating patients with comorbid conditions, including depression and/or anxiety, along with a chronic medical condition (e.g., diabetes, congestive heart failure) (Eghaneyan et al., 2014; Fortney et al., 2015; Robert Wood Johnson Foundation, 2011; Unützer et al., 2013). Hospital readmissions have been reduced by nearly 40%, with a significant decrease in associated costs of care (Epstein Becker Green, 2015).

The new generation of interprofessional teams. The concept of the interprofessional team is rapidly emerging in the literature. The Health and Medicine Division of the National Academies of Sciences, Engineering, and Medicine (formally the Institute of Medicine) discussed the obligation of academic health centers to conduct interdisciplinary education and patient care. This triggered an emphasis on interdisciplinary collaboration toward population health (Interprofessional Education Collaborative [IPEC], 2016).

Concerns have been raised about how the terminology of multidisciplinary, interdisciplinary, and related team approaches were used interchangeably. IPEC discusses Interprofessional Collaboration as the term of art and a unique domain (IPEC, 2016; Treiger and Fink-Samnick, 2016). The goal is to prepare health professions students for deliberately working together, with the common aim of building a safer and better patient-centered and population-oriented US health care system (IPEC, 2016).

Interprofessional teams refer to care delivered by intentionally created, usually relatively small work groups in health care. The teams are recognized by others, as well as by themselves, as having a collective identity and shared responsibility for a patient or group of patients. Examples include distinct teams for rapid response, palliative care, and primary care (IPEC, 2016). These teams are different from many teams found in interdisciplinary models, where members of only two different disciplines (such as nurses and doctors) might partner with or communicate with each other about the care of select patients. The four competencies identified for interprofessional teams are: values/ethics for interprofessional practice, roles/responsibilities, interprofessional communication, and teams and teamwork (IPEC, 2016).

Outcomes demonstrating the success of interprofessional teams are in the early stages, with the verdict still out on long-term acceptance across the industry. The implications for CM are vast, particularly with close alignment of its standards of practice with the IPEC principles. Sustainability will ultimately be driven by how the health care sector and its unique stakeholders interpret and operationalize the new term *interprofessional* as a construct (Treiger and Fink-Samnick, 2016). A number of demonstration projects are in process. Reports and funding opportunities are available on the IPEC website (https://www.ipecollaborative.org/about-ipec.html).

Competency-Based Models

In order for CM practice to progress in step with or ahead of general health care evolution, thought leaders must continuously generate theoretical frameworks and practical solutions to address the challenges of health care delivery, including definition of best practice, terminology (e.g., common language), dedication of resources (e.g., dosage), expected outcomes, and qualifications for professional practice (e.g., education, experience, credentials). In order to provide high quality care continuity, case managers need to speak the same language across the care continuum (Treiger and Fink-Samnick, 2016).

Rather than focus on care setting or organizational priorities as the driver of CM scope and practice, competency-based models approach practice through a lens of qualities and characteristics that contribute to practice excellence. As noted by the Case Management Society of America (CMSA, 2017b), case managers require specific knowledge of the CM process as well as a variety of skills in order to apply their expertise effectively. The most recognizable CM-specific competency framework is COLLABORATE.

The COLLABORATE model. This model builds and supports competent professional practice through the identification and application of essential skills, behaviors, and characteristics. Because it is a model based on characteristics and key elements, the paradigm integrates into existing CM processes and programs across the entire care continuum. COLLABORATE is an acronym identifying the competencies that are important to master for professional CM practice. The acronym stands for *C*ritical thinking, *O*utcomes-driven, *L*ifelong learning, *L*eadership, *A*dvocacy, *B*ig picture orientation, *O*rganized, *R*esource awareness, *A*nticipatory, *T*ransdisciplinary, and *E*thical–*L*egal (Treiger and Fink-Samnick, 2013; 2016).

Independent of health care's ongoing challenges, case managers must be sufficiently agile to frame (and reframe) professional practice in order to facilitate a client's best outcomes. This is why defining a competency-based CM model, which fits into any setting of care and applies to all populations, is essential. Ultimately, this competency-based model elevates the quality of practice and contributes to optimal CM and health care outcomes (Treiger and Fink-Samnick, 2013). Each competency and the associated key elements of the COLLABORATE model are displayed in Table 16.2.

Other Case Management Models

CM is practiced across the transitions of care, including but not limited to:

- ACOs,
- PCMHs,
- primary care,
- long-term care,
- rehabilitation,
- occupational health,
- workers' compensation, and
- pharmacies.

There are many care settings in which CM is practiced. However, a different setting of care does not necessarily mean another CM model has been created. In some models, the functions of CM, utilization review (UR), and disease management (DM) overlap. The overlap and distinctions between these areas result in organizational challenges. Policies, procedures, and processes are designed to clarify desired work flow in order to eliminate the risk of redundancy.

Insurance models may be divided into **brokerage, gatekeeper**, catastrophic, managed care, and government models. The brokerage model includes an emphasis on linkage to resources but with no provision of direct services. It is similar to the broker in other social work models except for a strong emphasis on conserving benefits utilization.

A **gatekeeper** model is defined as an informal, though widely used, primary care CM model health plan. In this model, all care from providers other than the primary care provider (except for true emergencies) must be authorized by the primary care provider before care is rendered (Kongstvedt, 2013). Cost savings are realized by managing care, including advocating for less costly but more appropriate services by not authorizing the requested higher-cost services. Rather than facilitating access, gatekeepers restrict access as a means to control utilization, which ostensibly controls costs but may just control short-term expenditures. Although there are variations in department configuration, many managed care plans have a medical management department under which a complex—also referred to as catastrophic—CM team exists.

Catastrophic CM is focused on complex and **catastrophic** illness or injury (e.g., spinal cord injury, traumatic brain injury, chronic degenerative neurological disease, medical–behavioral health dual diagnoses) and applies primarily to managed care, workers' compensation, and life-care planning. It is designed to manage and maximize insurance and health care benefits, which may be capped at a lifetime maximum. Screening, data mining, referrals, and other red flag strategies are leveraged to detect the potential for high-cost cases and to interact with clients and service providers proactively to optimize and economize the health services used (CMSA, 2016).

In **managed care** models, prospective or capitated reimbursement systems often place providers in the position of carrying financial risk. This creates pressure on providers to control total costs, provide and promote prevention-oriented services, and substitute lower-cost services, preferably without sacrificing quality. The type of managed care organization dictates the degree to which case managers directly interface with clients and providers.

In the **government model**, federal, state, and local agencies manage and reimburse health care via programs such as Medicare, Medicaid, and workers' compensation. Often management of these programs is handled by established health plans that create separate lines of business for government plans.

Case Management's Established Resources of Accountability

CM practice includes established resources of accountability that set both a context and hierarchy for CM practice. Included in this grouping are state licensure boards, accreditation organizations offering organizational credentialing, plus credentialing bodies, employers, and professional associations. This scope of this listing

TABLE 16.2 COLLABORATE Competencies and Key Elements

Acronym	Competency	Key Elements
C	Critical thinking	Out of the box creativity Analytical Methodical approach
O	Outcome driven	Patient outcomes Strategic goal setting Evidence-based practice
L	Lifelong learning	Valuing • Academia and advanced degrees • Professional development • Evolution of knowledge requirements for new and emerging trends (e.g., technology, innovation, reimbursement) • Practicing at top of licensure and/or certification • Acknowledging no one case manager can and does know all
L	Leadership	Professional identity Self-awareness Professional communication: verbal/non-verbal Team coordinator: a unifier rather than a divider
A	Advocacy	Patient Family Professional
B	Big picture orientation	Bio-psycho-social-spiritual assessment Macro (policy) impact on micro (individual) intervention
O	Organized	Efficient Effective
R	Resource awareness	Utilization management Condition/population specific Management of expectations per setting
A	Anticipatory	Forward thinking Proactive versus reactive practice Self-directed
T	Transdisciplinary	Transcending • Professional disciplines • Across teams • Across the continuum
E	Ethical–legal	Licensure Certification Administrative standards Organizational policies and procedures Ethical codes of conduct

Data from Treiger, T.M., & Fink-Samnick, E. (2016). *COLLABORATE for professional case management: A universal competency-based paradigm.* Philadelphia, PA: Wolters Kluwer.

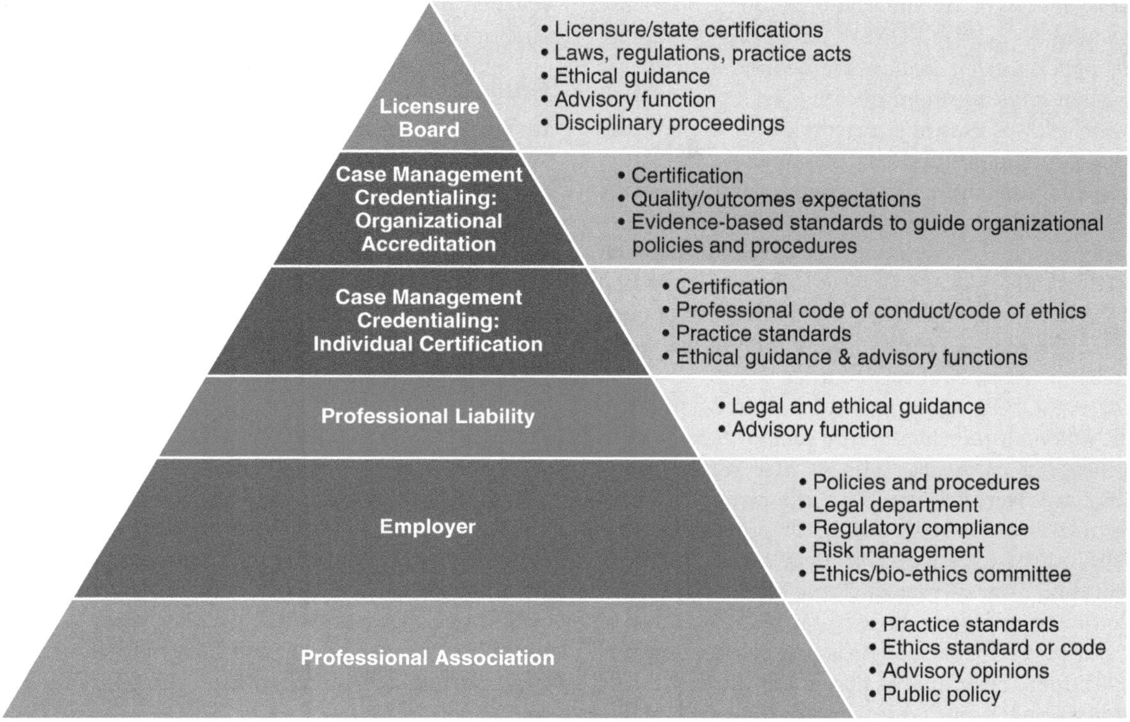

Fig. 16.1 Case management's hierarchy of authority oversight.

encompasses professional regulations and practice acts, codes of ethics, standards of practice, and employer policies and procedures. The actions of each entity inform the foundational pillars of CM practice (Fink-Samnick, 2019a). A graphic presentation of the official hierarchy of oversight for case managers appears in Fig. 16.1.

Case Management Practice Standards, Code of Conduct, and Program Accreditation

Practice Standards

CM practice has expanded at an accelerated rate in order to meet the evolving needs of health care and social services and proliferated across various health care and payer settings and practice models. As it grew and developed, it is essential to recognize that although these programs were frequently referred to as CM, the actual functions and activities of staff were often not reflective of the full scope of CM practice. Department and job titles were often grouped together within overarching care management strategies due, in part, to name recognition. It appears that little attention was given to ensuring CM departments and jobs were aligned with CM practice standards (Treiger and Fink-Samnick, 2013).

Two CM-specific **standards of practice** are offered by CMSA and the American Case Management Association (ACMA). Additional CM practice standards are offered by the US Department of Veterans Affairs (VA), which apply to CM practice within the VA system, and the NASW, which apply only to SWs. The American Nurses Association (ANA) offers overarching standards and scope of practice for nurses but does not offer CM-specific practice standards.

CMSA's *Standards of Practice for Case Management*, originally released in 1995, has undergone multiple revisions. Each revision was undertaken to address ongoing growth and expansion of CM across the continuum of care and into virtually every care setting. In addition to the standards, the document addresses definition, philosophy and guiding principles, practice settings, roles and responsibilities, and components of the CM process (CMSA, 2016).

ACMA developed professional standards resources for their certificants, holders of the Accredited Case Manager (ACM™) designation. The designation has regulatory oversight by the National Board for Case Management (NBCM). ACMA's *Standards of practice & scope of services for health care delivery system case management and transitions of care (TOC) professionals* (2013) includes professional principles for the areas of education, care coordination, compliance, transition management, utilization management, and standards of practice (including accountability, professionalism, collaboration, care coordination, resource management, and certification). ACMA focused on CM practiced within the health care delivery system, inclusive of transition management. As a result, the standards are applicable to a limited array of care settings.

In 2019, ACMA joined with 15 industry entities to publish *National transitions of care standards and a consensus measures crosswalk*. "The ACMA Transitions of Care Standards were designed with input from 15 collaborating organizations representing 10 practice settings across the industry: acute care, primary care, ambulatory, home care and hospice, managed care pharmacy, healthcare pharmacy, primary care, long-term care, behavioral health and payers." The standards include fundamental and aspirational benchmarks that guide successful care transitions. The consensus measures outline a method to assess a health care organization's performance as transitions are executed (Cobb, 2019).

Although adherence to practice standards is often considered to be voluntary, one exception is the Commission for Case Manager Certification's *Code of professional conduct* (CCMC, 2015). Adherence to this code is mandated for individuals possessing the Certified Case Manager (CCM) credential. It is important to recognize that in a situation where legal action against a case manager occurs, attorneys and the court look at practice standards (in addition to other documents and guidelines) as a means of determining whether the actions of a case manager were aligned with accepted practice. In the case of a nurse case manager, these additional documents include one's own state practice act or remote practice act (when practice involves the Nurse Licensure Compact), applicable nursing standards of practice, CM standards of practice, and organizational policies and procedures.

The most recognizable code of conduct for case managers is the *Code of professional conduct for case managers with standards, rules, procedures, and penalties*, produced by the CCMC (CCMC, 2015). The objective of the code is to protect the public interest. The code is divided into sections, including principles, rules of conduct, scope of practice, definitions, standards for board-CCM conduct, and procedures for processing complaints (CCMC, 2015).

Program Accreditation

In addition to individual certification, organizations, such as the National Committee for Quality Assurance (NCQA) and URAC, offer accreditation and/or distinction recognitions for CM programs. CM accreditation evaluates programs in provider, payer, or community-based organizations. There are also programs for CM rendered in the Long-Term Services and Supports (LTSS) sector. NCQA offers either full accreditation or distinction recognition depending upon the organization's need (NCQA, 2019).

The Case Management Process

The **CM process** focuses on the identification of individuals who would benefit from CM services and the activities of assessment, problem identification, care planning, care delivery, advocacy, monitoring, and evaluation of the care provided, specifically for its relevance to the needs of the patient and caregiver as well as for the health care team's ability to meet the desired outcomes and established goals (Tahan, 2017).

Although the process is presented as having a different number of phases, both CMSA and CCMC have supported following an organized iterative process. A consideration relating to the CM process is that of care setting. Care setting often dictates the type of interaction between case manager and client. For example, the acute care setting generally ensures face-to-face interaction, whereas the managed care setting varies and may be a combination of telephonic, face-to-face and/or Internet chat. The manner in which each case manager interacts with a client not only affects the ability to objectively assess that person but also influences how the relationship will evolve.

Commission for Case Manager Certification (CCMC)

CCMC defines the CM process as it applies to case managers who have achieved the CCM credential as being collaborative in nature. The phases of this process meld seamlessly and aim to support the patient, caregiver, support system, and care team members in addressing health and related issues (CCMC, 2016).

According to CCMC (2016), the process is divided into nine phases: screening, assessing, stratifying risk, planning, implementing (care coordination), following up, transitioning (transitional care), communicating post transition, and evaluating. The CCM navigates CM process being cognizant of the client and caregivers' cultural beliefs, interests, wishes, needs, and values. Because the CM process is an iterative cycle, each phase is revisited as necessary until desired outcomes are achieved and the client's interests are met (CCMC, 2016).

Case Management Society of America (CMSA)

CMSA also stipulates that the CM process is cyclical and recurrent, rather than linear or unidirectional. The CM process incorporates critical thinking and evidence-based knowledge and is carried out within the ethical and legal constructs of a case manager's scope of practice. The steps of the CM process as defined in the CMSA's *Standards of practice for case management* (2016) are client identification and selection, assessment and opportunity identification, development of the CM plan, implementation and coordination of CM plan interventions, monitoring and evaluation of the CM plan, and closing of the CM engagement. Table 16.3 elaborates the CM process phases and notes the similarities between CMSA, CCMC CM, and nursing processes.

Case Management Program Development and Implementation

Case Management Program Development

CM programs are structured around roles and functions of case managers. The case manager's role balances the

TABLE 16.3 Nursing and Case Management Processes

Nursing	CCMC	CMSA	Comments
	Screening	Client identification and selection	Screening and/or selection is specific to case management (CM) where access to a case manager is limited according to the capacity, policy, or practice scope of an organization or department.
Assessment	Assessing	Assessment and opportunity identification	
Diagnosis	Stratifying Risk		The CM process does not include a diagnosis phase, but there are some similarities that align in the opportunity identification and planning phases. • CCMC defines stratifying risk as the classification of a client into one of three risk categories (low, moderate, and high) in order to determine the appropriate level of intervention based on the client's situation and interests.* • In some CM settings, each client's stratification risk is set by the use of predictive modeling software. Subsequent risk score may be edited by the case manager based on client's current status (e.g., health, psychological health, social needs, complexity of care).
Outcomes/planning	Planning	Development of the CM plan	• Despite minute differences, a planning phase is intended to assimilate assessment findings into a workable plan of care for both nurse and case manager. • A CM plan includes overall goals and desired outcomes for identified needs.
Implementation	Implementing (care coordination)	Implementation and coordination of CM plan interventions	The implementation phase puts the plan into action.

CCMC, Commission for Case Manager Certification; *CMSA*, Case Management Society of America.
*Data from American Nurses Association (ANA). (2016). The nursing process. Retrieved May 22, 2016 http://www.nursingworld.org/EspeciallyforYou/StudentNurses/Thenursingprocess.aspx.; Commission for Case Manager Certification (CCMC). (2016). Case Management Body of Knowledge (CMBOK). Mount Laurel, NJ: Author. And Case Management Society of America (CMSA). (2016b). CMSA standards of practice for case management. Little Rock, AR: Author.

aspects of provider, care coordinator, and financial manager. Frequently identified case manager roles are advocate, facilitator, provider, liaison, coordinator, collaborator, broker, educator, negotiator, evaluator, communicator, risk manager, mentor, consultant, and researcher. CM functions are often identified as care coordination, facilitation and linkage, education, advocacy, discharge planning, resource management, and outcomes management.

For provider-based case managers, a CM program may be built based on CMSA's *Standards of practice for case management* (2016). The practice components identified in these standards are authoritative statements that are reflective of the unique roles and responsibilities for which case managers are held accountable. As a result, they can be used as an outline to establish step-by-step processes. In addition, the standards reflect how exclusive values and priorities of practitioners are operationalized and understood by mutual stakeholders (Treiger and Fink-Samnick, 2016).

CM programs are developed using a number of situation-specific elements. Two initial assessments are helpful: assessment of the organization and assessment of client populations. The *organizational assessment* focuses on identification of resources, whereas the client population assessment focuses on how care is experienced by clients and the characteristics of client populations served by the organizations. Box 16.2 lists related assessment questions. If CM is used for specific client populations, priority would go to clients who have a high rate of recidivism or frequent emergency department encounters; have unpredictable needs for care; have significant complications, comorbidities, or variances in usual care patterns; fall into high-risk profiles; and/or are high cost.

The general process for the development of a CM program is to:

1. Assess the organization and the client population served. This assessment provides a baseline for implementation.
2. Identify high-volume or high-risk case types. This assessment will indicate priority areas for care coordination.
3. Determine the usual client care problems, issues, or difficulties related to the high-volume or high-risk case types, with desired goals.
4. Form an interdisciplinary care team of the interrelated care providers who will be involved with the case types.

BOX 16.2 Case Management Assessment Questions

Organizational Assessment

- What clinical and support services are needed?
- When in the client experience are services most appropriately provided?
- How should services be provided?
- Where are services best delivered?
- Who are the most appropriate providers?
- Where and by whom are services best managed?

Client Assessment

- What are the major client populations served by the organizations—by volume, diagnosis, cost, payer mix, and high-intensity/resource use outliers?
- What is the service path followed by client populations—by entry point, internal flow, discharge, and recidivism?
- What groups of clients fall into high-risk categories—by volume?
- What clients are at risk for less-than-desired outcomes—by morbidity, mortality, infection rates, falls, and clinical outcomes?

5. Develop and design an interdisciplinary critical pathway for each selected case type. The path should outline and specify measurable clinical outcomes, key professional care processes, and exact corresponding timelines as based on practice patterns, professional standards of care, and length-of-stay parameters. The input and involvement of the client and each provider group needs to be clearly specified in relation to actions for achieving client outcomes. The pathway would mark the occurrence of routine treatments, tests, consults, client activities, medications, diet, educational interventions, and discharge planning. Variance from the path triggers analysis and intervention.
6. Develop a pilot program or trial site.
7. Evaluate the pilot program and consider system-wide implementation. Review the pilot program's articulation with the existing mode of nursing care delivery.

CM program development processes emphasize the potential of interprofessional team approaches by involving engaged disciplines in establishing treatment plans and completion of outcomes. They also highlight the importance of preparing patients, professionals, and the organization to facilitate success.

CM has become a popular and effective means to manage patients across populations and practice settings. In hospitals, it has decreased length of stay and secured important outcomes (Daniels, 2015; Watson, 2016). In the newest generation of CM settings, including primary care practices, ACOs, and PCMHs, quality and outcomes are being emphasized more than ever (Watson, 2016). Persuasive arguments exist for implementing CM programming. For example, close follow-up, continuous reinforcement, and systematic treatment adjustments facilitated by case managers contributed to improvement for adult clients with diabetes, heart failure, and comorbid physical and mental health conditions (Advancing Integrated Mental Health Solutions [AIMS] Center, 2019; Stellefson et al., 2013; Takeda et al., 2012; Unützer et al., 2013).

CM has equally been identified as a major strategy for cost containment, which also incorporates quality control. Given the vast financial impact for all practice settings, the case manager shoulders significant responsibilities for tracking both quality and outcomes in addition to targeting improvements. These actions are completed as a means to verify the case manager's own performance, the performance of the team, and to some extent the entire organization (Watson, 2016). Research has emerged over the past decade to substantiate savings from CM interventions, including studies on effectiveness from across the industry (Kolbasovsky et al., 2012; Stellefson et al., 2013).

Case Management Outcomes

Two basic outcomes categories to be captured are clinical outcomes and financial outcomes. For clinical outcomes, Braden (2002) identified these six direct outcomes of CM: (1) patient knowledge, (2) patient involvement, (3) patient participation in care, (4) patient empowerment, (5) patient adherence, and (6) coordination of care.

Improvement in a key indicator (e.g., patient knowledge) can be a direct measure of the clinical effectiveness of a CM intervention. The effectiveness of CM is further strengthened when the outcome of improved patient knowledge is linked to research evidence pertaining to improved patient knowledge reducing chronic relapse or use of health care resources.

Proving financial gain has been somewhat more problematic for CM, although the tide is turning. There has been acknowledged value and acceptance of CM in some areas, such as diabetes, congestive heart failure, and other chronic diseases (Kolbasovsky et al., 2012; Stellefson et al., 2013). In mental health and substance use, the outcomes are becoming more visible (Fortney et al., 2015; Unützer et al., 2013). A robust amount of literature has emerged courtesy of demonstration projects associated with the Collaborative Care Model out of the University of Washington's Advancing Integrated Mental Health Solutions (AIMS) Center (2019). A full listing of these programs is available on the AIMS Center website (http://aims.uw.edu/projects).

DISEASE MANAGEMENT

DM has been acknowledged as a payer strategy to prevent or manage one or more chronic conditions, improve care quality, and reduce costs (Ahmed, 2016; Walters et al., 2012). Since DM's entrance into the health care market, the term has experienced a fair level of transition. DM advanced from identification of persons at risk for one chronic condition to reflect a more comprehensive view of the customer base and is indicative of a global focus on care for entire populations (Ahmed, 2016; Goodman et al., 2014; Rushton, 2015; Walters et al., 2012).

The terms DM and PHM appear throughout this section. However, on the health care management continuum, the overall umbrella concept is better known as PHM. Both CM and DM are segments of the PHM spectrum.

History and Background

DM programs were developed and implemented largely as managed care health plan initiatives. The rise of DM occurred in the late 1980s and into the 1990s in the US health care delivery system. Nested within the general evolution of CM practice, managed care organizations and health plans began to look closely at DM after initial CM programs had been active for decades. Further refinements in program quality and cost savings were desired by employer group purchasers of health coverage. The unique challenges of chronic conditions occurring on a large scale needed to be addressed. Prior experiences with CM became the platform. In pharmaceutical companies, DM emerged as a way to encourage medication adherence.

Growth of Managed Care Systems and a Focus on Quality Care

Two major forces triggered the rise of a DM perspective: (1) a period of growth in managed care systems as a prevailing form of organized health care delivery (the influence of health plans), and (2) the national attention generated by *Crossing the quality chasm*, a health care quality initiative of the Institute of Medicine (IOM, now called the National Academies of Sciences, Engineering, and Medicine, Health and Medicine Division). Health plans led the charge to address the care coordination and service integration needs of clusters of members who had identifiable health conditions that are generally chronic in nature. In 1996, the Health and Medicine Division of the National Academies of Sciences, Engineering, and Medicine launched an ongoing effort focused on the assessment and improvement of the quality of health care in the United States. Their 2001 report *Crossing the quality chasm: A new health system for the 21st century* (IOM, 2001) highlighted the need for profound changes in the environment of care, including revamping practices that fragment the care system. The coordination of care across patient conditions, services, and settings was viewed over time as a major organizational challenge, yet a key dimension of patient-centered care.

DM evolved into proven and effective strategies to make groups of individuals who had a "disease" such as mental health or diabetes healthier while saving scarce health care coverage dollars. In the early 2000s, the federal government's Centers for Medicare & Medicaid Services (CMS, 2003) took notice of DM programs, sponsored DM demonstration projects, and encouraged contracting with DM vendors for outsourced medical management programs because DM was found to be effective in select populations.

Disease Management Transitions to Population Health Management

Moving into the 21st century, DM's identity shifted because of societal transitions. The community had become a more viable focus for health care services, prompting the need to expand DM's perspective. Social and economic pressures demanded that health care organizations focus on ways to provide cost-effective, population-based care. Roughly 40% of deaths were found to be caused by behaviors that could be modified by preventive, population-based intervention. Although these cases only accounted for a small percentage of health spending, the death and disability prevention aspects were important (Shaljian and Nielsen, 2013).

The next generation of health care began to explore the care process across the entire continuum. **Continuum of care** is a concept involving a system that guides and tracks patients over time through a comprehensive array of health services to span all levels and intensity of care (Young et al., 2014). The services incorporated in each patient's unique continuum vary based on the individualized health and/or behavioral health needs of each person.

Prevention and early detection programs (e.g., parenting, wellness), family and community services, pharmacies, behavioral health, and end-of-life care have also been incorporated as components of the continuum of care. Persons who are homeless and those on domestic and/or international travels are also factored into the equation, as are the services incurred during their experience (Young et al., 2014).

Building an effective continuum of care involves understanding the true health needs of an individual community. Emphasis on the health of a community is anchored in a rich history of innovations in community and public health methods and programs directed at reducing risk factor prevalence, decreasing acute and chronic disease burden and injury occurrence, and promoting health (Goodman et al., 2014). These factors also set a context and rationale for addressing the SDoH. As case managers often possess the prime responsibility in their organizations for care coordination, they face mounting pressures to reconcile client engagement, treatment adherence, and successful short and long-term wellness. As a result, attention to developing strategic partnerships with a responsive continuum of care will promote sound and effective CM intervention and contribute to more positive health outcomes (Fink-Samnick, 2019b).

Community health involves meeting the collective needs of a group or individual community by identifying problems and managing interactions both within the community and between the community and the larger society. Risk factors, health status indicators, functional ability levels, health promotion, health outcomes, and prevention of identified chronic diseases are the focus of data gathering, program planning, and implementation processes and activities. The term *community health* has experienced some evolution in recent years to account for the expansion into public health practice settings and the importance of community engagement as a core element (Goodman et al., 2014). The evolution is further understood by the need for health care professionals to focus more intentionally on both cultural diversity and the SDoH, which are key factors for successful patient engagement and activation (Ashford and LeCroy, 2017; Gillespie, 2016; Goodman et al., 2014; Hu et al., 2014).

As the scope of DM grew, a grander scale of attention beckoned for health care professionals interested in addressing societal trends and implications of chronic illness. In the emerging context of wellness and prevention for society, the term population provided a wider lens and presented as a more logical way to refer to the next wave of health management.

A **population** refers to a group of individuals—in contrast to the individuals themselves—organized in many different units of analysis, depending on the research or policy purpose. The **population health** perspective explores beyond a biomedical model of individual health and allows providers to consider what makes some groups of people healthier than other groups of people. The emphasis by the industry on the impact of socioeconomic factors on hospital readmissions speaks to a population health focus (Hu et al., 2014). Applying population health across the continuum entails the goals of (Nash et al., 2016, p. xvii):

1. Keeping the well, well
2. Reducing health risks
3. Providing quick access to care for acute illness so that health does not deteriorate
4. Managing chronic illness to prevent complications
5. Getting those with complex or catastrophic illness to centers of excellence or compassionate care settings

Accomplishing these goals involves both community participation and partnership, which are key concepts to PHM. Active participation in decision-making processes through a concerted and combined effort induces a vested interest in the success of any effort to improve the health of a community. For nurses, the concept of community as client directs the focus to the collective or common good instead of individual health. Population-based care draws on partnership and community-as-client concepts.

Chronic Health Conditions Align with Population Health Management

Chronic health conditions have long posed a formidable challenge to the health care delivery system. They affect almost half of the adult US population, with 25% having more than one chronic illness (Ward et al., 2013). The management of chronic conditions has been a particular burden for health care payers and employers. Chronic disease creates two particular difficulties for businesses. First, these conditions in the workforce lead to diminished productivity. Second, these conditions result in a greater portion of the business's revenue being diverted to health care expenditures. Further effects have an impact on the health care delivery system, society, and individuals' functioning and activities.

Population and health trends are tracked by governmental agencies such as the US Census Bureau, Centers for Disease Control and Prevention (CDC), Bureau of Labor Statistics (BLS), and Health Resources and Services Administration (HRSA), as well as private foundations and health care organizations. Clearly, health and health care delivery systems data are continually in flux. However, the available statistics are impressive. Costs are a considerable pressure, because on average individuals with chronic conditions cost 3.5 times as much to serve as others, and they account for a large proportion of services. According to the CDC (2019) chronic diseases, inclusive of heart disease, cancer, and diabetes, are the leading causes of death and disability in the United States. These illnesses affect approximately 133 million Americans, representing more than 40% of the total population of this country. These figures are projected to grow to an estimated 157 million, with 81 million having multiple conditions. Six out of 10 adults have at least one chronic disease, with 4 of 10 having two or more chronic diseases (CDC, 2019; National Health Council, 2014).

The chronic conditions that pose a particular economic burden but can be helped by PHM are characterized by high prevalence, high expense, relatively standardized treatment guidelines, and a significant role played by the individual's behavior on the progression of the condition. It is widely recognized that health care delivery can and must be improved. The pressures to provide access to care, maintain a high level of quality, and control expenditures are converging on a traditionally fragmented and acute care–focused system. Projections are that sociodemographic and economic tidal waves are set to converge in a "perfect storm" of crisis over health care in the near future. These tidal waves include the aging of the US population, the effect of the maturing of the baby boom generation, high pharmaceutical costs, advancing medical technology, dramatic increases in chronic health conditions, and US government budget deficits.

The solutions are not easy or obvious. However, PHM is now being viewed as a major health care strategy to improve health outcomes across multiple populations while lowering costs and improving patient satisfaction. It is one of the Institute for Healthcare Improvement's (2017) Triple Aims and is an important aspect of ACOs. PHM has demonstrated effectiveness across disease states, including integrated behavioral health, chronic illness (e.g., diabetes, congestive heart failure), and assorted payers (e.g., Medicare, Medicaid, third party populations) (Fortney et al., 2015; Lyles, 2016; Rushton, 2015; Sidorov & Romney, 2016). Attractive features include effective population management, coordination of care for chronic conditions, consistency of care for at-risk populations, customization of care support, encouragement of adherence to treatment, and proactive interventions. Although chronic diseases are among the most common and costly health problems, they are also among the most preventable. Adopting healthy behaviors such as eating nutritious foods, being physically active, and avoiding tobacco use can prevent or control the devastating effects of these diseases.

Population Health Management Practice Approaches

Early DM programs offered by health plans were developed in-house or purchased either from a vendor or another organization such as a hospital. The newest generation of PHM programs involves proactive outreach. Nursing outreach programs are the core element. Personal communications (usually via telephone) between an expert nurse and the health plan participant build a personal relationship, help identify knowledge deficits and counseling needs, facilitate close monitoring and progress toward goals, enhance treatment adherence, and promote clinical and cost stabilization.

Functioning as a personal health advisor, the health coach, case manager, or care coordinator establishes a single point of contact and coordination of care and service for patients having health problems and promotes a trusting relationship. Whether employed by a health plan or a contracted outside vendor, the PHM provided by nurses functioning as personal health advisors and advocates is central to effective outcomes.

The core of the DM concept was to comprehensively integrate care and reimbursement based on a disease or health condition's natural course. Both clinical and non-clinical interventions are timed to occur where and when they are most likely to have the greatest impact. This sequencing and targeting ideally prevents occurrences or exacerbations, decreases the use of expensive resources, and creates positive health outcomes through the use of prevention and proactive CM strategies. Chronic conditions are the focus, and the methods use systematic ways of delivering health care interventions to patients with similar characteristics. PHM models focus on the identification, standardization, and coordination of services across the continuum of care and for populations with the same or similar health care needs. Several program examples are discussed in the following sections.

The Population Care Coordination Process

Rushton's (2015) *Population care coordination process* provides a scalable framework for providers and/or organizations (e.g., single offices or larger ACOs) to provide multilevel care based on population- and patient-centered principles. It involves care coordination, CM, and PHM to maximize health outcomes and resource utilization for populations and the individuals within them. The process involves six phases to focus on coordinating care for the entire population with individualization of that care: data analysis, selection, assessment, multidisciplinary planning, implementation/intervention, and monitoring/evaluation (Rushton, 2015).

Care of Mental, Physical, and Substance Use Syndromes

Identified as one of the largest Collaborative Care population health implementation initiatives, the Care of Mental, Physical and Substance Use Syndromes (COMPASS) initiative included over 4000 Medicare and Medicaid patients across 187 clinics in seven states: California, Colorado, Massachusetts, Michigan, Minnesota, Pennsylvania, and Washington (Fortney et al., 2015). A core systematic case review (SCR) team intervened with chronically ill patients who were diagnosed with uncontrolled depression and uncontrolled diabetes and/or heart disease. The following program components were included:

- An initial evaluation to measure condition severity and assess the patient's readiness for self-management
- A computerized registry to track and monitor the patient's progress
- A care manager to provide patient education and self-management support, coordinate care with the

primary care physician and consultants, and provide active follow-up.

- A consulting psychiatrist and consulting medical physician to review cases with the care manager and recommend changes in treatment to the primary care physician
- Treatment intensification when there is a lack of improvement
- Relapse and exacerbation prevention

Overall aggregated results from all 18 participating regional groups demonstrated that goals were exceeded for depression, heart disease, and diabetes improvement (Advancing Integrated Mental Health Solutions, 2019; Fortney et al., 2015).

Evolving Practice Standards and Guidelines

Unlike the clear and prevalent industry practice standards for CM, PHM is just achieving its stride with respect to established professional guidelines. The *Population Health Alliance Outcomes Guidelines, Vol. 6* was released in 2015 and serves as a basis for many PHM programs throughout the industry (Population Health Alliance [PHA], 2015). For professional certification, the Chronic Care Professional (CCP) Certification has been offered since 2004 to eligible professionals working in health care or a health-related field. Non-clinical team members (e.g., community health educators, program leaders, or consultants who support health and chronic care improvement) may also apply (Health Sciences Institute, 2016).

Since 2002, The Joint Commission (TJC, 2019) has offered Disease-Specific Care (DSC) Certification to provide a framework for continuously reliable care. TJC accredited health care organizations may seek a 2-year certification for care and services programs that provide for a long list of chronic diseases or conditions. In addition, an advanced level of certification is available to programs that meet the requirements for DSC certification plus additional clinically specific requirements and expectations. The available advanced certification programs are listed by setting on the TJC website (https://www.jointcommission.org/accreditation-and-certification/certification/certifications-by-setting/).

The American Organization of Nurse Executives (now called the American Organization for Nursing Leadership [AONL]) (AONE, 2015) developed *Nurse executive competencies: Population health*. Leadership from the nurse executive is viewed as vital to the development, execution, and refinement of PHM programming. As an advocate for community health needs and patient populations, the nurse executive in his or her role as an agent of change is viewed as paramount (AONE, 2015).

The National Association of Chronic Disease Directors (NACDD, 2016) is a non-profit public health organization committed to serving chronic disease program directors of each state and US jurisdiction. NACDD works to provide educational and training, develop legislative materials, educate policymakers, provide technical assistance, develop partnerships and collaborations, and advocate for the use of epidemiological approaches in chronic disease services planning and chronic disease data. Moving forward, it is expected that the industry will see the further development and evolution of more standards, organizations, and certifications specific to PHM.

Disease Management Process, Program Development and Implementation

The goal of DM is to maintain or improve the current state of chronic disease(s) through the systematic use of evidence-based interventions. DM uses risk assessment, education, and risk factor reduction strategies to influence behaviors toward the goals of improving outcomes and reducing cost (Ahmed, 2016). DM has been a pivotal health care strategy for decades. However, unlike CM, there does not appear to be a single endorsed DM process that is consistently referenced in texts or journals. The general components associated with a DM program include population risk analysis, identification, stratification, enrollment and engagement, program delivery, outcomes and effectiveness evaluation, and reporting. Each of these components is displayed in Fig. 16.2 and is amplified further in this section.

Before identification of a specific population eligible for a DM program, health plans and DM companies analyze claims data to identify the conditions that are prevalent in a given population. This is completed using coding conventions such as the International Classification of Diagnosis (ICD) and Current Procedural Terminology (CPT). This, combined with claims expenditure data, reveals disease classifications that most affect a covered population. From this perspective an organization is able to determine its strategic and tactical priorities for program development.

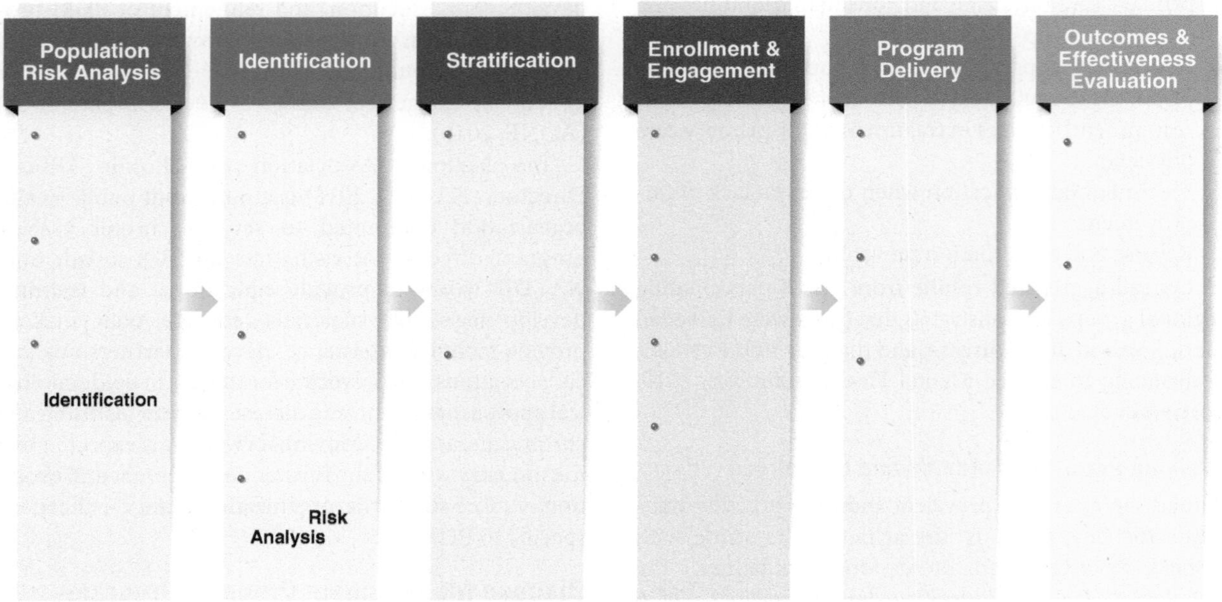

Fig. 16.2 Depiction of disease management program components.

Disease Management Program Components

Population Risk Assessment

The aggregate health care costs of chronic conditions increase yearly as individuals grow older. Older individuals tend to have chronic conditions that require complex care. It is estimated that one-third to one-half of all health care spending is consumed by the elderly. With the shift in demographic trends toward increasing numbers of elderly, there is a shift in the need for preventive care and chronic illness management services. To meet this challenge, managed care organizations have created infrastructures of population-based risk assessment, demand management (self-management and decision support systems such as call centers), DM, and CM.

To be effective at individual and population-based care management, both CM and DM programs need to identify, assess, and define the populations to be served early in the program planning effort. This component represents the effort to assess the health of a specific population (e.g., patient panel, enrollment). This assessment typically "triangulates" by drawing on available types of information (e.g., self-reported health questionnaires, health insurance claims, laboratory and pharmacy data, and clinician documentation). Once the population is defined, individuals within the population must be selected and assessed as to which program and level of intervention will optimally meet the most pressing needs. Factors that are included in an individual profile include age, number of chronic illnesses, and number of medications (Care Continuum Alliance [CCA], 2012a).

Identification

The participant identification process is driven by algorithms or other logic frameworks that are applied to claims data and look for specific diagnosis codes. In addition, predictive modeling tools (e.g., artificial intelligence, neural net logic) are leveraged to harvest information beyond simple diagnosis. *Predictive modeling* is "a commonly used statistical technique to predict future behavior. Predictive modeling solutions are a form of data-mining technology that works by analyzing historical and current data and generating a model to help predict future outcomes" (Gartner, 2016). Predictive models have been used in other industries and businesses, such as credit card companies and retailers, for years. In health care, these methodologies look for experience and other red flags that indicate an individual is at risk and to what extent. The case-finding techniques help to identify individuals who appear to be in most need of additional support in order to stem worsening health conditions and resource expenditures. The identified individuals are then screened by intake specialists to determine the best match between program intensity and client need (Ahmed, 2016).

Additional cycles of predictive modeling help to stratify each person's risk level (e.g., low, medium, high), as well as to look at care patterns and care gaps. These programs also have the ability to identify when an individual is not receiving optimal pharmaceutical therapy, is not having provider visits at the proper interval, or is not receiving the proper immunizations. This information is available to the DM nurse when reaching out to clients, providers, pharmacies, or other providers involved with the individual's care. These results also drive the intensity of intervention (e.g., reminders, risk reduction measures, DM program, or CM interventions) that an individual may be offered (Plocher, 2013).

Stratification

The next step in the population health process is to stratify patients into meaningful categories for patient-centered intervention targeting that uses information collected in health assessments (CCA, 2012a). In population health management, **stratification** has two meanings (PHA, 2015): a method of randomization and a process for sorting a population of eligible members into groups relating to their relative need for total population management interventions. Stratification may be based on the integration of a variety of data, if available, including claims, pharmacy, laboratory, health risks, or consumer-reported data such as health assessments. The stratification process harvests information that can be used to divide the patient population into different levels to ensure a return on investment (ROI) based on resources allowed.

Enrolment and Engagement

Once individuals are identified and stratified, those who appear to qualify for DM intervention receive an outreach notification (e.g., telephone call). The opportunity to enroll in a condition-specific program is offered during this initial contact. The program is explained, and consent to participate is requested. Although the enrollment process sounds straightforward, there are a number of barriers to overcome in getting individuals on-boarded into a program, such as inaccurate data, incorrect contact information, and outright refusal (Plocher, 2013).

One factor that is at the root of some non-enrolment is consumer mistrust of the insurance company's motives for contact. This concept contributes to unwillingness to participate in programs offered by the insurance company. Consumer mistrust is especially important when one considers the cost of delivering a DM program. The cost relating to a DM program is frequently reported at a per-member-per-month (PMPM) level. The expense of creating and maintaining such programs is borne by the insurance company regardless of whether the individual actively participates in the program (Ahmed, 2016).

Historically, program engagement has been a challenge, as typically only about 20% of those eligible participate in these programs (Brown et al., 2012). Despite these programs being established for decades, research on why people opt out or do not participate is limited (Hawkins et al., 2014).

The results of a 2014 study that examined factors driving engagement suggest that individuals most motivated to engage are those who are well informed of the program benefits and have a perceived need that would benefit from said program (e.g., living alone, needing a supportive person to discuss ideas) (Hawkins et al., 2014). Recruitment and engagement strategies continue to evolve, but the challenges facing this component of DM programming include privacy, meaningful engagement, and physician integration (Plocher, 2013).

Program Delivery

Whenever possible, the components of DM should be delivered by leveraging a variety of communications and interventions. This mixed mode approach optimizes the resources and outreach and accommodates the preferences and technological abilities of recipients with the ultimate goal of increased engagement and self-management (CCA, 2012b). This also takes into account that communication preferences vary based on generational differences. Although demographic splitting by age groups may not lead to absolute accuracy, it is generally accepted that communicating with a baby boomer versus a millennial requires consideration of a variety of channels (e.g., social media, hard copy print, telephone calls).

Interaction and management. Communication is a means of interaction and management for program delivery. It mostly involves the program participants, primary care providers, and program staff. There are a number of communication channels used to enhance interaction between the plan and both member and provider. The choice of modes used depends on the organization's ability to maintain compliance with the Health Insurance Portability and Accountability Act of 1996 (HIPAA) across each channel, financial resources to establish and maintain each channel, understanding of a given population's communication preferences, and other factors. Examples of communication options include (Plocher, 2013):

- Mailings
- Information to enrollee: welcome packet, interval updates and results, reminders
- Information to provider: orientation packet, periodic progress updates, periodic guideline recommendations
- Outbound telephone calls and interactive voice response (IVR) (e.g., initial welcome, assessments, progress checks, coaching)
- Inbound calls from participants to address condition and DM care plan questions
- Internet-based text and video chats for progress updates, reminders, condition and DM care plan questions
- Home telemonitoring devices for home device connection to monitor real time results. Frequently transmitted biometrics are weight, vital signs, and pulse oximetry.
- Medication adherence tools with pill box monitoring support for complex medication regimens
- Technology platforms (e.g., web portals) for secure messaging
- Face-to-face conversation for assessment, progress updates, and coaching

As technology continues to develop, so too will communication options. Technology is a core expectation of DM programs. Organizations have invested millions in developing technology to support DM programs from front (e.g., population assessment to identify prevalence, risk stratification) to back (e.g., reporting, effectiveness, outcomes analysis).

Outcomes and Effectiveness Evaluation

Program outcomes and effectiveness reports are an evolving source of information. Before-and-after program enrollment comparison is a common method of demonstrating program impact, but these often require at least a year of continuous participant enrollment to be deemed significant. In addition, the Healthcare Effectiveness Data Information Set (HEDIS®) requires this time span for data collection. These metrics look at testing frequency or certain drugs being prescribed, instead of test result improvement, such as hemoglobin A_1C, low density lipoprotein (LDL) cholesterol, appropriately prescribed angiotensin converting enzyme inhibitor, and appropriately prescribed beta blockers.

In today's lightning-fast, results-driven environment, waiting a full year to see results of an investment is difficult to sell. Metrics of interest include PMPM cost, episode-of-care cost, and utilization (e.g., hospital admissions, inpatient days) (Plocher, 2013). This imperative has spurred on the use of "big data" analytics. For example, at Geisinger Clinic in Pennsylvania, the big data approach was viewed as a way to better manage patients with chronic conditions. Big data is defined as the large volume of structured and unstructured data that swamps businesses on a day-to-day basis (SAS, 2016). Much of the data collected about patients lies dormant and is not used in routine analytic methods. Geisinger undertook a process redesign with its coronary artery disease (CAD) program that eliminated waste, automated processes where possible, and delegated tasks to appropriate staff. Geisinger accelerated the delivery of care through continuous use of data and informatics and addressed nine patient-oriented goals focused on improving the health of nearly 17,000 patients with CAD. The goals were measured in an "all or none" bundle to encourage team-based workflows rather than using measures that focused on a particular team member's performance (e.g., prescribing rate). The measures addressed care issues faced by all patients with CAD. The bundled approach to care measures realized a 300% improvement. The use of big data analytics was anticipated to harvest even more significant improvements in patient care (Graf et al., 2014). The use of big data is poised to flourish in all areas of health care, translating massive amounts of unusable data into useable information.

Reporting

In their 2015 joint report, the Health Enhancement Research Organization (HERO) and Population Health Alliance (PHA) published a core guide to metrics, the *Program measurement & evaluation guide: Core metrics for employee health management.* The categories included financial, health outcomes, participation, satisfaction, organizational support, productivity and performance, and value on investment framework. The report was framed by the following statement, "HERO and PHA are responding to employers who seek a greater level of clarity regarding the value of their wellness efforts. Thus we recommend an initial set of measures to assess the impact of the health management programs offered to employees. The results are better informed business decisions and boardroom discussions" (HERO-PHA, 2015). Although aimed at employer groups, these metrics are solid indicators of PHM program impacts. These metric categories may be applied in whole or in part to measure program impacts and as a means for classifying areas requiring further performance improvement.

When designing and implementing a DM program, use of a detailed project plan is essential to develop and maintain. This is done to track progress toward completion and hold stakeholders accountable for completing assigned tasks. Once implemented, in addition to program metrics, the project plan gives way to more simplified tools such as checklists. Table 16.4 depicts one such checklist. It is strongly recommended that tools such as this be customized to each unique program.

TABLE 16.4 Checklist to Evaluate Disease Management Programs

Component	Present (Yes); Absent (No)	Specific Method or Metric Used
Population identification and selection		
Risk assessment		
Risk stratification		
Use of evidence-based practice guidelines		
Type of practice model		
Collaborative mechanism		
Single discipline predominates (identify)		
Patient self-management		
Education		
Primary prevention		
Behavior modification		
Lifestyle change motivation		
Telephone contact		
Health advocates		
Compliance/adherence		
Surveillance		
Process, outcomes management		
Process identification and measurement		
Process evaluation		
Outcomes identification and measurement		
Outcomes evaluation		
Process and outcomes management		
Feedback loop		
Communication to:		
Patient		
Physician		
Health plan		
Ancillary providers		
Practice profiling		

From D.L. Huber. (2017). *Care for the total population.* Iowa City, IA.

LEADERSHIP AND MANAGEMENT IMPLICATIONS

Nurses who manage client care are clinical managers. The shift to managed care in integrated health systems and ever-expanding care settings (e.g., ACO, PCMH) highlights CM as a key strategy for nursing practice management and empowerment of nurses. It also has made care team collaboration an imperative. Leadership roles for nurses are essential because of the need for care continuity.

Future CM effectiveness is thought to be based on decisions about what types of organizational structures and nursing care delivery systems best enable nurse-managed client care and best support nurses in practice. One related question is, "How much management structure does a nurse require to be effective?" One assessment is the extent to which a nurse provides client care or manages the care of clients. CM is one specific approach to redesigning care delivery for client care improvement. This may mean that some traditional management practices need to be changed or discarded. CM has come to be a part of care delivery management that emphasizes the expertise of nurses.

CM is practiced beyond the walls of the acute care setting. There is no single way to go about identifying how much management structure is necessary because of the variety of care settings and associated bureaucracy. CM leader-managers need to examine the state of health care management in their organizations and develop strategies to implement coordination of care models to best meet client, organizational, societal, and professional priorities, often referred to as patient-and-family-centered models. Given the interdisciplinary nature of CM, model development and success may require a buy-in by other health care disciplines and other organizational stakeholders. Physicians and hospital administrators are crucial stakeholders for the success of CM programs. The CM leader-manager needs to master communication, collaboration, and advocacy skills in order to effect changes within their own department as well as across the organization.

Partnering With Human Resources

Another CM leader-manager challenge is the human resources department itself. Now more than ever the question "Who is qualified to be hired as a case manager?" is one that needs careful consideration. In today's outcomes-driven health care environment, it is important to have the right people in the right positions to maximize their experience, knowledge, and skills. In short, competence should be the driver of personnel changes.

The CM leader-manager works closely with a human resource specialist (HRS) to clarify department structure, mission, and vision. Job descriptions should clearly distinguish position types and grade levels. New position descriptions should provide the required experience, knowledge, and skills that a qualified candidate should possess. CM position descriptions need to reflect education level and credential requirements, being mindful to distinguish requirements from preferences so as to simplify the candidate screening process.

Individual Suitability for Case Management

CM leader-managers need to evaluate employees in existing positions who are considered as case managers. In many situations, job titles and/or responsibilities change over the years regardless of whether the employees are well suited for their new scope of work. In other instances, department reorganizations have allowed people to retain the coveted case manager job title despite the position's purpose having changed significantly. There needs to be an objective process in place in order to fairly evaluate existing employees. Reassignments may be necessary after such an evaluation process. The evaluation process is stressful on staff and management. The CM leader-manager needs to have a clear vision, strategy, and a proactive communication plan in order to move the department through the change management process.

It is important to clarify the requisite experience and credentialing required to fill the CM job. Certification is typically an official credential awarded to an individual by a nationally recognized professional organization based on eligibility and passing a standardized examination. The credential affirms a baseline degree of education, experience, and knowledge. Individual certification is a mark of professional achievement, and although it is difficult to attain, certification is a floor—not a ceiling—of achievement.

CURRENT ISSUES AND TRENDS

There are constant pressures that affect CM practice, including the lack of title protection, which allows misuse of the case manager designation; the inflow of unlicensed and inexperienced individuals performing CM tasks; and challenges with licensure portability affecting individuals' ability to work seamlessly to provide care coordination services across state lines. This section is devoted to select challenges currently challenging the CM workforce.

Branding and Lack of Universal Definition

Health care reform has amplified the number of career options for the CM workforce, especially with the expansion of ACOs, PCMHs, and integrated behavioral health programs. These opportunities span business models, practice settings, professional disciplines, and across the transitions of care. Yet a double-edged sword exists with regard to the vast number of CM-associated titles, roles, functions, and job descriptions that have followed suit. Experts challenge that this expansion has contributed to a paradoxical effect on CM's identity (Treiger & Fink-Samnick, 2013; 2016).

Patients and family caregivers, employers, and other stakeholders with a vested interest are consistently challenged to comprehend the similarities and differences among the many job titles for CM (e.g., case manager, care manager, geriatric care manager, care coordinator, case worker, care advocate, advanced life care planner, patient advocate, patient navigator, health care coach). This role multiplicity is one more obstacle to CM's maturity from advanced practice to established profession (Treiger & Fink-Samnick, 2013; 2016). It also serves to splinter rather than forge a strong foundation for professional CM practice.

Leveraging the Non-Clinical Workforce

Maintaining a workforce consisting primarily of licensed and/or certified clinical professionals is an expensive proposition. In spite of geographical variation, RNs and SWs are justifiably compensated for their clinical and health care system knowledge. Historically, organizations employed RNs and SWs in CM positions. Later, when organizations became more focused on cost-savings and efficiency, they began to use non-clinical staff to perform CM activities or applied the case manager job title indiscriminately in order to attract candidates with a desirable position. The impact of this staffing methodology on care quality or value for service delivered has not been clearly or consistently demonstrated (Treiger, 2011).

Organizations are recognizing the need to hire increasing numbers of non-clinical professionals to leverage the professional CM workforce. The influx of concrete and non-clinical service needs has prompted more primary level CM tasks (e.g., social service referrals, resource coordination, financial services, arranging transportation). To this end, the use of emerging roles, such as community health workers and health service coordinators, is being rapidly integrated into existing CM models across practice settings.

The economics of maintaining a workforce largely made up of clinical professionals continues to force review of hiring practices and raises questions pertaining to required qualifications of individuals working in CM. To reduce program costs, some organizations opt to hire individuals for care coordination positions who lack a professional degree and/or have limited if any clinical experience necessary to handle the complexity of CM functions. In one Midwestern health system, this hiring strategy was brought to an abrupt halt when leaders realized that the staff hired to coordinate care were not qualified to perform an independent assessment, unable to clearly identify patient care challenges and needs as an outcome of the independent assessment, and unqualified to develop a CM care plan to address individual challenges and needs. The failure was corrected by hiring appropriate staff (e.g., RN, SW) for CM positions. However, this was not without some pain and lost time in having to rework an otherwise well-considered corporate revitalization. CM leader-managers need to advocate for a tiered, yet collaborative CM workforce comprised of varying positions within their departments to best address both clinical and non-clinical needs of patient populations. Emphasis must also be on assuring sound partnerships among all members of the workforce to achieve successful patient outcomes.

Legislative and Regulatory Disruptors

Licensure Portability and the Nurse Licensure Compact

Current regulations continue to be grossly out of sync with practice realities for health care professionals, particularly nurses engaged in CM. Many case managers experience huge challenges and potential violations for practicing without a license in a state where the patient is located. The case manager may not be licensed to practice in that particular state and/or their scope of practice fails to allow for telehealth practice (Fink-Samnick & Muller, 2015). This has been a chronic issue, particularly for those nurses employed by national managed care and/or workers' compensation organizations, multihospital systems, or other health and behavioral health providers. For example, tele-management assessment is not permitted consistently across all professional disciplines or states. As a result, nurses are encouraged to check the websites for their respective individual professional state licensure boards and/or certifications on a regular basis to accurately define their individual scope of practice (Fink-Samnick & Muller, 2015).

The **Nurse Licensure Compact** (NLC) and the newer enhanced version, the eNLC, give multistate rights to RNs and licensed practical/vocational nurses (LPN/VN) residing in a member state. The eNLC addressed concerns voiced by several states that declined to join the Compact. The eNCL includes uniform licensure requirements, the authority to submit and obtain background checks, and reporting to participating in alternative to discipline programs in NURSYS® (National Council of State Boards of Nursing, 2016a). Advance practice nurses (APNs) maintain a separate compact. The eNLC allows nurses to have one multistate license with the ability to practice in both their home state and other compact states (National Council of State Boards of Nursing, 2016b). The advancement of the NLC across states has been a vital factor to promote the legal practice of CM across state lines. A current map of NLC member states is available at *https://www.ncsbn.org/nurse-licensure-compact.htm*.

Measuring and Sharing Case Management Outcomes

In 2010, the Agency for Healthcare Research and Quality (AHRQ) issued the comparative effectiveness report *Outpatient case management for adults with medical illness and complex care needs* (Hickam et al., 2013). The report focused on this single segment of practice and specific questions pertaining to CM as an intervention strategy for chronic illness outpatient management. The findings clearly note that there was a wide diversity in the included study populations, interventions, and outcomes. That notwithstanding, the overall conclusion was that CM demonstrated limited impact on patient-centered outcomes, quality of care, and resource utilization among patients with chronic medical illness (Hickam et al., 2013). It is important to sort out the conflicting literature on CM outcomes because direct cause-and-effect may not capture the actual importance of CM to clients and because cost reduction or ROI is hard to demonstrate when a labor-intensive service like CM is added.

These findings need to be leveraged to identify and implement program modifications as well as determine measures that accurately capture CM as value-added irrespective of monetary ROI. Sharing of program metrics across the health care continuum is one way in which research-generated evidence will influence practice moving forward. CM leader-managers undertaking quality and process improvements within a CM department must remain mindful of the importance of the evidence generated from these efforts because it is valuable to the entire CM community.

Treatment Adherence

Treatment adherence continues to be a driver of disease cost and a needed focus of intervention with patients. Medication adherence alone is estimated to have an annual cost of $100 billion in the United States (Lee, 2016). *Adherence* refers to the extent to which the patient continues a negotiated treatment. The topics of treatment adherence and patient engagement are major drivers in ensuring successful outcomes and establishing a PHM program's ROI.

Health risk behaviors (e.g., smoking, inactivity, poor diets, or nonadherence to prescribed therapies) significantly contribute to a population's overall morbidity, disability, mortality, reduced productivity, and escalating health care costs (Lee, 2016; Prochaska & Prochaska, 2016). Intense employer focus on wellness and prevention has escalated the importance of and growth of PHM programs. Studies show as many as 73% of companies are offering workplace or employee wellness to incentivize engagement in healthy lifestyles (Lee, 2016). Identified reasons for low ROI for early DM programs have included late identification of patients, turnover rate, lack of benefit coordination (especially when using an outside DM vendor), and the presence of comorbidities (Ahmed, 2016).

More engaged patients incur lower costs, whereas less engaged patients can generate up to 21% higher health care costs (Calhoun et al., 2016). Successful interventions with nonadherent patient populations include using the transtheoretical model of behavior change, which integrates advising, guiding, and supporting patients through the six stages of health behavior change: precontemplation, contemplation, preparation, action, maintenance, and termination. Key strategies and processes have been identified that work best at each stage to reduce resistance, facilitate progress, and minimize relapse (Prochaska & Prochaska, 2016).

There are planned updates to popular health risk assessments over the next few years toward a more conclusive assessment that takes into account determinants of health and performance (e.g., advances in technology, use of smartphones, and new research) (Edington et al., 2016). All health care professionals, especially nurses, can develop the skills to engage patients in the care process through leveraging meaningful use goals (e.g., health IT) and delivering adherence interventions (Calhoun et al., 2016; Prochaska & Prochaska, 2016).

CONCLUSION

Health care's strong fiscal imperatives have the industry well aligned with the business sector. Organizations strive to align overall goals, financial drivers of care, and department staffing in way that demonstrates ROI as a marker for financial viability. As a result, leaders need to ensure solid processes are in place to guide the development of department programming, provide clear job descriptions for those to be hired, and render a comprehensive means to identify and promote performance quality.

Despite the widespread dissemination of CM and DM as an intervention and system-wide strategy, a number of challenges remain specific to program development and implementation. Organizations struggle with a number of issues including whether and how to internally combine or separate functions. With an emphasis on financial viability or profit margin, CM and DM programs have been analyzed, challenged, redesigned, and reinvented under different labels in order to justify the allocation of scarce resources to them. Where CM is concerned, continued confusion over definitions, evolution and expansion of titles, and ongoing licensure and reimbursement challenges further contribute to constant changes within CM departments and programs.

RESEARCH NOTE

Source

Joo, J.Y., & Liu, M.F. (2019). Effectiveness of nurse-led case management in cancer care: Systematic review. *Clinical Nursing Research, 28*(8), 968–991.

Purpose

The purpose of this research article is to systematically examine the evidence for the effectiveness of nurse-led case management (CM) in adults with cancer. Because cancer is deadly, expensive, requires a high level of care, and care is often uncoordinated and fragmented, CM has been used to increase the efficiency and effectiveness of cancer care. CM has been shown to promote quality of life but is more commonly studied in high-risk or chronic illness populations.

Discussion

Using systematic review principles, the Cochrane processes and PRISMA statements were employed, and nine experimental studies published from 2008–2017 were retrieved from four electronic databases. Across all of the studies, CM interventions were palliative care, supportive services, and regular follow-ups. Three domains of outcomes were psycho-behavioral, hospital access, and health care costs. The results demonstrated that positive case management improved the quality of life for patients and significantly decreased hospital readmission rates. When looking at health care costs and other hospital access measures, the results were mixed. This demonstrates that there is some evidence for the effectiveness of nurse-led CM in cancer care.

Application to Practice

Consistent with other studies, when research is systematically reviewed, there is strong evidence for the fact that for patients with nurse-led CM interventions, there was improved quality of life and significantly decreased hospital readmission rates. Thus, CM is effective for these two outcomes. Other outcomes were mixed, and this may be due to imprecision in standardization of intervention protocols or in measurement of intervention effects on outcomes. Overall, nurse case managers play a pivotal role in cancer treatment, producing some important outcome results. The practice of nurse-led CM needs to be taught to nurses, nurse practitioners, and nurse managers.

CASE STUDY

Ramona St. Rose, RN, was hired to facilitate the Healthy Habits Advisory Group and Ministry at St. Patrick Church in Iowa City for a bilingual community. One third of the population was Latino and two-thirds were White Americans. She worked collaboratively with a team of parishioner volunteers. The team consisted of three physicians, a nurse attorney, two faculty members, prelicensure students in a public health practicum, and the mobile clinic at the local university. Pearl, one volunteer, offered a proactive role called the self-care transition coach. This role would allow discharged parishioners, especially those with chronic diseases, to contact her to manage their discharge instructions at home. The team identified, assessed, and defined the populations to be served early in the planning effort. What methods would Ramona use to define and assess the population? As the demand for services grows, what strategies can be used to avoid overwhelming Pearl and Ramona?

CRITICAL THINKING EXERCISE

Nurse Gloria Davis just got her dream job as a case manager for diabetes care in a large integrated delivery system. Nurse Davis is deeply committed to high-quality client care. She has structured an excellent teaching program that is administered through the ambulatory clinics. She has instituted population data collection using the SF-36 and Diabetes Quality of Life tools. Nurse Davis has begun to collect trend data on HbA_{1c} values and frequency of blood glucose instability or complications. The next outcome to measure is client satisfaction. Nurse Davis assumes that client satisfaction is related to adherence with treatment. The first step is a small focus group. In the focus group meeting, Nurse Davis discovers that client interactions with a health care provider are becoming more impersonal. The clients have fewer choices about to whom and where they can go for services, must get complicated authorizations, there is an increasing need to fill out more forms, listen to recorded messages, and are wait longer for appointments. On clinic days they wait a long time to see their provider briefly. The process of coming in for care actually makes many of these clients feel worse. Discuss the following questions based on the content presented:

1. Identify the problem(s).
2. Prioritize what Nurse Davis should do first, and why.
3. How should Nurse Davis analyze this situation?
4. How could Nurse Davis apply the COLLABORATE competencies to this situation?
5. How should Nurse Davis evaluate her final actions?
6. Outline leadership and management strategies that would be useful to Nurse Davis.

REFERENCES

Advancing Integrated Mental Health Solutions (AIMS) Center. (2019). *Our projects*. University of Washington, Psychiatry and Behavioral Sciences Division of Integrated Care and Public Health. http://aims.uw.edu/projects.

Affordable Care Act (ACA). (2010). *ACA the About*. https://www.hhs.gov/healthcare/about-the-aca/index.html.

Ahmed, O. I. (2016). Disease management, case management, care management, and care coordination: A framework and brief manual for care programs and staff. *Professional Case Management, 21*(3), 137–146.

American Association of Critical-Care Nurses (AACN). (2019). *AACN Synergy Model for patient care*. https://www.aacn.org/nursing-excellence/aacn-standards/synergy-model.

American Case Management Association (ACMA). (2013). *Standards of practice & scope of services for health care delivery system case management and transitions of care (TOC) professionals*.

American Organization of Nurse Executives (AONE). (2015). *Nurse executive competencies: Population health*.

Ashford, J. B., & LeCroy, C. W. (2017). *Human behavior in the social environment: A multi-dimensional perspective* (6th ed.): Cengage Learning.

Berger, C. S. (2015). Social work case management in medical settings. In K. Corcoran, & A. R. Roberts (Eds.), *Social workers' desk reference* (3rd ed., pp. 866–878). Oxford University Press.

Braden, C. J. (2002). *State of the science paper #2: Involvement/participation, empowerment and knowledge outcome indicators of case management*. Case Management Society of America.

Brown, R. S., Peikes, D., Peterson, G., Schore, J., & Razafindrakoto, C. M. (2012). Six features of Medicare coordinated care demonstration programs that cut hospital admissions of high-risk patients. *Health Affairs, 31*(6), 1156–1166.

Bullock, H. L., Waddell, K., & Wilson, M. G. (2017). *Knowledge synthesis: Identifying and assessing core components of collaborative-care models for treating mental and physical health conditions.* McMaster Health Forum.

Calhoun, C., Hall, L. K., & Kemper, D. (2016). Patient engagement: Engaging patients in the care process by leveraging meaningful use goals. In D. B. Nash, R. J. Fabius, A. Skoufalos, J. L. Clarke, & M. R. Horowitz (Eds.), *Population health: Creating a culture of wellness* (2nd ed., Chapter 7). Jones and Bartlett Learning.

Care Continuum Alliance (CCA). (2012a). *Implementation and evaluation: A population health guide for primary care models.* https://populationhealthalliance.org/population-health-guide-for-primary-care-models/.

Care Continuum Alliance (CCA). (2012). *Participant engagement and the use of incentives considerations.* https://populationhealthalliance.org/wp-content/uploads/2018/02/cca-incentives-document_1.pdf.

Carr, D. (2009). Building collaborative partnerships in critical care: The RN case manager/social work dyad in critical care. *Professional Case Management, 14*(3), 121–132.

Case Management Society of America (CMSA). (2016). *Standards of practice for case management.*

Case Management Society of America (CMSA). (2017a). What is a case manager? https://www.cmsa.org/who-we-are/what-is-a-case-manager/.

Case Management Society of America (CMSA). (2017b). *CMSA core curriculum for case management.*

Centers for Disease Control and Prevention (CDC). (2019). Chronic Diseases in America. https://www.cdc.gov/chronicdisease/resources/infographic/chronic-diseases.htm.

Centers for Medicare & Medicaid Services (CMS). (2003). Medicare program; Demonstration: Capitated disease management for beneficiaries with chronic illnesses. *Federal Register, 68*(40), 9673–9680.

Cline, B. G. (1990). Case management: Organizational models and administrative methods. *Caring: National Association for Home Care Magazine, 9*(7), 14–18.

Cobb, B. (2019). ACMA and 15 Collaborating Organizations Publish National Transitions of Care Standards and a Consensus Measures Crosswalk, Case Management. *Medical Management Plus, Inc.* http://mmplusinc.com/news-articles/item/acma-and-15-collaborating-organizations-publish-national-transitions-of-care-standards-and-a-consensus-measures-crosswalk.

Commission for Case Manager Certification (CCMC). (2015). *Code of professional conduct for case managers with standards, rules, procedures, and penalties.*

Commission for Case Manager Certification (CCMC). (2016). *Case management body of knowledge (CMBOK).*

Community Mental Health Act. (1963). *S. 1576.* https://www.govtrack.us/congress/votes/88-1963/h78.

Council on Social Work Education. (2015). *Educational policy and accreditation standards for baccalaureate and master's social work programs.* Alexandria: VA: Council on Social Work Education Commission on Accreditation, Commission on Educational Policy.

Daniels, S. (2015). Hospital case management: A new view from the C-Suite. *Professional Case Management, 20*(3), 156–158. https://doi.org/10.1097/NCM.0000000000000095.

Developmentally Disabled Assistance and Bill of Rights Act. (1975). *S. 462 (94th).* https://www.govtrack.us/congress/bills/94/s462.

Edington, D. W., Schultz, A. B., & Pitts, J. S. (2016). The future of population health at the workplace: Trends, technology, and the role of mind-body and behavioral science. In D. B. Nash, R. J. Fabius, A. Skoufalos, J. L. Clarke, & M. R. Horowitz (Eds.), *Population health: Creating a culture of wellness* (2nd ed., Chapter 20). Jones and Bartlett Learning.

Eghaneyan, B. H., Sanchez, K., & Mitschke, D. B. (2014). Implementation of a collaborative care model for the treatment of depression and anxiety in a community health center: Results from a qualitative case study. *Journal of Multidisciplinary Healthcare, 7*, 503–513. https://doi.org/10.2147/JMDH.S69821.

Ellsworth, J. (2015). Case managers: A key to reducing admissions. *Professional Case Management, 20*(3), 147–149.

Epstein Becker Green. (2015). *The challenges and rewards of integrating behavioral health into primary care.* Webinar. https://www.ebglaw.com/events/the-challenges-and-rewards-of-integrating-behavioral-health-into-primary-care-%e2%80%93-thought-leaders-in-population-health-webinar-series/.

Fink-Samnick, E. (2019). *The Essential Guide to Interprofessional Ethics for Healthcare Case Management*: HCPro.

Fink-Samnick, E. (2019). *The Social Determinants of Health: Case Management's Next Frontier* (1st ed): HCPro.

Fink-Samnick, E., & Muller, L. (2015). Case management practice: Is technology helping or hindering practice in legal and regulatory issues. *Professional Case Management, 20*(2), 98–102.

Forbes, M. A. (1999). The practice of professional nurse case management. *Nursing Case Management, 4*(1), 28–33.

Fortney J., Sladek R., Unützer J., Alfred L., Carneal G., Emmet B., et al. (2015). *Fixing behavioral health care in*

America: A national call for integrating and coordinating specialty behavioral health care with the medical system. The Kennedy Forum in Partnership with Advancing Integrated Mental Health Solutions (AIMS) Center, The Kennedy Center for Mental Health Policy and Research, Satcher Health Leadership Institute, Morehouse School of Medicine. Issue Brief. http://www.thekennedyforum.com.

Gartner, Inc. (2016). Predictive modeling. http://www.gartner.com/it-glossary/predictive-modeling/.

Gillespie, L. (2016). *Hospitals push Medicare to soften readmission penalties in light of socioeconomic risks.* Modern Healthcare. http://www.modernhealthcare.com/article/20160521/MAGAZINE/305219914.

Goodman, R. A., Bunnell, R., & Posner, S. F. (2014). What is "community health"? Examining the meaning of an evolving field in public health. *Preventive Medicine, 67*(Supp. 1), S58–S61. https://doi.org/10.1016/j.ypmed.2014.07.028 https://doi.org/.

Graf, T., Erskine, A., & Steele, G. D. (2014). Leveraging data to systematically improve care coronary artery disease management at Geisinger. *Journal of Ambulatory Care Management, 37*(3), 199–205.

Gupta, A. (2015). *Tech is driving collaboration in behavioral health.* TechCrunch. http://techcrunch.com/2015/09/19/tech-is-driving-collaboration-in-behavioral-health/.

Hawkins, K., Wells, T. S., Hommer, C. E., Ozminkowski, R. J., Richards, D. M., & Yeh, C. S. (2014). Factors driving engagement decisions in care coordination programs. *Professional Case Management, 19*(5), 216–223.

Health Enhancement Research Organization (HERO) and Population Health Alliance (PHA). (2015). *Program measurement & evaluation guide: Core metrics for employee health management.* https://populationhealthalliance.org/wp-content/uploads/2018/02/pha-hero-overview-handout_v4.pdf.

HealthCare.gov. (n.d.). *Chronic disease management.* https://www.healthcare.gov/glossary/chronic-disease-management/.

Health Sciences Institute. (2016). *Chronic care professional (CCP) certification.* http://healthsciences.org/Chronic-Care-Professional-Certification.

HealthyPeople.gov (2019a). *Approach to the social determinants.* https://www.healthypeople.gov/2020/topics-objectives/topic-social-determinants-of-health.

HealthyPeople.gov. (2019b). *About healthy people.* https://www.healthypeople.gov/2020/About-Healthy-People.

Herman, C. (2013). *The evolving context of social work case management: NASW releases revised standards of practice, practice perspective.* National Association of Social Workers.

Hickam D. H., Weiss J. W., Guise J-M., Buckley D., Motu'apuaka M., Graham E., et al. (2013). *Outpatient case management for adults with medical illness and complex care needs.* Comparative Effectiveness Review No. 99. (Prepared by the Oregon Evidence based Practice Center under Contract No. 290-2007-10057-I.) AHRQ Publication No.13-EHC031-EF. Rockville, MD: Agency for Healthcare Research and Quality. http://effectivehealthcare.ahrq.gov/index.cfm/search-for-guides-reviews-and-reports/?pageaction=displayproduct&productid=1369.

Hu, J., Gonsahn, M. D., & Nerenz, D. R. (2014). Socioeconomic status and readmissions: Evidence from an urban teaching hospital. *Health Affairs, 33*(5), 778–785. https://doi.org/10.1377/hlthaff.2013.0816 https://doi.org/.

Huber, D. L. (2005). The diversity of service delivery models. In D. Huber (Ed.), *Disease management: A guide for case managers* (pp. 55–67). Saunders.

Huber, D.L. (2017). *Care for the total population.* Iowa City, IA.

Improving Chronic Illness Care. (2006–2019). *The chronic care model.* http://www.improvingchroniccare.org/index.php?p=The_Chronic_CareModel&s=2.

Institute for Healthcare Improvement (IHI). (2017). *Triple aim for populations.* http://www.ihi.org/Topics/TripleAim/Pages/default.aspx.

Institute of Medicine (IOM). (2001). *Crossing the quality chasm: A new health system for the 21st century*: National Academies Press.

Interprofessional Education Collaborative (IPEC). (2016). *Core competencies for interprofessional collaborative practice: 2016 update.*

Kolbasovsky, A., Zeitlin, J., & Gillespie, W. (2012). Impact of point-of-care case management on readmissions and costs. *The American Journal of Managed Care, 18*(8), 300–306.

Kongstvedt, P. R. (2013). *Essentials of managed health care* (6th ed.). Jones and Bartlett.

Lee, J. (2016). Behavioral economics: How BE influences and changes health. In D. B. Nash, R. J. Fabius, A. Skoufalos, J. L. Clarke, & M. R. Horowitz (Eds.), *Population health: Creating a culture of wellness* (2nd ed., Chapter 8). Jones and Bartlett Learning.

Library of Congress (1975). *Education for all handicapped children act.* https://www.govtrack.us/congress/bills/94/s6/summary.

Lyles, C. A. (2016). The political landscape in relation to the health and wealth of nations. In D. B. Nash, R. J. Fabius, A. Skoufalos, J. L. Clarke, & M. R. Horowitz (Eds.), *Population health: Creating a culture of wellness* (2nd ed., Chapter 5). Jones and Bartlett Learning.

Milliman, Inc. (2014). *Economic impact of integrated medical-behavioral healthcare: Implications for psychiatry.* Milliman American Psychiatric Association Report. Denver, CO.

Nagasako, E., Waterman, B., & Dunagan, W. C. (2014). Adding socioeconomic data to hospital readmissions calculations may produce more useful results. *Health Affairs, 33*(5), 786–791. https://doi.org/10.1377/hlthaff.2013.1148.

Nash, D., Fabius, R. J., Skoufalos, A., Clarke, J. L., & Horowitz, M. R. (2016). *Preface. Population health: Creating a culture of wellness* (2nd ed.). Jones and Bartlett Learning.

National Association of Social Workers (NASW). (2013). *Standards for social work case management.*

National Association of Chronic Disease Directors (NACDD). (2016). *About NACDD.* http://www.chronicdisease.org/?page=AboutUs.

National Health Council (2014) About Chronic Diseases.

National Committee for Quality Assurance (NCQA). (2019). *About NCQA.* https://www.ncqa.org/about-ncqa/.

National Council of State Boards of Nursing (NCSBN). (2016a). *The nurse licensure compact: An overview.* https://www.ncsbn.org/9331.htm.

National Council of State Boards of Nursing (NCSBN). (2016b). *Nurse licensure compact.* https://www.ncsbn.org/nurse-licensure-compact.htm.

Older Americans Act. (1965). *42 U.S.C. 3056.* http://www.gpo.gov/fdsys/pkg/STATUTE-79/pdf/STATUTE-79-Pg218.pdf.

Patient Care and Affordable Care Act. (2010). *Public Law 111–148.* http://housedocs.house.gov/energycommerce/ppacacon.pdf.

Plocher, D. W. (2013). Fundamentals and core competencies of disease management. In P. R. Kongstvedt (Ed.), *Essentials of managed health care* (6th ed., Chapter 8). Jones and Bartlett.

Population Health Alliance (PHA). (2015). *2015 Population health alliance outcomes guidelines report.*

Population Health Alliance. (n.d.). *PHM-defined.* https://populationhealthalliance.org/research/understanding-population-health/.

Prochaska, J. O., & Prochaska, J. M. (2016). *Behavior change, population health: Creating a culture of wellness* (2nd ed.). Jones and Bartlett Learning.

Rice, S. (2016). Adjusting for social determinants in value-based payments still fuzzy. *Modern Healthcare.* http://www.modernhealthcare.com/article/20160112/NEWS/160119972.

Robert Wood Johnson Foundation. (2011). *Mental disorders and medical co-morbidity, research synthesis.* Report 21.

Rushton, S. (2015). The population care coordination process. *Professional Case Management, 20*(5), 230–238.

SAS. (2016). *What is Big Data?* http://www.sas.com/en_us/insights/big-data.html.

Shaljian, M., & Nielsen, M. (2013). *Managing populations, maximizing technology: Population health management in the medical neighborhood.* Patient-Centered Primary Care Collaborative.

Sidorov, J., & Romney, M. (2016). The spectrum of care. In D. B. Nash, R. J. Fabius, A. Skoufalos, J. L. Clarke, & M. R. Horowitz (Eds.), *Population health: Creating a culture of wellness* (2nd ed., Chapter 2). Jones and Bartlett Learning.

Social Security Act of 1935. (2013). *Legislative history.* http://www.ssa.gov/history/35act.html.

Stellefson, M., Dipnarine, K., & Stopka, C. (2013). The chronic care model and diabetes management in US primary care settings: A systematic review. *Preventing Chronic Disease, 10*, 1–21. https://doi.org/10.5888/pcd10.120180 https://doi.org/.

Summers, N. (2016). *Fundamentals of case management practice: Skills for the human services* (5th ed.). Cengage Learning.

Tahan, H. A. (2017). The case management process. In H. A. Tahan, & T. M. Treiger (Eds.), *CMSA core curriculum for case management* (3rd ed.). Wolters Kluwer.

Takeda, A., Taylor, S. J. C., Taylor, R. S., Kahn, F., Krum, H., & Underwood, M. (2012). Clinical service organisation for heart failure. *Cochrane Database of Systematic Reviews,* (9), CD002752. https://doi.org/10.1002/14651858.CD002752.pub3.

The Joint Commission (TJC). (2019). *Certifications by health care setting.* https://www.jointcommission.org/accreditation-and-certification/certification/certifications-by-setting/.

Treiger, T. M. (2011). Case management: Prospects in definition, education, and settings of practice. *The Remington Report, 19*(1), 46–48.

Treiger, T. M. (2012). Helping clients bridge gaps to self-advocacy, self-management. *Healthcare Intelligence Network.* [interview] http://hin.com/blog/2012/09/14/meet-healthcare-case-management-manager-teresa-treiger-helping-clients-bridge-gaps-to-self-advocacy-self-management.

Treiger, T. M., & Fink-Samnick, E. (2013). COLLABORATE: A universal competency based paradigm for professional case management, part I: Introduction, historical validation, and competency presentation. *Professional Case Management, 18*(3), 122–135.

Treiger, T. M., & Fink-Samnick, E. (2016). *COLLABORATE for professional case management: A universal competency-based paradigm*: Wolters Kluwer.

Unützer, J., Harbin, H., Schoenbaum, M., & Druss, B. (2013). *The collaborative care model: An approach to integrating physical and mental health care in Medicaid health homesCenter for Health Care Strategies and Mathematica Policy Research*: Centers for Medicare and Medicaid Services. CMS.

Walters, B. H., Adams, S. A., Nieboer, A. P., & Bal, R. (2012). Disease management projects and the Chronic Care Model in action: Baseline qualitative research. *BMC Health Services Research, 12*(1), 114. https://doi.org/10.1186/1472-6963-12-114.

Ward, B. W., Schiller, J. S., & Goodman, R. A. (2013). Multiple chronic conditions among US adults: A 2012 update. *Preventing Chronic Disease, 11*, E62.

Watson, A. (2016). Evaluating and measuring quality and outcomes: A new "essential activity" of case management practice. *Professional Case Management, 21*(1), 51–52.

Weil, M., & Karls, J. M. (1985). *Case management in human service practice: A systematic approach to mobilizing resources for clients*. Jossey-Bass.

World Health Organization (WHO). (2019). *About social determinants of health*. Retrieved from https://www.who.int/social_determinants/sdh_definition/en/.

Young, B., Clark, C., Kansky, J., & Pupo, E. (2014). *Health information exchange committee ambulatory toolkit*. Chicago, IL: Health Information Management and Systems Society (HIMSS).

17

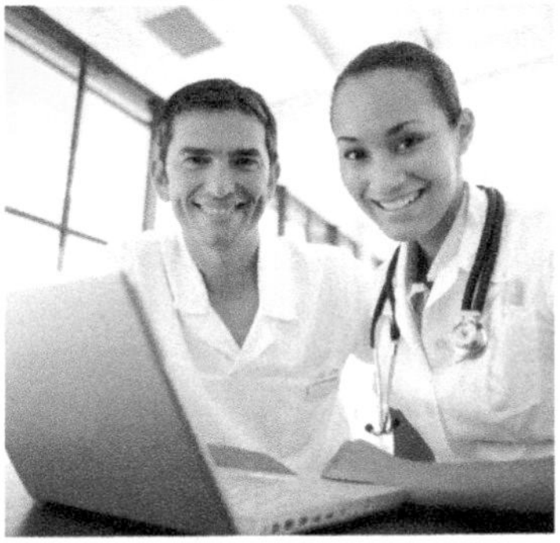

Nursing Leadership for Evidence-Based Practice

Laura Cullen, Kirsten Hanrahan, Erin M. Steffen, Michele Farrington, Cindy J. Dawson

http://evolve.elsevier.com/Huber/leadership

Nurse leaders have responsibility for building and expanding use of evidence-based practice (EBP) in care delivery to improve patient and organizational outcomes (Bunger et al., 2019; Gifford et al., 2018; Melnyk et al., 2016; Stetler et al., 2014). A number of models are available to provide direction for the EBP process. Implementing EBP changes as an organization and unit or clinic requires additional strategies for success. A growing body of research is available to build EBP programs within health care organizations and close the research-to-practice gap (Borsky et al., 2018). Application of EBP is the responsibility of every nursing leader, especially those in the nurse manager role. This chapter outlines the ways nurse leaders can grow the EBP culture in an organization and tactics to create a nurturing climate in the practice setting.

Processes to improve care include quality or performance improvement, EBP, and conduct of research. The best process to use depends on the question at hand, the intent (i.e., knowledge generation or local improvement), and the extent of research and other evidence available on the topic. For questions best addressed through quality improvement (e.g., efficient throughput), improvements may be brought directly to practice. EBP offers the benefit of using existing evidence for designing effective interventions, adapting them for local adoption, planning implementation, and guidance for avoiding unintended consequences. Clinical questions with little or no research that may include patient risk may be appropriate to answer by conducting research.

DEFINITIONS

An understanding of EBP and related concepts requires knowledge of a variety of terms. **Evidence-based practice** (EBP) is a process of shared decision-making in a partnership between patients and clinicians that involves the integration of research and other best evidence with clinical expertise and patient values and preferences in making shared health care decisions (Sackett et al., 2000; Sigma Theta Tau International Research Scholarship Advisory Committee, 2008). EBP is a scholarly process for improving health care quality and safety by building on what is learned from—and also influencing— the conduct of research and quality improvement.

Additional terms are also important to understand. **Knowledge translation** is defined as the process of putting scientific knowledge into practice (Harrison et al., 2013; Straus et al., 2011) and is synonymous with EBP in some regions across the globe. **Best practice** is a popular term, but the definition remains elusive. Use of the term may describe innovative practices that are recognized by peer organizations and that contribute to quality or fiscal goals. Although "best practice," "best evidence," and "evidence-based practice" are sometimes used interchangeably, the extent that "best practices" are based on "best evidence" is often unclear. To promote understanding, it is recommended that when using scientific evidence for guidance, the term evidence-based practice provides the most clarity.

Evidence-based interventions (EBI) are treatments that are supported by empirical evidence from research. EBI are expected to improve outcomes; if not, failure may be related to design of the practice change, related to a poor fit within the local context, not staying true to the treatment procedure (fidelity), or failed implementation.

A **clinical practice guideline** is a report designed to assist clinicians and clients in making decisions about appropriate health care for specific clinical circumstances (Institute of Medicine, 2011). Guidelines are systematically developed, link evidence with health outcomes (benefits and harms), and continue to require subjective judgments and local adaption to apply to patient care. Guidelines are developed with the intent to influence clinician behavior by making clear practice recommendations.

Implementation is the process of putting an idea or process change into practice. The implementation process uses strategies to promote adoption of EBP in a specific setting to improve outcomes (Brownson et al., 2018a). Integration involves the infusion of an innovation until that change is a practice routine. Implementation strategies are tactics used to impact the rate of integration into practice to achieve adoption and sustainability. Strategies that are data driven and evidence based are more likely to result in a sustainable practice change. A Precision Implementation Approach™ uses local data to drive selection of strategies for the most effective and efficient implementation, integration, and sustainability (Cullen et al., 2019b). After initial pilot implementation and evaluation, the boost used to promote integration of EBP is called **reinfusion**.

Implementation science is the "study of methods to promote the adoption and integration of evidence-based practices, interventions and policies, into routine health care and public health settings" (NIH, 2019), and offers great opportunity to learn effective strategies to promote EBP as the standard for health care delivery. Implementation research identifies enablers and barriers to effective health programming and policymaking (NIH, 2019), creating new knowledge that can be leveraged in the application of EBP.

Translation science may be a more confusing term, as it can be defined two ways (Rubio et al., 2010). First, to describe the process of moving knowledge from bench research to patient care (Titler, 2018), translational science is also defined as "the field of investigation focused on understanding the scientific and operational principles underlying each step of the translational process" (Institute of Translational Health Sciences, 2019a). The translation process, as defined by the Institute of Translational Health Sciences (ITHS), includes five interactive nonlinear phases (T_0–T_4):

> "T_0 is characterized by the identification of opportunities and approaches to health problems. T1 seeks to move basic discovery into a candidate health application. T2 assesses the value of application for health practice leading to the development of evidence-based guidelines. T3 attempts to move evidence-based guidelines into health care, through delivery, dissemination, and diffusion research. T4 seeks to evaluate the 'real world' health outcomes of population health practice" (Institute of Translational Health Sciences, 2019b).

The second definition is consistent with implementation science, testing the effect of interventions that promote the rate and extent of adoption of EBP by nurses, physicians, and other health care providers and describing organizational, unit, and individual variables that affect the use of evidence in clinical and operational decision-making (Institute of Translational Health Sciences, 2019a; Titler, 2018). Translational research provides guidance about what strategies are effective, for whom, and in what setting when implementing EBP. In this sense, *the term translational research* is often used interchangeably with implementation science. **Sustainment**, the goal of EBP implementation, is the long-term use of the practice recommendation and indicates the EBI has been hardwired as the new standard (Ament et al., 2015; NHS Institute for Innovation and Improvement, 2010). A comprehensive definition of **sustainability** encompasses five components: (1) the EBI or program, (2) that maintains a change in individual behavior, (3) over a defined time period, (4) in which the EBI may evolve or be adapted, but (5) continues to produce the expected benefits (Moore et al., 2017). Additional roll-out or **scaling up** is the systematic process used to expand the reach of effective clinical interventions in one setting to other similar areas or populations; whereas, **scaling out** refers to when EBIs are adapted either to new populations or new delivery systems, or both (Aarons et al., 2017).

In contrast to EBP are **sacred cows**, old practice habits considered routine, above dispute, and particularly resistant to change (Hanrahan et al., 2015). **De-implementation** or de-adoption is needed to reverse, stop, undo, or remove current practices that are not evidence-based, do not improve care, are ineffective, or may be harmful (Helfrich et al., 2018; Patey et al., 2018; Wang et al., 2018). Strategies needed for de-implementation may be different from implementation strategies; theories and research are just emerging.

Organizational context refers to the health system environment in which the proposed EBP is to be implemented. Six contextual features synergistically influence EBP implementation within an organization: (1) organizational culture (e.g., patient centered, innovative), (2) networks and communications (e.g., collaborations and teamwork), (3) leadership (e.g., transformational leadership that gives rise to clear role delineation and teamwork), (4) resources (including financial, staffing, time, and training), (5) evaluation, monitoring, and feedback (e.g., soliciting feedback and ongoing communication with point-of-care clinicians), and (6) champions (i.e., individuals with key attributes including EBP expertise, peer influence, and ability to troubleshoot) (Li et al., 2018).

BACKGROUND MODELS

A variety of knowledge translation theories, models, and frameworks exist to guide both application in practice (EBP) and implementation science (research) (Strifler et al., 2018). Nilsen (2015) described three overarching theoretical approaches in implementation science that aim to (1) describe or guide the EBP process (process models), (2) understand the determinants influencing implementation outcomes (determinant frameworks, classic theories, and implementation theories), and (3) evaluate implementation (evaluation frameworks) (Table 17.1). Process models give step-by-step guidance for planning and executing change. EBP process models may be best suited for guiding the team through organizational change. These models

TABLE 17.1 Select Evidence-Based Practice Models: Implementation Science Theories, Models, and Frameworks

Type	Examples	Citation	Sample of application
EBP Process Models	ACE Star Model of Knowledge Transformation	Stevens (2013)	Farra et al. (2015)
	Advancing Research and Clinical Practice Through Close Collaboration (ARCC) Model	Melnyk et al. (2017)	Little et al. (2017)
	Iowa Model Revised: Evidence-Based Practice to Promote Excellence in Health Care	Iowa Model Collaborative (2017)	Huether et al. (2016)
	Johns Hopkins Nursing Evidence-Based Practice (JHNEBP) Model	Dang & Dearholt (2017)	Pittman et al. (2019)
	Knowledge-to-Action Model (K2A)	Morton et al. (2018)	
	Stetler Model	Stetler (2001)	Stetler et al. (2014)
Determinant Frameworks	EBP Implementation Guide	Cullen & Adams (2012)	Abbott & Hooke (2017)
	Consolidated Framework for Implementation Research (CFIR)	Damschroder & Hagedorn (2011)	Damschroder & Lowery (2013)
	Promoting Action on Research Implementation in Health Services (PARIHS) Framework	Harvey & Kitson (2015)	Lewis et al. (2019)
Classic Theories	Diffusion of Innovation	Rogers (2003)	Zhao et al. (2018)
	Social Learning Theory	Bandura (1977)	Ishikawa et al. (2019)
Implementation Theories	Normalization Process Theory	May et al. (2009)	Mishuris et al. (2019)
	Capabilities, Opportunities, Motivations and Behaviour (COM-B) model	Michie et al. (2014)	Muhwava et al. (2019)

have been used successfully to improve adoption of EBP recommendations and improve patient and health care outcomes (Gawlinski & Rutledge, 2008; Strifler et al., 2018). For example, the *Iowa Model-Revised: Evidence-Based Practice to Promote Excellence in Health Care* (Iowa Model Collaborative, 2017) reflects the current environment in health care and uses implementation science to guide clinician decision-making in a variety of health care settings (Coleman et al., 2018; Huether et al., 2016). Additional details and comparisons of theories, models, and frameworks are summarized elsewhere (Camargo et al., 2017; Cullen et al., 2019a; Dang et al., 2019; Davis et al., 2015; Nilsen, 2015; Schaffer et al., 2013; Strifler et al., 2018).

The challenge for leaders is to identify a model that guides the EBP process and promotes successful adoption of EBP (Dang et al., 2019; Gawlinski & Rutledge, 2008). Adoption of one EBP model across an organization for interprofessional initiatives (Abbott & Hooke, 2017; Cullen et al., 2018a; Hanrahan et al., 2015; Huether et al., 2016) is one strategy for promoting continuous learning and coordination of efforts across a system. EBP models tend to follow a basic problem-solving process with step-by-step guidance, just as do some other quality improvement processes (e.g., Six Sigma). Senior leadership support for EBP can be leveraged by outlining the similarities between EBP and quality improvement processes, structures, and resources for comprehensive improvement in clinical and organizational outcomes (Djulbegovic et al., 2019; Mondoux & Shojania, 2019).

Determinant frameworks identify multi-level facilitators and barriers that influence implementation outcomes and are often linked to classic theories drawn from psychology, sociology, and organizational theory. For example, Cullen and Adams Implementation Strategies for EBP guide (Cullen & Adams, 2012), based on Rogers' Diffusion of Innovations Theory (Rogers, 2003) identifies strategies for clinicians and organizations across four phases of implementation (Fig. 17.1). A multitude of implementation theories and evaluation frameworks have been used to guide research, but most may lack the step-by-step guidance that clinicians need to achieve sustainability (Strifler et al., 2018).

STEPS FOR PERFORMING EVIDENCE-BASED PRACTICE

Nurses across the career continuum can learn and practice the basic steps for EBP. It begins with a question that arises out of practice (QSEN Institute, 2019). Formulate a purpose statement or clinical question by using the PICOT elements: P (patient population, problem, patient perspective, and pilot area), I (intervention), C (comparison), O (outcome desired). Including T is a variation some find helpful (T = time or anticipated completion date). Consider each of these elements in detail. Next, appropriate resources to search for evidence are determined and a search strategy developed. There are many bibliographic databases to use such as PubMed, MEDLINE, CINAHL, OVID, and the Cochrane Database of Systematic Reviews. Use keywords or Medical Subject Heading (MeSH) headings from the purpose statement to help focus the search. A librarian can be very helpful at this stage. If a librarian is not available, database websites often offer user-training modules. Once the search is conducted, there is a need to evaluate the yield from the search for further refinement, such as expanding or narrowing keywords.

Nurses need to have confidence in the evidence used for making decisions about practice. The search methodology that yields the best evidence changes as a clinical issue is analyzed. A focus on randomized controlled trials (RCT) and systematic reviews or meta-analysis for the most desirable study designs is often too limited. Instead, use a systematic process to evaluate the body of evidence in a stepwise manner, and consider appropriate research designs (Cullen et al., 2019a) as follows:

1. Prevalence of the issue—expect descriptive or cohort studies;
2. Risk or risk factors associated with this issue—look for descriptive or cohort studies;
3. Patients and caregiver perspectives, preferences, and values—likely reported in qualitative studies;
4. Assessment for accurate diagnosis—look for psychometric and descriptive studies;
5. Effective interventions—usually experimental and possibly RCT studies. Also consider synthesis reports such as clinical practice guidelines and systematic reviews;
6. Unintended consequences—often missed in RCT studies, look for these in descriptive and qualitative studies.

Implementation Strategies for Evidence-Based Practice

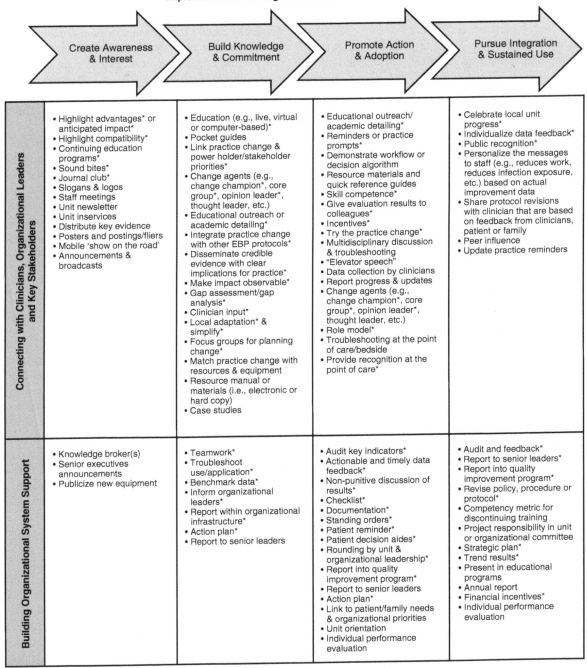

	Create Awareness & Interest	Build Knowledge & Commitment	Promote Action & Adoption	Pursue Integration & Sustained Use
Connecting with Clinicians, Organizational Leaders and Key Stakeholders	• Highlight advantages* or anticipated impact* • Highlight compatibility* • Continuing education programs* • Sound bites* • Journal club* • Slogans & logos • Staff meetings • Unit newsletter • Unit inservices • Distribute key evidence • Posters and postings/fliers • Mobile 'show on the road' • Announcements & broadcasts	• Education (e.g., live, virtual or computer-based)* • Pocket guides • Link practice change & power holder/stakeholder priorities* • Change agents (e.g., change champion*, core group*, opinion leader*, thought leader, etc.) • Educational outreach or academic detailing* • Integrate practice change with other EBP protocols* • Disseminate credible evidence with clear implications for practice* • Make impact observable* • Gap assessment/gap analysis* • Clinician input* • Local adaptation* & simplify* • Focus groups for planning change* • Match practice change with resources & equipment • Resource manual or materials (i.e., electronic or hard copy) • Case studies	• Educational outreach/ academic detailing* • Reminders or practice prompts* • Demonstrate workflow or decision algorithm • Resource materials and quick reference guides • Skill competence* • Give evaluation results to colleagues* • Incentives* • Try the practice change* • Multidisciplinary discussion & troubleshooting • "Elevator speech" • Data collection by clinicians • Report progress & updates • Change agents (e.g., change champion*, core group*, opinion leader*, thought leader, etc.) • Role model* • Troubleshooting at the point of care/bedside • Provide recognition at the point of care*	• Celebrate local unit progress* • Individualize data feedback* • Public recognition* • Personalize the messages to staff (e.g., reduces work, reduces infection exposure, etc.) based on actual improvement data • Share protocol revisions with clinician that are based on feedback from clinicians, patient or family • Peer influence • Update practice reminders
Building Organizational System Support	• Knowledge broker(s) • Senior executives announcements • Publicize new equipment	• Teamwork* • Troubleshoot use/application* • Benchmark data* • Inform organizational leaders* • Report within organizational infrastructure* • Action plan* • Report to senior leaders	• Audit key indicators* • Actionable and timely data feedback* • Non-punitive discussion of results* • Checklist* • Documentation* • Standing orders* • Patient reminder* • Patient decision aides* • Rounding by unit & organizational leadership* • Report into quality improvement program* • Report to senior leaders • Action plan* • Link to patient/family needs & organizational priorities • Unit orientation • Individual performance evaluation	• Audit and feedback* • Report to senior leaders* • Report into quality improvement program* • Revise policy, procedure or protocol* • Competency metric for discontinuing training • Project responsibility in unit or organizational committee • Strategic plan* • Trend results* • Present in educational programs • Annual report • Financial incentives* • Individual performance evaluation

*Implementation strategy is supported by at least some empirical evidence in health care.

Fig. 17.1 Evidence-based practice implementation guide. (Reproduced with permission from Laura Cullen, DNP, RN, FAAN, and the University of Iowa Hospitals and Clinics. From Cullen, L., & Adams, S. [2012]. Planning for implementation of evidence-based practice. Journal of Nursing Administration, 42[4], 222–230.)

Depending on the desired outcome and the situation, a search for documents from relevant professional organizations may be important.

Use the evidence to design the practice change and evaluation plan (Cullen et al., 2018b). When designing the EBI use the evidence to identify the core elements essential for achieving the desired outcome. Match the practice to patient preferences, values, and needs. Consider interprofessional perspectives, being broadly inclusive, to create a good fit for the local setting. Create a clear procedure, with specific inclusion and exclusion criteria, and decision points. Supporting documents—policies and algorithms—can be useful to promote adoption.

IMPLEMENTING AND SUSTAINING EVIDENCE-BASED PRACTICE CHANGES

Implementation of EBP changes can be challenging in complex health care settings. Baseline evaluation occurs before implementation so that baseline data can incorporate the evidence and locally adapted EBI can be used for implementation planning. Following a *Precision Implementation Approach*™ (Cullen et al., 2019b) leaders used baseline data to select implementation strategies matching local needs. For example, informational and educational strategies can focus specifically on a local clinician's knowledge gap. This avoids using resources on education where knowledge already exists. Likewise, implementation strategies can be selected to target local patient and clinician perceptions and behaviors. Data on outcomes and unintended consequences (balancing measures) can be used during implementation to identify if a midstream correction is warranted or if efforts can move toward integration and sustained use.

Strategies for implementing EBPs occur at the unit or clinic level (Moreno-Poyato et al., 2019), and also at the organizational/systems level (Hanrahan et al., 2015; Li et al., 2018; Sarkies et al., 2017; Stetler et al., 2014), as illustrated in the exemplar in the following section. A large variety of implementation strategies support adoption of EBP and need to target clinicians, patients, and the health care system (Cullen & Adams, 2012; Lewis et al., 2018; Perry et al., 2019; Powell et al., 2015; Rogers, 2003).

The Diffusion of Innovation Theory (Rogers, 2003) provides a well-recognized model with strong research support guiding the hard work of implementation (Davis et al., 2015; Goldstein & Olswang, 2017; Greenhalgh, 2018; Mohammadi et al., 2018). The *Implementation Strategies for Evidence-Based Practice* guide (see Fig. 17.1) was developed based on Rogers' Innovation-Decision Process Model to assist nurse leaders with planning for use of effective implementation strategies through a process of active diffusion: creating awareness and interest; building knowledge and commitment; promoting action and adoption; and pursuing integration and sustained use (Cullen & Adams, 2012).

Multiple interactive and reinforcing strategies, as outlined, promote adoption of EBP recommendations (Cullen & Adams, 2012; Cullen et al., 2018b; Mohammadi et al., 2018). Strategies to capture a busy clinician's attention are important to include early in the implementation. Nurse leaders can identify additional strategies when working across phases (Bunger et al., 2019). Strategies are added to create a cumulative and comprehensive implementation plan to garner momentum before, during, and after starting an EBP pilot change. The *Implementation Strategies for EBP* guide is a planning tool to be used in combination with an EBP process model (Cullen et al., 2018b).

Early in the EBP process, a fluid action plan is useful to keep the team on task and collectively moving forward (Gude et al., 2019). Implementation and creating sustainability are two of the most difficult steps in the EBP process. Common strategies used for sustaining EBP include adapting the practice recommendation, trending evaluative data, ongoing training, having champions and leaders across all levels, aligning project work with organizational priorities, having sufficient resources allocated, and communicating and partnering with stakeholders (Cullen et al., 2020; Li et al., 2018; Seneski & Stack, 2019; Valim et al., 2019).

Audit and feedback of key indicators remains a necessary component of an integration plan (Li et al., 2018). Key indicators to monitor are drawn from the pilot data and include process (i.e., knowledge, attitudes, and behaviors) and outcomes, including unintended consequences (Cullen et al., 2019b; Norton et al., 2016; Parry et al., 2018). Integration also requires linkages across the governance structure (Cullen et al., 2017, 2020). An important strategy is to link within the quality improvement infrastructure (Fleiszer et al., 2016; Harvey et al., 2019; Norton et al., 2016; Seneski & Stack, 2019) to promote essential influence needed from senior leaders (Li et al., 2018; Taylor et al., 2015).

Change can only be complete and sustained using a combination of implementation strategies (Cullen et al., 2018b; Hanrahan et al., 2015; Seneski & Stack, 2019; Staines et al., 2018; Valim et al., 2019). These principles are highlighted in the following EBP exemplar.

AN EVIDENCE-BASED PRACTICE EXEMPLAR

Title

Strategies for Reducing Reliance on Agency Nursing Staff Equate to $7.7 Million in Savings.

Purpose, Rationale, and Framework

The purpose of this strategic effort was to recruit and hire permanent nursing staff in fiscal year 18 in order to reduce the number of agency nursing staff and trim overall costs (Farrington et al., 2020). Faced with a 12% vacancy rate, a large academic health system opted to hire 224 full-time equivalent (FTE) agency nursing staff to fill the existing gaps while opening a new children's hospital and expanding adult inpatient bed capacity. Although this strategy helped to fill the short-term need, the expense was massive. At the time, the hourly rate the hospital paid for agency nursing staff ranged from $69 to $110, based on specialty. The organization's nursing team rallied to come up with innovative and creative solutions to reduce agency nursing staff to less than 75 FTEs, a two-thirds reduction, in just 6 months. The Iowa Model (Iowa Model Collaborative, 2017) provided the project framework.

Synthesis of Evidence

The ongoing nursing shortage, increasing vacancy rates, and need for expansion are a few challenges facing health care organizations today (Halter et al., 2017). To combat these challenges, hospitals often turn to agency nursing staff to fill the gaps (Warren et al., 2016; Xue et al., 2015). Competition between the public and private sectors to recruit and retain the same nurses forces employers to implement incentives such as higher pay, better benefits, and signing bonuses (Willis et al., 2016). Vacancy rates and replacing nurses place a financial burden on an organization and the health care industry (Huddleston & Gray, 2016b; Warren et al., 2016).

In May 2018 the median annual salary for a nurse in the United States was $71,730 (US Bureau of Labor Statistics, 2019). Using this number, combined with reports of turnover costs being 0.75 to 2 times the annual salary of a nurse, equates to a turnover cost between $53,798 and $143,460 per nurse. At the same time, lower nurse vacancy rates benefit health care consumers through improved patient outcomes and quality of care (Connor et al., 2018; Ducharme et al., 2017; Hairr et al., 2014; Kalisch & Lee, 2014; Martin, 2015). The conditions in which nurses work are critical, as shown by higher nurse retention occurring in "healthy work environments" (American Association of Critical-Care Nurses, 2005). Establishing and maintaining a healthy work environment requires organizations to make strategic investments aimed at improving care delivery, patient satisfaction, clinician satisfaction, patient safety/outcomes, and the culture of nursing practice (Ducharme et al., 2017; Huddleston & Gray, 2016a, 2016b; Huddleston et al., 2017).

There is currently no consistent strategy regarding how best to drive recruitment and retention (Gorman, 2019). A creative and comprehensive approach to recruitment and retention must be deployed at the organizational level and tailored to the unit or clinic.

Practice Change

A four-pronged recruitment approach was used. Focus was first placed on partnering with marketing and communications to improve the social media presence, next was website optimization, third hosting recruitment fairs with onsite interviews, and fourth considered the transition for nurses new to the organization. Since 2009 the organization has provided a nurse residency program (NRP), first accredited in 2012, to smooth the transition from school to hospital-based nursing practice (Hosking et al., 2016). Yet even the most experienced nurses may encounter stress and undergo a difficult professional transition to a new role. The Experienced Nurse Fellowship (ENF) program started in 2015 to support the transition of experienced nurses into new practice environments, increase job satisfaction, and reduce nursing turnover, all designed to positively impact patient outcomes. Advertising the availability of these programs for transitioning nurses, along with spotlighting the organization's Magnet® status as part of the recruitment efforts was critical.

New retention strategies focused on enhanced benefits for current and incoming permanent nursing staff including increased annual inpatient differential from $1000 to $2500; initiating reimbursement for moving expenses; creating a referral incentive for current nurses who recruited experienced nurses into the organization; and introduction of preceptor pay to recognize the time experienced nurses invested in training the incoming nurses.

Implementation Strategies

A comprehensive, phased approach to implementation (Cullen & Adams, 2012) was used as part of this initiative. Creating awareness and interest to get the attention of busy clinicians was accomplished by highlighting the advantages and compatibility; sharing the new initiatives at staff meetings, unit in-services, and in-unit newsletters; displaying posters and postings/fliers; and utilizing announcements and broadcasts by senior executives. Preparing clinicians for the change was critical to build knowledge and commitment. Implementation strategies in this phase included education, change agents, making the impact observable, gap assessment/gap analysis, clinician input, focus groups for planning change, teamwork, and reporting within the organizational infrastructure. Actual behavior change occurred during phase three as part of promoting action and adoption during the "go live" timeframes. Action and adoption strategies included reminders or practice prompts, resource materials and quick reference guides, reporting progress and updates, change agents, actionable and timely data feedback, reporting to senior leaders, and linking to patient/family needs and organizational priorities. In order to hardwire the process, the final stage of pursuing integration and sustained use involved celebrating local unit progress, individualizing data feedback, public recognition, personalizing the messages to staff based on actual improvement data, continuing to audit and provide feedback, reporting to senior leaders, trending results, and presenting in educational programs. The multifaceted content and messaging were widely disseminated via the well-established shared governance structure (Cullen et al., 2017).

Evaluation

Collective efforts resulted in the hiring of more than 800 registered nurses (RNs) in 1 year and reducing agency FTEs by 203 in a little over 5 months (Fig. 17.2), leading to a $7.7 million-dollar savings. Increasing the inpatient differential affected over 2100 RNs with a financial impact of almost $5 million dollars. Reimbursement for moving expenses impacted 21 newly hired nurses, who received almost $54,000. Twenty-four nurses benefited from the referral incentive, equating to $46,000, and 727 RNs financially benefited from disbursement of preceptor pay. The overall vacancy rate simultaneously fell to less than 5% by the end of the fiscal year and has been sustained since that time. Finally, the organization's annual turnover rate remains well below the NSI Nursing Solutions, Inc. benchmark (NSI Nursing Solutions Inc., 2019).

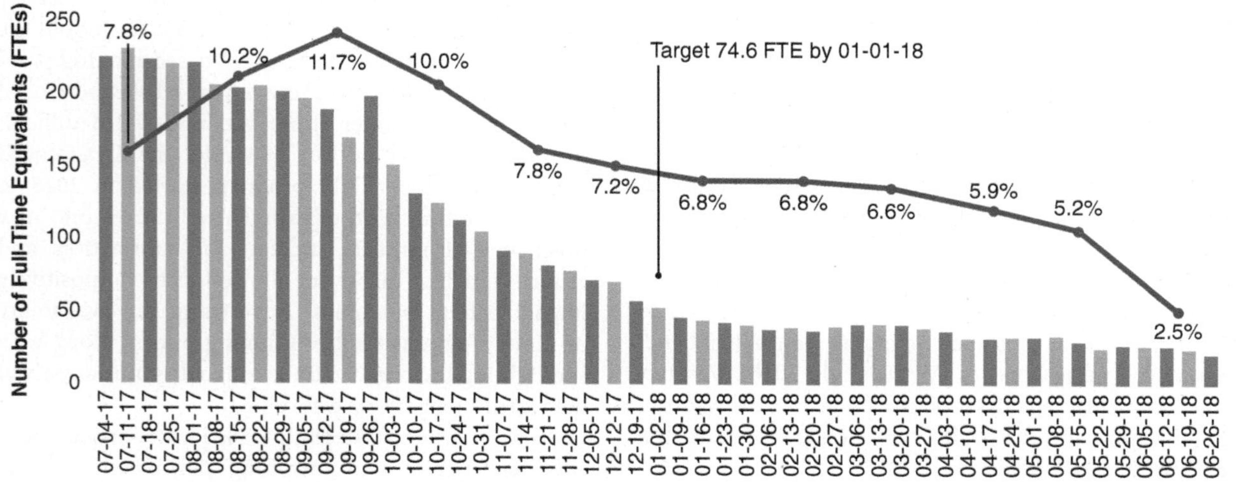

Fig. 17.2 Agency nursing staff by week and average registered nurse vacancy rate percent by month.

Conclusion

Collaborative efforts focused on innovative and aggressive recruitment and retention strategies leading to the reduction of agency nursing staff, recruitment of permanent nurses, and a cost savings of $7.7 million dollars in one fiscal year. These cost savings have allowed for ongoing strategic development in order to continue to positively impact recruitment and retention efforts throughout this large academic **health system**.

ORGANIZATIONAL INFRASTRUCTURE AND CONTEXT

Nurse leaders are in key positions responsible for developing and sustaining an organizational infrastructure and creating an environment that promotes adoption of EBPs and improves patient outcomes (McKay et al., 2018; Melnyk et al., 2016; Shuman et al., 2018; Stetler et al., 2014; Storey et al., 2019). In fact, organizational culture and climate are critical predictors of clinicians' knowledge of and attitudes towards EBP (Powell et al., 2017; Shuman et al., 2018; Yoo et al., 2019). A supportive organizational culture promotes use of evidence, values nurses questioning their practice, provides training about EBP, adopts an EBP model, and recognizes and rewards the work. Evidence-based decision-making is facilitated by roles that promote EBP within the organization, collaborative ties to researchers and networking with other opinion leaders outside the organization, a technical infrastructure to meet informational and data needs, and training programs for building capacity (Brownson et al., 2018b).

It is important to periodically evaluate the infrastructure and context for EBP in the organization. Assessment of EBP leadership, the work environment, and individual and organizational readiness for change may be helpful (Allen et al., 2017; Li et al., 2018; Pittman et al., 2019; Powell et al., 2017; Yoo et al., 2019). Standards for a professional practice environment, such as those outlined through the Magnet Recognition Program®, provide guidance when evaluating an EBP program (https://www.nursingworld.org/organizational-programs/magnet/). A strategic, systematic approach is needed for building EBP capacity (Everett & Sitterding, 2011; Fitzgerald & Harvey, 2015; Shuman et al., 2018; Stetler et al., 2014) at the organization or health system level, building the infrastructure, and creating a culture for change.

Mission, Vision, and Strategic Plan

A mission, vision, and strategic plan inclusive of EBP language provides a sturdy foundation for EBP work at all levels of the organization and begins the process of building a culture in which evidence-based care is the expected norm (Birken et al., 2018; Stetler et al., 2014). A **mission** statement defines the purpose and reflects the values of the organization. When a mission statement is developed, it should be clear that EBP and patient care outcomes are fundamental to why the organization exists (Gifford et al., 2018; Lahey & Nelson, 2020). The mission statement can create a foundation for a culture of inquiry and set the expectation that clinicians will make decisions based on evidence. The **vision** statement can further stretch the current boundaries by promoting EBP work that leads staff to reach for a higher standard. An example of a vision statement might be to develop a center of excellence for EBP within the organization or to be a leader in evidence-based care delivery. The **strategic plan** uses a continuous and systematic planning process to make the mission actionable and outcomes achievable. The strategic plan includes clearly articulated and measurable goals, objectives for meeting outcomes, metrics for measuring progress, a list of resources needed, and a timeline for completion. Attainment of strategic goals should be aimed at positioning the organization for success in a competitive, complex, rapidly changing health care environment (Robertson-Malt & Norton-Westwood, 2017). Goals and objectives should be consistent with the vision and values of the organization. Specific goals for EBP in the strategic plan provide structure for nurse leaders (Lahey & Nelson, 2020; Robertson-Malt & Norton-Westwood, 2017). Action steps are included for creating a culture that values inquiry and innovation and provides leaders with a foundation of support for EBP.

Shared Governance is designed to support the mission, vision, and strategic plan, and provides the infrastructure that integrates the work of EBP. A shared governance system is based on the belief that nurses own their practice and are best informed for making decisions about their practice (Clavelle et al., 2016; Goedhart et al., 2017; Stetler et al., 2014). The right committee or council structure will vary in each organization, but should include point-of-care clinicians and reflect the expertise, functions, and responsibility needed to promote EBP (Cullen et al., 2017; Stetler et al., 2014). Practice change is facilitated when documentation, policies and procedures, and education are based on EBP recommendations. Clinical experts can provide an excellent critique of a new policy or procedure and make recommendations so that policies link practices with evidence and support adaptation of evidence-based policies to fit the organization. Operationalizing communication within the governance structure creates internal peer networking to promote uptake of EBP (Gifford et al., 2018; Li et al., 2018). A clear path for communicating EBP work and necessary approvals between committees within the governance structure needs to be outlined (Cullen et al., 2017). Discussion during committee meetings can stimulate interest in—and use of—EBP, so include an EBP item on each agenda. Another key strategy is having a nurse leader on the Institutional Review Board and a clear process for determining research on human subjects, differentiated from EBP, with a clear process for organizational approvals (Cullen et al., 2018b; Lee et al., 2016; Office of Human Research Protections, U.S. Department of Health & Human Services, n.d.).

Performance Expectations and Appraisal

The value of EBP must be evident through the expected behaviors of nurses at every level in the organization (Taylor et al., 2015). Critical skills for shared governance committee members, include clinical experts, skill with appraisal and synthesis of the evidence, development of an implementation and evaluation plan, basic statistical analysis, and reporting of results (Cullen et al., 2017). Additional expertise can be developed through consultation and collaborations within a practice network, partnerships with academic institutions, or hiring nurse scientists (Sadeghnezhad et al., 2018). Performance appraisals based on job descriptions with EBP components are important for setting behavioral expectations. Inclusion of EBP components in performance appraisals across all job classifications—from top executives to the frontline—promotes positive reinforcement and priority setting in the busy work environment. Providing personal or group performance feedback helps clinicians have ownership of EBP and improves outcomes (Brown et al., 2019; Fleiszer et al., 2016; Hageman et al., 2015; Hysong et al., 2017).

Resources

EBP resources, including time, must be allocated by nurse executives, distributed fairly by managers, and be accessible to clinicians (Birken et al., 2018; Li et al., 2018). The organization can begin to build an EBP culture during orientation for new hires, competency review for current employees, and ongoing training for senior leaders and clinicians. Recruiting and hiring nurses with interest in EBP will help build the capacity. Orientation can contain basic EBP concepts and protocols, with new staff learning from colleagues who share experiences from EBP teamwork on their unit. This provides recognition for completed work, sets the expectation that EBP is important, and demonstrates that nurses have authority over their practice. New graduates have developed skills that support EBP (QSEN Institute, 2019). Nurses in new graduate residency programs can stimulate new—or support existing—EBP work using their creativity, technical skills, and dedicated work time (Hosking et al., 2016). Training opportunities for nurses and interprofessional teams across their career fosters improved outcomes (Cullen et al., 2020; Storey et al., 2019). EBP mentors can be developed from successful projects and used to nurture the next generation of clinical leaders (Abdullah et al., 2014; Gagliardi et al., 2014; Saunders & Vehvilainen-Julkunen, 2017; Spiva et al., 2017; Storey et al., 2019).

Organizational information systems need to be designed to incorporate EBP into clinical workflow if adoption for better outcomes is to be achieved (Renolen et al., 2018). Electronic documentation systems, designed to support clinical practice, need to capture essential elements of clinical practice guidelines that clinicians are expected to perform. The documentation system can serve as a reminder for new practices (Van de Velde et al., 2018). When done right, clinical decision support, such as order sets and interactive documentation prompts, facilitates integrating EBP into daily workflow, making EBP easy for clinicians (Fischer, 2016; Heekin et al., 2018; NAM, 2017; Patel et al., 2017).

Reporting

Internal and external dissemination of EBP results is essential to promote adoption, share learning, garner continued support, and recognize success from the institution's EBP program (Dembe et al., 2014; Esposito et al., 2015; Iowa Model Collaborative, 2017). Internal sharing of anticipated outcomes found in research reports can be helpful early in the EBP process by creating awareness and interest (Cullen & Adams, 2012). Outcomes that target patients and families, staff, and finances are valued by the team and organization, and need to be considered in evaluation planning (Cullen et al., 2018b; Dembe et al., 2014; Esposito et al., 2015; Institute for Healthcare Improvement, 2015; Parry et al., 2018). Cost savings or cost avoidance may not be achieved with every project but should be calculated and reported whenever possible (Sadler et al., 2009; Scott 2nd et al., 2019). Cost data may be available in the literature for estimating cost savings (AHRQ, 2017a; Hollenbeak & Schilling, 2018) and generating interest in EBP changes (Cullen et al., 2020).

Nursing leaders have a responsibility to clearly articulate EBP work in a way that will be heard by decision makers. Structural empowerment through shared governance has been associated with better patient outcomes (Goedhart et al., 2017). Shared governance provides a mechanism for sharing results with bidirectional communication among point-of-care nurses and senior leaders, so leaders can recognize great work while reporting the business case for EBP within governing boards (Abel & Hand, 2018; Murt et al., 2019). Communication with boards about EBP goals and initiatives is an important strategy (Cullen et al., 2017; Institute for Healthcare Improvement, 2016; Mason et al., 2013). Specific actions include sharing three to five brief talking points or take-away messages and including reporting of the links between EBP and the organization's mission, vision, values, and strategic plan.

Capturing EBP within the quality improvement program (Djulbegovic et al., 2019; Mondoux & Shojania, 2019) is another way to build a strong organizational context. EBP can use the existing quality improvement program's standardized forms, reporting system, and established goals for improving care processes (Allen et al., 2017; Cullen et al., 2017; Harvey et al., 2019). Using the quality improvement system for reporting EBP provides efficient communication within the existing organizational infrastructure. The quality improvement process also supports ongoing planning, monitoring, and reinfusion of expected care delivery, supporting successful integration of EBPs.

Rewards

EBP successes need to be recognized and rewarded along the way (Birken et al., 2018; Sveinsdottir et al., 2016). Celebrations help build a culture that supports and expects use of evidence in practice. Rewards need to include formal recognition from senior leaders, visibility for interprofessional teams and EBP change champions, and clear demonstration of the benefits of EBP. Celebrations provide an opportunity to put clinicians in the spotlight for doing great work and articulate the standard for excellence based on EBP. Recognition can highlight the benefits to, and commitment of, the organization and strengthens the foundation for future efforts.

LEADERSHIP ROLES IN PROMOTING EVIDENCE-BASED PRACTICE

Leaders play a critical role establishing operational support so nurses can learn about and implement EBP (Allen et al., 2017; Gifford et al., 2018; Kowalski et al., 2019; Warren et al., 2016). Leadership is essential to initiate EBP and facilitate sustained change (Li et al., 2018). Clinical nursing and leadership roles complement each other (e.g., chief nurse executives, nurse managers, advanced practice nurses, and point-of-care nurses) to promote EBP and achieve desired outcomes (Harvey et al., 2019). Core groups that include nurses in roles with local leadership can match needed skills with opinion leaders from relevant disciplines, creating an effective EBP team (Chauhan et al., 2017; Cullen et al., 2018a,b; Huether et al., 2016).

Point-of-Care Nurse

Patient care outcomes are directly impacted by point-of-care nurse engagement in EBP (Goedhart et al., 2017; Saunders & Vehvilainen-Julkunen, 2017). Point-of-care nurses are in the ideal position to question practice and identify patient and family needs. Having the confidence to challenge the status quo and ask the question "Why do we practice this way?" is foundational to the success of EBP changes in a continually changing environment (Porter-O'Grady & Malloch, 2008). Staying current in both EBP and a clinical specialty throughout the career continuum occurs through conference attendance, reading scholarly journal articles, continued academic coursework, and professional networking.

The success of many EBP initiatives is contingent on the knowledge, clinical expertise, and passion of the point-of-care nurses. Many organizations provide training opportunities so that point-of-care nurses can get guidance and mentoring through the EBP process (Gifford et al., 2018; Spiva et al., 2017; Storey et al., 2019). EBP training provides nurses with the knowledge and confidence to inquire about best evidence and pursue change, building upon clinical expertise, collaboration and problem-solving. Point-of-care nurses often identify creative solutions to improve adoption of EBP, and can function as EBP change champions and core group members (Chauhan et al., 2017; Cullen et al., 2018b, 2020). They can also engage the team in designing and integrating change into their practice (Chauhan et al., 2017). A positive working environment elevates point-of-care nurses to be able to provide evidence-based care and improve patient outcomes (Goedhart et al., 2017).

Clinical Nurse Leader

Ensuring EBP initiatives are in place to improve quality is a national standard (American Nurses Credentialing Center, n.d.; Royer et al., 2018; The Joint Commission, n.d.). To increase the adoption of EBI, it is important to have technical support and training from a designated leader (Leeman et al., 2017). A key role in bridging the gap between the point-of-care nurse and the leadership team is the clinical nurse leader (CNL) (Bender, 2016; Clavo-Hall et al., 2018). The CNL helps foster learning and supports implementation of an EBP change by using clinical expertise in conjunction with personal connections with the interprofessional team. CNL responsibilities include project management, leading the EBP process, evaluating the impact, and reporting to unit or clinic leaders. Doing so involves understanding opportunities for improvement, constructing interdisciplinary collaboration to create a team approach to improving care processes, role modeling, mentoring, and successfully sustaining the practice change (Bender, 2016).

Advanced Practice Registered Nurse

The Advance Practice Registered Nurse (APRN) (e.g., advanced registered nurse practitioners, clinical nurse specialists, unit practice leaders) plays a strong supportive role in promoting EBP among clinical teams (Patterson et al., 2017). Essential EBP steps offered by this role are helping the team to identify opportunities, successfully implement a practice change and provide ongoing mentorship to sustain the change (Patterson et al., 2017; Royer et al., 2018; Saunders & Vehvilainen-Julkunen, 2017). Having the evidence to support a change in practice is important; however, having the knowledge to implement the change successfully is also essential (Spiva et al., 2017). As a clinical expert and a respected resource, the APRN enhances the knowledge of team members and calls the team to continuously question practice and improve quality through the EBP process. The APRN can lead the EBP process, design the EBI, and provide project management (Stewart et al., 2017). Pivotal roles of APRNs are in the development of policies based on the best evidence and adapted to the local setting. They also serve as change agents with strong leadership skills and organizational knowledge to help motivate and support others delivering EBP (Hole et al., 2016). Active participation in mentoring and modeling the EBP change are important for facilitating change. Role modeling the change, being actively engaged, in addition to being in a leadership role on an interprofessional team, provides resources for point-of-care nurses and enhances the team's willingness to implement the change (Warren et al., 2016).

Nurse Manager

Point-of-care managers have a key role in making EBP the norm for their area (Gifford et al., 2018; Renolen et al., 2020; Shuman et al., 2018; Warren et al., 2016). In order for a team to successfully provide excellent care, managers need to support point-of-care nurses as drivers of change, while also giving and seeking input (Gifford et al., 2018). This promotes superior clinical performance, accountability, and ownership by the team (Porter-O'Grady & Malloch, 2008). Unit or clinic leaders have a responsibility to clear the path so clinicians can have ownership of their work in a way that makes EBP possible (Birken et al., 2018; Kouzes & Posner, 2012). The nurse manager juggles several roles including leading, coaching, addressing concerns, empowering, and overcoming obstacles (Birken et al., 2018; Gifford et al., 2018). Support from the nurse manager enables point-of-care nurses to use EBP by cultivating a shared vision for EBP, being transparent about the value of EBP, and providing resources for EBP (Caramanica & Spiva, 2018). The attitude of the nurse manager sets the tone for how EBP is perceived. It is important to help staff understand the reason for change associated with the EBP recommendations (Birken et al., 2018). In addition, staying mission driven with EBP means "keep the patient and family at the center of all your decisions and you'll always make the right decision" (C. Mentz, personal communication, April 14, 2017).

Managers leading EBP among point-of-care nurses promote a continuous culture of improvement that requires resources (i.e., people, training, supplies, and time) dedicated to EBP (Birken et al., 2018; Gifford et al., 2018). Learning to promote EBP is fostered by answering questions; guiding and resourcing before, during, and after piloting; describing the benefits; setting norms; and providing feedback to internal and external stakeholders (Birken et al., 2018; Gifford et al., 2018). Attention needs to be paid to building EBP into the daily workflow (Renolen et al., 2018). Actions include addressing EBP during daily huddles, staff meetings, and with the EBP team in conjunction with communicating regularly with stakeholders to promote both adoption and sustainability (Harvey et al., 2019), and addressing concerns and acknowledging efforts to change (Gifford et al., 2018). In addition, effectively communicating face-to-face with those hesitant about the change is most productive for addressing concerns and obtaining buy-in (Gifford et al., 2018; C. Mentz, personal communication, November 4, 2019).

By having a strong interest in EBP and being supportive of the time commitment, managers help by maintaining a positive perception of the process and impact (Jansson & Forsberg, 2016). Creating a culture of open dialogue and constructive, professional feedback is imperative. When unit leaders reinforce expectations and maintain priorities, the sustainability of EBP improves (Fleiszer et al., 2016).

Nurse Executive

Nurse executives are key to managers understanding and having ownership of EBP, while also allocating resources (Birken et al., 2018). The nurse executive has a unique opportunity to promote change, set expectations, provide resources and training, and open doors for successful EBP (Gifford et al., 2018). Aligning the infrastructure and strategic plan of the organization with EBP lays the groundwork for successful EBP implementation (Goedhart et al., 2017; Luckson et al., 2018; Stetler et al., 2014). To navigate the ever-changing paradigms of health care, the nurse executive needs to make EBP their priority and an expectation for clinicians, interprofessional teams, and the organization as a whole. By providing opportunities for EBP training, professional development, and growth along the career continuum, the institution can see sustained improvements while building the capacity for the future (Crawford et al., 2017).

Committed leadership and daily resources for EBP require support from senior executives (Balakas et al., 2013; Gifford et al., 2018; Luckson et al., 2018; Melnyk et al., 2016). Walking rounds encourage others and track progress through discussions with clinicians and patients (Harvey et al., 2019). When the nurse executive is passionate about EBP and has a consistent mission and philosophical goals to achieve excellence through EBP and incentivizes EBP, it is reflected in the nursing care provided (Leeman et al., 2017; Yoo et al., 2019). Additionally, it is important to support internal and external dissemination of the EBP work done through local, regional, national, and international oral and poster presentations, along with peer-reviewed publications.

LEADERSHIP AND MANAGEMENT IMPLICATIONS

Change is often difficult, yet challenges can be anticipated. Therefore use of a multifaceted approach by nurse leaders across roles is imperative to integrate and sustain EBP at the unit and organizational level. Empowering all nurses is pivotal to adoption. Transformational leadership can be used to focus nurses on being "leaders" to initiate and sustain EBP by fostering a culture and climate through leadership to provide EBP (Shuman et al., 2018).

Culture

The primary mechanism to drive culture is leadership, more specifically in how the leader "walks the talk." Culture is reinforced by the actions and behavior of the leader, what gets rewarded and punished, and where resources are allocated (Schein & Schein, 2016). Culture then translates to the expectations and behavioral norms that differentiate a work environment and shape the way in which employees' approach and prioritize their work (Glisson, 2015). The secondary drivers of culture are norms and expectations articulated in the organizational mission, vision, values, and documents such as policies and job descriptions (Schein & Schein, 2016; Shuman, 2017). A culture that expects the integration of EBP into practice to provide high-quality patient care is essential for nursing to thrive (Storey et al., 2019). Proficiency is based on having institutions with expectations to maintain the most current knowledge and skills to respond to the unique needs of their patients (Galdikiene et al., 2016; Glisson, 2015).

Climate

Climate refers to the shared perceptions created by employees of the psychological influence of their environment on their personal performance and well-being. Team perceptions represent personal assessments of the significance and value of their work, engagement, and functions (Galdikiene et al., 2016; Glisson, 2015). The EBP climate refers to the clinician's perceptions at the local unit or clinic level, which are influenced by expectations, rewards, and organizational support (Shuman, 2017). Having humble leadership creates a positive organizational climate with increased involvement, constructive feedback, and optimal outcomes (Aarons et al., 2017).

Transformational Leadership

Transformational leadership has been defined as leadership that empowers others, facilitates growth and learning of team members, translates EBP into practice with local application, critically reflects and communicates, and uses problem-solving (Fischer, 2016). Practices of transformational leaders have been described by Kouzes and Posner (2012) as modeling the way, inspiring a shared vision, challenging the process, enabling others to act, and encouraging the heart. Empowering nurses to provide EBP in their daily care through transformational nursing leadership includes a vision that drives organizational change (Hauck et al., 2013). Leaders use transformational leadership to motivate others and inspire their team to provide EBP (Gifford et al., 2018). Partnering with clinical staff to provide opportunities to learn about EBP in conjunction with time to execute new practices highlights the importance of and value placed on EBP. Using transformational leadership to commit to the culture and climate of a unit that supports EBP will achieve a return on investment for patients, families, nurses, and the organization.

Leaders influence an organization's capacity for EBP. Leadership that demonstrates and expects EBP will promote its use in clinical and operational decision-making at the unit or clinic and organizational level. Prioritizing and facilitating leaders' and clinicians' ownership of EBP work is essential. Helping clinicians provide EBP requires leaders to be change-oriented, communicate to build relationships, involve positive and influential team members, address concerns, and acknowledge efforts; management is required to distribute work, arrange for dedicated time, provide needed equipment, and monitor progress (Gifford et al., 2018).

CURRENT ISSUES AND TRENDS

There is a growing demand for evidence-based and patient-centered care, with increasing public accountability and transparency for quality and safety (Centers for Medicare & Medicaid Services, 2019). Reimbursement structures reflect the importance of system redesign to improve coordination, efficiency, and provision of EBP for improved population health. Pay for performance through the Centers for Medicare & Medicaid Services' value-based purchasing and accountable care organization alignment has mixed indications of improving quality and cost of care (Ouayogode et al., 2019; Rutledge et al., 2019; Zhang et al., 2019). Total waste in the US health care system is estimated to be $760–$935 billion, and an estimated 25% could be saved through providing evidence-based care (Shrank et al., 2019). National patient safety goals established by The Joint Commission include a growing number of evidence-based standards. For example, standards for catheter-associated urinary tract infections reflect a growing intolerance for hospital-acquired infections (The Joint Commission, 2016). Likewise, national benchmarks (https://data.medicare.gov/) promote transparency for quality. The financial pressure for provision of EBP will continue to grow with demand from payers and patients.

Patient engagement and provision of patient-centered care is central to the national and international health care agenda (AHRQ, 2017b, 2018; American Academy of Nursing, 2019; American Board of Internal Medicine, 2019). Research is still needed to understand how best to facilitate shared decision-making (Durand et al., 2014; Prochaska & Sanders-Jackson, 2016).

Doctoral preparation continues to grow, as nurse leaders want skills that improve application of scholarship and leadership (American Association of Colleges of Nursing, 2018a). The Doctor of Nursing practice final project is designed as EBP impacting quality in a local setting (American Association of Colleges of Nursing, 2018b). Student work is best done in coordination and with approval of the clinical setting. Integrating student work within the organizational system creates student learning about how organizations work and may facilitate sustainment of their practice changes. Unfortunately, these student projects often conclude with numerous key steps not completed (Minnick et al., 2019). In fact, as many as 82% of final student projects have been found to have insufficient rigor and even fatal flaws (Minnick et al., 2019; Roush & Tesoro, 2018). Basic standards have been published and work is needed to establish and apply standards for these EBP initiatives (Lee et al., 2013; SQUIRE, 2017). The result creates a win–win for students and organizations, which ultimately create a win for patients and families.

A continuing priority for implementation science is to better understand how nurse leaders can promote adoption of evidence-based health care to improve quality and reduce costs (Hollenbeak & Schilling, 2018; Sadler et al., 2009). Understanding how to scale up and sustain EBP improvements is a critical priority (Seneski & Stack, 2019; Valim et al., 2019).

Nurses want to work in an organization that promotes innovation and EBP. An exhaustive body of research consistently finds that leadership support is essential to an organization's ability to consistently use evidence in practice (Gifford et al., 2018; Kowalski et al., 2019). The organizational context within which clinicians work is a complex and dynamic culture unique to each practice setting. Leaders are responsible for providing resources, structures, and processes that move teams beyond barriers to facilitate EBP (Li et al., 2018). Research is still needed to better understand infrastructure design and effective strategies to affect organizational context and capacity, encouraging adoption and delivery of evidence-based care (Clavelle et al., 2016; Goedhart et al., 2017; Stetler et al., 2014).

CONCLUSION

Nursing has a long history of valuing and using the best evidence to improve care quality. However, there continue to be challenges in using evidence-based care within the current health care environment. Nurses in leadership positions have responsibility for supporting evidence-based clinical care and evidence-based operational decision-making. Models outline the process for updating practices when addressing clinical and operational issues. Implementation is one of the most challenging steps in the EBP process. A phased approach using multiple reinforcing and interactive strategies is needed for implementation and sustained improvement. An effective, data-driven implementation approach can be used to create a targeted and highly influential implementation plan.

Nursing leaders can systematically build a strong program supporting evidence-based care delivery. Implementing EBPs is best accomplished by understanding the interplay between organizational and unit factors supported through the organizational infrastructure. Nurse leaders need to connect their evidence-based initiatives to the organization's vision, mission, values, and infrastructure to garner support and resources for EBP care delivery. The leadership and infrastructure to support EBP is essential for creating the desired organizational culture, capacity, and unit climate. Communicating the business case for EBP will help nurses articulate their impact in a way that will be heard by senior leaders. Complementary skills are needed within all nursing roles to create effective EBP teams. Every nurse has a responsibility to lead evidence-based care delivery to improve outcomes for patients and their families, staff, and the organization.

RESEARCH NOTE

Source

Harvey, G., Gifford, W., Cummings, G., Kelly, J., Kislov, R., Kitson, A., et al. (2019). Mobilising evidence to improve nursing practice: A qualitative study of leadership roles and processes in four countries. International Journal of Nursing Studies, 90, 21–30. https://doi.org/10-1016/j.ijnurstu.2018.09.017.

Purpose

The purpose of this qualitative study was to describe senior and frontline leader roles in promoting evidence-based practice (EBP) and identify factors in the practice setting that influence leadership and the implementation process. Participants were nurse executives, nurse managers, and facilitators (i.e., educators or practice development specialists) within acute and community care settings in Australia, Canada, England, and Sweden.

Discussion

Varying roles and structures were used to support evidence-based health care in practice settings. Senior executives were strategic and visionary. Important elements of their role were to establish the infrastructure and create collaborations and processes that support

RESEARCH NOTE—cont'd

EBP. Executives had a local focus while also maintaining links at the regional and national level. Managers had a "gate keeper" role that is pivotal for operationalizing EBP, providing information and directions, role modeling, monitoring progress, and creating policies. The role of facilitation was to increase capacity for EBP and focus on support, including providing education, coaching, linking evidence to practice, providing skill development, and addressing barriers. Facilitators were important for communication and coordination while building practice networks.

The influence of national policy and regulatory monitoring varied across countries, reflecting the environment of the practice settings. Organizations supported EBP through a culture of continuous learning. Core to continuous learning was integration of quality improvement, benchmarks, and local data, as part of the evidence used to guide nursing practice, nursing standards, and accreditation. Inherent differences were reported when working in a health care organization compared with a person's home. Community care clinicians were challenged to audit use of EBP due to their responsiveness to the living situation of individual patients and a lack of electronic health records. Linking EBP to quality improvement processes facilitated adoption. Although participants could describe their role, educational preparation in implementation and the EBP process were limited. Other concerns were time and workload pressures, a deference to a dominant medical model, and focused adherence to policies that contributed to a lack of critical thinking by nurses.

Application to Practice

Leadership roles are complementary and cumulative, supporting evidence-based health care. Senior executives create a vision for the future, a culture of continuous improvement, and build an infrastructure and capacity to achieve EBP. Senior leaders provide support, resources, and training opportunities (Gifford et al., 2018). Managers' focus is operational and pivotal to enabling or obstructing EBP. Managers must commit to providing EBP with consistent messaging that links practice changes to organizational expectations. Managers are information conduits providing information and seeking input, while monitoring, encouraging, and recognizing clinicians (Gifford et al., 2018). Facilitator roles may fall under a variety of headings but were central to EBP capacity building, developing clinicians' knowledge and skills, and supporting ongoing learning, coaching, coordinating, and collaborating. Managers and facilitators should work consistently and collaboratively to garner commitment, navigate changing conditions, and encourage progress to provide evidence-based care (van der Zijpp et al., 2016).

From the perspective of the practice setting, there are several essential elements for EBP. The organization must provide training, resources, technology, expert facilitation, and a supportive infrastructure. Organizations must focus on continuous learning and integration of EBP within quality methods while using local data. Monitoring progress through audit and feedback are a foundational part of a comprehensive implementation plan (Brown et al., 2019; Phelan et al., 2018). The availability of guidelines, policies, practice registries, benchmarks, an electronic health record, and resources for training and development of local clinician leaders may be determined by government regulations.

CASE STUDY

Updated recommendations were published for cleaning endoscopes and preventing pathogen transmission, creating an opportunity to evaluate the organization's infection prevention policy related to cleaning, transporting, and storage. An ambulatory nursing leader recognized this as a chance to infuse evidence-based practice (EBP) into the Ambulatory Nursing division (Association for the Advancement of Medical Instrumentation—Endoscope Reprocessing Work Group, 2015; Office of Public Health Preparedness and Response, 2015). The following benefits were anticipated:

- Decreased risk of pathogen transmission
- Decreased endoscope cleaning time
- Decreased costs
- Empowered point-of-care nursing staff to use evidence-based recommendations
- Expanded culture in the Ambulatory Nursing division regarding use of evidence in daily practice

Next Steps

Essential steps are to recognize the need to form an interprofessional team; review and synthesize available evidence; revise the current policy and procedure; and create comprehensive implementation and evaluation plans. Collaborating with key stakeholders (e.g., nursing, infection prevention, central sterilizing services) throughout the

CASE STUDY—cont'd

organization was needed to match the skills and expertise required. The Nurse Manager (NM) of the Otolaryngology-Head and Neck Surgery Clinic had an identified need with over 700 patients getting scoped each month. The NM was already an opinion leader and ideally suited to lead the team. The team developed an action plan and divided responsibility for project work. Team members completed each of the following:

- Reviewed and synthesized the literature
- Developed a comprehensive implementation plan comprised of strategies to promote adoption of the practice change
- Developed an initial orientation and annual competency checklist where clinicians verbalize key components of the revised policy and procedure and completed a hands-on demonstration of the process for cleaning, transporting, and storing endoscopes
- Developed a standard workflow document for each type of endoscope
- Developed an educational presentation, visual learning tools, content for a just-in-time nursing education, and a poster based on the literature review
- Developed a process to monitor ongoing compliance with the practice change to ensure sustainability

The practice change involved precleaning endoscopes immediately following removal from patient care at the bedside or in the procedure or exam room. Clinicians performed hand hygiene and wore appropriate personal protective equipment, then used a lint-free sponge or towel to preclean the endoscope, which was placed in biohazard containers. In addition, endoscopes were not precleaned in handwashing sinks and only approved precleaning products were used. The date, time, and initials of the clinician performing the precleaning were written on the lid of the biohazard-labeled container. Finally, every endoscope was linked by a unique identification number to the patient's medical record number in the electronic health record.

Endoscopes were transported to the flexible endoscope reprocessing center to be reprocessed within 60 minutes of the completed precleaning procedure. After reprocessing, endoscopes were stored in unit- or clinic-based cabinets with continuous high-efficiency particulate air (HEPA) filtration, hung completely extended (no looping of insertion tubes), and not touching one another. Clean, ready-to-use endoscopes were used within 30 days or reprocessed.

This ambulatory nursing-led, and subsequent house-wide practice change required multiple strategies for implementation (Cullen & Adams, 2012). The team used the following implementation strategies: highlight anticipated impact; highlight compatibility; discuss at staff meetings/unit in-services/huddles; distribute key evidence; use posters and postings/fliers; publicize new equipment; use education, change agents, and gap assessment/gap analysis; match practice change with resources and equipment; troubleshoot use/application; have an action plan; create resource materials and quick reference guides; verify skill competence; audit key indicators; use actionable and timely data feedback, checklists, and documentation changes in the electronic health record; have unit orientation; and revise the current policy and procedure.

Process and outcome indicators were included in the evaluation (Cullen et al., 2019b; Institute for Healthcare Improvement, 2019; Parry et al., 2018). Data captured those performing the precleaning, the number of scopes processed per month for each clinical area, the number of scopes that required an extended reprocessing time each month, when no precleaning time was noted, when extra equipment was sent with the endoscope to the reprocessing center, and incidents of pathogen transmission, all of which were measured and trended.

This EBP filled a critical gap in patient safety related to properly maintaining, cleaning, and disinfecting endoscopes according to established industry guidelines and manufacturer's instructions. Identification of key stakeholders, who could continue to dedicate time to this practice change, was warranted to ensure sustainability and compliance with ever-evolving regulatory standards. To meet this need, the organization chose to form an Endoscope Life Cycle Committee. A revised process was introduced, and patient care improvements occurred through the EBP changes. The ambulatory NM facilitated project work and integration of the practice change by serving as the project director to establish the priority, find resources, and guide the team to maneuver through the system for adoption and dissemination (Dawson, 2012; 2013; 2016; 2018) of the practice change.

CRITICAL THINKING EXERCISE

As the nurse manager on a general surgery unit, questions about practice frequently come your way. At a staff meeting, a newer nurse, Emily, asks, "Why don't we perform end-tidal CO_2 ($EtCO_2$) monitoring for patients receiving opioid medications to help prevent opioid-induced respiratory depression? I have read about the benefits of $EtCO_2$ monitoring in the literature (Jungquist et al., 2019), and I think this would be a good fit for the patients on our unit. Plus, the current bedside monitors could easily be adapted to include the capnography component." Mary, an experienced nurse on the unit, states, "We already monitor our patients receiving opioid medications for unintended sedation and respiratory depression using a modified POSS (Pasero Opioid-Induced Sedation Scale) scale (Pasero, 2009). And, we do not want to hear more monitors alarming each shift just to say we are using more technology, especially when it is not needed." Others attending the staff meeting nod their heads in agreement with Mary. You ask those present if they know about the emerging evidence about the benefits of $EtCO_2$ monitoring that Emily referenced and if they are interested in learning more to ensure provision of safe, high-quality patient care while at the same time preventing adverse events. You realize this topic could result in an EBP initiative. How will you engage the team in this EBP project?

1. What issues do you anticipate with regards to an EBP project related to EtCO2 monitoring for postsurgical patients receiving opioid medications?
2. Who is an emerging leader, to assume the project director role and manage the project? Why was this person your top candidate to be the project director?
3. How can you help the project team determine whether $EtCO_2$ monitoring for postsurgical patients is a priority for the organization?
4. Who will be key stakeholders and potential team members?
5. How will you, as the nurse manager, be involved in the project?
6. What is the benefit of a current literature review specific to $EtCO_2$ monitoring for post-surgical patients receiving opioid medications?
7. Why is it important to adapt the practice change to fit into the unit workflow?
8. How might the core project team learn more about and incorporate patient and family preferences when designing the practice change and implementation?
9. After designing an EBP change to incorporate the use of $EtCO_2$ monitoring for post-surgical patients receiving opioid medications:
   a. How can you create awareness and interest about the need for a practice change?
   b. What education is needed and what other strategies would help you build knowledge and commitment among the health care team?
   c. How can the change agent role enhance adoption of the practice change?
   d. What key process and outcome indicators should be measured?
   e. How should the key indicators be measured?
   f. Who is going to provide actionable and timely data feedback to the frontline clinicians?
   g. Who can assist with ongoing monitoring of compliance with the practice change to ensure sustainability is achieved?

REFERENCES

Aarons, G. A., Ehrhart, M. G., Torres, E. M., Finn, N. K., & Beidas, R. S. (2017). The humble leader: Association of discrepancies in leader and follower ratings of implementation leadership with organizational climate in mental health. *Psychiatric Services, 68*(2), 115–122. https://doi.org/10.1176/appi.ps.201600062.

Aarons, G. A., Sklar, M., Mustanski, B., Benbow, N., & Brown, C. H. (2017). "Scaling-out" evidence-based interventions to new populations or new health care delivery systems. *Implementation Science, 12*(1), 111. https://doi.org/10.1186/s13012-017-0640-6.

Abbott, L., & Hooke, M. C. (2017). Energy through motion: An activity intervention for cancer-related fatigue in an ambulatory infusion center. *Clinical Journal of Oncology Nursing, 21*(5), 618–626. https://doi.org/10.1188/17.CJON.618-626.

Abdullah, G., Rossy, D., Ploeg, J., Davies, B., Higuchi, K., Sikora, L., et al. (2014). Measuring the effectiveness of mentoring as a knowledge translation intervention for implementing empirical evidence: A systematic review. *Worldviews on Evidence-Based Nursing, 11*(5), 284–300. https://doi.org/10.1111/wvn.12060.

Abel, S. E., & Hand, M. W. (2018). Exploring, defining, and illustrating a concept: Structural and psychological empowerment in the workplace. *Nursing Forum, 53*(4), 579–584. https://doi.org/10.1111/nuf.12289.

AHRQ. (2017a). *Estimating the additional hospital inpatient cost and mortality associated with selected hospital-acquired conditions*. https://www.ahrq.gov/hai/pfp/haccost2017-results.html.

AHRQ. (2017b). *Strategy 6I: Shared decisionmaking*. https://www.ahrq.gov/cahps/quality-improvement/improvement-guide/6-strategies-for-improving/communication/strategy6i-shared-decisionmaking.html.

AHRQ. (2018). *The guide to improving patient safety in primary care settings by engaging patients and families*. https://www.ahrq.gov/sites/default/files/wysiwyg/professionals/quality-patient-safety/patient-family-engagement/pfeprimarycare/pfepc-fullguide-final508.pdf.

Allen, J. D., Towne, S. D., Jr., Maxwell, A. E., DiMartino, L., Leyva, B., Bowen, D. J., et al. (2017). Measures of organizational characteristics associated with adoption and/or implementation of innovations: A systematic review. *BMC Health Services Research, 17*(1), 591. https://doi.org/10.1186/s12913-017-2459-x.

Ament, S. M., de Groot, J. J., Maessen, J. M., Dirksen, C. D., van der Weijden, T., & Kleijnen, J. (2015). Sustainability of professionals' adherence to clinical practice guidelines in medical care: A systematic review. *BMJ Open, 5*(12), Article e008073. https://doi.org/10.1136/bmjopen-2015-008073.

American Academy of Nursing. (2019). *Twenty-five things nurses and patients should question*. https://www.choosingwisely.org/societies/american-academy-of-nursing/.

American Association of Colleges of Nursing. (2018a). *2017–2018 enrollment and graduations in baccalaureate and graduate programs in nursing*. Author. Washington: DC.

American Association of Colleges of Nursing. (2018b). *Defining scholarship for academic nursing. Report from the task force for consensus position statement*. Author. Washington: DC.

American Association of Critical-Care Nurses (AACN). (2005). AACN standards for establishing and sustaining healthy work environments: A journey to excellence. *American Journal of Critical Care, 14*(3), 187–197.

American Board of Internal Medicine. (2019). *Choosing wisely*. https://abimfoundation.org/what-we-do/choosing-wisely.

American Nurses Credentialing Center. (n.d.). *Magnet recognition program*. https://www.nursingworld.org/organizational-programs/magnet/.

Association for the Advancement of Medical Instrumentation —Endoscope Reprocessing Work Group. (2015). *Flexible and semi-rigid endoscope reprocessing in health care facilities*. Arlington, VA: Association for the Advancement of Medical Instrumentation.

Balakas, K., Sparks, L., Steurer, L., & Bryant, T. (2013). An outcome of evidence-based practice education: sustained clinical decision making among bedside nurses. *Journal of Pediatric Nursing, 28*(5), 479–485. https://doi.org/10.1016/j.pedn.2012.08.007.

Bandura, A. (1977). *Social learning theory*. Englewood Cliffs, NJ: Prentice-Hall.

Bender, M. (2016). Clinical nurse leader integration into practice: Developing theory to guide best practice. *Journal of Professional Nursing, 32*(1), 32–40. https://doi.org/10.1016/j.profnurs.2015.06.007.

Birken, S., Clary, A., Tabriz, A. A., Turner, K., Meza, R., Zizzi, A., et al. (2018). Middle managers' role in implementing evidence-based practices in healthcare: A systematic review. *Implementation Science, 13*(1), 149. https://doi.org/10.1186/s13012-018-0843-5.

Borsky, A., Zhan, C., Miller, T., Ngo-Metzger, Q., Bierman, A. S., & Meyers, D. (2018). Few Americans receive all high-priority, appropriate clinical preventive services. *Health Affairs, 37*(6), 925–928. https://doi.org/10.1377/hlthaff.2017.1248.

Brown, B., Gude, W. T., Blakeman, T., van der Veer, S. N., Ivers, N., Francis, J. J., et al. (2019a). Clinical performance feedback intervention theory (CP-FIT): A new theory for designing, implementing, and evaluating feedback in health care based on a systematic review and meta-synthesis of qualitative research. *Implementation Science, 14*(1), 40. https://doi.org/10.1186/s13012-019-0883-5.

Brownson, R. C., Colditz, G. A., & Proctor, E. K. (2018a). *Dissemination and implementation research in health: Translating science to practice* (2nd ed.). Oxford: Oxford University Press.

Brownson, R. C., Fielding, J. E., & Green, L. W. (2018b). Building capacity for evidence-based public health: Reconciling the pulls of practice and the push of research. *Annual Review of Public Health, 39*, 27–53. https://doi.org/10.1146/annurev-publhealth-040617-014746.

Bunger, A. C., Birken, S. A., Hoffman, J. A., MacDowell, H., Choy-Brown, M., & Magier, E. (2019). Elucidating the influence of supervisors' roles on implementation climate. *Implementation Science, 14*(1), 93. https://doi.org/10.1186/s13012-019-0939-6.

Camargo, F. C., Iwamoto, H. H., Galvão, C. M., Monteiro, D. A. T., Goulart, M. B., & Garcia, L. A. A. (2017). Models for the implementation of evidence-based practice in hospital based nursing: A narrative review. *Texto & Contexto - Enfermagem, 26*(4), Article e2070017. https://doi.org/10.1590/0104-07072017002070017.

Caramanica, L., & Spiva, L. (2018). Exploring nurse manager support of evidence-based practice: Clinical nurse perceptions. *Journal of Nursing*

Administration, 48(5), 272–278. https://doi.org/10.1097/NNA.0000000000000612.
Centers for Medicare & Medicaid Services. (2019). *Sharing savings program*. https://www.cms.gov/Medicare/Medicare-Fee-for-Service-Payment/sharedsavingsprogram/index.
Chauhan, B. F., Jeyaraman, M. M., Mann, A. S., Lys, J., Skidmore, B., Sibley, K. M., et al. (2017). Behavior change interventions and policies influencing primary healthcare professionals' practice-an overview of reviews. *Implementation Science, 12*(1), 3. https://doi.org/10.1186/s13012-016-0538-8.
Clavelle, J. T., Porter O'Grady, T., Weston, M. J., & Verran, J. A. (2016). Evolution of structural empowerment: Moving from shared to professional governance. *Journal of Nursing Administration, 46*(6), 308–312. https://doi.org/10.1097/NNA.0000000000000350.
Clavo-Hall, J. A., Bender, M., & Harvath, T. A. (2018). Roles enacted by clinical nurse leaders across the healthcare spectrum: A systematic literature review. *Journal of Professional Nursing, 34*(4), 259–268. https://doi.org/10.1016/j.profnurs.2017.11.007.
Coleman, D. E., Kamai, S., & Davis, K. F. (2018). Impact of a collaborative evidence-based practice nursing education program on clinical operations. *Journal of Hospital Librarianship, 18*(4), 323–330. https://doi.org/10.1080/15323269.2018.1509194.
Connor, J. A., Ziniel, S. I., Porter, C., Doherty, D., Moonan, M., Dwyer, P., et al. (2018). Interprofessional use and validation of the AACN healthy work environment assessment tool. *American Journal of Critical Care, 27*(5), 363–371. https://doi.org/10.4037/ajcc2018179.
Crawford, C. L., Omery, A., & Spicer, J. (2017). An integrative review of 21st-century roles, responsibilities, characteristics, and competencies of chief nurse executives: A blueprint for the next generation. *Nursing Administration Quarterly, 41*(4), 297–309. https://doi.org/10.1097/NAQ.0000000000000245.
Cullen, L., & Adams, S. L. (2012). Planning for implementation of evidence-based practice. *Journal of Nursing Administration, 42*(4), 222–230. https://doi.org/10.1097/NNA.0b013e31824ccd0a.
Cullen, L., Baumler, S., Farrington, M., Dawson, C., Folkmann, P., & Brenner, L. (2018). CE: Oral care for head and neck cancer symptom management. *American Journal of Nursing, 118*(1), 24–34. https://doi.org/10.1097/01.NAJ.0000529694.30568.41.
Cullen, L., DeBerg, J., & Hanrahan, K. (2019a). *Turning the evidence pyramid upside down*. Poster session presented at the 2019 Fuld Institute for EBP National Summit. The Ohio State University.
Cullen, L., Hanrahan, K., Farrington, M., Anderson, R., Dimmer, E., Miner, R., et al. (2020). Evidence-based practice change champions program improves quality care. *Journal of Nursing Administration, 50*(3), 128–134.
Cullen, L., Hanrahan, K., Farrington, M., Deberg, J., Tucker, S., & Kleiber, C. (2018). *Evidence-based practice in action: Comprehensive strategies, tools and tips from the University of Iowa Hospitals and Clinics*. Iowa City: Sigma: Theta Tau International.
Cullen, L., Hanrahan, K., Tucker, S. J., & Gallagher-Ford, L. (2019b). Data-driven precision implementation approach. *American Journal of Nursing, 119*(8), 60–63. https://doi.org/10.1097/01.NAJ.0000577460.00222.32.
Cullen, L., Wagner, M., Matthews, G., & Farrington, M. (2017). Evidence into practice: Integration within an organizational infrastructure. *Journal of PeriAnesthesia Nursing, 32*(3), 247–256. https://doi.org/10.1016/j.jopan.2017.02.003.
Damschroder, L. J., & Hagedorn, H. J. (2011). A guiding framework and approach for implementation research in substance use disorders treatment. *Psychology of Addictive Behaviors, 25*(2), 194–205. https://doi.org/10.1037/a0022284.
Damschroder, L. J., & Lowery, J. C. (2013). Evaluation of a large-scale weight management program using the consolidated framework for implementation research (CFIR). *Implementation Science, 8*(51). https://doi.org/10.1186/1748-5908-8-51.
Dang, D., & Dearholt, S. L. (2017). *Johns Hopkins nursing evidence-based practice: model and guidelines* (3rd ed). Indianapolis, IN: Sigma: Theta Tau International.
Dang, D., Melnyk, B., Fineout-Overholt, E., Yost, J., Cullen, L., Cvach, M., et al. (2019). Models to guide implementation and sustainability of evidence-based practice. In B. Melnyk, & E. Fineout-Overholt (Eds.), *Evidence-based practice in nursing & healthcare: A guide to best practice* (4th ed.) (pp. 378–427). Philadelphia, PA: Lippincott, Williams & Wilkins.
Davis, R., Campbell, R., Hildon, Z., Hobbs, L., & Michie, S. (2015). Theories of behaviour and behaviour change across the social and behavioural sciences: A scoping review. *Health Psychology Review, 9*(3), 323–344. https://doi.org/10.1080/17437199.2014.941722.09.
Dawson, C. (2012, September). *An EBP project: High level disinfection of scopes*, Poster session presented at the 36th Annual Society of Otorhinolaryngology and Head-Neck Nurses Congress and Nursing Symposium, Washington, DC.
Dawson, C. (2013). *Cleaning and high-level disinfection (HLD) of flexible and rigid semi-critical medical scopes (without internal channels) using ortho-phthalaldehyde (Cidex OPA)*. Poster session presented at the 20th National Evidence-Based Practice Conference, University of Iowa Hospitals and Clinics, Iowa City, IA.

Dawson, C. (2016, September). *High level disinfection of scopes update*. Paper presented at the 40th Annual Society of Otorhinolaryngology and Head-Neck Nurses Congress and Nursing Symposium, San Diego, CA.

Dawson, C. (2018, October). *Disinfection and cleaning of scopes/instruments*. Paper presented at the 42nd Annual Society of Otorhinolaryngology and Head-Neck Nurses Congress and Nursing Symposium, Atlanta, GA.

Dembe, A. E., Lynch, M. S., Gugiu, P. C., & Jackson, R. D. (2014). The translational research impact scale: development, construct validity, and reliability testing. *Evaluation & the Health Professions, 37*(1), 50–70. https://doi.org/10.1177/0163278713506112.

Djulbegovic, B., Bennett, C. L., & Guyatt, G. (2019). Failure to place evidence at the centre of quality improvement remains a major barrier for advances in quality improvement. *Journal of Evaluation in Clinical Practice, 25*(3), 369–372. https://doi.org/10.1111/jep.13146.

Ducharme, M. P., Bernhardt, J. M., Padula, C. A., & Adams, J. M. (2017). Leader influence, the professional practice environment, and nurse engagement in essential nursing practice. *Journal of Nursing Administration, 47*(7/8), 367–375. https://doi.org/10.1097/NNA.0000000000000497.

Durand, M. A., Carpenter, L., Dolan, H., Bravo, P., Mann, M., Bunn, F., & Elwyn, G. (2014). Do interventions designed to support shared decision making reduce health inequalities? A systematic review and meta-analysis. *PLoS One, 9*(4), e94670. https://doi.org/10.1371/journal.pone.0094670.

Esposito, D., Heeringa, J., Bradley, K., Croake, S., & Kimmey, L. (2015). *PCORI dissemination and implementation framework*. Washington, DC: Patient-Centered Outcomes Research Institute. https://www.pcori.org/sites/default/files/PCORI-Dissemination-Implementation-Framework.pdf.

Everett, L. Q., & Sitterding, M. C. (2011). Transformational leadership required to design and sustain evidence-based practice: A system exemplar. *Western Journal of Nursing Research, 33*(3), 398–426. https://doi.org/10.1177/0193945910383056.

Farra, S. L., Miller, E. T., & Hodgson, E. (2015). Virtual reality disaster training: Translation to practice. *Nurse Education in Practice, 15*(1), 53–57. https://doi.org/10.1016/j.nepr.2013.08.017.

Farrington, M., Ward, E., & Dawson, C. (2020). Reducing Reliance on Agency Staff = $7.7 Million in Savings and Improved Nurse Engagement. *Journal of perianesthesia nursing : official journal of the American Society of PeriAnesthesia Nurses, 35*(3), 333–336. https://doi.org/10.1016/j.jopan.2020.02.006.

Fischer, S. A. (2016). Transformational leadership in nursing: A concept analysis. *Journal of Advanced Nursing, 72*(11), 2644–2653. https://doi.org/10.1111/jan.13049.

Fitzgerald, L., & Harvey, G. (2015). Translational networks in healthcare? Evidence on the design and initiation of organizational networks for knowledge mobilization. *Social Science & Medicine, 138*, 192–200. https://doi.org/10.1016/j.socscimed.2015.06.015.

Fleiszer, A. R., Semenic, S. E., Ritchie, J. A., Richer, M. C., & Denis, J. L. (2016). Nursing unit leaders' influence on the long-term sustainability of evidence-based practice improvements. *Journal of Nursing Management, 24*(3), 309–318. https://doi.org/10.1111/jonm.12320.

Gagliardi, A. R., Webster, F., Perrier, L., Bell, M., & Straus, S. (2014). Exploring mentorship as a strategy to build capacity for knowledge translation research and practice: A scoping systematic review. *Implementation Science, 9*, 122. https://doi.org/10.1186/s13012-014-0122-z.

Galdikiene, N., Asikainen, P., Rostila, I., Green, P., Balciunas, S., & Suominen, T. (2016). Organizational social context in primary health care. *Nordic Journal of Nursing Research, 36*(2), 103–111. https://doi.org/10.1177/2057158516628728.

Gawlinski, A., & Rutledge, D. (2008). Selecting a model for evidence-based practice changes: A practical approach. *AACN Advanced Critical Care, 19*(3), 291–300. https://doi.org/10.1097/01.AACN.0000330380.41766.63.

Gifford, W. A., Squires, J. E., Angus, D. E., Ashley, L. A., Brosseau, L., Craik, J. M., et al. (2018). Managerial leadership for research use in nursing and allied health care professions: A systematic review. *Implementation Science, 13*(1), 127. https://doi.org/10.1186/s13012-018-0817-7.

Glisson, C. (2015). The role of organizational culture and climate in innovation and effectiveness. *Human Service Organizations, Management, Leadership & Governance, 39*(4), 245–250. https://doi.org/10.1080/23303131.2015.1087770.

Goedhart, N. S., van Oostveen, C. J., & Vermeulen, H. (2017). The effect of structural empowerment of nurses on quality outcomes in hospitals: A scoping review. *Journal of Nursing Management, 25*(3), 194–206. https://doi.org/10.1111/jonm.12455.

Goldstein, H., & Olswang, L. (2017). Is there a science to facilitate implementation of evidence-based practices and programs? *Evidence-Based Communication Assessment and Intervention, 11*(3-4), 55–60. https://doi.org/10.1080/17489539.2017.1416768.

Gorman, V. L. (2019). Future emergency nursing workforce: What the evidence is telling us. *Journal of Emergency Nursing, 45*(2), 132–136. https://doi.org/10.1016/j.jen.2018.09.009.

Greenhalgh, T. (2018). *How to implement evidence-based healthcare*. Hoboken, NJ: Wiley & Sons.

Gude, W. T., Roos-Blom, M. J., van der Veer, S. N., Dongelmans, D. A., de Jonge, E., Peek, N., & de Keizer,

N. F. (2019). Facilitating action planning within audit and feedback interventions: A mixed-methods process evaluation of an action implementation toolbox in intensive care. *Implementation Science, 14*(1), 90. https://doi.org/10.1186/s13012-019-0937-8.

Hageman, M. G., Ring, D. C., Gregory, P. J., Rubash, H. E., & Harmon, L. (2015). Do 360-degree feedback survey results relate to patient satisfaction measures? *Clinical Orthopaedics and Related Research, 473*(5), 1590–1597. https://doi.org/10.1007/s11999-014-3981-3.

Hairr, D. C., Salisbury, H., Johannsson, M., & Redfern-Vance, N. (2014). Nurse staffing and the relationship to job satisfaction and retention. *Nursing Economic, 32*(3), 142–147.

Halter, M., Boiko, O., Pelone, F., Beighton, C., Harris, R., Gale, J., et al. (2017). The determinants and consequences of adult nursing staff turnover: A systematic review of systematic reviews. *BMC Health Services Research, 17*(1), 824. https://doi.org/10.1186/s12913-017-2707-0.

Hanrahan, K., Wagner, M., Matthews, G., Stewart, S., Dawson, C., Greiner, J., et al. (2015). Sacred cow gone to pasture: A systematic evaluation and integration of evidence-based practice. *Worldviews on Evidence-Based Nursing, 12*(1), 3–11. https://doi.org/10.1111/wvn.12072.

Harrison, M. B., Graham, I. D., van den Hoek, J., Dogherty, E. J., Carley, M. E., & Angus, V. (2013). Guideline adaptation and implementation planning: A prospective observational study. *Implementation Science, 8*(49). https://doi.org/10.1186/1748-5908-8-49.

Harvey, G., Gifford, W., Cummings, G., Kelly, J., Kislov, R., Kitson, A., et al. (2019). Mobilising evidence to improve nursing practice: A qualitative study of leadership roles and processes in four countries. *International Journal of Nursing Studies, 90*, 21–30. https://doi.org/10.1016/j.ijnurstu.2018.09.017.

Harvey, G., & Kitson, A. (2015). *Implementing evidence-based practice in healthcare: A facilitation guide*. London: Routledge.

Hauck, S., Winsett, R. P., & Kuric, J. (2013). Leadership facilitation strategies to establish evidence-based practice in an acute care hospital. *Journal of Advanced Nursing, 69*(3), 664–674. https://doi.org/10.1111/j.1365-2648.2012.06053.x.

Heekin, A. M., Kontor, J., Sax, H. C., Keller, M. S., Wellington, A., & Weingarten, S. (2018). Choosing wisely clinical decision support adherence and associated inpatient outcomes. *American Journal of Managed Care, 24*(8), 361–366.

Helfrich, C. D., Rose, A. J., Hartmann, C. W., van Bodegom-Vos, L., Graham, I. D., Wood, S. J., et al. (2018). How the dual process model of human cognition can inform efforts to de-implement ineffective and harmful clinical practices: A preliminary model of unlearning and substitution. *Journal of Evaluation in Clinical Practice, 24*(1), 198–205. https://doi.org/10.1111/jep.12855.

Hole, G. O., Brenna, S. J., Graverholt, B., Ciliska, D., & Nortvedt, M. W. (2016). Educating change agents: A qualitative descriptive study of graduates of a Master's program in evidence-based practice. *BMC Medical Education, 16*(71). https://doi.org/10.1186/s12909-016-0597-1.

Hollenbeak, C. S., & Schilling, A. L. (2018). The attributable cost of catheter-associated urinary tract infections in the United States: A systematic review. *American Journal of Infection Control, 46*(7), 751–757. https://doi.org/10.1016/j.ajic.2018.01.015.

Hosking, J., Knox, K., Forman, J., Montgomery, L. A., Valde, J. G., & Cullen, L. (2016). Evidence into practice: Leading new graduate nurses to evidence-based practice through a nurse residency program. *Journal of PeriAnesthesia Nursing, 31*(3), 260–265. https://doi.org/10.1016/j.jopan.2016.02.006.

Huddleston, P., & Gray, J. (2016a). Measuring nurse leaders' and direct care nurses' perceptions of a healthy work environment in an acute care setting, part 1: A pilot study. *Journal of Nursing Administration, 46*(7-8), 373–378. https://doi.org/10.1097/NNA.0000000000000361.

Huddleston, P., & Gray, J. (2016b). Describing nurse leaders' and direct care nurses' perceptions of a healthy work environment in acute care settings, part 2. *Journal of Nursing Administration, 46*(9), 462–467. https://doi.org/10.1097/NNA.0000000000000376.

Huddleston, P., Mancini, M. E., & Gray, J. (2017). Measuring nurse leaders' and direct care nurses' perceptions of a healthy work environment in acute care settings, part 3: Healthy work environment scales for nurse leaders and direct care nurses. *Journal of Nursing Administration, 47*(3), 140–146. https://doi.org/10.1097/NNA.0000000000000456.

Huether, K., Abbott, L., Cullen, L., Cullen, L., & Gaarde, A. (2016). Energy through motion: An evidence-based exercise program to reduce cancer-related fatigue and improve quality of life. *Clinical Journal of Oncology Nursing, 20*(3), E60–E70. https://doi.org/10.1188/16.CJON.E60-E70.

Hysong, S. J., Kell, H. J., Petersen, L. A., Campbell, B. A., & Trautner, B. W. (2017). Theory-based and evidence-based design of audit and feedback programmes: Examples from two clinical intervention studies. *BMJ Quality & Safety, 26*(4), 323–334. https://doi.org/10.1136/bmjqs-2015-004796.

Institute for Healthcare Improvement. (2015). *The Science of Improvement on a Whiteboard!*. http://www.ihi.org/education/IHIOpenSchool/resources/Pages/BobLloydWhiteboard.aspx.

Institute for Healthcare Improvement. (2016). *Governance Leadership of Safety and Improvement*. http://www.ihi.org/Topics/GovernanceLeadership/Pages/default.aspx.

Institute for Healthcare Improvement. (2019). *Family of Measures*. http://www.ihi.org/education/IHIOpenSchool/resources/Pages/AudioandVideo/Whiteboard15.aspx.

Institute of Medicine. (2011). *Clinical Practice Guidelines we can Trust*. Washington, DC: The National Acadmies Press.

Institute of Translational Health Sciences. (2019a). *Definitions of Clinical and Translational Research*. https://www.iths.org/investigators/definitions/definitions-of-clinical-and-translational-research/.

Institute of Translational Health Sciences. (2019b). *T-phases of Translational Health Record*. https://www.iths.org/investigators/definitions/translational-research/.

Iowa Model Collaborative. (2017). Iowa model of evidence-based practice: Revisions and validation. *Worldviews on Evidence-Based Nursing, 14*(3), 175–182. https://doi.org/10.1111/wvn.12223.

Ishikawa, S. I., Kishida, K., Oka, T., Saito, A., Shimotsu, S., Watanabe, N., et al. (2019). Developing the universal unified prevention program for diverse disorders for school-aged children. *Child and Adolescent Psychiatry and Mental Health, 13*(44). https://doi.org/10.1186/s13034-019-0303-2.

Jansson, I., & Forsberg, A. (2016). How do nurses and ward managers perceive that evidence-based sources are obtained to inform relevant nursing interventions?–An exploratory study. *Journal of Clinical Nursing, 25*(5-6), 769–776. https://doi.org/10.1111/jocn.13095.

Jungquist, C. R., Chandola, V., Spulecki, C., Nguyen, K. V., Crescenzi, P., Tekeste, D., et al. (2019). Identifying patients experiencing opioid-induced respiratory depression during recovery from anesthesia: The application of electronic monitoring devices. *Worldviews on Evidence-Based Nursing, 16*(3), 186–194. https://doi.org/10.1111/wvn.12362.

Kalisch, B., & Lee, K. H. (2014). Staffing and job satisfaction: Nurses and nursing assistants. *Journal of Nursing Management, 22*(4), 465–471. https://doi.org/10.1111/jonm.12012.

Kouzes, J. M., & Posner, B. Z. (2012). *The Leadership Challenge: How to Make Extraordinary Things Happen in Organizations*. San Franscisco, CA: Jossey-Bass.

Kowalski, M. O., Basile, C., Bersick, E., Cole, D. A., McClure, D. E., & Weaver, S. H. (2019). What do nurses need to practice effectively in the hospital environment? An integrative review with implications for nurse leaders. *Worldviews on Evidence-Based Nursing*. https://doi.org/10.1111/wvn.12401.

Lahey, T., & Nelson, W. (2020). A dashboard to improve the alignment of healthcare organization decisionmaking to core values and mission statement. *Cambridge Quarterly of Healthcare Ethics, 29*(1), 156–162. https://doi.org/10.1017/S0963180119000884.

Lee, M. C., Johnson, K. L., Newhouse, R. P., & Warren, J. I. (2013). Evidence-based practice process quality assessment: EPQA guidelines. *Worldviews on Evidence-Based Nursing, 10*(3), 140–149. https://doi.org/10.1111/j.1741-6787.2012.00264.x.

Lee, S. S., Kelley, M., Cho, M. K., Kraft, S. A., James, C., Constantine M., et al. (2016). Adrift in the gray zone: IRB perspectives on research in the learning health system. *AJOB Empirical Bioethics, 7*(2), 125–134. https://doi.org/10.1080/23294515.2016.1155674.

Leeman, J., Calancie, L., Kegler, M. C., Escoffery, C. T., Herrmann, A. K., Thatcher E., et al. (2017). Developing theory to guide building practitioners' capacity to implement evidence-based interventions. *Health Education & Behavior, 44*(1), 59–69. https://doi.org/10.1177/1090198115610572.

Lewis, A., Harvey, G., Hogan, M., & Kitson, A. (2019). Can oral healthcare for older people be embedded into routine community aged care practice? A realist evaluation using normalisation process theory. *International Journal of Nursing Studies, 94*, 32–41. https://doi.org/10.1016/j.ijnurstu.2018.12.016.

Lewis, C. C., Klasnja, P., Powell, B. J., Lyon, A. R., Tuzzio, L., Jones, S., et al. (2018). From classification to causality: Advancing understanding of mechanisms of change in implementation science. *Frontiers in Public Health, 6*(136). https://doi.org/10.3389/fpubh.2018.00136.

Li, S. A., Jeffs, L., Barwick, M., & Stevens, B. (2018). Organizational contextual features that influence the implementation of evidence-based practices across healthcare settings: A systematic integrative review. *Systematic Reviews, 7*(1), 72. https://doi.org/10.1186/s13643-018-0734-5.

Little, S. H., Dickerson, P. S., Randolph, G., Rocco, P., & Short, N. (2017). Using the ARCC model to implement the 2015 ANCC COA criteria: A North Carolina public health nursing project. *Journal of Continuing Education in Nursing, 48*(11), 501–507. https://doi.org/10.3928/00220124-20171017-07.

Luckson, M., Duncan, F., Rajai, A., & Haigh, C. (2018). Exploring the research culture of nurses and allied health professionals (AHPs) in a research-focused and a non-research-focused healthcare organisation in the UK. *Journal of Clinical Nursing, 27*(7-8), e1462–e1476. https://doi.org/10.1111/jocn.14264.

Martin, C. J. (2015). The effects of nurse staffing on quality of care. *Medsurg Nursing, 24*(2), 4–6 Suppl.

Mason, D. J., Keepnews, D., Holmberg, J., & Murray, E. (2013). The representation of health professionals on governing boards of health care organizations in New York City. *Journal of Urban Health: Bulletin of the New York Academy of Medicine, 90*(5), 888–901. https://doi.org/10.1007/s11524-012-9772-9.

May, C. R., Mair, F., Finch, T., MacFarlane, A., Dowrick, C., Treweek, S., et al. (2009). Development of a theory of implementation and integration: Normalization process theory. *Implementation Science, 4*(29). https://doi.org/10.1186/1748-5908-4-29.

McKay, V. R., Hoffer, L. D., Combs, T. B., & Margaret Dolcini, M. (2018). The dynamic influence of human resources on evidence-based intervention sustainability and population outcomes: An agent-based modeling approach. *Implementation Science, 13*(1), 77. https://doi.org/10.1186/s13012-018-0767-0.

Melnyk, B. M., Fineout-Overholt, E., Giggleman, M., & Choy, K. (2017). A test of the ARCC© model improves implementation of evidence-based practice, healthcare culture, and patient outcomes. *Worldviews on Evidence-Based Nursing, 14*(1), 5–9. https://doi.org/10.1111/wvn.12188.

Melnyk, B. M., Gallagher-Ford, L., Thomas, B. K., Troseth, M., Wyngarden, K., & Szalacha, L. (2016). A study of chief nurse executives indicates low prioritization of evidence-based practice and shortcomings in hospital performance metrics across the United States. *Worldviews on Evidence-Based Nursing, 13*(1), 6–14. https://doi.org/10.1111/wvn.12133.

Michie, S., Atkins, L., & West, R. (2014). *The behaviour change wheel: A guide to designing interventions.* London: Silverback Publishing.

Minnick, A. F., Kleinpell, R., & Allison, T. L. (2019). Reports of three organizations' members about doctor of nursing practice project experiences and outcomes. *Nursing Outlook, 67*(6), 671–679. https://doi.org/10.1016/j.outlook.2019.05.012.

Mishuris, R. G., Palmisano, J., McCullagh, L., Hess, R., Feldstein, D. A., Smith, P. D., et al. (2019). Using normalisation process theory to understand workflow implications of decision support implementation across diverse primary care settings. *BMJ Health & Care Informatics, 26*(1), Article e100088. https://doi.org/10.1136/bmjhci-2019-100088.

Mohammadi, M. M., Poursaberi, R., & Salahshoor, M. R. (2018). Evaluating the adoption of evidence-based practice using Rogers's diffusion of innovation theory: A model testing study. *Health Promotion Perspectives, 8*(1), 25–32. https://doi.org/10.15171/hpp.2018.03.

Mondoux, S., & Shojania, K. G. (2019). Evidence-based medicine: A cornerstone for clinical care but not for quality improvement. *Journal of Evaluation in Clinical Practice, 25*(3), 363–368. https://doi.org/10.1111/jep.13135.

Moore, J. E., Mascarenhas, A., Bain, J., & Straus, S. E. (2017). Developing a comprehensive definition of sustainability. *Implementation Science, 12*(1), 110. https://doi.org/10.1186/s13012-017-0637-1.

Moreno-Poyato, A. R., Delgado-Hito, P., Leyva-Moral, J. M., Casanova-Garrigos, G., & Monteso-Curto, P. (2019). Implementing evidence-based practices on the therapeutic relationship in inpatient psychiatric care: A participatory action research. *Journal of Clinical Nursing, 28*(9-10), 1614–1622. https://doi.org/10.1111/jocn.14759.

Morton, S., Wilson, S., Inglis, S., Ritchie, K., & Wales, A. (2018). Developing a framework to evaluate knowledge into action interventions. *BMC Health Services Research, 18*(1), 133. https://doi.org/10.1186/s12913-018-2930-3.

Muhwava, L. S., Murphy, K., Zarowsky, C., & Levitt, N. (2019). Experiences of lifestyle change among women with gestational diabetes mellitus (GDM): A behavioural diagnosis using the COM-B model in a low-income setting. *PLoS One, 14*(11), Article e0225431. https://doi.org/10.1371/journal.pone.0225431.

Murt, M. F., Krouse, A. M., Baumberger-Henry, M. L., & Drayton-Brooks, S. M. (2019). Nurses at the table: A naturalistic inquiry of nurses on governing boards. *Nursing Forum, 54*(4), 575–581. https://doi.org/10.1111/nuf.12372.

NAM. (2017). *Optimizing Strategies for Clinical Decision Support: Summary of a Meeting Series.* https://nam.edu/optimizing-strategies-clinical-decision-support/.

NHS Institute for Innovation and Improvemen. (2010). *Sustainability Model.* https://improvement.nhs.uk/documents/2174/sustainability-model.pdf.

NIH. (2019). *Implementation Science News, Resources and Funding for Global Health Researchers.* https://www.fic.nih.gov/ResearchTopics/Pages/ImplementationScience.aspx.

Nilsen, P. (2015). Making sense of implementation theories, models and frameworks. *Implementation Science, 10*(1), 53. https://doi.org/10.1186/s13012-015-0242-0.

Norton, S., Milat, A., Edwards, B., & Giffin, M. (2016). Narrative review of strategies by organizations for building evaluation capacity. *Evaluation and Program Planning, 58*, 1–19. https://doi.org/10.1016/j.evalprogplan.2016.04.004.

NSI Nursing Solutions Inc. (2019). *2019 National Health Care Retention & RN Staffing Report.* http://www.nsinursingsolutions.com/Files/assets/library/retentioninstitute/2019%20National%20Health%20Care%20Retention%20Report.pdf.

Office of Human Research Protections, U.S. Department of Health & Human Services. (n.d.). *Quality improvement activities FAQs.* https://www.hhs.gov/ohrp/regulations-and-policy/guidance/faq/quality-improvement-activities/index.html.

Office of Public Health Preparedness and Response. (2015). *Immediate need for healthcare facilities to review procedures for cleaning, disinfecting, and sterilizing reusable medical devices*. Atlanta, GA: U.S: Department of Health & Human Services.

Ouayogode, M. H., Mainor, A. J., Meara, E., Bynum, J. P. W., & Colla, C. H. (2019). Association between care management and outcomes among patients with complex needs in Medicare accountable care organizations. *JAMA Network Open, 2*(7), Article e196939. https://doi.org/10.1001/jamanetworkopen.2019.6939.

Parry, G., Coly, A., Goldmann, D., Rowe, A. K., Chattu, V., Logiudice, D., et al. (2018). Practical recommendations for the evaluation of improvement initiatives. *International Journal for Quality in Health Care, 30*(suppl 1), 29–36. https://doi.org/10.1093/intqhc/mzy021.

Pasero, C. (2009). Assessment of sedation during opioid administration for pain management. *Journal of PeriAnesthesia Nursing, 24*(3), 186–190. https://doi.org/10.1016/j.jopan.2009.03.005.

Patel, M. S., Volpp, K. G., Small, D. S., Wynne, C., Zhu, J., Yang, L., et al. (2017). Using active choice within the electronic health record to increase influenza vaccination rates. *Journal of General Internal Medicine, 32*(7), 790–795. https://doi.org/10.1007/s11606-017-4046-6.

Patey, A. M., Hurt, C. S., Grimshaw, J. M., & Francis, J. J. (2018). Changing behaviour 'more or less'-do theories of behaviour inform strategies for implementation and de-implementation? A critical interpretive synthesis. *Implementation Science, 13*(1), 134. https://doi.org/10.1186/s13012-018-0826-6.

Patterson, A. E., Mason, T. M., & Duncan, P. (2017). Enhancing a culture of inquiry: The role of a clinical nurse specialist in supporting the adoption of evidence. *Journal of Nursing Administration, 47*(3), 154–158. https://doi.org/10.1097/NNA.0000000000000458.

Perry, C. K., Damschroder, L. J., Hemler, J. R., Woodson, T. T., Ono, S. S., & Cohen, D. J. (2019). Specifying and comparing implementation strategies across seven large implementation interventions: A practical application of theory. *Implementation Science, 14*(1), 32. https://doi.org/10.1186/s13012-019-0876-4.

Phelan, S., Lin, F., Mitchell, M., & Chaboyer, W. (2018). Implementing early mobilisation in the intensive care unit: An integrative review. *International Journal of Nursing Studies, 77*, 91–105. https://doi.org/10.1016/j.ijnurstu.2017.09.019.

Pittman, J., Cohee, A., Storey, S., LaMothe, J., Gilbert, J., Bakoyannis, G., et al. (2019). A multisite health system survey to assess organizational context to support evidence-based practice. *Worldviews on Evidence-Based Nursing, 16*(4), 271–280. https://doi.org/10.1111/wvn.12375.

Porter-O'Grady, T., & Malloch, K. (2008). Beyond myth and magic: The future of evidence-based leadership. *Nursing Administration Quarterly, 32*(3), 176–187. https://doi.org/10.1097/01.NAQ.0000325174.30923.b6.

Powell, B. J., Mandell, D. S., Hadley, T. R., Rubin, R. M., Evans, A. C., Hurford, M. O., et al. (2017). Are general and strategic measures of organizational context and leadership associated with knowledge and attitudes toward evidence-based practices in public behavioral health settings? A cross-sectional observational study. *Implementation Science, 12*(1), 64. https://doi.org/10.1186/s13012-017-0593-9.

Powell, B. J., Waltz, T. J., Chinman, M. J., Damschroder, L. J., Smith, J. L., Matthieu, M. M., et al. (2015). A refined compilation of implementation strategies: Results from the expert recommendations for implementing change (ERIC) project. *Implementation Science, 10*(21). https://doi.org/10.1186/s13012-015-0209-1.

Prochaska, J. J., & Sanders-Jackson, A. (2016). Patient decision aids for discouraging low-value health care procedures: Null findings and lessons learned. *JAMA Internal Medicine, 176*(1), 41–42. https://doi.org/10.1001/jamainternmed.2015.7347.

QSEN Institute. (2019). *Quality and Safety Education for Nurses*. http://qsen.org/competencies/.

Renolen, A., Hjalmhult, E., Hoye, S., Danbolt, L. J., & Kirkevold, M. (2020). Creating room for evidence-based practice: Leader behavior in hospital wards. *Research in Nursing & Health*. https://doi.org/10.1002/nur.21981.

Renolen, A., Hoye, S., Hjalmhult, E., Danbolt, L. J., & Kirkevold, M. (2018). "Keeping on track"-Hospital nurses' struggles with maintaining workflow while seeking to integrate evidence-based practice into their daily work: A grounded theory study. *International Journal of Nursing Studies, 77*, 179–188. https://doi.org/10.1016/j.ijnurstu.2017.09.006.

Robertson-Malt, S., & Norton-Westwood, D. (2017). Framework of care: Communicating the structure and processes of care. *International Journal of Evidence-Based Healthcare, 15*(3), 82–89. https://doi.org/10.1097/XEB.0000000000000114.

Rogers, E. (2003). *Diffusion of innovations* (5th ed.). New York: The Free Press.

Roush, K., & Tesoro, M. (2018). An examination of the rigor and value of final scholarly projects completed by DNP nursing students. *Journal of Professional Nursing, 34*(6), 437–443. https://doi.org/10.1016/j.profnurs.2018.03.003.

Royer, H. R., Crary, P., Fayram, E., & Heidrich, S. M. (2018). Five-year program evaluation of an evidence-based practice scholars program. *Journal of Continuation Education in Nursing, 49*(12), 547–554. https://doi.org/10.3928/00220124-20181116-05.

Rubio, D. M., Schoenbaum, E. E., Lee, L. S., Schteingart, D. E., Marantz, P. R., Anderson, K. E., et al. (2010). Defining translational research: implications for training. *Academic Medicine, 85*(3), 470–475. https://doi.org/10.1097/ACM.0b013e3181ccd618.

Rutledge, R. I., Romaire, M. A., Hersey, C. L., Parish, W. J., Kissam, S. M., & Lloyd, J. T. (2019). Medicaid accountable care organizations in four states: Implementation and early impacts. *Milbank Quarterly, 97*(2), 583–619. https://doi.org/10.1111/1468-0009.12386.

Sackett, D. L., Strauss, S. E., Richardson, W. S., Rosenberg, W., & Haynes, R. B. (2000). *Evidence-based medicine: How to practice and team EBM* (2nd ed.). Edinburgh: Churchill Livingstone.

Sadeghnezhad, M., Heshmati Nabavi, F., Najafi, F., Kareshki, H., & Esmaily, H. (2018). Mutual benefits in academic-service partnership: An integrative review. *Nurse Education Today, 68*, 78–85. https://doi.org/10.1016/j.nedt.2018.05.019.

Sadler, B. L., Joseph, A., Keller, A., & Rostenberg, B. (2009). *Using evidence-based environmental design to enhance safety and quality*. IHI Innovation Series white Paper. Institute for Healthcare Improvement. www.IHI.org.

Sarkies, M. N., Bowles, K. A., Skinner, E. H., Haas, R., Lane, H., & Haines, T. P. (2017). The effectiveness of research implementation strategies for promoting evidence-informed policy and management decisions in healthcare: A systematic review. *Implementation Science, 12*(1), 132. https://doi.org/10.1186/s13012-017-0662-0.

Saunders, H., & Vehvilainen-Julkunen, K. (2017). Nurses' evidence-based practice beliefs and the role of evidence-based practice mentors at University Hospitals in Finland. *Worldviews on Evidence-Based Nursing, 14*(1), 35–45. https://doi.org/10.1111/wvn.12189.

Schaffer, M. A., Sandau, K. E., & Diedrick, L. (2013). Evidence-based practice models for organizational change: Overview and practical applications. *Journal of Advanced Nursing, 69*(5), 1197–1209. https://doi.org/10.1111/j.1365-2648.2012.06122.x.

Schein, E. H., & Schein, P. (2016). *Organizational culture and leadership* (5th ed.): Hoboken, NJ: John Wiley & Sons Inc.

Scott 2nd, R.D., Culler, S. D., & Rask, K. J. (2019). Understanding the economic impact of health care-associated infections: A cost perspective analysis. *Journal of Infusion Nursing, 42*(2), 61–69. https://doi.org/10.1097/NAN.0000000000000313.

Seneski, A., & Stack, A. M. (2019). A framework for maintenance and scaling of an evidence-based guideline program. *Pediatric Quality & Safety, 4*(2), e153. https://doi.org/10.1097/pq9.0000000000000153.

Shrank, W. H., Rogstad, T. L., & Parekh, N. (2019). Waste in the US health care system: Estimated costs and potential for savings. *JAMA, 322*(15), 1501–1509. https://doi.org/10.1001/jama.2019.13978.

Shuman, C. J. (2017). *Addressing the practice context in evidence-based practice implementation: Leadership and climate* (PhD thesis). Ann Arbor, MI: University of Michigan.

Shuman, C. J., Liu, X., Aebersold, M. L., Tschannen, D., Banaszak-Holl, J., & Titler, M. G. (2018). Associations among unit leadership and unit climates for implementation in acute care: A cross-sectional study. *Implementation Science, 13*(1), 62. https://doi.org/10.1186/s13012-018-0753-6.

Sigma Theta Tau International Research Scholarship Advisory Committee. (2008). Sigma Theta Tau International position statement on evidence-based practice February 2007 summary. *Worldviews on Evidence-Based Nursing, 5*(2), 57–59. https://doi.org/10.1111/j.1741-6787.2008.00118.x.

Spiva, L., Hart, P. L., Patrick, S., Waggoner, J., Jackson, C., & Threatt, J. L. (2017). Effectiveness of an evidence-based practice nurse mentor training program. *Worldviews on Evidence-Based Nursing, 14*(3), 183–191. https://doi.org/10.1111/wvn.12219.

SQUIRE. (2017). *SQUIRE 2.0 guidelines*. http://squire-statement.org/index.cfm?fuseaction=Page.ViewPage&PageID=471.

Staines, A., Vanderavero, P., Duvillard, B., Deriaz, P., Erard, P., Kundig, F., et al. (2018). Sustained improvement in hand hygiene compliance using a multi-modal improvement programme at a Swiss multi-site regional hospital. *Journal of Hospital Infection, 100*(2), 176–182. https://doi.org/10.1016/j.jhin.2018.04.010.

Stetler, C. B. (2001). Updating the Stetler Model of research utilization to facilitate evidence-based practice. *Nursing Outlook, 49*(6), 272–279. https://doi.org/10.1067/mno.2001.120517.

Stetler, C. B., Ritchie, J. A., Rycroft-Malone, J., & Charns, M. P. (2014). Leadership for evidence-based practice: strategic and functional behaviors for institutionalizing EBP. *Worldviews on Evidence-Based Nursing, 11*(4), 219–226. https://doi.org/10.1111/wvn.12044.

Stevens, K. R. (2013). The impact of evidence-based practice in nursing and the next big ideas. *OJIN: Online Journal of Issues in Nursing, 18*(2), 4.

Stewart, R. E., Adams, D. R., Mandell, D. S., Nangia G., Shaffer, L., Evans A. C., et al. (2017). Non-participant,s in policy efforts to promote evidence-based practices in a large behavioral health system. *Implementation Science, 12*(1), 70. https://doi.org/10.1186/s13012-017-0598-4.

Storey, S., Wagnes, L., LaMothe, J., Pittman, J., Cohee, A., & Newhouse, R. (2019). Building evidence-based nursing practice capacity in a large statewide health system: A multimodal approach. *Journal of Nursing*

Administration, 49(4), 208–214. https://doi.org/10.1097/NNA.0000000000000739.

Straus, S. E., Tetroe, J. M., & Graham, I. D. (2011). Knowledge translation is the use of knowledge in health care decision making. *Journal of Clinical Epidemiology, 64*(1), 6–10. https://doi.org/10.1016/j.jclinepi.2009.08.016.

Strifler, L., Cardoso, R., McGowan, J., Cogo, E., Nincic, V., Khan, P. A., et al. (2018). Scoping review identifies significant number of knowledge translation theories, models, and frameworks with limited use. *Journal of Clinical Epidemiology, 100*, 92–102. https://doi.org/10.1016/j.jclinepi.2018.04.008.

Sveinsdottir, H., Ragnarsdottir, E. D., & Blondal, K. (2016). Praise matters: The influence of nurse unit managers' praise on nurses' practice, work environment and job satisfaction: a questionnaire study. *Journal of Advanced Nursing, 72*(3), 558–568. https://doi.org/10.1111/jan.12849.

Taylor, N., Clay-Williams, R., Hogden, E., Braithwaite, J., & Groene, O. (2015). High performing hospitals: A qualitative systematic review of associated factors and practical strategies for improvement. *BMC Health Services Research, 15*(244). https://doi.org/10.1186/s12913-015-0879-z.

The Joint Commission. (2016). *R3 report issue 2: CAUTI.* https://www.jointcommission.org/standards/r3-report/r3-report-issue-2-cauti/.

The Joint Commission. (n.d.). ORYX performance measures. https://www.jointcommission.org/the_joint_commission_measures_effective_january_1_2019/.

Titler, M. G. (2018). Translation research in practice: An introduction. *OJIN: The Online Journal of Issues in Nursing, 23*(2). Manuscript 1. https://doi.org/10.3912/OJIN.Vol23No02Man01.

U.S. Bureau of Labor Statistics. (2019). *Occupational outlook handbook*. https://www.bls.gov/ooh/.

Valim, M. D., Rocha, I. L. S., Souza, T. P. M., Cruz, Y. A. D., Bezerra, T. B., Baggio, E., et al. (2019). Efficacy of the multimodal strategy for Hand Hygiene compliance: An integrative review. *Revista Brasileira de Enfermagem, 72*(2), 552–565. https://doi.org/10.1590/0034-7167-2018-0584.

Van de Velde, S., Heselmans A., Delvaux N., Brandt L., Marco-Ruiz L., Spitaels D., et al. (2018). A systematic review of trials evaluating success factors of interventions with computerised clinical decision support. *Implementation Science, 13*(1), 114. https://doi.org/10.1186/s13012-018-0790-1.

van der Zijpp, T. J., Niessen, T., Eldh, A. C., Hawkes, C., McMullan, C., Mockford, C., et al. (2016). A bridge over turbulent waters: Illustrating the interaction between managerial leaders and facilitators when implementing research evidence. *Worldviews on Evidence-Based Nursing, 13*(1), 25–31. https://doi.org/10.1111/wvn.12138.

Wang, V., Maciejewski, M. L., Helfrich, C. D., & Weiner, B. J. (2018). Working smarter not harder: Coupling implementation to de-implementation. *Healthcare (Amsterdam, Netherlands), 6*(2), 104–107. https://doi.org/10.1016/j.hjdsi.2017.12.004.

Warren, J. I., Montgomery, K. L., & Friedmann, E. (2016). Three-year pre-post analysis of EBP integration in a Magnet-designated community hospital. *Worldviews on Evidence-Based Nursing, 13*(1), 50–58. https://doi.org/10.1111/wvn.12148.

Willis, W. K., Muslin, I., & Timko, K. N. (2016). A house divided: Cooperative and competitive recruitment in vital industries. *Journal of Nursing Management, 24*(2), 253–260. https://doi.org/10.1111/jonm.12308.

Xue, Y., Chappel, A. R., Freund, D. A., Aiken, L. H., & Noyes, K. (2015). Cost outcomes of supplemental nurse staffing in a large medical center. *Journal of Nursing Care Quality, 30*(2), 130–137. https://doi.org/10.1097/NCQ.0000000000000100.

Yoo, J. Y., Kim, J. H., Kim, J. S., Kim, H. L., & Ki, J. S. (2019). Clinical nurses' beliefs, knowledge, organizational readiness and level of implementation of evidence-based practice: The first step to creating an evidence-based practice culture. *PLoS One, 14*(12), Article e0226742. https://doi.org/10.1371/journal.pone.0226742.

Zhang, H., Cowling, D. W., Graham, J. M., & Taylor, E. (2019). Five-year impact of a commercial accountable care Organization on health care spending, utilization, and quality of care. *Medical Care, 57*(11), 845–854. https://doi.org/10.1097/MLR.0000000000001179.

Zhao, Q., Yang, M. M., Huang, Y. Y., & Chen, W. (2018). How to make hand hygiene interventions more attractive to nurses: A discrete choice experiment. *PLoS One, 13*(8), Article e0202014. https://doi.org/10.1371/journal.pone.0202014.

18

Quality and Safety

Luc R. Pelletier

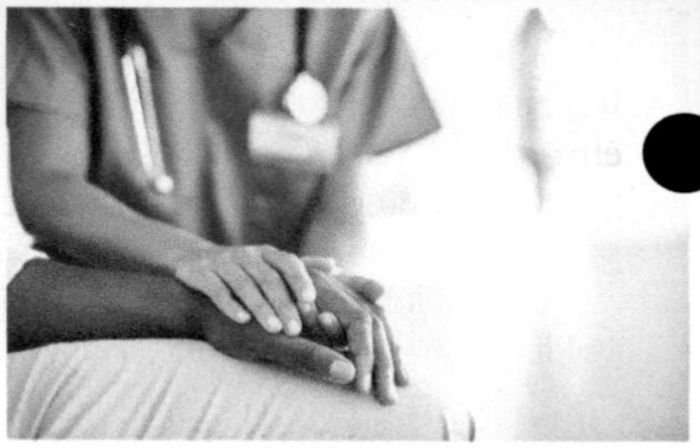

http://evolve.elsevier.com/Huber/leadership

Quality and safety share center stage in value-driven health care. Quality and safety principles and practices form the foundation of an accessible, reliable health care enterprise. Health care quality is an art and science that continues to evolve. Its relevance was heightened with ongoing reports from the American Academy of Nursing, National Academy of Medicine, and other national organizations related to health care and health care quality. Well before these reports were published, however, professional nurses assumed key roles in the business of measuring, monitoring, and improving health care quality and safety. Nurses have typically taken a leadership role in performance and quality improvement and continue to do so in their roles as board members, chief executives, experience officers, chief quality officers, health care quality professionals, enterprise risk managers, and safety officers. It is important to note that identifying opportunities for improvement and continuously improving services is every health care professional's responsibility. Patients and their families also have rights and responsibilities related to quality and safety. Where once there were dedicated quality departments in health care organizations, now best-in-class health care organizations train everyone in performance improvement models and techniques (e.g., *Plan-Do-Study-Act [PDSA]*, Lean, Six Sigma). It would be difficult to describe the entire field of health care quality and patient safety in one chapter. In this chapter a large amount of information and emerging trends have been distilled, and specific content has been targeted toward nurse leaders. This system overview includes definitions of commonly used terms; health care quality in a new millennium; interprofessional collaboration, patient engagement, and self-care as professional nursing imperatives; industrial models and standards of quality; quality and safety performance improvement models; costs associated with waste in health care; and issues and trends in leadership and management. Resources are provided throughout for nurse leaders to use in their everyday practice.

DEFINITIONS

There are many concepts and terms related to health care quality and safety. Definitions are as follows:

Benchmarking "includes routinely comparing indicators (structure, process, and outcomes) against best performance and seeking out ways to make improvements with the greatest impact on outcomes. Ideally, the reference point is a demonstrated best practice" (Rosati, 2018, p. 234).

Continuous quality improvement (CQI) is defined by the American Society for Quality (ASQ) as "a philosophy and attitude for analyzing capabilities and processes and improving them repeatedly to achieve customer satisfaction" (ASQ, 2019a, p. 71). **Evidence-based practice** was originally defined by Sackett et al. (1996) as "the conscientious, explicit, and judicious use of current best evidence in making decisions about the care of individual patients" (p. 71). A **fair and just culture** is defined as "organizational accountability for the systems they've designed and employee accountability for the choices they make" (Paradiso & Sweeney, 2019, p. 40).

Lean originated in manufacturing before being applied to health care. It is "a set of management practices to improve efficiency and effectiveness by eliminating waste. The core principle of lean is to reduce and eliminate non value-adding activities and waste" (ASQ, 2019b, p. 1). **Six Sigma** is achieved when the organization reaches an error or defect rate of 3.4 or less per one million. Six Sigma in health care "reduces the number of errors made by physicians, nurses and technicians; improving lab turnaround times; reducing appointment times; decreasing steps in the supply chain; accelerating reimbursement for insurance claims; and improving patient outcomes" (Villanova University, 2019, p. 5).

Patient engagement is defined as "the desire and capability to actively choose to participate in care in a way uniquely appropriate to the individual in cooperation with a healthcare provider or institution for the purposes of maximizing outcomes or experiences of care" (Higgins et al., 2017, p. 33). **Patient activation** describes the four degrees of engagement, including "Level 1—Disengaged and overwhelmed; Level 2—Becoming aware, but still struggling; Level 3—Taking action; and Level 4—Maintaining behaviors and pushing further" (Insignia Health, 2018, p. 1). Patient activation "is a proxy for terms such as self-care, self-management or readiness for discharge" (Stichler & Pelletier, 2020, p. 3).

Patient safety practices are "a type of process or structure whose application reduces the probability of adverse events resulting from exposure to the healthcare system across a range of diseases and procedures" (Shojania et al., 2001, p. 13).

A **performance measure** is "a quantitative tool (for example, rate, ratio, index, percentage) that provides an indication of an organization's performance in relation to a specified process or outcome" (The Joint Commission [TJC], 2019a, p. 110). A **performance measurement system** is a systems-based approach to quality and safety where "the organization uses evidence-based medicine and clinical decision support tools, engages in performance measurement and improvement, measures and responds to patient experiences and satisfaction, practices population health management, and publicly shares robust quality and safety data and improvement activities" (The Joint Commission, 2019b, p. 6).

A **performance/quality improvement program** is an overarching organizational strategy to ensure accountability of all employees, incorporating evidence-based health care quality indicators to continuously improve care delivered to various populations. It is the organization's blueprint for achieving and maintaining performance excellence. **PDSA** is an acronym for an improvement model for testing change, which includes "developing a plan to test the change (Plan), carrying out the test (Do), observing and learning from the consequences (Study), and determining what modifications should be made to the test (Act)" (Institute for Healthcare Improvement [IHI], 2020a, p.1).

Quality refers to characteristics of and the pursuit of excellence. **Health care quality** is classically defined as "the degree to which health services for individuals and populations increase the likelihood of desired health outcomes and are consistent with current professional knowledge" (Institute of Medicine, 2000, pp. 128–129). Inpatient **quality indicators** are "standardized, evidence-based measures of health care quality that can be used with readily available hospital inpatient administrative data to measure and track clinical performance and outcomes" (AHRQ, n.d.a., p. 3). The Agency for Healthcare Research and Quality (AHRQ) also has quality indicators for prevention, inpatient quality, patient safety, and pediatric care. A high **reliability organization** is "an organization operating in an industry that is complex and has high risk for harm that consistently performs at high levels of safety over long periods of time" (Pelletier & Beaudin, 2018, p. 252).

Risk adjustment is a process in which differences among clients or variables such as age or disease severity are weighted or adjusted for outcomes analyses or benchmarking efforts. **Enterprise risk management (ERM)** "in healthcare promotes a comprehensive framework for making risk management decisions which maximize value protection and creation by managing risk and uncertainty and their connection to total value" (Carroll, 2014, p. 5). An **ERM program** includes components of culture, strategy, objectives, appetite/tolerance, ERM structure and plans, communication and reporting plans, and oversight (Carroll, 2014, pp. 6–8).

A **sentinel event** "is a patient safety event that reaches a patient and results in any of the following: death, permanent harm, or severe temporary harm and intervention required. Such events are called 'sentinel' because they signal the need for immediate investigation and response" (TJC, 2019c, pp. 5–7).

Standards are defined as written value statements. These statements form the rules that apply to key processes and the results that can be expected when the processes are performed according to specifications.

The three basic types of standards for health care quality are (1) structure, (2) process, and (3) outcome, following Donabedian's (1980) quality framework. **Structure standards and measures** focus on the internal characteristics of the organization and its personnel. **Process standards and measures** focus on whether the activities within an organization are being conducted appropriately, effectively, and efficiently. **Outcome standards and measures** refer to a change in the patient's current or future health status that is attributed to antecedent health care and client attributes of health care.

BACKGROUND

HEALTH CARE QUALITY IN A NEW MILLENNIUM

Professional nurses have an obligation to reasonably ensure that the care they provide is evidence based (Sackett et al., 1996) and that work processes are consumer and family centric. Their interventions should be conscious and intentional (Waddill-Goad & Langster, 2016). Providing "quality" health care is "the degree to which health services for individuals and populations increase the likelihood of desired health outcomes and are consistent with current professional knowledge" (Institute of Medicine, 2000, pp. 128–129). As clinical leaders and managers, nurses have served as health care quality professionals and have promoted standardization, measurement, and continuous quality improvement in a variety of care delivery settings. Professional nurses have consistently held the practice of quality and safety management in high regard and have the effective care of clients and families as their primary focus. Nurses are bound by their professional association's *Code of Ethics* (American Nurses Association [ANA], 2015) and scope of professional standards to participate in the continuous improvement of the services they provide. Specifically, in Provision 3, the "nurse promotes, advocates for, and protects the rights, health, and *safety* of the patient" (Hegge, 2015, Set 2: slide 45). Recent health reform legislation serves as a call to action for professional nurses—from frontline clinicians to executives—to be actively involved in health care transformation. This includes nursing taking a leadership role in ensuring patients and families receive safe and effective person-centered health care (Institute of Medicine [IOM], 2011, p. 228).

Although the manufacturing industry has dutifully explored ways to enhance its business practices, health care has lagged behind, and only within the past half century has it embraced improvement concepts. Health care has borrowed and applied models of continuous quality improvement that contained principles and practices originally developed for the manufacturing industry. *Continuous quality improvement (CQI)* is defined by the American Society for Quality (ASQ) as "a philosophy and attitude for analyzing capabilities and processes and improving them repeatedly to achieve customer satisfaction" (ASQ, 2019a, p. 69). As industry has had its quality gurus, so too has the health care quality and safety movement been fostered by health care professionals who have focused on continuous improvement.

Donald M. Berwick, MD, coauthor of the book *Curing Health Care: New Strategies for Quality Improvement* (Berwick et al., 1990), was an early pioneer in identifying how the concepts of CQI programs could apply to health care. In 1991 the National Demonstration Project on Quality Improvement in Health Care was conducted as a collaboration between members of the John A. Hartford Foundation, the Harvard Community Health Plan, the Juran Institute, the Hospital Corporation of America, and other health care organizations (IHI, 2004). The goal was to apply the methods and tools of industrial quality improvement in a variety of organizations to determine whether they could apply to a service industry. Berwick was a principal investigator for this project. As a result of this endeavor, the IHI was founded and became an early advocate for the concepts of process improvement and team problem-solving in health care organizations. In 2010 Berwick was appointed by President Obama as administrator of the Centers for Medicare & Medicaid Services (CMS). He served for 18 months and was responsible for introducing the "Triple Aim": improving the patient care experience, improving population health, and reducing health costs (Berwick et al., 2008). In 2015, a fourth aim was introduced to rename it the "quadruple aim." This additional aim was proposed to address improving the experience of workforce environments, safety, and engagement (Sikka et al., 2015). Berwick's administration was also responsible for initiating major transformative changes under health reform legislation *(Affordable Care Act)*.

In the mid-1990s The Joint Commission (TJC), a health care accreditation organization, began incorporating the principles of CQI in its revised standards. Starting in 1996 the IOM, through its Committee on Quality of Health Care in America (CQHCA), convened the nation's quality leaders and other public and private stakeholders to assess and improve health care for all. These leaders have promoted CQI in health care through education, research, and evaluation. Tenets promoted by these health care leaders and organizations—and embraced by health care professionals—include:

- Processes and systems are the problems, not people.
- Standardization of core processes is key to managing work and people.
- Quality can be enhanced only in safe, nonpunitive, fair, and just work cultures.
- Quality and safety measurement, monitoring, and improvement are everyone's job.
- The impetus for quality monitoring is not primarily for accreditation or regulatory compliance, but as a planned part of an organization's learning culture to continuously enhance and improve its services based on continuous feedback from employees and customers.
- Consumers and stakeholders must be included in all phases of quality improvement planning.
- Consensus among all stakeholders must be gained to have an impact on quality and safety.
- Health policy should include a focus on continuous enhancement of quality and safety.

A framework for understanding health care improvement was proposed by the IOM Committee on Quality of Health Care in America (2001) (Box 18.1). These six aims for health care quality improvement propose that health care systems ensure that care is safe, effective, patient centered, timely, efficient, and equitable.

BOX 18.1 Institute of Medicine's Specific Aims for Health Care Quality Improvement

- *Safe:* "Patients should not be harmed by the care that is intended to help them, nor should harm come to those who work in health care" (IOM, Committee on the National Quality Report on Health Care Delivery, 2001, p. 47).
- *Effective:* "Refers to care that is based on the use of systematically acquired evidence to determine whether an intervention, such as a preventive service, diagnostic test, or therapy, produces better outcomes than do alternatives—including the alternative to do nothing" (IOM, Committee on the National Quality Report on Health Care Delivery, 2001, p. 49). Evidence-based practice requires that those who give care consistently avoid both underuse of effective care and overuse of ineffective care that is more likely to harm than help the patient (Chassin, 1997).
- *Patient-centered:* "Refers to health care that establishes a partnership among practitioners, patients, and their families (when appropriate) to ensure that decisions respect patients' wants, needs, and preferences; and that patients have the education and support they need to make decisions and participate in their own care" (IOM, Committee on the National Quality Report on Health Care Delivery, 2001, p. 50).
- *Timeliness:* "Refers to obtaining needed care and minimizing unnecessary delays in getting that care" (IOM, Committee on the National Quality Report on Health Care Delivery, 2001, p. 53).
- *Efficient:* "Refers to a health care system where resources are used to get the best value for the money spent" (Palmer & Torgerson, 1999, p. 1136). "The opposite of efficiency is waste; the use of resources without benefit to the patients a system is intended to help. There are at least two ways to improve efficiency: (a) reduce quality waste and (b) reduce administrative or production costs" (IOM, CQHCA, 2001, p. 54).
- *Equitable:* "Providing care that does not vary in quality because of personal characteristics such as gender, ethnicity, geographical location, and socioeconomic status" (IOM, CQHCA, 2001, p. 6).

From Pelletier, L.R., & Hoffman, J.A. (2002). A framework for selecting performance measures for opioid treatment programs. *Journal for Healthcare Quality, 24*(3), 25. Reprinted with permission from the National Association for Healthcare Quality.

LEADERSHIP AND MANAGEMENT IMPLICATIONS

Interprofessional Collaboration

Collaboration should be a goal of any interaction, regardless of the workplace or situation. Collaboration is an imperative set by the American Nurses Association (ANA). The ANA, in its current *Guide to the Code of Ethics for Nurses with Interpretive Statements*, proposed that "the nurse collaborates with other health professionals and the public to protect human rights, promote health diplomacy, and reduce health disparities" (Hegge, 2015, Set 3: slide 12). Collaborative partnerships are part of this imperative and shape the way professional nurses act clinically and how they participate in performance and quality improvement efforts. As the complexity of care increases, multidisciplinary and interprofessional teamwork is used to solve complex problems in practice. For example, nursing, medicine, pharmacy, and information technology (IT) personnel may form a team or committee to develop a risk screen and smart alert for patients at risk for delirium in hospital settings.

Collaboration is about relationships. Conflict may be the result of an undeveloped or poor interpersonal relationship with a colleague. To overcome conflicts, it is necessary to strengthen, not shy away from, the relationship of the two opposing parties. As early as the late 1990s, the Pew Health Professions Commission (PHPC) talked about practicing relationship-centered care as one of 21 health profession competencies for the twenty-first century (O'Neil & PHPC, 1998). Relationship-centered care in this context surely involves nurse and client/family interactions, but it also stresses the importance of collaborative interprofessional relationships. These 21 competencies are necessary ingredients for effective professional relationships and can become guideposts for successful professional working relationships within a continuous improvement framework.

The 21 competencies also include a professional nurse's responsibility and accountability for health care quality. The specific statements related to health care quality include "take responsibility for quality of care and health outcomes at all levels" and "contribute to continuous improvement of the health care system" (O'Neill & PHPC, 1998, p. vii) (Box 18.2). Four core competencies specific to interprofessional collaborative practice have also been developed (Interprofessional Education Collaborative, 2016, p. 10). They include:

1. *Values/ethics for interprofessional practice:* work with individuals of other professions to maintain a climate of mutual respect and shared values.

BOX 18.2 Twenty-One Competencies for the Twenty-First Century

1. Embrace a personal ethic of social responsibility and service.
2. Exhibit ethical behavior in all professional activities.
3. Provide evidence-based, clinically competent care.
4. Incorporate the multiple determinants of health in clinical care.
5. Apply knowledge of the new sciences.
6. Demonstrate critical thinking, reflection, and problem-solving skills.
7. Understand the role of primary care.
8. Rigorously practice preventive health care.
9. Integrate population-based care and services into practice.
10. Improve access to health care for those with unmet health needs.
11. Practice relationship-centered care with individuals and families.
12. Provide culturally sensitive care to a diverse society.
13. Partner with communities in health care decisions.
14. Use communication and information technology effectively and appropriately.
15. Work in interdisciplinary teams.
16. Ensure care that balances individual, professional, system, and societal needs.
17. Practice leadership.
18. Take responsibility for quality of care and health outcomes at all levels.
19. Contribute to continuous improvement of the health care system.
20. Advocate for public policy that promotes and protects the health of the public.
21. Continue to learn and help others learn.

From O'Neil, E.H., & the Pew Health Professions Commission (PHPC). (1998). *Recreating health professional practice for a new century: The fourth report of the Pew Health Professions Commission.* San Francisco, CA: PHPC.

2. *Roles/responsibilities:* use the knowledge of one's own role and those of other professions to appropriately assess and address the health care needs of patients and to promote and advance the health of populations.
3. *Interprofessional communication:* communicate with patients, families, communities, and professionals in health and other fields in a responsive and responsible manner that supports a team approach to the promotion and maintenance of health, and the prevention and treatment of disease.
4. *Teams and teamwork:* apply relationship-building values and the principles of team dynamics to perform effectively in different team roles to plan, deliver, and evaluate patient/population-centered care and population health programs and policies that are safe, timely, efficient, effective, and equitable.

Patient Engagement

Health care reform brings a heightened focus on accountability for health care professionals. A critical component of reform includes an emphasis on patient-centered care and patient engagement. The American Academy of Nursing has declared patient engagement and activation a health reform imperative for nursing (Pelletier & Stichler, 2013). *Patient engagement* is defined as "the desire and capability to actively choose to participate in care in a way uniquely appropriate to the individual in cooperation with a healthcare provider or institution for the purposes of maximizing outcomes or experiences of care" (Higgins, et al., 2017, p. 33). Emphasis is on the actions of patients and families and their self-care behaviors. Engaging patients in their own care can affect inpatient safety in psychiatric inpatient settings (Pelletier, 2015; Polacek et al., 2015). Patient engagement in this context involves an active process of synthesizing health information, recommendations of health care professionals, and personal beliefs and preferences to manage one's illness.

Nurse leaders continue to play an important role in designing care delivery systems that promote patient and family engagement (Pelletier & Stichler, 2014a). Various toolkits have been developed to assist staff nurses and managers who desire to engage patients and their families in hospitals (AHRQ, 2017a; AHRQ, 2017b; Pelletier & Stichler, 2014b), and ambulatory and primary care (Caplan et al., 2014; Robert Wood Johnson Foundation, 2014). *Patient activation* describes the four degrees of engagement, including "Level 1—Disengaged and overwhelmed; Level 2—Becoming aware, but still struggling; Level 3—Taking action and gaining control; and Level 4—Maintaining behaviors and pushing further" (Insignia Health, 2020, p. 1). Patient activation "is a proxy for terms such as self-care, self-management or readiness for discharge" (Stichler & Pelletier, 2019, p. 3). Patient/consumer satisfaction is but one common outcome measure of patient engagement, along with desired clinical outcomes.

Self-Care and Resilience

Aligned with the quadruple aim of healthy workplaces (Sikka et al., 2015), burnout is seen as an "unrecognized threat to safe, quality care" (Dyrbye et al., 2017, p. 791). Burnout, compassion fatigue, and secondary trauma are all personal consequences of caregiving (Kelly, 2020; McCann et al., 2013). Clinician burnout can negatively influence levels of patient satisfaction, clinical outcomes, and patient safety (Brigham et al., 2018). The National Academy of Medicine Action Collaborative on Clinician Well-being and Resilience has developed resources, including a conceptual model and evidence-based solutions, to promote clinician well-being and reduce burnout (National Academy of Medicine, 2019). The Joint Commission also published a brief on developing resilience to combat nurse burnout. They identified five leadership empowering behaviors to promote workplace empowerment. These include:

1. Enhancing the meaningfulness of work;
2. Fostering opportunity to participate in decision-making;
3. Expressing confidence in high performance;
4. Facilitating the attainment of organizational goals;
5. Providing autonomy and freedom from bureaucratic restrictions (The Joint Commission, 2019c, p. 2).

The Advisory Board (2018) proposed that unmet needs form "cracks in the foundation" of health care. They targeted four "cracks" and recommended specific nurse manager/executive strategies to foster nurse resilience to prevent burnout as follows:

1. Since violence and point-of-care safety threats are now commonplace, reduce response time to routine point-of-care threats.
2. Since nurses feel they have to make compromises in care delivery, surface and address frontline perceptions of "unsafe" staffing.

3. Since staff bounce from traumatic experiences to other care activities with no time to recover, make emotional support "opt-out" only.
4. Since new technology, responsibilities, and care protocols cause nurses to feel "isolated in a crowd," reconnect nurses through storytelling (pp. 1–4).

Nurse leaders can use these resources, concepts, assessment tools, and methods in ensuring an engaged, well, and effective workforce.

INDUSTRIAL MODELS OF QUALITY

Industrial models have heavily influenced the way quality is currently understood and measured in health care settings across the continuum. Industry leaders who have influenced nursing's understanding of health care quality include Walter Shewhart, Joseph Juran, Philip Crosby, and W. Edwards Deming. These leaders provided blueprints from which nursing performance and quality improvement programs have been derived. Understanding quality in health care is enhanced by understanding the development of industrial models of quality.

Shewhart explored causes of variation in core work processes. He quantified these variations, categorizing variables as common or special cause. His *Plan, Do, Check, Act (PDCA)* model was updated to the PDSA cycle and is probably the most frequently used improvement tool in health care quality settings today, as follows (Fig. 18.1): developing a plan to test the change (Plan), carrying out the test (Do), observing and learning from the consequences (Study), and determining what modifications should be made to the test (Act) (IHI, 2020a, p. 1). Shewhart also provided the industrial community with statistical process control techniques that are used widely today. Deming (2000a, b) adopted his work and refined it.

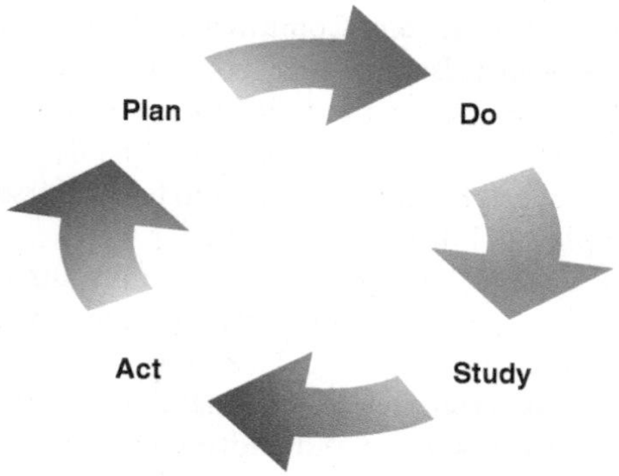

Fig. 18.1 PDSA (Plan, Do, Study, Act) cycle.

Juran (1989) defined quality as "fitness for use." In his work, quality was defined as freedom from defects plus value and continuously meeting customer expectations. His approach to quality centered on the use of interdisciplinary teams that used diagnostic tools to understand why industrial processes produce a product not fit for use. His framework included a three-pronged approach: quality planning, quality control, and quality improvement. Quality planning "establishes the design of a product, service, or process that will meet customer, business, and operational needs to produce the product before it is produced. Quality planning follows a universal sequence of steps, as follows:

- Identify customers and target markets
- Discover hidden and unmet customer needs
- Translate these needs into product or service requirements: a means to meet their needs (new standards, specifications, etc.)
- Develop a service or product that exceeds customers' needs
- Develop the processes that will provide the service, or create the product, in the most efficient way
- Transfer these designs to the organization and the operating forces to be carried out." (Juran Institute, 2009, pp. 1–2).

Crosby viewed quality in production terms of zero defects and measured quality in relation to conformance to requirements. He believed that the results or products of a company are made by people. He focused on systems and the consequences of poor quality. He emphasized doing the right thing the first time to prevent waste. Waste and rework were seen as costly, and good managers were those who prevented costly mistakes. The cost of waste in health care is discussed later in this chapter.

In addition to PDSA, Deming focused on statistical process control techniques and on continuous quality improvement through a culture of quality. He is credited as being influential in the success of Japanese industries post–World War II. He proposed 14 points to help management understand and commit to quality. These points are listed in Box 18.3 (Deming, 2000a, b) and have heavily influenced health care's adoption of quality and safety improvement principles.

BOX 18.3 Deming's 14 Points for Quality

1. Create constancy of purpose toward improving products and services.
2. Adopt the new philosophy.
3. Cease dependence on inspection to achieve quality.
4. End the practice of awarding business on the basis of cost alone.
5. Improve constantly and forever every process for planning, production, and service.
6. Institute training on the job.
7. Adopt and institute leadership aimed at helping people do their jobs better.
8. Drive out fear by promoting two-way communication.
9. Break down barriers between departments.
10. Eliminate exhortations for the workforce in such forms as posters and slogans; these methods tend to create adversarial relationships.
11. Eliminate numerical quotas for productivity; instead have leaders promote continuous quality improvement (CQI).
12. Permit pride of workmanship by removing the barriers that prevent this.
13. Encourage education and self-improvement for all workers.
14. Define management's commitment to CQI and their obligation to implement these points.

From Deming, W.E. (2000a). *The new economics for industry, government, education.* Cambridge, MA: MIT Center for Advanced Engineering Studies; and Deming, W.E. (2000b). *Out of the crisis.* Cambridge, MA: MIT Center for Advanced Engineering Studies.

STANDARDS OF QUALITY

Donabedian (1980) developed the initial theoretical model of health care quality standards: structure, process, and outcomes, which identified that quality can be measured using these three aspects. Donabedian's framework is the most widely referenced model of quality; professional nurses have used this model to develop performance and quality improvement programs and conduct evidence-based improvement studies and nursing research. *Standards*, or written value statements, essentially define quality, against which performance and outcomes are measured. Standards and measures are typically developed from *benchmarking* activities and reviews of best practices in best-in-class organizations. Therefore the selection of standards and measures is a critical activity in the performance and quality improvement process. Actually, standards establish the baseline against which measurement and evaluation are conducted. It is also critical to decide who determines the standards and which standards are selected to define quality. Over the past 70 years, national groups have been formed to gain consensus on health care performance standards and measures. One such entity is the National Quality Forum (NQF), a not-for-profit, public–private membership organization created in 1999 to develop and implement a national strategy for health care quality measurement and reporting.

Structure Standards and Measures

Structure standards and measures focus on the internal characteristics of the organization and its personnel. They answer the following questions. Is an infrastructure in place and tools accessible to allow quality to exist? Is the structure of the organization set up to allow for the effective, efficient delivery of services? For example, a structural standard for a long-term care facility might be to have an adequate mix of registered nurses (RNs), licensed vocational/practical nurses (LVNs, LPNs), and nursing assistants on site to ensure that comprehensive care is delivered. For specialized areas, structure standards may address whether there are enough specialists, hospitalists, or intensivists to ensure quality care. Certain committees, policy statements, rules and regulations, or manuals, forms, or contracts may be needed. Structure standards regulate the environment to ensure quality. Human, organizational, and physical resources, and environmental characteristics, are examples of structure elements.

Process Standards and Measures

Process standards and measures focus on whether the activities within an organization are being conducted appropriately, effectively, and efficiently. Process measures focus on the behaviors of the professional nurse as a provider of care. The interventions recommended in a clinical practice guideline or best practice are examples of process standards. They relate to what the nurse will be doing and the process the nurse should follow to ensure effective, *evidence-based care*. Process standards look at activities, interventions, and the sequence of caregiving events, sometimes referred to as workflow. Typically, processes are assessed by audits, observational studies, or workflow analyses. Examples of process standards include the following: a nursing assessment is completed within 24 hours of admission, client calls are returned within 1 hour of the initial call, or a face-to-face assessment is completed within 1 hour by appropriate personnel for seclusion and restraints in a behavioral health setting.

Outcome Standards and Measures

Outcome standards and measures refer to whether the services provided by the organization make any difference. Were they effective? They answer important questions about the services that nurses provide. Did those services make a difference to the clients or to the health status of the population? Outcome standards address physical health status, mental health status, social and physical function, health attitudes/knowledge/behavior, utilization of services, and the client's perception and satisfaction with the care received. *Outcome process and measures* refer to a change in the current or future health status attributed to antecedent health care and client attributes of health care. Outcome standards present the possibility of measuring the effectiveness, quality, time, and resources allocated for care. Outcomes are reported as a rate per unit of measurement. Examples of outcome measures include the following: percentage of patients whose activities of daily living have improved by 80%, percentage of clients who have stopped smoking after 12 weeks of intensive psychoeducational therapy, and falls with injury per 1000 patient days.

In measuring quality, both structure and process parameters are important, but they are not sufficient in determining whether the care led to an effective outcome or whether the client learned, recovered, or improved his or her health status. Over the years, the emphasis on structure, process, and outcome aspects of health care has varied. Ultimately, various stakeholders are interested in knowing whether care resulted in a positive, expected clinical outcome, based on objective, measurable criteria.

When developing a quality and safety improvement program, nurse leaders are cautioned not to start by creating new standards and measures. Rather, locating the evidence through a literature search or finding a systematic review will most likely yield measures from which to choose. These measures have typically been tested for reliability and validity and have been piloted in the field. National repositories of quality and safety performance measures can be found at:

- Centers for Medicare & Medicaid Services Quality Measures
- The Joint Commission
- National Database for Nursing Quality Indicators (NDNQI) and the CALNOC Registry (Press Ganey, 2020)
- National Quality Forum Quality Positioning System
- National Committee for Quality Assurance Health Effectiveness Data and Information Set (Health plans)
- Leapfrog Group
- The Cochrane Library
- Specialty professional associations and societies (American Psychiatric Association, American Nurses Association).

Selection criteria can then be adopted and measures chosen for a specific intervention or program. A number of selection criteria guideline statements have been developed, including the performance measurement evaluation criteria from the NQF (2012a). The performance measurement attributes common to these entities' guideline statements have been reported in the set of criteria proposed to be used for a national health care quality report (Institute of Medicine [IOM], Committee on the National Quality Report on Health Care Delivery, 2001). Common performance measurement selection criteria are listed in Box 18.4 (Pelletier & Hoffman, 2002). The adoption of these performance measurement selection criteria is the first step in developing a comprehensive *performance measurement system*, which is a systems-based approach to quality and safety where "the organization uses evidence-based medicine and clinical decision support tools, engages in performance measurement and improvement, measures and responds to patient experiences and satisfaction, practices population health management, and publicly shares robust quality and safety data and improvement activities" (The Joint Commission, 2019b, p. 6).

BOX 18.4 Common Performance Measurement Selection Criteria*

- *Relevance:* The measure should address features of the health care system applicable to health professionals, policy makers, and consumers.
- *Meaningfulness and interpretability:* The measure should be understandable to at least one of the audiences. It should help inform them about the important issues or concerns.
- *Scientific or clinical evidence:* The measure should be based on evidence documenting the links between the interventions, clinical processes, and/or outcomes it addresses.
- *Reliability or reproducibility:* The measure should produce the same results when repeated in the same population and setting.
- *Feasibility:* The measure should be specified precisely. Collection of data for the measure should be inexpensive and logistically feasible.
- *Validity:* The measure should make sense (face validity), correlate well with other measures of the same aspects of care (construct validity), and capture meaningful aspects of care (content validity).
- *Health importance:* The measure should include the prevalence of the health condition to which it applies, and the seriousness of the health outcomes affected.

*Criteria are listed in order of their frequency, with the one mentioned most often listed first. The same label for a criterion can have different meanings depending on the framework, because the criteria are not standardized. The definitions, rather than the labels, were used to construct the figure. Feasibility was used as a category covering several criteria in some of the frameworks and as a single criterion in others. Parts of this figure were adapted from NCQA's list of desirable attributes for HEDIS measures (IOM, Committee on the National Quality Report on Health Care Delivery, 2001, p. 81).
From Pelletier, L.R., & Hoffman, J.A. (2002). A framework for selecting performance measures for opioid treatment programs. *Journal for Healthcare Quality, 24*(3), 26. Reprinted with permission from the National Association for Healthcare Quality.

QUALITY AND SAFETY PERFORMANCE IMPROVEMENT MODELS

A number of industry-based models for quality and safety performance management have been adopted by the health care industry. These include Six Sigma, Lean, the Baldrige National Quality Award, high-reliability organizations, American Nurses Credentialing Center's Magnet Recognition Program®, and Planetree. These models are briefly described in the following sections.

Six Sigma

A strategy developed by Motorola and implemented successfully at General Electric (GE) and AlliedSignal Companies provided an innovative approach to reduce variation and error rates. Not surprisingly, the Six Sigma approach that these companies use is similar to tried-and-true approaches historically deployed by health care quality professionals. In the Six Sigma breakthrough strategy, errors are measured in defects per million opportunities (dpmo). *Six Sigma* is achieved when the organization reaches an error or defect rate of 3.4 or less per one million. Application of Six Sigma in health care "reduces the number of errors made by physicians, nurses and technicians; improving lab turnaround times; reducing appointment wait times; decreasing steps in the supply chain; accelerating reimbursement for insurance claims; and improving patient outcomes" (Villanova University, 2019, p. 5). The Six Sigma strategy of **d**efine, **m**easure, **a**nalyze, **i**mprove, and **c**ontrol (DMAIC) (Harry & Schroeder, 2000) is remarkably similar to Juran's problem-solving strategy (Plsek & Omnias, 1989) that has been applied to health care. Table 18.1 illustrates these similarities (Pelletier, 2000).

Lean

Lean is a model of quality measurement that was originally associated with Deming, but was reintroduced to the United States by Womack in the mid-1990s (Jones & Womack, 2003). The premise of this model is that operational waste in an organization needs to be eliminated. *Lean* originated in manufacturing before being applied to health care. It is "a set of management practices to improve efficiency and effectiveness by eliminating waste. The core principle of lean is to reduce and eliminate non value-adding activities and waste" (ASQ, 2019b, 1). With a focus on core processes, "a perfect process creates precisely the right value for the customer. In a perfect process, every step is valuable (creates value for the customer), capable (produces a good result every

TABLE 18.1 Comparison of Six Sigma Breakthrough Strategy and Juran's Problem-Solving Strategy

SIX SIGMA BREAKTHROUGH STRATEGY		JURAN'S PROBLEM-SOLVING STRATEGY	
Stage	**Step (Objective)**	**Phase**	**Step**
Identification	1. Recognize 2. Define (Identify key business issues)	Project definition and organization	1. List and prioritize problems 2. Define project and team
Characterization	1. Measure 2. Analyze (Understand current performance levels)	Diagnostic journey	1. Analyze symptom 2. Formulate theory of causes 3. Test theories 4. Identify root causes
Optimization	1. Improve 2. Control (Achieve breakthrough improvement)	Remedial journey	1. Consider alternative solutions 2. Design solutions and controls 3. Address resistance to change 4. Implement solutions and controls
Institutionalization	1. Standardize 2. Integrate (Transform how day-to-day business is conducted)	Holding the gains	1. Check performance 2. Monitor control system

From Pelletier, L.R. (2000). On error-free health care: Mission possible! (Editorial). *Journal for Healthcare Quality, 22*(3), 9. Reprinted with permission from the National Association for Healthcare Quality.

time), available (produces the desired output, not just the desired quality, every time), adequate (does not cause delay), flexible, and linked by continuous flow" (IHI, 2005, p. 6). When any of these components are missing, the result is waste, which must be eliminated because it is costly. Lean has wide applicability in health care where there are many opportunities to improve processes such as supply chain management or medication administration. By challenging and analyzing any work process, obvious wasteful rework is flushed out and then the process is redone to be both more efficient and effective. Nurses find it rewarding to reduce or eliminate unnecessary effort; it gives them more time to spend at the bedside.

Baldrige National Quality Award Program

The Baldrige National Quality Award (BNQA) established a set of performance standards that define a total quality organization. Named after the Secretary of Commerce, the BNQA "was established by Congress in 1987 to enhance the competitiveness and performance of US businesses" (Baldrige Foundation, 2020, p. 3). The standards in seven areas of excellence are (1) leadership, (2) strategic planning, (3) customer and market focus, (4) information and analysis, (5) human resource focus, (6) process management, and (7) business results. A study completed in 2011 found that a return on investment of money spent to implement the Baldrige criteria vis-à-vis economic benefit was 820:1 (Link & Scott, 2011). Organizations committed to quality improvement choose to adopt the BNQA approach as another means of defining and improving their organizational processes to achieve quality outcomes. Manufacturing, service, and small business were the original award categories, but education and health care were added in 1999. With the trend in health care of adopting industry applications and measure sets for quality improvement, it was fitting that the health care industry was recognized as one that could benefit from participating in this program. It is appropriate for health care entities to strive to achieve internationally recognized standards for performance excellence that enable them to benchmark their "best practices" with others in the field. The first health care organization to apply and be awarded the BNQA in health care was the SSM system in St. Louis, MO, in 2002. The most recent health care awardees include Adventist Health White Memorial in Los Angeles, CA and Mary Greeley Medical Center in Ames, IA (National Institute of Standards and Technology, 2019, p. 3). The Alliance for Performance Excellence is a network of national, state, and local Baldrige-based organizations helping institutions achieve performance excellence using the Baldrige criteria (https://www.baldrigealliance.org/). Various states have also developed quality awards based on the BNQA criteria.

High-Reliability Organizations

In their book *Managing the Unexpected* (2007), Weick and Sutcliffe described high reliability as involving anticipation and containment. They believed that an organization's "collective mindfulness" (Chassin & Loeb, 2013) ensured that potential problems are anticipated and that strategies are in place should an unexpected event occur, and responses are early enough to prevent catastrophic consequences (AHRQ, 2019a, p. 2).

- Anticipation has three elements: (1) preoccupation with failure—being mindful of how complex their operations are and the fact that errors do occur, (2) reluctance to simplify—requiring staff to dig deep in understanding the cause of error versus overly simplified explanations (e.g., staff education), and (3) sensitivity to operations—be aware of structure and processes that are in place to effect desired patient outcomes.
- Containment has two elements: (1) commitment to resilience—having systems in place to return to normal operations quickly, and (2) deference to expertise—relying on and listening to frontline staff for their intimate knowledge about daily operations (Chassin & Loeb, 2013; Weick & Sutcliffe, 2007).

A high reliability organization is "an organization operating in an industry that is complex and has high risk for harm that consistently performs at high levels of safety over long periods of time" (Pelletier & Beaudin, 2018, p. 252). The Institute for Healthcare Improvement (IHI; 2020b), The Joint Commission (Joint Commission Center for Transforming Healthcare, 2020) and AHRQ's Patient Safety Network have a multitude of resources for helping healthcare entities implement HRO concepts and principles (AHRQ, 2019a).

American Nurses Credentialing Center Magnet Designation

The American Nurses Credentialing Center's (ANCC) Magnet Recognition Program® recognizes health care organizations for aligning "their strategic goals to improve the organization's outcomes" (ANCC, n.d., p. 2). Magnet-designated hospitals "attract" staff and retain them due to their characteristics or "forces of magnetism," such as the quality of nursing leadership, professional models of care and quality of care, nursing research, and evidence-based practice (ANCC, n.d.). The Magnet model includes the following components: transformational leadership, structural empowerment, exemplary professional practice, new knowledge, innovations and improvements, and empirical quality outcomes. Hospitals that embark on the Magnet journey first must assess where they are related to preestablished Magnet standards. Typically, nursing leadership staff complete a gap analysis to identify opportunities for improvement before submitting their application for designation. Organizations have used the journey to effect higher patient ratings of their hospital experience (Stimpfel et al., 2016), lower mortality (Bekelis et al., 2017; Missios & Bekelis, 2018), lower central line-associated bloodstream infection rates (Barnes et al., 2016), lower RN turnover (Park et al., 2016), and lower length of stay (Bekelis et al., 2017; Missios & Bekelis, 2017).

Planetree

Since 1978 Planetree has designated health care organizations for person-centered excellence. The Planetree model proposes that "Person-centered care yields internal, external, financial and cultural benefits to healthcare organizations. It engages patients, aligns with today's mandates for better population health management and improves organizational performance in quality, safety and experience" (Planetree, 2018, p. 1). Its standards help organizations increase patient activation, staff engagement, and foster staff and leadership development. Recently a Planetree Higher Education Advisory Council convened to develop person-centered care standards of excellence for universities and colleges preparing the next generation of health care providers. National University in California was one of the first universities to receive Planetree recognition in 2017 (National University, 2020).

COSTS ASSOCIATED WITH WASTE IN HEALTH CARE

According to Shrank et al. (2019), the cost associated with waste in health care ranges from $760 to $935 billion annually and plagues every sector in the health care industry. Berwick and Hackbarth (2012) listed categories of waste as: failures of care delivery, failures of care coordination, overtreatment, administrative complexity, pricing failures, and fraud and abuse. Shrank and colleagues further stated that policy experts have proposed that this waste represents 25% of total health care spending, estimated to be $3.82 trillion in 2019. They believe that aligning payers and providers through current value-based care initiatives can help cut waste.

The number of medical errors was described as unacceptable in *To Err Is Human: Building a Safer Health Care System* (Kohn et al., 2000), an IOM report that has been referenced widely in the professional and consumer press since its release. The IOM report reached the highest levels in the federal government, but response to its findings and recommendations have been lackluster. Health care organizations were slow to adopt its recommendations fully even 20 years later. Several reports on health care quality and safety have followed this landmark report.

The IOM (now called the National Academies of Sciences, Engineering, and Medicine, Health and Medicine Division) reports defined specific strategies that could inform the development and refinement of health care safety systems nationwide. An important component of these reports is the mention of the error-reduction techniques of other industries. The federal reports provided another opportunity to advocate for patients, families, and populations. They gave health care quality professionals the evidence and research with which to defend a quality management budget, enhance information systems and technologies to monitor and track errors, and further develop quality activities and studies using proven tools and techniques. The reports are also models in defining and describing cost/benefit analyses and return-on-investment scenarios for quality and performance improvement programs. In essence, they provided a business case for quality and safety.

The IOM *report Crossing the Quality Chasm: A New Health System for the 21st Century* (IOM, Committee on Quality of Health Care in America [CQHCA], 2001, p. 11) recommended that Congress establish a Health Care Quality Innovation Fund "to support projects targeted at (1) achieving the six aims of safety, effectiveness, patient-centeredness, timeliness, efficiency, and equity; and/or (2) producing substantial improvements in quality for the [15] priority conditions." The overall goal of the funding would be to produce a "public-domain portfolio of programs, tools, and technologies of widespread applicability" (p. 11). The report recommended an initial investment of $1 billion over three to five years to support this goal (p. 11). Health care organizations could take the lead either by enhancing the current resources dedicated to quality and performance improvement in their organizations, or by using the funds to finance regional collaborative health care quality projects. These successes could then be described in the literature for wider application.

Leadership by Example: Coordinating Government Roles in Improving Health Care Quality, the third in a series of IOM quality chasm reports, was released in 2002 (Corrigan et al., 2002). The original charge of the IOM Committee on Enhancing Federal Healthcare Quality Programs (CEFHQP) was to acknowledge that "The current federal quality oversight programs represent a patchwork of requirements and processes that have evolved over the last 30 to 35 years" (IOM, CEFHQP, 2002, p. 1). The committee was convened "to re-examine the various federal quality improvement and oversight programs to assess whether changes are needed to (1) provide adequate protection to beneficiaries, (2) provide strong incentives to providers to improve quality, and (3) improve the efficiency of the oversight processes by reducing redundancy" (IOM, CEFHQP, 2002, p. 1). In doing their work, the committee held workshops to obtain perspectives and information from various stakeholders with expertise in the fields of quality measurement, improvement, oversight, and research on ways to improve current federal programs (e.g., Medicare, Children's Health Insurance Program, Tricare, and Veterans Affairs).

These findings were not a surprise to many nurses and health care quality professionals who have been burdened with duplicative reporting such as licensing and accreditation for years. The positive message was that strong recommendations from this committee were sent to the federal government's leadership, asking them to attack these problems with a good deal of muscle to shape performance measurement for the whole health care sector. Standardization of protocols and measures is not a new idea (Pelletier, 1998). Reducing administrative burden and duplicative reporting would provide more time for clinical responsibilities and direct health care services to individuals, families, and populations/communities.

Clinical standardization has become the focus of efforts to reduce variability in practice and health care costs. However, a lack of centralization and absence of enforced universal standards have led to the development of guidelines not based on evidence (Benavidez & Frakt, 2019, p. 6). These authors proposed two steps to strengthen clinical practice guidelines: (1) restore funding for the Agency for Healthcare Research and Quality's National Guideline Clearinghouse, or establish a similar central guidelines repository, and (2) enforce a rigorous, universal methodology for creating guidelines (pp. 22–28).

CURRENT ISSUES AND TRENDS

Mission, Vision, and Core Values

An organization that adopts and nurtures a continuous quality and safety improvement culture (and rewards those who identify opportunities for improvement and their solutions) recognizes that change is an everyday event. One of the ways that change can be managed is to acknowledge it and make it a part of the organization's strategic planning process. Just as an organization defines its mission, vision, and core values, so too must change agents and teams define the purpose of the change (expected outcomes), the mission and vision of the change process, and the core values of the group that will be responsible for managing the change.

An organization's mission is a concise statement that answers the question: What business are we in today? For example, Sharp HealthCare, a San Diego-based not-for-profit integrated regional health care delivery system that was the recipient of the BNQA in 2007, stated that its mission is "to improve the health of those we serve with a commitment to excellence in all that we do. Our goal is to offer quality care and programs that set community standards, exceed patients' expectations and are provided in a caring, convenient, cost-effective and accessible manner" (Sharp HealthCare, 2020, p. 1). The Visiting Nursing Service of New York's (VNSNY) mission is "to improve the health and well-being of people through high-quality, cost-effective healthcare in the home and community" (VNSNY, 2020, p. 1).

An organization's vision should accurately depict what the company is striving to become. For example, Sharp HealthCare's vision is "to be the best health system in the universe" (Sharp HealthCare, 2020, p. 2). VNSNY's vision "...continues to draw strength from this mission to care for vulnerable individuals and families. We strive to be the most significant, best-in-class, not-for-profit community-based health care organization, providing superior care coordination and health care services to vulnerable New Yorkers across a broad regional footprint" (VNSNY, 2020, p. 2).

It is critical for mission and vision statements to be communicated effectively and widely to internal stakeholders (employees and management personnel) and to external stakeholders (investors, clients, patients, vendors, and accreditation agencies). In this way the statements keep employees on a path to an attainable goal such as quality outcomes. Mission, vision, and value statements form the foundation for quality and safety and their management and improvement. Departmental mission and vision statements need to be aligned with the organization's core value statements.

Core value statements frame the organization's culture in the same way mission and vision statements do; they remain constant in an ever-changing landscape. "Values are operational qualities used by organizations to maintain or enhance performance" (Harmon, 1997, p. 246). Values consciously and unconsciously guide a professional nurse's personal and professional behavior. His Holiness the Dalai Lama and Cutler (1998) said the following about values: "Higher stages of growth and development depend on an underlying set of values that can guide us. A value system that can provide continuity and coherence to our lives, by which we can measure our experiences. A value system that can help us decide which goals are truly worthwhile and which pursuits are meaningless. Values help us with the challenges of everyday life" (pp. 192–193).

Nurses' personal and professional values come from the experiences they have shared with others in interpersonal exchanges at work and at home. To identify a group's core values, investigate these questions: Which three people have had the greatest influence in your personal and professional life? What are the three most important values these influential people taught you? The answers to these questions can help inform the development of mission, vision, and core value statements. An example is a set of core values or "core principles" from the Mayo Clinic, as outlined in Table 18.2.

TABLE 18.2 Mayo Clinic Value Statements

These values, which guide Mayo Clinic's mission to this day, are an expression of the vision and intent of our founders, the original Mayo physicians, and the Sisters of Saint Francis.	
Respect	Treat everyone in our diverse community, including patients, their families, and colleagues with dignity.
Integrity	Adhere to the highest standards of professionalism, ethics, and personal responsibility, worthy of the trust our patients place in us.
Compassion	Provide the best care, treating patients and family members with sensitivity and empathy.
Healing	Inspire hope and nurture the well-being of the whole person, respecting physical, emotional, and spiritual needs.
Teamwork	Value the contributions of all, blending the skills of individual staff members in unsurpassed collaboration.
Innovation	Infuse and energize the organization, enhancing the lives of those we serve, through the creative ideas and unique talents of each employee.
Excellence	Deliver the best outcomes and highest quality service through the dedicated effort of every team member.
Stewardship	Sustain and reinvest in our mission and extended communities by wisely managing our human, natural, and material resources.

From Mayo Foundation for Medical Research and Education. (2020). *About Mayo Clinic: Mayo Clinic mission and values.* Rochester, MN: Author. http://www.mayoclinic.org/about-mayo-clinic/mission-values.

A Nurse Leader's Health Care Quality Toolbox

Along with the paradigm shift from quality assurance to organizational performance improvement came the expectation that accredited organizations become skilled at the art and science of CQI. This included the concepts of leadership involvement, a commitment to customers' needs (i.e., patients and families), an understanding of the principle of process versus people, a devotion to data collection and analysis as the foundation for problem-solving, and the recognition that interprofessional study teams are the experts and are best equipped to drive change and improvement.

Nurses are frequently tapped to participate in organization-wide improvement teams designed to address overarching problem resolution or process redesign projects. Many of the early quality leaders received training in facilitation and group meeting techniques in addition to the performance and quality improvement (PQI) tools. This enabled them to promote the team-based model of cross-functional and interprofessional problem-solving that became the standard for most organizations. Nurses in the new millennium continue to need skills and expertise in the concepts of team building, conflict resolution, statistical process control, customer service, and process improvement.

Nurse leaders in accredited organizations are expected to learn principles and tools for quality improvement, educate all staff on these techniques, collaboratively identify improvement opportunities on nursing units, and use data analyses to demonstrate the impact of change initiatives.

Nurses at all levels are affected by organizational quality efforts. Knowledge through continuous learning forms the backdrop for quality and safety. New nurses in nurse residency programs may undertake a small-scale, unit-based quality initiative, or change projects. Often the impetus arises from seeing a problem in practice and then pursuing an evidence-based quality improvement approach (Melnyk et al., 2015), and using PQI tools to analyze, plan, and take action through interprofessional teams and shared governance structures.

Health care quality professionals and nurses involved in quality and safety improvement activities have an enormous set of resources available to them as they plan for an enterprise-wide quality and safety program. Tools and techniques that nurses can readily use are shown in Table 18.3 and Figs. 18.2 through 18.7, which illustrate examples of templates and forms to be included in a nurse leader's quality "toolbox."

Two excellent resources for hospital-based and ambulatory quality programs are the National Database of Nursing Quality Indicators (NDNQI) and the CALNOC Registry, owned by Press Ganey (Press Ganey, 2020). NDNQI was originally developed by the ANA. This database is composed of nurse-sensitive indicators collected at the nursing unit level and provides the ability for participants to benchmark performance with national

TABLE 18.3 A Nurse Manager's Health Care Quality Toolbox

Tool	Description of the Tool	Example
Data-collection tools	Check sheets and checklists facilitate the gathering of data for eventual analysis and reporting. Good data collection tools can help to count and categorize data.	Sample data collection sheet for a nurse manager's quality toolbox (see Fig. 18.2).
Control chart	This tool includes data points and their placement on a graph to depict variation. Its purpose is to illustrate whether the process variation is expected ("common cause") or an unexpected or unusual variation ("special cause"). Included are three lines—the mean, an upper control limit (UCL), and a lower control limit (LCL). Generally, a process is considered "out of control" when the data points stray outside of the control limits or a series of data points follow a defined pattern that illustrates a lack of control in the process.	Sample control chart for a nurse manager's quality toolbox (see Fig. 18.3).
Cause-and-effect (or fishbone) diagram	This tool resembles diagramming sentences. The "effect" is illustrated in a box at the end of a midline (or "head" of the fish). The "causes" are generally four or five categories of elements that might contribute to the effect (e.g., machines, methods, people, materials, and measurements) and the specific activities. Under each of these category headings, individual items that might lead to the effect are listed. By diagramming all of the possible contributors, the predominant or root causes may be found more readily.	Sample cause-and-effect diagram for a nurse manager's quality toolbox (see Fig. 18.4).
Detailed flowchart	Using various shapes, this tool is used to depict a work process, from start to finish, illustrating all of the processes' action steps, decision points, handoffs, or waiting stages. Flowcharts form the cornerstone of process improvement planning and analysis. The entire process must first be accurately defined to identify problems or process improvement opportunities.	Sample detailed flowchart for a nurse manager's quality toolbox (see Fig. 18.5).
Pareto chart	This bar graph can help depict the "80/20" rule. In the nineteenth century, it was used to show that 80% of the wealth was held by 20% of the people. In health care, typically 20% of the issues cause 80% of the problems. The use of this tool allows a performance improvement team to focus on the "vital few" causes of the problems in a process under study.	Example of a Pareto chart for a nurse manager's quality toolbox (see Fig. 18.6).
Scatter diagram	This graph describes the relationship between two variables that are continuous. It is used when the potential causes of effects under study cannot be easily categorized, such as in a Pareto chart or cause-and-effect diagram. Data points are plotted along the vertical and horizontal axes of the graph, and a correlation between the two variables can either be weak or strong, based on the pattern of the data points.	Example of a scatter diagram for a nurse manager's quality toolbox. (see Fig. 18.7).

Data Collection Sheet

Organization/Unit: ______________________ Date: __________

Process: ____

MEASURE	DATE	TIME	WHERE	WHEN

Fig. 18.2 Sample data collection sheet for a nurse manager's quality toolbox.

averages. The CALNOC Registry is the first database registry of inpatient and ambulatory nurse-sensitive quality indicators, now managed by Press Ganey, a company that partners with more than 26,000 organizations to better the patient experience. The NQF, in collaboration with the Robert Wood Johnson Foundation, has developed nurse-sensitive performance measures under its Core Measures for Nursing Care Performance Project (NQF, 2012a). Some of these measures have since been endorsed by the NQF. They include falls and falls with injury, hospital-acquired pressure ulcers, health care–associated infections, nursing care hours per patient day, nursing care hours, nursing turnover, physical restraints, RN engagement survey, and skill mix (Press Ganey, 2020). These "nurse-sensitive" indicators refer to the structure, process, and outcomes of professional

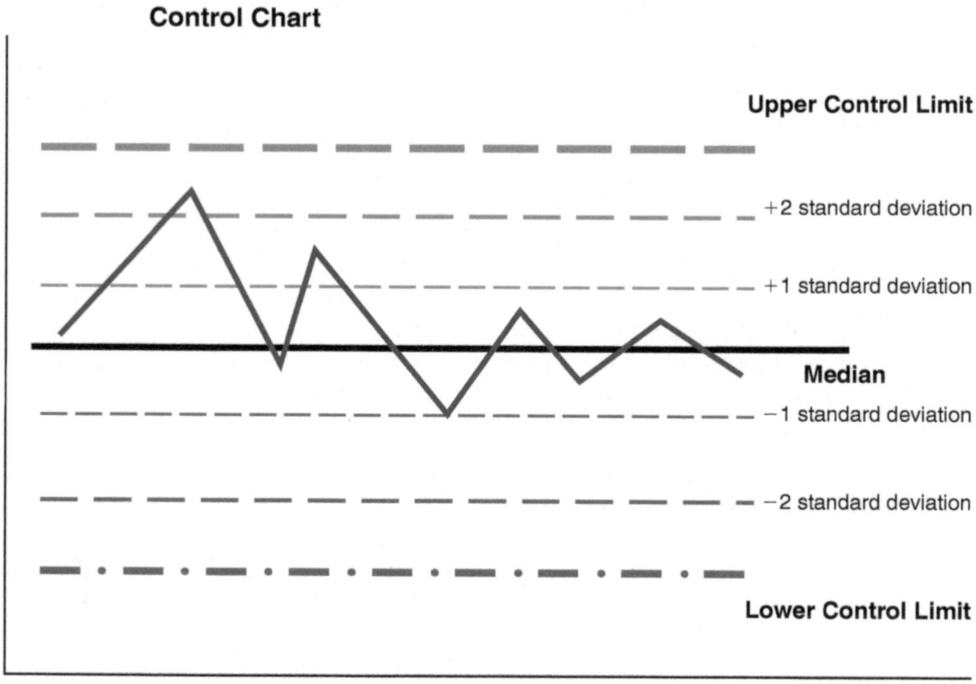

Fig. 18.3 Sample control chart for a nurse manager's quality toolbox.

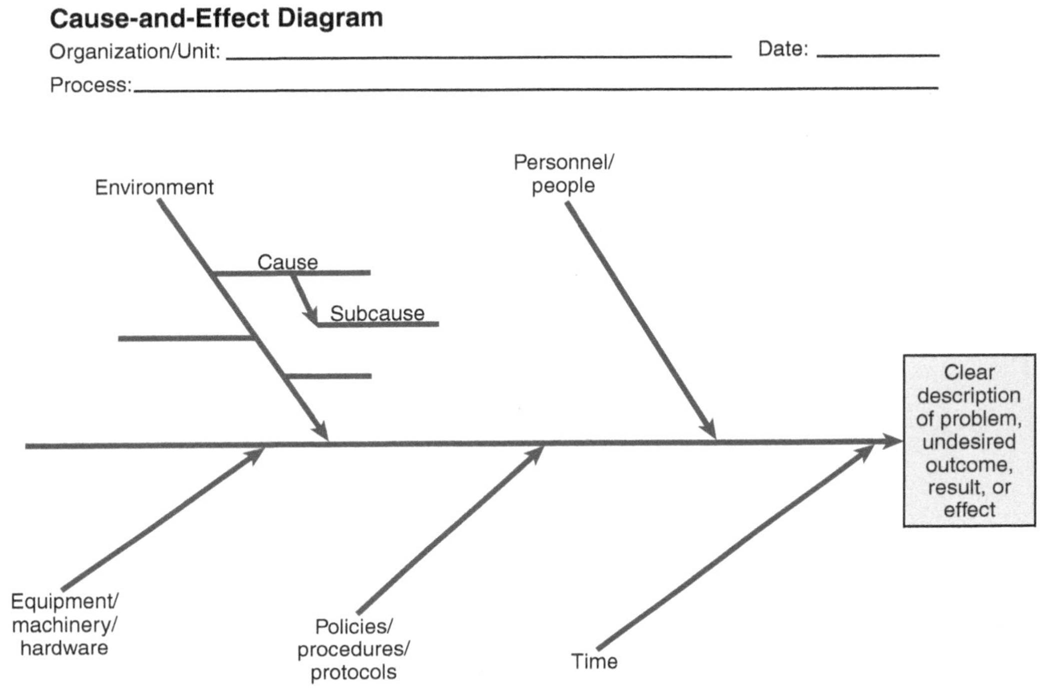

Fig. 18.4 Sample cause-and-effect diagram for a nurse manager's quality toolbox.

nursing care. Because nursing care influences these outcomes (positively or negatively), they are called nurse sensitive.

The most frequently cited factor in medical errors is poor or inadequate communication. TeamSTEPPS 2.0, an evidence-based teamwork system, was designed for health care professionals by the US Department of Defense and the Agency for Healthcare Research and Quality (AHRQ) to improve communication and teamwork skills among health care professionals

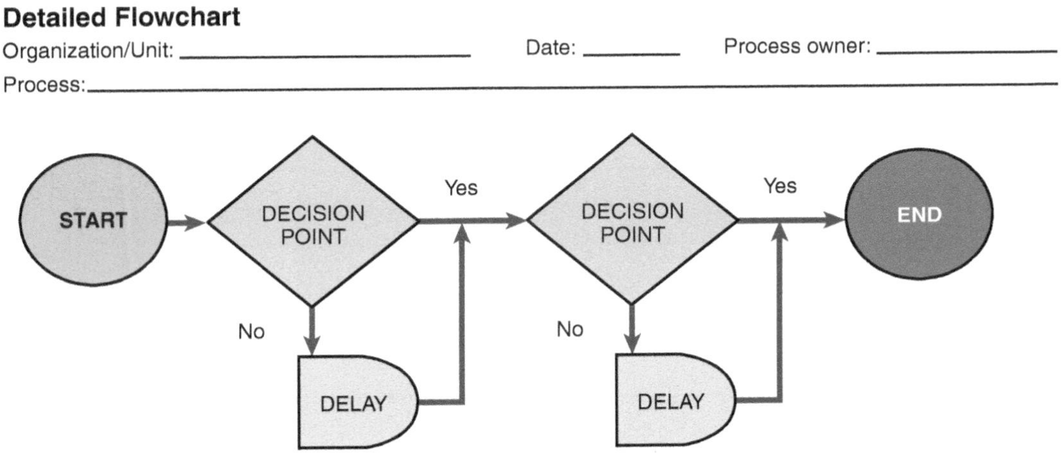

Fig. 18.5 Sample detailed flowchart for a nurse manager's quality toolbox.

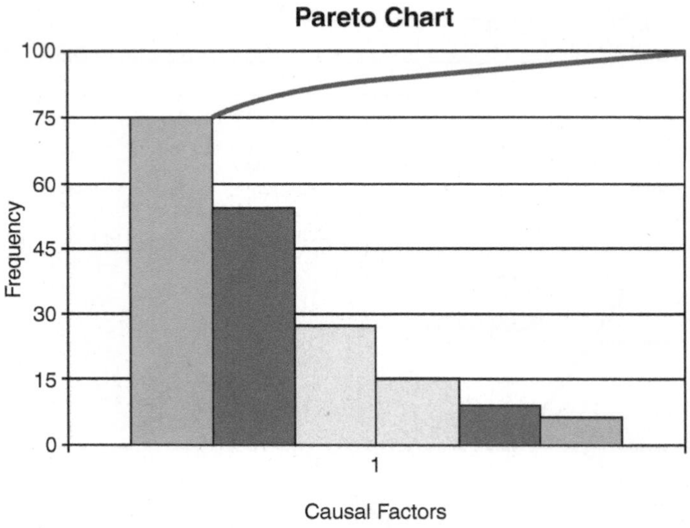

Fig. 18.6 Example of a Pareto chart for a nurse manager's quality toolbox.

(AHRQ, n.d.b.). The program provides a comprehensive suite of ready-to-use materials and a training curriculum to successfully integrate teamwork principles in all areas of a health care system. In addition, the Internet can provide professional nurses with administrative and clinical tools to support a quality and performance improvement program regardless of the delivery setting. A health care quality glossary can also assist professional nurse managers in navigating the health care quality field. A glossary of frequently used terms in this chapter is discussed in the Definitions section.

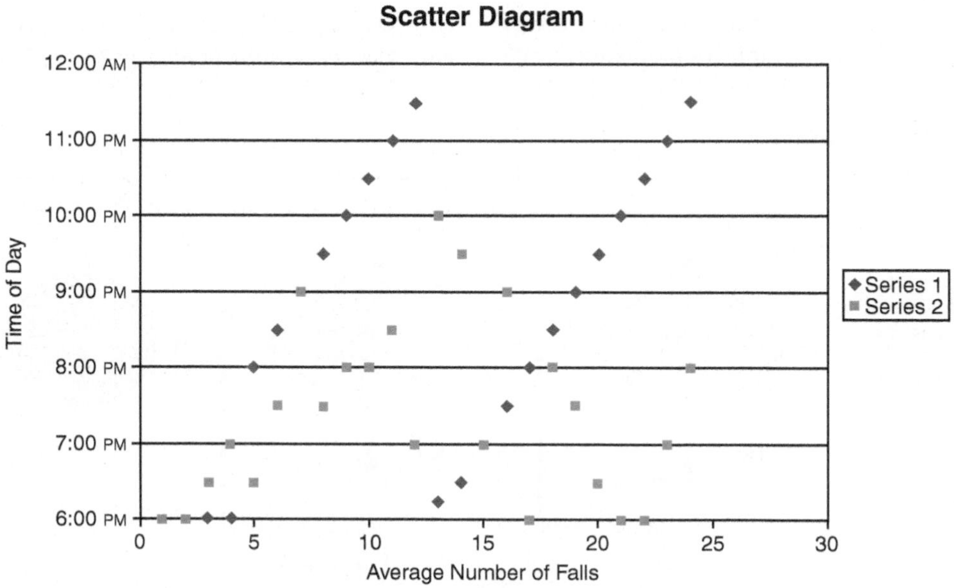

Fig. 18.7 Example of a scatter diagram for a nurse manager's quality toolbox.

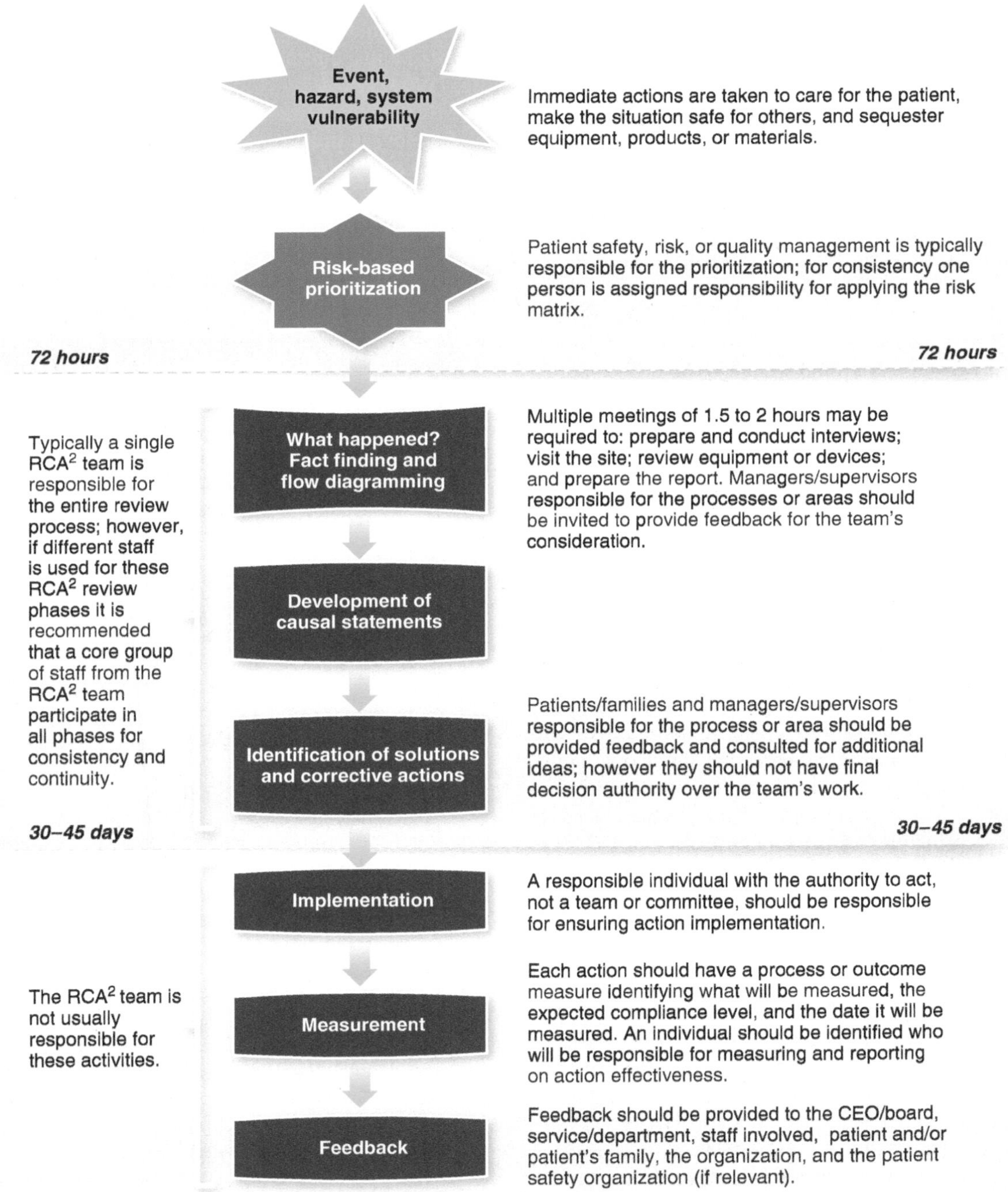

Fig. 18.8 NPSF Root Cause Analysis and Action (RCA^2) Process. Reprinted from www.IHI.org with permission of the Institute for Healthcare Improvement, ©2019.

Patient Safety

A landmark report from the IOM launched a major national focus on the safety of health care systems and processes. In fact, the conclusion that 98,000 deaths in health care organizations were preventable was considered a call to action not only by health care providers but also by business and government. Not surprisingly, health care safety became the focus as a key component of the accreditation process. Soon after the start of this millennium, new standards were established by TJC and other accrediting, regulatory, private, and public organizations to address the issue of safety within health care organizations.

Since 2001 standards require all hospitals accredited by TJC to establish and implement a formal patient safety program. Additional standards have been added over time to integrate health care safety programs in organization-wide processes. The components of a health care safety program are listed in Box 18.5. Those individuals and organizations committed to health care safety initiatives believe that a rigorous, ongoing, and proactive approach to the identification of risks will result in the prevention of errors and provide the framework to respond most effectively when errors do occur.

Just as a paradigm shift was required to move from a quality assurance mindset to one of performance improvement, the new paradigm for health care safety requires that organizations create a nonpunitive culture for error reporting. Systems that single out, blame, and punish caregivers who commit errors are no longer viable. More importantly, nurse leaders need to learn the principles of the nonpunitive approach (i.e., they applaud and commend staff for reporting errors or "near misses"). In fact, in some industrial models, those managers or staff who detect and report errors or system failures in their areas are rewarded.

Human resources management regarding safety practices has generated the concept of a *fair and just culture* (Wise, 2014). A fair and just culture is defined as "organizational accountability for the systems they've designed and employee accountability for the choices they make" (Paradiso & Sweeney, 2019, p. 40). Everyone throughout the organization is aware that medical errors are inevitable, but all errors and unintended events are reported—even when the events may not cause patient injury. This culture can make the system safer as it recognizes that competent professionals make mistakes and acknowledges that even competent professionals develop unhealthy norms (shortcuts or routine rule violations), but it has zero tolerance for reckless behavior. Health care organizations that have adopted a just culture typically have these characteristics (Wise, 2014):

- Mission and value statements are clear.
- Employees protect the organization's values by the choices they make and how they accomplish their duties.
- The organization has designed a system that catches errors before they become critical and designs recoveries to stop or reduce bad outcomes.

BOX 18.5 Components of a Health Care Safety Program

- Leadership commitment as evidenced through the allocation of resources for health care safety
- Assignment of individual(s) to manage the program
- Interdisciplinary (cross-organizational) participation, coordination, and communication about safety activities
- Education and involvement of patients and families in health care safety issues
- Disclosure of unanticipated outcomes of care to patients and families
- Education of staff on safety-related topics and training in team communication techniques
- Data collection and analysis in safety-related areas, including the following:
  - Incident/variance reporting
  - Medication errors, near misses
  - Infection surveillance and prevention; outbreak management
  - Facility/environmental surveillance
  - Staff willingness to report errors
  - Staff perceptions of and suggestions for improving safety
  - Patient and family perceptions and/or suggestions for improvement regarding safety
- Definition of terms related to safety, including sentinel events, "near misses," and what is reportable, and the development of policies and procedures to address each category of patient safety event
- Management of sentinel events
- Adherence to The Joint Commission National Patient Safety Goals
- Establishment of a risk reduction process to include Healthcare Failure Modes Effects Analysis (HFMEA)

- The organization continuously refines its core processes from employee feedback and is always learning; employees feel safe in reporting errors or potential errors.

Health care organizations that embrace a fair and just culture identify and correct the systems or processes of care that contributed to the medical error or near miss. Nurse leaders believe that more health care professionals will report more errors and near misses when they are protected by a nonpunitive culture of medical error reporting, and this will further improve patient safety through opportunities for improvement and lessons learned (Paradiso & Sweeney, 2019). The American Nurses Association has endorsed just culture as a means of ensuring safe care (ANA, 2010).

The Veterans Affairs (VA) National Center for Patient Safety (NCPS) is an example of a large organization that has created health care safety programs. The NCPS is committed to the reduction of error and improvement of quality through proactive approaches to risk reduction (US Department of Veterans Affairs, 2018a). This is accomplished through focusing on prevention, creating nonpunitive environments, and conducting safety research through such concepts as human factors analysis, and studying HROs in other industries such as aviation and nuclear energy.

In 1998 the VA created a VA Quality Scholars Program to train leaders and scholars in health care improvement for the VA who are prepared to lead change nationally and internationally. The program consists of 11 sites across the United States and has affiliate sites in Toronto and Canada. Each site in the US consists of a partnership between a VA hospital and an academic institution. It has an interprofessional emphasis with physicians, nurses educated nurses to doctoral level, clinical psychologists, and pharmacists as fellows and faculty (US Department of Veterans Affairs, 2018b). The VA has created numerous educational programs through the NCPS and freely shares them with all health care providers who want to learn about health care safety tools and techniques. They have taken the lead in adopting the methodology and tools of Healthcare Failure Modes and Effects Analysis (HFMEA).

The National Quality Forum is a consortium of public–private organizations that work collaboratively to address health care quality and safety. In 2003 the NQF published a list of 30 consensus standards to address safe practices that, if implemented, would yield improvements in the safety of health care. Examples of this initial list included establishment of a culture for safety, adoption of protocols to prevent wrong-side surgery, and implementation of effective admission assessments to identify and treat underlying conditions early in the care process. The NQF Safety Practices were updated in 2006, and a total of 34 practices were included in 2009 Safe Practices. New Safe Practices in the 2009 set were added in areas such as pediatric imaging, glycemic control, organ donation, catheter-associated urinary tract infection, and multidrug-resistant organisms. A number of previously endorsed practices were updated based on new evidence, including the pharmacist's role in medication management, pressure ulcers, and an entire chapter on health care associated infections (NQF, 2012b). Current safety topics that the NQF has endorsed and recommend include implementation of effective handoff communication, initiation of rapid response teams, and management of methicillin-resistant *Staphylococcus* aureus (MRSA) infection.

Nurses and nurse leaders can personally create an environment that is devoted to health care safety by doing the following:

- Learning the concepts and tools related to risk identification, analysis, and error reduction;
- Adopting and embracing the concept of nonpunitive error reporting;
- Advocating for the establishment of a nonpunitive culture if it is not currently a strong ideal within the organization;
- Encouraging staff to be constantly vigilant in identifying potential risks in the care environment;
- Creating a sense of partnership with patients and families to promote communication about safety concerns and soliciting their suggestions to correct and prevent potential risks;
- Being a role model and coach for staff and peers in practicing health care safety concepts.

National Patient Safety Goals

Since the late 1990s, TJC has collected data on sentinel events and the outcomes of their root cause analyses (RCAs) for the purpose of sharing those data with health care organizations to prevent similar sentinel events from occurring. The results of the aggregation of these data are published by TJC in a series of newsletters titled *Sentinel Event Alerts*. These *Sentinel Event Alerts* address events such as preventing unintended retained foreign objects, preventing infection from the misuse of vials, safe use of health information technology, preventing falls and fall-related injuries in health care facilities, and detecting and treating suicide ideation in all settings (TJC, 2020c). The original intent of these alerts was for health care organizations to review the "lessons learned" from facilities that had experienced these sentinel events. With the emphasis on health care patient safety (including the adoption of their own set of patient safety standards), the impact of the IOM reports, and the industry-wide emphasis on error prevention as a backdrop, TJC formalized the information contained in their sentinel event database into a new accreditation requirement called the *National Patient Safety Goals* (TJC, 2020d).

In 2002 TJC's Board of Commissioners approved an initial list of six National Patient Safety Goals (NPSGs) that represented the most commonly occurring and/or serious events from its sentinel event database, combined with the recommendations of an interdisciplinary task force. Each goal has evidence-based or expert-based recommendations to define how to implement the goal successfully. The Joint Commission board reevaluates the goals annually. New goals are added to the list if necessary, and/or existing goals may be replaced with new goals that reflect processes in which there are safety concerns (e.g., hand hygiene, goals for medication reconciliation and handoff communications, and a goal for anticoagulation therapy). Each organization must demonstrate compliance with all applicable NPSG recommendations during the time of their accreditation survey (there are specific goals for ambulatory health, behavioral health, critical access hospitals, home care, hospitals, laboratories, nursing care centers, and office-based surgery centers). These goals have become the underpinning of the survey process. Those organizations that effectively implement the NPSGs find that they are more apt to have a successful survey outcome in this era of unannounced surveys.

Nurse leaders can serve as role models by fully committing to the NPSGs on their units/departments and communicating their belief that implementation of these standards leads to safer patient care. They are key to successful design and implementation of processes to address NPSGs.

Accreditation and Regulatory Influences on Quality and Safety

Quality and safety are crucial aspects of health care delivery. Yet how do consumers know if an organization is safe and of high quality? Health care organizations have always been required to meet standards for federal and state reimbursement regulations (Medicare and Medicaid) and state licensure rules and regulations in order to operate. These regulations have traditionally defined requirements for quality. However, the private accreditation process has probably had the most significant impact on the development of quality improvement systems in health care. It has been through organizations such as The Joint Commission (TJC), Accreditation Association for Ambulatory Health Care (AAAHC), Community Health Accreditation Partner (CHAP), The American Osteopathic Association's Healthcare Facilities Accreditation Program (HFAP), CARF International, URAC, and the National Committee for Quality Assurance (NCQA) that performance standards have been promulgated and universally adopted. In each of these accreditation processes, the concept of system-wide quality improvement provides the framework for the standards. Although accreditation is not mandatory, eligibility to participate in and receive reimbursement from managed care organizations or federal and state program funding sources such as Medicare is often tied to the achievement of accreditation by one or more of the voluntary accreditation organizations.

Of all of these voluntary accreditation programs, TJC has had the greatest degree of impact on the health care industry. Founded in 1951, it led the way in establishing a set of performance standards for hospitals to follow to become accredited. Over the years its accreditation standards and programs have evolved to reflect the many types of providers that now constitute the health care system, thus expanding its role beyond hospital accreditation. Currently TJC sponsors accreditation programs for organizations that provide services in the areas of ambulatory care, assisted living, behavioral health, critical access hospitals, health care networks, hospitals, home care, laboratory, long-term care, and office-based surgery.

TJC has continually adjusted its performance standards for quality throughout its evolution. During the 1980s and the early 1990s, TJC promoted a "10-Step Process for Quality Assurance" that provided the framework for quality in hospitals. In 1994 TJC identified the need to enhance overall quality of care via an improvement in its own accreditation processes, and it completely revised the accreditation standards for all programs. Instead of chapters organized by department, the new approach revised and reorganized the requirements into cross-functional processes of care and services (e.g., Patients' Rights, Patient Assessment, Patient Family Education) to more appropriately reflect the manner in which care is delivered. A new chapter titled "Improving Organizational Performance" was introduced that created specific standards focused on quality that were based on the principle of continuous improvement rather than on preestablished thresholds for performance of individual health care quality indicators. This change reflected the influence of the industrial quality movement on health care in the early 1990s.

With this major restructuring of TJC standards, the new era of thinking in terms of *process improvement* rather than quality assurance began not only for TJC-accredited organizations, but also for other accrediting bodies. The description for this organization-wide programmatic approach, or *performance improvement* (PI), established the expectation that quality initiatives in the organization were no longer the responsibility of a single quality assurance nurse or department but instead the responsibility of the enterprise's leaders. Standards in the newly developed "Leadership" chapter established the expectation that the outcomes of performance improvement measures be elevated to review by the administrative and clinical leaders of the organization. This review of performance measurement at senior levels of the organization supplies the information that leaders require to provide oversight to the quality of care being delivered to all patients and families (customers).

The Joint Commission's PI standards delineate specific requirements for data collection in high-risk areas such as medication management, restraints, and blood transfusions. Beyond these mandatory quality indicators, the leaders of each organization are expected to set their own priorities for measurement that reflect the types of services provided to the various populations served by the organization. The PI and Leadership standards also expect that the outcomes of data analysis and the actions taken to address improvement opportunities should be communicated to staff. It is in this arena that a nurse leader can make the PI process come alive for nursing staff. Staff can relate to and understand data outcomes that are based on measurement of the everyday processes in which they work. The nurse leader needs to involve staff in identifying relevant and significant data collection measures for their unit/department that will have a direct impact on changing and continuously improving care processes. A sample data collection sheet is displayed in Fig. 18.2.

Nurse leaders need to stay abreast of changes in the standards of their organization's primary accrediting and state and federal regulatory agencies to ensure that quality outcome measures for their units/departments remain current and viable. In addition to keeping up with these requirements, as previously described, many hospitals are pursuing or have plans to pursue Magnet designation of their hospital's nursing practice as awarded by the American Nurses Credentialing Center through its Magnet Recognition Program® (ANCC, n.d.). To be positioned to score well on an application for the Magnet Recognition Program, nurse leaders need to take an active role in the management (monitoring and improving) of robust and effective quality measures (nurse-sensitive patient outcomes, patient and staff satisfaction and engagement, etc.). A step further might be to participate in local, regional, and national committees that set performance standards. This can be done through professional associations such as the American Nurses Association, the National Association for Healthcare Quality and the American Society for Professionals in Patient Safety. Certification programs are available through these professional associations.

Policies and procedures and guidelines of care at the unit/department level must be updated and/or revised as new standards are introduced, either through participation in voluntary accreditation programs or because of regulatory requirements. Staff need to be educated about the impact and meaning of the standards that are applicable to the care they provide. Documentation requirements may change, and this may affect the outcome of clinical data measures and/or reimbursement. Nurse managers need to provide leadership in adopting and adapting to ongoing changes in these arenas. Many organizations do not have the luxury of devoting one individual or department solely to managing accreditation or regulatory compliance processes. At best, in those organizations that have dedicated individuals or departments for this purpose, they serve as facilitators and coaches for the accreditation and licensing processes. TJC conducts accreditation surveys on an unannounced basis. This requires that leaders and managers throughout the organization be in a continual state of readiness (i.e., to have their departments and staff in compliance with all applicable standards at all times). Thus the onus of responsibility and accountability for continuous readiness has moved from a single regulatory or quality department to all leaders and managers in the organization.

Data Collection and Public Reporting of Quality Outcomes

TJC requires accredited organizations to participate in its core measure initiative. This program requires accredited health care organizations to select outcome measures that reflect the operations of their organizations and to choose a performance measurement vendor to aggregate and analyze the data and submit them on a quarterly basis to TJC. Similarly, the National Committee for Quality Assurance's (NCQA) Healthcare Effectiveness Data and Information Set (HEDIS) outcomes have been an integral part of the NCQA accreditation process for health plans. Of note, CARF International has required both program evaluation and quality outcomes measurement as components of its accreditation process since the 1980s, about a decade before the other accreditors.

An initial drawback to TJC's initial performance measurement process—and that of the quality reporting required by other accreditors—was an inability to compare performance outcomes across and among health care organizations. This was due primarily to the variability allowed in selection of measures and reporting systems. To remedy this critical flaw, TJC devised its Core Measures program. The initial measures in 2001 were acute myocardial infarction (AMI), community-acquired pneumonia (PN), and heart failure (HF) and comprised 10 process measures, often referred to as the "starter set." The current Core Measure sets include: cardiac care, emergency department, health care staffing services, hospital outpatient department, hospital-based inpatient psychiatric services, immunization, palliative care, perinatal care, stroke, substance use, tobacco treatment, total hip and knee replacement, and venous thromboembolism (TJC, 2020a); see Box 18.6 for sample Core Measures from the Hospital Compare database (CMS, n.d.). Consumers are able to access these data and compare hospital performance.

CMS has historically mandated data submission programs for health care organizations to qualify for participation in their Medicare programs. *The Specification Manual for National Hospital Inpatient Quality Measures* is a guide that combines both the CMS measures and the TJC Core Measure sets "to minimize data collection efforts for these common measures and focus efforts on the use of data to improve the health care delivery process" (TJC, 2020a, p. 3). For long-term care hospitals (LTCH), CMS requires the submission

BOX 18.6 Selected Measures Reported on the Hospital Compare Website

Survey of Patients' Experiences
- ***Hospital Outpatient Department Consumer Assessment of Healthcare Providers and Systems (CAHPS)***
- Patients who reported that staff definitely gave care in a professional way
- Patients who reported that staff definitely communicated about what to expect during and after the procedure
- Patients who reported YES they would definitely recommend the facility to family or friends

Timely and Effective Care
Sepsis Care
- Percentage of patients who received appropriate care for severe sepsis and septic shock
- ***Heart Attack Care***
- Average (median) number of minutes before outpatients with chest pain or possible heart attack who needed specialized care were transferred to another hospital

Complications & Deaths
Infections
- Catheter-associated urinary tract infections (CAUTI) in ICUs and select wards
- Surgical site infections (SSI) from colon surgery

Payment and Value of Care
- ***Value of care for heart attack patients***
- Death rate for heart attack patients
- Payment for heart attack patients

From Centers for Medicare & Medicaid Services. (CMS, n.d.). *Hospital Compare: Compare hospitals*. https://www.medicare.gov/hospitalcompare/search.html.

of data through its LTCH Quality Reporting Program. For home health care, CMS requires submission of data to the Home Health Quality Reporting Program, which includes data from the Outcome and Assessment Information Set (OASIS; patient outcome measures) and the Home Health Consumer Assessment for Healthcare Providers and Systems (HHCAHPS; patient survey results) (CMS, 2019a). In both these initiatives, the results for individual health care organizations also were not originally made public. In fall 2001 the US Secretary of Health and Human Services announced the George W. Bush administration's commitment to quality health care through the publication of consumer information. Various Centers for Medicare & Medicaid Services quality programs allow consumers to make informed choices about their health care providers and encourage providers to improve their care.

In 2011 CMS developed the Hospital Value-Based Purchasing Program. Under the program, CMS makes value-based incentive payments to 2700 acute care hospitals based either on how well the hospitals perform on certain quality measures or how much the hospitals' performance improves on certain quality measures from their performance during a baseline period. Reimbursement is based on quality of care, not quantity. The higher a hospital's performance or improvement during the performance period for a fiscal year, the higher the hospital's value-based incentive payment for the fiscal year (FY) would be (CMS, 2019b). The measurement domains for FY2020 are clinical outcomes, safety, person and community engagement, and efficiency and cost reduction. It is estimated that $1.9 billion is available for value-based incentive payments in FY2019 (CMS, 2019c, p. 3).

Initially health care providers were resistant and concerned about issues such as data integrity and the lack of risk adjustments that would ensure that the results were comparable. They were convinced that without safeguards built into state reporting systems, their organizations might look bad to the public. Data analysis systems have evolved and improved over the years to address these concerns. A majority of states have now enacted legislation requiring public reporting. With federal reporting requirements increasingly linked to reimbursement, providers must participate in data submission for public reporting or risk losing accreditation, income, and community status. As an example, organizations must be diligent in documentation of initial patient assessments, because care for patients with poor outcomes (e.g., skin breakdown) that are not recorded as being present on admission (POA), are no longer reimbursed. Terms like "never events" represent a category of adverse outcomes that, in the view of insurers, should never happen and for which they are no longer willing to pay.

Nurses need to be cognizant of the variety of measures being collected for state, federal, and accreditation purposes that apply to their units and patients. Nurse leaders and their staff often have to participate in the data collection effort and discuss outcomes at unit practice council and/or quality improvement committees. Nurse managers, leaders, and executives are held accountable to implement corrective action plans focused on their unit/department to address issues of noncompliance with quality indicators such as Core Measures (e.g., not documenting education about smoking cessation or offering tobacco replacement therapy for patients with AMI). In the future, patients and families may inquire about the organization's publicly reported outcomes (for example, from Hospital Compare or the Leapfrog Group), so it is imperative that all nurses are engaged in quality initiatives and that managers are conversant with this topic.

Health Care Enterprise Risk Management

The Joint Commission has traditionally required a risk management program for the entire organization as a part of its quality improvement efforts. Risk management is an integral component of an organization's quality and safety programs and a risk manager is one of the "first responders" in a serious or sentinel event situation. A new concept and process called *Enterprise Risk Management* (ERM) addresses the evaluation of all risks confronting an organization in order to maximize safety and risk reduction. The idea is to prevent undesirable events from happening and to minimize the impact of unpreventable risks. The concept of enterprise risk management dovetails with the overall requirements of a comprehensive organization-wide approach to patient safety. ERM "promotes a comprehensive framework for making risk management decisions which maximize value protection and creation by managing risk and uncertainty and their connection to total value" (Carroll, 2014, p. 5). *An ERM program* includes components of culture, strategy, objectives, appetite/tolerance,

ERM structure and plans, communication and reporting plans, and oversight.

- **Culture:** A culture supporting ERM, including programs such as High Reliability Organizations (HROs), Crew Resource Management (CRM), TeamSTEPPS, Just Culture, and Mindfulness.
- **Strategy:** Management's game plan for strengthening enterprise performance, with an organizational strategy that is linked to vision, mission, goals, and objectives.
- **Objectives:** Ensuring that ERM objectives are SMART—specific, measureable, achievable, realistic, and timely.
- **Appetite/tolerance:** Determining the desired level of risk the organization will take vis-à-vis its mission and threshold or qualitative range of risks taken in pursuit of the organization's strategy (tolerance).
- **ERM structure and plans:** Organization-wide communication and education plans that describe key roles and committee structures, employee engagement strategies, techniques to update employees on the progress of ERM initiatives, key performance and key risk indicators, and scenarios that highlight the value of ERM to the organization.
- **Oversight:** Acknowledging that the governing body is responsible for ERM oversight, leadership ensures that the governing body is regularly apprised of progress on risk strategies, status of key performance indicators (KPIs) and key risk indicators (KRIs), emerging risks, and recommendations for new projects (Carroll, 2014, pp. 6–8).

Patient Safety Event Reporting

Tools for ongoing risk identification and reporting, incident or variance reports, form the core of organizational reporting from a risk management perspective. An important tool is an incident/variance report. This report provides factual accounting of a patient safety incident or adverse event to ensure that all facts surrounding the incident are recorded. Key attributes of an effective incident reporting system include the following: (1) institution must foster a supportive environment for event reporting that protects the privacy of staff who report occurrences, (2) reports should be received from a broad range of personnel, (3) summaries of reported events must be disseminated in a timely fashion, and (4) a structured mechanism must be in place for reviewing reports and developing action plans (AHRQ, 2019b, p. 3). A successful incident reporting process is one in which the majority of all appropriate incidents/adverse outcomes are reported by various health care professionals.

Fear of disciplinary action continues to be a reason for not reporting, and organizations put an emphasis on data collection versus participative learning (Macrae, 2016, p. 74). Aguilar stated that "healthcare still has a prevalent culture of silence. Frontline workers worried about litigation or job loss cover up mistakes and leaders fail to address medical errors even in a pre-emptive fashion..." (Aguilar, 2019, p. 34). Frequent reporting is more apt to be achieved in those organizations that have adopted a learning, nonpunitive, fair and just culture for reporting errors. Further, "a culture of empowerment enables an organization's frontline staff—the people with the most timely exposure to potential medical errors—to signal the presence of an error or defect and work together with their teams to resolve it" (Virginia Mason Institute, 2016, p. 1).

The data contained in an incident/variance report also alert the nurse leaders and risk managers about facts and circumstances that may contribute to a potential malpractice or lawsuit claim. Similar to quality improvement activities, the analysis of incident reports is the responsibility of the nurse leaders in many organizations. The incident/variance reporting system provides the nurse manager with the opportunity to investigate all serious situations immediately. Data from incident reports are collated, analyzed, and used by unit nurse managers and risk managers to identify risk areas that have ongoing trends or to point to areas that have emerging risk potential. These data can inform the choices that the organization's leaders make in the selection of processes to target for HFMEA projects or to "drill down" further via an RCA to study an adverse outcome or "near miss" more fully. Aggregated data from the organization's health care ERM program are reported through the performance improvement and safety reporting systems to coordinate information about overall organizational risks. New performance measures defined in the action plan resulting from an RCA or HFMEA can be incorporated in a unit's/department's set of quality measures. Nurse managers can set the expectation for reporting of all risk events and "near misses" or "close calls" on their units/departments. Through diligent follow-up and the adoption of a nonpunitive culture, managers can set the tone for a truly proactive and responsive ERM program.

In addition to internal reporting, many states (most via their health care licensure agencies, such as a department of health) have implemented mandatory adverse event reporting requirements, resulting in a new role for many health care risk managers. In organizations in these states, the risk manager is often accountable for the reporting of incidents that are on the mandated list. Most of these mandatory reporting programs also require the submission of formal RCAs as a follow-up to the initial report, including actions taken and assessment of the effectiveness of those actions. If the regulatory agency determines that the organization has not appropriately responded to the identified risks, it may result in further requirements for reporting and follow-up. This expanded role of the health care risk manager in external reporting creates a need for collaboration with the quality professionals in the organization. Working together as a team, the risk manager and quality manager will often share responsibilities for facilitation of RCA and HFMEA teams to meet all of the internal and external accreditation and regulatory reporting requirements.

Sentinel Events

Organizational response to sentinel events is one element included in TJC standards in both the Leadership and Performance Improvement chapters. A *sentinel event* is defined by TJC as "a patient safety event that reaches a patient and results in any of the following: death, permanent harm, or severe temporary harm and intervention required. Such events are called 'sentinel' because they signal the need for immediate investigation and response" (TJC, 2019d, pp. 5–7).

Since 1999 TJC has required health care organizations to respond to sentinel events in a systematic and formal way such as conducting a RCA. The purpose of the RCA is to "drill down" to the most common cause(s), using flowcharting and cause-and-effect diagramming, for the event and determine what process improvements can be made to prevent the sentinel event from occurring in the future.

The detailed requirements for reporting and submitting RCAs are contained in the Sentinel Event policy and can be found on the TJC website (https://www.jointcommission.org/resources/patient-safety-topics/sentinel-event/sentinel-event-policy-and-procedures/). Specific sentinel event outcomes are considered "reviewable" by TJC. Reviewable sentinel events are events that have resulted in an unanticipated death, permanent harm, or severe temporary harm. Examples of events that are considered sentinel:

- Suicide of any patient receiving care, treatment, and services in a staffed-around-the-clock care setting or within 72 hours of discharge, including from the hospital's emergency department (ED)
- Unanticipated death of a full-term infant
- Discharge of an infant to the wrong family
- Abduction of any patient receiving care, treatment, and services
- An elopement (unauthorized departure) of a patient from a staffed-around-the-clock care setting (including the ED), leading to death, permanent harm, or severe temporary harm to the patient
- Administration of blood or blood products having unintended ABO or non-ABO incompatibilities, hemolytic transfusion reactions, or transfusions resulting in severe temporary harm, permanent harm or death
- Rape, assault, or homicide of any patient receiving care, treatment, and services while on site at the hospital
- Rape, assault, or homicide of a staff member, licensed independent practitioner, visitor, or vendor while on site at the hospital
- Surgery or other invasive procedure performed on the wrong site, on the wrong patient, or that is the wrong (unintended) procedure for a patient
- Unintended retention of a foreign object in a patient after an invasive procedure, including surgery
- Severe neonatal hyperbilirubinemia (bilirubin >30 mg/dl)
- Prolonged fluoroscopy with cumulative dose >1500 rads to a single field or any delivery of radiotherapy to the wrong body region or >25% above the planned radiotherapy dose
- Fire, flame, or unanticipated smoke, heat, or flashes occurring during direct patient care caused by equipment operated and used by the hospital
- Any intrapartum (related to the birth process) maternal death
- Severe maternal morbidity (not primarily related to the natural course of the patient's illness or underlying condition) when it reaches a patient and results in any of the following: permanent harm or

severe temporary harm (TJC, 2019d, Hospital, pp. SE1–SE3).

Time frames for concluding this analysis and guidelines for conducting a *thorough* and *credible* process are outlined in the current accreditation standards.

The action plan that results from the RCA must be robust and must be strong enough to sustain the prevention of such events from occurring in the future. The VA NCPS has developed an action hierarchy that outlines strong, intermediate, and weak actions (Box 18.7; US Department of Veterans Affairs, 2015, p. 28).

The National Patient Safety Foundation has also developed a definitive guide on conducting RCAs (NPSF, 2016), which has been endorsed by TJC and other public and private patient safety organizations. The document provides teams with effective techniques to conduct comprehensive systematic reviews (RCAs) and develop sustainable actions to prevent their future occurrence (see Fig. 18.8 for the *NPSF Root Cause Analysis and Action* [*RCA*^{2}] Process).

Organizations that have initiated comprehensive and robust safety programs are committed to the process of ongoing risk identification and prevention. These organizations encourage the staff to identify potential errors and report any "near misses" or "close calls" that occur. Even if an adverse event is not considered reviewable, such organizations conduct RCAs on these identified risks to prevent similar errors from occurring in the future.

The Joint Commission accreditation standards also require that organizations go a step beyond the RCA process in their health care risk reduction and management programs. A set of standards in the Patient Safety Systems chapter of the accreditation manual (TJC, 2016) encourages leaders to maintain a safety system by promoting learning and motivating staff to uphold a fair and just safety culture, providing a transparent environment in which quality measures and patient harms are freely shared with staff, modeling professional behavior, removing intimidating behavior that might prevent safe behaviors, and providing the resources and training necessary to take on improvement initiatives (TJC, 2020b).

One of the methods for proactive risk assessment that accredited hospitals are expected to implement is the process of HFMEA. The expectation is that an HFMEA will be performed on at least one identified high-risk process annually. The HFMEA is conducted by an interdisciplinary team of professionals who own the process being studied and is facilitated by someone with knowledge and skills in quality improvement tools. The HFMEA begins with flowcharting the steps of the process being studied. The team assesses risk points within the process steps, and these key risk points are ranked in terms of their impact on the potential failure of the system. Scores for severity and probability are calculated to give a "hazard" score to the identified breakdown, and detectability of the failure mode is factored into the analysis of its impact on the overall process. The team then "designs out" the most critical of the potential failures and recommends process improvements for prevention of the failures. Once these prevention strategies are identified, action plans for implementing them are reported to the

BOX 18.7 VA National Center for Patient Safety Action Hierarchy

Stronger Actions
- Architectural/physical plant changes
- New devices with usability testing before purchasing
- Engineering control, interlock, forcing functions
- Simplify the process and remove unnecessary steps
- Standardize on equipment or process or care maps
- Tangible involvement and action by leadership in support of patient safety

Intermediate Actions
- Redundancy/back-up systems
- Increase in staffing/decrease in workload
- Software enhancements/modifications
- Eliminate/reduce distractions
- Checklist/cognitive aid
- Eliminate look- and sound-alikes
- Enhanced documentation/communication

Weaker Actions
- Double checks
- Warnings and labels
- New procedure/memorandum/policy

From US Department of Veterans Affairs, VA National Center for Patient Safety, 2015b. http://www.patientsafety.va.gov/docs/joe/rca_tools_2_15.pdf.

enterprise leaders and endorsed for implementation (US Department of Veterans Affairs, 2019).

Educating Nurses about Quality and Safety

Academia has confronted the challenge of educating nurses about quality and safety by developing formal curricula. Quality and Safety Education for Nurses (QSEN), originally funded by the Robert Wood Johnson Foundation, and now managed by the Frances Payne Bolton School of Nursing at Case Western Reserve University, is a comprehensive resource for faculty to help new health care professionals learn the knowledge and skills necessary to lead and support quality and safety initiatives in health care organizations (QSEN Institute, 2020). QSEN has identified six core knowledge, skills, and attitude competencies related to quality and safety:

> *"1) Patient-centered care: Recognize the patient or designee as the source of control and full partner in providing compassionate and coordinated care based on respect for patient's preferences, values and needs; 2) Teamwork and collaboration: function effectively within nursing and interprofessional teams, fostering open communication, mutual respect, and shared decision-making to achieve quality patient care; 3) Evidence-based practice (EBP): Integrate best current evidence with clinical expertise and patient/family preferences and values for delivery of optimal health care; 4) Quality improvement (QI): Use data to monitor the outcomes of care processes and use improvement methods to design and test changes to continuously improve the quality and safety of health care systems; 5) Safety: Minimizes risk of harm to patients and providers through both system effectiveness and individual performance; and 6) Informatics: Use information and technology to communicate, manage knowledge, mitigate error, and support decision making" (QSEN Institute, 2020, pp. 5–11).*

Regional education sessions have provided the opportunity for the content to spread throughout nursing academia.

Acknowledging the critical role that nurses play in improving the quality and safety of patient care, the AHRQ published *Patient Safety and Quality: An Evidence-Based Handbook for Nurses*, a comprehensive compendium of health care quality resources. Readers are provided with proven techniques and interventions they can use to enhance patient care outcomes (Hughes, 2008).

The Institute for Healthcare Improvement provides an "Open School" for health professionals to learn about quality and safety. The IHI Open School for Health Professions is an interprofessional educational community that gives students the skills to become change agents in health care improvement (IHI, 2020c).

Advancing Quality and Safety Policy

The Nursing Alliance for Quality Care (NAQC) was established in 2010 at the George Washington University School of Nursing and managed by the American Nurses Association since 2013. "It has become the 'go-to' organization in the field for advancing high quality, patient-centered healthcare" (ANA/NAQC, n.d., p. 1). NAQC members include nursing professional associations and consumer groups such as ANA, American Association of Colleges of Nursing, National Council of State Boards of Nursing, American Academy of Nursing, and Mothers Against Medical Error. The group proposes to set policy related to nursing's pivotal role in health care transformation.

CONCLUSION

Clearly, nurses have been accountable for health care quality and safety since the profession's inception. Over the years, nurses have assumed roles in various health care settings for oversight of quality and safety improvement, as well as health care ERM. The IOM reports, the CMS requirements for public data reporting, and recent health care reform legislation initiatives have raised public awareness about quality and safety outcomes in health care organizations. These quality and safety issues have challenged health care quality professionals and nurse leaders for decades. A heightened public awareness, combined with increasingly stringent standards for reporting quality and safety outcomes, are driving the need for health care organizations to address these issues. Professional nurses in direct care and leaders in managerial and executive roles need to continue to be at the forefront, leading the charge in adoption of quality and safety initiatives that continuously enhance the quality of care and services provided to patients/clients, families, and populations/communities.

RESEARCH NOTE

Source

Stichler, J.F., & Pelletier, L.R. (2019). Psychometric testing of a patient empowerment, engagement, and activation survey. *Journal of Nursing Care Quality, 35*(4), E49–E57.

Purpose

Patient or person-centered care has become a widely used philosophical framework and yet has varying definitions and characteristics. Person-centered care has recently been conceptualized as patient empowerment, engagement, and activation with studies citing positive outcomes. This study reports the psychometric properties of the Patient Empowerment, Engagement, and Activation Survey.

Discussion

An instrument development and testing approach was used. A 21-item survey was developed demonstrating respectable Cronbach α coefficients for the total scale ($\alpha = 0.88$) and for each subscale: Empowerment ($\alpha = 0.71$), Engagement ($\alpha = 0.81$), and Activation ($\alpha = 0.76$). A regression analysis with 1 item, "I am ready to be discharged" as the dependent variable and all other items as independent variables explained 65% of the variance in readiness for discharge ($P < .001$). Limitations of the study included: small sample size, not testing the survey in combination with other valid and reliable instruments. This study validates the predictive strength of empowerment and engagement on activation similar to other studies.

Application to Practice

Professional nurses need to be aware of the patient's level of empowerment, engagement, and activation and how these influence outcomes of care. It is also important to be aware of any barriers that may impede the patient's level of empowerment, engagement, and activation (limited health literacy, severe medical illness, altered psychological states, language, and cultural), and determine ways to alleviate these barriers. The Patient Empowerment, Engagement, and Activation Survey (PEEAS) can be used to evaluate patients' perspectives of care quality (empowerment and engagement) and readiness for discharge (activation). Used within 24 hours of discharge, the survey can be used to measure the patient's readiness to leave the hospital and assume responsibility for their own care. Future research could combine this new survey with other similar instruments to gauge convergent and divergent validity of the instrument. Additionally, if this type of scale was programmed within the electronic health record, it could trigger various learning strategies in the individualized plan of care based on the patient's level of empowerment, engagement, and activation.

CASE STUDY

Nurse Manager Jaxson has been asked by his Chief Nursing Officer to spearhead a group to evaluate self-injurious behavior (SIB) on a child and adolescent psychiatric unit. Prevention of injury is aligned with the organization's patient safety goals. Based on incident/variance reports, he determines that there is indeed an improvement opportunity, and he selects nurses and a mental health associate (MHA) for the project team. He asks a pharmacist and physician to join the project team to represent the interprofessional aspects of the issue. Jaxson recruits a family member of one of the patients on the child and adolescent unit to provide their perspective. Jaxson then applies the Define, Measure, Analyze, Improve, and Control (DMAIC) improvement model to conduct a quality and safety improvement project.

- **Define phase:** Jaxson and the project team research the scientific and nursing literature to determine the prevalence of SIB. They also determine that patient safety is a national imperative and review The Joint Commission statements related to self-injurious behavior. They propose an aim of "zero harm" from self-injurious injuries, which has been described in the patient safety literature.
- **Measure phase:** Jaxson and the project team request incident/variance data from the Clinical Effectiveness Department for the past year. They request that the data be stratified by time of day, age of patient, location of incident, type of injury, and whether or not the injury required medical intervention.
- **Analyze phase:** The project team analyzes the data they received from the Clinical Effectiveness

CASE STUDY—cont'd

Department. They use flowcharting to visually illustrate a typical SIB episode. Next the team brainstorms a list of all of the problems that are associated with these incidents. From this list, Jaxson directs the team to categorize these factors in five or six groups using an affinity diagram. Once the categories are defined, the team uses a cause-and-effect (fishbone) diagram to identify all of the potential causes that lead to the eventual effect of a self-injurious injury. From this fishbone diagram, specific factors are considered as potential root causes (e.g., lack of safety check on admission, incomplete admission assessment, poor observation in some areas of the unit, lack of consistent evening programming, staffing and staffing mix, lack of consistent staffing during visiting hours, patient's lack of safety awareness, and poor impulse control). The project team used a Pareto chart to visually illustrate the most frequently occurring problems in descending order. By using this technique, they find that lack of safety check on admission, inadequate admission assessment, poor observation in some areas of the unit, and lack of consistent evening programming are the most common factors in SIB incidents. They also use Pareto charts to further define the stratification categories. When using this tool, they find that female teenagers with a presenting problem of suicidal ideation on admission are the most likely to self-injure. Most of the occurrences are on the evening shift.

- **Improve phase:** Jaxson and the project team design a checklist for nursing assessments, highlighting the admission safety check and admission assessment and reassessments. They collect data for 2 months; they meet to analyze the data to find that compliance with admission assessment processes have improved. They meet with Plant Operations to discuss "blind spots" on the unit; those areas that are hard to observe because of physical barriers. They discuss a plan for unit renovations; renovations are completed in 6 months. The project team discuss barriers to meeting expectations for evening programming. They identify a lack of knowledge in leading groups. Jaxson meets with the Unit Psychologist, who will provide education on leading and managing groups; the plan is to complete education in 2 months. After education has been completed, the project team develop an evening programming audit to determine which groups were completed weekly; data are collected for a month. Barriers to offering evening programming are also identified. Jaxson hires a 0.5 FTE MHA to ensure evening programming occurs as scheduled. The audit results show that evening programming has improved 90% over the last 6 months.
- **Control phase:** The team reconvenes to evaluate the data collected in the Improve phase. Since they found a 75% improvement in assessments, they plan to implement the assessment checklist once per quarter for 6 months to "hold the gains." They also plan to implement the evening programming audit 1 week per quarter for 6 months. The project team plans to look at incident/variance data for the year to determine if their rates have decreased due to their patient safety interventions.

Jaxson shares the data with the hospital's nursing leadership group using control charts to demonstrate the outcomes. They also present their DMAIC project at the hospital's Quality Council. Jaxson applies for an annual Quality Award based on their successful project. He and his Director have also submitted their project as a poster presentation at the next American Psychiatric Nurses Association annual meeting. They also plan on disseminating their work in a peer-reviewed publication in the near future.

CRITICAL THINKING EXERCISE

Nurse Manager Adeline has been in her current position for 6 months. Her hospital is preparing for their first Magnet designation, and her Director would like Adeline to work on improving nursing engagement on her unit. The Director gives Adeline last year's results of the National Database of Nursing Quality Indicators (NDNQI) RN Engagement Survey (see following table). Since Adeline is not familiar with the Magnet standards, she asks her Director for the standard requirements and information about the survey.

Results of RN Engagement Survey

	Autonomy	Professional Development	Leadership Access & Responsiveness	Interprofessional Relationships	Fundamentals of Quality Nursing Care	Adequacy of Resources & Staffing	RN–RN Teamwork & Collaboration
Adeline's Unit	3.85	3.17	3.63	4.19	4.15	3.85	4.27
National Benchmark	3.44	3.83	3.82	3.30	3.74	3.73	3.50

1. What should Adeline do first to address this issue (what additional information does she need before she can plan a course of action)?
2. What domains of RN engagement should she target (which domains received scores below the national benchmark)?
3. Should she do a literature search on RN engagement?
4. Who should she include on a team to address RN engagement on her unit?
5. Describe the interventions she will employ to enhance RN engagement on her unit based on a literature review, addressing the domains that have scored below the benchmark.
6. Describe the reports she will write about the project and to whom she would send the reports.

REFERENCES

Advisory Board. (2018). *Cracks in the foundation undermine nurse resilience*. https://www.advisory.com/research/nursing-executive-center/resources/posters/nurse-resilience.

Agency for Healthcare Research and Quality (AHRQ). (2017a). *Guide to patient and family engagement in hospital quality and safety*. http://www.ahrq.gov/professionals/systems/hospital/engagingfamilies/index.html.

Agency for Healthcare Research and Quality. (2017b). *Strategy 3: Nurse bedside shift report implementation handbook*. Rockville, MD: AHRQ. http://www.ahrq.gov/professionals/systems/hospital/engagingfamilies/strategy3/index.html.

Agency for Healthcare Research and Quality (AHRQ). (2019a). *High reliability*. https://psnet.ahrq.gov/primer/high-reliability.

Agency for Healthcare Research and Quality (AHRQ). (2019b). *Patient safety primer: Reporting patient safety events*. https://psnet.ahrq.gov/primer/reporting-patient-safety-events.

Agency for Healthcare Research and Quality (AHRQ). (n.d.a.). *AHRQuality indicators*. https://www.qualityindicators.ahrq.gov/.

Agency for Healthcare Research and Quality (AHRQ). (n.d.b.). *TeamSTEPPS: National implementation*. http://teamstepps.ahrq.gov/.

Aguilar, A. (2019). Culture of silence contributes to lack of progress on patient safety. *Modern Healthcare, 49*(44), 34.

American Nurses Association (ANA). (2010). *Position statement: Just culture*. http://nursingworld.org/psjustculture.

American Nurses Association (ANA). (2015). *Code of ethics for nurses with interpretive statements*. Silver Spring, MD: ANA.

American Nurses Association/Nursing Alliance for Quality Care (NAQC). (n.d.). *About NAQC*. https://www.nursingworld.org/practice-policy/naqc/.

American Nurses Credentialing Center (ANCC). (n.d.). ANCC Magnet Recognition Program®. https://www.nursingworld.org/magnet.

American Society for Quality (ASQ). (2019a). *Quality glossary – C*. https://asq.org/quality-resources/quality-glossary/c.

American Society for Quality (ASQ). (2019b). *What is lean?* https://asq.org/quality-resources/lean.

Baldrige Foundation. (2020). *Baldrige – America's best investment*. https://baldrigefoundation.org/who-we-are/history.html.

Barnes, H., Rearden, J., & McHugh, M. D. (2016). Magnet hospital recognition linked to lower central line-associated bloodstream infection rates. *Research in Nursing & Health, 39*(2), 96–104. https://doi.org/10.1002/nur.21709.

Bekelis, K., Missios, S., & MacKenzie, T. A. (2017). Association of Magnet status with hospitalization outcomes for ischemic stroke patients. *Journal of the American Heart Association, 6*(4), Article e3005880. https://doi.org/ 10.1161/JAHA.117.005880.

Benavidez, G., & Frakt, A. B. (2019). Fixing clinical practice guidelines. *Health Affairs Blog*. https://www.healthaffairs.org/do/10.1377/hblog20190730.874541/full/. https://doi.org/10.1377/hblog20190730.874541.

Berwick, D. M., Godfrey, A. B., & Roessner, J. (1990). *Curing health care: New strategies for quality improvement*. San Francisco, CA: Jossey-Bass.

Berwick, D. M., & Hackbarth, A. D. (2012). Eliminating waste in US health care. *Journal of the American Medical Association, 307*(14), 1513–1516. https://doi.org/10.1001/jama.2012.362.

Berwick, D. M., Nolan, T. W., & Whittington, J. (2008). The triple aim: Care, health and cost. *Health Affairs, 27*(3), 759–769. https://doi.org/10.1377/hlthaff.27.3.759.

Brigham, T., Barden, C., Dopp, A. L., Hengerer, A., Kaplan, J., Malone, B., et al. (2018). *A journey to construct an all-encompassing conceptual model of factors affecting clinical well-being and resilience*. Washington, DC: National Academy of Medicine.

Caplan, W., Davis, S., Kraft, S., Berkson, S., Gaines, M. E., Schwab, W., & Pandhi, N. (2014). Engaging patients at the front lines of primary care redesign: Operational lessons for an effective program. *The Joint Commission Journal on Quality and Patient Safety, 40*(12), 533–540. https://doi.org/10.1016/s1553-7250(14)40069-2.

Carroll, R. (2014). *Enterprise risk management: A framework for success*. Chicago, IL: American Society for Health Risk Management.

Centers for Medicare & Medicaid Services (CMS). (2019a). *Home health quality measures*. https://www.cms.gov/Medicare/Quality-Initiatives-Patient-Assessment-Instruments/HomeHealthQualityInits/Home-Health-Quality-Measures.

Centers for Medicare & Medicaid Services (CMS). (2019b). *The hospital value-based purchasing program*. https://www.cms.gov/Medicare/Quality-Initiatives-Patient-Assessment-Instruments/Value-Based-Programs/HVBP/Hospital-Value-Based-Purchasing.

Centers for Medicare & Medicaid Services (CMS). (2019c). *CMS hospital value-based purchasing program for fiscal year 2020*. https://www.cms.gov/newsroom/fact-sheets/cms-hospital-value-based-purchasing-program-results-fiscal-year-2020.

Centers for Medicare & Medicaid Services (CMS). (n.d.). *Hospital Compare: Compare hospitals*. https://www.medicare.gov/hospitalcompare/search.html.

Chassin, M. R. (1997). Assessing strategies for quality improvement. *Health Affairs, 16*(3), 151–161. https://doi.org/10.1377/hlthaff.16.3.151.

Chassin, M. R., & Loeb, J. M. (2013). High-reliability health care: Getting there from here. *The Milbank Quarterly, 91*(3), 459–490. https://doi.org/10.1111/1468-0009.12023.

Corrigan, J. M., Eden, J., & Smith, B. M. (Eds.). (2002). *Leadership by example: Coordinating government roles in improving health care quality*. Washington, DC: National Academies Press.

Deming, W. E. (2000a). *The new economics for industry, government, education*. Cambridge, MA: MIT Center for Advanced Engineering Studies.

Deming, W. E. (2000b). *Out of the crisis*. Cambridge, MA: MIT Center for Advanced Engineering Studies.

Donabedian, A. (1980). *Explorations in quality assessment and monitoring: The definition of quality and approaches to its assessment* (Vol.1). Ann Arbor, MI: Health Administration Press.

Dyrbye, L. N., Shanafelt, T. D., Sinsky, C. A., Cipriano, P. F., Bhatt, J., Ommaya, A., et al. (2017). Burnout among health care professionals: A call to explore and address this unrecognized threat to safe, quality care. Discussion Paper, *NAM Perspectives*. Washington, DC: National Academy of Medicine.

Harmon, F. G. (1997). Future present. In F. Hesselbein, M. Goldsmith, & R. Beckhard (Eds.), *The organization of the future* (pp. 239–247). San Francisco, CA: Jossey-Bass.

Harry, M., & Schroeder, R. (2000). *Six Sigma: The breakthrough strategy revolutionizing the world's top corporations*. New York: Currency/Doubleday.

Hegge, M. (2015). *Faculty pak: Guide to the code of ethics for nurses with interpretive statements: Development, interpretation and application*. American Nurses Association. http://www.nursingworld.org/MainMenuCategories/EthicsStandards/CodeofEthicsforNurses/Faculty-Pak.

Higgins, T., Larson, E., & Schnall, R. (2017). Unravelling the meaning of patient engagement: A concept analysis. *Patient Education and Counseling, 100*(1), 30–36. https://doi.org/10.1016/j.pec.2016.09.002.

His Holiness the Dalai Lama, & Cutler, H. C. (1998). *The art of happiness*. New York: Penguin Random House, Riverhead Books.

Hughes, R. G. (2008). *Patient safety and quality: An evidence-based handbook for nurses*. Rockville, MD: (AHRQ Publication No. 08-0043). http://archive.ahrq.gov/professionals/clinicians-providers/resources/nursing/resources/nurseshdbk/nurseshdbk.pdf.

Insignia Health. (2020). *Patient activation measure*. https://www.insigniahealth.com/products/pam-survey.

Institute for Healthcare Improvement (IHI). (2004). *About IHI*. http://www.ihi.org/about/Pages/default.aspx.

Institute for Healthcare Improvement (IHI). (2005). *Going lean in health care*. Cambridge, MA: IHI.

Institute for Healthcare Improvement (IHI). (2020a). *Plan-Do-Study-Act (PDSA) worksheet*. http://www.ihi.org/resources/pages/tools/plandostudyactworksheet.aspx.

Institute for Healthcare Improvement (IHI). (2020b). *High reliability* (search). http://www.ihi.org/sites/search/pages/results.aspx?k=high+reliability.

Institute for Healthcare Improvement (IHI). (2020c). IHI Open School: *Overview*. http://www.ihi.org/education/ihiopenschool/overview/Pages/default.aspx.

Institute of Medicine. (2000). *Medicare: A strategy for quality assurance* (Vol.2). Washington, DC: National Academies Press.

Institute of Medicine (IOM), Committee on Enhancing Federal Health Care Quality Programs (CEFHQP). (2002). *Enhancing federal health care quality programs*. https://www8.nationalacademies.org/onpinews/newsitem.aspx?RecordID=0309086163.

Institute of Medicine (IOM), *Committee on Quality of Health Care in America (CQHCA)*. (2001). *Crossing the quality chasm: A new health system for the 21st century*. Washington, DC: National Academies Press.

Institute of Medicine (IOM), Committee on the National Quality Report on Health Care Delivery. (2001). *Envisioning the national health care quality report*. Washington, DC: National Academies Press.

Institute of Medicine (IOM), Committee on the Robert Wood Johnson Foundation Initiative on the Future of Nursing. (2011). *The future of nursing: Leading change, advancing health*. Washington, DC: National Academies Press.

Interprofessional Education Collaborative. (2016). *Core competencies for interprofessional collaborative practice: 2016 update*. https://hsc.unm.edu/ipe/resources/ipec-2016-core-competencies.pdf.

Joint Commission Center for Transforming Healthcare. (2020). *High reliability in health care is possible*. https://www.centerfortransforminghealthcare.org/en/high-reliability-in-health-care/.

Jones, D., & Womack, J. (2003). *Lean thinking: Banish waste and create wealth in your corporation, revised and updated*. New York: Free Press.

Juran, J. M. (1989). *Juran on leadership for quality: An executive handbook*. New York: Free Press.

Juran Institute. (2009). *Product store*. https://www.juran.com/resources/.

Kelly, L. (2020). Burnout, compassion fatigue, and secondary trauma in nurses: Recognizing the occupational phenomenon and personal consequences of caregiving. *Critical Care Nursing Quarterly, 43*(1), 73–80. https://doi.org/10.1097/CNQ.0000000000000293.

Kohn, L. T., Corrigan, J. M., & Donaldson, M. S. (Eds.). (2000). *To err is human: Building a safer health care system*. Washington, DC: National Academies Press.

Link, A. N., & Scott, J. T. (2011). *Planning report 11-2: Economic evaluation of the Baldrige Performance Excellence Program*. National Institute of Standards and Technology, US Department of Commerce. https://www.nist.gov/system/files/documents/2017/05/09/report11-2.pdf.

Macrae, C. (2016). The problem with incident reporting. *BMJ Quality & Safety, 25*, 71–75. https://doi.org/10.1136/bmjqs-2015-004732.

McCann, C. M., Beddoe, E., McCormick, K., Huggard, P., Kedge, S., Adamson, C., et al. (2013). Resilience in the health professions: A review of the recent literature. *International Journal of Wellbeing, 3*(1), 60–81. https://doi.org/10.5502/ijw.v3i1.4.

Missios, S., & Bekelis, K. (2018). Association of hospitalization for neurosurgical operations in Magnet hospitals with mortality and length of stay. *Neurosurgery, 82*(3), 372–377. https://doi.org/10.1093/neuros/nyx203.

Melnyk, B., Buck, J., & Gallagher-Ford, L. (2015). Transforming quality improvement into evidence-based quality improvement: A key solution to improve healthcare outcomes. *World Views of Evidence Based Practice, 12*(5), 251–252. https://doi.org/10.1111/wvn.12112.

National Academy of Medicine. (2019). *Action collaborative on clinician well-being and resilience*. https://nam.edu/initiatives/clinician-resilience-and-well-being/.

National Institute of Standards and Technology. (2019). *Six health care, nonprofit and education organizations win Baldrige awards for performance excellence*. https://www.nist.gov/news-events/news/2019/11/six-health-care-nonprofit-and-education-organizations-win-baldrige-awards.

National Patient Safety Foundation. (2016). RCA^2 *Improving root cause analyses and actions to prevent harm*. https://www.ashp.org/-/media/assets/policy-guidelines/docs/endorsed-documents/endorsed-documents-improving-root-cause-analyses-actions-prevent-harm.ashx.

National Quality Forum (NQF). (2012a). *Nursing-sensitive care: Initial measures*. http://www.qualityforum.org/Projects/n-r/Nursing-Sensitive_Care_Initial_Measures/Nursing_Sensitive_Care__Initial_Measures.aspx.

National Quality Forum (NQF). (2012b). *Measure evaluation criteria*. http://www.qualityforum.org/Measuring_Performance/Submitting_Standards/Measure_Evaluation_Criteria.aspx.

National University. (2020). *Planetree*. https://www.nu.edu/planetree/.

O'Neil, E. H., & The Pew Health Professions Commission (PHPC). (1998). *Recreating health professional practice for a new century: The fourth report of the Pew Health Professions Commission*. University of California, San Francisco, CA: PHPC.

Palmer, S., & Torgerson, D. J. (1999). Definition of efficiency. *British Medical Journal, 318*, 1136.

Paradiso, L., & Sweeney, N. (2019). Just culture: It's more than policy. *Nursing Management, 50*(6), 38–45. https://doi.org/10.1097/01.NUMA.0000558482.07815.ae.
Park, S. H., Gass, S., & Boyle, D. K. (2016). Comparison of reasons for nurse turnover in Magnet and non-Magnet hospitals. *Journal of Nursing Administration, 46*(5), 284–290. https://doi.org/10.1097/NNA.0000000000000344.
Pelletier, L. R. (1998). Guest editorial: Standardization. *Journal of Nursing Care Quality, 13*(1), vii.
Pelletier, L. R. (2000). On error-free health care: Mission possible! [Editorial]. *Journal for Healthcare Quality, 22*(3), 2, 9.
Pelletier, L. R. (2015). Commentary on "Engagement as an element of safe inpatient psychiatric environments". *Journal of the American Psychiatric Nurses Association, 21*(3), 191–194. https://doi.org/10.1177/1078390315593061.
Pelletier, L. R., & Beaudin, C. L. (2018). *HQ solutions: Resource for the healthcare quality professional (4th ed.).* Philadelphia: Wolters-Kluwer Health.
Pelletier, L. R., & Hoffman, J. A. (2002). A framework for selecting performance measures for opioid treatment programs. *Journal for Healthcare Quality, 24*(3), 24–35. https://doi.org/10.1111/j.1945-1474.2002.tb00430.x.
Pelletier, L. R., & Stichler, J. F. (2014a). Ensuring patient and family engagement: A professional nurse's toolkit. *Journal of Nursing Care Quality, 29*(2), 110–114. https://doi.org/10.1097/NCQ.0000000000000046.
Pelletier, L. R., & Stichler, J. F. (2014b). Patient-centered care and engagement: Nurse leaders' imperative for health reform. *The Journal of Nursing Administration, 44*(9), 473–480. https://doi.org/10.1097/NNA.0000000000000102.
Pelletier, L. R., & Stichler, J. F. (2013). Action brief: Patient engagement and activation: A health reform imperative and improvement opportunity for nursing. *Nursing Outlook, 61*(1), 51–54. https://doi.org/10.1016/j.outlook.2012.11.003.
Planetree. (2018). *Creating a standard of person-centered care.* https://www.planetree.org/how-we-help.
Plsek, P., & Omnias, A. (1989). *Juran Institute quality improvement tools: Problem solving/glossary.* Wilton, CT: Juran Institute.
Polacek, M. J., Allen, D. E., Damin-Moss, R. S., Schwartz, A. J., & Sharp, D., et al. (2015). Engagement as an element of safe inpatient psychiatric environments-. *Journal of the American Psychiatric Nurses Association, 21*(3), 181–190. https://doi.org/10.1177/1078390315593107.
Press Ganey. (2020). *Capture nursing-specific measures.* https://www.pressganey.com/solutions/clinical-excellence/capture-nursing-specific-measures.
QSEN Institute. (2020). *QSEN competencies.* http://qsen.org/competencies/pre-licensure-ksas/.
Robert Wood Johnson Foundation. (2014). *Aligning forces for quality: Patient engagement toolkit.* http://forces4quality.org/node/6319.html.
Rosati, R. (2018). Health data analytics. In L. R. Pelletier, & C. L. Beaudin (Eds.), *HQ Solutions: Resources for the Healthcare Quality Professional.* Philadelphia, PA: Wolters Kluwer.
Sackett, D. L., Rosenberg, W. M. C., Gray, J. A. M., Haynes, R. B., & Richardson, W. S. (1996). Evidence-based medicine: What it is and what it isn't. *British Medical Journal, 312*(7023), 71. https://doi.org/10.1136/bmj.312.7023.71.
Sharp HealthCare. (2020). *Mission, vision and values. http://www.sharp.com/about/our-story/mission-vision-values.cfm.*
Shojania, K. G., Duncan, B. W., McDonald, K. M., & Wachter, R. M. (2001). *Making health care safer: A clinical analysis of patient safety practices.* Evidence Report/Technology Assessment No. 43. https://archive.ahrq.gov/clinic/ptsafety/pdf/ptsafety.pdf.
Shrank, W. H., Rogstad, T. L., & Parekh, N. (2019). Waste in the US health care system: Estimated costs and potential for savings. *New England Journal of Medicine, 322*(15), 1501–1509. https://doi.org/10.1001/jama.2019.13978.
Sikka, R., Morath, J. M., & Leape, L. (2015). The quadruple aim: Care, health, cost and meaning in work. *BMJ Quality and Safety Online.* http://qualitysafety.bmj.com/content/qhc/24/10/608.full.pdf.
Stichler, J. F., & Pelletier, L. R. (2019). Psychometric testing of a patient empowerment, engagement, and activation survey. *Journal of Nursing Care Quality, 35*(4), E49–E57. https://doi.org/10.1097/NCQ.0000000000000452.
Stimpfel, A. W., Sloane, D. M., McHugh, M. D., & Aiken, L. H. (2016). Hospitals known for nursing excellence associated with better hospital experience for patients. *Health Services Research, 51*(3), 1120–1134. https://doi.org/10.1111/1475-6773.12357.
The Joint Commission (TJC). (2016). *Comprehensive accreditation manual for hospitals: Patient safety systems (Update 2).* http://www.jointcommission.org/assets/1/18/PSC_for_Web.pdf.
The Joint Commission (TJC). (2019a). *Specifications Manual for Joint Commission National Quality Measures.* https://manual.jointcommission.org/releases/TJC2019A1/.
The Joint Commission (TJC). (2019b). *Primary Care Medical Home Certification Program.* https://www.jointcommission.org/accreditation-and-certification/certification/certifications-by-setting/hospital-certifications/primary-care-medical-home-certification/#6013d8e234884e60a1326022ca98c9e4_ae0c115936bd43f98842cd6001c8145f.
The Joint Commission (TJC). (2019c). *Quick Safety: Developing resilience to combat nurse burnout. Issue 50.* Oakbrook Terrace, IL: TJC. https://www.

jointcommission.org/resources/news-and-multimedia/news/2019/07/the-joint-commission-issues-quick-safety-advisory-on-combating-nurse-burnout-through-resilience/.

The Joint Commission (TJC). (2019d). *Sentinel event policy and procedures*. https://www.jointcommission.org/resources/patient-safety-topics/sentinel-event/sentinel-event-policy-and-procedures/.

The Joint Commission (TJC). (2020a). *Measures*. https://www.jointcommission.org/en/measurement/measure/, https://www.jointcommission.org/en/measurement/specification-manuals/chart-abstracted-measures/.

The Joint Commission (TJC). (2020b). *Joint Commission urges healthcare leaders to develop cultures of safety*. https://www.fiercehealthcare.com/healthcare/healthcare-leaders-must-develop-a-culture-safety-joint-commission-says.

The Joint Commission (TJC). (2020c). *Sentinel event alert newsletters*. https://www.jointcommission.org/resources/patient-safety-topics/sentinel-event/sentinel-event-alert-newsletters/.

The Joint Commission (TJC). (2020d). *National patient safety goals*. http://www.jointcommission.org/standards_information/npsgs.aspx.

US Department of Veterans Affairs. (2015). *Root cause analysis tools*. http://www.patientsafety.va.gov/docs/joe/rca_tools_2_15.pdf.

US Department of Veterans Affairs. (2018a). *VA National Center for Patient Safety*. http://www.patientsafety.va.gov/index.asp.

US Department of Veterans Affairs. (2018b). *VA Quality Scholars*. https://www.vaqs.org.

US Department of Veterans Affairs. (2019). *Healthcare failure mode and effect analysis (HFMEA)*. http://www.patientsafety.va.gov/professionals/onthejob/hfmea.asp.

Villanova University. (2019). *A look at Six Sigma's increasing role in improving healthcare*. https://www.villanovau.com/resources/six-sigma/six-sigma-improving-healthcare/.Virginia Mason Institute. (2016). *Leader tools to prevent medical errors*. https://www.virginiamasoninstitute.org/2016/03/health-care-leaders-can-stop-medical-errors/.

Visiting Nursing Service of New York (VNSNY). (2020). *Vision and mission*. https://www.vnsny.org/who-we-are/about-us/mission-vision/.

Waddill-Goad, S. M., & Langster, H. J. (2016). *Nurse burnout: Planning intentional quality and safety*. https://www.reflectionsonnursingleadership.org/features/more-features/Vol42-1-nurse-burnout-planning-intentional-quality-and-safety.

Weick, K. E., & Sutcliffe, K. M. (2007). *Managing the unexpected (2nd ed.)*. San Francisco, CA: Jossey-Bass.

Wise, D. (2014). *Getting to know just culture*. https://www.outcome-eng.com/getting-to-know-just-culture/.

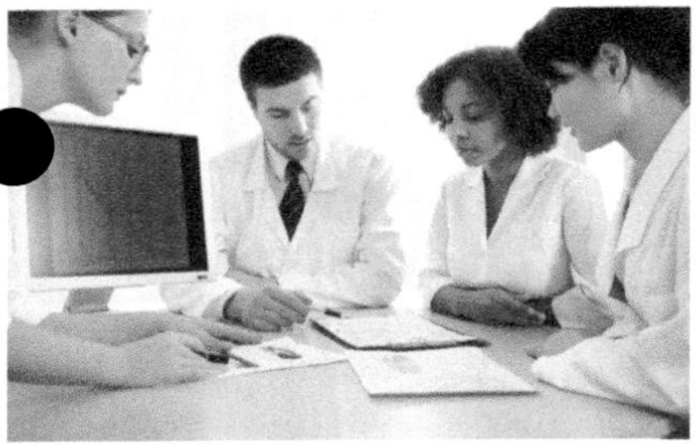

Measuring and Managing Outcomes

Christina Dempsey, Mary Jo Assi

http://evolve.elsevier.com/Huber/leadership

Achieving and sustaining quality outcomes is a goal in every health care organization. This effort requires the companion efforts of measuring and managing outcomes as a guide. Measuring important outcomes helps decision makers draw conclusions about new programs, tests, or procedures, and whether to promote the adoption of these new innovations. For example, Wu and colleagues' (2018) literature synthesis indicated that the effectiveness of telehealth interventions in diabetes management was supported by evidence. This bolsters support for advocating for telehealth interventions to policy and decision makers.

Rising costs and demands for accountability in the health care system have led to an increased focus on measuring quality (National Quality Forum [NQF], 2015). Porter (2010) framed outcomes as a key part of value in health care. He defined value as the patient outcomes obtained in a health care setting divided by the costs incurred in providing the services, which places outcomes measurement and management at the heart of health care leadership. In 2001 The Institute of Medicine (IOM) established six aims for care: safe, effective, timely, equitable, patient-centered, and efficient (Agency for Healthcare Research and Quality [AHRQ], 2018). Outcomes research examines variations in the delivery and results of health care services that have particular relevance for clinicians and leaders alike. Health care leaders and researchers understand that quality outcomes related to safety, clinical excellence, and experience of care for both patients and caregivers require a continued effort to quantify the contribution of nurses and nursing interventions in databases that enable benchmarked nursing-related outcomes across units, institutions, systems, regions, and even countries (Jeffs et al., 2015a; Loan et al., 2011; Zrelak et al., 2012). Moreover, Jones (2016) demonstrated that measuring outcomes is part of the social contract nurses have with the community as stewards of health care resources and done to meet the six aims articulated by the IOM. Furthermore, this social obligation to move the profession beyond a task-based, checklist-oriented practice to one that is outcomes-based demonstrates that the value of nursing care depends upon data and evidence (Jones, 2016). This chapter provides an overview of definitions, key concepts in outcomes and outcomes management, defines outcomes research and the challenges it involves, elements of outcome research, leadership and management implications, and current issues and trends.

DEFINITIONS

Key terms related to outcomes and their measurement and management include outcomes, indicators, common data elements (CDEs), measures, nurse-sensitive care, nursing outcomes research, and high reliability.

An **outcome** is the result or results obtained from the efforts to accomplish a goal. In proposing a three-part model of health care quality, Donabedian (1985) described outcomes as changes in the actual or potential health status of individuals, groups, or communities, and contrasted outcomes with processes (what occurs in the delivery of health care) and structures (the organizational context and "raw materials" of health care delivery). Donabedian's classic framework is useful for understanding the relationship between outcomes and the structures and processes that have produced them. This suggests that nurses and nurse managers need to attend to structure and process factors as precursors to patient outcomes (Donabedian, 2005). A patient-focused definition of outcomes considers them "the results people care about most when seeking treatment, including functional improvement and the ability to live normal, productive lives" (International Consortium for Health Outcomes Measurement [ICHOM], 2016; Porter, 2010).

Indicators: Indicators can be used to measure all three of Donabedian's (1985) domains of quality: structure, process, and outcomes. Specifically, structure indicators include the supply, skill level, education, and certification levels of nursing staff; process indicators measure methods of patient assessment and nursing interventions; and outcome indicators reflect both patient clinical and experience outcomes, such as pressure ulcers and falls, and nurse outcomes such as job satisfaction or turnover. Although patient outcomes are the focus of this chapter, other indicators are key to understanding and managing variations in outcomes. AHRQ (2016) has listed a set of three broad desirable attributes of a quality indicator: (1) importance to stakeholders in the health care system, (2) meets rigorous survey science requirements, and (3) feasibility of collection. A variety of accreditation and regulatory bodies and a number of trade and professional associations—as well as health care quality assessment organizations (sometimes alliances of stakeholders)—have developed sets of standardized health care performance indicators for measuring outcomes (see Chapter 18). For example, in 2003 the AHRQ developed a series of measures that help hospitals to identify potential adverse events and provide the opportunity to assess both adverse events and complications through data analysis of the patient record. "Following the seminal 'To Err is Human' report from the Institute of Medicine, the Agency for Healthcare Research and Quality (AHRQ) developed measures that health providers can use to identify potential in-hospital patient safety problems for targeted institution-level quality improvement efforts" (Centers for Medicare & Medicaid Services [CMS], 2019).

Measures: "These Patient Safety Indicators (PSIs) are comprised of 26 measures (including 18 provider-level indicators) that highlight safety-related adverse events occurring in hospitals following operations, procedures, and childbirth. CMS developed the PSIs after a comprehensive literature review, analysis of available International Classification of Diseases (ICD) codes, review by clinical panels, implementation of risk adjustment, and empirical analyses" (CMS, 2019). Table 19.1 illustrates the 18 provider-level indicators that specify preventable adverse events and complications that patients may experience in their contacts across the health care continuum (CMS, 2019). Although the primary focus and interest of stakeholders is actual outcomes related to care, it is important to note that quality measurement sets in health care have been critiqued for an excessive focus on processes rather than patient outcomes (Porter, 2010).

Nursing-sensitive care measures: Measures to assist in quantifying nursing's contribution to quality and safety; there have been long-standing efforts to develop indicator sets addressing outcomes of care that are believed to be especially nursing specific or nursing sensitive (Doran et al., 2011; Jeffs et al., 2015b; Loan et al., 2011). Among these nursing-sensitive measures are institutionally acquired pressure injuries (formerly pressure ulcers) and falls with injuries. These indicators are called nursing sensitive because there is evidence that they reflect nursing availability, attention, and nurses' clinical judgment. The National Quality Forum (NQF) endorsed (and subsequently re-endorsed) a set of voluntary consensus standards for nursing-sensitive care that quantify the contribution of nursing to patient safety, health care outcomes, and the professional work environment (Frith et al., 2010; Naylor, 2007; NQF, 2004). Expanding measure sets that are potentially linked with nursing may help clinicians and administrators focus on areas of performance possibly tied to the organization of nursing services and processes of care. Outcomes depend largely on the structure that underlies a nursing organization and the scope and standards of its practice. Nursing structure comprises many distinct elements, including staffing ratios, education and certification, availability of resources, nurse engagement, team culture, and skill mix. These elements combine to shape nurses' work environment, which is the foundation for their success. Defects or dysfunction in the nursing work environment can lead to minor local disruptions or major systemic consequences, both of which influence the quality, safety, cost, and patient experience of care.

Common data elements (CDEs): CDEs are defined as variables that are operationalized and measured in identical ways in similar settings and contexts to enable

TABLE 19.1 Centers for Medicare & Medicaid Services' Quality Measure Domains

Quality Domain	Examples of Structures/Processes/Outcomes in the Domain
Clinical care	"Clinical care measures reflect clinical care processes closely linked to outcomes, based on evidence and practice guidelines from professional clinical societies, or can be measures of person-centered outcomes of disease conditions, including PROMs and measures of functional status."
Safety	"Safety measures reflect the safe delivery of clinical services in all health care settings. These measures address a structure or process that is designed to reduce risk of harm or the occurrence of an untoward outcome in the delivery of health care, such as an adverse event. Safety measures also address complications of procedures, treatments, or similar interventions during health care delivery. Measures of inappropriate use that could harm a patient."
Patient and caregiver experience	"The domain of patient and caregiver experience includes measures that focus on the potential to improve person-centered care and family and caregiver experiences. For example, this domain includes measures of organizational structures or processes that foster the inclusion of persons and family members as active members of the health care team and collaborative partners with clinicians and provider organizations. This domain also includes PROMs that assess patient-reported experiences and outcomes that reflect involvement of persons and families in the care process and demonstrate knowledge, skill, and confidence to self-manage health care."
Care coordination	"Measures assigned to the care coordination domain focus on appropriate and timely sharing of information with patients, caregivers, and families and coordination of services among health professionals. The measures in this domain may also reflect outcomes of successful coordination of care [e.g.] admissions and readmissions to the hospital."
Population health and prevention	"Population health is defined as the health outcomes of a group of individuals, including the distribution of such outcomes within the group. Measures in this domain reflect the use of clinical and preventive services and the achievement of improvements in the health of the population served. Included in this domain are outcome measures that reflect the health of a population or community and process measures that focus on the primary prevention of disease or screening for early detection of disease that is unrelated to a current or prior condition."

PROMs, Patient-reported outcome measures.
Data from Centers for Medicare & Medicaid Services (CMS). (2016). *CMS quality measure development plan: supporting the transition to the merit-based incentive payment system (MIPS) and alternative payment models (APMs)*. https://www.cms.gov/Medicare/Quality-Initiatives-Patient-Assessment-Instruments/Value-Based-Programs/MACRA-MIPS-and-APMs/Final-MDP.pdf, pp. 36-40.

comparison of data across datasets or studies in ways that would otherwise be impossible (National Institutes of Health [NIH], 2016; Redeker et al., 2015). CDEs are both a research tool and elements that inform standardized formats for electronic health records to provide comparison data for quality improvement initiatives.

Outcomes management: Outcomes management is a process used to assist managers and others in making rational patient care-oriented decisions based on what is known about the effect of those choices on patient outcomes (Ellwood, 1988). It is defined as "a multidisciplinary process designed to provide quality health care, decrease fragmentation, enhance outcomes, and constrain costs. The core idea of outcomes management is the use of care process activities to improve outcomes" (Huber & Oermann, 1998, p. 4). In outcomes management, information about client experiences or other endpoints of care is assembled, trends are identified, departures from expectations are examined, and needed modifications are identified. To understand outcomes the process of care across the entire continuum of care needs to be carefully examined, and variations must be analyzed. Outcomes management is a five-step process: (1) data are collected about outcomes, (2) trends are identified from data analysis, (3) variances are investigated, (4) potential service delivery changes are explored and selected, and (5) changes are implemented and their impacts evaluated.

Management of care: Potential changes in care delivery or the management of care are intended to optimize care or reduce undesirable variances in care for a group of patients or a larger population. This is the analytical management of care delivery. Goals of optimization include robust quality improvement within a framework of high reliability and risk reduction (Fig. 19.1). For nurses, variations of interest may mean departures from anticipated clinical trajectories for some or all patients. Variances may be positive or negative, but identifying them is critical.

Outcomes research: a subfield of health services research that "seeks to understand the end results of particular health care practices and interventions" (AHRQ, 2000) or the extent to which services achieve the goals of health care. What makes outcomes research distinct from other bodies of research that examine end points in patients (i.e., much clinically oriented research) is that outcomes researchers seek to tease out the effects of patient-level care and systems-level environments from the background demographic, psychosocial, and clinical characteristics of patients as influences on end points. The goal is to understand which patients or clients fare well and which do not in relation to treatments selected and/or the organizational context of care delivery (Kane, 2006). Examples of variables that might be investigated as a predictor of patient outcomes might be the provider's professional or educational background (e.g., physicians versus advanced practice nurses, registered nurses [RNs] versus licensed practical or vocational nurses [LPNs/LVNs]), or the characteristics of care settings).

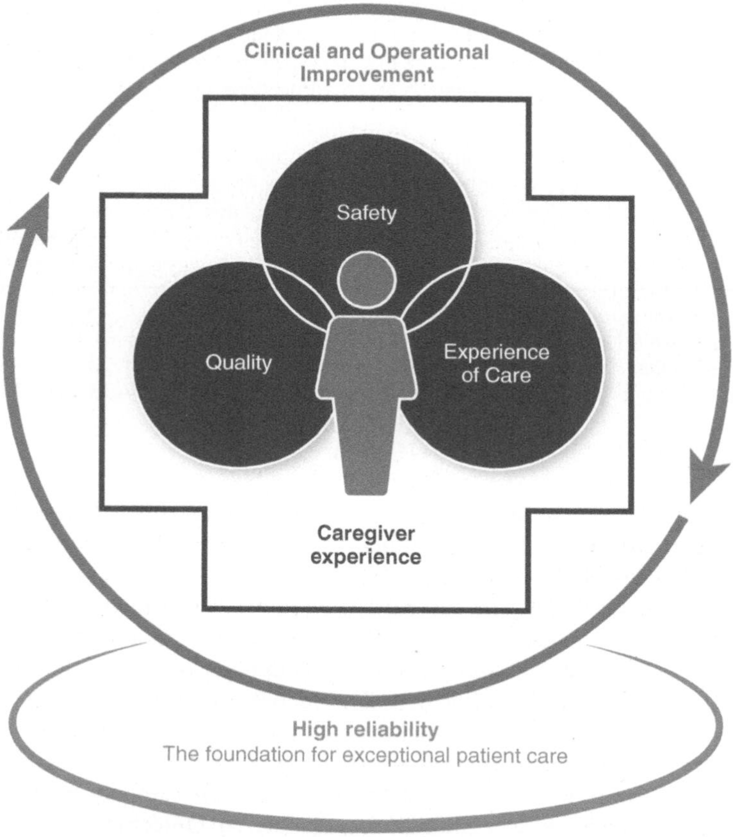

Fig. 19.1 High reliability operating model.

Comparative effectiveness research: A broadening of outcomes research has been the use of comparative effectiveness research (CER) and patient-centered outcomes studies, which include the effects of treatment on health outcomes in different patient populations. The goal is to produce new knowledge and reduce uncertainty about the effects on patient health outcomes of treatments, prevention, or other interventions by investigating on a large scale.

Nursing outcomes research: This is a subspecialty within the larger field of health outcomes research that focuses on determining the effect of different contexts and conditions that are related specifically to nurses and nursing care on the health status of patients. Nursing outcomes researchers are often interested in the structures or management strategies for nursing care delivery and the mix of health care workers best equipped to care for them or the types of patients who benefit most from certain nursing interventions.

Outcomes research: This strategy can help identify interventions that may be the most useful in improving patients' health status, sometimes leading to changes not only in care in the clinic or hospital but also in preparation and coaching of patients for self-management. Ideally clinical care or the management of health services is at least partially guided by research evidence. Although outcomes research has a great deal in common with other forms of research, it involves some special elements. For example, outcomes researchers are especially concerned about understanding "real" (clinically or practically important) differences between expected and observed outcomes and between outcomes on different units, in different institutions, or at different points in time. Outcomes research can provide key data for managerial decision-making to improve quality of care. Data derived from outcomes research can be used to answer the following types of questions:

- What mix of staff types (including education levels among RNs) is most likely to achieve optimal outcomes for a clinical population with a particular level of services?
- Which technologies and blends of technology and staff achieve the best outcomes for high-risk patients?
- What are the optimal organizational structures to maintain efficiency, safety, and patient satisfaction at institutions that provide high volumes of services?

Although the answers to each of these questions depend on individual and institutional contexts and economic considerations, data from outcomes research can be used to inform decision-making. For example, nurse practitioners may be interested in accomplishing outcomes for patients that improve their health yet also reduce costs. Thus they may investigate interventions such as pharmacogenetics testing and profiling to identify the best metabolized pain medication versus those that provide an individual little benefit at a given dose.

BACKGROUND

To measure and manage outcomes, approaches are needed that use appropriate measures and include the experience of care to lead to optimal outcomes for patients and nurses, and in turn, provide a return on investment that aligns with value-based purchasing initiatives driving reimbursement in today's health care environment. Influences on outcomes, measurement of outcomes, and elements of outcomes research will be discussed.

INFLUENCES ON OUTCOMES

It is critical that consumers of outcomes data, including clinical nurses and nurse leaders, understand how to interpret outcomes measures. Nurses and nurse leaders are obviously most interested in the impact of clinical care on patient and population health outcomes. For nurses, the focus is usually on outcomes related to the care delivered by clinical teams and often encompasses the actions of the entire multidisciplinary health team.

MEASUREMENT OF OUTCOMES

Other outcomes indicators incorporate a broader impact of disease and its management on patients' lives. These outcomes, often measured through surveys of patient perceptions and experiences, include quality of life, functional status, health status, and patient experience of care. There are also provider and organizational outcomes. Provider-focused outcomes can include measures of processes and outcomes of care for individual professionals as well as health care work as experienced by workers reflected in such phenomena as nurse burnout, turnover, job satisfaction, work environment, and occupational injuries. Organization-focused outcomes may include patient or provider outcomes that are aggregated to the organizational level, such as rates of hospital-wide inpatient or 30-day mortality, errors, hospital acquired conditions, and other adverse events; or they may examine aspects of the performance of a system that are more of concern to managers than to clinicians or patients. For instance, cost of care indicators are commonly measured at the organizational (hospital-wide) or unit level. A number of health system-level outcomes are also receiving increased attention and include measures of successful movements of patients across settings (i.e., care transitions) (Dusek et al., 2014) and readmission rates (Berkowitz et al., 2013). There is a growing body of evidence linking outcomes to practice environment characteristics such as workplace culture, staffing levels, skill mix, interprofessional collaboration, job satisfaction, burn-out to care quality, productivity, and experience (Aiken et al., 2011; Hinno et al., 2012; McHugh et al., 2011; Nantsupawat 2011; Roche et al., 2012; Trinkoff et al., 2011; Twigg et al., 2013; Van Bogaert et al., 2014; You et al., 2013). Given the breadth of the evidence linking nursing care to patient and organizational outcomes, and the financial stakes associated with value-based incentives and penalties tied to patient outcomes and engagement, the business case for scrutinizing and optimizing nurse work environments is strong (Press Ganey, 2015).

ELEMENTS OF OUTCOMES RESEARCH

Indicators can highlight areas for improvement in structures and processes of nursing care and justify various investments in human and material resources needed to improve outcomes. Nurses can turn to research that has formally examined specific indicators for guidance to understand indicators, how they vary across settings, and the factors that most strongly influence them. Areas to pay particular attention to in outcomes research include the choice of specific measures or variables to address quality and the role of risk adjustment. In addition, the advent of value-based purchasing and values-based reimbursement have added quality and outcomes measures that also drive reimbursement across the continuum of care.

Variable Selection

When interpreting outcomes research, nurses need to be aware that researchers face considerable challenges when selecting outcome measures. For instance, outcomes can either be generic or broadly applicable to many patient groups, or be condition-specific, but they must be clearly defined. An outcome that is not clearly associated with a precise method for gathering and processing of data to measure it is difficult to interpret. Conclusions or decisions based on research results from those data may be flawed. Nurses also need to consider the sources of data used. For example, when evaluating a study examining the association of workload with nurse injuries, it would be important to know whether the injury data were gathered from nurse self-reports, an injury database, manager reports, insurance records, or some other source—and to be aware of the potential limitations or biases of each of these sources.

Risk Adjustment

Risk adjustment analyses of outcomes across groups are meaningful only if relevant individual differences in the patients examined are taken into consideration. Risk adjustment accounts for patient factors, such as the intrinsic risks that a patient brings to the health care encounter in the form of clinical and/or demographic factors, before drawing conclusions about the meaning of different values for indicators. Comparisons of outcomes across settings or time periods are meaningful only when potential differences in the characteristics of patients cared for are taken into account. Risk adjustment can be complicated but is important, because if key patient factors are not considered then differences across units, hospitals, or time periods may or may not be reflective of variations in quality of care. It is important to note that certain types of outcomes are so dramatic and so closely tied to systems failures (e.g., transfusion errors, severe pressure injuries) that risk adjustment is unlikely to alter the interpretation of the relevant indicators. The literature contains some excellent references that discuss the state of the science in risk adjustment techniques (Iezzoni, 2013; Kane, 2006).

LEADERSHIP AND MANAGEMENT IMPLICATIONS

Evidenced-Based Informed Decisions

Health care leaders are accountable for ensuring high quality services that achieve a variety of desired outcomes, including the Institute for Healthcare Improvement's Triple Aim of improving the patient experience of care, improving the health of populations, and reducing the per capita cost of health care. Many organizations have added a fourth aim: attaining joy in work of health care providers (Bodenheimer, 2014; Institute for Healthcare Improvement [IHI], 2016). Outcomes research can provide nurse leaders with evidence to guide decisions around resource allocation and ongoing monitoring of patient safety, quality care outcomes, and a positive work environment for nurses and interprofessional teams (NQF, 2015; Rosen et al., 2018; Westra et al., 2015,). Correctly analyzed and interpreted, local outcomes data help leaders make evidence-based informed decisions around creating healthier work environments and conditions for nurses to provide effective and efficient care, for positive outcomes and experiences for all stakeholders. Managers and executives today have a wealth of information available to them, and they are charged with determining which data indicate a need for action. A significant body of literature from nursing outcomes research continues to grow and is a valuable resource and reference point. For example, a large body of literature suggests that lower staffing levels and skill mix in acute care hospitals are associated with increased risk of negative outcomes. For example, the RN4CAST study involving nine European countries extended earlier findings, and reported that an increase in a nurse's workload by one patient increased the likelihood of an inpatient dying within 30 days of admission by 7% (Aiken et al., 2014). This study also reported that every 10% increase in the proportion of RNs holding bachelor's degrees was associated with a decrease in the likelihood of an inpatient dying within 30 days of admission by 7%. However, the specific context of the care environment and the patient population of interest call for continual monitoring of outcomes against internal and external benchmarks. Several data systems support the monitoring of nursing-sensitive outcomes. For example, the American Nurses Association (ANA) developed a proprietary national database of quality indicators and measures called the National Database for Nursing Quality Indicators (NDNQI). This database, along with the Collaborative Alliance for Nursing Outcomes (CALNOC), both acquired by Press Ganey Associates, LLC in 2013 and 2019 respectively, provide a deep benchmark for unit-specific data on nursing-sensitive indicators. Agencies as diverse as the Centers for Medicare & Medicaid Services (CMS), The Joint Commission, and the Magnet Recognition Program® of the American Nurses Credentialing Center (ANCC) now have outcomes-based reporting requirements that focus on a variety of indicators and outcomes. Many believe that mandated quality reporting has greater potential to improve quality than voluntary reporting (Mukamel et al., 2015). Nurses need to ensure that data-driven patient care improvement strategies are foundational to transformational efforts within organizations (Jeffs et al., 2015b; Murphy et al., 2013; Reichert & Furlong, 2014). Nurse leaders need to guide how nursing data is captured and used. Evidence may be used for (1) improving nursing operations and advancing nursing practice, (2) improving patient, and population health outcomes, and (3) ensuring that data regarding structures, processes, and outcomes of nursing care be integrated into Big Data architecture to facilitate the translation of Big Data into actionable information (Garcia et al., 2015). Nurse leaders also have a critical role in ensuring that nursing perspectives and priorities are represented in collecting, understanding, interpreting, and using performance measures (Murphy et al., 2013), and they are well positioned to develop infrastructure to ensure data are being used to inform decisions about care delivery in health care organizations (Murphy et al., 2013).

High-Reliability Organizations

Press Ganey's research demonstrated the impact of nurse managers on safety, quality, and experience of care. This quantitative and qualitative study found that high performing nurse managers have an unwavering focus on safety and quality, build a culture of respect and interprofessional teamwork, utilize huddles for communication and team building, leverage data for practice, and utilize safe and appropriate staffing (Press Ganey, 2015). High-reliability organizations are those that exhibit these elements of culture. The Agency for Healthcare Research and Quality (AHRQ) defined a highly reliable organization as one that operates in a complex, hazardous environment for extended periods of time without serious accidents or catastrophic failures (AHRQ, 2018). Highly reliable organizations have a proactive approach in which problems are anticipated. There is a preoccupation with failure so that problems are identified early and addressed early enough to prevent catastrophic consequences. These organizations are identified by five characteristics: preoccupation with failure; reluctance to simplify explanations for operations, successes, and failures; situational awareness; deference to frontline expertise; and a commitment to resilience (AHRQ, 2018).

When operating on a foundation of high reliability, health care organizations utilize a skill-based approach to standardizing leader and employee work that enhances communication and ensures consistency in the application of best practices known to improve quality, safety, and the experience of care. Practices that support consistency and standardization include the use of daily management boards, standard leader work, and daily safety huddles. A primary goal of high-reliability organizations, and critical to success, is an enterprise-wide adoption and enculturation of new habits and behaviors that are laser focused on improving quality and safety across all domains of the system.

Big Data Applications

Big Data is a term that is being used to encompass artificial intelligence (AI) and machine learning (the application of AI) as well as predictive analytics. It functions on the principle that collecting and analyzing large amounts of data will allow for relationships that may have been unknown to be identified and studied, thus allowing nurses to make better and more informed decisions (Marr, 2017). With the advent of electronic health records, discrete data points about patient demographics, clinical processes, and outcomes are available. Data from wearables like fitness bands and monitors provide real-time information. Drug and other specialty kinds of databases like that of American College of Cardiology also contribute to the amount of data. In addition, CMS has the Consumer Assessment of Healthcare Providers and Services (CAHPS) programs that offer data relative to the patient's perception of the care they received. Patient reported outcomes measures (PROMS) promises to provide data and insights into the patient's own perceptions of their functional status. With Natural Language Processing (NLP), it is also possible to use patient's comments or sentiment analysis to add to this body of data (Bresnick, 2018). Harnessing all of this data and turning it into insights and improvement is the key. Data without measurement is simply numbers. Measurement without insight is a fool's errand and leads to nothing. Insight without action is stagnation.

Performance Scorecards and Dashboards

Managers and executives often struggle to find a manageable number of data elements and indicators to collect and track to satisfy payers and regulators as well as meet the needs for managing quality related to safety, clinical quality, and the experience of care for both patients and caregivers. Balanced scorecards and dashboards are often used in health care as a part of continuous quality improvement. Balanced scorecards were first introduced in 1992 in the business sector by Kaplan and Norton as a way to review performance more broadly. A balanced scorecard links financial measures with operational measures such as patient experience and outcomes that drive future financial performance. Balanced scorecards help leaders to understand performance by answering four key questions. (1) Financial: What is our financial situation? (2) Internal business: What must we excel at? (3) Innovation and learning: How will we continue to improve and create value? (4) Customer perspective: How do customers see us? (Kaplan & Norton, 1992).

By reviewing measures in this way, leaders are more able to see the interrelationships necessary for success. Dashboards allow clinicians and leaders to view and synthesize multiple sources of data and information simultaneously for improvement efforts. When thoughtfully designed, scorecards and dashboards provide a visual display of critical information so that leaders can quickly grasp performance across multiple domains (Fig. 19.2). Coupled with internal and external best-practice structures and process benchmarks, dashboards provide a robust framework for targeting, implementing, and evaluating improvement activities (Baker, 2015).

CURRENT ISSUES AND TRENDS

Mitigating Cost-Containment Requests

More than ever, decisions involving nursing services need to be justified in terms of their impact on organizational outcomes. Cost-containment strategies sometimes involve targeting human resources expenditures by dropping staff coverage or reducing the proportion of RNs in staff mixes without forethought to the potential consequences for patient outcomes. Outcomes research will be vital for understanding the consequences of deploying various care-delivery models and configurations of staff in different circumstances, especially if circumstances arise where traditional models of care are no longer viable because sufficient numbers of the certain types of nursing staff are no longer available or affordable. Outcomes research can shape the policy environment and can ultimately influence constraints under which managers operate. Since 1999 when California Governor Gray Davis signed Assembly Bill 394 (AB 394)

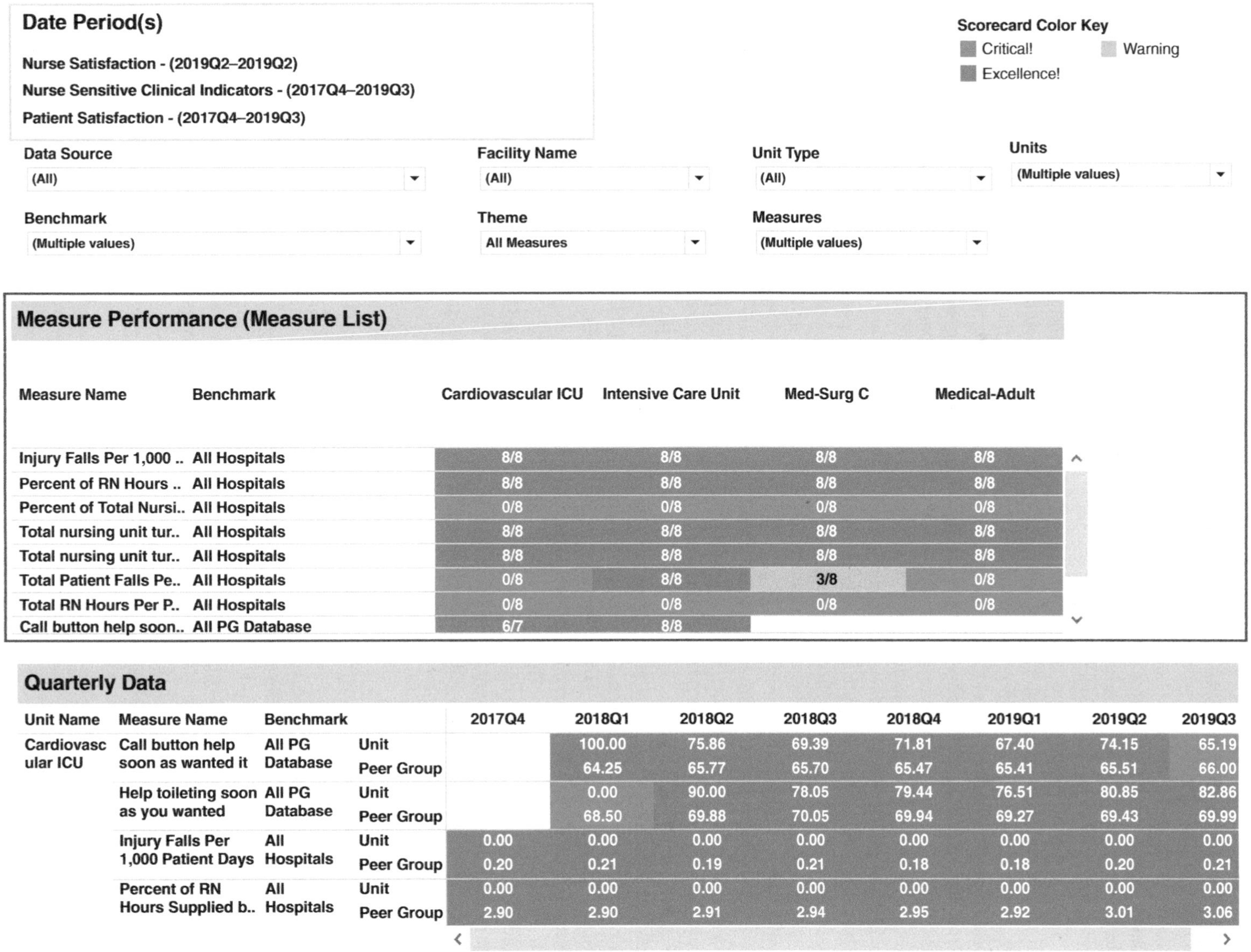
Date Period(s)
Nurse Satisfaction - (2019Q2–2019Q2)
Nurse Sensitive Clinical Indicators - (2017Q4–2019Q3)
Patient Satisfaction - (2017Q4–2019Q3)
Scorecard Color Key
Critical!
Warning
Excellence!
Data Source
(All)
Facility Name
(All)
Unit Type
(All)
Units
(Multiple values)
Benchmark
(Multiple values)
Theme
All Measures
Measures
(Multiple values)
Measure Performance (Measure List)
Measure Name
Benchmark
Cardiovascular ICU
Intensive Care Unit
Med-Surg C
Medical-Adult
Injury Falls Per 1,000 .. All Hospitals 8/8 8/8 8/8 8/8
Percent of RN Hours .. All Hospitals 8/8 8/8 8/8 8/8
Percent of Total Nursi.. All Hospitals 0/8 0/8 0/8 0/8
Total nursing unit tur.. All Hospitals 8/8 8/8 8/8 8/8
Total nursing unit tur.. All Hospitals 8/8 8/8 8/8 8/8
Total Patient Falls Pe.. All Hospitals 0/8 8/8 3/8 0/8
Total RN Hours Per P.. All Hospitals 0/8 0/8 0/8 0/8
Call button help soon.. All PG Database 6/7 8/8
Quarterly Data
Unit Name
Measure Name
Benchmark
2017Q4
2018Q1
2018Q2
2018Q3
2018Q4
2019Q1
2019Q2
2019Q3
Cardiovascular ICU
Call button help soon as wanted it
All PG Database
Unit 100.00 75.86 69.39 71.81 67.40 74.15 65.19
Peer Group 64.25 65.77 65.70 65.47 65.41 65.51 66.00
Help toileting soon as you wanted
All PG Database
Unit 0.00 90.00 78.05 79.44 76.51 80.85 82.86
Peer Group 68.50 69.88 70.05 69.94 69.27 69.43 69.99
Injury Falls Per 1,000 Patient Days
All Hospitals
Unit 0.00 0.00 0.00 0.00 0.00 0.00 0.00 0.00
Peer Group 0.20 0.21 0.19 0.21 0.18 0.18 0.20 0.21
Percent of RN Hours Supplied b..
All Hospitals
Unit 0.00 0.00 0.00 0.00 0.00 0.00 0.00 0.00
Peer Group 2.90 2.90 2.91 2.94 2.95 2.92 3.01 3.06

Fig. 19.2 Integrated dashboard.

into law requiring the California Department of Health Care Services to adopt regulations establishing minimum nurse-to-patient ratios, there has been widespread discussion of similar legislation at both the state and federal levels across the United States and elsewhere. The legislative intent behind the California initiative was to improve quality of care, patient safety, and nurse retention. Then and now, proposals to regulate nurse staffing in some way, for example, requiring the reporting of staffing levels, submission of staffing plans, or mandating specific ratios, cite the body of evidence from outcomes research demonstrating links between low nurse staffing and poor outcomes. Evaluation of the impacts of the California experiment continues, and results in terms of net benefits to patients and the state's health care system have been decidedly mixed (Serratt, 2013a, b). Although the continued dialogue does reflect ongoing interest in tracking and perhaps regulating structural elements in health care settings such as staffing, it is important to note that research supports the importance of staffing in the context of the broader work environment. A Press Ganey study (2015) examined the influence of staffing and factors of the work environment on nurse and patient outcomes. And although significant correlations were seen between staffing and nurse and patient outcomes, correlations to the same outcomes were influenced more strongly by factors of the work environment. There is a significant opportunity to evolve and expand research activity to more deeply explore the elements of nursing care, care-delivery models, and factors of the practice and work environment that most strongly impact nurse and patient outcomes.

Population Health

Another trend is heightened interest in measuring and managing outcomes in populations. Population health management is *proactive* care, delivered on an individualized basis. By emphasizing prevention and customization, it optimizes quality while lowering cost and improving value. Population health management is a key feature of the *Affordable Care Act* (ACA). Under this legislation, providers across the health care continuum may form Accountable Care Organizations (ACOs), taking responsibility for a patient population, including the costs and quality of its care. According to Abrams and colleagues, at the Commonwealth Fund (2015), the ACA established the Medicare Shared Savings Program that encouraged the development of ACOs so that if they met quality benchmarks and kept spending below budget, they would receive half the savings achieved, with the remainder going back to CMS. Policymakers hoped that this kind of bundled payment program would encourage continuity and coordination of care, prompting organizations to focus more on health promotion and disease prevention, which would in turn drive costs down. According to a *Harvard Business Review* profile (Porter & Kaplan, 2016), the bundled payment holds everyone on the health care team accountable for achieving outcomes that matter to patients. This entails the forward-looking management of care. The risk adjustment of bundled payments incentivizes providers to care for even difficult cases. If organizations do not provide care efficiently, or if they provide it inappropriately, the government penalizes them financially. Policymakers hoped that if they held providers accountable for outcomes that encompassed the entire continuum of care, organizations would add new services, interventions, or diagnostic tests that improved outcomes or lowered the cost of care. Porter and Kaplan (2016) suggested that costs could potentially decrease by up to 20% or 30% without compromises in quality.

Management of Nursing Outcomes

As consumers, regulators, and payers increase their focus on outcomes, nurses need to proactively manage outcomes and participate in the ongoing development and implementation of indicators related to nursing care and services. Awareness of advances in outcomes measurement and familiarity with outcomes research findings are essential and will continue to be critical for effective nursing leadership. As health care systems become increasingly outcomes driven, nurse managers and leaders must be involved and spearhead the development of outcomes tracking and management systems appropriate to the setting. The integration of Big Data from electronic health records and other information systems provides opportunities to predict patient outcomes and resource utilization that can be used to guide improvements in patient safety and other outcomes (Westra et al., 2015). Further, Big Data offers a more comprehensive and synthesized understanding of health data across populations that can lead to discovering new knowledge that positively affects nurses and the people they serve with improved health care (Healthcare Information and Management Systems Society [HIMSS], 2015; Westra et al., 2015). Specifically, the profession and its leadership need to contribute to Big Data initiatives by (1) offering definitions and context for data elements, (2) providing expertise in the use of theories to organize variables and interpret analysis results, and (3) creating interventions that assist patients in interpreting and acting on the information afforded through data science investigations (Brennan & Bakken, 2015).

This is crucial to the measurement and management of outcomes. Widespread use of common data elements and measures provides opportunities to compare results across studies and supports the goal of disseminating and translating information into practice (Cohen et al., 2015).

CONCLUSION

Meaningful measurement is key to helping organizations understand what is working well and where opportunities for improvement still exist. For many reasons, outcomes measurement has emphasized health care processes and outcomes that reflect the values and priorities of health professionals, researchers, and administrators. More recently, there has been an important movement by health care thought leaders toward measuring outcomes from the patient's standpoint, especially experiences in receiving health care and quality of life issues (Porter et al., 2016). Researchers and health care leaders are now being pushed to collect meaningful data that can enhance decision-making by health care leaders and policymakers as well as provide patients, families, and the clinicians who work with them with data that can inform treatment choices. The 2015 CMS Quality Measure Development Plan identified the patient and caregiver experience as one of the five quality domains along with clinical care, safety, care coordination, and population health and prevention to be targeted in quality-oriented reforms to payment structures (CMS, 2015). Integrating these datasets has been a challenge, but tools are evolving that will allow for more sophisticated analytics across different databases that help to demonstrate the impact that safety, quality, experience, and engagement has collectively and in parallel. This integration helps to target improvement efforts in the most effective and efficient manner that can mitigate organizational initiative fatigue—a common pain point for health care leaders and clinicians. Nurse leaders seeking to involve their organizations in indicator benchmarking will have to participate in data-sharing initiatives to align such participation with meaningful quality improvement efforts and other organizational priorities.

Most organizations identify improvement opportunities through data analysis and synthesis. These improvement efforts are often thwarted when they are not sustainable. The evolution of high-reliability science, a well-known framework in the aviation, nuclear, and manufacturing industries, has also moved into the health care arena. In high-reliability organizations scores are not the goal; they are a tool. Meaningful measurement is key to achieving patient, nurse, and organizational outcomes.

RESEARCH NOTE

Source

Press Ganey (2015). *Nursing special report: The influence of nurse work environment on patient, payment and nurse outcomes in acute care settings.* http://healthcare.pressganey.com/2015-Nursing-SR_Influence_Work_Environment

Purpose

As survey science related to the patient and caregiver experience has evolved, so has data analysis methodology. Cross-domain analytics provide organizations with important insights into key drivers and correlations across multiple domains, including patient experience, engagement, safety, and clinical quality. Nursing leaders and clinical nurses can easily articulate current barriers to creating and sustaining an engaged workforce, as well as challenges that interfere with the ability to provide safe, quality patient-centered care. Today as in the past, nurse staffing continues to be a significant pain point for nurses in many different roles and settings. Responding to overwhelming consensus from the Press Ganey CNO Advisory Council, a study was undertaken in 2015 to better understand critical factors related to staffing, the practice, and the work environment that impact both patient and nurse outcomes.

Discussion

This study combined data from the National Database of Nursing Quality Indicators (NDNQI) and the Press Ganey

Continued

RESEARCH NOTE—cont'd

Patient Experience database to conduct cross-domain analytics to determine the impact of nurse staffing and factors of the work environment on selected outcomes. Key findings demonstrated that overall, although staffing does significantly impact RN perception of quality and job satisfaction, the patient experience global measure (Likelihood to Recommend), clinical outcome measures (i.e., falls, CLABSI, and CAUTI), and key components of the work environment (i.e., nurse intent to remain in current position and perceived status of nursing) are significantly more impactful on nurse and patient outcomes.

Application in Practice

Achieving and sustaining quality outcomes is a goal in every health care organization. Given the vast amount of data that leaders are expected to process and understand at a granular level, improvement efforts can get mired down by initiative fatigue—an ongoing concern of many health care leaders. Thinking about data more holistically, and understanding how factors across the domains of patient experience, clinical quality, engagement and safety influence one another, provides nurse leaders with insights that can focus improvement efforts across all domains.

CASE STUDY

Margaret, the director of quality in an inpatient rehabilitation facility (IRF), recognized a trend upward in the number of patient falls. Data were reviewed to determine opportunities for improvement. She knew that a review of the data was important in order to determine next steps in improvement. After a review of the incident reports she found the following.

Data were stratified by the IRF to evaluate trends by day of week, time the fall occurred, the day of the stay, the fall risk score, diagnosis, whether the policy was enforced, and what the patient was doing prior to the fall. The lowest fall rate by month occurred in December with four falls, while the highest number was in October with 34 falls. These both appeared to be outliers in the data. Average monthly fall volume was 12.5 falls per month or 11.74 with outliers removed. Fall rates by month demonstrated that the fall rate had been less than 8% for three out of six months: January, May, and June. However, the rates for February at 11.64%, March at 11.07%, and April at 16.98% were significantly higher. The breakdown of falls by day of week demonstrate that 40% of patient falls occurred on Tuesdays and Sundays, Wednesdays had the fewest falls at 6%, Mondays accounted for 17% of falls, Thursdays for 10%, and both Friday and Saturday at 13% each. In terms of hour of day, 22% of patient falls occurred between the hours of 3 pm and 6 pm; only 6% occurred between midnight and 3 am; 17% between 6 am and 9 am; 15% for both 9 am to noon and noon to 3 pm; 16% for 6 pm to 9 pm; 2% from 9 pm to midnight. Falls on day of stay 0–11 accounted for 63% of falls, with 28% of these falling between day 8 and day 11. Of note, this corresponded with the average length of stay of 11 days. Cerebral vascular accident (CVA) diagnosis accounted for 49% of falls but was also the highest volume diagnosis for the facility. The next highest was traumatic brain injury at 17% of falls. Patient falls from a wheelchair occurred in 38% of falls, and 33% fell during transfer or ambulation. Unwitnessed falls accounted for 56% of falls. Fortunately, only two falls with injury were reported from January to June. Despite the policy to perform a post-fall huddle, only 41% of falls had a huddle documented post-incident.

1. What other data should Margaret obtain?
2. Who should be involved in the data review and improvement strategies?

Leaders and clinical staff agreed to completely reframe their approach and thinking by adopting a philosophy of zero harm, which, in turn, required an absolute goal of zero falls. Leaders clearly articulated that the goal of zero harm is a journey and that incremental reductions in falls from the average of 12.5 per month will be expected. The aim was to reduce patient falls in this inpatient rehabilitation hospital from the average of 12.5 per month to at or below the stated goal of 6 per month or less than 8% within 90 days after improvement implementation for the patient population as a first step, and zero falls by the end of the calendar year.

Is this a reasonable aim? Why or why not?

CRITICAL THINKING EXCERCISE

Utilizing the fundamentals of high-reliability organizations, a staff-driven falls team was convened for the inpatient rehabilitation facility noted in the case study. Data were shared demonstrating trends that illustrated the need to reduce falls, and a comprehensive assessment was completed that identified cultural challenges and a lack of consistent processes. The falls team identified and prioritized a bundled approach to nonnegotiable tactics including safety huddles, room signage, patient contracts, transfer training, and purposeful rounding. A skills fair was conducted to include all staff within the facility that focused on each of the bundle components. Further, stark concerns relative to the nursing transfer abilities were identified during the skills fair allowing for changes to orientation and ongoing training. Particular components of rounding were also identified as opportunities for all staff to understand how to keep patients and staff safe. Falls were reduced during the project with a low of 8.29% in March, closely approximating the goal of 8% and demonstrating a downward trend in falls over the course of the project. The staff-driven nature of this work provided a model that the organization will continue to use for performance improvement going forward.

1. What data measurement and management strategies should be employed to drive sustainability of this work?
2. Describe how the five characteristics of a high-reliability organization were utilized with the proposed change?

REFERENCES

Abrams, M. K., Nuzum, R., Zezza, M. A., Ryan, J., Kiszla, J., & Guterman, S. (2015). *Delivery system reforms: A progress report at five years*. Commonwealth Fund. http://www.commonwealthfund.org/publications/issue-briefs/2015/may/aca-payment-and-delivery-system-reforms-at-5-years.

Agency for Healthcare Research and Quality (AHRQ). (2000). *Outcomes research fact sheet*. http://archive.ahrq.gov/research/findings/factsheets/outcomes/outfact/outcomes-and-research.html.

Agency for Healthcare Research and Quality (AHRQ). (2016). *Desirable attributes of a quality measure*. https://www.qualitymeasures.ahrq.gov/tutorial/attributes.aspx.

Agency for Healthcare Research and Quality (AHRQ). (2018). *Six domains of health care quality*. https://www.ahrq.gov/talkingquality/measures/six-domains.html.

Aiken, L. H., Sloane, D. M., Bruyneel, L., Van den Heede, K., Griffiths, P., Busse, R., et al. (2014). Nurse staffing and education and hospital mortality in nine European countries: A retrospective observational study. *Lancet, 383*(9931), 1824–1830.

Aiken, L. H., Cimiotti, J. P., Sloane, D. M., Smith, H. L., Flynn, L., & Neff, D. F. (2011). Effects of nurse staffing and nurse education on patient deaths in hospitals with different nurse work environments. *Medical Care*, (*12*), 1047–1053.

Baker, J. D. (2015). Language of improvement: Metrics, key performance indicators, benchmarks, analytics, scorecards, and dashboards. *AORN Journal, 102*(3), 223–227.

Berkowitz, R. E., Fang, Z., Helfand, B. K., Jones, R. N., Schreiber, R., & Paasche-Orlow, M. K. (2013). Project ReEngineered Discharge (RED) lowers hospital readmissions of patients discharged from a skilled nursing facility. *Journal of the American Medical Directors Association, 14*(10), 736–740.

Bodenheimer, T., & Sinsky, C. (2014). From triple to quadruple aim: Care of the patient requires care of the provider. *Annals of Family Medicine, 12*(6), 573–576.

Brennan, P. F., & Bakken, S. (2015). Nursing needs big data and big data needs nursing. *Journal of Nursing Scholarship, 47*(5), 477–484.

Bresnick, J. (2018). *EHR users want their time back, and artificial intelligence can help*. Health IT Analytics. https://healthitanalytics.com/features/ehr-users-want-their-time-back-and-artificial-intelligence-can-help.

Centers for Medicare & Medicaid Services (CMS). (2015). *CMS quality measure development plan: Supporting the transition to the merit-based incentive payment system (MIPS) and alternative payment models (APMs)*. https://www.cms.gov/Medicare/Quality-Initiatives-Patient-Assessment-Instruments/Value-Based-Programs/MACRA-MIPS-and-APMs/Draft-CMS-Quality-Measure-Development-Plan-MDP.pdf.

Centers for Medicare & Medicaid Services (CMS). (2019). *CMS Patient Safety Indicators PSI 90 (NQF #0531) National Quality Strategy Domain: Patient Safety*. https://innovation.cms.gov/Files/fact-sheet/bpciadvanced-fs-psi90.pdf.

Cohen, M. Z., Thompson, C. B., Yates, B., Zimmerman, L., & Pullen, C. H. (2015). Implementing common data elements across studies to advance research. *Nursing Outlook, 63*(2), 181–188.

Donabedian, A. (1985). *The methods and findings of quality assessment and monitoring: An illustrated analysis* (Vol 3). Ann Arbor, MI: Health Administration Press.

Donabedian, A. (2005). Evaluating the quality of medical care. (1966. *Milbank Quarterly, 83*(4), 691–729.

Doran, D., Mildon, B., & Clarke, S. (2011). Towards a national report card in nursing: A knowledge synthesis. *Nursing Leadership, 24*(2), 38–57.

Dusek, B., Pearce, N., Harripaul, A., & Lloyd, M. (2014). Care transitions: A systematic review of best practices. *Journal of Nursing Care Quality, 30*(3), 233–239.

Ellwood, P. M. (1988). Shattuck lecture—Outcomes management: A technology of patient experience. *New England Journal of Medicine, 318*(23), 1549–1556.

Frith, K. H., Anderson, F., & Sewell, J. P. (2010). Assessing and selecting data for a nursing services dashboard. *Journal of Nursing Administration, 40*(1), 10–16.

Garcia, A., Caspers, B., Westra, B., Pruinelli, L., & Delaney, C. (2015). Sharable and comparable data for nursing management. *Nursing Administration Quarterly, 39*(4), 297–303.

Healthcare Information and Management Systems Society (HIMSS). (2015). *HIMSS CNO-CNIO vendor roundtable guiding principles for Big Data in nursing: Using Big Data to improve the quality of care and outcomes*. http://www.himss.org/sites/himssorg/files/FileDownloads/HIMSS_Nursing_Big_Data_Group_Principles.pdf.

Hinno, S., Partanen, P., & Vehviläinen-Julkunen, K. (2012). Nursing activities, nurse staffing and adverse patient outcomes as perceived by hospital nurses. *Journal of Clinical Nursing, 21*(11-12), 1584–1593.

Huber, D., & Oermann, M. (1998). The evolution of outcomes management. In D. L. Flarey & S. S. Blancett (Eds.), *Cardiovascular outcomes: Collaborative, path-based approaches* (pp. 3–12). Gaithersburg, MD: Aspen.

Iezzoni, L. I. (Ed.). (2013). *Risk adjustment for measuring health care outcomes* (4th ed.). Chicago, IL: Health Administration Press.

Institute for Healthcare Improvement (IHI). (2016). *Triple Aim for populations*. http://www.ihi.org/Topics/TripleAim/Pages/default.aspx.

International Consortium for Health Outcomes Measurement (ICHOM). (2016). *ICHOM's mission*. http://www.ichom.org/why-we-do-it/.

Jeffs, L., Doran, D., Hayes, L., Mainville, C., VanDeVelde-Coke, S., Lamont, L., & Boal, A. S. (2015a). Implementation of the National Nursing Quality Report initiative in Canada: Insights from pilot participants. *Journal of Nursing Care Quality, 30*(4), E9–E16.

Jeffs, L., Nincic, V., White, P., Hayes, L., & Lo, J. (2015b). Leveraging data to transform nursing care: Insights from nurse leaders. *Journal of Nursing Care Quality, 30*(3), 269–274.

Jones, T. (2016). Outcome measurement in nursing: Imperatives, ideals, history, and challenges. *OJIN: The Online Journal of Issues in Nursing, 21*(2).

Kane, R. L. (2006). Introduction: An outcomes approach. In R. L. Kane (Ed.), *Understanding health care outcomes research* (2nd ed.), (pp. 3–22). Burlington, MA: Jones & Bartlett.

Kaplan, R. S., & Norton, D. P. (1992). The balanced scorecard–measures that drive performance. *Harvard Business Review, 70*(1), 71–79.

Loan, L. A., Patrician, P. A., & McCarthy, M. (2011). Participation in a national nursing outcomes database: Monitoring outcomes over time. *Nursing Administration Quarterly, 35*(1), 72–81.

Marr, B. (2017). *Data strategy: How to profit from a world of big data, analytics and the internet of things*. London: Kogan Page Publishers.

McHugh, M. D., Kutney-Lee, A., Cimiotti, J. P., Sloane, D. M., & Aiken, L. H. (2011). Nurses' widespread job dissatisfaction, burnout, and frustration with health benefits signal problems for patient care. *Health Affairs, 30*(2), 202–210.

Mukamel, D. B., Ye, Z., Glance, L. G., & Li, Y. (2015). Does mandating nursing home participation in quality reporting make a difference? Evidence from Massachusetts. *Medical Care, 53*(8), 713–719.

Murphy, L. S., Wilson, M. L., & Newhouse, R. P. (2013). Data analytics: Making the most of input with strategic output. *Journal of Nursing Administration, 43*(7–8), 367–370.

Nantsupawat, A., Srisuphan, W., Kunaviktikul, W., Wichaikhum, O. A., Aungsuroch, Y., & Aiken, L. H. (2011). Impact of nurse work environment and staffing on hospital nurse and quality of care in Thailand. *Journal of Nursing Scholarship, 43*(4), 426–432.

National Institutes of Health (NIH). (2016). *Common data element (CDE) resource portal*. https://www.nlm.nih.gov/cde/.

National Quality Forum (NQF). (2004). *National voluntary consensus standards for nursing-sensitive care: An initial performance measure set—a consensus report*. Author. http://www.qualityforum.org/Publications/2004/10/National_Voluntary_Consensus_Standards_for_Nursing-Sensitive_Care__An_Initial_Performance_Measure_Set.aspx.

National Quality Forum (NQF). (2015). *Data needed for systematically improving healthcare.* http://www.qualityforum.org/Publications/2015/07/Data_for_Systematic_Improvement_Final_White_Paper.aspx.

Naylor, M. D. (2007). Advancing the science in the measurement of health care quality influenced by nurses. *Medical Care Research & Review, 64*(Suppl. 2), S144–S169.

Porter, M. E. (2010). What is value in health care? *New England Journal of Medicine, 363*(26), 2477–2481.

Porter, M. E., Larsson, S., & Lee, T. H. (2016). Standardizing patient outcomes measurement. *New England Journal of Medicine, 374*(6), 504–506.

Porter, M. E., & Kaplan, R. S. (2016). How to Pay for Health Care. *Harvard Business Review, 94*(7-8), 88–134.

Press Ganey. (2015). Nursing special report: The influence of nurse work environment on patient, payment and nurse outcomes in acute care settings. http://healthcare.pressganey.com/2015-Nursing-SR_Influence_Work_Environment.

Redeker, N. S., Anderson, R., Bakken, S., Corwin, E., Docherty, S., Dorsey, S. G., et al. (2015). Advancing symptom science through use of common data elements. *Journal of Nursing Scholarship, 47*(5), 379–388.

Reichert, J., & Furlong, G. (2014). Five key pillars of an analytics center of excellence, which are required to manage populations and transform organizations into the next era of health care. *Nursing Administration Quarterly, 38*(2), 159–165.

Roche, M., Duffield, C., Aisbett, C., Diers, D., & Stasa, H. (2012). Nursing work directions in Australia: Does evidence drive the policy? *Collegian, 19*(4), 231–238.

Rosen, M. A, Diaz-Granados, D., Dietz, A. S., et al. (2018). Teamwork in healthcare: Key discoveries enabling safer, high-quality care. *The American Psychologist, 73*(4), 433–450.

Serratt, T. (2013a). California's nurse-to-patient ratios, Part 2: 8 years later, what do we know about hospital level outcomes? *Journal of Nursing Administration, 43*(10), 549–553.

Serratt, T. (2013b). California's nurse-to-patient ratios, Part 3: Eight years later, what do we know about patient level outcomes? *Journal of Nursing Administration, 43*(11), 581–585.

Trinkoff, A. M., Johantgen, M., Storr, C. L., Gurses, A. P., Liang, Y., & Han, K. (2011). Nurses' work schedule characteristics, nurse staffing, and patient mortality. *Nursing Research, 60*(1), 1–8.

Twigg, D. E, Geelhoed, E. A., Bremner, A. P., & Duffield, C. M. (2013). The economic benefits of increased levels of nursing care in the hospital setting. *Journal of Advanced Nursing, 69*(10), 2253–2261.

Van Bogaert, P., Van Heusden, D., Timmermans, O., & Franck, E. (2014). Nurse work engagement impacts job outcome and nurse-assessed quality of care: model testing with nurse practice environment and nurse work characteristics as predictors. *Frontiers in Psychology,* (5), 1261.

Westra, B., Clancy, T., Sensmeier, J, Warren, J. J., Weaver, C., & Delaney, C. W. (2015). Nursing knowledge: Big data science—implications for nurse leaders. *Nursing Administration Quarterly, 39*(4), 304–310.

Wu, C., Wu, Z., Yang, L., Zhu, W., Zhang, M., Zhu, Q., et al. (2018). Evaluation of the clinical outcomes of telehealth for managing diabetes: A PRISMA-compliant meta-analysis. *Medicine, 97*(43), e12962. doi:10.1097/MD.0000000000012962.

You, L. M., Aiken, L. H., Sloane, D. M, et al. (2013). Hospital nursing, care quality, and patient satisfaction: Cross-sectional surveys of nurses and patients in hospitals in China and Europe. *International Journal of Nursing Studies, 50*(2), 154–161.

Zrelak, P. A., Utter, G. H., Sadeghi, B., Cuny, J., Baron, R., & Romano, P. S. (2012). Using the agency for healthcare research and quality patient safety indicators for targeting nursing quality improvement. *Journal of Nursing Care Quality, 27*(2), 99–108.

20

Workplace Violence and Incivility

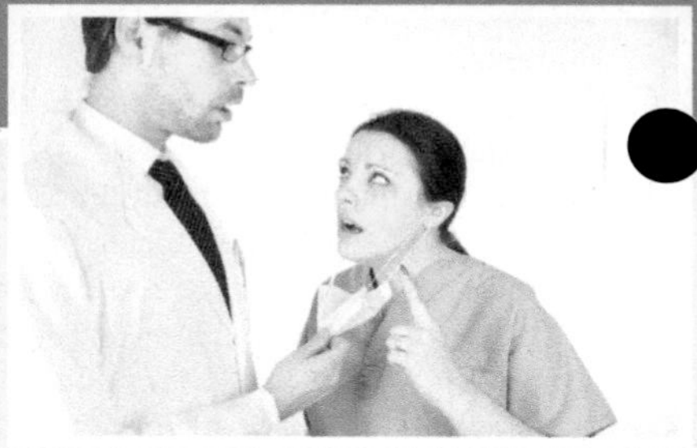

Palma D. Iacovitti

http://evolve.elsevier.com/Huber/leadership

Nurses expect to be safe at work, especially in health care organizations. Surprisingly, nurses encounter workplace violence and incivility far too commonly. It is important to begin with a general concept of workplace violence and its subsets, workplace bullying and incivility, because they are terms used interchangeably and contain various elements under their definitions. For the purpose of this context, a workplace can be described as a health care organization or setting of any size, location, and type of health care service provided. This also includes care performed outside the health care organization, such as ambulance services or home health care. Any place where such health services are performed will be considered a workplace.

The American Psychological Association (APA, 2020) defined **violence** as an extreme form of aggression, such as assault, rape, or murder. Violence has many causes including, but not limited to, frustration, anger, exposure to violent media, and violence in the home. Certain circumstances can provoke the risk of violent behavior, such as alcohol, drugs, slurs and other irritations, and environmental influences (APA, 2020). This chapter discusses forms of employee violence, health care regulatory bodies to manage violence, leadership roles and responsibilities, de-escalation methods, and current legislation.

DEFINITIONS

The basic terms used in relation to workplace violence and incivility are violence, workplace incivility, workplace violence, and workplace bullying.

Violence is assault, battery, manslaughter, or homicide.

Workplace incivility is violent acts, including physical assaults and threats of assault, directed to persons at work or on duty (Occupational Safety and Health Administration [OSHA], 2015a, p. 1).

Workplace violence is the act or threat of violence, ranging from verbal abuse to physical assaults directed toward persons at work or on duty (National Institute of Occupational Safety and Health [NIOSH], 2019).

Workplace bullying is a situation in which "anyone who uses his perceived strength or power to intimidate another person who he or she think is weaker in order to gain power over that person." (Ciocco, 2018, p. 39).

BACKGROUND

Workplace violence comes in multiple forms. It is defined as the act or threat of violence, ranging from verbal abuse to physical assaults directed toward persons at work or on duty (NIOSH, 2019). There are four types of workplace violence based on the perpetrator's relationship to the workplace. Table 20.1 outlines the types and their description. Health workers all over the world are subject to workplace violence. Between 8% and 38% of health workers are likely to endure physical violence at work. This percentage does not include those who are intimidated or subjected to verbal assault. Most violence is committed by patients and visitors. Groups of health workers who are at high risk, especially in emergency services, include nurses and ancillary staff directly involved in patient care, emergency room staff,

TABLE 20.1 Types of Workplace Violence and Perpetrator Relationship to Workplace

Type	Description	Example
I (Criminal intent)	Perpetrator has no legitimate relationship to the business or its employees	A nurse assaulted in the hospital parking garage.
II (Customer/patient) Most common in healthcare environments	Perpetrator is a customer or patient of the workplace or employee	Patient with paranoid schizophrenia kicks nursing personnel.
III (Customer/patient) Commonly referred to as lateral or horizontal violence	Perpetrator is current or former employee	Employee assaults supervisor after receiving performance evaluation.
IV (Personal relationship)	Perpetrator has a relationship to the employee outside of work, no relationship with the organization	Spouse of an employee follows him/her to work, places ultimatums, and makes threats that pose harm.

Source: National Institute of Occupational Safety and Health (NIOSH). 2019. *Occupational violence*. https://www.cdc.gov/niosh/topics/violence/default.html.

and paramedics (World Health Organization, 2020). Workplace violence is a major concern for employers and employees nationwide.

Every year the number of workers who report being a victim of some type of workplace violence increases. In 2017 assaults resulted in 18,400 injuries and 458 fatalities. Seventy-one percent of the assaults occur in health care and social services, amounting to 9% of the US workforce, according to the National Safety Council (NSC, 2019). Further data reveal a median of 5 days of absences for injuries occurring to head, upper extremities, and trunk (NSC, 2019). Fig. 20.1 provides a graph of nonfatal injuries and time away from work trends.

Nurses are at risk for verbal or physical assaults every day. There is a major crisis in our society when nurses are having to confront this type of peril on a regular basis. According to the Bureau of Labor Statistics (BLS, 2019a), the rate of fatal injury overall for hospitals for 2018 was 0.4 per 100,000 full-time equivalent workers. Data are not available by event type. The data further reveal that hospitals in 2018 had a total of 7720 nonfatal reported cases, an incident rate of 19.4 over the year, and employees were off work an average of 6 days (BLS, 2019b).

Risk factors for violence in health care organizations include patient, client, and setting-related risk factors such as (1) working with people who have a history of violence, (2) transporting patients, (3) working alone with patients, (4) unsafe building and parking lot design, (5) lack of means of emergency communication, and (6) availability of items that can be used as weapons. Other risk factors are organizational such as (1) lack of facility policies and training, (2) working when understaffed, (3) high worker turnover, (4) inadequate security personnel, (5) long waits for patients and clients in overcrowded waiting rooms, (6) unrestricted access by the public, and (7) a perception that violence is tolerated (OSHA, 2015b). In addition, an inadequate facility design may contribute to the penetration of violent incidents. Box 20.1 provides a checklist to develop new facilities or mitigate issues with facility designs (OSHA, 2015b).

Regulatory Bodies

Occupational Safety and Health Administration

The Occupational Safety and Health Act of 1970 created the Occupational Safety and Health Administration (OSHA) in the US Department of Labor. This legislation declared that employers have a general duty to provide safe and healthy working conditions. OSHA followed up on the general duty requirement in 1989 with voluntary generic safety and health program management guidelines for all employers to use as a foundation for their safety and health programs. However, the guidelines were not regulations. Nevertheless, under the OSHA Act, employers face fines if an incident of workplace violence occurs. OSHA made it clear that safety and

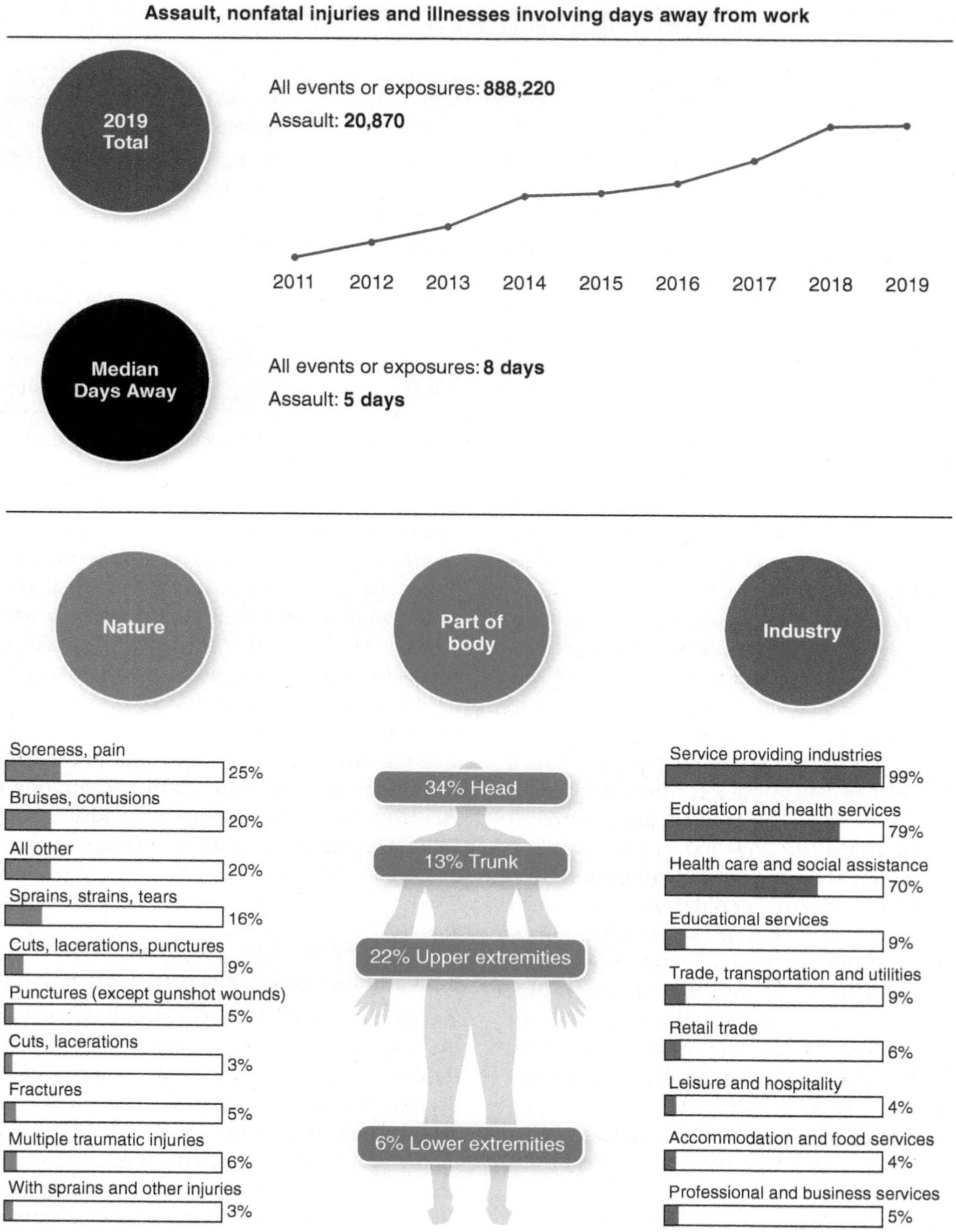

Fig. 20.1 Assault, nonfatal injuries, and illnesses involving days away from work. Permission to reprint/use granted by the National Safety Council © 2020. https://injuryfacts.nsc.org/work/safety-topics/assault/.

BOX 20.1 Facility Design Checklist

- Are there enough exits and adequate routes of escape?
- Can exit doors be opened only from the inside to prevent unauthorized entry?
- Is the lighting adequate to see clearly in indoor areas?
- Are there employee-only work areas that are separate from public areas?
- Is access to work areas only through a reception area?
- Are reception and work areas designed to prevent unauthorized entry?
- Could someone hear a worker call for help?
- Can workers observe patients or clients in waiting areas?
- Do areas used for patient or client interviews allow co-workers to observe any problems?
- Are waiting and work areas free of objects that could be used as weapons?
- Are chairs and furniture secured to prevent their use as weapons?
- Is furniture in waiting and work areas arranged to prevent workers from becoming trapped?
- Are patient or client areas designed to maximize comfort and minimize stress?
- Is a secure place available for workers to store their personal belongings?
- Are private, locked restrooms available for staff?

Modified from Occupational Safety and Health Administration (OSHA) US Department of Labor. (2015b). *Guidelines for preventing workplace violence for healthcare and social service workers*. OSHA publication 3148-04R 2015. https://www.osha.gov/Publications/osha3148.pdf.

health programs could be construed to include workplace violence prevention programs. In 1998 OSHA built on the 1989 generic workplace safety and health guidelines by announcing guidelines designed to identify common risk factors. They also included policy recommendations and practical corrective methods to help prevent and mitigate the effects of workplace violence in the health care industry (OSHA, 2015b). According to OSHA (2015a) an effective workplace violence prevention program includes:

1. **Management commitment and employee participation.** Commitment of all C-suite executives, leaders, and management for a violence prevention initiative including employee feedback in the development process.
2. **Worksite analysis:** Perform needs assessment to gauge an organization's susceptibility to violence.
3. **Hazard prevention and control:** Implement appropriate controls to eliminate or reduce hazards identified through Evaluation of Physical Environment.
4. **Safety and health training:** Strongly recommended for all employees. Content should include but not limited to: definition of workplace violence, prevention policies, risk and warning signs, and de-escalation. NIOSH (2019) offers a video that discusses sensible actions for identifying risk factors for violence at work and tactical actions that can maintain safety.
5. **Record-keeping and program evaluation:** Records maintenance is essential, including data of work-related injuries and illnesses, workers' compensation records, education records, safety committee minutes, and the identification and correction of recognized hazards.

National Institute for Occupation Safety and Health

The Occupational Safety and Health Act of 1970 also created the National Institute for Occupation Safety and Health (NIOSH), located within the Centers for Disease Control & Prevention (CDC) in the Department of Health and Human Services. Through this act, NIOSH was charged with drafting and recommending occupational safety and health standards (NIOSH, 2015).

NIOSH recognized that workplace violence is an issue in the health care industry and recommended the following violence prevention strategies for employers: environmental designs, administrative controls, and behavior modifications. Environmental designs include signaling systems, alarm systems, monitoring systems, security devices, security escorts, lighting, and architectural and furniture modifications to improve worker safety. Administrative controls include (1) adequate staffing patterns to prevent personnel from working alone and to reduce waiting times, (2) controlled access, and (3) development of systems to alert security personnel when violence is threatened. Behavior modifications provide all workers with training in recognizing and managing assaults, resolving conflicts, and maintaining hazard awareness (OSHA, 2015c). NIOSH (2013) has produced a free course on workplace violence prevention that earns three continuing education unit credits for nurses (http://www.cdc.gov/niosh/topics/violence/training_nurses.html). The American Nurses Association also offers education and several resources related to workplace violence (https://www.

nursingworld.org/practice-policy/work-environment/violence-incivility-bullying).

The Joint Commission

The Joint Commission (TJC, 2020a) is an independent, not-for-profit organization that accredits and certifies nearly 21,000 health care organizations and programs in the United States. The mission of TJC is "to continuously improve health care for the public, in collaboration with other stakeholders, by evaluating health care organizations and inspiring them to excel in providing safe and effective care of the highest quality and value." Toward this end, TJC requires the reporting of incidents and causes of workplace violence in the Sentinel Event Database (TJC, 2020b). TJC has recently updated Sentinel Event Alert 45: Preventing violence in the health care setting. It modified causal factors, high-risk areas, prevention strategies, and suggested actions, with emphasis on reporting workplace violence (TJC, 2019a).

Regulatory guidelines for the prevention of workplace violence derive from OSHA, NIOSH, and TJC. OSHA establishes that leaders have a general responsibility to create an awareness, take measures to prevent workplace violence, and promote safety and health in the work environment. NIOSH, OSHA, and TJC all make recommendations for standards to protect workers from violence. All these bodies, including BLS, continuously collect data on injuries, fatalities, and workplace violence. Given the economic strain of workplace violence and the potential legal liability, leaders of health care organizations have a financial responsibility to prevent workplace violence and provide a safe environment in which employees can speak up.

LEADERSHIP AND MANAGEMENT IMPLICATIONS

Leadership Responsibility for Workplace Violence

Organizational leaders have an obligation to protect employees from workplace violence. They must first acknowledge that a risk exists, then be committed to adopting TJC, OSHA, and NIOSH recommendations to increase awareness and implement workplace violence programs, policies and procedures, proper consequences for breaching policies, and encouragement of staff to report any type of workplace violence.

Employees should feel safe going into work without fear of being hurt physically or emotionally. OSHA (2015c) stated, "All employees can bring important knowledge and perspectives to the workplace violence prevention program—especially caregivers who interact directly with patients. A joint management–employee committee can foster a participatory approach where employees and management work together on worksite assessment and solution implementation". This includes (1) acknowledging the value of a safe and healthful, violence-free workplace, (2) distributing appropriate authority and resources to all accountable groups, (3) assigning responsibility and authority for the various aspects of the workplace violence prevention program to ensure that all managers and supervisors understand their duties, (4) maintaining a system of accountability, (5) supporting and implementing appropriate recommendations from safety and health committees, (6) developing medical and psychological therapy and debriefing for employees who have been affected by violent incidents, and (7) creating policies that certify the reporting, recording, and monitoring of incidents and near misses that protect the employee from retribution.

In the 2019 American Nurse Today's third annual Nursing Trends and Salary Survey (Spader, 2019), there were 5262 registered nurse respondents. Over fifty respondents were victims of violence, verbal assault, sexual harassment, or bullying in the workplace. Fifty-nine percent reported verbal assault by a patient in the past 24 months, 43% were verbally assaulted by a patient's family member or visitor, 23% of respondents were physically assaulted by a patient (a 3% increase compared with 2018). Forty-four percent reported being unsatisfied in the management of the events. In the same 2019 survey, 90% of those surveyed reported that policies had been implemented within their organization for workplace violence, 76% have received de-escalation education, with 83% declaring it is beneficial, and 73% were able to apply de-escalation techniques (Spader, 2019).

De-escalation

TJC (2019b) described de-escalation as a combination of strategies, techniques, and methods intended to reduce a patient's agitation and aggression. These can include communication, self-regulation, assessment, actions, and safety maintenance in order to reduce the risk of harm to patients and caregivers, and the use of restraints or seclusion. Annual training should include all employees at all levels within the organization. Additional training is recommended for those staff working in high-risk areas such as hospitals, schools, and food service places. TJC recommended three de-escalation models and four tools for managing workplace violence.

De-escalation models (TJC, 2019b)

- *The Dix and Page* model consists of three interdependent components: assessment, communication, and tactics (ACT).
- *Turnbull et al.* model is similar to Dix and Page's model. However, it describes how the de-escalator evaluates the aggressor's response to their use of de-escalation skills by constantly monitoring and evaluating feedback from the aggressor.
- *Safewards Model* begins with delimiting the situation by moving the patient or other patients to a safe area and maintaining a safe distance, clarifying the reasons for the anger using effective communication, and resolving the problem by finding a mutually agreeable solution.

Tools to Recognize Risk of Workplace Violence

- *STAMP* (Staring, Tone and volume of voice, Anxiety, Mumbling, and Pacing) is a validated tool for use in the emergency department (ED).
- *Overt Aggression Scale* (OAS) is a tool for use in the inpatient setting for children and adults.
- *Broset Violence Checklist* (BVC) is a validated checklist for use in the adult inpatient psychiatric unit.
- *Brief Rating of Aggression by Children and Adolescents* (BRACHA) is a valid tool for the ED to determine the best placement for children and adolescents on an inpatient Psychiatric unit.

A study using questionnaires was conducted by Arnetz and colleagues (2018) to examine the effect of work stress, staff interaction, and safety climate on self-reported workplace violence (see conceptual model, Fig. 20.2). Descriptive and correlational analyses were conducted. Results indicated interpersonal conflict was a risk factor for verbal violence, low work efficiency was a risk factor for physical violence, and poor violence prevention climate was a risk factor for verbal and physical violence. The researchers recommended that interventions should aim at enhancing employee interactions, work efficiency, and management endorsement of a violence prevention environment.

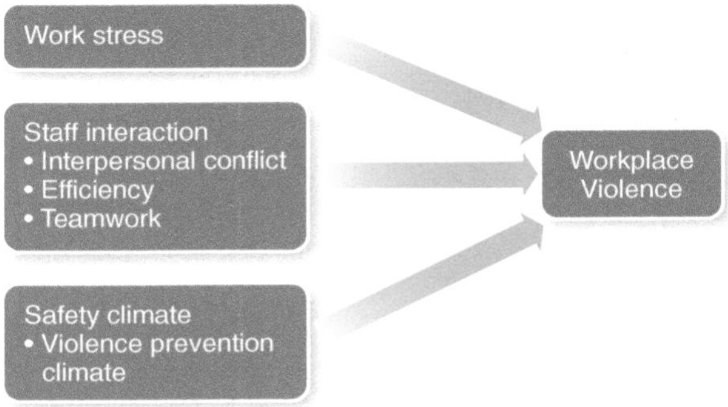

Fig. 20.2 A conceptual model of workplace violence. Source: Arnetz, J., Hamblin, L. E., Sudan, S., & Arnetz, B. (2018). Organizational determinants of workplace violence against hospital workers. *Journal of Occupational and Environmental Medicine, 60*(8), 693–699. https://doi.org/10.1097/JOM.0000000000001345.

Workplace Incivility

Incivility is "one or more rude, discourteous, or disrespectful actions that may or may not have a negative intent behind them" (American Nurses Association [ANA], 2015). The behaviors can be either intentional or unintentional, having the potential to cause long-term effects on the victim. It is a mild form of bullying and unlike incivility, bullying is considered a type of violence. If incivility is not managed in a timely and appropriate manner, it has the potential to escalate into bullying. It is everyone's responsibility to create a culture of safety and well-being. The following behaviors define incivility (Ciocco, 2018):

- Covert
- Direct and blatant aggression
- Overt—more subtle behaviors such as sarcasm, gossiping, or gesturing
- From one person to another or between a group and a targeted person ("mobbing"); this is when a specific person is the victim of rude and discourteous behavior from two or more persons
- Displaying favoritism
- Making verbal insults

Workplace Bullying

Bullying is defined as "anyone who uses his or her perceived strength or power to intimidate another person

TABLE 20.2 Roles in Bullying

Roles	Definitions
Bully/perpetrator	Someone invoking repeated, malicious, intentional arrogant, underhanded behavior
Victim/target	Someone who is the recipient of bully's behavior (unwanted, repeated, malicious, intentional behavior) causing physical and emotional harm
Bystander	Someone who witnesses bullying
Upstander	Someone who witnesses bullying and intervenes

Source: Ciocco, M. 2018. *Fast facts on combating nurse bullying, incivility and workplace violence.* New York: Springer: Pelletier, P. (2015). *Workplace bullying: It's just bad for business.* (p. 54). Diversity Publishing.

who, he or she thinks, is weaker in order to gain power over that person" (Ciocco, 2018, p. 39). Definitions vary among researchers and experts on the topic. However, the underlying themes are similar. The ANA (2015) described bullying as "repeated, unwanted harmful actions intended to humiliate, offend, and cause distress in the recipient, including those that harm, undermine, and degrade." Research on workplace bullying started in the late 1980s in Sweden with Heinz Leymann's seminal works. Subsequently the fields of psychology, occupational health and medicine, epidemiology, violence, and management research have contributed to the knowledge of this area.

Bullying occurs in any type of occupation, not just health care (Namie, 2017); 60.4 million Americans are affected by bullying, and 61% of Americans are aware of abusive conduct in the workplace. Causes of bullying include work culture, workforce mix, and the employer's response to bullying. According to Glambeck and colleagues (2018), bullying can include all members of a team. In addition, intense workplaces promote the greatest occurrences of bullying. In a recent study, these researchers noted that bullying behaviors dismissed by leadership increased the risk of continued abuse by perpetrators (Glambeck et al., 2018). There are various types of bullying including:

- **Verbal bullying:** Slandering, ridiculing, or maligning a person or their family; persistent name-calling that is hurtful, insulting, or humiliating; using a person as the butt of jokes; abusive and offensive remarks.
- **Physical bullying:** Pushing, shoving, kicking, poking, tripping, assault or threat of physical assault, and damage to a person's work area or property.
- **Mobbing:** Mobbing is the bullying or social isolation of a person through collective unjustified accusations, humiliation, general harassment, or emotional abuse.
- **Cyberbullying:** Cyberbullying is bullying that takes place over digital devices like cell phones, computers, and tablets. Cyberbullying includes sending, posting, or sharing negative, harmful, false, or mean content about someone else. It can include sharing personal or private information about someone else causing embarrassment or humiliation.
- **Exclusion:** Socially or physically excluding or disregarding a person in work-related activities.

There are various roles assumed by individuals in the bullying process. These include perpetrator, target, bystander, and upstander. Table 20.2 shows terms and definitions for specific roles in bullying (Cioccio, 2018; Pelletier, 2015).

Pelletier (2015) identified common attributes of victims or targets (Box 20.2). These include independence, technically skilled, go-to workers to whom new staff turn for guidance, successful, better social skills

BOX 20.2 Common Attributes of Victims (Targets)

- Targets are independent
- Targets are more technically skilled than their bullies
- They are the "go-to" workers to whom new staff turn for guidance
- Targets are better liked
- They are successful
- They have more social skills and possess greater emotional awareness and maturity
- Targets are ethical and honest
- Targets are people with personalities founded on a nurturing and social orientation—a desire to help, heal, teach, develop, and nurture others

Pelletier, P. (2015). *Workplace bullying: It's just bad for business.* (p. 54). United States of America: Diversity Publishing.

with a nurturing and social orientation. Ciocco (2018) described bullying in further detail: (1) it can be physical or verbal; (2) it may include threats, exclusion, or violence; (3) it can take place in a single occurrence or over a period of time, by the same person or by a group; (4) it occurs throughout all age ranges and in all places: schools, workplace, and social settings; (5) it can include recurrent efforts to include physical injury, emotional and mental harm; (6) it can occur between strangers, work peers, acquaintances, or friends; (7) it is intentional; (8) it focuses on a specific target or targets; (9) it includes psychological cruelty and well-thought out actions; and (10) it is disruptive and interferes with work.

Organizational Role

Organizational leaders have an instrumental role in managing workplace bullying. Bullying can be perpetrated by nurses on others, or by others on nurses. Although leaders may be aware of toxic behaviors, very little is done to address it. There are multiple reasons for this. Some reasons are due to education, little experience or self-confidence with having difficult conversations with staff, fear of being a victim themselves, or they may have a personal relationship with the bully. All of these factors make it very difficult to promote civility in work environments. In a 2019 survey (Spader, 2019) 35% of respondents had been verbally assaulted by a health care provider in the past 24 months, as compared to 36% in 2018. A total of 64% of respondents reported the event, and only 25% perceived that the issue was well managed. Approximately 46% of nurses spoke up when bullying was witnessed, 77% reported the incident, and less than 50% were content with how the incident was handled (Spader, 2019). Although workplace bullying is widespread, some behaviors do not constitute bullying:

- Reasonable management practices, including performance management and disciplinary procedures;
- A direction to carry out reasonable duties and instructions.

An OSHA report provided through TJC stated that "over 50 percent have been verbally abused (a category that included bullying) in a 12-month period and 59 percent experienced verbal abuse during a seven-day period" (TJC, 2016). Destructive acts cause unhealthy work environments impacting patient care, quality outcomes, and financial loss in organizations. Bullying increases feelings of anxiety and depression, reduces job satisfaction, and increases organizational nursing turnover. Perpetrators thrive on control. They often focus on individuals who are perceived weak, have stronger skills sets, or are well liked by others. Bullying has financial ramifications to organizations, among the array of negative consequences overall for organizations.

The public views nursing as the most trusted, ethical, and honest profession. Behind closed doors, nurses are losing trust and reverence for one another. Bullying is a hidden epidemic. It poses jeopardy to financial stability, job security, and employees' health and well-being. There are health-related risks to bullying such as anxiety, depression, posttraumatic stress disorder, insomnia, panic attacks, and migraine headaches. Because of psychosocial and physical harm to employees, it leads to absenteeism, poor morale, and decreased job satisfaction, which affects hospital outcomes and patient care.

Bullying and incivility in health care are being addressed by many regulatory agencies such as TJC. They published the following Sentinel Alerts:

- Sentinel Event Alert 40 in 2008: Behaviors that undermine a culture of safety,
- Sentinel Event 24 in 2016: Bullying has no place in health care,
- Sentinel Event Alert 57 in 2017: The essential role of leadership in developing a safety culture,
- Sentinel Event Alert 59 in 2018: Physical and verbal violence against health care workers, and the recently updated,
- Sentinel Event Alert 45 in 2019: Preventing violence in the health care setting.

The Magnet® Recognition program within the American Nurses Credentialing Center (ANCC) has taken steps to address these issues. In 2017, within the domain of Exemplary Professional Practice (EP), a culture of safety EP criterion was developed for physical and verbal violence in health care systems. The EP15EO expects organizations pursuing Magnet designation to demonstrate strong data and strategies regarding workplace violence, bullying, and incivility towards nursing (Thompson, 2019, p. 25).

Impact of Workplace Bullying

Hostile work environments can harm patients and the organization's status, decrease employee satisfaction, and greatly affect a company's bottom line due to increased turnover and absenteeism. An unhealthy work culture can lead to increased rates of insomnia, high blood pressure, anxiety, headaches, posttraumatic stress disorder, depression, gastrointestinal disorders, strained personal relationships, mistrust, substance abuse, eating disorders, and suicidal ideations (Ciocco, 2018). Bullying results in companies losing more than $250 million every year from not only employee turnover but lost productivity, workers' compensation claims, recruitment, orientation of new staff, and court costs (American Psychiatric Association Foundation, 2020; Herschcovis et al., 2015).

Employment Assistance Programs

Employee assistance programs (EAPs) provide a range of services to help employees cope with stressors that occur at home and at work. Family counseling might be useful in reducing domestic violence that can spill over into the workplace. Programs that counsel both the victim and the abuser could be instrumental in initiating needed interventions to defuse domestic violence situations that could affect the worksite. Furthermore, individual counseling can help employees cope with personal stressors that might contribute to unpredictable or violent behaviors. EAPs can be useful in preventing or mitigating loss caused by domestic violence that extends to the workplace.

CURRENT ISSUES AND TRENDS

Active Shooter

The deadliest situations involve an active shooter. US Department of Homeland Security (DHS) defined active shooter as someone "actively engaged in killing or attempting to kill people in a confined and populated area" (National Safety Council [NSC], 2019). During a chaotic situation involving an active shooter, DHS suggested avoiding knee-jerk reactions, remaining calm, and doing one of three options (NSC, 2019):

1. If there is an accessible escape route, leave belongings and get out.
2. If evacuation is not possible, find a hiding place where you won't be trapped should the shooter find you, lock and blockade the door, and silence your phone.
3. As a last resort and only when your life is in imminent danger, attempt to incapacitate the shooter by throwing items, improvising weapons, and yelling.

Many organizations have recognized and adopted strategies to navigate active shooters. The following actionable framework is commonly promoted for decision-making during active shootings: (1) run and escape if possible, (2) hide if escape is not possible, or (3) fight as a last resort (see Box 20.3 for more details).

Active shooter training has not only been strongly encouraged by DHS, but it is an expectation by OSHA, TJC, and NIOSH. Active shooter incidents frequently end within 10 to 15 minutes. Therefore prior to law enforcement arrival to the incident, employees need to be trained mentally and physically to cope with an active shooter situation (OSHA, 2019d). DHS has developed a protocol for dealing with an active shooter: https://www.dhs.gov/xlibrary/assets/active_shooter_booklet.pdf

Legislation

The American Nurses Association (ANA, 2015) developed a Position Statement on Incivility, Bullying, and Workplace Violence. Position statements by the (Professional Issues Panel on Incivility, Bullying, and Workplace Violence 2015) include:

- The nursing profession will not tolerate violence of any kind from any source.
- Nurses and employers must collaborate to create a culture of respect.
- The adoption of evidence-based strategies that prevent and mitigate incivility, bullying, and workplace violence; and promote health, safety, and wellness and optimal outcomes in health care.
- The strategies employed are listed and categorized by primary, secondary, and tertiary prevention.
- The statement is relevant for all health care professionals and stakeholders, not exclusively to nurses.

Lawmakers have taken steps to protect health care workers from violence in the workplace. The US House of Representatives proposed the *Healthcare Workplace Violence Prevention Act* in March 2018 titled H.R. 5223. The bill would have guided OSHA to develop a criterion that required and encouraged health care organizations to develop workplace violence prevention plans. Although the bill did not move forward, it was reintroduced in February 2019 as H.R. 1309. The current bill "requires the Department of Labor to address workplace violence in the healthcare and social service sectors" (Henkel, 2019). This bill will encourage employees to speak up, decreasing fear of retaliation as they would be protected from such acts. On November 21, 2019 the

BOX 20.3 Protocol for Dealing with an Active Shooter

Be Informed
- Sign up for an active shooter training.
- If you see something, say something to an authority right away.
- Sign up to receive local emergency alerts and register your work and personal contact information with any work sponsored alert system.
- Be aware of your environment and any possible dangers.

Make a Plan
- Make a plan with your family, and ensure everyone knows what they would do, if confronted with an active shooter.
- Look for the two nearest exits anywhere you go, have an escape path in mind, and identify places you could hide.
- Understand the plans for individuals with disabilities or other access and functional needs.

During
RUN and escape, if possible
- Getting away from the shooter or shooters is the top priority.
- Leave your belongings behind and get away.
- Help others escape, if possible, but evacuate regardless of whether others agree to follow.
- Warn and prevent individuals from entering an area where the active shooter may be.
- Call 911 when you are safe, and describe shooter, location, and weapons.

HIDE, if escape is not possible
- Get out of the shooter's view and stay very quiet.
- Silence all electronic devices and make sure they won't vibrate.
- Lock and block doors, close blinds, and turn off lights.
- Don't hide in groups—spread out along walls or hide separately to make it more difficult for the shooter.
- Try to communicate with police silently. Use text message or social media to tag your location, or put a sign in a window.
- Stay in place until law enforcement gives you the all clear.
- Your hiding place should be out of the shooter's view and provide protection if shots are fired in your direction.

FIGHT as an absolute last resort
- Commit to your actions and act as aggressively as possible against the shooter.
- Recruit others to ambush the shooter with makeshift weapons like chairs, fire extinguishers, scissors, books, etc.
- Be prepared to cause severe or lethal injury to the shooter.
- Throw items and improvise weapons to distract and disarm the shooter.

After
- Keep hands visible and empty.
- Know that law enforcement's first task is to end the incident, and they may have to pass injured along the way.
- Officers may be armed with rifles, shotguns, and/or handguns and may use pepper spray or tear gas to control the situation.
- Officers will shout commands and may push individuals to the ground for their safety.
- Follow law enforcement instructions and evacuate in the direction they come from, unless otherwise instructed.
- Take care of yourself first, and then you may be able to help the wounded before first responders arrive.
- If the injured are in immediate danger, help get them to safety.
- While you wait for first responders to arrive, provide first aid. Apply direct pressure to wounded areas and use tourniquets if you have been trained to do so.
- Turn wounded people onto their sides if they are unconscious and keep them warm.
- Consider seeking professional help for you and your family to cope with the long-term effects of the trauma.

Source: Department of Homeland Security (DHS). (2020). *Active shooter.* https://www.ready.gov/active-shooter.

bill passed the House with a 251–158 vote (Congress. Gov, 2019–2020). H.R. 1309 remains in the House as of this publication. California has the most thorough legislation affecting health care workers. Beginning April 2017, senate bill 1299 required hospitals to create, implement, and educate employees on comprehensive workplace violence prevention plans (Henkel, 2019).

Bullying Prevention

Eradicating bullying is an enormous undertaking. Solutions can happen simultaneously, and each takes effort, patience, dedication, and time. The following are recommendations for leaders: (1) acknowledge bullying is occurring then establish a consistent process to collaboratively examine and manage nurse bullying so that staff can work in a healthier workplace, (2) C-suite executives should collaborate with staff and human resources to enforce a "No Tolerance" or code of conduct policy, and (3) behaviors of bullying and incivility should be clearly delineated in policies, and perpetrators are to be held accountable for their behavior and take responsibility for their actions by making amends to those affected, (4) create a reporting system that prevents retaliation, (5) encourage staff to speak when bullying actions are witnessed without fear of retribution, and (6) provide awareness, education, and training.

Organizations should develop workplace bullying policies and guidelines as directed by TJC, NIOSH, and OSHA. Collaborating with risk management, human resources, employee health, leaders, and educators would be advisable to encourage staff to report bullying conduct through an incident reporting system for tracking and trending. The language should be clear and concise with a strong message on consequences when policies are not followed; how to report bullying; and how to appropriately document the event, investigate, and follow-up. Employees need to be provided psychological safety for reporting bullying. Bullying goes under-reported for fear of retaliation or that nothing will be done about it. Leaders have a great opportunity to change a negative work environment by promoting a culture of civility through their own behavior. When leaders do nothing, this sends a negative message to employees that uncivil behavior is condoned. Inaction will make employees feel that they cannot trust their leaders to uphold a culture of safety and well-being. Leaders must support employees by reinforcing the importance of speaking up. Management of this population and related destructive behaviors begins with awareness and education. Education is key for addressing workplace bullying given the current prevalence.

Cognitive rehearsing (CR) described by Longo (2017) allows staff to effectively practice communication to recognize and respond to bullying behavior in the workplace. CR is reported to decrease toxic work environments, create a healthy workplace, and improve staff satisfaction (Longo, 2017). CR decreases the fear of dealing with perpetrators who are verbally condescending, insulting, and intimidating. It cultivates a nurse's confidence by identifying a bully and mentally preparing for when they are confronted with bullying behaviors. In a study conducted by Razzi and Bianchi (2019) with nurses in a community hospital, it was identified that the nurses felt more empowered to confront an uncivil situation through the CR education and training. When nurses are given techniques to face a bully and stop destructive behavior, it minimizes the probability of a perpetrator targeting others.

Taking into consideration the universal nursing shortage, attempts need to be made to safeguard seasoned and newly licensed professional nurses to clinical practice by encouraging bully-free conditions, aiding their positions in the workforce. To counter the culture of bullying in their work environments, organizations need to (1) determine what types of bullying are occurring, (2) endorse training, continuing education, and awareness of what bullying is and the characteristics of the perpetrators of bullying, (3) respond to signs of bullying, (4) identify staff in jeopardy for other emotional or performance issues, and (5) develop the skills needed to create safe workplaces to provide early interventions and detection of risky behaviors by perpetrators. It would be advantageous to identify work units at high risk, determine what types of bullying are occurring, and identify what kind of education is needed to increase a healthier work environment.

Legal Implications

Bullying is legal in every US state. To counteract this, nearly 30 states and two territories have introduced some version of the Healthy Workplace Bill (HWB) on antibullying (Healthy Workplace Bill, 2019; Namie, 2019). Fig. 20.3 illustrates those states with an antibullying bill.

"Bullying potentially violates the law if it is proven that the bullying falls within the clearly defined terms of

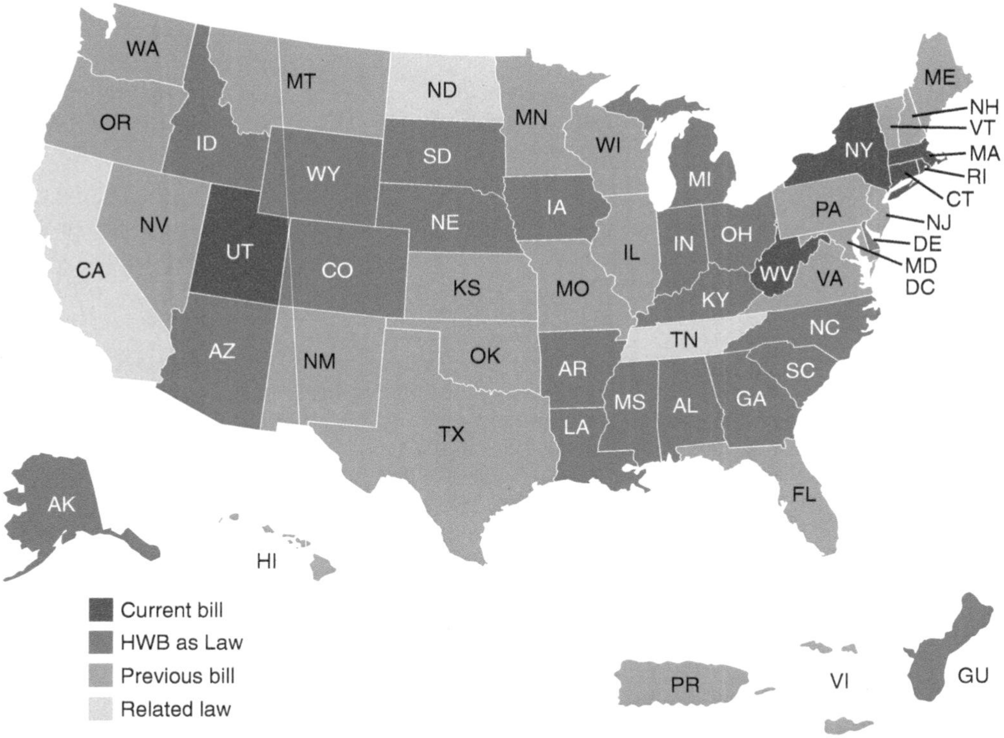

Fig. 20.3 Healthy Workplace Bill Locations, 2019. Source: Healthy Workplace Bill. (2019). *Healthy workplace campaign*.https://healthyworkplacebill.org/.

the legislation" (Pelletier, 2015, p. 59). Basic provisions of the model HWB legislation, developed and introduced by David Yamada in 2000, include a clear definition of an "abusive work environment." These bills offer a way to obtain legal compensation for being exposed to a toxic work environment. Employees would be allowed to prosecute the bully as an individual and hold the employer answerable to a cruel work environment and compensation for lost wages and benefits, forcing the employer to make changes to institutional processes (HWB, 2019).

CONCLUSION

Stamping out bullying will create a healthier, happier, more satisfying, and positive workplace for all employees and patients; decrease the risk of harm to patients; and shield seasoned and newly licensed nurses to practice under safe conditions to avoid needless distractions of being bullied.

Workplace bullying and violence add stress factors to an employee's longevity in their current work environment. Addressing bullying reduces the risk of losing veteran bedside nurses, reduces the financial impact on organizations, reduces the risk of increasing hospital-acquired infections, and most importantly places perpetrators accountable for their pathological and unforgivable behavior. Regardless of whether an employee enjoys their work or not, the income provides families with housing, food on the table, transportation, and increased access to health care.

The struggle to come to work every day in a hostile environment, being psychologically assaulted, is agonizing. Nurse bullying increases the threat of losing skilled and experienced bedside nurses, decreases intent to stay in the organization and nursing, and increases patients at risk for harm. Everyone has a right to work in a bully-free environment. Therefore taking actions to expose and stop workplace bullying is imperative.

RESEARCH NOTE

Source

(Bambi, S., Guazzini, A., Piredda, M., Lucchini, A., De Marinis, M., & Rasero, L. 2019). Negative interactions among nurses: An explorative study on lateral violence and bullying in nursing work settings. *Journal of Nursing Management, 27*(4), 749–757.

Purpose

Lateral violence and bullying have an effect on nurses' professional and health status. The purpose of this research was to investigate prevalence and risk factors of lateral violence and bullying among Italian nurse peers in different work settings, both inside and outside hospitals.

Discussion

Data were collected via a web survey using the 17-item "Negative Interactions Among Nurses Questionnaire" and a cross-sectional method. Emails were sent to 5009 nurses in three Tuscan public health care institutions. The response rate was 18.6% (n = 930). Twenty-six respondents were removed as they reported working with no peer colleagues. Negative interactions were experienced by 35.8% (n = 324), 42.3% (n = 137) of whom were bullied, with intensity being moderate and wide variability of prevalence. Psychophysical consequences of negative interactions were reported by 59% (n = 191). Victims who thought of leaving nursing were 21.9% (n = 71).

The main interventions implemented to confront these problems were sensitizing nurses, managers and administrators; prevention education events; acquisition of communication and conflict management skills; zero tolerance strategies; and codes of conduct that explicitly condemn unacceptable behaviors. However, there is no evidence of effectiveness for many of these interventions.

Application to Practice

Of note is that lateral violence and bullying among nurses were consistently present in all studied settings. Nurse managers could play a crucial role in preventing negative interactions among nurses. Strategies could include continuing education programs to promote awareness of this problem, implementation of an anonymous reporting system for bullying, introduction of occupational psychologists in wards with larger numbers of reported negative interactions and bullying, and increasing changes in staff composition within shifts.

The results suggest the need for an important cultural change by increasing the awareness of lateral violence and bullying among peers, which could be maintained through continuing education programs for nurses employed in all institutions and positive leadership by head nurses to promote healthy work environments with lower conflicts and psychosomatic complaints among nurses. In parallel, nurse managers need to monitor the work climate to break the occurrence of lateral violence and its escalation towards bullying.

CASE STUDY

Kelly, nurse manager (NM) of 15 years, oversees a busy 28-bed solid organ transplant unit in a large city hospital. Patients who have end-stage kidney failure get transported there to the dialysis unit for treatment. The transplant nurses needed to get clarity on whether nurses can administer antibiotics to patients who are receiving dialysis. Kelly reached out via email to Nurse Charlie, who had a long history with the dialysis nursing practice at this institution, to inquire when and if nurses can initiate orders for antibiotics in dialysis. Kelly wanted to make sure she understood some of the background history of what nurses in dialysis can and cannot do in regard to initiating orders that originated from the transplant team versus a nephrologist, so that she had some background information prior to then contacting Michael, NM of the dialysis unit. When Charlie replied to the email, he included Michael the dialysis NM and Marge, the nurse administrator, and the charge nurse in the dialysis unit. Michael noted that a patient being treated in dialysis is technically under the care of the nephrologist. This was new knowledge for Kelly. Dialysis nurses are not permitted to administer any medication to patients unless ordered by the nephrologist. If medication must be administered, the primary physician would need to contact the nephrologist. Kelly shared this information with her nursing staff.

CASE STUDY—cont'd

That same day nurse administrator Marge emailed Kelly and Kelly's nurse administrator regarding the recent inquiry. She accused Kelly of purposely going around Michael, the dialysis NM, to make him look bad. Kelly personally called Marge to explain that was not her intent. Kelly did not have a strong background in dialysis practice and was seeking information. Nurse Charlie was a historian regarding the dialysis unit. Kelly thought he would be a great resource to understand policies and procedures in that area. Once she got the information she needed, it may not have been necessary to reach out to NM Michael to report any potential delays of medication administration by his nurses. Marge insisted that Kelly purposely had malicious intent. That call led to an immediate meeting with Kelly's administrator, Allison. Allison accused Kelly of blindsiding Michael and purposely avoiding him, so he looked bad to his subordinates. Kelly sunk into the office chair in disbelief. Kelly was given a verbal warning. Allison began spreading rumors about Kelly to her peers and colleagues regarding her lack of self-awareness, poor teamwork, unprofessionalism, and sabotaging Michael's stellar reputation. Kelly did not know what to do. She was accused of things that were false. This caused her peers to avoid her, she often sat alone, and was removed from two committees.

At a meeting a few days later, she saw Michael. She decided to apologize for any misunderstanding regarding the inquiry she made about medication administration. Michael looked confused. Kelly shared that she was under the impression she had purposely made him look bad. He assured Kelly that was absolutely false. Michael was supportive about Kelly reaching out to Charlie and was not offended in the least.

Kelly tried to make every effort to clear the air about this matter. It weighed heavy on her and negatively impacted her reputation and working relationship with her peers. Kelly contacted administrators Allison and Marge. She shared the positive conversation she had with Michael. Marge thanked her for the update. Allison, on the other hand, wrote Kelly up for insubordination. Kelly was clearly being bullied by her administrator. Allison was being completely unreasonable; she told Kelly that Kelly would not be successful in this organization if she had anything to do with it. Kelly stated that she would have no choice but file a grievance with human resources (HR) to settle this matter. Allison said, "Good luck, they won't believe you over me."

Kelly did go to HR, and Allison was correct in that they did not believe her. Their comment was "if you don't like the way this played out, this organization may not be the right place for you." Kelly did some research on this type of behavior. She was experiencing isolation, gaslighting, false accusations, emotional abuse, professional sabotage, and intimidation. Kelly felt alone, depressed, and defeated. She went onto social media and found several bullying support groups that provided her with good information on how to cope with workplace bullying. Those resources led to others. All these resources gave her the needed strength to understand bullies and why and how they target certain types of people as their victim. As Kelly gained strength and confidence from information and supportive colleagues, she took positive and affirming steps to diminish the effects of bullying and to better counter negative behaviors at work.

1. How would you feel if you were Kelly?
2. Would you have done anything differently in this situation?
3. Having support is important to survive bullying. What other resources would you have used and why?
4. If you were a witness to this type of bullying, how would you provide Kelly support? Would you too isolate yourself from her for fear of being a target?
5. What have you identified as the characteristics of the bully and target?

CRITICAL THINKING EXERCISE

Two East evening shift has been having constant turnover. The director Shelly was concerned since there was a need for continuity on the Dedicated Diabetes Care Unit. Patients on that unit would typically be readmitted for diabetic ketoacidosis or infections.

When Shelly attended a conference she met Beth, a Certified Diabetes Educator. She convinced Beth to interview to ensure that there was an experienced person to hire to reduce the constant turnover that was very concerning to her. Beth had worked for an Outpatient Diabetes Setting for 10 years and was very excited about the new role.

During her orientation, she felt highly supported and provided her preceptor with tips to better manage acute patients. After the orientation, Beth was assigned to the 3–11 shift. On her first 3–11 shift the other nurses seemed very reserved. During the break time, Beth felt isolated from the other nurses. She felt that she was being excluded. At times, she thought it may be her imagination, but it continued, and she observed it happening with selected people on the unit. After work she would return home and feel anxious at bedtime.

Beth decided she would speak to Shelly about the hostility she was experiencing. She scheduled an appointment with Shelly and brought a list of her experiences and that of her peers.

1. If you were Shelly, what additional information would you want from Beth?
2. Should Shelly take Beth's word for the situation?
3. As a leader, what is the first action you would take?
4. What is the evidence base for Shelly's leadership actions?
5. How can Shelly track turnover after she takes action?

REFERENCES

American Nurses Association (ANA). (2015). *Incivility, bullying, and workplace violence: ANA position statement.* https://www.nursingworld.org/practice-policy/nursing-excellence/official-position-statements/id/incivility-bullying-and-workplace-violence/.

American Psychiatric Association Foundation. (2020). *Bullying.* http://workplacementalhealth.org/Mental-Health-Topics/Bullying.

American Psychological Association (APA). (2020). *Violence.* https://www.apa.org/topics/violence/index.

Arnetz, J., Hamblin, L. E., Sudan, S., & Arnetz, B. (2018). Organizational determinants of workplace violence against hospital workers. *Journal of Occupational and Environmental Medicine, 60*(8), 693–699. https://doi.org/10.1097/JOM.0000000000001345.

Bambi, S., Guazzini, A., Piredda, M., Lucchini, A., De Marinis, M., & Rasero, L. (2019). Negative interactions among nurses: An explorative study on lateral violence and bullying in nursing work settings. *Journal of Nursing Management, 27*(4), 749–757.

Bureau of Labor Statistics (BLS). (2019a). *Census of Fatal Occupational Injuries (CFOI) for 2018,* Bureau of Labor Statistics Injuries, Illnesses, and Fatalities. https://www.bls.gov/iif/oshcfoi1.htm#rates.

Bureau of Labor Statistics. (2019b). *Survey of Occupational Injuries and Illnesses (SOII) for 2018.* Bureau of Labor Statistics Injuries, Illnesses, and Fatalities. https://www.bls.gov/respondents/iif/.

Ciocco, M. (2018). *Fast facts on combating nurse bullying, incivility and workplace violence.* New York: Springer.

Congress.Gov, 116th Cong. (2019–2020). *H.R.1309–Workplace Violence Prevention for Health Care and Social Service Workers Act.* https://www.congress.gov/bill/116th-congress/house-bill/1309/actions?KWICView=false.

Department of Homeland Security. (2020). *Active shooter.* https://www.ready.gov/active-shooter.

Glambeck, M., Skogstad, A., & Einarsen, S. (2018). Workplace bullying, the development of job insecurity and the role of laissez-faire leadership: A two-wave moderated mediation study. *Work and Stress: An International Journal of Work, Health & Organisations,* 32(3), 1–16. https://doi.org/10.1080/02678373.2018.1427815.

Healthy Workplace Bill. (2019). *Healthy workplace campaign.* https://healthyworkplacebill.org/.

Henkel, S. (2019). *Threat assessment strategies to mitigate violence in healthcare.* IAHSS Foundation. https://iahssf.org/assets/IAHSS-Foundation-Threat-Assessment-Strategies-to-Mitigate-Violence-in-Healthcare.pdf.

Longo, J. (2017). Cognitive rehearsal. Learn a strategy for addressing incivility and bullying in nursing. *American Nurse Today, 12*(8), 41–44. https://www.americannursetoday.com/cognitive-rehearsal/.

Namie, G. (2017). *2017 WBI US Workplace Bullying Survey.* Workplace Bullying Institute. http://www.workplacebullying.org/wbiresearch/wbi-2017-survey/.

Namie, G., (2019). *WBI frequently asked questions.* https://www.workplacebullying.org/faq/#14.

National Institute for Occupational Safety and Health (NIOSH) Centers for Disease Control and Prevention, US Department of Health and Human Services. (2013). *Workplace violence prevention for nurses*: DHHS, NIOSH Publication. No. 2013–155. https://www.cdc.gov/niosh/topics/violence/training_nurses.html.

National Institute for Occupational Safety and Health (NIOSH) Centers for Disease Control and Prevention, US Department of Health and Human Services. (2015). *Notable milestones in NIOSH history.* https://www.cdc.gov/niosh/timeline.html.

National Institute of Occupational Safety and Health (NIOSH). (2019). *Occupational violence.* https://www.cdc.gov/niosh/topics/violence/default.html.

National Safety Council (NSC). (2019). *Assaults fourth leading cause of workplace deaths.* https://www.nsc.org/work-safety/safety-topics/workplace-violence.

Occupational Safety and Health Administration (OSHA). (2015a). *Preventing workplace violence: A roadmap for healthcare facilities.* https://www.osha.gov/Publications/OSHA3827.pdf.

Occupational Safety and Health Administration (OSHA). (2015b). *Workplace violence in healthcare*. https://www.osha.gov/Publications/OSHA3826.pdf.

Occupational Safety and Health Administration (OSHA). (2015c). *Guidelines for preventing workplace violence*, pp. 6–7. https://m.afscme.org/issues/health-safety/resources/document/osha3148.pdf.

Occupational Safety and Health Administration (OSHA). (2019d). *Emergency preparedness and response: Getting started*. https://www.osha.gov/SLTC/emergencypreparedness/gettingstarted_evacuation.html.

Pelletier, P. (2015). *Workplace bullying: It's just bad for business* (p. 54). Vancouver, CA: Diversity Publishing.

Professional Issues Panel on Incivility, Bullying, and Workplace Violence. (2015). *Incivility, bullying, and workplace violence position statement*. http://www.nursingworld.org/DocumentVault/Position-Statements/Practice/Position-Statement-on-Incivility-Bullying-and-Workplace-Violence.pdf.

Razzi, C., & Bianchi, A. (2019). Incivility in nursing: Implementing a quality improvement program utilizing cognitive rehearsal training. *Nursing Forum*, *54*(4), 526–536. https://doi.org/10.1111/nuf.12366.

Spader, C., (2019). *2019 Nursing Trends and Salary Survey results*. https://www.myamericannurse.com/2019-nursing-trends-and-salary-survey-results/.

The Joint Commission (TJC). (2016). *Quick Safety Issue 24: Bullying has no place in health care*. https://www.jointcommission.org/-/media/tjc/documents/newsletters/quick_safety_issue_24_june_2016pdf.pdf.

The Joint Commission (TJC). (2019a). *Sentinel Event Alert 45: Preventing violence in the health care setting*. https://www.jointcommission.org/resources/patient-safety-topics/sentinel-event/sentinel-event-alert-newsletters/sentinel-event-alert-issue-45-preventing-violence-in-the-health-care-setting/.

The Joint Commission (TJC). (2019b). *Quick Safety Issue 47: De-escalation in health care*. https://www.jointcommission.org/resources/news-and-multimedia/newsletters/newsletters/quick-safety/quick-safety-47-deescalation-in-health-care/.

The Joint Commission (TJC). (2020a). *Resources for consumers*. https://www.jointcommission.org/resources/for-consumers/.

The Joint Commission (TJC). (2020b). *Sentinel event alert and quick safety newsletters*. https://www.jointcommission.org/resources/patient-safety-topics/workplace-violence-prevention/sentinel-event-alert-and-quick-safety-newsletters/.

Thompson, R. (2019). *Enough! Eradicate bullying & incivility in healthcare: Strategies for front line leaders* (p. 25). United States of America: Incredible Messages Press.

World Health Organization (WHO). (2020). Violence against healthcare workers. https://www.who.int/violence_injury_prevention/violence/workplace/en/.

21

Nursing Workforce Staffing and Management

Therese A. Fitzpatrick

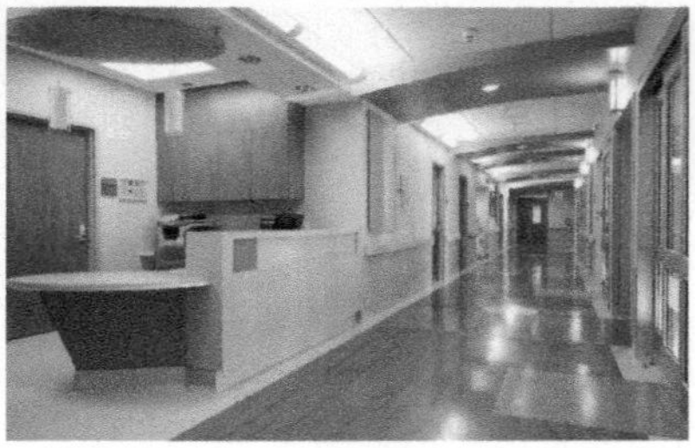

http://evolve.elsevier.com/Huber/leadership

Staffing and scheduling are perennial concerns for nurses. Nursing is essential in the delivery of health care to society. According to the Gallup organization, for the past 18 consecutive years more than four in five Americans (84%) rated the nursing profession's honesty and ethical standards as very high or high, earning nurses the top spot among a diverse list of professionals (Brenan, 2018; Thew, 2020) The American Nurses Association's (ANA) *Nursing's Social Policy Statement* reflects the societal contract for the provision of safe and quality nursing care and services for all people in every health care setting (ANA, 2010). Therefore, staffing management is a critical contributor to achieving the societal contract. Staffing management is one of the most crucial yet highly complex and time-consuming activities for nurses and nurse leaders at every level of the health care organization today.

Although nursing's goals remain focused on providing patients the right nursing resources to achieve the best clinical outcomes for a reasonable cost, the environment in which leaders contend has becoming increasingly complex and chaotic. Evolving payment reform initiatives such as value-based care, bundled payments, and various shared savings programs all consider the quality and efficiency of services delivered to patients, both in the inpatient and outpatient settings. Although the notion of value is still being defined by the Centers for Medicare & Medicaid Services (CMS) and various professional organizations, generally it is defined as the quality of care (numerator) divided by the cost of care (denominator) or stated simply, patient health outcomes achieved by dollar spent (Shi & Singh, 2019). These developments in payment methods will continue to place the utilization of all resources, both labor (including nursing) and non-labor under significant scrutiny and pricing pressure.

The seminal work of Aydelotte (1973) stated that the aim of staffing is to provide, at a reasonable cost, a standard of nursing care acceptable to its clientele and the nursing staff serving it. This continues and remains as a critical issue affecting the quality, safety, and cost of health care (Aiken et al., 2002, 2003, 2014, 2016; Blegen et al., 1998; Kane et al., 2007a,b; Litvak et al., 2005; Mensik, 2014; Needleman et al., 2002, 2006, 2011; Unruh, 2008).

Emerging knowledge suggests that we begin to examine staffing as a complex adaptive system. Clancy (2007) posited that as organizations evolve, they become more complex over time, which means the traditional methods to measure and manage these complex systems must also evolve. By their very nature, complex systems are a dynamic network of many elements acting in parallel, and constantly acting and reacting to what other agents are doing. The planning and deployment of nursing resources is an example of such a complex system and includes the need to predict demand, synchronize complex work rules, control costs, and manage fluctuating labor markets while simultaneously being mindful of staff's personal preferences.

What is needed is the means to measure and manage the confluence of competing and dynamic interests using a system of staffing influenced by a changing external environment, data, many interacting agents (work rules, work load, work flow, and financial imperatives), and individual factors such as schedules, personal preferences, communications, and policies. These forces all influence how one staffs optimally (Gavigan et al., 2016). In addition, the nursing workforce is undergoing transformation and is being affected by generational differences, diversity, new lifestyles, family lives, cultural differences, technological skills, and the need for greater integration of work life into personal life. These traditions, emerging knowledge, and workforce transformations call for the profession of nursing to fulfill its societal contract and envision staffing methodologies to inform the future (Flanders & Carr, 2016; Joseph & Fowler, 2016; National Council of State Boards of Nursing [NCSBN], 2016).

The major goal of staffing management is to provide the right number of nursing staff with the right qualifications to deliver safe, high-quality, and cost-effective nursing care to a group of patients and their families as evidenced by positive clinical outcomes, satisfaction with care, and progression across the care continuum (Eck Birmingham, 2010). Additionally, in an effort to fulfill the responsibilities as leaders in the creation of innovative systems and processes of care and as full participants in the governance of our organizations, nursing resource allocation needs to also reflect the critical activities that support direct care as well as our professional development. The ANA (2016a) noted that nurses are the largest clinical subgroup in hospitals and a common target for cost containment by reducing nursing hours. However, "appropriate safe nurse staffing and skill mix levels are essential to optimize quality of care" (ANA, 2016a), and this determination is challenging yet essential.

Staffing management is one of the most critical yet highly complex and time-consuming activities for nurse leaders at every level of the health care organization. How well or poorly nursing leaders execute staff management affects the safety and quality of patient care including minimizing complications and unnecessary readmissions, the financial results, and organizational outcomes, such as job satisfaction and retention of registered nurses (RNs). The purpose of this chapter is to assist students, nurses, and nursing leaders at all levels to understand the complex issues associated with staffing management in patient care. A framework for staffing management is presented, and critical components of the staffing management plan are described. New evidence that fosters an understanding of just-in-time service delivery, big data analytics, technology, and algorithmically driven applications are presented for optimal and effective staffing.

DEFINITIONS

Staffing terminology in nursing is multifaceted and often confusing, with a specific set of terms used.

Admissions, discharges, and transfers (ADT): ADT refers to the patients who are admitted, discharged, and transferred. The ADT factor has also been referred to as a churn or turnover of patients. ADT is associated with increased care or workload to meet the standard of care for the patient and with safe and effective RN-to-RN communication or handoff regarding the patient's condition and plan of care. The movement of patients in, out, or between units has a significant impact on scheduling and assignment of clinical resources because this is time-consuming work.

Average daily census (ACD): The average number of inpatients on any given day, calculated by dividing the number of patients cared for per day over a certain period by the number of days in a period is the ADC. It may be an actual ADC or a budgeted (anticipated) ADC. It is important to note when creating a budget or staffing plan for a unit that there may be additional categories or classification of patients cared for on an inpatient unit and that volume must be accounted for in the plan. For example, patients in an outpatient, observation, or phase 2 recovery status may be placed on an inpatient unit. For departments outside of acute care the average workload may be measured in other types of mathematical units such as surgical minutes in the operating room, or average daily visits (ADV) in ambulatory settings or emergency departments. It is important to note that emergency department patients waiting for an inpatient bed in order to be admitted or transferred still need to be included in the emergency department's workload.

Average length of stay (ALOS): ALOS is the average number of days each patient is in the hospital. It is determined by dividing the total number of patient days by the total number of admissions (Finkler et al., 2013; Fitzpatrick & Brooks, 2010). Patient and organizational needs are evolving based on improved care models, technology, advanced pharmacology, and payer mandates. As a result, lengths of stay are significantly decreasing. Therefore, encounters with a hospital, whether inpatient or outpatient, may be measured in hours rather than days.

Human resources staffing strategy: This is process that determines human resource needs; links to the strategic plan, recruits, selects, and retains qualified applicants; and meets the needs of the organization by ensuring that there is appropriate, sufficient, qualified, and competent staff. The human resource strategy also supports professional development and succession planning processes.

Nurse staffing: Nurse staffing refers to the process of identifying and allocating nursing staff on a shift to a patient care area. It typically is a daily operations function. "Appropriate nurse staffing is a match of registered nurse expertise with the needs of the recipient of nursing care services in the context of the practice setting and situation. The provision of appropriate nurse staffing is necessary to reach safe, quality outcomes; it is achieved by dynamic, multifaceted decision-making processes that must take into account a wide range of variables" (ANA, 2012, p. 6). The geography of a nursing unit may also impact staffing. Examples include blind spots, hallway separations, or sheer size. Any of these limitations may need to be mitigated by adjusting staffing.

Nurse staffing management plan: This is a structured approach to the process of identifying and allocating unit-based personnel resources to optimize care needs, quality outcomes, and effectiveness.

Nursing direct-care hours: Direct-care hours are the number of nursing staff hours that are assigned to provide direct care to a patient or groups of patients for a specified period; the most common direct-care staff include the RN, licensed practical nurse (LPN)/licensed vocational nurse (LVN), and unlicensed assistive personnel (UAP). The hours are typically calculated per patient day or nursing hours per patient day (NHPPD).

Nursing indirect-care hours: Indirect-care hours are the number of staff hours that are assigned to complete organization business such as performance improvement activities, staff development, committee work, or shared governance participation. Indirect-care hours may also include nurses in support roles such as preceptors that support either the direct-care staff or the business of the organization or department.

Nurse-to-patient ratio: The RN-to-patient ratio reflects the actual patient care assignment, model of care, or a state-mandated regulatory requirement for an RN-to-patient assignment. The number of RNs assigned to care for a certain number of patients is stated as a ratio. For example, 1:2 is a common ratio for one RN to care for two patients in an intensive care unit (ICU) and may be changed based on the condition of the patients.

Nursing workload: Nursing workload is the patient care plus non-patient care activities (direct and indirect) performed by a nurse and includes the time, complexity of skill mix, patient dependency, and severity of illness (intensity in terms of effort required) of the work a nurse performs within a given period (Morris et al., 2007). It is typically measured by units of service. For most inpatient departments care requirements are defined as hours per patient day (HPPD). When multiplied by the expected patient volume, the total number of care hours is determined and used to create a personnel budget. In the operating room (OR) surgical minutes or numbers of cases drive the workload calculation; in ambulatory areas such as the emergency room, an hours per patient visit (HPPV) calculation is used as the measure of the workload.

Optimizing a staffing strategy: The planning of staffing is predicated on predictions of the future state of a system and is highly dependent on describing its current state. The ability to analyze demand is a powerful means to describe and understand the behavior of the system, and the results of these analyses form the basis of an optimal strategy. This requires an understanding of a variety of data, the interactions and dependencies of those data elements, statistical analysis, and the quantification of patient need, specifically acuity. Mathematical optimization produces the best result or option given the myriad of competing factors.

Innovative organizations are now beginning to consider multidisciplinary, patient-needs driven, unit-based care models. For example, it may be more effective and efficient to add physical therapists to a direct care team on an orthopedic unit or include a respiratory therapist in a critical care team. As a result, the measurement of direct care hours beyond just nursing will need to evolve as well.

Scheduling: Scheduling is the process of determining a set number and type of staff for a future time period by assigning individual personnel to work specific hours, days, or shifts and in a specific unit or area over a specified period of time.

Skill level: Skill level is a function of education and competency for the job. In nursing, it is determined by the licensure (e.g., RN, LPN, LVN) or certification (e.g., UAP, NA) of a staff member.

Skill mix: Skill mix is the range of types and levels of ability and preparation of the workforce. In nursing it is the proportion of direct-care RNs to total direct-care nursing staff expressed as a percentage of RNs to total nursing staff. For example, a medical surgical patient care unit may have a skill mix of 60% RNs and 40% UAP. A skill mix ratio is typically budgeted for at the patient care unit level but must also be examined at the shift level during the scheduling process. The determination of an appropriate skill mix requires the understanding and examination of the specific care requirements of a group of patients and a responsible determination of those activities that can be safely delegated to UAP or other care providers. Those elements of care that may be delegated are often outlined in the State's Nursing Practice Act.

Staffing is composed of four distinct and interdependent processes, including (1) budgeting, (2) scheduling, (3) deployment, and (4) assignment making. Box 21.1 displays these definitions. In the discussion of staffing, it is important to specify which subprocess is the topic of focus. For example, if a leader determines that a department is understaffed, is the root cause a budget that does not reflect the actual demand within the department, whether insufficient resources were scheduled for a particular day, whether there was a lack of adequate backfill to accommodate a sick call, or was an assignment created that did not reflect the actual care requirements for a specific group of patients. Not unlike correcting a clinical misstep, isolating the root cause of a problem is required before an appropriate intervention can be deployed.

BOX 21.1 Definitions of Staffing Processes

1. **Budgeting:** A formal plan established by leaders that compares expected revenues with expenses. It requires an understanding of the expected demand for care by patient type, specific care requirements, anticipated cost of that care, and specific human resources required to provide that care, including the appropriate mix of staff.
2. **Scheduling:** The procedural plan to inform nurses and other providers of the days and hours/shifts when they are expected to work. Schedules are typically created several weeks or months in advance and reflect the variety of work rules determined by the organization, department, or as designated in a collective bargaining agreement. Examples of work rules are number of consecutive shifts permitted, weekend rotations, and shift length. Schedules may be created using advanced technology applications that allow the staff remote access to the schedule, standard spreadsheet applications, or even paper-based in smaller departments or organizations such as surgical centers.
3. **Deployment:** After the schedule has been created, the immediate or real time allocation of personnel to a department is called deployment. This process typically occurs immediately prior to the start of a shift when demand is reassessed, the numbers and types of scheduled resources assessed, staff is reassigned, or additional staff are assigned based on patient requirements or to supplement scheduled staff. This process may also include the assignment of nurses in a float pool or other flexible resources.
4. **Assignment:** The process by which a department leader allocates the right care giver, with the right competencies, at the right time to a specific patient or group of patients based on clinical requirements. Modifications to assignments may occur throughout the course of a shift based on dynamic patient needs.

Staffing effectiveness: An evaluation of the effect of nurse staffing on clinical quality and patient, financial, organizational, and professional nursing outcomes.

Staffing pattern: A staffing pattern lists the total number of direct-care staff by skill level scheduled for each day and each shift. For example, for a 12-hour day shift for a pediatric unit on Mondays, there may be six RNs and two UAP for direct care. An additional RN assigned to care for children being admitted or discharged may be scheduled from 3 to 6 pm, during this peak time where children are returning from the OR or going home.

BACKGROUND

Staffing strategies reflect the organization's mission, annual strategic goals, and service line strategies and are executed to meet the staffing management plan of an organization. In hospitals, chief nursing officers are accountable to establish and translate staffing management strategies for the overall patient care areas. The nurse manager who is accountable for a patient care unit or area executes staffing management strategies to yield an optimal health experience and clinical outcomes for patients and their families; a healthy, satisfying work environment; and cost-effective staffing model for the organization. Nursing leaders at all levels are challenged to fairly balance staffing management and adopt technologies that provide the real-time tools to execute, measure, and achieve desired outcomes. Direct-care nurses are involved in the responsibility for coverage of patient care needs, determining patient acuity and intensity, and making patient assignments.

Direct care nurses are increasingly called to participate in the creation of staffing strategies. This strategic work may happen through involvement in professional shared governance committees, organizational advisory panels, or even through state mandated committees. For example, as an alternative to state mandated staffing ratios, the state of Illinois in 2007 passed the Nurse Staffing by Acuity Law (Public Act 09509491). This legislation requires every hospital within the state to create a Nursing Care Committee with 50% of its membership to be composed of staff nurses. These groups are charged with reviewing staffing plans and providing feedback for the selection, implementation, and evaluation of staffing levels (Fitzpatrick et al., 2013). This suggests the importance of staff nurses understanding the science of budgeting; the quantification of clinical requirements; and the creation, execution, and evaluation of staffing plans. These types of committees or panels give staff an important seat at the table along with operational and finance executives in creating and evaluating staffing plans. This requires that nurses develop the vocabulary and the skills to be able to communicate the impact of various staffing strategies on clinical outcomes when conversing with key decision makers.

FRAMEWORK FOR STAFFING MANAGEMENT

Nurse staffing can be determined in multiple ways. The three main models of nurse staffing are (1) budget based: nurse staff are allocated according to NHPPD, which is a financial metric; (2) nurse–patient ratio: this is the number of nurses per number of patients or patient days, which is a mathematical workload balancing; and (3) patient acuity (or intensity) based. Patient characteristics are used to determine staffing needs, which is a determination of the need for care and not based on raw numbers of patients (Mensik, 2014). Staffing management is complex and challenging because of the numerous dependencies and interrelated organizational processes. A conceptual framework provides logic and order to complex processes for administrators and scientists to consider (Edwardson, 2007). A conceptual framework for staffing management is proposed and illustrated in Fig. 21.1.

This conceptual framework is adapted from Donabedian's (1966) framework for the evaluation of quality of care, relating various structures (e.g., hospital characteristics) that affect various processes (e.g., actual staffing) and subsequently influence various outcomes (e.g., patient quality, patient satisfaction, and staff satisfaction). Multiple staffing studies have adapted this framework to organize the variables of interest (Edwardson, 2007; Kane et al., 2007a,b; Mark et al., 2007). In the proposed framework, structures represent the various nursing strategies—both internal and external to the organization—that directly influence an organization's ability to effectively manage processes for staffing. The processes are a series of defined stages with outputs that directly affect subsequent stages of staffing. Finally, the outcomes of staffing management are multidimensional and measured in terms of organizational outcomes including patient, fiscal, and staff outcomes. The staffing management framework is not intended to address all possible variables, but instead is intended to provide a guide for nursing leaders to assess staffing management in their organizations.

STRATEGIES INFLUENCING STAFFING MANAGEMENT

It is important for all nursing leaders to remain current on both the internal and external influences affecting staffing management. Some major influences are (1) professional resources and recommendations, (2) patient acuity and intensity, (3) nursing care delivery models, (4) The Joint Commission (TJC) and other regulatory agencies' regulations, (5) local state legislation, and (6) nurse union agreements.

American Nurses Association's Principles for Nurse Staffing

The ANA is the professional organization that speaks for the profession of nursing and develops and maintains scope and standards of practice and ethics. ANA has published guiding documents that serve as resources to understand the complex staffing issues associated with creating a nursing unit schedule, preparing an organization-wide staffing plan, or meeting staffing legislation. *ANA's Principles for Nurse Staffing* (ANA, 2012) identified the major elements needed for achieving optimal nurse staffing. The document first defines appropriate nurse staffing and presents the core components of nurse staffing. It then groups the principles into five areas: (1) the health care consumer, (2) RNs and other staff,

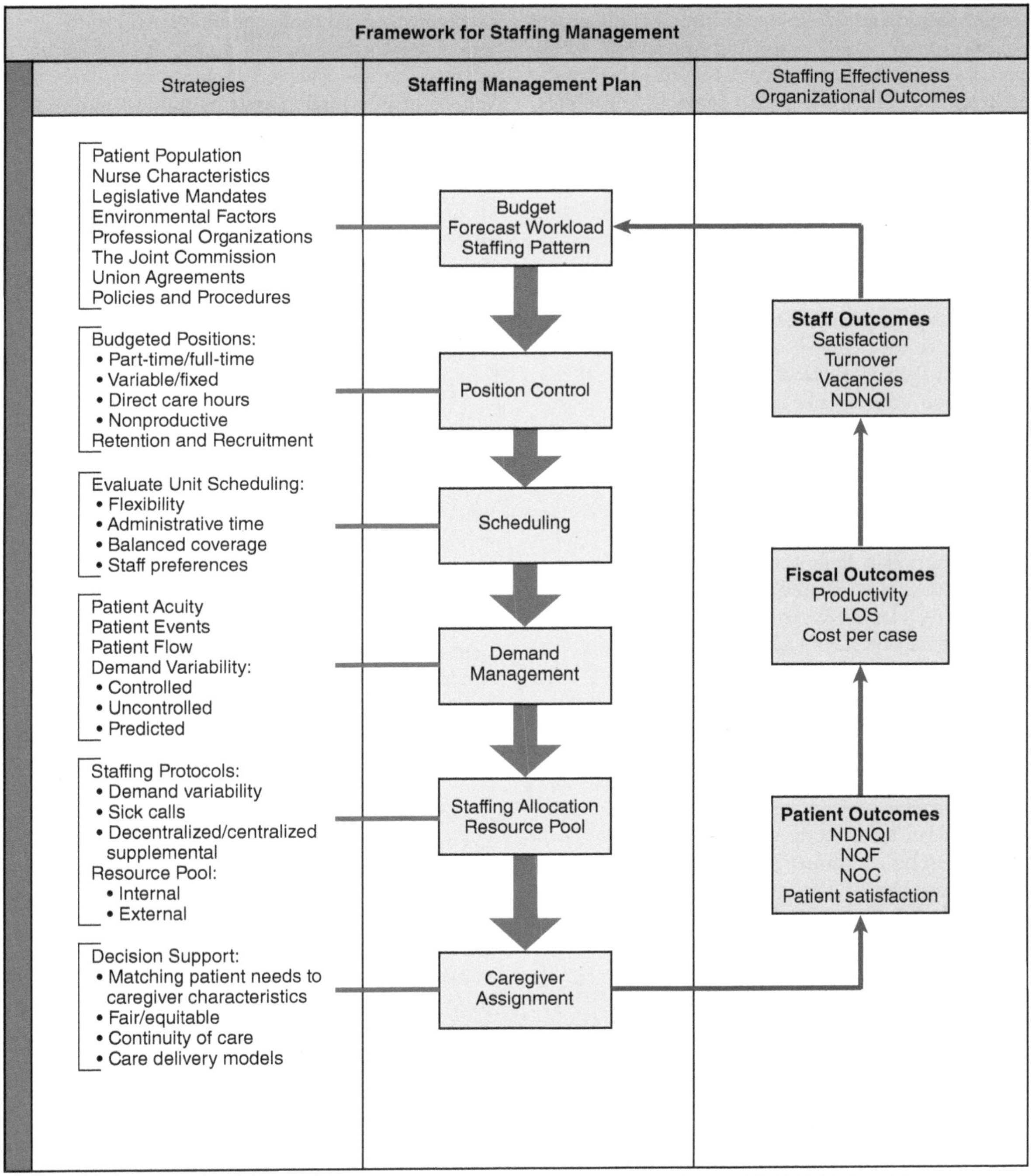

Fig. 21.1 Framework for staffing management. *LOS*, Length of stay; *NDNQI*, National Database of Nursing Quality Indicators; *NOC*, nursing outcomes classification; *NQF*, National Quality Forum.

(3) organization and workplace culture, (4) the practice environment, and (5) staffing evaluation. ANA emphasized their use of evidence to drive the development of the principles, which serve as guidelines for RN staffing solutions.

In its second edition, ANA (2012) noted that since the initial publication of the original *Principles for Nurse Staffing*, the evidence has grown supporting the link between adequate nurse staffing and better patient outcomes. Under principles related to the practice environment, ANA (2012, p. 10) stated, "Registered nurses should be provided a professional nursing practice environment in which they have control over nursing practice and autonomy in their workplace," and "routine mandatory overtime is an unacceptable solution to achieve appropriate nurse staffing. Policies on length of shifts; management of meal and rest periods; and overtime should be in place to ensure the health and stamina of nurses and prevent fatigue-related errors." This is an area where staff can provide valuable input as their insights and experience will assure that staffing plans are practical, implementable, and achieve desired clinical outcomes.

ANA's Principles for Nurse Staffing (ANA, 2012) has been augmented by ANA's advocacy for the proposed Registered Nurse Safe Staffing Act, which would require Medicare-participating hospitals to establish and publicly report unit-by-unit staffing plans. These plans would establish adjustable minimum numbers of RNs; have input from RNs; be based on patient numbers and variable intensity of care needed; consider elements such as education, training, and experience levels of RNs and staffing recommendations from professional organizations; ensure RNs are not forced to float to areas where they have no experience; have whistleblower protections; and require public reporting (ANA, n.d.).

American Organization for Nursing Leadership

The American Organization for Nursing Leadership (AONL, formerly called American Organization of Nurse executives, AONE), a subsidiary of the American Hospital Association, is a national organization whose mission is to represent nurse leaders. This key leadership group published *Staffing Management and Methods: Tools and Techniques for Nurse Leaders* (AONE, 2000), which presents an introduction to evolving staffing measures. It has a chapter dedicated to staffing management approaches in each of four hospital types: the large academic medical center, an integrated health care system, a small community hospital, and a rural hospital setting. The final chapter discusses how various innovations in information systems support nurse staffing. AONL continues to be involved in advocacy, policy, and issues around nurse staffing.

Staffing Recommendations by Professional Organizations

Adoption of staffing recommendations in clinical settings by relevant professional organizations is endorsed in the *Principles of Nurse Staffing* (ANA, 2012) and frequently seen written into staffing plans. Nursing leaders in specialty practice need to encourage identification and discussion of the position statement or guidelines promulgated by the relevant specialty professional organization during the annual staffing plan review. Several professional nursing specialty organizations have published position statements for nurse staffing to offer evidence-based guidelines for specialty practice. For example, the National Association of Neonatal Nurses (2014) has a staffing position statement. Recommended staffing ratios are also described in the *Guidelines for Perinatal Care* (American Academy of Pediatrics [AAP] and the American College of Obstetricians and Gynecologists [ACOG], 2012). The ratios delineate care provided for women and newborns in the antepartum, intrapartum, and postpartum settings, as well as the newborn nursery. The Association of Women's Health, Obstetric and Neonatal Nurses (AWHONN, 2010) described the specific staffing recommendations for women in the various stages of normal labor and labor with complications.

Similarly, the Association of Perioperative Registered Nurses (AORN, 2014) has a position paper addressing key staffing issues in the OR, and the Emergency Nurses Association (ENA, 2015) has published recommendations for staffing in emergency departments. The American Academy of Ambulatory Care Nursing (AAACN, 2005) published an annotated bibliography summarizing the ambulatory nurse staffing literature. Although they do not offer a position paper or guidelines, research continues in staffing models in ambulatory care, where staffing needs to be highly related to the problems, complexity, and needs of patient populations (Haas et al., 2016).

Patient Acuity and Nursing Intensity

Patient acuity is a concept commonly referenced but without specificity or consistency (Habesevich, 2012).

In a concept analysis, Brennan and Daly (2008) defined acuity as the severity of the physical and psychological status of the patient, while the intensity attribute of acuity indicates the nursing care needs and the corresponding workload required. Essentially, patient acuity is a measure of the severity of illness of the patient, whereas nursing intensity is the number of nursing hours with associated costs and total time and staff mix of nursing personnel resources consumed by an individual patient during the episode of care under review (Thompson & Diers, 1985; Welton & Dismuke, 2008). According to Unruh and Fottler (2004), estimation of staffing should be considered based on work intensity. The authors defined two indicators for nurse intensity: patient acuity and patient turnover. Because nursing accounts for the highest expenditures in hospitals, Welton and Dismuke (2008) called for a nursing billing model. A billing model based on the intensity of care allows appropriate reimbursement and thus allows for appropriate staffing and a way to capture the direct value of nursing. Despite changes in health care reimbursement structures, nurses still need to demonstrate value, which is determined by a fair and accurate method that shows nurses' work.

Patient classification systems aimed at adjusting staffing for acuity have been plagued with an inability to accurately and reliably measure patient care variability. Further, they have lacked organizational credibility and added documentation burden to the direct-care nurse. The Health Information Technology for Economic and Clinical Health (HITECH) Act, enacted as part of the American Recovery and Reinvestment Act of 2009, was signed into law on February 17, 2009, to promote the adoption and meaningful use of health information technology. This health care reform and meaningful use legislation has catapulted the advancement of health information technology into widespread adoption of electronic medical records (EMR) in the United States (http://www.hipaasurvivalguide.com/hitech-act-summary.php). These advances additionally offer nursing leaders technologies that leverage the automated patient assessment information entered in the patient EMR by nurses to generate accurate measurements of patient acuity (Eck Birmingham et al., 2011). The electronic patient assessment information is translated not only into workload information at the patient level but also standardized outcomes of care that may assist the nurse and care team in tracking patient progression to the Medicare Severity Diagnosis Related Groups (MS-DRGs) and length of stay (LOS) (Eck Birmingham, 2010). The objective patient acuity information generated as a by-product of routine clinical documentation allows frontline charge nurses to make informed patient care assignment decisions. From the chief nurse's perspective, new acuity technologies help build the business case for acuity-adjusted staffing for both improved quality and cost outcomes (Dent & Bradshaw, 2012).

There are three basic types of patient classification/acuity measurement (PCAS) methodologies, each predicated on a different philosophical assumption. Each type defines nursing care and the fluctuations in that care and connects to or informs the staffing and scheduling systems. Box 21.2 describes these three types of PCAS methods.

BOX 21.2 Three Types of PCAS Methods

Prototype Tools

This methodology generally describes different patient care levels in terms of subject categories of *minimum, moderate, or maximum* care requirements. When classifying a patient, the nurse subjectively compares their assessment of the patient's needs to prototypical vignettes describing patients with similar care needs. Often these systems do not accommodate the rapidly changing needs of a patient throughout the day.

Summative Task Tools

These measures are task and frequency based and are predicated on the assumption that care requirements are best expressed through a series of observable activities. Each task is assigned a time-based weight and points are added, converted to hours, and eventually computed to nurses required per shift. A task-based methodology presumes each task is discrete and often not reflective of the critical thinking upon which a task is based. A nurse may be performing multiple assessments along with a specific task making it difficult to quantify. The reality of clinical practice is frequent multi-tasking.

Care Interaction Tools

This approach to acuity measurement presumes that care is more complex than simply a series of tasks but rather is a combination of qualitative and quantitative attributes. Using professional judgment, the interaction between various subjective and objective critical predictors of care, such as the type, frequency, duration, and complexity of care requirements, are documented. This system accepts that patient care is greater than the sum of its parts (American Nurses Association, 2020).

Nursing Care Delivery Models

Nursing care delivery models significantly influence staffing management. Care delivery models are the operational mechanisms by which care is actually provided to patients and families. Specific nursing care delivery models are discussed in Chapter 15.

Person (2004) described the four fundamental elements of any nursing care delivery model as follows: (1) nurse/patient relationship and decision-making, (2) work allocation and patient assignments, (3) communication among members of the health team, and (4) management of the unit or environment of care. Translating the nursing care delivery model's elements and inherent values to staffing management is a key role for nursing leaders. One common element among care models is the value of the nurse and patient/family relationship. Patient assignment technology offers charge nurses access to real-time data in order to match the right nurse (i.e., competency, expertise) with the right patient and provide continuity of care during an episode of care. A second common trend is the evolving role of the charge nurse as a hospital's frontline leader with responsibility to coordinate patient flow with expert communication among health care team members as well as serving as a key resource and expert advisor to staff and the interdisciplinary care team.

Increasingly a charge nurse is appointed as a resource, managing patient flow and supporting novice nurses, and thus does not always assume a direct-care assignment. In this role, the charge nurse works closely with patient placement or transfer centers in managing efficient throughput as well as with central staffing or resource centers to assure adequate resources to provide safe and effective care. In large health care systems, these command centers may manage patient flow across multiple organizations. The charge nurse may also coordinate communication with the interdisciplinary team, including facilitation of discharges and post-acute care.

Three nursing care delivery models of relationship-based care (RBC) influence staffing management: the synergy model, case management, and the clinical nurse leader (CNL). RBC is a common model used in care delivery (Koloroutis, 2004) that supports achieving recognition by the Magnet Recognition Program® (Guanci & Felgen, 2016).

The Synergy Model for Patient Care was developed by the American Association of Critical-Care Nurses (2016) and is a patient-centered model focused on the needs of the patient, the competencies of the nurse, and the synergy created when the needs and competencies match. Synergy—or optimum patient outcomes—results when the needs and characteristics of the patient and clinical unit or system are matched with a nurse's competencies. Patient assignment technology may assist in defining—and thereby aligning—patient needs with the nurse's abilities, a concept that is central to the model.

Case management is defined by the Case Management Society of America (CMSA) as "a collaborative process of assessment, planning, facilitation, care coordination, evaluation, and advocacy for options and services to meet an individual's and family's comprehensive health needs through communication and available resources to promote quality, cost-effective outcomes" (CMSA, 2016). Case management can be coupled with demand management to best coordinate care and resources to achieve positive patient outcomes, transitions of care coordination, and hospital reimbursement (Pickard & Warner, 2007).

Complementing these models, the American Association of Colleges of Nursing (AACN, 2007) has introduced a new professional nurse role, the clinical nurse leader (CNL), in current care delivery models. The CNL role integrates various aspects of previous roles in nursing, such as the case manager and clinical nurse specialist. The CNL vision statement notes that the CNL champions innovations to improve patient outcomes, ensure quality care, and reduce health care costs. The CNL leads this effort to enhance patient care. The CNL is an advocate for putting best practices into action (AACN, 2007). CNLs are master's prepared and are being used at the unit level to provide knowledge, clinical expertise, and skill in evidence-based practice implementation.

Nursing leaders often utilize other resources in the creation of their staffing plans, most frequently benchmarks, whereby they can compare themselves to other organizations and units with similar characteristics and patient types to determine how like organizations are staffed. The National Database of Nursing Quality Indicators (NDNQI), which was acquired by the Press Ganey organization in 2014, is a popular resource. NDNQI was founded by the ANA in 2001 and had been managed by the University of Kansas School of Nursing. The NDNQI database is utilized by 2000 hospitals nationwide, and participation is a requirement for Magnet designation. On a monthly basis, participants submit to the database nurse-sensitive quality data as well as financial and staffing related data such as hours per patient day, skill mix, direct and indirect care hours, direct care responsibilities, and contract labor utilization. Organizations are then able to extract robust comparative data to assist in planning staffing strategy, developing budgets, and as a periodic performance monitor (NDNQI, 2011).

The staffing management plan should reflect the values and roles established in the care delivery model that will ultimately influence patient and organizational outcomes. Both the care delivery model and staffing plan within the context of patient populations in the health care organization are critical to the overall annual strategic plan for nursing.

Systemic changes in the national health care system, including evolving payer schemes as well as dynamic market forces, require that nurses continue to innovate new models of care. There are significant efforts underway in hospitals and health care systems and within professional organizations to leverage the full interdisciplinary team to create systems and processes of care that are more efficient and cost effective. There is recognition that inpatient utilization will continue to decline as ambulatory care becomes increasingly sophisticated. The health care industry now finds itself in competition with new entrants into the health care market, including large employers and technology companies with significant resources. These organizations have created an Internet-savvy consumer market expecting real-time, 24/7 convenience, and coordination of services. Nurses will need to leverage creativity to respond to and lead model of care innovative efforts.

The Joint Commission Staffing Regulation

Private regulatory agencies such as TJC are widely used by hospitals today to conduct external reviews for quality of care and patient safety. TJC standards include the human resources function of verifying that nurses are qualified and competent to ensure that the hospital determines the qualifications and competencies for staff positions based on its mission, populations, care, treatment, and services. Hospitals must also provide the right number of competent staff members to meet the patients' needs (TJC, 2016). TJC human resource standards clearly outline the complex requirements associated with staffing management and include, but are not limited to, the adequacy of staff numbers, mix of staff levels, licensure, education, certification, experience, and continuing education.

Det Norske Veritas (DNV) Staffing Regulation

Several health care organizations are now utilizing Det Norske Veritas (DNV) as their external consultancy to help provide regulatory oversight in assuring there are systems and processes in place to provide safe, quality care as well as ensuring general safety for staff and visitors. Not unlike other regulatory organizations, DNV, which has been awarded deemed status by CMS, has developed written standards and interpretative guidelines and conducts periodic onsite inspections. Their standard related to Nursing Services requires a plan to assure adequate staffing with qualified personnel and further requires a periodic assessment of skill mix and nurse to patient ratios that deliver safe and effective care that meets service users' physical, emotional, and social needs (DNV, 2019).

Collective Bargaining Agreements and Staffing Management

Provisions in the ANA Code of Ethics articulate the rights of nurses to address work conditions through collective action (ANA, 2015a). The two largest nursing and health care unions are (1) National Nurses United, a branch of the ANA; and (2) the Service Employees International Union (SEIU) District 1199. Nursing unions are organizations that represent nurses for the purpose of collective bargaining, which has been defined as "the performance of the mutual obligations of the employer and the representative of the employees to meet at reasonable times and confer in good faith with respect to wages, hours, and other terms and conditions of employment … such obligation does not compel either party to agree to a proposal or require the making of a concession" (National Labor Relations Board, 2016, Section 8b, paragraph 7d).

In nursing, there is a process of negotiation between the health care employer and the union representatives of nurse employees to reach a written agreement regarding certain terms of employment. The mandatory terms of employment vary widely, but they include subjects such as, but not limited to, wages, hours, overtime, low census call-off procedures, recall, floating, use of UAP, seniority, sick leave, discharges, and leaves of absence.

The National Labor Relations Board has legislated these as mandatory subjects of bargaining, stating that issues related to wages, hours, and other conditions of employment, when introduced into negotiations, must be bargained (Fried & Fottler, 2008; NLRB, 2020) These employment subjects have significant implications for staffing management and vary in their specificity regarding nurse staffing and scheduling.

Nursing leaders working in settings with collective bargaining units need to have detailed knowledge of the relevant contractual implications for staffing management and incorporate them into the staffing technologies for compliance monitoring. Collective bargaining environments are compatible with professional nursing practice. Porter (2010) described a successful model of professional practice labor partnerships. Lawson et al. (2011) described a program to recognize nurse professional growth and development and its implementation in a collective bargaining environment.

LEADERSHIP AND MANAGEMENT IMPLICATIONS

Legislative Impact on Staffing Management

Evidence has accumulated over the years to indicate that low nurse staffing levels have an adverse effect on patient outcomes and that there is an association between higher levels of experienced RN staffing and lower rates of adverse patient outcomes (ANA, 2016b). This is seen, for example, in the work of Kane et al. (2007a,b) and multiple studies by Aiken et al. (e.g., Aiken et al., 2002, 2003, 2007, 2014, 2016). At issue are safety, attainment of outcomes, and patient and nurse satisfaction.

Nurse dissatisfaction and concern for adequate staffing to provide quality nursing care to patients and their families arose from hospital cost-reduction initiatives throughout the 1990s. Armed with quality-of-care concerns, nurses began to organize and craft proposed staffing legislation in many states. The historical context that led to quality-of-care concerns continues to affect legislation today. Throughout the 1990s, hospital administrators relied on consultants to implement work redesign to promote patient-focused care as a method of cost reduction. The central labor reduction approach in patient-focused care was reducing the number of RNs and increasing the number of UAP. This approach for decreasing nursing RN skill mix was implemented in a "one size fits all" approach across organizations and often lacked evaluation of the skill mix change and other changes on the quality of care and nurse job satisfaction and retention (Norrish & Rundall, 2001). This was most apparent in California, where a leaner RN skill mix was tried by Kaiser Permanente Northern California in the early 1990s. Skill mix was reduced from 55% RNs to 30% RNs in 1995 (Robertson & Samuelson, 1996). The changes in skill mix led to widespread real and perceived increases in RN workload, patient safety concerns, and nurse and consumer complaints (Norrish & Rundall, 2001; Seago et al., 2003). This is partially because the workload element of supervision responsibility of the RN for UAP was not accounted.

Despite patient complaints and reports of nurse dissatisfaction, little was done until 1999. Only then did the California legislature pass Assembly Bill 394 (AB 394) to mandate minimum nurse staffing ratios and acuity-adjusted staffing. The mandating of minimum nurse-to-patient ratios legislated in California ignited great debate, controversy, and study. Nurse scientists and policy experts have presented compelling arguments against mandated ratios and note that local nursing leaders are in the best position to determine the actual staffing required by the patient population (Clarke, 2005). However, the bold action of the California state legislative mandate stimulated focused attention on addressing nurse staffing issues.

Since the late 1990s, state legislation regarding nurse staffing issues has been commonplace, and 14 states have various regulations (ANA, 2016b). There are three general models of state staffing laws: (1) require a nurse-driven staffing committee to create staffing plans, (2) mandate specific nurse-to-patient ratios (California is the only one, but Massachusetts passed a law specific to intensive care units), or (3) require disclosure of staffing levels to the public and/or a regulatory body (ANA, 2016b). ANA supports the first model (nurse-driven staffing plans). Primary areas of focus for state legislation include limiting or precluding mandatory overtime, requiring staffing committees with direct-care nurse input, whistleblower protection, mandated public access to staffing information, and a requirement that implementation of patient acuity methodologies must adjust for staffing workload. State nurse staffing legislation has a significant impact on staffing management through regulation. The economic downturn in 2008 following the end of the George W. Bush administration shifted political attention to jobs and the economy and stalled further legislative nurse staffing mandates. However, the reductions in nursing budgets and challenges of the nurse shortage have resulted in fewer nurses and longer hours of work under the burden of care for sicker patients. The result is compromised care and exacerbation of the nurse shortage due to the environment of care. ANA (2015b) urged passage of the Registered Nurse Safe Staffing Act (H.R. 2083/S. 1132), national legislation to require all Medicare-participating hospitals to establish RN staffing plans using a committee.

THE STAFFING MANAGEMENT PLAN

The staffing management plan provides the structured processes to identify patient needs and then to deliver the staff resources as efficiently and effectively as possible. An effective plan first focuses on stabilizing the unit core staffing. In many organizations the staffing management plan also includes the creation of a float pool or flexible team of nurses available for deployment to cover various leaves, unscheduled absences, vacations, or an unanticipated surge in demand. This ability to augment core staffing requires a robust orientation and training infrastructure to assure that these nurses possess the competencies required to work on multiple units.

A staffing pattern, or core coverage, is determined through a forecasted workload and a recommended care standard (e.g., HPPD). Hiring to the associated position complement and developing balanced and filled schedules without holes are essential building blocks for efficient and cost-effective daily resource allocation. This also allows nurses to have predictable schedules to support work life balance. Balanced and complete schedules also enable leaders to more effectively manage the unit's finances.

Daily staffing allocation requires managing a variable staffing plan, measuring and predicting demand, and then providing balanced workload assignments to ensure that the correct caregivers are best matched to patient needs (ANA, 2012). A successful staffing management plan incorporates the policies of the organization, patient care unit, and nurse population including union and contracting affiliations. Kane and colleagues (2007a,b) suggested that nurse staffing policies should address both patient care units and organizations, such as shift rotation, overtime, full-time/part-time mix, and weekend staffing. The traditional emphasis in staffing planning has been on hospital settings. However, with shifts to primary care as the predominant site of care delivery, staffing planning is equally critical there and in all settings where nurses practice.

Forecasted Workload and Staffing Pattern (Core Coverage)

Forecasting nursing workload for each patient care area is typically carried out at least once a year and as part of the annual budgeting process or when the patient characteristics, services, and/or volume changes. The amount of work performed by a unit is referred to as its workload, and *workload* volume is measured in terms of units of service. The unit of service is specific to the type of unit, such as the number of patients, patient days, deliveries, clinic or home visits, treatments, encounters, or procedures.

Not long ago, demand forecasting, or deciding on the units of service to anticipate during the next budget cycle, was primarily focused on the current year's performance coupled with an educated guess of what the following year might hold. More sophisticated organizations examined local market trends, refreshed strategic plans, and met with key providers for their opinions.

In the contemporary health care organization, however, teams of data scientists can harness significant computational and mathematical power to analyze large data sets to more accurately predict future demand, resources requirements, and create sophisticated scenario models of financial performance. The term *big data* does not just refer to large data sets. Big data is characterized by three V's: velocity, meaning acquisition of the data is rapid; variety, meaning that there are many data types used, and volume, meaning there is a vast amount of information. Some authors suggest a fourth V that is veracity, or that data are correct and error free, as well as a fifth V of value (Rambur & Fitzpatrick, 2017, Roski, Bo-Linn & Andrews, 2014 & Rubenfire, 2017).

Fig. 21.2 describes the evolution of big data analysis. Although these types of analyses continue to evolve, they are becoming increasingly more refined. Nurse executives, in partnership with interdisciplinary teams of data scientists, mathematicians, and operations research scientists, are optimizing operational performance and developing innovative staffing models, often through the use of management simulation models that can be shared with staff for their valuable input.

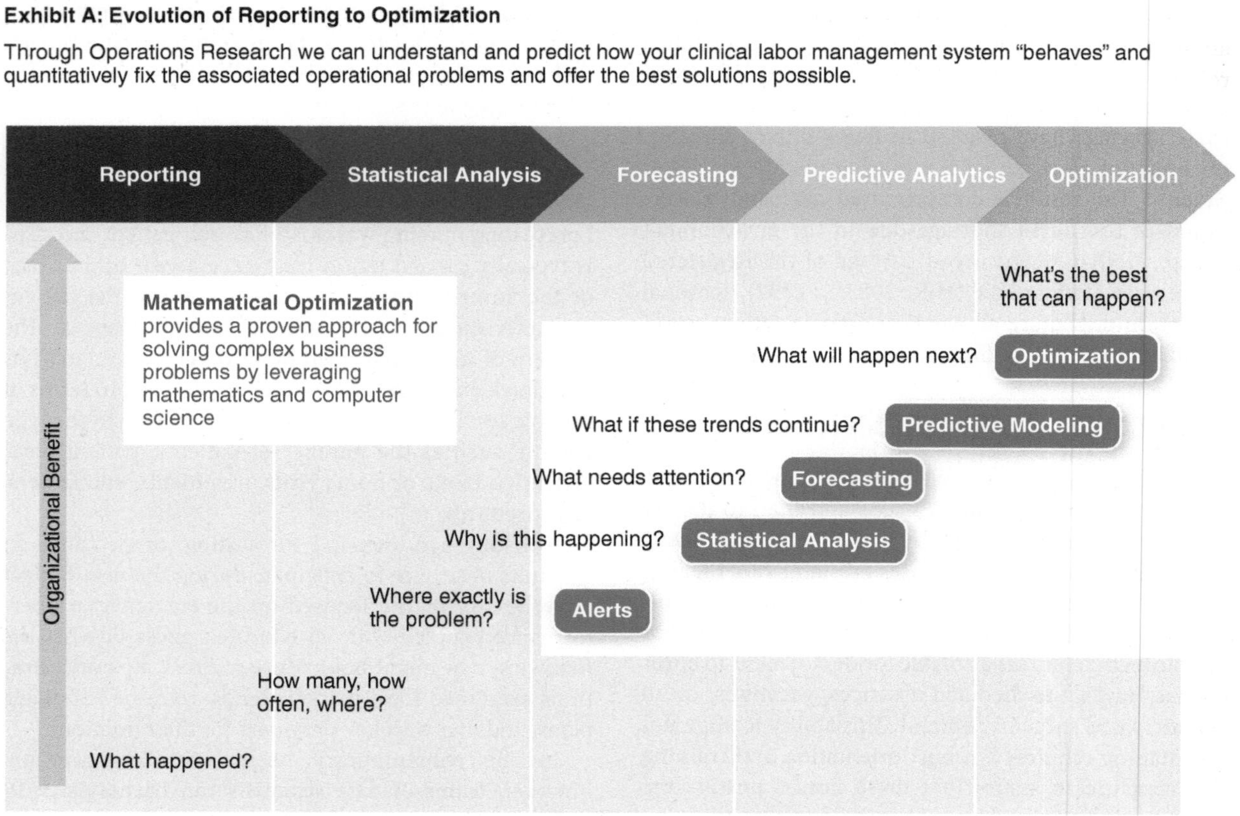

Fig. 21.2 Exhibit A: Evolution of reporting to optimization.

Staffing planners often presume patient demand patterns are somewhat random and, as a result, often plan staffing for "what if" scenarios. By analyzing big data sets that contain multiple years of patient census data at the hourly level, seasonal, daily, and even hourly patterns emerge. This allows staffing plans to go from "what if" to "what's best." These advanced computational methods simultaneously consider multiple and often disparate variables such as staffing to demand while accommodating work rules such as weekend requirements or shift lengths.

Once the unit of service is determined, the number of units of service that will be provided in the coming year must be forecasted. Total patient days are commonly used in inpatient hospital areas. This is calculated by multiplying the ALOS and the ADC. The workload standard commonly used is NHPPD, although the validity of this measure is disputed. In outpatient settings, balanced workload, patient waiting times, and staff overtime are measures used. There are intensity/acuity tools in ambulatory settings to establish appropriate staffing levels (Liang & Turkcan, 2016).

However, not all patients require the same number of care hours, and the total number of patient days may be inadequate for planning purposes. Finkler and colleagues (2013) suggested using adjusted units of service. For example, a nursing unit can be adjusted using a system for classifying patients, such as a patient acuity system, based on the resources each classification category is expected to use. Segregating patients into acuity classifications allows the staffing pattern to be developed based on the resource requirements of the specific mix of patients forecasted for the unit. Similar calculations can be made in ambulatory and primary care by using a method to classify patients into different categories to estimate the average resource required for patients in each category (Finkler et al., 2013).

Nursing's work is complex and measuring nursing care requires sophisticated methods. Malloch (2015) presented a nursing workforce staffing model that aimed for accurate and reliable determination of the required time for care needs aligned with the appropriate nurse competencies and available time. Clear identification of care needs leads to required staff for nurse interventions, which leads to a matching process and then to value-based outcomes. High variability and intensity (or acuity) are complex patient scheduling and nurse assignment factors in clinic settings (Liang & Turkcan, 2016).

In addition to workload adjustment based on acuity, patient turnover on the unit is an important factor in patient care workload measurement. Reduced LOS in hospitals or higher patient turnover require intensive periods of higher resources for patient admissions, transfer, discharge, and other 1:1 activities that will affect overall workload, such as when the RN accompanies an unstable patient off the unit for a test or procedure.

Outside of state-mandated nurse staffing ratios, there is no one gold care standard or recommended process to determine nursing workload. Inconsistent operational definitions and methods of measuring care have been a challenge both for benchmarking resources across organizations and for research analysis related to adequate nursing care (Kane et al., 2007a,b). Therefore, each organization must document and provide rationale regarding how staffing standards are determined within each patient care area. Once the annual workload is forecasted, the skill mix required on each shift is determined.

There are two general staffing methods: (1) with *fixed staffing*, staffing is built around a fixed projected maximum workload requirement, and the staffing pattern is based on maximum workload conditions; (2) with *variable staffing*, units are staffed below maximum workload conditions and staff is then supplemented when needed. An effective staffing pattern requires clear definitions for productive time, non-patient care or "nonproductive" time (i.e., benefits time, work for the organization, knowledge-related projects), worked time, paid full-time equivalents (FTEs), and hours per unit of service. In addition, staff roles must be clearly defined as to whether they are fixed or variable. The necessary number of FTEs to yield the desired care standard for the forecasted number of patients in each department must be calculated. In addition, the number of FTEs to replace staff members when they use non-patient care, such as benefit time, must be accounted for in the model. Finkler and colleagues (2013) described the method for calculating a staffing pattern as follows:

1. Determine the number of paid hours per FTE.
2. Determine the percentage of productive hours to total paid hours.
3. Multiply the number of paid hours per FTE by the percentage of productive hours to find the number of productive hours per FTE.
4. Divide the required care hours by productive hours per FTE to find the required number of FTEs.
5. Divide the required care hours by the number of days per year that the unit has patients to find care hours/day.
6. Divide that result by hours per shift to find the number of person shifts needed per working day.
7. Assign staff by employee type and among required shifts per day.

Box 21.3 refers to an example of variable staff calculation. Table 21.1 provides a sample staffing pattern that includes the final step of allocating total FTEs across shifts and by skill mix. In many patient care areas, the staffing pattern may be different by day of week. For example, a post-surgical unit may have a lower patient census on weekends because of the lack of a surgical schedule, thus a different staffing pattern may apply (McKinley & Cavouras, 2000).

BOX 21.3 Variable Staff Calculation

- 2080 paid hours per full-time equivalent (FTE)
- 80% productive hours to total paid hours
- 2080 × 0.8 = 1664 productive hours per FTE
- 71,830 care hours ÷ 1664 = 43.17 FTEs
- 71,830 care hours ÷ 365 days per year = 197 hours of care per day
- 197 hours of care per day ÷ 8-hour shifts = 24.6 person shifts

Mathematical Staffing Optimization: The Next Evolution of Staffing Science

As organizational capabilities around big data analysis evolve, approaches to predicting workload and planning staffing have become increasingly sophisticated and precise. Utilizing averages such as a department's average daily census, typically marked at midnight, in budget

TABLE 21.1 Sample Staffing Pattern for a Wednesday for a Medical Surgical Unit (39 Beds)

Staff Type	7 am–7 pm Shift	7 pm–7 am Shift	Skill Mix	Total
Fixed 8-hour day staff				
Nurse manager	1			1
Nurse educator—shared	0.5			0.5
Lactation specialist	1			1
Variable staff				
Charge nurse	1*			1
RN	8	7	75% RN	15.0
LPN/LVN	0	1	5% LPN	1
UAP	2	2	20% UAP	4
HUC	1	1		2

* Charge nurse on day shift without a direct-care assignment.
HUC, Health unit coordinator; *LPN/LVN*, licensed practical nurse/licensed vocational nurse; *RN*, registered nurse; *UAP*, unlicensed assistive personnel.

and staffing calculations is imprecise and often leads to either significant over- or understaffing.

> "Approaches that use advanced and predictive analytics to anticipate customer demand and proactively improve productivity are now common in grocery stores, automotive plants, and even professional sports to solve common yet seemingly unsolvable problems. While nascent in healthcare, productivity approaches that leverage data to predict volume and other clinical challenges have the potential to make redesigning patient care and safety, managing hospital throughput, and improving clinician and patient satisfaction more science and less art. This data-driven approach also helps align and embed workforce optimization and planning with overall hospital strategic and operational planning" (Fitzpatrick et al., 2018, p. 3).

The midnight census has long been the cornerstone for determining how many nurses are needed for each shift, applying the number of patients on the unit at midnight for the entire 24-hour period. This measure is then lined up to the nursing unit's target for HPPD to determine the minimum number of nurses needed on the unit at any given time. The dynamic ADT activity experienced throughout the course of a day cannot be accurately represented by a midnight census.

When the logic of this exercise is examined, flaws emerge. How does the unit adjust to variations in patient demand throughout the day, and how do we know the census at midnight is not the lowest point of the day when applying it as an average? Given these caveats, potential understaffing or overstaffing is likely. Fig. 21.3 illustrates this "flaw of averages" on a surgical unit that has budgeted staffing based on an ACD of 25. As these data demonstrate, adjustments to staffing are required to accommodate actual demand, meaning that staff are sent home on Tuesday and costly premium labor such as overtime may be required on Thursdays (Fitzpatrick et al., 2018).

Big data analysis allows a view of demand data or patient census at the hourly level over the course of several years by extracting data directly from the electronic medical record (EMR). Understanding the census on a surgical unit at 2 pm on Tuesdays or 8 pm on Wednesdays over the course of several years provides valuable insight not only for staffing but will also inform multiple other operational processes such as surgical throughput, surgeon block scheduling, the delivery of supplies to the unit, and OR utilization, to name a few. This valuable census data, when combined with acuity data, will produce schedules that are significantly more accurate and predictable, requiring less

Exhibit B: Average Daily Census

Example
Tuesday and Thursday have the same **average demand** of 25, but Tuesday fluctuates between **18 and 32**, whereas Thursday fluctuates only between **22 and 28**. What is the "right" level of staffing?

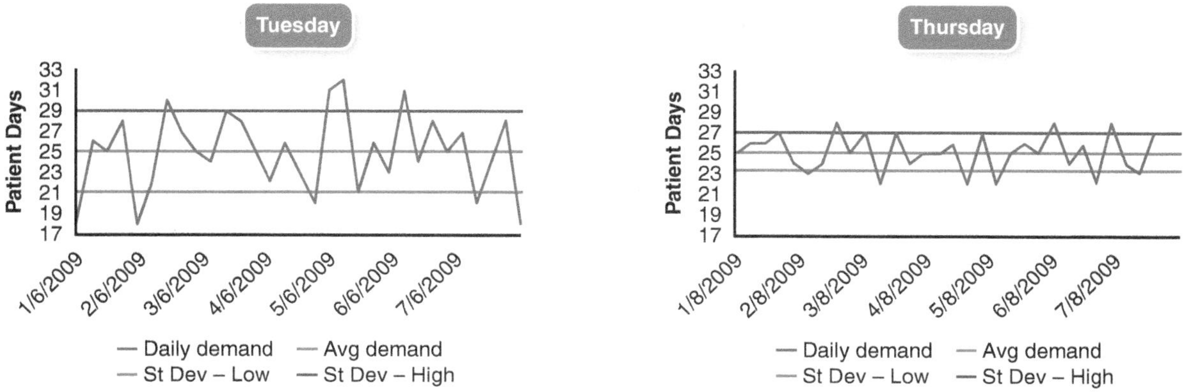

Fig. 21.3 Exhibit B: Average daily census.

last-minute adjustment. Seasonal, monthly, weekly, and daily demand patterns emerge that can provide the basis for aligning schedules and staffing patterns with demand. For example, in areas of the country impacted by seasonal weather patterns that may increase inpatient utilization, staffing can be adjusted upward to assure appropriate nurse availability.

How Does Optimization Work?

Optimization modeling based on linear programming is a computational methodology that not only solves this difficult problem with a single solution but also provides the *best* solution from a myriad of possibilities—often millions of possible solutions. The process of modeling is best described as mathematically representing every nuance or constraint and variable in the scheduling process, including demand, staffing models, and the quantification of every work rule.

To mathematically represent the staffing business problem, the optimization model illustrated in Fig. 21.4 includes the following:

- The business objectives, including the staffing model or desired ratio minimizing overall cost (best coverage at the lowest cost);

Exhibit C: What is optimization?

Optimization takes decision making from **what-if** to **what-is-best** solutions by applying sophisticated modeling to produce a staffing strategy **optimized** to **best coverage at the lowest cost**, while accommodating unique organizational and staff needs

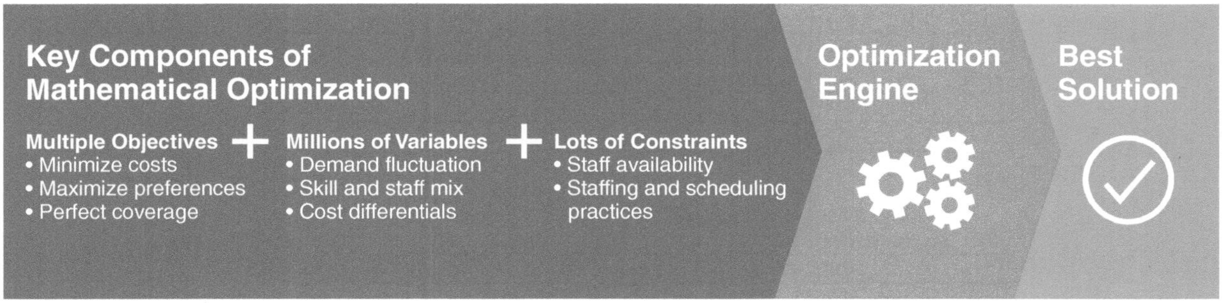

Fig. 21.4 Exhibit C: What is optimization?

- The decision variables such as skill mix, demand fluctuations, and the various costs of the staff (full time, part time, flexible staff);
- The business constraints such as staff availability, time off requirements, and various work rules or scheduling practices.

When conceptualizing this model, it is helpful to envision a giant Rubik's Cube, whereby every small square on the cube represents a distinct demand value or an individual work rule, practice, or process. The model is then dropped into a solver that essentially arranges the cube to produce the *best* answer for the business objective. For example, if a nurse could work no more than three consecutive 12-hour shifts, needed to be scheduled every other weekend, and needed to be paid overtime for hours over 40 each week, what is the optimal size and configuration of the position roster for this unit? Imagine the complexity of calculating this when considering the hourly demand patterns (Fitzpatrick, 2014; Fitzpatrick & Brooks, 2010; Gavigan et al., 2016).

When optimizing staffing, however, demand is only one of the myriad of complex variables that need to be considered. Work rules, policies, or terms within a labor contract also play a significant role in determining accurate staffing. Fig. 21.5 illustrates the significant impact of just the one work rule of weekend requirements. In this simple example, two nurses need to be scheduled for each day of the week. In the "every third weekend" example, in order to provide two nurses per day, two full-time (0.9) nurses are required in addition to four part-time (0.6) nurses. This model requires a total of six employees. By contrast, when the staff works every second weekend, four full-time (0.9) and only one part-time (0.6) nurses are required. During a period of nursing shortages, or if there are other prevailing market conditions, it is extremely important that the implications of various work rules are quantified as they relate to staffing plans as well as the overall staffing strategy (Brian J. Cole, personal communication, July 17, 2019).

Exhibit D: Weekend Pattern Work Rule Overview

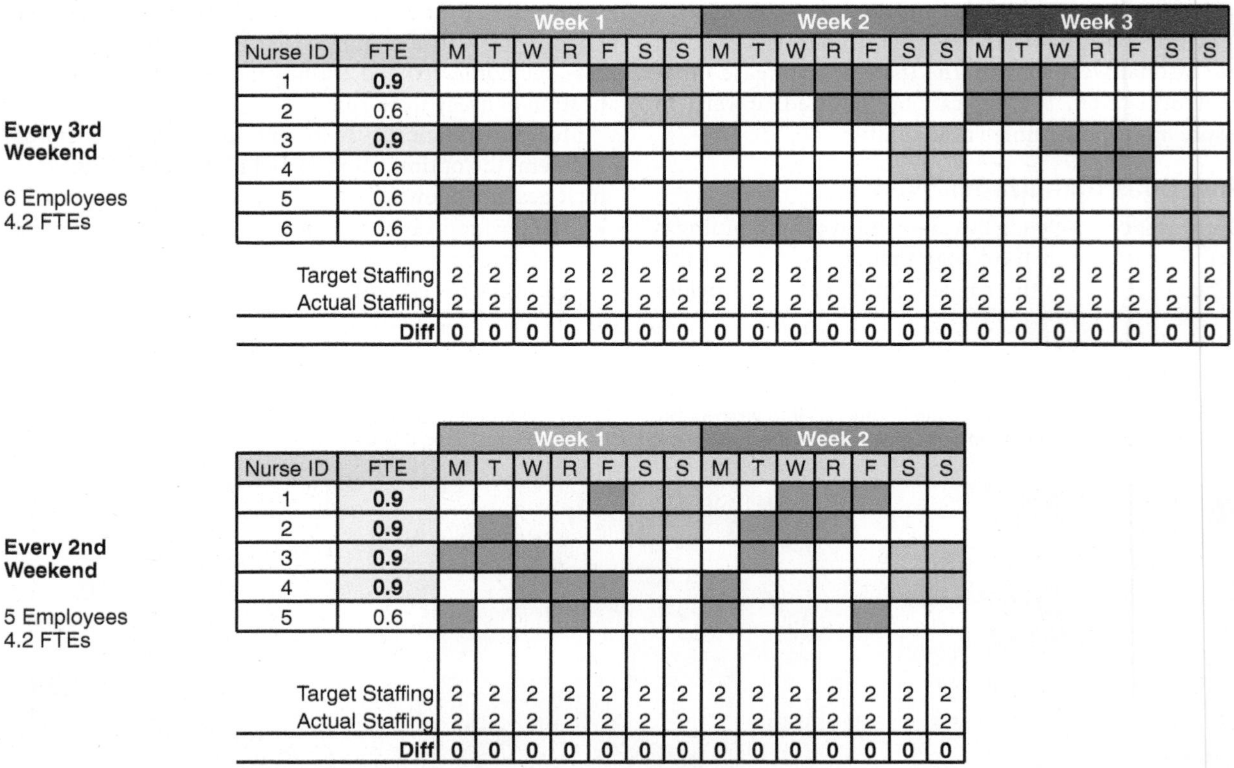

Fig. 21.5 Exhibit D: Weekend pattern work rule overview.

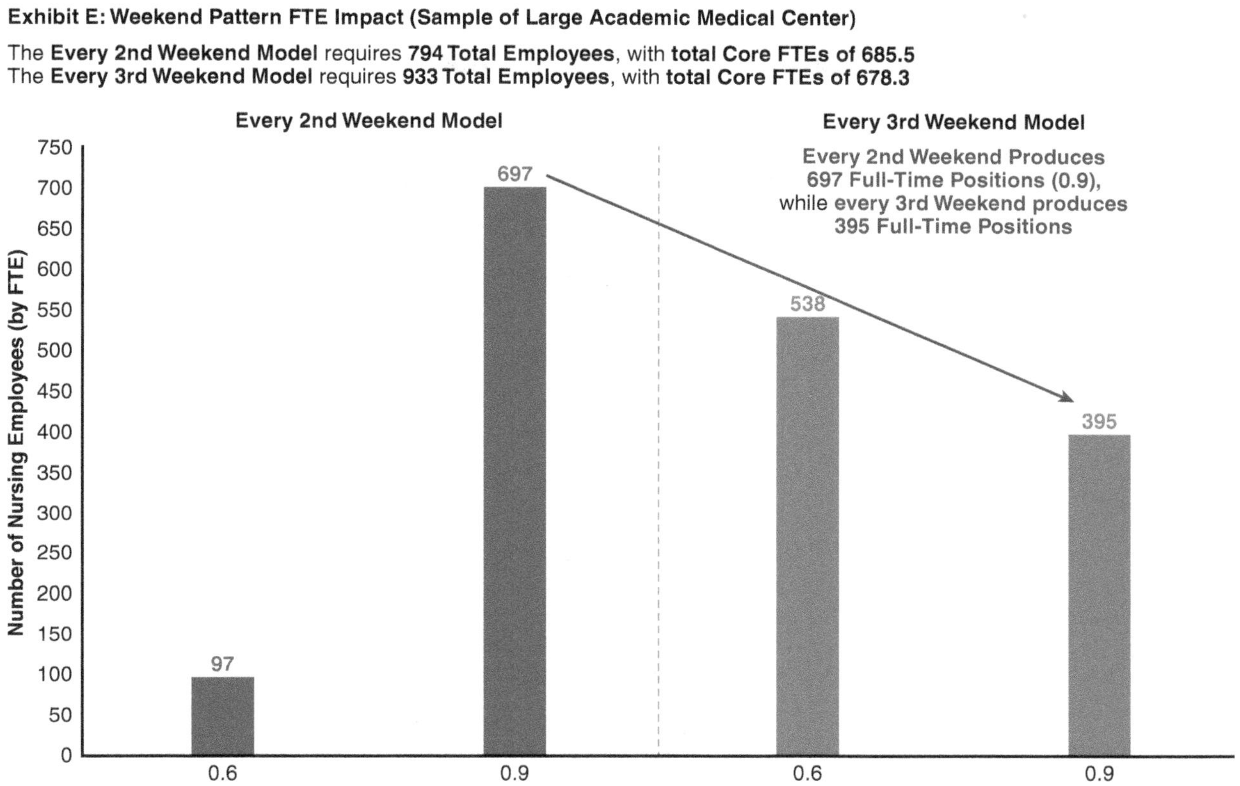

Fig. 21.6 Exhibit E: Weekend pattern FTE impact (sample of large academic medical center). *FTE*, full time equivalent.

Fig. 21.6 is another poignant example of the impact of various work rules on the overall staffing strategy. As illustrated, the weekend requirement changes the need for full-time (0.9) nurses by almost half. If this hospital were in a market where there were significantly more nurses preferring full-time employment, there would be negative consequences for their recruitment strategy (Brian J. Cole, personal communication, February 25, 2019).

More precise modeling of staffing to actual demand helps health care organizations meet staffing and scheduling challenges. Organizations using this scientific approach have seen significant improvement in their ability to have the appropriate nursing resources available when required, reduced staffing costs and demonstrating an improvement in staff satisfaction with the scheduling process. Using these big data analyses provides the evidence required to continue to innovate around staffing strategies, recognizing the complexity of this leadership responsibility.

Position Control

Irrespective of the methodology utilized to create a staffing strategy, once the staffing pattern for each unit has been established, the next step for safe staffing coverage is to provide a structured measurement and evaluation of position control. Future schedule coverage and adequate staffing first require that unit staff are available to work the needed shifts. Therefore, the hours of care requirement on a unit must be converted to the correct number of FTE positions. Position control, which can be thought of as the means to operationalize a budget, is the process of providing and measuring the correct FTE, or complement, to adequately staff a given area. Full-time and part-time mix, shift lengths, weekend commitments, and available contingency, or flex staff, are components to be analyzed to produce the ideal complement. The correct complement of full-time and part-time employees requires an understanding of the institution's non-patient care time and other budgeted activities (e.g., new staff orientation, continuing education) that are not included in the direct patient care hours required for the staffing pattern. An ideal measure of nursing staff adequacy considers intensity. A staffing adequacy measure needs to indicate the volume of nurses of a certain skill level needed for a given volume of patients and the given intensity of nursing care required for those patients.

Once position control is established to support the staffing patterns, vacancy and turnover rates need to be managed. A strategy for developing a recruitment pipeline and covering future vacant positions needs to be identified to prevent the use of costly, last-minute staff resources. For example, one organization reported actual cost savings by over-recruiting by 1.0 FTE in the ICU area, which resulted in lower use of more expensive contingency and external staff resources (Cipriano & Cutruzzula, 2007). With fiscal and human resources support, managers need to recruit and retain the FTE complement of the full-time and part-time mix needed for each staffing level. This will then increase the available resource pool to respond to higher-than-budgeted patient volume. Filled positions are the foundation for adequate, balanced work schedules.

Scheduling

Best practice for scheduling is a system that is automated, provides data-driven targets for core coverage, and engages staff members to participate in working specific shifts, hours, and days in their clinical area. The schedule typically spans a period of 4 to 6 weeks into the future. Staff members are usually hired by the organization with a commitment to work a number and type of hours (e.g., 36 hours, rotating day and night shifts). Balanced, flexible, and predictable work schedules are powerful human resource strategies for recruitment and retention, because, for nurses, choice over work schedules is one of the most important aspects of a healthy work environment (MacPhee & Borra, 2012). There is some controversy over the advantages of flexible self-scheduling versus fixed scheduling. Koning (2014) advocated for the freedom to organize shifts worked around nonwork commitments using self-scheduling; Kullberg and colleagues (2016) advocated for fixed scheduling because it lowered overtime. Whether utilizing a fixed or variable approach, creating predictability around schedules is of great benefit to the nurse in planning personal time as well as for the manager to assure adequate qualified resources for the unit.

An assessment of scheduling procedures should include the manager's role and time spent in scheduling. A recent strategy to better align the nurse manager's role to the accountabilities of the role included providing support through technology, staffing office assistants, and having staff members on scheduling committees. The manager's role is accountable for the oversight of the scheduling process, approval of the final complete schedule, and to assure that the schedule aligns with the budget. The final schedule then needs to be accessible electronically to all staff members, whether at work or remotely from home or on their cell phone. Maintaining a consistent annual schedule of the precise dates for each scheduling request period and for when the final schedule is available is a best practice for staff satisfaction and work–life balance. The managerial role shifts from time-consuming scheduling tasks to a role approving a complete schedule that meets the guidelines of the organization and *ANA's Principles for Nurse Staffing* (ANA, 2012).

The definition or perception of a "complete" schedule is likely as variable as nursing staff member satisfaction with staffing. Direct-care nurses, however, expect when a schedule is electronically submitted to their home computer or cell phone that is it complete. Specifically, the staff expects that RNs, LPNs/LVNs, UAP, unit secretaries, and key staff are scheduled to their target number for every shift of the schedule. Sharing the patient census and acuity trends by month, day of week, and time of day with the staff will foster mutual understanding in how targets are established. Dialogue about nurse staffing for patient care is credible when it is data driven. Direct-care nurses expect that there will be a clinical expert on every shift and that new graduates are distributed across shifts with their preceptors. These are a few examples of how nursing leaders at all levels may engage staff to develop value statements and data-driven guidelines that serve to explicitly and transparently articulate the organization's scheduling process. Many scheduling committees have developed such documents to reflect values such as a shared commitment to safe and excellent nursing care for all patients and families, support for staff members' pursuit of education leading to a bachelor of science in nursing, fairness in scheduling the major holidays (e.g., Thanksgiving, Christmas, and New Year), fiscal stewardship to not pre-schedule overtime, guidelines for numbers of staff vacations at one time by role, clarity in self-service dates for scheduling and communication, fatigue management guidelines, and a fair on-call schedule.

Demand Management

Demand management as a discipline focuses on (1) measuring, predicting, and understanding demand for an institution's products and services; (2) deploying resources and management to ensure that demand is met in the way the consumer's wants and needs are satisfied; and (3) directing demand as feasible to optimize patient placement, workload, and throughput, along with operational needs. For hospitals, a key component of the "product and service" equation is high-quality, safe patient care, with the goal of having the patient leave the hospital with the best care experience, in the shortest amount of time and at the lowest cost care (Pickard & Warner, 2007). McDonough (2013) described an evidence-based optimum staffing method based on patient demand with a focus on work activities. Time observations determined nursing work activities and were then matched to patient demand by hour of day and day of the week.

An often-overlooked strategy for creating predictable and cost-effective staffing is the need to staff according to real-time patient information or to make staffing decisions that facilitate individual patients moving through their stay as quickly as possible with high-quality, safe care (throughput or patient flow initiatives). Because most staffing plans staff to average forecasted care levels, periods of higher patient volume and/or acuity levels or peaks may create serious stressors for both patients and nurses. Severe stress occurs with sustained peaks of volume or acuity. Litvak and colleagues (2005) described the following three types of stress intrinsic to daily operations:

- Flow stress, representing the rapid rate of patients presenting for hospital care
- Clinical stress, which is expressed in the variability in type and severity of disease
- Stress caused by competing responsibilities of health care providers.

System stress introduced by demand for nurses to care for more or sicker patients has been shown to be a leading cause of adverse patient outcomes (Litvak et al., 2005). When variability is minimized and/or better predicted, a hospital has greater resources for the remaining patient-driven peaks in demand over which it has no control. Effective staffing requires an assessment of demand variability or the required hourly nursing care for each day on each unit. Ways to control variability (and hence decrease peaks and valleys) include better planning for scheduled events such as elective OR procedures, physician vacations or major conferences, seasonal variations, integration to patient flow and bed management systems, better control over bed assignments based on current unit workload, and improved planning for discharges—all of which decrease the demand and stress for nursing resources.

Computer technologies and big data analysis that continuously track and predict demand assist managers with variability analysis and prospective planning for predicted variability. These data support managerial decisions for non-traditional shorter shifts for the care areas that have high requirements at select predictable portions of the day. Predictive modeling can forecast unplanned patient and staff events, such as admissions by day of week and unplanned sick calls. These data are also helpful in understanding patient movement through the system, including inter-institutional transfers in large health systems.

Several examples driven by data include higher cesarean section rates in a labor and delivery unit may necessitate two RNs in the OR; infant births that are higher in the evening than during the day may require a shift of resources from days to evenings; or late-afternoon patient transfers from the recovery room after neurosurgery on Tuesdays and Thursdays may require an increase in RN staff for those days and specific hours in a neurosurgical ICU.

Pickard and Warner (2007) outlined the essential components for effective demand management as the following 10 principles:

1. Being based on patient outcomes (how well they are progressing)
2. Being focused on the individual patient
3. Incorporating progress goals for each patient throughout their stay with which actual progress may be compared
4. Continuously measuring progress in real time so that decisions can be made as the patient's needs change (rather than once a shift or once a day, which inherently bases decisions on information that is typically 8 to 16 hours old)
5. Being projected into the near future (several days ahead) to allow time for optimal staffing decisions to be made while there is still time for numerous

choices among available caregivers and cost-effective options
6. Being able to be embedded in a decision support system
7. Being acceptable to all stakeholders, especially administration and finance, to avoid organizational polarity
8. Producing a need for care in terms of not only quantity and skill but also the caregiver attributes necessary to provide optimal care for the patient
9. Using outcomes-driven acuity system based on an established taxonomy for assessing and documenting patient care on outcomes
10. Incorporating all presently and planned electronically available data to reduce nursing time in data gathering and provide as much real-time, valid data as possible

"Incorporating these elements is not a simple task but doing so offers significant advantages and benefits. By focusing on the individual patient, with individual outcome progress goals for each patient, hospitals can achieve results not previously addressed with traditional models" (Pickard & Warner, 2007, p. 31). In addition, this allows organizations to be informed and responsive when a select population of patients typically cared for in one location is housed in a new location. These results include (1) best-practice staffing protocols based on what is called "true (outcomes-oriented) demand" and the optimal staffing levels to move a patient through each phase of their stay as quickly as possible, (2) early identification of patients who are not moving through their hospital stay as planned, and (3) improved near-term projection and prediction of staffing needs. These data are a vital part of service line management, which may include various venues of care, both inpatient as well as ambulatory.

Staffing Allocation and Resource Pool

Even with the best planning and most accurate prediction of supply and demand, uncontrolled events such as unexpected high demand and sick calls are intrinsic to the health care environment and overall personnel management. Key to effective staffing are protocols and processes for daily staffing decision support that are aligned with a budget-sensitive variable staffing plan. In a decentralized model, individual department managers and directors are responsible for daily staffing allocation. Units with decentralized staffing are typically units in which volume and/or acuity may be most unpredictable and the nursing competencies are unique to that area (e.g., emergency department, labor and delivery, critical care). However, a decentralized model places a higher level of staffing responsibility on managers, which may take them away from other more strategic responsibilities.

In contrast, centralized staffing is filtered through a central staffing office, which maintains responsibility for ensuring adequate staffing for multiple units or for multiple hospitals or business units in larger systems. Centralized staffing offers the benefit of being able to view supply and demand from an enterprise perspective. With patient acuity, nursing competencies, and available staff viewed across multiple units, staffing resources can be optimized by increasing staff in one area and reducing staff in another to accommodate variable patient demand. Staffing protocols for obtaining supplemental staff can be standardized, such as procedures for using internal staff, per diems, and external sources (e.g., travelers and agency). The staffing office can relieve nurse managers and/or charges nurses of the time-consuming administrative task of responding to sick calls and obtaining supplemental staff. In addition, the central staffing office provides a command center with protocols and information to manage disasters in which staff must be quickly obtained and deployed.

The downside to relying solely on a centralized staffing office is that it can become too remote from the unit, thus losing some of the intelligence that may be considered when making staffing decisions (Lauw & Gares, 2005). Policies and procedures clearly define the roles and responsibilities and communication among areas. But as with any of these staffing models, the key to eliminating chaotic, last-minute staffing decisions is to adopt predictive tools and move more of the staffing decisions to the near future or the next 2 to 4 days (Pickard & Warner, 2007). Assessment and analysis of staffing needs in the near future provide more available options, including more competent staff, at optimal costs.

Computerized staffing systems play a pivotal role in providing what is described as a "single version of the truth" and offering decision support such as staffing variances across units, workload indicators, employee competencies, and decision costs. Many of these systems interface with time and attendance systems and therefore provide various productivity reports, dashboards, or other performance metrics required by managers.

Information for staffing decisions must be readily available and accurate. Staffing systems serve as a communication tool for all staffing "stakeholders," including employees, unit managers, centralized staffing office, and executives. Staffing systems also offer automated open-shift management, which posts open shifts electronically to qualified staff. Protocols direct which personnel are the best qualified and the most cost effective to fill needed shifts. The staffing system measures and reports the staffing management performance at both unit and organization levels, providing staffing effectiveness data for the organization.

Access to nurses outside the unit to cover transient shortages is critical to meet last-minute, unplanned nurse shortages, such as sick calls, and high patient demand. Supplemental staffing resources—frequently referred to as the *staffing pool*—are defined as a group of nurses who supplement the core unit staffing. This includes per diem nurses, float pool nurses, part-time nurses desiring additional hours, seasonal nurses, agency nurses, and traveling nurses. The scope of clinical competency, pay rates, and contractual arrangements varies among these internal and external pools of nurses as well. For example, select nurses may be competent to work on all of the adult medical–surgical units, whereas other specialty nurses may be competent to work in several areas, such as perioperative practice sites, or only one area, such as labor and delivery, the emergency department, or the dialysis unit.

Supplemental staffing resource guidelines need to be established to direct the use of additional resources detailing the data for decision-making and algorithms for staffing. These guidelines are designed to prevent depletion of supplemental resources for core staff coverage and instead to reserve them for unexpected intervals of high acuity or transient shortages. For example, a guideline may direct the use of a part-time nurse who has signed up to work extra shifts to fill a sick call, then to use a supplemental float pool nurse, and finally to use an external agency nurse if previous resources are unavailable. The option for overtime is also a consideration based on policy regarding the fatigue associated with excessive hours in a day or days worked in a row and cost. The costs associated with each resource progression are then inherently built into the staffing decision model. Additional strategies for covering long-term family medical leaves are also needed to meet core coverage. Strategies for covering these longer-term shortages are critical, otherwise a manager is depleting the resource pools intended for last-minute and transient shortages.

Operational metrics for the supplemental resource pool are not only defined for daily staffing allocation but also may be defined during the scheduling stage. The operational total nurse vacancy rate for scheduling purposes is defined as all budgeted nurse positions that are vacant during the scheduling period, including the unfilled or vacant positions and positions for which nurses are on short-term or long-term leaves of absence (e.g., Family and Medical Leave Act [FMLA], workers' compensation). For example, if a unit has an operational RN vacancy rate of 5% to 10%, it may be approved to cover the shortage with part-time nurses working additional shifts and possibly overtime but would not be approved for agency nurses. Alternatively, a unit with a 22% operational RN vacancy rate may be approved for longer-term contracted higher labor expense (e.g., travelers). Defining operational vacancy rates and incremental resource actions are important aspects of consistently managing staff shortages and ensuring a standard of care delivery. As such, protocols driven by operational vacancy rates generate consistency in how higher labor costs are aligned with the greatest need. In addition, wages, benefits, transfers, and work policies of supplemental internal float pools should be carefully designed so that the stability of unit-based core nursing staff is not compromised.

Fitzpatrick and Brooks (2010) and Gavigan and colleagues (2016) called for the optimization of human capital as a staffing consideration. These authors believe that there is a need to build a scaffolding structure to allow for optimal mathematical optimization for best staffing solutions. Box 21.4 lists criteria to optimize modeling of staffing for best solutions.

BOX 21.4 Criteria for Optimization of Staffing

1. Multiple objectives

   +

2. Variables

   +

3. Constraints

Optimization Modeling for Best Solutions

From Fitzpatrick, T., & Brooks, B. (2010). The nurse leader as logistician: Optimizing human capital. *Journal of Nursing Administration, 40*(2), 69–74.

Patient Assignments

Nurse managers are responsible not only for forthcoming schedules and immediate staffing but also for ensuring that the patient care assignments reflect appropriate use of personnel considering scope of practice, competencies, patient needs, and complexity of care. Patient assignment in hospitals is defined as the task of assigning the scheduled staff to specific patients for the shift duration. Nurse managers in hospitals typically delegate assignment making to the charge nurse in the patient care area. The charge nurse is responsible for matching the qualified caregivers to meet the patients' needs and for providing a balanced workload across caregivers. Often the nursing care delivery model articulates the value of nurse-to-patient continuity across time. A balanced workload enables nurses to provide reasonable equity in nursing care delivery to patients and their families. In addition, the staff members expect the charge nurse to create equitable assignments as a valued measure of fairness in workload distribution. Many organizations require an annual charge nurse competency review and peer feedback demonstrating effective assignment making.

In the staffing management framework, the patient assignment is the point at which individual patients are linked with individual nurses. Welton (2010) identified this as a critical new level of analysis to examine the relationship between staffing and clinical quality and cost that may better inform operational decision-making.

ORGANIZATIONAL OUTCOMES

Staffing Effectiveness

ANA says that identifying and maintaining the appropriate number and mix of nursing staff are central to the provision of quality care (ANA, 2016b). Optimal nurse staffing is fiscally responsible and appropriate to patients' needs. Hospital organizations examine the relationships between staffing and nurse-sensitive outcomes to meet TJC staffing effectiveness requirements showing that there is the appropriate number, competency, and skill mix of staff in relation to the provision of needed care and treatment. However, staffing for effectiveness, including cost effectiveness, is highly complex and a critical issue for nurse leaders.

The Staffing Evidence on Quality

The link between nurse staffing and quality of care is evidence based and long-standing. Better RN staffing has been shown to reduce patient mortality, enhance outcomes, and improve nurse satisfaction (Mensik, 2014). Over a decade of rigorous studies and a summary of current research conducted by the Ruckelshaus Center at the University of Washington concluded that "fewer patients per nurse or more NHPPD is associated with fewer adverse outcomes—in particular mortality, failure to rescue, and some specific adverse events among surgical patients" (Mitchell, 2008, p. 30). Comprehensive reviews of staffing evidence and sentinel works are available (Aiken et al., 2002, 2003, 2014; Blegen et al., 1998; Needleman et al., 2002, 2006, 2011; Unruh, 2008). These studies and a meta-analysis by Kane and colleagues (2007a,b) demonstrated the strong evidence linking inadequate staffing with adverse events and failure to rescue. Frith and colleagues (2010) found that higher RN staffing was associated with a reduced LOS among community hospitals. These findings suggest the direct fiscal impact that nurses have on hospital margin today (Bogue, 2012). A body of research over at least the past decade has shown that sufficient nurse staffing levels and favorable work environments function to facilitate nurses' effectiveness as a surveillance system. Sufficient numbers of RNs are necessary to manage complex patient care needs and identify and intervene when something goes wrong (McHugh et al., 2016). Because research continues to confirm the many associations of nurse staffing with outcomes, innovative and technology-based strategies are being employed to more precisely manage staffing for quality outcomes.

Hospitals routinely employ supplemental nurses to provide additional resources to cover transient shortages. However, little is known about this nurse workforce and its relationship to quality of care. Aiken and colleagues (2007) examined the characteristics of supplemental nurses and the relationships of the supplemental staff to nurse outcomes and adverse events. Their findings suggested that widely held negative perceptions of temporary nurses may be unfounded. However, the effect on the organization's culture is unknown but suspected to be disruptive. The employment patterns of nurses and their effect on cost and quality is an important area needing further study.

Nurse leaders at all levels are called to action to incorporate relevant scientific findings in staffing administrative policy and practice and to lead the evaluation of all innovations in care delivery. Balancing these decisions with organizational fiscal constraints and conducting cost-effectiveness analyses are the current challenges for organizations and nurse leaders.

CURRENT ISSUES AND TRENDS

There is an increasing call to use technology and innovate with scheduling. Fitzpatrick (2015) suggested nurses reflect on the airline industry and how they have managed to coordinate flights, maintenance, staggering across different time zones, and weather conditions. These industries use logistics science and a form of mathematical modeling called optimization to solve scheduling problems. Logistic science offers new insights in planning and deployment of clinical workers because it recognizes the complexities and interconnectedness of the systems and processes involved in scheduling and deploying nurses (Joseph & Fowler, 2016).

Fitzpatrick (2015) illustrated how the field of nursing has started to transition from standardized, computerized scheduling to the use of sophisticated, algorithmically driven applications like how the airline industry used logistics science and a form of mathematical modeling called optimization to solve scheduling problems. To ensure optimization of staffing modeling, the author calls for three key variables: (1) business objectives such as staffing costs and ensuring adequate coverage, (2) decision variables such as skill mix and cost differences, and (3) business constraints such as vacancy rates, work rules (e.g., weekend requirement), and cultural issues such as being off for Mother's Day. The use of optimization can move decision-making from "what-if" to "what is the best" solution. When all these factors are considered, there is more precise modeling of staffing to actual demands, allowing health care organizations to meet staffing and scheduling challenges. Additionally, the process of optimization cuts the time spent on scheduling by 50%. Nurse leaders need to reflect on how they have mastered modeling with care processes such as medication administration and use that experience as a requisite to optimize problems with staffing and scheduling (Fitzpatrick, 2015).

In the quest to validate nursing's value, the next two discussions illustrate good examples of how the appropriate data can guide administrators with appropriate decision-making for staffing. Pappas and colleagues (2015) called for greater precision with staffing. The authors demonstrated that approaches to minimize patient risks are needed to avoid unwanted clinical and subsequent negative financial outcome. The authors advocated for staffing models that are based on unit-specific data that incorporate the nurse's view of the amount of surveillance to prevent hospital-acquired harm and the associated costs.

Pruinelli and colleagues (2016) stated that the emergence of Big Data for data analytics is poised to influence the value of nurses' work. Their recent article advocates for the use of the nursing management minimum data set (NMMDS) in conjunction with staffing systems in electronic health systems. The NMMDS is an evidence-based tool that defines and measures the context of care within and across all enterprise settings. Use of the NMMDS provides data about variables affecting the delivery of timely, cost-effective care. This knowledge is critical to maintain clinical and operational excellence. The authors advocated for integration of data from multiple sources because this helps nurse leaders to balance workloads, thus improving patient outcomes and nurse satisfaction. Technology that integrates elements of the NMMDS for staffing or other complex management decisions can return valuable hours to the nurse leaders. This is the emergence of Big Data for data analytics.

A health care system in Oregon underwent a transformation to define and implement staffing and scheduling by using software to optimize scheduling. The criteria included a simple and easy-to-use network, remote and mobile access, integration of personal calendars, and time and attendance. Intelligence included definitions, predictive staffing, acuity-based scheduling, and patient acuity. Customization included staffing based on skill mix, with customization of reports, shifts, and dashboards. Bonus features were ease of build, maintenance, upgrades, and successful integration.

The Magnet Recognition Program® continues to be a driver of current staffing trends. For more than 20 years, Magnet designation has been associated with healthier work environments (better staffing—excluding California, where there is a state-mandated ratio; lower burnout; lower turnover; and improved RN–MD collaboration) (Kelly et al., 2011) and higher-quality patient care. Achieving Magnet designation has been increasingly associated with quality. It is now incorporated in the scoring for *U.S. News & World Report's* Best Hospitals in America Honor Roll and earns full credit for Safe Practice Standard #9 Nursing Workforce in the Leapfrog Hospital Survey, which scores hospitals on their commitment to staffing with highly trained nurses. A number of the hospital financial credit rating agencies utilize Magnet designation in their evaluation of an organization's operating performance.

Given the advent of value-based purchasing (VBP) and the CMS provision 1533-F, health care leaders have been incentivized to focus on improving care processes. CMS provides health care coverage for 80 million Americans via Medicaid, Medicare, and state children's programs and represents the largest payer in the world, administering more than $800 billion in benefits annually. Many of the clinical processes and patient satisfaction measures under VBP are directly affected by the quality and quantity of nursing care, and the outcomes will have a significant impact on the key metrics that will drive hospital reimbursements (Bogue, 2012).

Since CMS provision 1533-F became effective on October 1, 2008, hospitals are not being reimbursed for hospital-acquired conditions (HACs). These are conditions such as skin pressure ulcers, urinary tract infections, ventilator-acquired pneumonia, and falls with injury that occurred within the hospital stay and were not present on admission (POA). Among the 14 HACs in the provision, at least nine of the conditions are sensitive to nursing care intervention. Thus, hospitals have new financial incentives to support both nursing education and appropriate staffing to prevent HACs, reduce costs, and increase reimbursement. In addition, the Patient Protection and Affordable Care Act (ACA) mandates 2% of hospitals' Medicare payment will be at risk under value-based payments in 2017. Penalties for certain 30-day admissions began in 2012. The LOS and readmissions financial penalties are the most compelling incentives for hospitals to support the appropriate amount of nursing care that is of high quality because of the known positive effect of nursing care and coordination on patients' transitions of care and acute care LOS (Frith et al., 2010). The nurse's inherent role in discharge planning with the interdisciplinary team, linkages to community services, and effective medication, symptom, and disease management teaching in all care settings is becoming increasingly important to organizational outcomes.

There are national policy initiatives to identify and make visible nursing care in the US health care reimbursement system. It has long been known that nursing care historically has been bundled within the "room and board" hospital charges, which do not capture the variability in nursing care costs. Given the variability in nursing care intensity and cost of nurse staffing, this traditional costing system has resulted in cost compression and distortion in the inpatient prospective payment system (Dalton, 2007). A proposed solution separates nursing care from the room and board charges and accounts for this care as a variable, direct cost within the billing system based on actual nursing time delivered to patients (Welton & Harris, 2007; Welton et al., 2006). Finkler and colleagues (2013) describe this as nursing as a revenue center and explain the use of variable billing. Even in a bundled payment system, nurses need both cost and productivity data to better manage care for both efficiency and effectiveness. Welton (2010) suggested a new value-based nursing care model, including (1) allocating nursing cost and intensity to each patient, (2) new metrics that link nursing-specific outcomes to individual patients, and (3) moving the focus from staffing to the assignment of caregivers to individual patients. Simpson (2012) further called to action the adoption of technology at the point of care to achieve value-based nursing care.

These current issues in health care policy raise the visibility and importance of nursing care in society and create a climate to advocate for safe, cost-effective, high-quality nursing care for all. Current issues and trends in staffing and scheduling demonstrate that nursing has transformed its thinking and approaches based on the evolving science of systems theory, technology, advanced mathematics, and logistics science—as well as human capital and social theory—to optimize its staffing needs.

RESEARCH NOTE

Purpose

The Affordable Care Act's Readmission Reduction Program penalizes hospitals based on excess readmission rates among Medicare beneficiaries. Many evidence-based interventions that reduce readmissions are grounded in the fundamentals of basic nursing care. Hospitals with higher nurse staffing had 25% lower odds of being penalized compared with similar hospitals with lower staffing.

Discussion

Effective October 2012, the Centers for Medicare & Medicaid Services (CMS) implemented a policy under the Affordable Care Act intended to curb the estimated $15 billion Medicare spends annually on preventable readmissions. The logic behind the Hospital Readmissions Reduction Program (HRRP) is that hospitals can reduce readmissions by implementing evidence-based practice standards of care, specifically focused on single disease-based populations such as heart failure. Many of these interventions, known to reduce complications and readmissions, such as discharge planning, care coordination, and patient education are clearly within the scope and responsibility of nursing. Further evidence suggests that hospitals that staff for manageable nurse workloads have lower readmission rates.

These researchers studied the impact of nurse staffing on readmission penalties by analyzing the CMS HRRP data for fiscal year 2012 and compared these data to nurse staffing as reported in the American Hospital Association (AHA) Annual Survey for the same time period. Staffing was measured as the ratio of registered nurse hours per adjusted patient day. Full time equivalent registered nurse staffing was multiplied by 1768 and divided by adjusted patient days to determine average hours per adjusted patient day.

Adjusting readmissions for other factors such as racial, ethnic, and socioeconomic factors, the researchers observed a significant and consistent difference in readmission penalties when nurse staffing levels were higher. In fact, their estimates suggest that each additional nurse hour per adjusted patient day was associated with 10% lower odds of being penalized.

Application to Practice

This important work adds to the growing literature that describes the implications of nurse staffing on multiple clinical outcomes including surgical complications, falls, and hospital acquired infections, to name a few. Understanding how to define adequate staffing by patient type continues to be a challenge, however, yet the ramifications of not doing so create significance consequences for individual patients and the financial health of organizations generally. The mechanism by which better staffing affects readmissions is multifactorial considering the presence of and need for nursing care across the duration of patients' hospitalizations. Nurses are responsible for the core processes that have been widely associated with readmissions: discharge planning, patient and family education, complication surveillance and intervention, knowledge assessment, and care coordination. By focusing on a system factor such as nurse staffing, leaders may be able to address multiple quality issues while reducing their likelihood of penalties for readmissions. Policy makers also may be able to gain traction on complications and attendant costs through policy that creates a care environment sufficiently staffed and resourced to allow nurses to do their important work more effectively.

NEXT-GENERATION NCLEX® EXAMINATION-STYLE CASE STUDY

Nurse Manager Dan's budget has been cut and is projected to have increasing cuts over the next two years due to COVID-19 implications. He made the decision to not hire new employees and use the existing employees to cover staffing needs. Employees on his unit are feeling overworked. Many employees are being asked to do mandatory overtime without adequate compensation. Dan's director was told by human resources that employees are feeling overwhelmed with the increasing staffing demands without adequate compensation. The director pulls Dan's non- salary YTD expense report to examine where opportunities may exist to reallocate funds towards staffing.

NEXT-GENERATION NCLEX® EXAMINATION-STYLE CASE STUDY—cont'd

Question

Utilizing the non-salary expense report, the director makes the recommendation for Dan to redirect dollars from some itemized items in the budget. Dan decides to redirect budgetary dollars. Which indicate an effective strategy to fund staffing? **Select all that apply.**

1. Redirect dollars from food service to staffing
2. Redirect dollars from equipment rental to staffing
3. Redirect dollars from departmental supplies to staffing
4. Redirect dollars from travel to staffing
5. Redirect dollars from other expenses to staffing

YTD Non-Salary Expense Report

Non-salary expense	Actual	Budget	Var%	Prior
Purchase Professional	350	0	0.0%	0
Patient Nonchargeable (e.g., Kleenex, bath wipes, deodorant)	100,655	60,656	(65.0%)	59,999
Drugs	0	178	100.0%	0
Food service	6,252	4,200	(48.0)%	4,736
Medical supplies	0	449	100.0%	0
Department Supplies	8,668	8,546	(1.4)%	5,429
Forms and access to databases	1,025	1,255	18.3%	1,204
Minor equipment (e.g., vital signs machine, I.V. vein finder)	0	1,080	100%	0
Equipment Rental (e.g., wound VAC, low bed, bariatric bed)	6,148	6,800	9.5%	1,529
Publications	350	50	(600)%	44
Dues and Memberships	0	8	100%	0
Travel	567	1,058	46.4%	1,325
Other Expenses (e.g., outside catering, holiday parties, recognition trophies)	0	8000	100%	3,000
Total Non-salary expenses	124,015	92,280	34.3%	77,266

CRITICAL THINKING EXCERCISE

Gizelle Guadalupe is a new manager on the busiest medical and surgical unit in a tertiary hospital. There are 39 beds on 9 Tower, which has a high volume of diabetic and other patients with multisystemic clinical conditions requiring complex care planning. She is excited to improve the quality and outcomes on this unit. During her interview, she learned that under the previous leadership the quality was deteriorating, as reflected in the Hospital Consumer Assessment of Healthcare Providers and Systems (HCHAPS) scores, staff absenteeism, and increasing turnover rates. It was costing the unit between $42,000 to $65,000 to replace a nurse, including the cost of recruitment and temporarily filling the vacancy at premium labor costs, as well as the immeasurable costs to quality outcomes.

While making rounds, Manager Guadalupe observed complaints about missed nursing care from all shifts and decided to make staff accountable for ensuring that patient care is completed. She asked a Clinical Nurse Leader (CNL) to monitor the types of patient care activities that were being omitted. After 1 week, the CNL stated that it was difficult to make that determination because everyone had a different opinion on which interventions were being omitted. Additionally, she reported that staffing was an issue. The manager's initial response was, "What's wrong with staffing? Why would you blame staffing for omissions in patient care?"

1. Based on documented evidence in the literature, does staffing and resource allocation play a role in clinical outcomes, including the omission of various elements of patient care?
2. What types of quantitative data would you look at to determine if indeed nursing care was inadvertently being omitted? Additionally, what types of analyses would you perform to understand the root cause of missed care?
3. What questions could you pose to frontline nurses to understand how their staffing experience related to missed care?
4. Whom will you engage institutionally to understand the issue fully? Why them?
5. Which qualitative data elements may be required to build a case for staffing and missed nursing care?
6. What ideas would you propose to administration to reverse the financial effects and improve HCHAPS scores?
7. Presuming you receive support to implement your ideas, how would you measure and monitor the outcomes of your plans?

REFERENCES

Aiken, L. H., Clarke, S. P., Cheung, R. B., Sloane, D. M., & Silber, J. H. (2003). Educational levels of hospital nurses and surgical patient mortality. *Journal of the American Medical Association, 290*(12), 1617–1623.

Aiken, L. H., Clarke, S. P., Sloane, D. M., Sochalski, J., & Silber, J. H. (2002). Hospital nurse staffing and patient mortality, nurse burnout, and job dissatisfaction. *Journal of the American Medical Association, 288*(16), 1987–1993.

Aiken L. H., Sloane D. M., Bruyneel L., Van den Heede K., Griffiths P., Busse R., et al. (2014). Nurse staffing and education and hospital mortality in nine European countries: A retrospective observational study. *Lancet, 383*(9931), 1824–1830.

Aiken L. H., Sloane D. M., Griffiths P., Rafferty A. M., Bruyneel L., McHugh M., et al. (2016). Nursing skill mix in European hospitals: Cross-sectional study of the association with mortality, patient ratings, and quality of care. *BMJ Quality & Safety*, 1–10. http://qualitysafety.bmj.com/content/early/2016/11/03/bmjqs-2016-005567.full.pdf+html.

Aiken, L. H., Xue, Y., Clarke, S. P., & Sloane, D. M. (2007). Supplemental nurse staffing in hospitals and quality of care. *Journal of Nursing Administration, 37*(7–8), 335–342.

American Academy of Ambulatory Care Nursing (AAACN). (2005). *Ambulatory care nurse staffing: An annotated bibliography*. Author.

American Academy of Pediatrics (AAP) and the American College of Obstetricians and Gynecologists (ACOG). (2012). *Guidelines for perinatal care* (7th ed.). March of Dimes.

American Association of Colleges of Nursing (AACN). (2007). *White paper on the education and role of the clinical nurse leader*. Author.

American Association of Critical-Care Nurses. (2016). *AACN synergy model for patient care*. http://www.aacn.org/wd/certifications/content/synmodel.pcms?menu=certification.

American Nurses Association (ANA). (n.d.). *Safe staffing: The registered nurse safe staffing act HR 876/S.58*. http://www.nursingworld.org/SafeStaffingFactsheet.aspx.

American Nurses Association (ANA). (2010). *Nursing's social policy statement: The essence of the profession* (3rd ed.). Author.

American Nurses Association (ANA). (2012). *ANA's principles for nurse staffing* (2nd ed..) Author.

American Nurses Association (ANA). (2015a). *Code of ethics for nurses with interpretive statements*. Author.

American Nurses Association (ANA). (2015b). *The registered nurse safe staffing act HR2083/S.1132*. https://www.nursingworld.org/news/news-releases/2018/ana-applauds-nurse-staffing-legislation/.

American Nurses Association (ANA). (2016a). *Nurse staffing*. https://www.nursingworld.org/practice-policy/nurse-staffing/.

American Nurses Association (ANA). (2016b). *Nurse Staffing*. https://www.nursingworld.org/practice-policy/nurse-staffing/nurse-staffing-advocacy/.

American Nurses Association (2020). *Patient Acuity/Classification Systems (PCAS)*. https://www.nursingworld.org/practice-policy/nurse-staffing/workforce-management-pcas.

American Organization of Nurse Executives (AONE). (2000). *Staffing management and methods: Tools and techniques for nurse leaders*. Author.

Association of Perioperative Registered Nurses (AORN). (2014). *AORN position statement on perioperative safe staffing and on-call practices*. Author. https://www.aorn.org/guidelines/clinical-resources/position-statements.

Association of Women's Health, Obstetric and Neonatal Nurses (AWHONN). (2010). *Guidelines for professional registered nurse staffing for perinatal units*. Author.

Aydelotte, M. K.. *Nurse staffing methodology: A review and critique of selected literature*. US Department of Health,

Education and Welfare, Division of Nursing. Publication No. (NIH) (1973) Government Printing Office pp. 73–433.
Blegen, M. A, Goode, C. J., & Reed, L. (1998). Nurse staffing and patient outcomes. *Nursing Research, 47*(1), 43–50.
Bogue, R. J. (2012, May 29). Nurses: Key to making or breaking your future margin. *Hospitals and Health Networks.*
Brenan, M. (2018, December 20). Nurses again outpace other professions for honesty, ethics. *Gallup*. https://news.gallup.com/poll/245597/nurses-again-outpace-professions-honesty-ethics.aspx.
Brennan, C. W., & Daly, B. J. (2008). Patient acuity: a concept analysis. *Journal of Advanced Nursing, 65*(5), 1114–1126.
Case Management Society of America (CMSA). (2016). *What is a case manager?* Little Rock, AR: Author. http://www.cmsa.org/Home/CMSA/WhatisaCaseManager/tabid/224/Default.aspx.
Cipriano, P., & Cutruzzula, J. (2007). Over-recruiting: Breaking the short staffing and turnover cycle. *Nurse Leader, 5*(6), 28–32.
Clancy, T. R. (2007). Planning: what we can learn from complex systems science. *Journal of Nursing Administration, 37*(1), 436–439.
Clancy, T. R. (2007). Organizing: new ways to harness complexity. *Journal of Nursing Administration, 37*(12), 534–536.
Clarke, S. P. (2005). The policy implications of staffing-outcomes research. *Journal of Nursing Administration, 35*(1), 17–19.
Dalton, K. (2007). *A study of charge compression in calculating DRG relative weights*. Centers for Medicaid & Medicare Services (CMS): Contract no. 500-00-0024-TO18 Baltimore, MD: CMS.
Dent, R. L., & Bradshaw, P. (2012). Building the business case for acuity-based staffing. *Nurse Leader, 10*(2), 26–28.
DNV. (2019). *DNV GL- Healthcare NIAHO accreditation requirements, interpretive guidelines and surveyor guidance*. https://www.dnvgl.us/assurance/healthcare/standards/niaho-ac-dl.html.
Donabedian, A. (1966). Evaluating the quality of medical care. *Milbank Memorial Fund Quarterly, 44*(3), 166–206.
Eck Birmingham, S. (2010). Evidenced-based staffing: The next step. *Nurse Leader, 8*(3), 24–26, 35.
Eck Birmingham, S., Nell, K., & Abe, N. (2011). Determining staffing needs based on patient outcomes vs. patient interventions. In P. Cowan, & S. Moorhead (Eds.), *Current issues in nursing* (8th ed., pp. 391–404): Mosby Elsevier.
Edwardson, S. (2007). Conceptual frameworks used in funded nursing health services research projects. *Nursing Economics, 25*(4), 222–227.
Emergency Nurses Association (ENA). (2015). *Staffing and productivity in the emergency care setting.* https://www.ena.org/docs/default-source/resource-library/practice-resources/position-statements/staffingandproductivityemergencydepartment.pdf?sfvrsn=c57dcf13_8.
Finkler, S. A., Jones, C. B., & Kovner, C. T. (2013). *Financial management for nurse managers and executives* (4th ed.). Saunders.
Fitzpatrick, T. A. (2014). Does the package delivery industry hold the answer to our scheduling problems? *American Nurse Today, 9*(3), 48–54.
Fitzpatrick, T., & Brooks, B. (2010). The nurse leader as logistician: Optimizing human capital. *Journal of Nursing Administration, 40*(2), 69–74.
Fitzpatrick, T., Goetz, K., & Cole, B. (2018). Advanced analytics must drive the next round of productivity initiatives. *Healthcare Cost Containment (Newsletter of the Healthcare Financial Management Association)*, 1–4.
Fitzpatrick, T., Anen, T., & Martinez-Soto, E. (2013). Nurse staffing: The Illinois experience. *Nursing Economics, 31*(5), 221–229.
Fitzpatrick, T. (2015, June 24). *Clinical labor optimization: Managing supply and demand in a dynamic environment.* International webinar innovations for advancing nursing administration [Webinar]..
Fitzpatrick, T. A., & Brooks, B. A. (2010). The nurse leader as a logistician: Optimizing human capital. *Journal of Nursing Administration, 40*(2), 69–74.
Flanders, K., & Carr, D. (2016). Staffing by acuity: Building a bridge to support nursing effectiveness. *Voice of Nursing Leadership, 14*(5), 12–14.
Fried, B. J., & Fottler, M. D. (2008). *Human resources in healthcare*: Health Administration Press.
Frith K., Anderson F., Caspers B., Tseng F., Sanford K., Hoyt N., et al. (2010). Effects of nurse staffing on hospital-acquired conditions and length of stay in community hospitals. *Quality Management in Health Care, 19*(2), 147–155.
Gavigan, M., Fitzpatrick, T., & Miserendino, C.
Effective staffing takes a village: Creating the staffing ecosystem. *Nursing Economics, 34*(2), 58–65.
Gavigan, M., Fitzpatrick, T. A., & Miserendino, C. (2016). Effective staffing takes a village: Creating the staffing ecosystem. *Nursing Economics, 34*(2), 58–65.
Guanci, G., & Felgen, J. (2016). How relationship-based care supports the Magnet journey. *Nursing Management, 47*(1), 9–12.
Haas, S. A., Vlasses, F., & Havey, J. (2016). Developing staffing models to support population health management and quality outcomes in ambulatory care settings. *Nursing Economics, 34*(3), 126–133.
Habasevich, B. (2012, July 26). *Re: Defining acuity* [Online forum blog]. https://www.mediware.com/rehabilitation/blog/defining-acuity/.
Joseph, M. L., & Fowler, D. (2016). Innovating traditional nursing administration challenges. *Journal of Nursing Administration, 46*(3), 120–121.

Kane, R., Shamliyan, T., Mueller, C., Duval, S., & Wilt, T. (2007a). *Nurse staffing and quality of patient care.* US Department of Health and Human Services AHRQ Publication No. 07-E005. Author.

Kane, R., Shamliyan, T., Mueller, C., Duval, S., & Wilt, T. (2007b). The association of registered nurse staffing levels and patient outcomes. *Medical Care, 45*(12), 1195–1204.

Kelly, L. A., McHugh, M. D., & Aiken, L. H. (2011). Nurse outcomes in Magnet and non-Magnet hospitals. *Journal of Nursing Administration, 41*(10), 428–433.

Koloroutis, M. (Ed.). (2004). *Relationship-based care: A model for transforming practice.* Creative Health Care Management.

Koning, C. (2014). Does self-scheduling increase nurses' job satisfaction? An integrative literature review. *Nursing Management, 21*(6), 24–28.

Kullberg, A., Bergenmar, M., & Sharp, L. (2016). Changed nursing scheduling for improved safety culture and working conditions-patients' and nurses' perspectives. *Journal of Nursing Management, 24*(4), 524–532.

Lauw, C., & Gares, D. (2005). Resource management: What's right for you. *Nursing Management, 36*(12), 46–49.

Lawson, L. D., Miles, K. S., Vallish, R. O., & Jenkins, S. A. (2011). Recognizing nursing professional growth and development in a collective bargaining environment. *Journal of Nursing Administration, 41*(5), 197–200.

Liang, B., & Turkcan, A. (2016). Acuity-based nurse assignment and patient scheduling in oncology clinics. *Health Care Management Science, 19*(3), 207–226.

Litvak, E., Buerhaus, P., Davidoff, F., Long, M., McManus, M., & Berwick, D. (2005). Managing unnecessary variability in patient demand to reduce nursing stress and improve patient safety. *Journal on Quality and Patient Safety, 31*(6), 330–338.

MacPhee, M., & Borra, L. S. (2012). *Flexible work practices in nursing. International Council of Nurses.*

Malloch, K. (2015). Measurement of nursing's complex health care work: Evolution of the science for determining the required staffing for safe and effective patient care. *Nursing Economics, 33*(1), 20–25.

Mark, B. A., Harless, D. W., & Berman, W. F. (2007). Nurse staffing and adverse events in hospitalized children. *Policy, Politics, and Nursing Practice, 8*(2), 83–92.

McDonough, K. S. (2013). Development of the McDonough Optimum Staffing Method: Evidence-driven recommendations based on patient demand. *Virginia Nurses Today, 21*(2), 8–11.

McHugh M. D., Rochman M. F., Sloane D. M., Berg R. A., Mancini M. E., Nadkarni V. M., et al. (2016). Better nurse staffing and nurse work environments associated with increased survival of in-hospital cardiac arrest patients. *Medical Care, 54*(1), 74–80.

McKinley, J., & Cavouras, C. (2000). Evolving staffing measures. In American Organization of Nurse Executives (AONE). *Staffing management and methods: Tools and techniques for nurse leaders*, 1–33. Jossey-Bass.

Mensik, J. (2014). What every nurse should know about staffing. *American Nurse Today, 9*(2), 1–11.

Mitchell, P. (2008). *Nurse staffing—A summary of current research, opinion and policy* (pp. 1–37). The William D. Ruckelshaus Center.

Morris, R., MacNeela, P., Scott, A., Treacy, P., & Hyde, A. (2007). Reconsidering the conceptualization of nursing workload: Literature review. *Journal of Advanced Nursing, 57*(5), 463–471.

National Association of Neonatal Nurses (NANN). (2014). *RN staffing in the neonatal intensive care unit.* NANN Position Statement No. 3061. Author.

National Council of State Boards of Nursing (NCSBN). (2016). A changing environment: 2016 NCSBN environmental scan national council. *Journal of Nursing Regulation, 6*(4), 4–37.

National Database of Nursing Quality Indicators version 9.3. (August 2011). Kansas City: University of Kansas School of Nursing.

National Labor Relations Board (NLRB). (2016). *National Labor Relations Act.* Author. https://www.nlrb.gov/how-we-work/national-labor-relations-act.

National Labor Relations Board. (2020). Bargaining in good faith with employees' union representative (Section 8 (d) & 8 (a)(5). https://www.nlrb.gov/rights-we-protect/whats-law/employers/bargaining-good-faith-employees-union-representative-section.

Needleman, J., Buerhaus, P., Mattke, S., Stewart, M., & Zelevinski, K. (2002). Nurse-staffing levels and the quality of care in hospitals. *New England Journal of Medicine, 346*(22), 1715–1722.

Needleman, J., Buerhaus, P., Pankratz, S., Leibson, C., Stevens, S., & Harris, M. (2011). Nurse staffing and inpatient hospital mortality. *New England Journal of Medicine, 364*(11), 1037–1045.

Needleman, J., Buerhaus, P. I., Stewart, M., Zelevinsky, K., & Mattke, S. (2006). Nurse staffing in hospitals: Is there a business case for quality. *Health Affairs, 25*(1), 204–211.

Norrish, B. R., & Rundall, T. G. (2001). Hospital restructuring and the work of registered nurses. *Milbank Quarterly, 79*(1), 55–79.

Pappas, S., Davidson, N., Woodard, J., Davis, J., & Welton, J. (2015). Risk-adjusted staffing to improve patient value. *Nursing Economics, 33*(2), 72–87.

Person, C. (2004). Patient care delivery. In M. Koloroutis (Ed.), *Relationship-based care: A model for transforming practice* (pp. 159–182). Creative Health Care Management.

Pickard, B., & Warner, M. (2007). Demand management: A methodology for outcomes-driven staffing and patient flow management. *Nurse Leader, 5*(2), 30–34.

Porter, C. (2010). A nursing labor management partnership model. *Journal of Nursing Administration, 40*(6), 272–276.

Pruinelli, L., Delaney, C., Garcia, A., Caspers, B., & Westra, B. L. (2016). Nursing management minimum dataset: Cost effective tool to demonstrate the value of nurse staffing in the Big Data science era. *Nursing Economics, 34*(2), 66–89.

Rambur, B., & Fitzpatrick, T. (2017). A plea to nurse educators: Incorporate big data use as a foundational skill for undergraduate and graduate nurses. *Journal of Professional Nursing, 34*(3), 176–181.

Robertson, R., & Samuelson, C. (1996). Should nurse patient ratios be legislated? Pros and cons. *Georgia Nursing, 56*(5), 2.

Roski, J., Bo-Linn, G., & Andrews, T. (2014). Creating value in healthcare through big data: Opportunities and policy implications. *Health Affairs, 33*(7), 1115–1122.

Rubenfire, A. (2017). Understanding value at the crossroads of cost and outcomes. *ModernHealthcare. http://www.moderhealthcare.com/article/20170601/SPONSORED/170609999.*

Seago, J. A., Spetz, J., Coffman, J., Rosenoff, E., & O'Neil, E. (2003). Minimum staffing ratios: The California workforce initiative survey. *Nursing Economics, 21*(2), 65–70.

Shi, L., & Singh, D. (2019). *Essentials of the U.S. health care system*. Burlington, MA: Jones & Bartlett.

Simpson, R. (2012). Technology enables value-base nursing care. *Nursing Administration Quarterly, 36*(1), 85–87.

The Joint Commission (TJC). (2016). *Joint Commission FAQ page*. Author. https://www.jointcommission.org/about/jointcommissionfaqs.aspx.

Thew, J. (2020, January 9). *Nursing tops Gallup's most honest and ethical professions list*. https://www.healthleadersmedia.com/nursing/nursing-tops-gallups-most-honest-and-ethical-professions-list.

Thompson, J. D., & Diers, D. (1985). DRGs and nursing intensity. *Nursing & Health Care, 6*(8), 434–439.

Unruh, L. (2008). Nurse staffing: Patient, nurse, financial outcomes. *American Journal of Nursing, 108*(1), 62–71.

Unruh, L., & Fottler, M. D. (2004, June). *Patient turnover and nursing staff adequacy*, Paper presented at Academy Health Annual Research Meeting.

Welton, J. M. (2010). Value-based nursing care. *Journal of Nursing Administration, 40*(10), 399–401.

Welton, J. M., & Dismuke, C. E. (2008). Testing an inpatient nursing intensity billing model. *Policy, Politics, & Nursing Practice, 9*(2), 103–111.

Welton, J. M., & Harris, K. (2007). Hospital billing and reimbursement: Charging for inpatient nursing care. *Journal of Nursing Administration, 30*(6), 309–315.

Welton, J. M., Zone-Smith, L., & Fischer, M. H. (2006). Adjustment of inpatient care reimbursement for nursing intensity. *Policy, Politics, & Nursing Practice, 7*(4), 270–280.

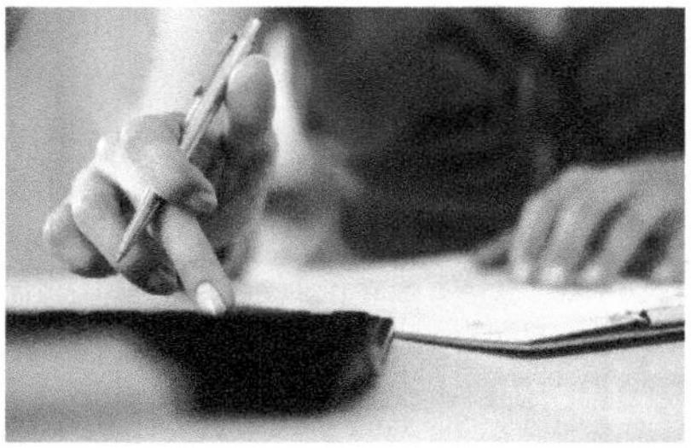

22

Budgeting, Productivity, and Costing Out Nursing

Linda B. Talley, Diane H. Thorgrimson

http://evolve.elsevier.com/Huber/leadership

National Health Expenditures (NHEs) are a measure of spending for health care in the United States. In 1998 NHEs exceeded $1 trillion for the first time. By 2027, NHEs are projected to increase to $6 trillion. Considered from another perspective, by 2027, this level of health care spending will exceed Gross Domestic Product (GDP) (the value of all the goods and services produced in the US in 1 year) growth by 0.8 percentage points, representing 19.4% of the GDP. In 2014 NHEs represented 17.5% of the GDP. Health care spending is projected to increase at a rate of 5.8% per year for the next 10 years (Centers for Medicare & Medicaid Services [CMS], 2019). Projections for insured and Medicare enrollment growth used to forecast the above expenditure increases do not include potential changes to federal health care legislation that may significantly increase the percentage of insured individuals in the United States.

Under a new rule of the Patient Protection and Affordable Care Act, which was signed into law March 2010, effective January 1, 2019, CMS required all hospitals to post prices on line in efforts to provide patients more cost information related to their health care (Gander, 2018). Price categories for posting include stays, procedures, services, drugs, and supplies. Given the complexities of health care billing and reimbursement, this transparency of pricing may not immediately drive down costs. Consumers of health care have multiple avenues to explore related to health care pricing and providers before making knowledgeable and significant changes to their practices (Viviano, 2019). From a provider perspective, this new transparency highlights the importance of nursing staff at all levels in identifying and understanding health care costs and cost drivers.

The magnitude of these expenditure increases—along with the changes in practice related to the Affordable Care Act—emphasizes that nurses, as members of the largest health care profession, need to understand the implications of these data for clinical practice. Understanding budgeting, productivity, and costing out nursing and relating that knowledge to the management of professional nursing is a leadership skill that will serve the nursing profession in an era of accelerating health care expenditures.

BACKGROUND

Staff nurses, new and experienced, may not recognize their important role in identifying and managing budgeted resources for patient care and the related outcomes to patient and staff satisfaction. Through transformational leadership a staff nurse can contribute to changes in patient care and financial practices and innovations across the organization. This transformative work places the staff nurse "at the table" where discussions focusing on the responsible management of financial resources address, but are not limited to, patient care, patient acuity, patient flow, workforce measures, workforce productivity, staff training, and supplies. As nurses across an organization improve their individual and collective knowledge of health care financial management to guide their decision making, outcomes related to resource allocation, patient care, and staff satisfaction will be achieved (Nurses First Solutions, 2018).

Budgeting is a major aspect of an organization's or unit's planning processes. A budget is a plan that is specified in dollar amounts. This plan becomes a guiding framework for organizational activities. It conveys management's intentions and financial expectations regarding revenues and expenditures. An organization-level budget compares expected revenues with expected expenses to forecast profit (margin) or loss (deficit). Budgeting is a cyclical process of planning, implementing, and evaluating.

Budgets are designed to be planning documents, but one often hears the statement "we don't have the budget for that" or "the budget won't allow it." It is crucial to understand that the budget is a tool created by humans. To be useful, it must be flexible and have processes in place to modify it when necessary. Individuals and organizations should not become so constrained by the approved budget that they hesitate to take appropriate actions or make appropriate decisions that vary from, or were unanticipated in, the budget process.

DEFINITIONS

A **budget** is defined as a written financial plan aimed at controlling the allocation of resources. It functions as both a planning instrument and an evaluation tool useful for financial management. A budget is used to manage programs, plan for goal accomplishment, measure change, and control costs.

Expenses are defined as the costs or prices of activities undertaken in the organization's operations.

Income (or profit) is the excess of revenues over expenses, or revenues minus expenses.

Revenue is defined as income or amounts owed for purchased services or goods. *Total operating expenses* are the result of summing the costs of all resources (e.g., labor, patient consumable supplies, small medical equipment, utilities, office supplies, and other related miscellaneous fees and materials) used to produce services.

Total operating revenues are the result of multiplying the volume of services provided by the charges (rate) for the services.

A **variance** is the difference between the budgeted and the actual amounts. A variance may be favorable or unfavorable relative to the budget amount. A budget developed to provide resources for direct patient care, such as nursing budgets, will use actual volumes (units of service) to interpret favorable or unfavorable variances.

There are three main types of organizational budgets, as follows:

1. *Capital budget:* This budget is the plan for the purchase of major equipment or assets. Each organization will define its own capital dollar threshold limits.
2. *Operating budget:* The operating budget is the annual plan for the unit's or organization's daily functioning revenue and expenses for a single year. For nursing units, this is a plan that lays out what it is going to cost to run the unit in the coming year. It includes such things as consumable and non-consumable supplies, small medical equipment, telephones, postage, paper, personal electronic devices for staff, printers, and copy machines. In addition, there may be a cost allocation for such things as heat, light, and housekeeping. Inflation projections for goods need to be factored into each year's budget.
3. *Personnel budget:* This is the staffing budget of the cost center (department or unit). It may be developed as part of the operating budget, or it may stand alone. Personnel budgets must include expenses related to productive and nonproductive time as well as projected replacement time. Use of premium pay—to include, but not be limited to, overtime and shift differential—is to be included in all personnel budgets. A good personnel budget contains fiscal resources to flex up staffing during periods of high inpatient census and/or patient volumes.

THE BUDGET PROCESS

Each institution establishes standard budgetary formats and processes. Because employees of a cost center will have to implement the budget decision, it is imperative that they have input in the process. This is often done in staff meetings where the manager uses the opportunity to teach about the process, present financial and volume data, and solicit staff input. Nursing and administrative leadership rounds also provide a forum for staff nurses to share their observations and recommendations regarding the many factors that affect resource use related to direct patient care on their unit and/or across the organization. Such factors may include quality and safety concerns, patient acuity, volumes, staffing, patient throughput, average length of stay, and patient experience.

The annual budgeting cycle process is complex and requires the completion of several related documents. It may be compared with income tax preparation, where an individual gathers all the necessary data and receipts, completes all of the required forms, and submits them to the Internal Revenue Service. Like tax preparation, the budget process may require multiple revisions.

A typical budget process follows the priorities identified in the organization's strategic plan and supports the organization's mission and vision. This is done to ensure that resources are appropriately aligned with key organizational initiatives. The budget process consists of three periods:

1. *Preparation:* As a beginning point, the manager reviews the organization's strategic plan and the last year's budget for the cost center (including budget and current year projected). The strategic plan will aid in writing budget justifications and links requests to organizational priorities. The prior year's budget for the cost center will help the manager to identify volume projections and changes in the past year and potential changes in the coming year. In concert with nursing leadership, the organization's finance staff and other members of the leadership team will often establish the next year's budgeted volumes through analysis of relative internal and external environmental factors and activity. Such analysis includes input from key departments such as strategy, managed care, case management, and reimbursement. Hospitals that employ physicians will also include physicians in budget volume projection work. In the hospital, patient days and adjusted patient days are the usual volume measurement. For example, if the manager of a surgical unit knows that two general surgeons are being recruited to the organization, it is reasonable to project an increase in patient days. With a review of the previous year's data, an informed projection can be made about the increase that can be anticipated. Similarly, the manager may be aware of factors that will decrease the volume of patient days, such as a new hospital being built nearby. In ambulatory care, the volume unit of measurement is clinic visits. If a new nurse practitioner (NP) is being hired, how will that affect the volume of visits projected? Volume measurements, or units of service, are determined by the type of service provided. For example, in the operating room (OR), budgets are based on resources required for OR minutes; in an outpatient setting, budgets are based on resources required for a patient visit.
2. *Completing the forms:* Typically, the manager will have access to sophisticated budget software for use in preparing the cost center budget. The software includes embedded formulas that compute differential pay, premium pay, productivity, and other summary statistics, thereby reducing human error and promoting consistency across the organization. Firm due dates are assigned for the completion of this first draft of the budget. Typically, a margin target is assigned to each cost center to guide managers in preparing their first draft. The finance department then "rolls up" the unit budget into the organizational budget.
3. *Revise and resubmit:* As budget documents go through review by senior management, requests tend to exceed the available resources. This necessitates review, adjustment, and appeal. This is when competition for available resources enters the process. Managers may be asked to reduce their unit budget by a dollar percentage, leaving the question of where to cut as the manager's decision. At other times, a manager may be directed to reduce the personnel budget by a number of full-time equivalents (FTEs), thereby reducing labor expenses and addressing productivity. This is the point at which the nurse manager needs to skillfully advocate for patient care to ensure safety and quality.

The nurse manager's knowledge of clinical care processes may be in conflict with directives of a financial administrator who lacks clinical expertise. This is when nurses need to be prepared to "speak finance" to effectively respond to budget challenges. The nurse manager must be able to speak to the variable needs of a patient care budget, for example, the ability to flex up direct-care nursing (variable) staff when patient volumes surge and/or patient acuity increases and the ability to flex down nursing staff when patient volumes and acuity decrease. The nurse manager needs to be sure that budgets include adequate expenses for reasonable productive and non-patient care paid hours for all staff. Non-patient care hours include sick, vacation, holiday, family leave, jury duty, and other types of leave as well as time spent away from the patient care area in education programs or working on administrative assignments and meetings. Failure to ensure that non-patient care labor expenses are budgeted appropriately will lead to a budget bust as well as staffing difficulties and other issues related to patient care, patient outcomes, patient experience, and employee relations.

An often-overlooked aspect of the labor budget is anticipated turnover. Turnover will typically generate additional labor expenses through replacement of exiting staff with premium pay labor. In addition, expenses related to training new staff can extend through several months to a year. To this end, those areas that experience significant turnover need to focus on staying ahead of the turnover through an "over-hired" or "rightsizing" strategy. There may be multiple iterations of budget drafts before the final budget is approved.

Capital Budget Development

Capital budget preparation is usually the first step in the annual budget cycle. The organization will define a capital expense in terms of a dollar amount and the anticipated life span of the purchase. For example, capital expenditures may be "items costing over $10,000 and having a life span of 5 years." Items of this magnitude are not placed in the operating budget.

The specific process used to create a capital budget will vary from organization to organization, but most organizations require extensive background material to support capital budget requests. The background or supporting material required will probably include vendor quotes for costs of purchase, installation, staff education and training, and a justification or explanation of the reasons that the capital expenditure is needed. The justification must relate the expenditure to the organization's strategic goals or objective. For capital construction projects, architectural plans, regulatory considerations, and other supporting materials may also be required as part of the capital budget preparation process.

After each unit submits the capital expenditure list to the finance department, a compiled list is generated and typically prioritized by senior management. This is a period of intense negotiation. Given that there are rarely enough financial and/or labor resources to meet all of the requests, difficult decisions must be made.

Operating Budget Development

The *operating* budget covers a specific period, called a *fiscal year*. The fiscal year may begin July 1, may correspond to the calendar year beginning January 1, or may follow the federal government year that starts on October 1. Regardless of the fiscal year start date, the operating budget is the budget plan for day-to-day service delivery operations. It has at least two parts: the labor budget and the expense budget for costs other than labor. Expense budgets typically include consumable and non-consumable patient supplies, office supplies, pharmacy, and nutrition expenses. Use of budget software easily allows for the sharing of information regarding historical or trend data, expenses, and revenues. Typically, the revenue associated with a nursing unit reflects charges for room and board services. Room and board charges represent a bundling of hospital expenses related to patient care that are not individually billed elsewhere. Such expenses may include nursing and non-nursing labor, utilities, housekeeping, linen, and miscellaneous administrative services. All nursing service areas will adopt a unit of service measure that reflects the type of service provided. Inpatient nursing units measure patient volumes in the form of daily room and board charges or observation hourly charges. The OR measures volumes in terms of OR minutes, and ambulatory settings measure volume in terms of patient visits. Use of units of service measures comes into play when productivity analyses are conducted for budgeting, trending, benchmarking, regulatory reporting, and other purposes. The nurse manager who conducts his or her budget performance analysis referencing units of service can better represent their budget performance to hospital administration and finance. An astute manager will look for multiple ways to interpret budget performance.

The specific process used to develop operating budgets will vary considerably from one organization to another. The nurse manager's and/or nurse executive's role in developing operating budgets for nursing units and services will typically include input on or determination of volume projections, development of associated expense projections (including supplies, equipment, and salary/labor expenses), and some form of revenue projection. Many organizations develop and disseminate a set of budget assumptions that are to be used by managers and leaders in developing the operating budget. These assumptions may include such items as pre-established increases in labor or salary expenses based on contractual obligations, adjustments that must be made based on economic forecasts for supply charge changes (e.g., increased utility rates, increased cost of pharmaceuticals), or factors that will affect patient volume, such as the addition of a new service line. The nurse manager who can share benchmark comparisons, both internal and external, demonstrates greater knowledge of the impact of required resources throughout the budget process.

Projected Volume

The foundation of the development of the operating budget at the unit level is based on the projected volume of work for the coming year. The workload aspect often is measured in units of service. Key units of service need to be identified, the number of units predicted, and related expenses and staffing calculated accordingly. Activity reports such as historical census and average length of stay identify trends related to volume of activity. The unit of service often needs to be adjusted to the case or patient mix, which is a proxy for severity of illness or need (Jones et al., 2019). Given that a budget is a plan prepared several months before implementation, budget assumptions can be proven wrong throughout the budget year. In this event, budget variances—the measure between actual and budget—are often demonstrated. The successful nurse manager will know when and why budget assumptions have been incorrect and can speak to the related impact and possible adjustments required for the current and or following budget year.

Tables 22.1 and 22.2 show sample volume budget flow sheets. Historical trend data are needed (e.g., occupancy percentages by time frames such as weekly or monthly) to determine growth projections and any impact of seasonality. Table 22.1 displays volume changes on Unit X by month for 1 fiscal year, with variances clearly demonstrated. Table 22.2 shows volume changes on Unit X over 4 fiscal years, with variances rolled up to yearly values for comparison purposes. The volume of services delivered for a year may be expressed as patient days, visits, procedures, or other units of service. Effects on volume are environmental effects such as reimbursement changes, new programs, process improvements, new technology, and marketing. If volume projections depend on another service or department, it is important for the two departments to communicate closely so that similar assumptions are used in establishing volume projections.

TABLE 22.1 Volume Budget Flow Sheet

Fiscal Year Y; Volumes for Unit X

Month	Patient Days Budgeted	Patient Days Actual	Variance	% Variance
July	650	667	17	2.6%
August	668	652	−16	−2.4%
September	652	680	28	4.3%
October	667	692	25	3.7%
November	700	665	−35	−5.0%
December	752	721	−31	−4.1%
January	691	682	−9	−1.3%
February	683	692	9	1.3%
March	667	671	4	0.6%
April	665	652	−13	−2.0%
May	667	674	7	1.0%
June	673	685	12	1.8%
TOTAL	**8135**	**8133**	**22**	**0.0%**

TABLE 22.2 Volume Budget Flow Sheet

Fiscal Year Trends; Volumes for Unit X

Fiscal Year	Patient Days Budgeted	Patient Days Actual	Variance	% Variance
FY A	8021	8650	629	7.8%
FY B	8210	8689	479	5.8%
FY C	7658	7789	131	1.7%
FY D	7432	7652	220	3.0%
TOTAL	**31,321**	**32,780**	**1459**	**4.7%**

Staffing Calculation

Once the volume projection has been completed, the manager can determine the *personnel services* (or *staffing/labor budget*) portion of the expense budget. Calculation of staffing in a variable environment is complex and given that staffing expenses generally are the largest portion of the nursing operating budget, nurse managers and nurse executives need to have a consistent and well-defined approach to estimating staffing expenses. The methodology and/or terminology used will likely vary from organization to organization.

Rundio (2016) described the following method that may be used to estimate staffing expenses. For inpatient nursing units, the first step in budgeting variable staffing expenses is to know the number of planned patient days. This number can be presented on an annual basis or daily basis, known as average daily census (ADC). The next step is to determine the number of required hours, by discipline, for each patient day. For instance, based on projected patient acuity for Unit X, it is determined that each patient will require an average of 9.0 direct nursing care hours each day. This is stated as 9.0 direct registered nurse (RN) hours per patient day (HPPD). Note that this is a calculated average, not actual needs. To determine the number of FTEs required on Unit X, the nurse manager will multiply 9 hours by the projected number of patient days (8021) and find that 72,189 hours of direct RN care are required for patient care. Dividing the 72,189 hours by 2080 hours (1 FTE), the nurse manager will conclude that 34.71 direct-care RN FTEs are required to deliver safe patient care. The unit manager will next add in nonproductive time to determine the number of required budgeted RNs for Unit X. Should the manager determine that nonproductive time equals 13% per each RN FTE, the total number of "replacement" RNs equals 4.51 FTEs. Therefore, Unit X needs to budget for a total of 39.22 RN FTEs for direct patient care.

Salary Calculations

Table 22.3 displays a sample budget expense sheet for salaries based on the total unit. Similar tables can be created for subgroups, such as direct-care RNs. Table 22.4 demonstrates how personnel budgets might be displayed. Salary increases might also be included as another column. These are examples to show how data might easily be displayed as a report. Today's sophisticated budget software has reduced the effort once required for these calculations. The software will calculate salary expenses in an expeditious manner, working from historical data related to pay rates, use of premium pay, and differentials. Table 22.5 demonstrates the percentage variance when measuring actual staffing against target staffing, developed by multiplying budgeted HPPD against actual census.

TABLE 22.3 Budgeted Salary Expense Flow Sheet

Salaries and Wages: Unit X for Fiscal Year Y

	Budget	Actual	Variance	% Variance
Regular				
Overtime				
Differential				
Holiday				
Vacation				
Sick				
Education				
Administrative				
Other				
TOTAL				

TABLE 22.4 Personnel Budget Flow Sheet

Fiscal Year Y; Personnel Budget for Unit X

Position	FTE	Average Hourly Rate	Annual Salary
Unit Manager	1.0	40.00	83,200
Direct-Care RN	22.3	37.00	1,716,208
RN Education	1.0	34.00	70,720
Patient Care Tech	4.7	19.00	185,744
Unit Clerk	5.2	17.00	183,872
	34.2	31.49	2,239,744

FTE, Full-time equivalent; *RN,* registered nurse.

Supply and Revenue Budgets

Supply budgets are a major component of the operating budget. Similar to labor, many supply items are variable (the amount used will vary based on the volume of service provided). Other supply costs are fixed and will be incurred at the same level no matter the volume of service that is provided. Items such as office supplies, intravenous (IV) solutions, instruments, linens, gloves and other personal protective equipment, medical/surgical supplies, and drugs are examples of supplies that would vary with a higher volume of patient days. Leases, maintenance contracts, staff education funds for travel to conferences or meetings, and books and subscriptions are all examples of supply items that would not vary with a higher volume of patient days. Dollar amounts are assigned based on historical projections and any known or anticipated adjustments resulting from inflation, contractual increases, or other factors as specified in the organization's budgetary assumptions. The operating budget will also need to include expenses for overhead, depreciation, utilities, telecommunications services, and other related facility expenses. Finance will typically guide nurse managers in budgeting for these overhead expenses.

Revenue budgets are based on a set of calculations that determine expected receipts that will result from charging patients and payers for services. Nursing services are often not viewed as revenue-generating

TABLE 22.5 Measures of Productivity

Fiscal Year Y; Productivity for Unit X

	Budget	Actual	Variance	% Variance
Total productive hours/patient day	12.2	13.1	0.9	–7.4%
Total productive direct-care RN hours/patient day	9.0	9.2	0.2	–2.2%
Salaries and wages/patient day	621.2	643.2	21.9	–3.5%
Contract hours/day	12.0	36.0	24.0	–200.0%
Contract expenses/day	600.0	1980.0	1380.0	–230.0%
Total supplies/patient day	32.0	35.3	3.3	–10.3%

RN, registered nurse.

departments, but in many organizations the patient days and related charges are used as a proxy for revenue. Revenue projections are based on volume projections. Factors such as payer mix and contractual rates will affect the overall revenue that is received. Contractual allowances (discounts), bad debt, and indigent care all become reductions of gross revenue and generally are not under the nurse manager's control (Jones et al., 2019).

TRACKING AND MONITORING OF BUDGETS

The budget process is continual. It is not an event that occurs once a year and then ends until the next budget development process begins. Although "formal" budget development may occur once a year, the budget sets the stage for ongoing monitoring and evaluation of the organization's financial performance related to the budget projection (plan) as well as external benchmarking. Regular budget analyses (e.g., quarterly or monthly) are used for monitoring, feedback, and managerial control. The variance (difference) between budgeted and actual revenue and expenses is determined to identify problem areas, enhance control, and ensure timely adjustments. Variances between actual and budgeted (planned) performance need to be analyzed to determine the cause so that nurses and managers can take the appropriate action. Variances can be favorable or unfavorable. Most organizations now use electronic reporting formats that automatically calculate variance rates, but it is important that nurses understand the reasons for the variances. Variances can result from a single cause (e.g., volume of patients or a rate change such as salary, usage, or price) or from a combination of causes.

Nurse executives often require nurse managers to document their analysis of budget variances on a monthly basis. Many nurse managers also find it is useful to share variance reports and the reasons for budget variances at unit meetings with their nursing staff. If, for example, the overtime was 4% over the budget rate, staff can engage in discussing the reasons for this expense and perhaps how it may be managed differently in the future. It may be that acuity was very high or that there were sick calls that required nurses to "work short," resulting in overtime. This will enhance the nursing staff's awareness of the unit's financial performance. Engaging unit staff in discussions about the unit's financial performance will also provide nursing staff the opportunity to suggest cost-saving strategies to control costs at the unit level. Some managers post and present unit financial data monthly. This way, all nurses and staff better understand and can be a part of generating solutions to financial issues. Use of a dashboard tool to review monthly financial performance measures is helpful to the manager and staff. In addition to tracking of expenses and revenues, related workforce measures such as premium pay, vacancy rate, turnover, and absenteeism assist the manager in telling their story. Working together as a team, nurse managers can better understand and guide activities that influence budget development and fiscal performance.

LEADERSHIP AND MANAGEMENT IMPLICATIONS

Nursing services make up the single largest aggregate expense in most health care organizations because they represent a large personnel component and control a large share of supplies and equipment. This is both an advantage and a vulnerability. It is a strength and advantage because nurses clearly manage the organization and system, especially at the operational unit level. With powerful and accurate data and analysis support, unit-level management becomes effective and efficient. However, many organizations simply do not provide a nurse-friendly support structure.

It is a vulnerability to be the largest aggregate expense because quick, short-term economic gains can be made by ratcheting down resources allocated to nursing services. This often occurs at the expense of strategy, long-term gains, staff satisfaction, group cohesion, patient experience, quality, and safety. Because health care generally faces strict fiscal constraints, both staff nurses and nurse managers need to be knowledgeable and skilled in anticipating financial fluctuations and trends and in making bold decisions based on rapid analysis of information. Staff nurses often will be handling day-to-day budgetary decisions; thus they must be aware of the unit's budget, the financial status of the unit and the organization, and the impact of their decisions about supply and resource (staff) utilization on the financial performance of the unit. Nurse leaders are more involved with strategic or long-range financial planning and decision making, but they may track unit productivity carefully.

The budgeting process requires a broad range of leadership and management skills. Resources are limited. This fact is difficult for some nurses, especially if they believe they should be able to do everything for every patient under every circumstance. Some professionals think that their job is to provide the maximum quantity and quality of service and that cost consciousness should not be a concern of direct-care providers. Nurses are familiar with managing clinical care delivery. These skills can be transferred to the management of money as a necessary component of providing care. However, the management of any scarce resource such as money includes balancing competing interests and making difficult decisions.

Leadership is involved in influencing others to achieve the group's goals within the constraints of scarce resources. Leaders need to be actively involved in setting the vision for how to accomplish goals through budget planning. Ethical considerations such as fairness, transparency, and reasonable targets are part of leadership decision making. Leaders can influence employee morale and organizational culture through role modeling and the decision-making process. Organizational culture can be engaged to diminish negative aspects of budgeting and financial management. There is an opportunity for innovation to occur in a way that eases financial pressures. For example, with the use of data, a better schedule may be devised that deploys the same RN and assistive personnel in a new configuration that better addresses peaks and flows and the needs of patients for nursing care.

Fiscal Responsibility for Clinical Practice

Continuous change in the health care delivery and reimbursement systems has created a challenge to controlling costs while continually improving the quality of care. The programs of the Affordable Care Act, designed to improve patient care quality and control costs, utilize the expanding transformative leadership role of the staff nurse and nurse executive to guide changes in health care practice and fiscal responsibility. Today's nurse is positioned to lead fiscal responsibility and innovation through a unique skill set that includes expertise in wellness, population care, patient-centered care, care coordination, data analytics, and quality improvement (Salmond & Echevarria, 2017).

Being fiscally responsible means that the nurse manager makes responsible resource allocation decisions. Some decisions a nurse manager might need to make include the following:

- Staff time: Are there sufficient budgeted HPPD to provide quality care?
- Staff assignments: Which member of the patient care team can care for the patient in a cost-effective manner?
- Discharge planning: Is there a process in place to avoid delays in discharges to nursing homes?
- Costs of human resources: How can you evaluate workforce metrics and track the impact of turnover, onboarding, and orientation as related to the budget?
- Professional growth and development: How do you support continual growth and professional development of nursing staff across the continuum in equitable and diverse ways?

There are also multiple opportunities for staff nurse nurses to demonstrate fiscal responsibility. For a client with poor skin integrity, perhaps the most expensive tape should be used because the tape needs to stick and be waterproof. However, in a routine situation, can a lower-cost item be substituted with equal results? Nurses cannot help reduce costs unless they know the per-item cost of the supplies they use, and then use this information to evaluate substitutions. Even small cost reductions can be significant if they are applied to high-volume items. Immediately apparent is the costliness of inappropriate use of items (e.g., wiping up spills with a sterile pad; opening a sterile pack in the OR "to be ready just in case" or to use only one of the instruments). Convenience versus cost trade-off must be considered (e.g., bag baths may be convenient or necessary in a staffing shortage but are an expensive supply cost).

Evaluation of Budget Expenditures

The public is becoming increasingly knowledgeable regarding the quality and safety of health care. Health care consumers and payers expect that money for new initiatives will result in added value in terms of improved quality, safety of care, and patient experience. Business plans must include specific metrics that will be used to measure the impact of expenditures on clinical outcomes, quality, safety, and patient experience, as well as on cost. Metrics should specify the impact on nurse-sensitive indicators when feasible to further validate the significant role that nurses play in improving the health status of patients.

Costing Out Nursing Services

Accurately determining the costs of providing nursing service is an important budgetary function. Nurses need to know their costs to plan better and negotiate more effectively. Nursing has historically been seen as a cost center but not a revenue generator. One strategy proposed to compensate for nursing's revenue disparity was to cost out nursing services. This idea became popular for a while but lost attraction as capitated reimbursement systems gained prominence. With a "per member per month" flat payment structure, many felt that efforts to cost out for purposes of charging a fee for service were useless. Therefore, costing out nursing services was abandoned by some. However, the unintended consequence was that the value of knowing precisely what it costs to deliver nursing services was lost.

Costing out nursing services is defined as the determination of the costs of the services provided by nurses. By identifying the specific costs related to the delivery of nursing care to each client, nurses have data to identify the actual amount of services received. In reviews of the literature related to costing out nursing services, a variety of variables were examined, such as length of stay, nursing care costs, direct-care costs, patient acuity, and diagnosis-related group (DRG) reimbursements. Analyses of cost data continue to expand in correlation with increasing sophistication of related software products. Understanding costs through data and measurements allows leaders to achieve improved productivity for both variable and fixed expenses. Today's sophisticated software products provide data that ultimately links costs to patient acuity, scheduling and staffing, volumes, supply management, workforce management, care delivery decisions, and other benchmarking metrics (Bannow, 2019).

The process of costing out nursing services provides data for productivity comparisons. Activity-based costing (ABC) is one approach to service costing that may be useful in multiple settings. The key advantage of ABC is that it reflects what it costs to provide services and identifies why costs were incurred. The first step in ABC is to identify all the cost drivers associated with a specific service. For example, if the service is a preschool physical examination provided by a nurse practitioner, here are some potential costs associated with the service:

- Nursing assistant (NA): 5 minutes to room the patient and 5 minutes to clean the room after the visit. The NA is paid $15 per hour with a 35% benefit rate and works 52 weeks per year, 40 hours per week. The cost of the NA time is $31,200 + $10,920 = $42,120/2080 (number of hours in a year), for an hourly cost of $20.25, or $20.25/60, $0.3375 per minute or $1.69 cost per visit.
- One-half hour of NP time: The nurse is paid $86,000 per year and associated benefits at 35% ($30,100); the NP works 52 weeks (40 hours per week) per year. The cost of the time of the NP is ($116,100/2080) = $55.86 cost per hour or $27.91 cost per NP time.
- All other costs are identified in the same manner: equipment, such as stethoscope, tongue depressor, and linens on examination table; cost of electronic health record (EHR); costs of a billing clerk.

Once this process is completed, the costs are aggregated, yielding what it costs to provide one unit of one nursing service—providing a preschool physical examination. The next step is to assign activities to cost centers, service lines, or programs. In the previous example, the cost of the service may be placed in a pediatric well-child clinic program.

A more sophisticated and rapidly expanding approach to collecting nursing's cost data is using *acuity*, or patient classification systems. The premise is that nursing care needs to be based on patients' actual needs for care, not on historical allocation of nursing time. *Acuity* is defined as a measure of the severity of illness of an individual patient or the aggregate patient population on a unit. The acuity of patients has increased dramatically in the past 10 to 15 years. Formerly, patients were admitted for diagnostic tests and for additional preparation before surgery. They typically remained in the hospital until they were able to care for themselves, often through a lengthy convalescence. A nurse was able to provide care to larger numbers of these patients because they required less care, assessment, and monitoring. Today, these patients are receiving care in other settings and only very ill patients remain in the hospital. Utilization review experts have stated that the only reason a patient is in the hospital is because they need monitoring and assessment by an RN. If these skills are not needed, patients can probably be safely cared for in a less expensive setting. The increased acuity seen today decreases the number of patients for whom a nurse may safely provide care. This results in what might look like (on paper) a decrease in productivity. Any measure of the productivity of nursing staff that does not consider the acuity level of patients is seriously flawed and would probably result in a gross underestimation of the output. Nurse executives reflect that patient acuity increases year after year, creating increased demand for additional direct-care RNs.

Many of the classifications share a similar approach to the determination of the workload based on the required hours of nursing care. This is intuitively attractive because it can be assumed that a ventilator-dependent patient in an intensive care unit (ICU) will require more care than a patient who has had a total knee replacement. If the nurse manager uses a classification system whereby, for example, type 1 patients receive 2 to 4 hours of nursing care per day and type 2 patients receive 5 to 8 hours per day, these data can be used in constructing a personnel budget when it is linked to the volume indicator of patient days. If the nurse manager predicts that the unit will provide 800 days of type 1 patients, this information can be used to predict the staffing requirements for that patient group. Multiple commercial patient classifications systems are available for purchase. Some involve entering nurse-collected patient data in a software program, yet increasingly this information can be extracted from electronic medical records to calculate objective scores for acuity. One caveat to this process is that, when used to create staffing ratios, the judgment of an expert nurse clinician must override an empirical system and be based on patients' needs in real time.

Various approaches are used to determine this acuity level and then relate it to staffing needs. Patient classification software is available from vendors. These systems attempt to categorize the levels of nursing care required by patients and then project appropriate nursing and ancillary staff. Some of these may be expensive to purchase and then modified to meet the needs of a specific hospital; they may also be costly to install and maintain. Critics argue that such systems cannot capture the invisible knowledge work of nursing. The systems often inadequately adjust for the experience level and varied expertise of RNs, such as a new graduate versus an experienced senior nurse.

In general, too little effort has been devoted to isolating actual nursing costs and determining the costs of nursing and the provision of care. With actual data, nurses are in a better position to demonstrate the economic value of their service, and nurse managers will have appropriate information with which to accurately manage nursing services.

PRODUCTIVITY

Understanding the concept of productivity and relating it to the management of professional nursing is a leadership skill that will serve nursing in an era of accelerating health care expenditures. Based on this understanding, the nurse manager will be able to determine the costs associated with providing nursing care. Productivity is defined as the relationship between output and the goods and services used to produce them.

Measures of Productivity

Various measures of productivity exist, but all involve relationships between volume of inputs and cost. Nurses' time is the critical input in the production of nursing care. Home health agencies measure their productivity in patient home visits and hours of care, hospitals measure patient days, and clinics measure the number of patient visits. The cost measure is the cost of the nursing time required to produce this care. Table 22.5 displays some productivity measures that track and benchmark unit performance and assist the unit manager in presenting unit-related fiscal outcomes to nurse executives and hospital leadership.

The oldest method of measuring nursing productivity is the analysis of HPPD. The input is the nursing hours worked. The number of hospitalized patient days is the output. This index is imprecise because of the wide variation in patient acuity, with the result that the measure of patient days is not equivalent across cases. Patient "churn" further complicates this calculation. The number of heads in a bed at midnight (midnight census) is often less than what is seen at noon or 4 pm. Table 22.6 shows staffing variance calculations, measuring actual staffing against budgeted staffing based on actual census.

A variety of data sources and productivity indices can also be considered. In nursing, productivity has been tightly linked to staffing numbers. For example, staffing—calculated as the total number of hours of a given staff for a given time period—can be compared with patient volume or census. Using this method, if the output (patient days) increased while staffing remained the same, then strictly speaking the productivity would be increased. This typically happens in hospitals, for example, when the influenza season is severe and a large number of geriatric patients are admitted to the hospital. In this short-term staffing crisis, the same numbers of staff are available to care for the high census, and productivity temporarily increases. However, the gains may be short lived in that the short-staffing situation may result in nurse burnout, overtime, and resignations. To this end, during the budget process, it is important that the nurse executive advocate for expenses to fund a flexible workforce (as needed, float pool, overtime, and contract staff). Some organizations track productivity and quickly adjust for when it is both too high and too low.

No one measure of productivity adequately captures the knowledge-based work of nursing. Productivity measurement is complex for several reasons. The causal linkages between nursing interventions and patient outcomes are not always well established. There is little research that addresses economic efficiency—that is, what is the least cost combination of inputs required to produce an outcome.

Enhancing the productivity of nurses while protecting the quality of patient care will continue to be a major challenge for nurse leaders. As outcomes research continues, the nurse executive needs to share this information with hospital leadership to support increased nursing expenses.

CURRENT ISSUES AND TRENDS

Evaluation of Budget Expenditures

The public is becoming increasingly knowledgeable regarding the quality and safety of health care. Health care consumers and payers expect that money for new initiatives will be well invested and that a significant return on investment will be realized in terms of improved quality or safety of care. Business plans must include specific metrics that will be used to measure the impact of expenditures on clinical outcomes, quality, safety, and cost. Metrics should specify the impact on nurse-sensitive indicators when feasible to further validate the significant role that nurses play in improving the health status of patients.

TABLE 22.6 Staffing Variance

Bud HPPD	Act Census	Target Hrs/Day	Target RNs/Day	Act RNs/Day	Staffing Variance
11.86	29	343.9	14.3	26	−81%
11.86	34	403.2	16.8	36	−114%
9.1	49	445.9	18.6	39	−110%
9.1	54	491.4	20.5	38	−86%

HPPD, hour per patient day; *RN*, registered nurse.

Nurse Workforce Participation

The continuing nurse shortage and related nurse workforce participation issues carry ramifications for budgeting and financial management. Two trends to watch are nurses nearing retirement and the educational capacity available for the nurse workforce. The concern is with the number of projected nurses retiring, although to date the projections have not been realized, possibly due to economic pressures. However, it appears to be a matter of time.

For replacement prospects, the job of an RN is attractive for its employment potential. The Bureau of Labor Statistics (2015) noted the positive job outlook for RNs: "Employment of registered nurses is projected to grow 16% from 2014 to 2024, much faster than the average for all occupations. Growth will occur for a number of reasons, including an increased emphasis on preventive care; growing rates of chronic conditions, such as diabetes and obesity; and demand for health care services from the baby-boom population, as they live longer and more active lives."

Educational capacity is a concern due to the finite number of slots in schools and colleges of nursing plus an even more severe nurse faculty shortage, which limits student capacity. The age of nursing faculty is an acute issue due to impending retirements. Strategies are needed to address the nurse faculty shortage.

It is possible that increased use of technology will be a partial solution to increasing nursing productivity. Computerized documentation and medication administration systems are widespread applications of technology that have resulted in time savings and subsequent increased productivity for nurses. Information technology is another enhancement to nurses' productivity. Medical records are easily accessed from multiple sites, results of diagnostics tests are communicated instantly, and monitoring devices detect deviations from normal limits and communicate these to the nurse as they occur. However, as the EHR captures key nursing data related to quality, safety, staffing, patient engagement, and satisfaction, it must do so in concert with the nursing process in order to avoid stress burnout and "death by data entry" (O'Brien et al., 2015).

Another responsibility of nurse leaders related to productivity is ensuring a future workforce by participating in the recruitment of future nurses. One conference speaker reported that as a colleague leaves her home for work each day, she tells her young children, "Mom is going to go to the hospital to save lives today." Although nursing does not *always* offer that level of drama, it certainly speaks of the importance of the work that nurses do. That importance needs to be communicated to the pool of potential nurses.

Integration of Economics in Clinical Practice

The incorporation of economic evaluation in clinical practice is important to productivity because health care resources are limited and choices must—and will—be made. In the years preceding managed care, health care providers acted as if health care resources were infinite, with the result that health care costs spun out of control. Today, providers are faced with difficult decisions about "who gets what." Although rationing health care is inherently unacceptable to most of the US population, it is true that rationing is occurring. Currently, rationing is done based on the ability to pay for health care, with the uninsured receiving less health care. Well-educated nurse leaders who understand economics and finance are in a unique position to bring the values of nursing to decision making about the allocation of health care resources.

Nurses are able to tap into their full skill set to assess, educate, intervene, and evaluate the care they provide to increasing numbers of patients. Care providers are evaluated in their ability to provide efficient and quality care, and their reimbursements are directly related to their ability to demonstrate best practices. Their results are compared with others, and performance that varies from agreed-on outcomes will not be reimbursed. This means nurses are encountering more patients than ever before, but the reimbursement for these services is negotiated and often times less than in the past.

Simply put, nurses need to commit to continued learning and professional development over the course of their careers, seek collaborative and productive partnerships with all members of the provider team and beyond with members of the community at large, and become increasingly comfortable using data to measure outcomes, demonstrate achievements, and drive improvements across the continuum.

RESEARCH NOTE

Source

DiMattio, M. J. K., & Spegman, A. M. (2019, April 30). Educational preparation and nurse turnover intention from the hospital bedside. *OJIN: The Online Journal of Issues in Nursing, 24*(2). https://doi.org/DOI:10.3912/OJIN.Vol-24No02PPT22.

Purpose

Although there is a lot of evidence about why nurses leave their jobs, there has been little clear understanding about turnover from the hospital bedside as a specific setting for practice. The purpose of this article was to examine the relationship between educational preparation and turnover intent, defined as intention to leave the hospital bedside as a practice setting, and gain a better understanding of the relationship between registered nurse (RN) educational preparation and turnover intentions.

Method

Data were obtained from a larger study of career trajectories of nurses at an integrated health system in Pennsylvania focusing only on direct patient care nurses. A cross-sectional, comparative design using a non-probability sample of 424 RNs who identified their primary work setting to be at the point of care was used. Study measures included turnover intent, educational preparation, clinical expertise, years of experience, and practice environment. Results showed that having a baccalaureate degree or more and current enrollment in school independently predicted turnover intention from the hospital bedside as a practice setting. Hospitals with a higher percentage of Bachelor of Science in Nursing prepared nurses might unwittingly set themselves up for turnover.

Discussion

Turnover of baccalaureate nurses negatively impacts both safe patient care and hospital costs. Staff churn, inadequate staffing, decreased continuity of care, and adverse events are attributed to RN turnover. Documented nurse satisfaction scores among this group of highly educated direct patient care nurses trends higher as a reflection of "hard" work and exhaustion experienced. The need for nurses in expanded roles provides an incentive for career advancement, and it has been reported that nurses seek to advance their education as a means to leave or "escape" the hospital bedside. In light of career mobility available to the higher educated staff nurses and the associated costs of nurse turnover, researchers have suggested that the employment of associate degree nurses may produce a more consistent and less expensive RN workforce. Current patterns indicate that hospitals are training newly graduated baccalaureate nurses who have the intention of leaving that organization once they master certain bedside skills. The authors advocated for deliberate and intentional re-envisioning of the acute care hospital setting as one specialty among others with commensurate hiring practices, recognition, and advancement opportunities that include salary adjustments as a way to retain these nurses. It is suggested that future research focus on the impact of turnover when more advancement and educational opportunities are available, thus allowing the nurse to become a specialist.

Application to Practice

To support safe patient care through decreasing baccalaureate RN turnover, nurse leaders need to creatively re-envision bedside direct care nursing as a specialty. This includes recognizing nurses as human capital needing advanced education to meet the complexity and critical thinking needed in clinical care.

CASE STUDY

Medical Center A has a 47-bed intensive care unit (ICU) budgeted for an average daily census (ADC) of 35.2, with nursing hours per patient day (HPPD) of 21.5. Based on historical experience, budgeted patient days were spread in a bell shaped curve with "high census" months, November through February (fiscal year months 5 through 8), budgeted at an ADC of 45. The budgeted ADC for non-peak months averaged 22 to 35. Three months into the fiscal year, the ICU was experiencing a consistently strong ADC of 35, with many days reaching peak ADC levels of 40 and above.

As the unit's variable workforce is budgeted to meet average budgeted volumes, it is expected and planned that premium pay staff will be used during budgeted high census months. Unfortunately, those early months in the fiscal year, not budgeted at peak volumes, used up increasing amounts of premium pay labor to meet the experienced census levels of 40 and above.

CASE STUDY—cont'd

Since early in the fiscal year, unit and nursing leaders have been managing the increasing workforce needs in the ICU through multiple measures, such as floating nurses from other critical care units, deploying large numbers of float pool nurses to the intensive care unit, using contract nursing assignments, use of an extra shift bonus, and use of overtime pay. Unfortunately, the income from operations for the ICU has been marginalized at the per-unit of service level. During the early months of the fiscal year, the levels of premium pay required to meet patient care needs were not placed in the budget based on the lower patient day volumes. Although the ICU is aggressively hiring and onboarding new nurses, the time required for these activities coupled with normal attrition cannot fully solve staffing needs. At present, the unit is limited to hiring at budgeted levels only.

1. How many additional nurses above budget are required to meet actual patient levels experienced during the first 4 months of the fiscal year? How many additional nurses above budget are required to meet budgeted patient levels during the time period of November through March?
2. As Chief Nursing Officer, what information and metrics would you share with finance to support the need for increased nurses in the intensive care unit? If you were granted an "ask," how many nurses would you ask to hire outside of the budget?
3. To onboard additional nurses, what plans, programs, and strategies do you need to develop and implement in order to achieve your workforce goals?

CRITICAL THINKING EXERCISE

As manager of the Surgical Care Unit (SCU), Ms. Dawson has identified a trending increase in unit-related RN patient care staffing challenges, which are correlating with changing patterns in patient case mix. To this end, Ms. Dawson has shared with the nursing leadership team that several new surgical care attending physicians have joined the organization over the past nine months. These surgeons, national experts in colorectal and pelvic reconstruction and orthopedic specialties, such as spinal infusions, are adding new and expanded service lines to the organization.

Although the SCU has not experienced an RN shortage in over 3 years, Ms. Dawson is preparing a review of the SCU's budgeted hours per patient day, with the goal of demonstrating a need for an increase in budgeted nursing hours during the next budget cycle.

1. What guiding principles should frame the review?
2. What are the key components and metrics Ms. Dawson should address in her review?
3. What external benchmarks would help support Ms. Dawson's position? Please explain.
4. What financial outcomes/measures would interest the chief finance officer?
5. Should the SCU not receive increased nursing hours in the next budget year, what would be Ms. Dawson's next steps?

REFERENCES

Bannow, T. (2019). More hospitals calculating actual cost of care. *Modern healthcare*. May 18. https://www.modernhealthcare.com/finance/more-hospitals-calculating-actual-cost-care.

Bureau of Labor Statistics. (2015). *Occupational outlook handbook: Registered nurses*. https://www.bls.gov/ooh/healthcare/registered-nurses.htm.

Centers for Medicare & Medicaid Services (CMS). (2019). *National Health Expenditure Fact Sheet 2018–2027*. Centers for Medicare & Medicaid Services (CMS.Gov). cms.gov/Research-Statistics-Data-and-Systems/Statistics-Trends-and-Reports/NationalHealthExpendData/NHE-Fact-Sheet.

Gander, K. (2018, December 27). Hospital prices: Full cost lists must be published from January 1, new federal rule says. *Newsweek*. https://www.newsweek.com/end-hidden-costs-january-1st-all-us-hospitals-must-publish-price-lists-all-1272328.

Jones, C., Finkler, S. A., Kovner, C. T., & Mose, J. (2019). *Financial management for nurse managers and executives*. Amsterdam, NL: Elsevier, Inc. E-Book on Vital Source.

Nurses First Solutions. (2018, January 20). https://nursesfirstsolutions.com/patient-and-staff-satisfaction-on-a-budget/.

O'Brien, A., Weaver, C., Settergren, T., Hook, M., & Ivory, C. (2015). EHR documentation: The hype and the hope for improving nursing satisfaction and quality outcomes. *Nursing Administration Quarterly*, *39*(4), 333–339.

Rundio, A. (2016). *The nurse managers guide to budgeting & finance*. Indianapolis, IN: Sigma Theta Tau International.

Salmond, S., & Echevarria, M. (2017). Healthcare transformation and changing roles for nursing. *Orthopedic Nursing*, *36*(1), 12–25.

Viviano, J. (2019, January 7). Hospitals post prices online to meet federal requirement. *The Columbus Dispatch*. https://www.dispatch.com/news/20190107/hospitals-post-prices-online-to-meet-federal-requirement.

23

Performance Appraisal

Barbara Seifert

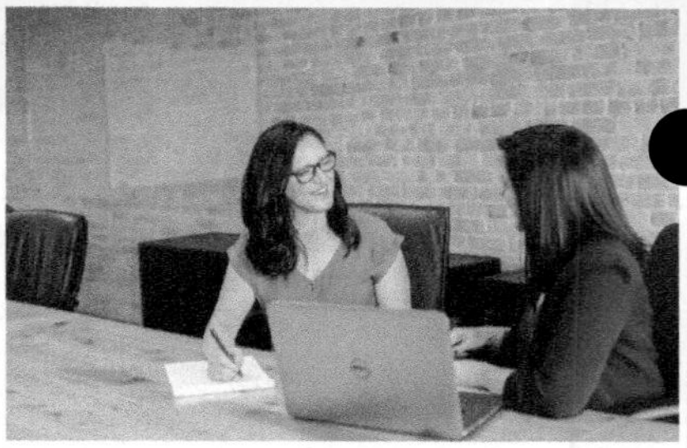

http://evolve.elsevier.com/Huber/leadership

Insight into one's job performance is a critical component of not only keeping that job, but also for job satisfaction and promotional opportunities. The way to ensure that a nurse's performance is meeting, or exceeding, organizational standards, is through performance appraisal, which is a function of human resource management (HRM) systems. Appraisals guide managerial and administrative decisions that affect staffing and ensure competency for patient care standards, which are tied to organizational goals.

The purpose of an appraisal is to evaluate and improve the employee's performance, which in turn will enhance organizational effectiveness. Nursing leadership is in charge of guiding this process. In this chapter, the appraisal process, approaches to performance appraisals, developmental approaches to drive performance, and organizational goals will be discussed.

DEFINITIONS

In order to understand the concept of performance management, it is necessary to know the various meanings that underlie it.

360 review: A formal process whereby employees receive feedback on their behavior or outcomes from various individuals they regularly interact with. It is useful to assess individual, department, or team performance (360pev.com, 2013).

Coaching: A means of "partnering with clients in a thought-provoking and creative process that inspires them to maximize their personal and professional potential" (International Coach Federation, n.d.).

Feedback: "Information about reactions to a product or a person's performance of a task, which is used as a basis for improvement" (Lexico Dictionary, n.d.).

Peer-review: "The process by which practicing registered nurses systematically access, monitor, and make judgments about the quality of nursing care provided by peers as measured against professional standards of practice.... Peer review implies that the nursing care delivered by a group of nurses or an individual nurse is evaluated by individuals of the same rank or standing according to established standards of practice" (Haag-Heitman & George, 2011).

Performance: The accomplishment of a specific action; it is getting people to do the things we ask them to in a way that contributes to the goals of the business (Benedictine University, n.d.).

Performance appraisals: The process through which supervisors assess, after the fact, the job-related performance of their supervisees and allocate rewards to the supervisees based on that assessment (Capelli & Conyon, 2018); "the systematic evaluation of the performance of employees and to understand the abilities of a person for further growth and development" (Juneja, 2020).

Performance improvement plan (PIP): A formal performance action plan that is used as a tool to facilitate conversation in the form of constructive discussion between staff members and their managers or supervisors in order to clarify work performance and needed improvements (Heathfield, 2016). A PIP outlines specific goals to work towards, specific improvement steps to take, and specific time frames for improvements to be made.

Performance management: "A wide variety of activities, policies, procedures, and interventions designed to help employees to improve their performance. These programs begin with performance appraisals but also include feedback, goal setting, and training, as well as reward systems" (DeNisi & Murphy, 2017, p. 421).

Performance management systems/human resource information systems (HRIS): A software or online solution that is used for data entry, data tracking, and data management of all human resources (HR) operations of an organization, which aids in effective HRM and planning (Ghosh, 2019).

Self-evaluation: The aspect of performance appraisal whereby employees are asked to do their own evaluation of their job performance, which includes "evaluating progress towards pre-defined annual objectives and performance standards" (Performance-appraisals.org, 2018).

PURPOSE OF PERFORMANCE APPRAISALS

Administrative

Performance appraisals serve several administrative functions to meet compliance standards and organizational goals. These functions include helping to strengthen the appraisal process, improving employee performance, meeting compliance standards, and assisting with HR workforce planning, such as recruiting, compensation, and succession planning (Iqbal, 2017). HR can work in conjunction with administration to develop competencies and standards that lead to fair and effective evaluation with compensation tied to them. Appraisals help the nurse manager in updating personnel records and making decisions on staffing, including hiring, scheduling, promotions, or terminations. Another function is to assist with the culture, or "positive organizational climate, in which problems and grievances can be easily detected and handled" which leads to fairness and employee satisfaction" (Iqbal, 2017, p. 49).

Another administrative function of performance appraisal is that they function as psychological contracts, which is an unwritten agreement between employees and the organization (Geise & Thiel, 2015). This contract sets expectations for what the employer will provide, such as fair treatment, acceptable working conditions, and feedback on their job performance. As a result, employee expectations are to "demonstrate a good attitude, follow directions, and show loyalty to the organization" (Robbins & Judge, 2018, p. 140). Performance appraisals are a way to ensure that these unwritten expectations are carried out by the manager and employee.

Measurement

A second purpose for performance appraisals is to evaluate an employee's performance, which is done through various types of measurement standards. This helps the manager to determine if performance goals are met or if further development of the employee needs to be implemented. Performance measures should be tied to job duties and roles as well as to departmental and organizational goals. For example, a hospital that is working to win a Joint Commission Certification for Disease Management in Orthopedics, which sets standards and expectations for providing reliable care (The Joint Commission, n.d.), would have measurements that address pre-and post-operative care and how the nurse meets those standards to provide excellent, quality patient care. Processes such as these can determine if the measures are valid and reliable and actually measuring what they were intended to do.

Development

Employee development is a necessity from both the employee and employer. A worker can become complacent in their skills and duties, which can affect patient care and liability; the organization is able to identify and plan for developmental needs, such as training, certifications, or other resources to aid in employee development.

An appraisal allows for an employee to see their work from an external perspective, which they may not often see. An appraisal is a first step in ensuring legal compliance. Through observational feedback, the manager can make recommendations to advance the employee, such as by sending them to classes or for certifications that would build on their skills and lead to higher performance. It also allows for identification of potential leadership opportunities. However, when deficits are identified, it gives both the manager and the employee the ability to come up with a plan for improving either skills, behaviors, and/or attitudes. It also provides the manager with the opportunity to ensure formal documentation for employee improvements or hard decisions, such as by termination.

Relationships

Performance appraisal involves providing feedback to the employee (i.e., nursing staff) about their performance, with the intent of recognizing achievements and offer developmental opportunities. Therefore, the appraisal should not do harm to the relationship between the nurse manager and nursing staff. Research has shown that trust is an essential factor to moderate a positive relationship when providing feedback and leads to a positive interaction and feedback acceptance, with the belief that performance was accurately characterized. When specific feedback is provided, it moderates a positive relationship with trust and feedback acceptance which, in turn, leads to greater job satisfaction and involvement (Moon, 2019). The appraisal process should be conveyed as an open, positive experience by the manager. "Managers who take time outside of the formal performance appraisal process to seek common ground, practice reciprocity, understand their employees and provide informal feedback will develop trust and support that will enhance workforce productivity" (Teckchandani & Pichler, 2015, p. 16).

ISSUES IN PERFORMANCE MANAGEMENT

A long-held focus, by both researchers and HR practitioners, is the accuracy and measurements used in performance appraisals. Are they valid? Do they reflect actual performance? These questions will be addressed in this section.

What Is Being Measured in the Performance Appraisal?

Traits

Traits are characteristics that one possesses, such as initiative or work ethic. The Big Five Model is a highly recognized tool to identify five basic dimensions of one's personality. They are a predictor for how one behaves in a variety of situations and the stability of those behaviors. The five dimensions include: conscientiousness, emotional stability, extraversion, openness to experiences, and agreeableness (Robbins & Judge, 2018, p. 67). This rating scale has positive relationships with both empathy and ethical decision-making. Other traits that may be rated include decision-making, ability to resolve conflict, or time management. Trait resilience is the ability to handle high levels of stress; individuals who possess this type of resiliency have been shown to handle higher workloads to either exceed standards and are aware of monetary and promotional results, as well as to avoid any negative consequences, such as discipline or termination.

Critics of trait models are against the use of these types of assessments as they may not be reflective of the worker as it puts them in a category that may not necessarily be accurate. Trait studies have been inconclusive in demonstrating whether trait results are actually indicative of performance. For instance, extroverts are often seen as leaders, due to their outgoing nature, but this does not always translate to effectiveness in a leader role, as some studies show that introverts are just as capable because they tend to think before reacting (Farrell, 2017).

Another issue with using a trait model is the rater's interpretation of the meanings of them, making them subjective in nature. One nurse might rate Agreeableness as a 2 if they had a conflict with that nurse, while another might give a rating of 5 if their interactions were positive. Although raters can be trained in trait assessments as to its meaning, there still can be misunderstanding and confusion as to how traits translate to performance.

Behaviors

Behaviors are more easily tied to performance appraisals when they are observable, thus reducing the subjectivity found in trait models. Employees are rated either by the frequency or the quantity of specific work actions. Examples include exhibits positive interactions with coworkers or patient's family members, willingness to stay to help the team, and responds to patient concerns in a timely manner. There are several means to formulate a behavioral rating; these can vary from a simple checklist or rating scale, based on 1–5 scale for each behavior, to structured assessments, such as the Behavioral Observation Scale (BOS) (Latham & Wexley, 1977) or the Behavioral Expectation Scale, also known as the Behaviorally Anchored Rating Scale (BARS) (Smith & Kendall, 1963).

Although researchers show that behavior models hold more validity than using traits, there are still some problems that can occur in their use. Behaviors are observable, yet the rater may not see every behavior an employee has, thus it can skew their assessment. It can lead the rater to rely on specific observations or from opinions of others. Another issue with this type of rating is that behaviors can change over time, thus requiring the evaluations to change and increase in their frequency. This can be confusing, costly, and time consuming for managers and staff.

Competencies

Competency-based models are commonly used in appraisals today. Schub (2014) defined competencies as the ability to perform a task based on clinical skills, knowledge, education, and experience. Competencies relate to demonstrating skills, knowledge, and abilities that enable and improve the efficiency of job performance. The focus is on behaviors and how they relate to a job task. Competencies should be evaluated regularly to assess and maintain the nurse's skills to achieve the best patient outcomes and within their scope of practice. Some examples of competencies are conducting a patient assessment, medication management, or proper hygiene procedures.

Competency assessments should relate back to specific behaviors of the job and be tied to goals of the department and the organization. There are nursing bodies that have developed competency-based assessments, such as the American Nurses Association (ANA), Association for Rehab Nurses (ARN), and National League for Nurses (NLN). States can independently develop their own nursing competences, such as the Massachusetts Nurse of the Future Core Competencies. Massachusetts core competencies is behaviorally based. It relies on individual perception by the rater, which can leave room for interpretation and bias.

Results

Results-based measures can be used to reduce any bias that may occur during the performance evaluation. The focus is on what is to be accomplished on the job versus observing traits or on-the-job behaviors. The focus is recognizing both quantitative and qualitative outcomes as it relates to the nurse's performance. These outcomes may result in compensation based on goal attainment. Robbins and Judge (2018) based this type of evaluation on the work of Peter Drucker (1954) and his Management by Objectives (MBO), which bases performance on set goals that are "tangible, verifiable, and measurable" (Drucker, 1954, as cited in Robbins & Judge, 2018, p. 107). Since results-based measures have clear objectives and outcomes, the nurse can work to fulfill these goals.

This method has its flaws. Due to its focus on goals, it can miss many other performance indicators or leave an employee only focusing on reaching the goals of results-based measures. This may cause employees to neglect other parts of their work, sometimes causing them to seem ineffective. This focus may lead to unrealistic expectations on all sides as to what can actually be accomplished. In addition, there may be circumstances that can occur outside of the scope of the nurse that may have an impact on their actual performance, such as if the pharmacy is taking too long to deliver a patient's medication (Weirks, 2007).

Which Performance Measurement Should be Used?

There is no uniform measure for performance appraisals. Each is developed based on an organization's needs. A tiered rating standard is utilized, either by a Likert scale of 1–5, or ratings of Meets Standards, Exceeds Standards, or Does Not Meet Standards. The intent is two-fold: (1) to review past employee performance, and (2) set a direction for future performance and development. Usually, a past appraisal is used to determine the progress on goals and improvements.

Rating Accuracy: Can We Measure It Accurately?

The question arises whether performance reviews are accurate in assessing performance and a person's abilities and effectiveness in their job role. There has been much research done to perfect the system, but problems still exist.

Rater Bias

Rater bias is an error in judgment when the rater uses their predetermined judgments and biases to affect their evaluation and decisions related to an employee. This is a big factor in ensuring accurate measurements. Bernardin et al. (2016, p. 325-325) found that: "a managers attributes may affect the importance attached to the various goals that can be pursued in the context of performance appraisal activities and that the relative importance raters assign to these various goals may in

TABLE 23.1 Definitions of Rater Bias Types

Rater Bias Term Definition
• **Central tendency:** The rater does not want to give too high a score, believe anyone merits the highest score, or want to be too strict and give a low score, so everyone is rated in the middle, or "average."
• **Contrast effect:** The rater bases their score on comparison with another employee, either overvaluing or undervaluing.
• **Halo effect:** The rater focuses only on a positive experience and rates all areas based on that measure.
• **Horns effect:** The rater focuses on a negative experience and rates on that measure
• **Leniency:** Ratings are higher than the employee deserves.
• **Recency of events error:** The rater considers only more recent events, rather than what occurred since the last evaluation period.
• **Severity, or strictness:** Awarding lower ratings than the employee deserves.
• **Similar to me:** The rater scores more highly those who are like them, such as gender, age, race, personality.

Reiken, J. (2018). *8 Rater biases that are affecting your performance management.* Trakstar https://www.trakstar.com/blog-post/8-rater-biases-impacting-performance-management/.

turn affect the levels of performance appraisal competencies manages develop and sustain".

This affirms that rater bias does occur, which is subjective to each rater. Some common types of rater bias are presented in Table 23.1.

The performance appraisal system should include rater training. This will help to mitigate and/or avoid biases, provide oversight by managers, and give accountability to the rater to ensure they are using fair practices in the evaluation. Rater training has been shown to increase a rater's understanding of the evaluation process, including potential biases, leading to more accurate performance assessments (Sanchez et al., 2019).

Political Motivations

Political motivations or influencing occurs with particular individuals or groups and does exist in the performance evaluation process (Dello Russo et al., 2017). This can include envy of another's occupational status or accomplishments (Henniger, 2016), personal feelings of affection for a favorite employee, or affinity bias (Include-empower.com, 2018). The opposite is also true, namely, to "punish" a difficult employee, or for financial compensation.

Larsen (2019) found that political motivations are intentional to favor one person or group, either positively or negatively, which leads to inaccuracies that may or may not be reflective of the nurse's performance. Rater training enhances the knowledge and understanding of performance measures and lessens the risk of any adverse motivations that may affect a fair evaluation. More research must be done in this area to examine raters' use of political motivation.

Who Should Do the Rating?

The manager is responsible for evaluation and providing feedback on results. There have been improvements in recent years to involve others in the process. As the possibility for bias exists with a manager's rating, having the input from others is now becoming more the norm. Peer review and 360-degree feedback are two common techniques.

Peer-Reviewed

Many health care systems use a peer-review system to evaluate their staff. This can take the form of one-to-one review or with a panel. A peer review may involve observations or a skills test. The format involves feedback from peers regarding skills, performance, attitude, and competencies. The benefits of this format are that it can give the manager a more well-rounded view of the employee's strengths and challenges. The feedback will be used toward employee development such as training, competency acquisition, or building on their strengths.

A peer-review system can help provide feedback to individuals with high potential who do not seek recognition. However, these systems may have a negative effect. Peers may provide biased ratings, depending on their relationships with each other.

If employees receive negative feedback or strong criticism from the appraiser, an employee's relationship with their employer is more likely to be impacted. Employees might become reluctant to forge new working relationships, collaborate with colleagues, and might feel the pressure to provide feedback based on a group's consensus (Steele, n.d.). Negative reviews can also lead an employee to "adjust their roles to be around people who will give them more-positive reviews" (Berinato, 2018, p. 1). Worrying about potential feedback can increase stress levels of staff and have a detrimental result on performance, productivity, and team cohesion.

360-Degree Feedback

The 360-Degree Feedback is a tool that more organizations are beginning to use in the performance appraisal process. It has long been used for leadership development but is now becoming more popular as a tool for all employee levels in recent years. This appraisal involves multiple individuals who interact with the employee, specifically, the supervisor, peers, patients, families, staff from other departments, and outside vendors. The employee also completes a self-assessment (Chopra, 2017). The results are then discussed, and feedback is provided to compare and contrast results. This type of feedback provides a more rounded view of the employee, which does reduce bias to some extent.

There are both benefits and limitations to the 360-degree appraisal. Some limitations include expenses, timeliness, and the involvement of multiple people. Other issues may include raters having other duties, raters rushing through the evaluation to get it done quickly, raters able to over-or underinflate their results. When employees get to choose who is involved in the evaluation, bias can occur. Benefits of a 360 are that they give a more-rounded view of the employee because data are from multiple sources. In addition, (1) it gives the employee more recognition and validation of their duties, which can raise their confidence in their role; (2) it increases accountability to raise performance; (3) it promotes continuous improvement; and (4) it can change the culture through openness, accountability, and empowerment for role responsibility and professional development (Chopra, 2017).

DEVELOPING EMPLOYEES THROUGH THE PERFORMANCE APPRAISAL AND REVIEW

The Manager as Coach

The use of coaching by organizations is becoming more common, with the manager taking the role of the coach, where managers "give support and guidance rather than instructions, and employees learn how to adapt to constantly changing environments in ways that unleash fresh energy, innovation, and commitment" (Ibarra & Scoular, 2019, para 3). Managerial coaching can be described as empowering employees to exceed their performance and providing the tools and resources that allows them to do so (Ladyshewsky & Taplin, 2018).

Coaching has been found to raise self-awareness, self-confidence, and self-leadership while positively facilitating relationships with others. According to the International Coach Federation (ICF), 80% of those who received coaching reported an increase in self-confidence with 70% reported improved work performance and more effective communication skills. Organizations would benefit from training managers on the use of coaching as a leadership strategy (Institute of Coaching, n.d.).

Performance Improvement Plans

What happens if a nurse is not performing up to standards or has a critical incident that is averse to patient care or the team? A PIP is the first step to take before any major consequences occur, such as termination. The PIP gives the manager the opportunity to correct any actions in a formalized manner, as it is a tool that provides the opportunity for the nurse to make performance corrections. It should be used to help the employee improve and is not to be used as a punitive measure. It does not always mean that a termination is imminent, but it is the first step if it does occur (Society for Human Resource Management [SHRM], n.d.).

The PIP needs to be very detailed, with specific examples of identified problems, to avoid any confusion by the employee; it should also include specific and measurable goals and outcomes with a time frame for improvements to be made. The manager then meets with the employee to discuss reasons for the plan, improvements to be made, support needed, and if any resources, such as training or tools to accomplish job expectations. According to Kirkpatrick (2005), any adverse actions by the manager should also be identified in the root-cause of the problem, such as not keeping the employee updated on information or not clarifying what is needed for the job.

PIPs should be tied to job duties in the performance appraisal and should focus on employee strengths and overcoming challenge areas. Once signed by the employee, frequent check-ins should be made to see how the employee is performing and meeting their goals and if any revisions need to be made. A PIP can be extended if improvements are being observed to allow the employee the time to develop. If no improvements are observed, then moving to termination is the last step.

LEADERSHIP AND MANAGEMENT IMPLICATIONS

Elements of a Successful Performance Review

Managers drive the performance appraisal process, although they may bring in supervisors or others with whom the nurse has interacted. The manager will gather relevant data related to the employee, which can include notes, previous evaluations, and interviews with staff. This data should be collected on a continuous basis, lessening the chance of any bias. The manager then develops a written plan and writes an assessment according to the organization's appraisal format. The manager would include any observations on performance, recommendations that would continue to develop the nurse in skills, classes or certifications to take, or suggestions for behavioral change (such as improvement in documentation). Finally, an overall rating is tallied.

Now the manager can meet with the nurse to discuss the outcomes and recommendations and any compensation attached to the rating. The tone of this meeting is set by the manager so the more positive and open it is, the more positive the review process is looked at from both sides.

If the nurse was involved in the evaluation (self-rating), this is brought into the meeting and compared against the manager's evaluation. It is in this conversation that the nurse is allowed the opportunity to express views and concerns and any desired goals to attain over the next evaluation period, such as a desire to move into a new role.

Stress and Burnout

The effect of performance appraisals on the work effort of employees to meet performance standards can lead to performance pressure, or the urgency to achieve performance levels with rewards and consequences attached. This often leaves employees feeling the need to work harder and longer. This can compound the stress level of a nurse, who may already be under pressure to provide the highest level of care in dealing with staff and families and encountering pressure to meet regulatory compliance. Nurses must also regulate their own emotions in their work to calm patients and families and in carrying out their duties. Kim (2020) distinguished between deep acting and surface acting. Deep acting is changing one's emotions to meet demands of the job, and surface acting refers to hiding one's emotions. Both types of acing can lead to more stress and, eventually, burnout.

Job stress "results when the requirements of the job do not meet the capabilities, resources, or needs of workers" (National Institute for Occupational Safety and Health (NIOSH), 2009, p. 6). The American Institute of Stress (2019) reported that 40% of workers experience job stress, although that number continues to climb higher. Adverse effects of stress include physical problems and can lead to aggressive behavior (https://www.stress.org). This topic has many layers and implications, outside the scope of this chapter, but it is critical for health care organizations to be more aware of the emotional health of workers and for managers to have "check-ins" with staff to determine how they are doing, as well as providing tools and resources to address staff emotional reaction or level. Nurse managers who are aware of the signs and symptoms of stress are better able to assess the emotional needs of staff and mitigate adverse effects, such as absenteeism or inadequate patient care.

CURRENT ISSUES AND TRENDS

There is a growing trend to eliminate the current use of performance appraisals and move to a performance management system. According to a Gallup report (Wigert & Harter, 2017) about 14% or only 2 in 10 employees feel that performance appraisals motivate them to make improvements. As a subsequent, Sutton and Wigert (2019) concluded that the current system is ineffective.

Performance management systems benchmark employees to set standards that one either meets, exceeds, or needs improvement on. The set-up includes the use of a technology-based platform, or Human Resource Information Systems (HRIS). In this platform or system, job roles are entered, benchmarks for each of those roles, and thresholds to meet national standards. Goals are set to meet those thresholds, and feedback is done through an ongoing process. This process benefits both the manager and employee, as feedback is done in real time so problems can be immediately addressed, and corrective action taken. This benefits the nurse and the organization overall.

Along with benchmarks, many organizations are adding coaching, either from an internal coach or external coach. Coaching has been shown to help an employee to meet their goals faster by setting expectations, increasing communication skills, and attaining goals through accountability (Sherpa Coaching, 2019). Once benchmarks are set, the coach then works with the employee to meet required standards, and coaching has been shown to get them there faster (Sherpa Coaching, 2019). Training managers in coaching principles, as part of the HRIS system, would lead to faster development of employees in meeting work expectations.

Many major corporations have changed their performance appraisal system, or eliminated them entirely, and are setting the trend for other companies to follow. Netflix is a prime example. Netflix changed its performance management system in 2009 to a context environment, where the focus is less on goal setting and more on helping employees understand the context, specifically, "organizational goals, the priority of those goals, level of refinement required, key stakeholders, and the definition of success" (Cognology, n.d.). In this appraisal model, it is the responsibility of the manager to set the environment for employees to succeed. If an employee makes a mistake, the context and environment are first examined to determine whether they were conducive for goal attainment.

Netflix also moved to a continuous feedback system, as opposed to a yearly review, which led to better performance. Google uses a continuous feedback system as well, but it is based on a peer-review system: employees are not promoted if they do not get good reviews from their peers. Zappos is also based on feedback; however, half of their ratings focus on the relationship with the organization's culture and values (Cognology, n.d.). These companies are discovering, through continuous feedback, that employees have higher performance and better alignment with core values, which leads to delivering high quality products, services, and customer service.

Agile Performance Management

Agile Management has been around for a long time, but it is mainly used in manufacturing and defense agencies. It is about efficiency, so services and resources are utilized in the most energetic and productive way. Due to that focus, health care organizations are now beginning to see the value and adopt this strategy. Agile Performance Management is a collaborative, continuous, and developmental strategy that is focused on processes that evaluate an employee over a period of time, such as 6-months to a year. "Agile Performance Management focuses on both the process and end goal. Continuous improvement is key" (Pawar, 2016). There are three processes in this model: (1) continuous feedback, (2) communication, and (3) coaching. Health care organizations are using this model to improve the quality of services and their competitive advantage: Mayo Clinic uses Agile with streamlining Information Technology (IT) functions to improve processes and systems without compromising patient care (Pool et al., 2019). Benefits of using the Agile model include: (1) increased accountability, (2) collaboration, and (3) communication through supportive leadership.

Deficit Versus Strengths Model

The new paradigm focuses on the strengths of an employee versus their deficits. Current feedback tends to focus on what an employee has done wrong and then sets the goals for improvement. However, this approach does not lead to improvement. This new paradigm is based on the model of Appreciative Inquiry, which is an organizational development process that has shifted from deficits to strengths, affirms past and present strengths, and acknowledges successes and the individual's potential (Cooperrider & Srivatsa, 1987). The employee (i.e., nurse) is then asked how they will apply their past behavior to current or future situations, thereby, bestowing accountability on them. By focusing on strengths and past successes, more awareness and accountability is given to the nurse who can override challenges they face. This is a much more positive experience in the feedback process for both the nurse and manager.

SUMMARY

The development of employee competencies leads to quality patient care or positive organizational outcomes based on the organizations mission. This is augmented through the performance appraisal system. This process allows managers to assess the knowledge, skills, and abilities of employees to aid in their development and future needs. Understanding various factors that make up the appraisal process will lead to a fair assessment and feedback that aligns the employee to individual, departmental, and organizational goals. Managers with an employee development mindset have the knowledge to drive the appraisal process to build relationships (i.e., with nurses and support staff) and have continuous feedback into their development. This allows the employee to be conscientious and take more responsibility in meeting set goals. Hospitals can meet organizational goals and standards of care through supporting a strong performance management system.

RESEARCH NOTE

Source

Setiawati, T., & Ariani, I. D. (2020). Influence of performance appraisal fairness and job satisfaction through commitment on performance. *Review of Integrative Business and Economics, 9*(3), 133–151.

Purpose

This quantitative study discussed the influence of performance appraisal fairness and job satisfaction through commitment on job performance among respondents working in a hospital in Indonesia.

Research

Purpose

The study aims were to determine the influence of performance appraisal fairness and job satisfaction through commitment on job performance. This study used a survey design with a questionnaire using a six-point Likert scale that was mailed to 187 people. Returned were 155 questionnaires. Participants were between the ages of 26 and 79 years old.

Discussion

Four key variables were used to operationalize the study. These include performance appraisal fairness, job satisfaction, commitment, and job performance. The authors tested nine hypotheses. Proven hypotheses included: (1) performance appraisal fairness has a positive effect on commitment, (2) job satisfaction has a positive effect on commitment, (3) commitment has a positive effect on job performance, (4) performance appraisal fairness has a positive effect on job performance, (5) job satisfaction has a positive effect on job performance, (6) performance appraisal fairness and job satisfaction have a positive effect on commitment, and (7) performance appraisal fairness and job satisfaction have a positive effect on job performance. Two unproven hypotheses were: (1) indirect influence of performance appraisal fairness on job performance with commitment as the intervening variable is greater than the direct influence, and (2) indirect influence of performance appraisal fairness on job performance with commitment as the intervening variable is greater than the direct influence.

Application to Practice

Similar studies have been done in other industries such as banking and hotels. These new findings are specific to health care. The authors have concluded that performance appraisal fairness and job satisfaction had positive effects on job performance. Therefore, these findings can inform health care in an era of nursing shortages and an increasing aging population.

With the increasing need to hire and develop staff, an effective way to do so is through an efficient performance management system. Fairness in the appraisal system will lead to equity and job satisfaction. Enhancing these can lead to higher performance, which this study proved. Although commitment was not supported, independently it can lead to higher levels of commitment to the job and ensure quality patient care.

CASE STUDY

Stephanie is a nurse manager in a large hospital system, where she is in charge of several departments, including two medical-surgical units that serve general medicine and orthopedics, with over 40 staff. Stephanie has been in nursing leadership for over 10 years and considers herself a caring manager. As she works to develop relationships with her employees to ensure their satisfaction, she knows that will result in high quality care.

Through the "grapevine," Stephanie heard that several of her nurses are unhappy, and unit level metrics indicate that there has been a higher rate of turnover in the last 6 months. Performance appraisals are done in the short-term, and Stephanie worries how the feedback will further affect her staff, considering that several of the nurses have been under-performing. She worries that there will be more staff dissatisfaction and, worse, more turnover.

Stephanie is a caring and involved leader. She reads about the latest trends, not just in nursing, but also in other fields. During her research to assess problems and identify solutions, she discovered information about how some companies are implementing newer, best practices that focus on an employee's strengths, rather than on problems, and use benchmarks to develop employees, one of which is providing continuous feedback. Stephanie decides to work on implementing this practice by having regular meetings with each staff member to let them know how they are performing, to share information on events in the hospital, and to also get their feedback on how she is doing and for any ideas/or recommendations for improvements.

By collaborating with Human Resources (HR), Stephanie restructured the performance management program in her department. This made the process more fulfilling both for her employees and for her as the leader. The new program was well received by staff. She now intends to present the new program to her leadership for consideration to adopt enterprise-wide.

CRITICAL THINKING EXERCISE

Maxine has been in nursing for 30 years. She started as a floor nurse then expanded her skills in several specialties. For the last 5 years she worked in a nursing home and decided to return to a hospital setting, where she functions in the role of nurse manager for a medical-surgical unit.

Maxine is enjoying her new role but tends to be critical of newer nurses who she feels are not as dedicated as she is and tend to circumvent many practices in day-to-day events. She gets along with tenured nurses, and has difficulty relating to younger nurses. Maxine has upcoming performance appraisals in the next month and is feeling a bit awkward.

This "disconnect" is causing Maxine stress as she attempts to write fair appraisals. For the past month, she has been diligently working on them, despite feeling uneasy. HR has given her the schedule to receive their reviews. To her dismay, Maxine finds one of the young nurses is the first for a performance review, which includes not just writing the review, but meeting with them in person. Maxine now finds herself procrastinating and finding excuses to not write the appraisal. She realizes she needs to proceed with the meeting but has delayed it twice and now has heard from both HR and her immediate manager that the appraisal is past due.

1. What is the problem?
2. What is the cause, or causes, which could be leading to Maxine's behavior?
3. If you were Maxine's supervisor, what interventions would you take to address her delay in getting the appraisals completed?
4. What recommendations would you make to Maxine to get through the appraisals successfully?

REFERENCES

360pev.com. (2013). *Here you will find all you need to know about a 360 feedback*. http://360performanceevaluation.com/.

American Institute of Stress. (2019). *Workplace stress*. http://www.stress.org/workplace-stress/.

Benedictine University. (n.d.). *What is performance and how does it relate to culture?* https://online.ben.edu/programs/msmob/resources/what-is-performance.

Berinato, S. (2018). Negative feedback rarely leads to improvement: Mr. Green, defend your Research. *Harvard Business Review*, *96*(1), 32–33.

Bernardin, J., Thomason, S., Buckley, M. R., & Kane, J. S. (2016). Rater rater-level bias and accuracy in performance appraisals: The impact of rater personality, performance management competence, and rater accountability. *Human Resource Management*, *55*(2), 321–340.

Capelli, P., & Conyon, M. J. (2018). What do performance appraisals do. *ILR Review*, *71*(1), 88–116.

Chopra, R. (2017). 360 degree performance assessments: An overview. *Global Journal of Enterprise Information System*, *9*(3), 102–105.

Cognology. (n.d.). *What can Netflix, Hubspot, Zappos and Google teach you about the future of performance management.* https://www.cognology.com.au/can-netflix-hubspot-zappos-google-teach-future-performance-management/.

Cooperrider, D. L., & Srivasta, S. (1987). Appreciative inquiry in organizational life. *Research in Organizational Change and Development*, *1*, 129–169.

Dello Russo, S., Miraglia, M., & Borgogni, L. (2017). Reducing organizational politics in performance appraisal: The role of coaching leaders for age-diverse employees. *Human Resource Management*, *56*(5), 769–783. https://doi.org/10.1002/hrm.21799.

DeNisi, A. S., & Murphy, K. R. (2017). Performance appraisals and performance management. *Journal of Applied Psychology*, *102*(3), 421–433.

Drucker, P. F. (1954). *The practice of management*, New York, NY: Harper & Row.

Farrell, S. (2017). Leadership reflections: Extrovert and introvert leaders. *Journal of Library Administration*, *57*(4), 436–443.

Geise, K., & Theil, A. (2015). The psychological contract Chinese-African informal labor relations. *International Journal of Human Resource Management*, *26*(14), 1807–1826.

Ghosh, P. (2019). What is HRIS? System, model, and application. *HR Technologist*. https://www.hrtechnologist.com/articles/performance-management-hcm/what-is-hris/.

Haag-Heitman, B., & George, V. (2011). Nursing peer-review: Principles and practice. *American Nurse Today*, *6*(9), 48–52. https://www.mghpcs.org/eed_portal/Documents/ProfDev/Nursing-Peer-Review-Article.pdf.

Heathfield, S. M. (2016). *Performance improvement plan: Contents and sample form*. https://www.thebalance.com/performance-improvement-plan-contents-and-sample-form-1918850.

Henniger, N. (2016). *Appraisals and envy: The influence of situational factors on envious feelings and motivation*. (Doctoral dissertation). University of San Diego. California. https://escholarship.org/uc/item/823902nj.

Ibarra, H., & Scoular, A. (2019). The leader as coach. *Harvard Business Review*, *97*(6), 110–119. https://hbr.org/2019/11/the-leader-as-coach.

Include-empower.com. (2018). *Explaining affinity bias: Preferring people like us*. https://cultureplusconsulting.com/2015/06/19/explaining-affinity-bias/.

Institute of Coaching. (n.d.). *Benefits of coaching*. https://instituteofcoaching.org/coaching-overview/coaching-benefits.

International Coach Federation (ICF). (n.d.). *Current competency model*. https://coachfederation.org/core-competencies.

Iqbal, M. Z. (2017). Expanded dimensions of the purposes and uses of performance appraisals. *Asian Academy of Management Journal*, *17*(1), 41–63.

Juneja, P. (2020). *Performance appraisal*. Management Study Guide. https://www.managementstudyguide.com/performance-appraisal.htm.

Kim, J.- S. (2020). Emotional labor strategies, stress, and burnout among nurse: A path analysis. *Journal of Nursing Scholarship*, *52*(1), 105–112.

Kirkpatrick, D. L. (2005). *The performance improvement plan. Improving employee performance through appraisal and coaching* (2nd ed.). New York, NY: American Management Association (pp. 66–78).

Ladyshewsky, R. K., & Taplin, R. (2018). The interplay between organizational learning culture, the manager as coach, self-efficacy and workload on employee work engagement. *International Journal of Evidence Based Coaching and Mentoring*, *16*(2), 3–19.

Larsen, D. A. (2019). Using the elaborate likelihood model to explain performance appraisal inaccuracies. *Journal of Practice and Policy Management*, *20*(4), 65–77.

Latham, G. P., & Wexley, K. N. (1977). Behavioral observation scales for performance appraisal purposes. *Personnel Psychology*, *30*, 255–268.

Lexico Dictionary (n.d.). *Feedback*. https://www.lexico.com/definition/feedback.

Moon, K. (2019). Specificity of performance appraisal feedback, trust in manager, and job attitudes: A serial mediation model. *International Journal of Social Behavior and Personality*, *47*(6), 2–12.

National Institute for Occupational Safety and Health (NIOSH). (2009). *Stress…at work*: DHHS (NIOSH) Publication No. 99–101. https://www.cdc.gov/niosh/docs/99-101/default.html.

Pawar, Y. (2016). Traditional versus agile performance management. *Uprise Together*. https://upraise.io/blog/traditional-vs-agile-performance-management/.

Performance-appraisals.org. (2018). *What is employee self-appraisal?* http://performance-appraisals.org/faq/selfappraisals.htm.

Pool, E. T., Poole, K., Upjohn, D. P., & Fernandez, J. S. (2019). Agile project management proves effective, efficient for Mayo Clinic. *American Association for Physician Leadership*. https://www.physicianleaders.org/news/agile-project-management-proves-effective-efficient-mayo-clinic.
Reiken, J. (2018). *8 Rater biases that are affecting your performance management*. Trakstar. https://www.trakstar.com/blog-post/8-rater-biases-impacting-performance-management/.
Robbins, S. P., & Judge, T. A. (2018). *Essentials of organizational behavior* (14th ed.). Upper Saddle River, NJ: Pearson.
Sanchez, C. R., Diaz-Cabrera, D., & Hernandez-Fernaud, E. (2019). Does effectiveness in performance appraisal improve with rater training? *PLoS One*, *14*(9), 1–20. https://doi.org/10.1371/journal.pone.0222694.
Schub, E. (2014). *Clinical competencies assessment*. Cinahl Information Systems. https://www.ebscohost.com/images-nursing/assets/ClinicalCompetenceAssessment.pdf.
Sherpa Coaching. (2019). *Executive Coaching Survey Report 2019*: Sasha Corporation. https://www.sherpacoaching.com/pdf_files/2019_Executive_Coaching_Survey_Summary_Report.pdf.
Smith, P. C., & Kendall, L. M. (1963). Retranslation of expectations: An approach to the construction of unambiguous anchors for rating scales. *Journal of Applied Psychology*, *47*, 149–155.
Society for Human Resource Management (SHRM). (n.d.). *How to establish a performance improvement plan*. https://www.shrm.org/resourcesandtools/tools-and-samples/how-to-guides/pages/performanceimprovementplan.aspx.
Steele, D. (n.d.). Pros and cons of peer-review in the workplace. Council for Adult and Experiential Learning. https://www.cael.org/blog/pros-and-cons-of-peer-review-in-the-workplace.
Sutton, R., & Wigert, B. (2019). *More harm than good: The truth about performance reviews*: Gallup Organization. https://www.gallup.com/workplace/249332/harm-good-truth-performance-reviews.aspx.
Teckchandani, A., & Pichler, S. (2015). Quality results in performance management. *Industrial Management*, *57*(4), 16–20.
The Joint Commission. (n.d.). *Orthopedic certification: Pathways to excellence in patient care*. https://www.jointcommission.org/-/media/enterprise/tjc/imported-page-assets/tjc-ortho-cert-brochure-v4pdf.pdf?db=web&hash=189A318A66F917F27AA76B3C901DAF36.
Weirks, T. G. D. (2007). *Behavior and result-based performance management and the performance of business management: An examination of the mediating relationships between proactive behavior between performance management and performance*. Tillburg, Netherlands: Tillburg University Master's thesis.
Wigert, B., & Harter, J. (2017). *Re-engineering performance management*: Gallup Organization. https://www.gallup.com/workplace/238064/re-engineering-performance-management.aspx.

24

Emergency Management and Preparedness

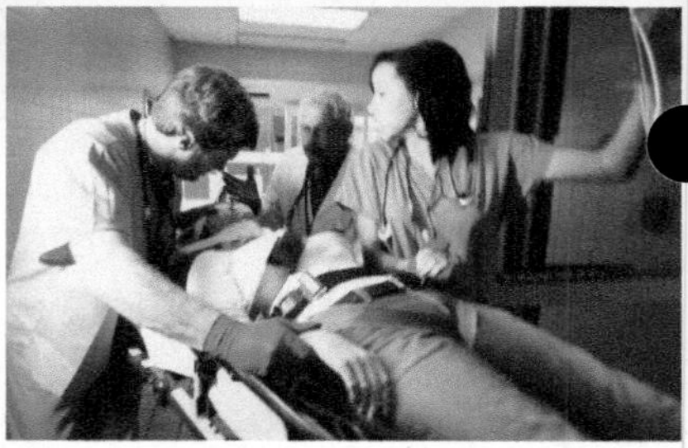

Kimberly K. Hatchel, Melinda Hirshouer

http://evolve.elsevier.com/Huber/leadership

Editors' note: In early February 2020, when this chapter was prepared and submitted, we all were unaware of what was about to happen: a severe worldwide coronavirus pandemic. Although COVID-19 was a new virus, it had been some 17 years since the last severe coronavirus outbreak (SARS). As this book goes into production, we are watching the responses by governments and organizations in real time. The need for emergency management and preparedness has been brought into sharp focus in the pressing urgency of what is now unfolding.

TRANSITIONING THEORY INTO PRACTICE FOR ALL-HAZARDS PREPAREDNESS

The events of September 11, 2001, a tragic day in history, changed Americans' perception of a "safe" world. In the years that followed the world has experienced numerous catastrophic events with causes across a continuum. A new disaster preparedness narrative has emerged as a result of the diversity, magnitude, and frequency of these events. People of all backgrounds have been forced to consider preparation in their homes, at their church, schools, and work environments for the eventuality of a disaster. It was once assumed that people were knowledgeable about how to prepare for potential natural disasters within their local regions. As disasters have impacted larger groups of people and events are impacting the same geographical areas including large rural and isolated areas in shorter periods of time, preparation has changed. Appropriate planning has become more crucial than ever. A list of man-made possibilities is endless: biological exposures, chemical spills, gun violence, radiological exposures, nuclear blasts, conventional bombings, agricultural contamination, cyber viruses, and other unforeseen cataclysmic nature events may also occur. Thus developing a contingency plan for most types of disasters, including bioterrorism, is most appropriately termed **all-hazards disaster preparedness.**

Since the occurrence of major disasters such as the attack on the World Trade Center, Hurricane Sandy in 2012, and the devastating tornado in Joplin, Missouri in 2011, key community stakeholders such as local governments, fire and rescue workers, and hospitals have been focused on sharing information from a variety of resources, developing collaborative response plans, and preparing for a probable disaster. However, there are still gaps in the possession and execution of emergency preparedness knowledge. In a 2008 study, Niska and Shimizu (2011) found that while greater than 95% of hospitals had emergency preparedness plans for chemical, biological, or natural disasters, considerably fewer facilities were prepared for radiological-nuclear or explosive-incendiary incidents. Additionally, only 73% of facilities were prepared for loss of utilities. The American College of Emergency Physicians (ACEP) has recommended that hospitals use their Emergency Operations Plan (EOP) to develop their training plan and that they execute situational drills to ensure that the staff has retained knowledge and that the training remains a valuable tool for the hospitals. Of the 88% of facilities that had prepared plans to continue operations during an emergency, 15% of these hospitals had to enact these plans for an actual incident in 2007. Additionally, only 47% of hospitals were prepared to manage and shelter mobility or cognitively impaired patients (Niska & Shimizu, 2011). In 2014, there were 84 federally declared disasters in the United States and that is only a small portion of the emergency events that a hospital may encounter (Federal Emergency Management Agency, 2016).

In order to close some of these gaps, The Joint Commission (TJC) has advanced hospital efforts through the development of six crucial areas for emergency preparedness: communication, safety and security, resources and assets, staff responsibilities, utilities management, and patient clinical and support activities (TJC Resources, 2008, 2020). These crucial areas create a framework for all-hazards disaster preparedness planning. Hospitals must prepare for a variety of internal or external events that cause enough disruption that the normal operations are forced into crisis mode. If the employees chosen to lead the hospital in its response to casualties, property damage, or suspending patient care are unprepared or make ineffective decisions, the crisis will quickly escalate to a disaster (Sternberg, 2003). TJC requires hospitals to have a written EOP (TJC, 2020). The EOP must include how the hospital trains, prepares, and responds to potential events. What is certain is that patients and their family members will expect the hospital to continue to provide normal operations regardless of internal or external circumstances.

Health care executives across the country understand the need to dedicate resources to support effective all-hazards preparedness. The Health Insurance Portability and Accountability Act (HIPAA) and TJC require all health care facilities to have detailed all-hazard preparedness plans. Nursing leaders are an integral part of the planning process and should have knowledge of the national Emergency Response Plan promulgated by the Federal Emergency Management Agency (FEMA) (https://www.ready.gov/business/implementation/emergency), as well as state and local disaster response plans. Effective planning and evaluation skills for all-hazards preparedness is an essential management competency for nursing leaders. The ability to receive federal response grants must be compliant with the National Incident Management System (NIMS) (US Department of Homeland Security [DHS], 2020). Additionally, TJC requires hospitals to practice elements of their EOP and evaluate areas of success and opportunity (2016).

This chapter describes how to orchestrate a multilevel plan for a health care facility. A comprehensive all-hazards preparedness plan will assist in establishing (1) an organized hospital-based plan for both internal and external disasters at the department/unit level, (2) an interhospital plan for effectively collaborating with other hospitals within a health care system and within the vicinity, (3) a community plan that will integrate the hospital plan with other external community plans, and (4) a national plan that will guide nurse leaders in accessing financial assistance from federal and state all-hazards preparedness resources.

DEFINITIONS

From a health care perspective, a **disaster** is "a type of emergency that, due to its complexity, scope, or duration, threatens a health care center's capabilities … and requires outside assistance to sustain patient care, safety, or security functions" (TJC, 2008, p. 2). There are a wide variety of types and causes of disasters, including sudden onset (severe weather events or chemical spills) and slow-onset events (progressive disease outbreaks) (World Health Organization [WHO], 2013). Although often triggered by nature, disasters can be caused by human acts, including chemical, biological, radiological, nuclear, or explosives (CBRNE). Wars and civil disturbances that destroy homelands and displace people are included among man-made disasters. Causes of natural disasters include severe weather events such as blizzards, wildfires, floods, tsunamis, volcanic eruptions, earthquakes, tornadoes, hurricanes, and the devastation caused by Hurricane Sandy in 2012 or the earthquake and resulting tsunami in Japan in 2011. Disasters can be *internal*, such as a catastrophic event that occurs within a facility, such as a loss of utilities or an unplanned extended downtime of the electronic health record, making it difficult to maintain operations (TJC, 2012); or *external*, such as a catastrophic event that affects the community that may or may not affect the facility, such as the 2020 coronavirus 2019 (COVID-19) worldwide viral pandemic.

Other disaster-related definitions are:

- *All-hazards*: A general term that is descriptive of all types of natural and/or human terrorist events.
- *All-hazards disaster preparedness*: An effective and consistent response to any disaster or emergency regardless of the cause (Wright State University, 2016).
- *Crisis standards of care*: "Substantial change in the usual healthcare operations and the level of care it is possible to deliver … in a public health emergency, justified by specific circumstances, declared by a state government in recognition that crisis operations will be in effect for a sustained period" (Institute of Medicine [IOM], 2012).

- *CBRNE*: Chemical, biological, radiological, nuclear, explosives (US Department of Defense, 2015).
- *Biological disaster*: Disease epidemics and insect/animal plagues or an incident occurring as a result of the deliberate or unintentional release of biological materials that may adversely affect the health of those exposed (International Federation of Red Cross and Red Crescent Societies [IFRC], 2016; US Department of Defense, 2015).
- *Chemical disaster*: The deliberate or unintentional release of poisonous vapors, liquids, or solids that have a toxic effect on people, plants, and animals (Ready.gov, 2016).
- *Radiological/nuclear disaster*: Radiological or nuclear emergencies may be intentional (caused by terrorists) or unintentional (accidents that may result from accidents within a facility, e.g., the departments of nuclear medicine and radiation oncology or from external sources involving vehicles transporting radioactive materials) (Centers for Disease Control and Prevention [CDC], 2014).
- *Explosives*: A catastrophic event caused by the use of weapons such as guns, bombs, missiles, or grenades.
- *Cyber disaster*: A catastrophic event that results from an attack initiated from one computer against another computer with the purpose of compromising the information stored on it (Arnand, 2014).
- *Hazard vulnerability analysis*: An exercise that is a systematic approach to recognizing hazards and identifying an organization's potential emergencies, the likelihood of the event occurring, and the impact it would have on the organization. The risks associated with each hazard are analyzed to prioritize planning, mitigation, response, and recovery activities (California Hospital Association, 2011).
- *Mass casualty incident*: A natural or manmade event generating large numbers of patients requiring medical care and that overwhelms a health care facility and prevents it from delivering medical services that are consistent with accepted standards (Agency for Healthcare Research and Quality [AHRQ], 2012).

BACKGROUND

GETTING STARTED: FIRST STEPS

Starting any systems project can be complex and difficult. Beginning the work of establishing a comprehensive all-hazards preparedness plan is no exception. Historically, most hospitals have had some type of disaster plan in place. Evaluating the hospital's existing EOP while focusing on maintaining a state of constant readiness can be a complicated process. One of the first steps to gaining participation from appropriate stakeholders and moving the evaluation process forward is the creation of an emergency management oversight committee, or an all-hazards preparedness task force. Based on the American Organization of Nurse Executive's (AONE, 2016) *Role of the Nurse Leader in Crisis Management,* the nurse executive—often called the *chief nursing officer (CNO)*—will play a pivotal role in facilitating the initial committee. The AONE guiding principles include:

- Nurse leaders are trained in media relations and understand the tenets of good communication.
- Leaders are skilled critical thinkers, collaborative, and able to manage ambiguity.
- Nurse leaders project calm, confidence, and authority in all situations. They also are empathetic to how people react to loss, challenges, and uncertainty.
- Nurse leaders are prepared to review and practice the organization's crisis readiness plan with nursing staff.
- The CNO is a member of the senior leadership team, whose role is clearly defined and sought by colleagues, particularly during a crisis.

Creating an Emergency Management Committee

As many nurses understand, effective projects start with the basic nursing process: assessment, planning, implementation, evaluation, and, if necessary, modification. The emergency management committee will follow a similar process when developing an emergency management plan, which will incorporate mitigation of potential hazards (assessment), developing a plan of what to do should the event occur (planning), responding to the actual event (implementation), and assisting the hospital and the community in the short- and long-term recovery that will follow (evaluation). Developing an original plan is best accomplished by establishing a high-level administrative committee whose purpose will be oversight of the multilevel emergency management plan development. Whether the hospital is part of a larger health care system or is a freestanding, independent hospital, the committee will function similarly.

Health care systems with multiple facilities are very familiar with the complexity and intricacies of trying to establish a standardized system-wide approach to care needs. In organizations such as these, system-wide executive administrators need to be part of the committee. Having a senior executive administrator of the health care system serve as the chairperson of the committee will provide the leadership needed to communicate the importance of emergency preparedness as a system priority. A representative CNO and emergency medicine physician, serving as co-chairs with the senior executive administrator, can create a dynamic team that is uniquely prepared to tackle any issues that arise. A project facilitator is helpful in getting the committee started and operational. The project facilitator can also serve in a pivotal maintenance role, keeping the emergency management plan current and in the forefront of the administration's strategic planning over time.

Establishing the committee requires that all departments be committed to the tasks at hand and cognizant of the need for consensus building and standardization of processes. Multidirectional communication is imperative. The standing membership should be composed of stakeholders representing all areas of the organization, both clinical and non-clinical. Because not all departments can logistically be on the committee, the members will have large areas of oversight and communication. Committee membership might typically look like that outlined in Table 24.1.

TABLE 24.1 Emergency Management Committee Membership Responsibilities

Responsibility Area(s)	Position Title	Detail of Area Covered
Executive owner (chair)	Executive administrator	Leads the emergency management committee as chair. If the hospital is part of a health care system, this person will be a system-wide senior administrator. If the hospital is a freestanding, independent facility, this person will be the hospital's chief operating officer.
Clinical operations (co-chair)	Chief nurse officer	Represents all nursing and clinical departments; co-chairs the emergency management committee.
Chemical, biological, radiological, nuclear, or explosives (CBRNE) threats (co-chair)	Emergency department/ medical director	Represents all aspects of emergency medicine and physician needs related to all-hazards preparedness. This person also will co-chair the committee.
Physician liaison(s)	Department chiefs	Serve as spokespersons for physician needs with regard to disaster preparedness. Facilitate communication of timely information should an event occur. Have oversight for physician credentialing in times of a disaster. Assist in approval of medical standards established for various types of disasters.
Chief operating officers (COOs) from health care system facilities	Chief operating officer(s)	Represent the needs of their facilities in establishing an effective all-hazards preparedness plan. Facilitate system-wide collaboration in standardizing practices and communicate essential information to employees.
Security	Safety and security director	Serves as liaison for system-wide safety and security departments in the system. Coordinates and synchronizes efforts of all departments as related to all-hazards preparedness. Responsible for rapid "lock-down" of all entrances and flow of people in the event of a disaster.
Communications	Chief information technology officer	Oversees successful operation of the integrated information system, including telephones, radios, and computers and satellite technology, during times of instability. Creates and maintains redundant systems to ensure an ability to communicate within facilities, outside to other hospitals, and partners with community.

TABLE 24.1 Emergency Management Committee Membership Responsibilities—cont'd

Responsibility Area(s)	Position Title	Detail of Area Covered
Messages/media	Marketing director/ information officer	Plays an active role in communicating the all-hazards preparedness message to all employees, patients, and community. Acts on behalf of the health care system or hospital in speaking with press about impending or actual disaster situations.
Human resources	Human resources director	Serves as the staff's voice in meeting the needs of employees during a disaster. Creates manuals to guide staff in preparing for and responding to a disaster. Manages the human resources pool when the incident command center is active.
Financial reimbursement	Chief financial officer	Leads efforts in monitoring financial expenses related to establishing an effective all-hazards preparedness plan. Seeks out state/federal reimbursement opportunities for planning.
Government funding	Government affairs director	Serves as a vital link to local, state, and federal boards representing the system financial and operational needs regarding all-hazards preparedness. Advocates for funding related to all-hazards preparedness.
Biological threats	Infectious disease medical director	Serves as the liaison for all infection control (IC) departments in the system.
Infection control	Infection prevention and control practitioner	Coordinates and synchronizes efforts of all IC departments as related to all-hazards preparedness. Responsible for development, dissemination, and understanding of procedures related to biological events.
Legal	Executive attorney	Advises all-hazards preparedness task force in legal matters related to establishing an effective all-hazards preparedness plan.
Education planning	Education director	Has oversight for planning and implementing educational efforts for staff and patients. As needed, coordinates "just in time" training for any arising incident and is an integral partner in planning and implementing internal and external disaster drills.
Logistics	Pharmacy director	Serves as the liaison for all system pharmacies. Has oversight for stockpiling medications for use in a disaster. Establishes par levels of drugs for use in "patient surge" situations. Establishes contracts with pharmaceutical vendors to ensure adequate supply of medications in the event of a disaster. Has oversight for any medical supply trucks ready for deployment in times of a disaster (e.g., stocking par level of drugs used in a chemical disaster).
Logistics	Materials management director	Serves as an active participant on the task force. This liaison is the system representative for all materials management departments. Is very involved in setting par levels for supplies and equipment on the units at the time of a disaster. Establishes contracts with materials management vendors to ensure adequate supply of medications in the event of a disaster (e.g., stocking a supplemental supply truck for use in a disaster).
Logistics	Engineering	Directs any operational building redesign needed to prepare hospital for handling a disaster (e.g., decontamination showers).

Note: This assessment tool was developed by Inova Health System based on a bioterrorism preparedness survey created by a committee consisting of representatives from Baylor University's Graduate Program in Healthcare Administration, the US Army Center for Healthcare Education and Studies, and the University of Texas Health Science Center at San Antonio. (For more information, see Drenkard et al., 2002.) Courtesy Inova Health System, Falls Church, VA.

As the team evolves in its work, ad hoc members can be added as needed. Internal ad hoc members might include radiology, facility engineering, telecommunications, volunteer support, chaplain services, physician chairs, social work, case management, and dietary, respiratory, and laboratory services. External ad hoc members might include representatives from the local public health department, government liaison, police, fire and rescue, public school system, representatives from the faith community, community physicians, and even vendor representatives who can be contracted to provide such things as oxygen, ice, food, cots, and linens in the event of a disaster.

During the start-up, the system-wide committee will need to meet frequently. To begin, the committee should perform a hazard vulnerability analysis (HVA). The HVA will be used as a starting point to create an EOP that identifies risks and prioritizes likely emergencies in order to mitigate them when possible and develop strategies for preparedness (TJC Resources, 2016). For specific details on the HVA process, there are several resources available, including the FEMA and TJC Resources websites.

Performing an Effective Gap Analysis

There are many ways to perform an all-hazards preparedness gap analysis, and a multitude of online reference websites exist, including these examples:

- FEMA: https://www.fema.gov/media-library/assets/documents/27403.
- Office of Emergency Management, US Department of Health and Human Services: https://www.phe.gov/about/oem/Pages/default.aspx; the American Hospital Association (AHA): https://www.aha.org/2006-05-10-emergency-readiness-1.
- CDC: https://www.cdc.gov/.
- Agency for Healthcare Research and Quality (AHRQ): https://www.ahrq.gov/.
- Clinics and Community Health Centers (CCHC) Emergency Preparedness Gap Analysis: https://docplayer.net/2969385-Cchc-emergency-preparedness-gap-analysis.html.

The guiding principle for creating a hospital-specific all-hazards gap analysis is to keep it simple. One example of a simple way to assess the current state is to create an emergency preparedness survey that is easy to read and requires the department directors to answer in simple checklists one of two ways: (1) "Yes, we have it," or (2) "No, we don't have it." Survey questions need to be concise and clear. The goal is to begin by identifying the areas where there are gaps in the facility's preparedness plans. Questions should be addressed to appropriate departments who then assess the items and determine the current state. A review of the literature and online searches will assist the team in identifying the areas of assessment (Federal Emergency Management Institute (FEMA), 2014; Joint Commission Resources, 2008, 2016). Examples of questions to ask in the survey might include those listed in Box 24.1.

BOX 24.1 Hospital Gap Analysis Survey: Sample Questions

General

- Has your organization conducted a thorough hazard vulnerability analysis (HVA)?
- Does your organization have an emergency operations plan (EOP) that specifically addresses the four disaster phases?
- Does your EOP identify how to activate an emergency response and who is in charge of the command center in a disaster?
- Does your facility have an operational command center to coordinate the hospital's response to a disaster?
- Does your department staff know the chain of command in an emergency?
- Does your department know their role in each type of disaster?
- Does your hospital know their role in the community in an emergency situation?
- Are there specific plans for chemical, biological, radiological, nuclear, or explosives (CBRNE) emergencies?
- Is there a bed and staffing plan for surge capacity for 50 patients? 100 patients? 250 patients? Do you have the necessary supplies and equipment for use in a surge situation?

Human Resources

- Does your department staff know how to prepare themselves, their significant others, and pets in the event of a disaster?
- Is there a credentialing plan for health care professionals who come to the nearest facility in a disaster to volunteer their services?

BOX 24.1 Hospital Gap Analysis Survey: Sample Questions—cont'd

Safety and Security

- Does your facility have the following during an emergency:
- A lockdown plan?
- A plan for facility traffic flow and staff entry?
- Multi-language signage to direct people where to go?

Communication

- Does your hospital have emergency-powered phones in case of a disaster?
- Does your facility have a backup radio system and volunteer staff to run it?
- Does your facility have a tiered paging system that can reach multiple staff simultaneously?
- Does your department know the central command center telephone number (if there is one)?
- Is there an on-call procedure for notifying the administrator on-call and opening the command center in the event of a disaster?
- Are there established linkages to the external community (e.g., other hospitals in the region, fire department, police, emergency medical system, public schools, public health)?
- Is there a procedure for how to link patients and families both in your facility and in the community should a disaster occur?

Logistics

- Does your facility have:
- Backup emergency supplies, pharmaceuticals, and equipment?
- The ability to release and send pharmaceuticals, medical supplies, and equipment such as respirators to the areas in need in the event of a chemical or biological emergency?
- Prearranged plans with physicians, ambulances, nearby churches, and nursing homes to clear beds in an emergency? (What sites can take patients?)
- Contracts with vendors to bring in food, ice, oxygen, and other needed supplies?
- Is there an established written psychosocial role for social work, chaplains, psychiatry, employee health, and case management in the event of a disaster?
- Are there contingency plans for 4 to 5 days of no power, no water, no computers, and/or no food?
- Are there contingency plans for staff to report to nearest facility to work?
- Are there contingency plans for childcare during an emergency so that parents can work?
- Is there common nomenclature used during an emergency so that everyone understands what is happening and who has what responsibility?

Clinical Operations

- Does your facility have:
  - Procedures established to maximize staff safety in the event of a disaster?
  - Procedures for respiratory mask fit testing and training for personal protective equipment for staff?
  - The ability to track patients until discharge, admission, or death using HIPAA guidelines?
  - Clear established policies and procedures to respond to CBRNE emergencies?
  - A decontamination area and detailed step-by-step procedures on how to work in this area?
  - A backup staff to assist with people/patients arriving to the hospital?
- Does your facility have procedures for how to:
  - Track available beds, arriving patients, and discharges?
  - Track regular and volunteer staff and direct them to a designated area?
  - Operate every department of the hospital during an emergency?
  - Handle surge capacity situations including an understanding of crisis standards of care?
  - Handle operating room cases in the event of an emergency?
  - Track biological, chemical, or nuclear events and report them to authorities?

Financial

- Is there an established plan for tracking costs and submitting them for reimbursement or claims during an emergency?

Messages/Media

- Is there an established communication plan in case of an emergency?
- Is there an established communication script in the event of an emergency?
- Is there an alternative communication plan if wi-fi, power, telephones, and radios are not working?

Courtesy Inova Health System. From Drenkard, K., & Rigotti, G. (2002, updated 2016). *Inova Health System survey*. Falls Church, VA: Inova Health System.

Once the survey is created, it should be distributed to all stakeholders. Directors should be challenged to complete and return it within an appropriate deadline so that work can be initiated to address outstanding issues. The committee should review the survey results and start an issues list to address deficiencies. Nursing leaders will play key roles in creating aggressive timelines for resolving issues identified. Most resolutions will be modified and enhanced over time as the committee gains more knowledge about all-hazards planning. For issues that require multiple steps to correct, commonly seen with widespread education efforts, the use of SMART (specific, measurable, actionable, realistic, and time-bound) goals should be used.

From the gap analysis, the committee needs to establish high-level, multifaceted standards of practice and system-wide goals for all-hazards preparedness. These standards and goals will be implemented at the facility level and department level as directed by the chief operating officer (COO), CNO, and emergency department (ED) medical director. At this point, there is latitude for departments to design and implement the standards and goals based on the unique needs of the populations served. Annual review and evaluation of goals is an effective project management activity, with new goals being created based on the HVA, changing regulatory requirements, new threats, and the results of gaps identified during drills. Sustaining attention and focus on disaster preparedness efforts becomes a key role of the nurse executive in ensuring a constant state of organizational readiness. The project facilitator assists the nurse executive in researching new and evolving initiatives in the discipline of all-hazards preparedness, determining the importance of new trends to the effective operations of the health care organization's all-hazard plan, and implementing relevant enhancements that support the strategic vision for preparedness within the organization.

Keeping the Momentum Going

Once the gap analysis is completed and the issues are identified, development of a comprehensive plan is a critical next step. The work can appear daunting, and it is hard to know where to start. It is at this point that nursing leadership has the opportunity to take charge of the process. Even though the gap analysis may show a multitude of areas for improvement, issues are solvable one step at a time. The CNO and nurse leaders can help focus the committee and department directors. Efforts should be directed toward creating a streamlined, comprehensive internal emergency management plan that will set the foundation for later steps when the hospital begins to work externally with the community.

Action Items List

Over the next phase, the development of an action items list will become the working action plan used to prioritize and organize work to be done. Subgroups made up of members from the task force who are content experts can be assigned to lead efforts to resolve issues. Issues need to be constantly added and resolved as the facility refines the plan. Reports from subgroups on their progress should be regularly submitted to the committee. The committee needs to have oversight of the subgroups and should strive to clear the road for subgroup progress as needed. Hospitals may need to address common issues such as allocation of resources, including funds to educate staff. Although the immediate return on investment may not be seen or may have a negative effect on productivity numbers during the training, Arbon et al. (2013) found that disaster training did positively influence an employee's willingness to report to work following a disaster. Nurses, in particular, were four times more likely to report to work if they had any pre-existing disaster knowledge or skills, and they were also more likely to respond during a disaster if they perceived their peers and employers were prepared (Arbon et al., 2013). Educating the nursing workforce will be critical to promote an effective disaster response. Planning and education will reduce variability and increase reliability in times of uncertainty.

Establishing a Common Nomenclature, Structure, and Role Definition for Writing All-Hazards Preparedness Plans

When working with the community, using common language becomes especially important for promoting interagency communication in crisis situations. Therefore the NIMS was created by the US DHS (2020) Secretary in response to specific deadlines first identified in Homeland Security Presidential Directive 5 after the September 11 terrorist attacks to further standardize and integrate response practices nationally (Committee on Homeland Security of the House of Representatives, 2008).

> *The NIMS is a systematic, proactive approach to guide departments and agencies at all levels of government, nongovernmental organizations, and the private sector to work together seamlessly and manage incidents involving all threats and hazards—regardless of cause, size, location, or complexity—in order to reduce loss of life, property and harm to the environment. The NIMS is the essential foundation to the National Preparedness System (NPS) and provides the template for the management of incidents and operations in support of all five National Planning Frameworks. (FEMA, 2016)*

In the past, the limited focus of the disaster plan on file at a hospital usually related specifically to safety and security preparedness. Today the primary responsibility for the safety and security department, in conjunction with nursing leadership, is to develop or refine the hospital's EOP for incidents based on the HVA. The safety and security department need to have assigned oversight for facility security, quick lockdown or controlled access, and management of people flowing into and out of the hospital. This not only includes the time the incident is occurring but also during the time that family members are seeking reunification.

Nursing leadership needs to ensure that all facility departments understand their role in a disaster situation. Nurse leaders are the coordinators in synchronizing department plans so that everything fits together to meet the essential needs of the staff, patients, hospital, and community. Once the comprehensive emergency management plans are complete, every department should understand its identified written role.

Creating Procedural Annexes to All-Hazards Preparedness Plans

In addition to overall all-hazards preparedness plans, the hospital will need to define procedures regarding what will be done in any CBRNE disaster and what the surge capacity needs will be related to any of these events. *Surge capacity* is a measurable representation of the ability to manage a sudden influx of patients (ACEP, 2011). These specific procedures are added separately to the plan and are called annexes. The committee can assign the creation of each of these procedures to a subgroup. These teams are often led by nursing leadership and the emergency medicine director, with appropriate ad hoc participation. For example, the infection prevention and control department, in partnership with public health, can co-lead the biological planning efforts; the radiology department can co-lead the nuclear/radiological efforts partnering closely with local authorities; and nursing, pharmacy, and emergency medicine can co-lead the explosives, chemical, and surge capacity efforts, partnering closely with police, fire, and rescue. The goal with these procedural annexes is to create easy, step-by-step action plans, fact sheets, and algorithms for identifying, intervening, and notifying the appropriate authorities. As with most all-hazards preparedness literature, the most current references will be online. Some essential websites to assist in writing specific hospital procedures include the CDC, the DHS), and the US Department of Labor's Occupational Safety and Health Administration (OSHA).

In establishing procedural annexes and the overall all-hazards disaster preparedness plan, TJC's emergency management accreditation standards call for hospitals to sustain disaster operations for at least 96 hours should an external disaster occur that affects the local area or region (TJC, 2012). Lessons learned from Hurricane Katrina illustrate just how long it can take before assistance is available. This means surge capacity planning must go beyond the traditional areas of the ED and operating rooms. Hospital leadership needs to make sure every operating unit and department is prepared. The following are only a few examples of what hospitals will need:

- A conservative stockpile of essential antibiotics for biological threats
- Antidotes for chemical exposures
- Basic food and bottled water surpluses for environmental contamination events
- Preplanned contracts with local supply companies and businesses for ice, oxygen and other gases, and emergency power
- Alternative communication methods and plans, both internal and external, in case of power outage
- Staff and volunteer credentialing and identification procedures
- Established entrances for staff during lockdowns or controlled access situations
- Patient identification and tracking systems for families in search of loved ones

- Downtime procedures for cyber threats (with the ability to function up to 5 days)
- Accommodations for staff to bring in their children for care while they are working
- Mutual aid agreements to assist with levels of care not usually available (e.g., pediatrics) or to assist in accelerating discharges or post-acute placements.

Creating a Planning Subgroup

Even with comprehensive emergency management plans and annexes, the unexpected will happen, such as in threats and incidents involving anthrax, severe acute respiratory syndrome (SARS), smallpox, potentially harmful H1N1 influenza, and the Ebola and Zika viruses. Initially no one will know whether these are true terrorist threats or isolated spontaneous incidents. The hospital must be ready to respond at all times. An ongoing emergency management planning group needs to be formed at the local level and chaired by a nurse executive who sits on the system emergency management committee along with key stakeholder membership (including ED, employee health staff, and infection prevention and control). Based on the changing needs of the events, this planning group will enable the facility to respond quickly to the "just in time" educational needs of the staff, allow for rapid procedural planning for community needs, and ensure appropriate authority notification in the event of a disaster. For example, the staff will be expected to recognize the symptoms and presentation of Ebola and respond by critical thinking, as follows:

- Triaging and isolating the patient on admission to the ED and placing the patient in the hospital or facility's negative pressure room if available
- Obtaining and having the staff don and doff appropriate personal protective equipment (PPE)
- Controlling access to the ED and possibly the entire hospital
- Identifying (name, address, telephone number) all patient contacts, transport services (emergency medical services [EMS]), staff, and patients in the waiting room
- Notifying the infection prevention and control practitioner, hospital/facility infectious disease physician or epidemiologist, public health officials, and police

Biological and chemical terrorism are examples of unexpected severe events needing a strategic plan for preparedness and response. The CDC (2001) provided recommendations for biological and chemical terrorism. They noted that:

> *Terrorist incidents in the United States and elsewhere involving bacterial pathogens (3), nerve gas (1), and a lethal plant toxin (e.g., ricin) (4), have demonstrated that the United States is vulnerable to biological and chemical threats as well as explosives. Recipes for preparing "homemade" agents are readily available (5), and reports of arsenals of military bioweapons (2) raise the possibility that terrorists might have access to highly dangerous agents, which have been engineered for mass dissemination as small-particle aerosols. Such agents as the variola virus, the causative agent of smallpox, are highly contagious and often fatal. Responding to large-scale outbreaks caused by these agents will require the rapid mobilization of public health workers, emergency responders, and private health-care providers. Large-scale outbreaks will also require rapid procurement and distribution of large quantities of drugs and vaccines, which must be available quickly.*

There are numerous potential biological and chemical agents. Attacks with biological agents are more likely to be covert. There are three categories of biological agents, with the highest priority agents including emerging pathogens that could be engineered for mass dissemination in the future. Chemical agents that might be used by terrorists range from warfare agents to toxic chemicals commonly used in industry: nerve gas, blood agents, blister agents, heavy metals, volatile toxins, pulmonary agents, incapacitating agents, pesticides, polychlorinated biphenyls (PCBs), nitro compounds, flammable gasses and liquids, poisons, and corrosive acids and bases.

Managing causes of biological or chemical mass casualty or terrorism events includes strategies for preparedness and prevention, detection and surveillance, diagnosis and characterization of biological and chemical agents, and response and rapid deployment in the event of an overt attack. Hospitals and hospital systems will need to make sure they are aware of how to access national or system stockpiles should the need arise, because an organization can quickly become overwhelmed with a surge of patients. Effective communication is also an essential element. For example, educational materials need to be prepared to inform the public during and after an attack. The initial detection of a covert biological or chemical attack will probably occur at the local level. Thus disease surveillance systems at state and local health agencies need to be capable of detecting unusual patterns of disease or injury, including those caused by unusual or unknown threat agents (CDC, 2001). Early identification and notification of the threat to emergency medical services and hospitals must also be provided in order to maintain surveillance.

Despite the best PPE guidance by the CDC (https://www.cdc.gov/vhf/ebola/healthcare-us/ppe/index.html), the Ebola crisis highlighted serious issues in the health care delivery system, such as gaps in training, the cost of PPE, and a story reported by *60 Minutes* about a company accused of providing faulty surgical gowns to US hospitals and the US strategic national stockpile, although the company denied the allegations (CBS News, 2016). Because Ebola is so lethal, these gaps and the ways organizations responded to protect their employees came to the forefront. Nurses and other health care workers were directly affected. PPE availability quickly became a critical issue in the COVID-19 pandemic.

Developing a Command Center

In the event of a disaster, the hospital would need a dedicated centralized command center where all department directors can report for instructions. The four essential elements of a command center, explained in more detail in later sections, are as follows:

1. Setting up the room
2. Developing processes in the command center
3. Establishing the hospital's role in the community
4. Testing the all-hazards preparedness plans and command center functionality

Setting Up the Command Center Room

The location of the incident command center will depend on the organization's physical layout, but it often is located near the safety and security department. It is commanded by the on-call administrator along with the CNO, the ED medical director, and the safety and security director, although if the event occurs outside of normal business hours, the command center may be opened by personnel pre-designated by administration or by the employee with the best set of qualifications to handle the event. Not knowing when a disaster may occur makes it essential for the emergency management oversight committee to involve leaders at all levels of the organization and determine what training each leadership level will require. TJC has determined a basic set of training requirements in order to work within the command center. The following equipment should be available in the room:

- Multiple telephones/telephone lines with speed dial for frequently called numbers
- Computer access (with both intranet and Internet capabilities)
- Printing capability
- Batch copying capabilities
- Alternative phone options (e.g., 800 MHz radio technology and/or Voice over Internet Protocol [VoIP] technology—a phone system that operates over Internet lines with functioning antenna) and people trained to use them
- Tiered paging capability
- Television access
- Office-related supplies such as paper, pens, easels, dry erase boards, worktables, phone books, and reference materials such as the all-hazards preparedness plans for each hospital area

The command center should be available at a moment's notice and fully functional within minutes. A common scenario is that the call comes into the ED, but many internal disasters, such as utility failures, may come from other sources. When an external disaster occurs, nursing leadership staff in the ED, along with medical staff, will determine the gravity of the situation and decide whether the incident can be handled in the ED or whether the hospital administrator needs to be contacted. Internal disasters function in a similar manner with the affected unit escalating concerns through the appropriate channels and contacting the hospital administrator if necessary. If it is deemed appropriate to contact the hospital administrator, there will be dialogue among nursing leadership, medical leadership, and the administrator to decide whether the command center should be opened. If the command center is to be opened, the hospital administrator will start the process and call in the additional staff necessary to assist with incident command operations. In the event that the disaster involves the area where the command center is located, the hospital will have to have a predetermined plan to establish a backup command center in another location. In the case of a multifacility system, the alternate command center could be at another hospital.

Developing Processes in the Command Center

Because one of the rotating on-call administrators may be called on to open the command center, the creation of a simple, step-by-step, short document (one to two pages) of how to open, operate, and close down the command center is important. A more extensive manual can also be created, but in times of a disaster, the short "How to Open the Command Center" document is crucial. If the facility does not have an on-call administrator list, one should be established, and staff must know how to reach the on-call person(s). A clear decision matrix should be in place outlining when to open the command center and who needs to be notified. It may be helpful to create a communication tree identifying the process for quickly notifying the administrative team and emergency management committee members. Using a group paging function can be helpful for rapid notification of the leadership team.

To facilitate the incident command structure during a disaster, many hospitals have adopted the Hospital Incident Command System (HICS) for their all-hazards preparedness plans, because it allows logical standardization with common nomenclature that is understood both in the hospital environment and in the community setting (US Department of Health & Human Services, 2012). In addition, the HICS organizational chart provides a comprehensive structure that is scalable to the size of the event and has standardized role descriptions. Techniques such as using vests to identify people in charge during a disaster, with a one-page job action sheet in each vest pocket, are essential in a crisis situation. Color-coded vests may also be useful in identifying the role of each leader based on the incident command structure utilized. All hospital and department all-hazards preparedness plans must be on hand and clearly labeled in the command center, along with in-house phone and pager directories.

Testing the Emergency Management Plans and Command Center

The benefits of conducting biannual emergency drills, both announced and unannounced, includes being able to test the EOP, the command center, and staff roles and responsibilities. Announced drills have the added benefit of teaching opportunities. Tabletop exercises test a group's ability to cooperate and their readiness to respond to a disaster situation (FEMA, 2015a). There are many types of drills, including:

- *Internal drills* to test specific department and/or hospital responses. Examples include setting up and operating the command center, recognizing a biological event both in the ED and on the units, locking down the hospital entrances, simulating decontamination processes, using downtime procedures during a communications or cyber disaster event, and handling various surge capacity situations.
- *External drills* in collaboration with community agencies and departments involving patients (police, fire, and rescue; public health); tabletop drills simulating an unknown biological, nuclear/radiological, or chemical scenario and prioritizing the response by departments; and surge capacity drills testing a community's ability to respond to overwhelming demand. Joint command centers and mutual aid agreements may also be tested.

All of these drills offer great insight into the merit of the all-hazards preparedness plan and allow facilities the opportunity to modify plans to improve processes. Regardless of the type of drill or who is involved, the drill should always be set up as a safe place where participants are encouraged to ask questions and be provided an opportunity to learn from any mistakes.

Establishing the Hospital's Role in the Community

The hospital will play an important role in the community in the case of a disaster. Knowing how the hospital fits in the all-hazards disaster response plan from the perspective of such entities as the police and fire departments, EMS, public health department, and the local school system will be important in coordinating efforts. The emergency management committee will be instrumental in defining the hospital's role locally in the community and nationally to meet federal government expectations and regulatory compliance. Additionally, the public expects the same level of competent care to be provided at all times regardless of the situation.

On a local level, the lead person of the committee (often this will be a designated hospital administrator) will partner with public health, local police, fire departments, EMS, community physicians, regional alliances with other health care facilities, and local emergency management agencies/councils. It will be important to define the hospital's and community's role in emergency situations. Testing of plans using local community disaster drills, often biannually, is essential to continually improve processes. The hospital should strive to test its internal all-hazards preparedness plans whenever there is a planned community drill in order to get a full picture of its ability to respond in a disaster in step with the community response.

Nationally, each hospital will play an important role in the political arena by helping local and federal government personnel understand that hospitals, like police and fire departments, are first responders in a disaster. The materials, equipment, and training required for hospitals to prepare adequately for their role in responding to disasters are very expensive. Capital expenditures will be required to create decontamination facilities; purchase PPE; train and educate staff on effective all-hazards preparedness; stockpile emergency equipment, supplies, and pharmaceuticals; ensure adequate isolation rooms; and outfit a hospital command center. Replacement of expired supplies and pharmaceuticals will also need to be considered. Hospitals need financial assistance to do this well, and the committee members can be advocates for federal and state funding. It is helpful to establish a financial subgroup whose mission will be to develop a set plan for capturing costs related to the event as the disaster unfolds. The financial subgroup can also partner with individual units to develop a business continuity plan that can be incorporated into the EOP. This will enable the hospital to submit immediately for any reimbursement funding that becomes available after the event. This may include business disruption insurance. In addition, the subgroup can identify potential federal grants or public funding that might be available to support costly financial expenditures.

Helping Staff Overcome Fear Associated With Disaster and All-Hazards Preparedness

It is important to know that the first rule of disaster preparedness is to keep staff safe. In a disaster, the paradigm of keeping the patient safe first must be modified to focus on helping staff members (and their families) feel as safe as possible. This may be a shift in thinking, but the reality is that if staff members do not feel comfortable coming to work, then the patients' needs cannot be met.

Nursing leadership, in partnership with human resources and the education department, will need to develop educational tools to assist staff in creating personal disaster preparedness plans for themselves and their significant others. Many websites and mobile apps are available to assist in developing educational tools, such as the FEMA and America Red Cross websites. Tools such as personal disaster preparedness plans should be effectively communicated so that employees know that the organization's first priority in a disaster is to keep staff safe. Arrangements will need to be made for 24-hour childcare somewhere close to the hospital or on-site. Employee assistance programs need to be available at all times to help employees cope with fear related to a disaster. It is important that nurse leaders understand the psychological impact of a disaster on the victims as well as the staff (Tillman, 2011), so that staff can positively influence victims of a disaster. This requires educating nurses about how to provide care during extreme conditions.

CRISIS STANDARDS OF CARE

During times of crisis in health care delivery, it may become necessary to make decisions about allocating resources. When the number of patients exceeds the available supplies, equipment, and medications, health care organizations may have to change the way they use their resources in order to deliver the best care to the most people. In 2012 the Institute of Medicine (IOM, now called the National Academies of Science, Engineering, and Medicine, Health and Medicine Division) developed *Crisis Standards of Care* to help with this decision-making process with the understanding that these decisions are complex and must be made using fair and equitable principles (Hodge et al., 2013). The framework for these decisions works to inspire fairness and trust and includes heightened ethical sensitivity, understanding what is at stake ethically, adequate planning and policy-making, and flexibility (McLean, 2013). *Crisis Standards of Care* have specific applications based on changing situations. The decisions are often difficult for caregivers but are designed to be consistent in their execution across all disciplines. This type of framework allows for ethical decision-making based on caring for the community as a whole in a disaster situation (McLean, 2013).

LEADERSHIP AND MANAGEMENT IMPLICATIONS

Moving Into the Future With Confidence

Nursing leaders can effect change and ensure that a fully functional emergency management plan for the hospital is developed within 6 to 12 months. Nursing leadership competencies in disaster planning and crisis management are invaluable, and fortunately they have been developed by a collaborative group led by the Department of Veterans Affairs, Office of Nursing Services. These disaster competencies are categorized into four domains: assessment of the disaster scene, technical skills, risk communication, and critical thinking (Coyle et al., 2007).

Clearly, nurse executives are in a position to take a greater role in planning and implementing a disaster response for their organizations. Nursing leaders, from charge nurses through nursing executives are called on to take charge, make decisions, successfully implement protocols, and then modify their action plans based on routine evaluation. Expectations exist that nursing leaders at all levels will act in their patients' best interests and will follow appropriate procedures. In addition, being willing to take risks is an important attribute of the nursing leader. Nurse executives are in a unique position to forge new pathways in the arena of emergency management because of their combination of clinical skills, strong organizational ability, networking expertise, and training in clinical crises. If the emergency management committee is not diligent in its efforts to keep everyone continually focused on preparedness, a sense of complacency about refining the emergency management plan may result. With strong nursing leadership at the managerial and executive level, the oversight of disaster planning can be proactively addressed, and a constant state of readiness can be achieved. Engagement of staff nurses—often through shared governance committees or organization-wide all-hazards disaster preparedness planning—is essential for keeping readiness high. Participation in disaster drills is one example of action learning.

CURRENT ISSUES AND TRENDS

Current nursing and medical literature is focused on specific departments and how they are establishing their unique roles and responsibilities in a disaster. Nurse leaders can use these benchmark articles to motivate units and departments to move forward in fully assessing and defining their roles in all-hazards preparedness. For instance, making decisions about consolidating care sites may require closing clinics, emergency care centers, and community health programs during a disaster to free up clinical staff to assist in a hospital's surge capacity planning in a disaster, provide staff for vaccination teams in a biological event, or help with decontamination in a chemical exposure event. Allocation of staff may be required to build capacity in outpatient and community arenas depending on the disaster threat. Decisions about alternate care sites should be considered well ahead of an event and often require regional collaboration across many disciplines and agencies. Clinical staff may need to flex up or assume roles not usual to their job assignment.

All-hazards preparedness has become a way of life, and knowledge about the level of alertness is an everyday expectation. Hospital staff and leadership have begun to settle in at a heightened state of preparedness. In April 2011, the federal government implemented a new alert system, the National Terrorism Advisory System (NTAS), which replaced the colored-coded system implemented by the DHS. The new two-level system will alert the American public about an "elevated threat" in the event of a credible terrorist threat or an "imminent threat," if a credible and specific terrorist threat is about to occur (US DHS, 2011).

One area of all-hazards preparedness that has not been fully developed, yet has great potential in disaster planning, is the role of various community resources such as outpatient centers, schools, and even churches. The nurse executive can facilitate the establishment of partnerships between the hospital and the community facilities. Once established, these partnerships can be used to set up communication centers where people can congregate to receive support and obtain information about the disaster situation or family and friends who may have been injured.

To effectively manage large-scale events, networking beyond the hospital will be critical to create partnerships with other facilities, hospitals, community agencies, and local, state, and federal departments. To assist in this process, it may be helpful to have a signed agreement or memorandum of understanding (MOU) with community organizations and businesses for assistance. A trend is underway, as evidenced by a growing alliance between regional hospitals and the community at large throughout the United States, to strategically plan for allocation and sharing of federal and state resources in the event of a disaster. As an example, in Virginia, a Regional Hospital Command Center (RHCC) has been established in which 14 northern Virginia hospitals have been networked to more effectively respond in a disaster. This is accomplished via radio communication and a shared web-based bed availability tracking system displaying each hospital's ability to take varying levels of patient acuities. These hospitals can directly link with hospitals in Washington, DC, to coordinate efforts during an event and communicate effectively with fire, police, EMS, public health, the emergency operating center (a local command center for overseeing the event), and the field incident commander in coordinating the disaster response. Similar to the Virginia RHCC just mentioned, cohorts of hospitals, firefighters, EMS, law enforcement, schools, public health, and businesses are joining together to form regional alliances and collaborations to leverage their capability to respond in a coordinated manner.

Under the direction of FEMA, incident management assistance teams (IMATs) were created to provide rapidly deployable (within 2 hours) supplemental assistance to the region affected by a disaster. These teams consist of trained personnel from different departments, organizations, agencies, and jurisdictions, activated to support incident management at major or complex emergency incidents. IMATS function as an initial interface with regional and state responders (FEMA, 2015b).

Building on the idea of partnering with the community to strengthen preparedness, in 2012 FEMA established a community-based assistance program called FEMA Corps. FEMA Corps is dedicated to disaster preparedness, response, and recovery. It is designed to help communities prepare for, respond to, and recover from disasters by supporting disaster recovery centers; assisting in logistics, community relations, and outreach; and performing other critical functions (Corporation for National & Community Service, n.d.). The FEMA Corps provides a pool of trained personnel and pays long-term dividends by adding depth to existing workforce reserves. Hospital executives need to stay abreast of these newly emerging resources and explore ways to partner with them. These types of programs will be pivotal in providing extra human resources and support services desperately needed for hospitals to function effectively in times of crisis.

One other emerging issue that challenges care during a disaster is allocation of scarce resources when the system is overwhelmed. This need was directly experienced in the United States during the Hurricane Katrina and Sandy events, was also witnessed with the Haiti earthquake, with devastating tornadoes in Joplin, Missouri, and with the COVID-19 pandemic. As a result of these catastrophic events, both state and national disaster preparedness leaders examined planning needs for response requirements when resources are scarce. These efforts include substantial planning efforts to address immediate needs, including ethical considerations and planning assumptions, as well as management issues regarding responder protection, with the health care workforce as a primary concern. In recommendations of the Ethics Subcommittee of the Advisory Committee to the Director, CDC, ethical guidelines were outlined for pandemic planning (CDC, 2007) and are a useful resource. To maximize the level of national and regional preparedness, these principles included the identification of clear overall goals, principles of transparency in decision-making, public engagement and involvement in the process, use of sound scientific evidence for decision-making, and thinking in a global context.

The guidelines recommended early planning efforts that balance utilitarian concepts with respect of persons, nonmaleficence, and justice. The recommendations gave examples of distribution criteria that will need to be considered well ahead of the time of an actual event. The development of triage criteria for allocation of scarce resources has been documented in several articles (Hick & O'Laughlin, 2006; Kraus et al., 2007). Further, adopting standards of care under altered conditions has been described and addressed in numerous documents from states and associations seeking to offer guidelines to care providers (American Nurses Association, 2008; New York State Department of Health Task Force on Life and the Law, 2007; Phillips & Knebel, 2007). Each nursing leader and team needs to understand these guidelines and begin the planning process at both the local and regional levels for developing protocols to allocate scarce resources and implementing triage criteria for care in overwhelming events. Implementing periodic tabletop discussions regarding how to allocate resources in a time of scarcity will prove to be a powerful tool in setting the stage for what to do if such an event occurs. Collaborative professional staff and hospital leadership discussions about scarce resource allocation will present ethical dilemmas that need to be thoughtfully considered in a planning time that is devoid of emotion. Questions to be discussed at the tabletop include the following: (1) Which hospital and/or clinical leader will make the final decision about ventilator allocation and other scarce resource distribution? (2) What are the criteria used to determine which patients receive aggressive treatment and which will receive palliative care, both imminently and long term, as other life-threatening complications ensue? (3) How are prophylactic pharmaceutical dissemination plans going to be activated to protect staff and their families? Knowing the hospital's approach to handling these types of scenarios will be a critical precursor in implementing an effective plan in the event of a disaster that is compounded by a shortage of resources.

RESEARCH NOTE

Source

Arbon, P., Ranse, J., Cusack, L., Considine, J., Shaban, R. Z., Woodman, R. J., et al. (2013). Australasian emergency nurses' willingness to attend work in a disaster: A survey. *Australasian Emergency Nursing Journal: AENJ*, 16(2), 52–57.

Purpose

All types of hospital staff would be required to show up for work during an internal or external disaster and many hospitals consider staffing shortages as a barrier to efficiently operationalize their response plans. Identifying factors that would encourage willingness of the staff to be present in times of disaster would mitigate some of the family and other external factors that place employees into conflict. The purpose of this research was to confirm if previously identified factors that influenced nurse absenteeism could be mitigated and to develop strategies for sufficient staffing for use during times of disaster.

Discussion

A 10-minute survey was designed and distributed to greater than 1000 emergency nurses in the country of Australia. Characteristics of the individuals in addition to their willingness to come to work under different types of circumstances were analyzed. Out of the 451 participants who submitted the survey, the majority were female with a mean age of 39.8 years. Although there was a general willingness to attend work during a disaster, participants were 23.9 times more likely to be willing to come to work for events such as earthquakes and fires versus pandemics and chemical events. Gender and level of nursing education/licensure did not influence willingness to be present during time of disaster, but employment status measured by full time equivalents did. Nurses who had different types of disaster training or perceived that their peers and leaders were prepared for a disaster were also more likely to be willing to come to work. Although the participants who lived with children at home were the most likely to be unwilling to attend work during a disaster, those who had a personal disaster plan were almost eight times more likely to be willing to work.

Application to Practice

Health care facilities will need to consider individual, family, and workplace factors that may influence a nurse's willingness to come to work during a disaster. Proactive personal disaster planning and the ability to communicate with loved ones during these times appeared to have the biggest influence. Hospitals can develop mitigation strategies by encouraging nurses to develop personal plans using disaster preparedness checklists and having crucial conversations prior to any events with their support systems. Educating nurses to use these checklists to develop plans for their families or others that they care for outside of the work environment can also provide peace of mind and increase willingness to come to work if they feel their families are cared for. Hospitals can also work to provide disaster education at the workplace for nurses, allied health, and hospital leaders as the perception of peer and workplace readiness also increased willingness to work. Implementing strategies around these types of practices provide hospitals an opportunity to mitigate staffing shortages during times of crisis.

CASE STUDY

Shooting Incident

Day 1 (Sunday)

At approximately 10:05 pm on the final evening of a 3-day music festival held in a large metropolitan city and known for being a world-renowned tourist attraction, more than 1000 shots were fired over a 15 minute time-frame, with shooting occurring in the concert venue. The venue was outdoors, on a flat area of nearly 15 acres. Approximately 22,000 concert goers were in attendance over the course of the event. The hospitals servicing the area were a mix of for-profit and not-for profit facilities with Level 1 and Level 2 trauma centers within miles of the concert venue.

The shooter was across the street from the venue and began shooting down from about 30 stories, and about 300 yards away. The crowd was initially disoriented by

CASE STUDY—cont'd

the sound and assumed it was part of the show. When people in the crowd began to fall from gun-shot wounds, the crowd began to run for their lives. All points of egress became quickly over-run, and some began jumping over temporary barriers, including fencing meant to outline the concert boundaries.

Utilizing all resources available to them, concert goers began to stabilize wounds, stop bleeding, and help as many of the injured as possible escape the area and seek shelter or emergency care. That night 31 people were killed before reaching a hospital, and an additional 800 were injured. Fleeing on foot the crowd expanded beyond the 15-acre site an additional 4 miles into the densely populated city.

Day 1–2 (Post Incident–After Midnight–Pre-Hospital)

There were about 800 injured patients. The injured eventually found their own transportation to surrounding hospitals. Many were routed to medical care through the use of smartphones or mapping applications. The Emergency Medical Personnel were responding to approximately 20 sites around the perimeter of the event to treat or transport the wounded who had fled on foot. It is reported that each site had as few as 3 patients and as many as 40 patients. To complicate communication there were multiple calls being placed to law enforcement regarding potential additional active shooters. The massive use of cell phones quickly overwhelmed already heavily utilized cell towers.

Day 1–2 (Post Incident–After Midnight–Hospital)

The occurrence of the event on a Sunday night and other events discussed above created unique circumstances around patient arrivals. Many hospitals reported not having supplies restocked or having already flexed off extra staff. It was at this time that the surge of patients started coming in. Carloads, truck loads, Uber drivers, and taxi drivers were arriving without prior notice. The closest hospitals to the concert began to receive the largest number of patients and began to manage the volume as a mass casualty. No prior field triage or formal pre-hospital care had occurred, and hospitals reported lines longer than a quarter of a mile. For example, one of the hospitals received 200 patients in need of treatment within 8 hours of the event.

Questions for Reflection

1. How do you plan for the following areas of potential impact on patients arriving via privately owned vehicles in large numbers with no forward notification?
2. How does EMS respond to more than 20 locations in a 15-acre area with some order and priority?
3. How should orchestrated communication occur when cell phone towers are overwhelmed?

Mass Casualty Disaster Plan Implementation

Communications	**Day 1:** Check and test redundant communications systems (telephone, VoIP, radio, satellite, Internet). Communicate with hospital leadership and established community partners regarding the hospital's emergency plan. **Day 1:** Open the incident command center and review action plans for the next 24 to 48 hours. Open the manpower pool to communicate with staff, including surgeons, to be prepared to stay at the hospital and work extra shifts if necessary. Notify community partners regarding the plan for the duration of the mass casualty event. Prepare spaces for staff to change clothes if soiled and be able to get back to work quickly. **Day 4:** The incident command center should be fully staffed and operational. Review internal surge plan specific to bed capacity, discharges, and staff. Communicate the plans to physicians and leadership. The appointed media relations personnel will provide accommodations for media. Communicate with local, state, regional, and federal resources for support including supplies, personnel, and infrastructure. Provide frequent situational updates to staff and visitors. Receive frequent updates from department leadership for effective decision-making. Request support from state and/or local authorities to help transport personnel to the hospital to relieve on-duty staff if possible. **Day 5:** Connect with local and regional partners to update your situation, request help if needed, and offer assistance if possible.

(continued)

CASE STUDY—cont'd

Safety and security	**Day 1:** Complete a facility safety survey regarding incoming patient surge and potential visitor surge. **Day 3:** Do frequent facility surveys inside and outside to check communication infrastructures. **Day 4:** Prepare for an influx of patients in the emergency department. Set up a space for the "worried well" (community members who are not ill but are distressed about the mass casualty). Monitor patients and visitors for stress-related behavioral problems. **Day 5:** Monitor the exterior building and grounds for any safety hazards. Including where you will set up extra morgue sites.
Resources and assets	**Day 1:** Inventory supplies including food, fuel, water, medical supplies, and staff. Order for any shortages from vendors. **Day 3:** Organize emergency supplies for rapid deployment to units. Food service changes to surge-level meal planning. **Day 4:** Consider allocating resources and medical supplies according to crisis standards of care. Request any needed supplies from the central warehouse if available. **Day 5**: Inventory supplies, food, water, linens, and pharmaceuticals. Begin restocking units with available supplies.
Staff responsibilities	**Day 1–2:** Remind staff to prepare to be able to respond to the hospital's needs as essential personnel. This includes arranging for child, elder, or pet care; securing their homes against damage; and having adequate supplies for their families. Be certain that you communicate with employees to be proactive for Day 2 and continue care. **Day 1–2:** Work to arrange timely discharge for appropriate patients and receive new admits from the emergency department. **Day 2:** Staff should be prepared for the possibility of working in an area other than their home unit. Prepare for "just in time" training. **Day 2:** Alter the nurse/patient ratio to accommodate surge levels and train personnel who will work in a different area. Coordinate patient tracking with EMS.
Utilities management	**Day 1:** Check and test redundant utilities systems including having a 96-hour supply of fuel. **Day 3:** Transfer all essential equipment to emergency outlets. Continue to check utility operations frequently including outside the facility for infrastructure problems. **Day 4:** Monitor fuel supply, equipment operations, and infrastructure. Respond to any internal or external damage. **Day 5:** Restore equipment to main power source. Arrange generator fuel delivery, and test that systems are functioning adequately including air handlers, water, and lighting.
Clinical and support activities	**Day 1:** Consider discharging appropriate patients and canceling elective surgeries to increase bed capacity. **Day 1–2:** Consider a discharge holding area for patients who are discharged but not able to go home. **Day 1–2:** Incident commander orders surge capacity plan in effect. Open surge beds. Incident commander and medical director review *Crisis Standards of Care* for possible implementation. Monitor blood supply and storage capability. Inventory pharmaceutical supplies and consider using the emergency supply if necessary. **Day 1–2:** Arrange for discharges to accommodate emergency department patients.

CASE STUDY—cont'd

After Action

An after-action meeting is necessary to evaluate the hospital's response to the emergency event. Leaders will discuss what went well and what did not, what could have been done better, and how to plan for the next event. It is also an opportunity to evaluate and make needed updates or changes to the emergency operations plan. Some common questions for this meeting may include:

1. Did your incident command team maintain planning using the six critical areas of preparedness (communications, resources and assets, safety and security, staff responsibilities, utilities management, and patient clinical and support activities)?
2. Did you document every action over the past 6 days, with time, date, and names?
3. Were communications effective?
4. Were you able to integrate your response with state, regional, and local authorities?
5. How could you have improved your response to the surge situation?
6. Were the crisis standards of care decisions consistent and decided using fair and equitable principles?

CRITICAL THINKING EXERCISE

It is a Friday evening in the middle of winter. Cold and influenza season continues. The Centers for Disease Control & Prevention has just confirmed a small outbreak, less than 10 patients, in your city of a novel virus that has symptoms listed as influenza-like illnesses. You have been working in health care for greater than 10 years and remember the outbreaks of H1N1 and different corona viruses that created surge capacity events in areas throughout North America and other parts of the world. The emergency department (ED) is staffed with nine registered nurses, three ED physician providers, and one emergency medical technician. Information continues to change rapidly, including the inclusion criteria for testing. Your infection prevention department has told you to isolate symptomatic patients and place them in droplet and contact precautions. On a normal day, the ED sees 150–200 patients, and you know that an increase in symptomatic patients or even the walking well will easily create a surge event. You have concerns about the ability to triage patients quickly while keeping staff and others from contracting the virus. The ED team has requested other areas of the hospital be available as secondary triage and the ability to fast track confirmed admissions.

Planning process: Epidemic planning process for a novel virus.

Purpose: To prepare and educate all staff on a surge capacity event and plan for staffing shortages resulting from community impact on social services including day cares and schools.

Background information: You are one of several nursing directors at a 400-bed hospital with a 30-bed emergency room in a large metropolitan city. There are multiple hospitals in the city who are also anticipating surge events. The staff at the hospital have done drills for emerging diseases after SARS and Ebola events, and have identified and trained a group of initial responders for positive cases. You are the administrator on duty and have been tasked with leading the effort to quickly develop a plan for surge capacity.

1. How and where can the ED screen the walking well while maintaining all of the elements of Emergency Medical Treatment and Labor Act (EMTALA)?
2. What triage and safety considerations need to be put in place for separating influenza like illness apart from other non-infectious chief complaints?
3. What considerations will need to be addressed for personal protective equipment (PPE)?
4. How will you manage staffing shortages that may occur from surge, fear, or employees that have to stay home to care for loved ones?
5. What education needs to be provided to staff? Is this different by discipline?
6. How do you manage additional foot traffic, including visitors and vendors?
7. What should be done to secure the campus and manage media requests?
8. Do you have enough respiratory equipment including ventilators? What is your process for securing more if needed?
9. Are positive patients appropriate to cohort? What is your first area for admission placements and where do you expand to if additional beds are needed?

10. Are there additional or potential disruptions in the supply chain? How will you manage scare resources or items affected by backorders?
11. Can non-essential staff be redeployed to assist in other areas?
12. How will you maintain your processes should the surge event last longer than 7 days?

REFERENCES

Agency for Healthcare Research and Quality (AHRQ). (2012). *Allocation of scarce resources during mass casualty events*. https://effectivehealthcare.ahrq.gov/products/mass-casualty-events-scarce-resources.

American Nurses Association (ANA). (2008). *Adapting standards of care under extreme conditions: Guidance for professionals during disasters, pandemics, and other extreme emergencies*. https://www.aft.org/sites/default/files/ept_sect2_ana-care-standards.pdf.

American Organization of Nurse Executives (AONE). (2016). *AONE guiding principles: Role of the nurse leader in crisis management*. https://www.aonl.org/sites/default/files/aone/role-of-the-nurse-leader-in-crisis-management.pdf.

Arbon, P., Ranse, J., Cusack, L., Considine, J., Shaban, R. Z., Woodman R. J., et al. (2013). Australasian emergency nurses' willingness to attend work in a disaster: A survey. *Australasian Emergency Nursing Journal: AENJ*, *16*(2), 52–57.

Arnand, K. (2014). *Cyber attacks—Definition, types, prevention*. Retrieved from http://www.thewindowsclub.com/cyber-attacks-definition-types-prevention.

California Hospital Association. (2011). *Emergency preparedness: Hazards vulnerability analysis*. http://www.calhospitalprepare.org/hazard-vulnerability-analysis.

CBS News. (2016). *60 Minutes investigates medical gear sold during Ebola crisis*. http://www.cbsnews.com/news/60-minutes-investigates-medical-gear-sold-during-ebola-crisis/.

Centers for Disease Control and Prevention (CDC). (2007). *Ethical guidelines in pandemic influenza*. https://www.cdc.gov/od/science/integrity/phethics/panFlu_Ethic_Guidelines.pdf.

Centers for Disease Control and Prevention (CDC). (2001). *Biological and chemical terrorism: Strategic plan for preparedness and response*. https://www.cdc.gov/mmwr/preview/mmwrhtml/rr4904a1.htm.

Committee on Homeland Security of the House of Representatives. (2008). *Compilation of homeland security presidential directives (HSPD) (updated through 39 December 31, 2007): Prepared for the use of the committee on homeland security of the House of Representatives*: US Government Printing Office.

Corporation for National & Community Service. (n.d.). *What is FEMA Corps?* https://www.nationalservice.gov/programs/americorps/americorps-programs/fema-corps/fema-corps-faqs#12439.

Coyle, G., Sapnas, K., & Ward-Presson, K. (2007). Dealing with disaster. *Nursing Management*, *38*(7), 24–29.

Drenkard, K., & Rigotti, G. (2002, updated 2016). *Inova Health System survey*. Falls Church, VA: Inova Health System.

Drenkard, K., Rigotti, G., Hanfling, D., Fahlgren, T., & LaFrancois, G. (2002). Healthcare system disaster preparedness, part 1: Readiness planning. *Journal of Nursing Administration*, *32*(9), 461–469.

Federal Emergency Management Agency. (2006). *NIMS Implementation Activities for Hospitals and Healthcare Systems* (pp. 1–26) (United States of America, Department of Homeland Security, Federal Emergency Management Agency). http://www.fema.gov/pdf/emergency/nims/06_training.pdf.

Federal Emergency Management Agency (FEMA). (2015a). *Emergency planning exercises*. https://www.fema.gov/emergency-planning-exercises.

Federal Emergency Management Agency (FEMA). (2015b). *Fact sheet: Incident management assistance teams*. http://www.fema.gov/media-library-data/1440617086827-f6489d2de59dddeba8bebc9b4d419009/IMAT_July_2015.pdf.

Federal Emergency Management Agency (FEMA). (2016). *National incident management system*. http://www.fema.gov/national-incident-management-system.

Federal Emergency Management Institute (FEMA). (2014). *Academic emergency management and related courses (AEMRC) for the higher education program: Comparative emergency management book*. https://training.fema.gov/hiedu/aemrc/booksdownload/compemmgmtbookproject/.

Hick, J. L., & O'Laughlin, D. T. (2006). Concept of operations for triage of mechanical ventilation in an epidemic. *Academic Emergency Medicine*, *13*(2), 223–229. http://dx.doi:10.1197/j.aem.2005.07.037.

Hodge, J. G., Jr., Hanfling, D., & Powell, T. (2013). Practical, ethical, and legal challenges underlying crisis standards of care. *Journal of Law, Medicine, and Ethics*, *41*, 50–55, 2012. Public Health Law Conference: Practical Approaches to Critical Challenges, Spring 2013.

Institute of Medicine (IOM). (2012). *Crisis standards of care—A systems framework for catastrophic disaster response*. National Academics Press. http://hmd.nationalacademies.org/hmd/Activities/PublicHealth/DisasterCareStandards.aspx.

International Federation of Red Cross and Red Crescent Societies (IFRC). (2016). *Biological hazards: Epidemics*. http://www.ifrc.org/en/what-we-do/disaster-management/about-disasters/definition-of-hazard/biological-hazards-epidemics.

Joint Commission Resources. (2008). *Emergency management in health care: An all-hazards approach*. Oakbrook Terrace, IL: Author.

Joint Commission Resources. (2016). *Emergency management in health care: An all-hazards approach* (2nd ed.). https://store.jointcommissioninternational.org/emergency-management-in-health-care-an-all-hazards-approach-4th-edition/.

Kraus, C. K., Levy, F., & Kelen, G. D. (2007). Lifeboat ethics: Considerations in the discharge of inpatients for the creation of hospital surge capacity. *Disaster Medicine and Public Health Preparedness*, *1*(1), 51–56. http://dx.doi:10.1097/DMP.0b013e318065c4ca.

McLean, M. R. (2013). Allocating resources—A wicked problem. *Health Progress*, *94*(6), 60–67.

New York State Department of Health Task Force on Life and the Law. (2007). *Allocation of ventilators in an influenza pandemic*. www.health.state.ny.us/diseases/communicable/influenza/pandemic/ventilators/.

Niska, R. W., & Shimizu, I. (2011). *Hospital preparedness for emergency response United States, 2008*. US Dept. of Health and Human Services, Centers for Disease Control & Prevention, National Center for Health Statistics.

Phillips, S. J., & Knebel, A.(Eds.). (2007). *Mass medical care with scarce resources: A community planning guide*. (Prepared by Health Systems Research, Inc., an Altarum company, under contract No. 290-04-0010. AHRQ Publication No. 07-0001). Agency for Healthcare Research and Quality. http://archive.ahrq.gov/research/mce/mceguide.pdf.

Ready.gov. (2016). *Chemical threats*. https://www.ready.gov/chemical.

Sternberg, E. (2003). Planning for resilience in hospital internal disaster. *Prehospital and Disaster Medicine*, *18*(4), 291.

The Joint Commission (TJC). (2008). *Accreditation program: Hospital emergency management*. Author. https://store.jcrinc.com/2020-comprehensive-accreditation-manual-for-hospitals-pdf-manual-/ebcah20/.

The Joint Commission (TJC). (2012). *Comprehensive accreditation manual for hospitals 2012: Emergency management accreditation standards*. Author.

The Joint Commission. (2016). Joint Commission Resources Portal. Retrieved February 20, 2016 from https://e-dition.jcrinc.com/Frame.aspx.

The Joint Commission. (2020). *Joint Commission resources portal*. https://e-dition.jcrinc.com/Frame.aspx.

Tillman, P. (2011). Disaster preparedness for nurses: A teaching guide. *The Journal of Continuing Education in Nursing*, *42*(9), 404–408. http://dx.doi:10.3928/00220124-20110502-02.

US Department of Defense. (2015). *DOD dictionary of military terms*. https://www.jcs.mil/Portals/36/Documents/Doctrine/pubs/dictionary.pdf.

US Department of Health & Human Services. (2012). *Emergency management and the incident command system*. https://www.phe.gov/preparedness/planning/mscc/handbook/chapter1/Pages/emergencymanagement.aspx.

US Department of Homeland Security. (2011). *NTAS public guide*. https://www.dhs.gov/xlibrary/assets/ntas/ntas-public-guide.pdf.

US Department of Homeland Security. (2020). *National incident management system (NIMS)*. https://www.fema.gov/national-incident-management-system.

World Health Organization (WHO). (2013). *Emergency response framework*. Geneva, Switzerland: WHO. http://apps.who.int/iris/bitstream/10665/89529/1/9789241504973_eng.pdf.

Wright State University. (2016). *Emergency preparedness*. https://www.wright.edu/police/emergency-preparedness.

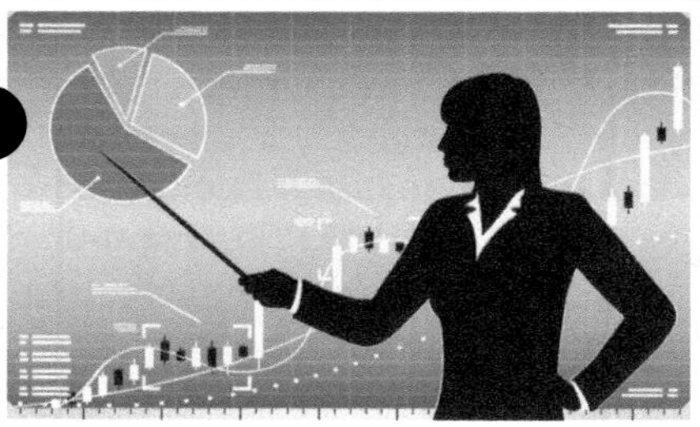

25

Nursing Informatics for Leaders in Clinical Nursing

Karen Dunn-Lopez, Lisa Janeway, Michele A. Berg

Nursing informatics is a subspecialty of nursing that applies computer, data, and information science to nursing science and practice, and emerged as a subspecialty in nursing in the mid-1970s. For those who did not understand the need for the subspecialty, in the early 1990s, Norma Lang articulated the importance saying, "If we cannot name it, we cannot control it, practice it, teach it, finance it or put it into public policy" (Clark & Lang, 1992, p. 128). Today, given the vast array of clinical care activities, data recorded, and rule-based prompts mediated by computers, software, and other technologies, informatics plays an increasingly prominent role in nursing. In fact, the American Association of Colleges of Nursing (AACN) requires that nurses at all levels outside the subspecialty of informatics, including nurse leaders, have basic competencies in nursing informatics (AACN, 2019).

The business of health care information technologies is evolving rapidly in all settings where people spend time, including schools, work settings, homes, and where they shop. Management of the health care industry and care delivery relies extensively on not only the device capture, collection, and analysis of data, but also on the workflow process for what, when, where, who, and how the data are captured. Data about the patient, provider, outcomes, and processes of care delivery are collected from many individuals practicing in different specialties and must be standardized, integrated, coordinated, and managed. Moreover, widespread demand to use these data for performance measurement and reporting to accountable care customers, regulators, and accrediting/certification bodies comes at a time when reimbursement and incentive payments to providers and health care institutions are linked with performance on selected patient outcome measures. Whereas the imperative in nursing used to be that nurses needed their nursing-specific data, now a subspecialty of nursing informatics has become rooted and is growing in clinical care management as nurses migrate to using their data for care management. The purpose of this chapter is to delineate what clinical nursing informatics is and discuss informatics competencies, regulatory and policy issues, current trends, and the implications that all these areas have for clinical nursing leaders.

DEFINITIONS

What Is Nursing Informatics?

Informatics is a multidisciplinary field defined by the American Medical Informatics Association (AMIA) as applying principles of computer and informatics science to advance life science research, health professions education, patient care, and public health (AMIA, 2020). The application of informatics knowledge is applied by clinical informaticists who facilitate the delivery of health care.

The field of **nursing informatics** has been defined in multiple ways in the past decades, including technology-, conceptual-, and role-focused definitions. Staggers and Thompson (2002) articulated one of the most encompassing versions of the definition as follows:

> *Nursing informatics is a specialty that integrates nursing science, computer science, and information science to manage and communicate data, information, and knowledge in nursing practice. Nursing informatics facilitate the integration of data, information, and knowledge to support patients, nurses, and other providers in their decision-making in*

all roles and settings. This support is accomplished through the use of information structures, information processes, and information technology. (Staggers & Thompson, 2002, p. 260)

The language of data management and clinical informatics contains many acronyms and specific technical terminology. Selected terms are:

Clinical informatics: The area of informatics that is applied to facilitate the delivery of health care.

Clinical nursing informatics: The area of informatics that is applied to facilitate the delivery of nursing care.

Contingency plans: Preparations to continue the safe care of patients throughout the continuum in case electronic health records or technology systems are not available for use.

Data set: A collection of patient specific variables.

Electronic health records: A longitudinal record of patient information that is stored electronically that crosses encounters and the continuum of care.

Electronic medical records: An electronic version of a medical record that contains medical information from one provider or health care facility.

End users: Persons who are the intended and actual user of a product or technology.

Information blocking: Blocking of information by health care providers, organizations, or developers that interferes or prevents health information from being exchanged and is punishable by law.

Interoperability: The ability of an information system to accurately exchange information with another system.

Medical device integration: A method that allows medical devices to flow patient data from one system to another using software programs known as middleware or interface engines.

mHealth: Patient health care and wellness that is supported by mobile devices such as mobile phone, wearable monitors, and other wireless devices.

Ransomware: A threat where a malicious software causes system access issues and a monetary threat to organizations, holding patient data hostage.

Usability: The degree to which a technology is easy to learn and remember, and efficient and pleasant to use. In addition, technologies that are useable have limited errors that are easy to detect and recover from.

BACKGROUND

Nursing informatics can best be described, understood, and contextualized using the *Data, Information, Knowledge, and Wisdom (DIKW)* Framework (Nelson, 2019). The model (Fig. 25.1) includes four major constructs defined in Table 25.1. Although it may seem that nursing informatics focuses on health information technologies used by nurses, the DIKW framework demonstrates increasing levels of critical thinking or "knowledge work" at each level.

Although this framework provides an important lens to understand nursing informatics broadly, we propose a new informatics area, **Clinical Nursing Informatics**. In contrast to those nursing informatics scientists who focus on the creation of generalizable knowledge about nursing informatics using scientific methods, we believe that clinical nursing informatics focuses on optimizing quality and safety of patients using information and communication systems through the delivery of nursing care. Although it is necessary to have clinical informatics departments in health systems, this alone is not adequate to ensure that informatics solutions will be applied that optimize nursing's unique role in health care. Rather, organizations need to have a well-educated cadre of clinical nursing informaticist nurses who specialize in *nursing* informatics, along with nurse leaders and bedside nurses who have robust competencies in nursing informatics.

Nursing Informatics Competencies

Professional nursing organizations have developed, and regularly revise, competencies for the profession, including competencies in nursing informatics for all clinical roles. AACN develops competencies to guide faculty members to develop and integrate curricula that support these competencies at the prelicensure through graduate levels. Of interest, the AACN is currently in the process of re-envisioning its essentials (AACN, 2019). Early drafts suggest an increasing emphasis on informatics. The Quality and Safety Education for Nurses Institute (QSEN) focuses on preparing nurses to improve the quality and safety of the organizations they work in (QSEN, 2020). A core area for this initiative is informatics.

Other leading interdisciplinary organizations (e.g., Health Information Management Systems Society's TIGER Initiative and AMIA) have also developed competencies. Table 25.2 highlights some of the competencies that focus on informatics skills for nurses. This is an important distinction. We believe nurses who have nursing informatics competencies are likely to have a more focused impact on advancing the profession

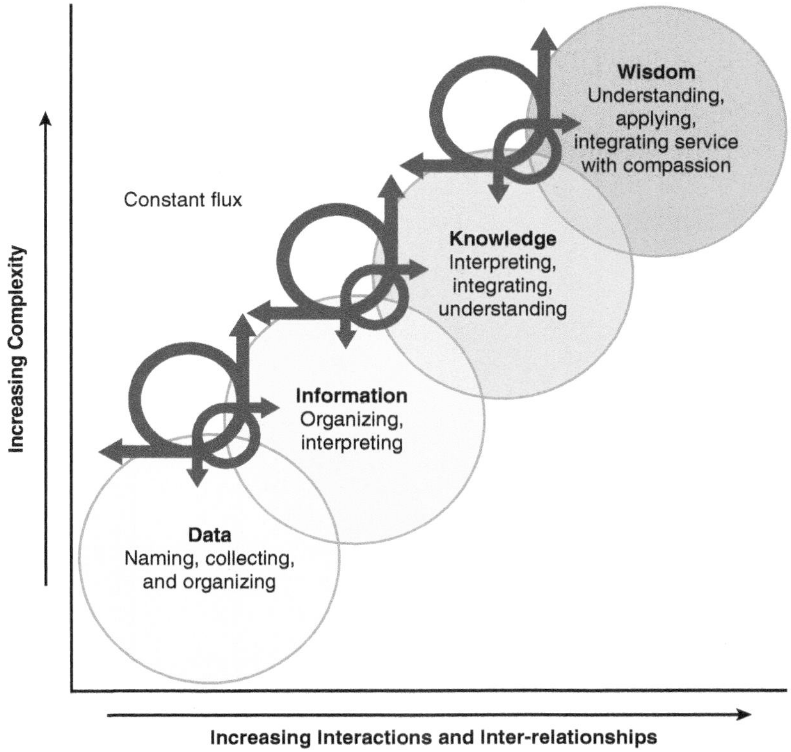

Fig. 25.1 Data, Information, Knowledge, Wisdom, Framework. Source: Nelson, R. (2019). Informatics: evolution of the nelson data, information, knowledge and wisdom model: part 1. *OJIN: The Online Journal of Issues in Nursing, 23*(3). https://ojin.nursingworld.org/MainMenuCategories/ANAMarketplace/ANAPeriodicals/OJIN/Columns/Informatics/Informatics-Evolution-of-Nelson-Model-Part-1.html.

TABLE 25.1 Data, Information, Knowledge, Wisdom Core Constructs

Construct	Definition	Example
Data	Single uninterpreted variables	Weight, blood pressure, body temperature
Information	A group of variables that are organized in a manner that meaning can be interpreted	Body mass index is a measure of body size based on height, weight and gender
Knowledge	The formalization of relationship and rules between data and information	Knowledge that patients with cancer are often at risk for infection guides the action to check patients' body temperature when they exhibit chills
Wisdom	The application of data, information and knowledge to make decisions with compassion to meet the needs of the patients, families, and communities	Providing highly immunosuppressed cancer patient exhibiting signs of infection with rapid assessments, mobilization of the needed members of the health care team, while providing interventions to decrease their fever and ease their discomfort.

Source: Nelson, R. (2019). Informatics: evolution of the nelson data, information, knowledge and wisdom model: part 1. *OJIN: The Online Journal of Issues in Nursing, 23*(3). https://ojin.nursingworld.org/MainMenuCategories/ANAMarketplace/ANAPeriodicals/OJIN/Columns/Informatics/Informatics-Evolution-of-Nelson-Model-Part-1.html.

TABLE 25.2 Nursing Informatics Competencies Across Levels of Clinical Nurses

AACN Informatics Related Competencies[a-c]	QSEN Informatics Knowledge Competencies[d]
Bachelors Essential IV	**Prelicensure**
1. Demonstrate skills in using patient care technologies, information systems, and communication devices that support safe nursing practice.	1. Explain why information and technology skills are essential for safe patient care
2. Use telecommunication technologies to assist in effective communication in a variety of health care settings.	2. Identify essential information that must be available in a common database to support patient care
3. Apply safeguards and decision-making support tools embedded in patient care technologies and information systems to support a safe practice environment for both patients and health care workers.	3. Contrast benefits and limitations of different communication technologies and their impact on safety and quality
4. Understand the use of CIS systems to document interventions related to achieving nurse sensitive outcomes.	4. Describe examples of how technology and information management are related to the quality and safety of patient care
5. Use standardized terminology in a care environment that reflects nursing's unique contribution to patient outcomes.	5. Recognize the time, effort, and skill required for computers, databases and other technologies to become reliable and effective tools for patient care
6. Evaluate data from all relevant sources, including technology, to inform the delivery of care.	
7. Recognize the role of information technology in improving patient care outcomes and creating a safe care environment.	
8. Uphold ethical standards related to data security, regulatory requirements, confidentiality, and clients' right to privacy.	
9. Apply patient care technologies as appropriate to address the needs of a diverse patient population.	
10. Advocate for the use of new patient care technologies for safe, quality care.	
11. Recognize that redesign of workflow and care processes should precede implementation of care technology to facilitate nursing practice.	
12. Participate in evaluation of information systems in practice settings through policy and procedure development.	
Master's Essential V	**Graduate**
1. Analyze current and emerging technologies to support safe practice environments, and to optimize patient safety, cost-effectiveness, and health outcomes.	1. Contrast benefits and limitations of common information technology strategies used in the delivery of patient care. Evaluate the strengths and weaknesses of information systems used in patient care.
2. Evaluate outcome data using current communication technologies, information systems, and statistical principles to develop strategies to reduce risks and improve health outcomes.	2. Formulate essential information that must be available in a common database to support patient care in the practice specialty. Evaluate benefits and limitations of different communication technologies and their impact on safety and quality.

(Continued)

TABLE 25.2 Nursing Informatics Competencies across Levels of Clinical Nurses (cont'd)

3. Promote policies that incorporate ethical principles and standards for the use of health and information technologies.	3. Describe and critique taxonomic and terminology systems used in national efforts to enhance interoperability of information systems and knowledge management systems.
4. Provide oversight and guidance in the integration of technologies to document patient care and improve patient outcomes.	
5. Use information and communication technologies, resources, and principles of learning to teach patients and others.	
6. Use current and emerging technologies in the care environment to support lifelong learning for self and others.	
Doctorate in Nursing Practice Essential V 1. Design, select, use, and evaluate programs that evaluate and monitor outcomes of care, care systems, and quality improvement including consumer use of health care information systems.	
2. Analyze and communicate critical elements necessary to the selection, use, and evaluation of health care information systems and patient care technology.	
3. Demonstrate the conceptual ability and technical skills to develop and execute an evaluation plan involving data extraction from practice information systems and databases.	
4. Provide leadership in the evaluation and resolution of ethical and legal issues within health care systems relating to the use of information, information technology, communication networks, and patient care technology.	
5. Evaluate consumer health information sources for accuracy, timeliness, and appropriateness.	

[a] (American Association of Colleges of Nursing, 2008).
[b] (American Association of Colleges of Nursing, 2011).
[c] (American Association of Colleges of Nursing, 2006).
[d] (Quality and Safety Education for Nursing, 2020).
Source: Based on AACN's Essentials for Baccalaureate, Master's and Doctorate in Nursing practice Education and QSEN Informatics Competencies. https://qsen.org/competencies/pre-licensure-ksas/.

and practice of nursing as compared to nurses who are trained primarily in the interdisciplinary informatics context, because nurses who are primarily trained in interdisciplinary informatics are more likely to be pulled away from nursing to lead overarching informatics programs and projects, and may become disconnected from nursing care.

Regulatory and Policy Issues Related to Clinical Informatics

Recent federal policy initiatives have had a wide range and transformative impact on clinical informatics. In 2009 the United States government enacted the *Health Information Technology Act* (HITECH) as part of the

American Recovery and Reinvestment Act (ARRA). HITECH required organizations to adopt electronic health records, offering incentives for meaningful use (MU). MU focused on three key areas of clinical data: capture and storage, advancing clinical processes, and improving outcomes (Adler-Milstein & Jha, 2017). The overarching goal of the HITECH act was to use technology to arm providers with the tools to be able to manage care better in a safe and secure methodology, and improve the quality of care (O'Grady et al., 2016). Electronic health records (EHRs) have the technology to share information electronically across multiple organizations through health information exchanges and are equipped with interoperability, a method to communicate information between systems. However, systems must be secure, and patient information must be private. *The Health Insurance Portability and Accountability Act* (HIPAA) of 2009 was instituted to protect patients' privacy in electronic records (Cohen & Mello, 2018).

As the nation moved beyond meaningful use, there were new provisions following the Medicare Access and Children's Health Insurance Program (CHIP) that have had an impact on clinical informatics. *The Reauthorization Act* of 2015 (MACRA) changed the reimbursement landscape, adding a quality payment program (QPP) under the premise of value, quality, and better care (Kahn & Baum, 2020). The new payment model will impact organizations as metrics will drive reimbursement rates and create a potential need to modify electronic health records systems and report outcomes.

The 21st Century Cures Act (2015) amends the HITECH Act and became public law in 2016 (Lye et al., 2018). The Office of the National Coordinator for Health Information Technology (ONC, 2016) is responsible for implementing parts of the act through "delivery, advancing interoperability, prohibit information blocking and enhancing the usability, accessibility and privacy and security of HIT." Unintended consequences of health information technology (HIT) have led to new problems enfolding, including security threats in the form of ransomware, an increase in the burden of documentation, usability problems, and safety concerns. New regulatory policies, which often have implications for the delivery of nursing care, are in constant development to address these problems. It is imperative for clinical leaders in nursing to stay informed and be responsive to this changing landscape.

CURRENT ISSUES AND TRENDS

Nursing informatics is a current issue and trend. Nurses comprise the majority of the workforce in health care are the most abundant "end-users" of EHRs. Technological advances to improve patient care and safety during the delivery of care are continuing to develop at a fast pace. Several current issues and trends impacting the profession of nursing are described next.

Dashboards and Reports

There is now a vast amount of information stored from all of these systems and available to provide data analytics in the form or reports or dashboards to nurse leaders. Nurse leaders need to take part in the development of these reports to ensure data validity and be able to understand the output of the reports for monitoring and decision-making. Examples of analytical reports are bar code compliance, late medication administration, and missing or late documentation. Dashboards can be specific and group information together, such as capacity management, quality and safety metrics, and staffing information. Information can also be reused in the form of complex algorithms and decision trees to make predictions based upon a data set, for example, for sepsis, falls, and readmissions (Alexander et al., 2019).

Clinical Decision Support Systems

Clinical decision support systems (CDS) is a method embedded in electronic systems, providing actions and relevant information for clinicians to make decisions related to patient care (Lowry et al., 2012). Clinical decision support is represented in the form of active and passive alerts, banners, icons, or order entry. These interventions must be carefully designed and developed using best practices to increase adoption, reduce over-dependency, over-warning, and linked to measurable goals and monitored (Osheroff, 2012). Before implementing CDS, nurse leaders need to ensure that decisions are for the right reason, have clear measurable objectives, and a plan to monitor. Using a framework such as the Five Rights of clinical decision support (Osheroff, 2012), in collaboration with key stakeholders and governance, will lessen potential pitfalls.

The Five Rights consider:

1. **What:** The right information provides clear direction to the clinicians about the next steps to consider.
2. **Who:** The right person ensures that the CDS is aimed at the correct provider.

3. **How:** The right format is the type of tool used.
4. **Where:** The right channel describes the place information is delivered.
5. **When:** The right time ensures that the intervention occurs in the precise moment of the workflow.

Patient Education

Informatics tools are shaping the way patients engage in learning. These informatics tools have flipped the format of nurse-only led patient education to allow for asynchronous on-demand education for patients and their caregivers. Nurses play a pivotal role in ensuring that the education is evidence-based, culturally sensitive, and addresses health literacy for patients. Nurses should be involved in vetting the materials to ensure they are written at or below a fifth-grade reading level (Stossel et al., 2012). Usability is also a high priority action (Dunn Lopez & Fahey, 2018) that nurses can engage in to ensure patients can easily log in to these applications and navigate through learning materials.

In addition to the reading level and usability, ensuring the patient understands the material presented remains a critical role of nurses. Nurses need to follow up with the patient using teach-back and/or validation methods via verbal understanding. Nurse leaders and clinical nurse educators need to evaluate which tools best fit their IT infrastructure and the long-term costs associated with maintaining such systems. For example, patients may prefer watching videos compared to reading from a handout, and can review the content multiple times.

Clinical Documentation Burden

In February 2020 the ONC finalized the report on reducing regulatory and administrative burden relating to the use of health IT and the EHR (United States Department of Health and Human Services, 2020). There are three primary goals:

1. Reduce the effort and time required to record information in the EHR
2. Reduce the effort and time needed to meet regulatory reporting requirement for clinicians, hospital and health care organizations
3. Improve the functionality and intuitiveness.

The ONC has put forth three major strategies (Table 25.3) to reduce documentation burden that has important implications for nurses. Nursing leaders should be familiar with the strategies and collaborate with informatics and operations personnel to implement local level strategies and processes to reduce the burden of documentation.

Mobile Health

Mobile health applications (known as mHealth) are on the rise in the health care industry as more patients have access to smartphones, tablets, and wearable sensor technologies (e.g., smart watches, etc.). mHealth apps contain multimodal interventions such as diaries, patient-entered data, education, reminders, symptom and activity trackers, and text messages, and can be connected to wearables or other external devices such as scales, glucometers, or blood pressure devices (Alexander et al., 2019). Less common, but expected to rise, are feedback loops to providers that can be interfaced to electronic health records and can inform providers of patients' changes real time, to modify treatment plans or intervene without an office visit. Like technologies to support patient education, nurses need to be aware of the quality of mHealth their patients may be using. Assessment of quality should include how readable and useable the app is, the degree to which the information is guided by high quality evidence, and whether the mHealth secures patient privacy.

Mobile Devices in Clinical Settings

Mobile devices are also used by clinicians at the point-of-care to enter information, place orders, and review patient records. Electronic health record vendors are developing applications to supplement computer-based charting and increasing functionality. Examples include bar code scanning of medication, blood, and infusion pumps. The advantage of this technology is to reduce the burden on nursing of having a toolkit of hardware to perform safe and quality care. Mobile devices also allow nurses to look up reference information. As organizations deploy these types of devices, there are cost and security implications. Middleware software must be deployed to form a bridge between the devices to other systems and still be secure.

Bring Your Own Device and Medical Device Management (MDM)

Due to the cost of commercial mobile devices, some organizations are allowing nurses to bring their own device (BYOD). The convenience of performing such activities on devices, however, requires strict mobile device management to ensure HIPAA compliance and security.

TABLE 25.3 Clinical Documentation Burden: Strategies and Recommendations for Nurse Leaders

ONC Strategy[a]	Recommendations for Nurse Leaders
Reduce regulatory burden around documentation requirements for patient visits	Recognize that this policy is a major driver of nursing documentation. Identify ways to align documentation practice with documentation policies. Engage nurse users in analysis for streamlining documentation processes. Identify and remove redundant nursing documentation. Develop best practice for copy and paste or copy forward. Use nursing governance structures to manage these changes.
Continue to partner with clinical stakeholders to encourage adoption of best practices related to documentation requirements	Implement training programs that focus on both on both quality and efficiency of documentation. Identify potential outside resources via professional organizations for documentation best practices for nurses. Engage with vendors to improve the usability of vendors' documentation in the EHR. Partner with vendors and clinical implementation teams to address documentation redundancies. Build cross-institutional interdisciplinary teams who meet on a regular basis to evaluate performance metrics after large changes. Advocate at the federal level for high quality nursing documentation for outcomes related to patient safety and care quality.
Leverage health IT to standardize data and processes around ordering services or equipment and related prior authorization processes	Integrate supply chains and order sets for equipment used by nursing. Evaluate other workflow factors related to the burden of nurse ordered equipment.

[a] (United States Department of Health and Human Services, 2020).

There are implications for nursing leadership when nurses are using mobile devices to deliver care and should include policies to ensure the data and information are secure. Whether the device is issued by the organization or brought by the staff, hospitals may decide to manage the device encryption and applications on the phones in-house, or via a third-party MDM provider. Devices must be encrypted, and employees are required to "opt in" or consent to organizational security policies when using personal phones. Employees will sign a consent to the security and enrollment policies set forth by the IT department. For example, if a phone is lost or stolen, the applications associated with patient data can be removed using a remote "wipe" function. Adding to the complexity, all devices need to run the same operating system defined by the organization. This ensures each device can support the applications and resources. Organizations may find that supplying company owned devices is less cumbersome than managing applications and security on personal phones. An example of how to ensure this security includes disabling the phone from taking screenshots of patient information and limiting what is stored on the mobile device within the application.

Nurse Communication Systems, Middleware, and Alarm Management

Nurse call and communications systems are now integrated into mobile devices, which push physiologic alarms and calls from patient rooms to nurses' phones. Alarms can originate from the patient monitor, their ventilator, intravenous pump, or any connected device. This decentralization of monitoring from the nursing station to the phone allows the nurse to manage multiple patients and their physiological alarms on the go.

Middleware serves as a bridge that connects the patient monitor and call light to the phone. Nurse leaders should plan for future applications and select middleware that will connect any other device they anticipate using. For example, middleware used for inpatient systems may need to integrate or work with the outpatient middleware if they serve similar functionality. Extreme caution and care must be followed to ensure any system is programmed with safety in mind and that nurses are educated on the policies and procedures used to mitigate risk. These include and are not limited to defining time limits for answering alarms, defining alarm priority (critical versus warning alarms), standardizing default alarm settings and sounds, planning for backup if systems fail, and ensuring alarms for the patient population are appropriate. For example, when making staff assignments, nurse managers should have a method of communicating which patients are at the most risk for deterioration based on their alarm frequency and clinical history. Nursing leaders should lean on the shoulders of others and understand what has worked in their clinical setting based on the existing and progressing literature from patient safety organizations such as ECRI (https://www.ecri.org/) and the Association for the Advancement of Medical Instrumentation (https://www.aami.org/).

Usability

As organizations have adopted electronic health records and emerging technologies are on the rise, a new problem has arisen that impacts nursing. Technologies that are not easy to use can cause unintended consequences such as documentation mistakes, workarounds, interpretation errors, missing information, decrease in productivity, delay in patient care, increased cognitive load, patient safety concerns, and dissatisfied users (Coiera et al., 2016).

Nursing informaticists play a vital role in assessing the usability of technologies. Along with nursing informaticists, nurse leaders need to ensure that the voices of frontline nursing staff, who are the primary users of systems, are heard (Dunn Lopez & Fahey, 2018), that systems are highly useable, and avoid unintended consequences that compromise patient safety.

Patient Acuity and Staffing Systems

Patient acuity and staffing systems assist management in determining patient acuity levels, workload intensity, and the type of care needed by nurses through electronic systems. Organizations have the ability to track and monitor expenses and resources to promote patient care with patient acuity systems. These systems can also assist with forecasting future trends and strategize on changing market trends (Hawkins et al., 2019). One of the advantages of having systems for patient acuity and staffing is to monitor and improve nurse patient staffing levels and provide documentation for regulatory agencies. On the other hand, some external staffing systems require manual intervention to update, are not real time, and increase organizational costs to maintain. Also, the information is typically entered by resources not in the direct care of the patient, which can lead to subjective information that does not account for patient complexity. More forward-thinking tools can predict nurse staffing needs based on existing nursing documentation of the nurses' assessment of patient outcomes (Garcia & Lovett, 2018).

Nursing Documentation

For many EHRs have moved from adoption to optimization. Nurses are interested in leveraging the EHR to make nursing work more efficient, data driven, transferable, shareable, and measurable, to improve quality and outcomes. Others want to be able to conduct queries to understand what nursing interventions will lead to the highest quality outcomes in a given patient population. However, in order to leverage nursing documentation, it must be based on the use of valid, reliable, interoperable nursing terminologies.

There are five standardized nursing terminology sets endorsed by the American Nurses Association that represent the nursing process, three of which are comprehensive and can be used across patient care populations. This include: (1) NANDA-I, Nursing Outcome Classification (NOC) and Nursing Intervention Classification (NIC) that include linkages to each other for nursing diagnosis, interventions, and outcomes; (2) The International Classification of Nursing Practice (ICNP), and (3) Clinical Care Classification (Macieira et al., 2019). Of note, all of these comprehensive terminology sets can be integrated into EHRs for interoperable flow of nursing information, but there is greater evidence supporting the successful integration of NANDA-I, NIC, and NOC (Macieira et al., 2019).

Electronic Health Record Downtime

With the implementation of the EHR system, downtime presents challenges to organizations and especially nurses who are accustomed to having systems available. Downtime is used to describe the inability to access information systems and can be scheduled or unplanned. There are multiple reasons that outages occur with EHR, including system maintenance, upgrades, hardware failure, software problems, loss of power, security threats, and natural disasters. Nursing workflow can be disrupted by not having patient-level data information easily accessible, the ability to document electronically, and the operation of clinical decision support systems (CDS) results, medication information, and provider order entry.

System downtime, either planned or unplanned, can lead to unintended consequences causing a decrease in productivity, medication errors, delays in patient care, and safety and quality issues resulting in adverse effects. Nurse and other organizational leaders need to be prepared for downtime by having policies and procedures in place, contingency plans, and operational readiness. System outages can last one hour or up to days. It is essential that information systems (IS) work in partnership with Nursing Departments to ensure the plan encompasses all aspects of patient care and workflow. Downtime documentation forms are important to accreditors (e.g., The Joint Commission and Centers for Medicare & Medicaid Services) and should be readily available in designated areas so patient care and documentation are not interrupted. Some departments chose to create "safety stations" with binders of documentation forms and emergency preparedness workflows.

According to the ONC, a recommended practice is to have downtime and reactivation policies that are complete, available, and reviewed regularly. The policies should describe when a downtime should be called, who will be in charge, notifications, and how orders will be executed (ONC, 2016). Not only are downtime procedures important but equally imperative is the reactivation procedures. According to the Safer Guides, Safety Assurance Factors for EHR Resilience (ONC, 2016), organizations should regularly conduct downtime simulations or drills.

Nursing leaders need to consider incorporating downtime training for new hires and annual competencies for nursing staff. Formal training related to downtime procedures and policy will allow nurses to be more efficient, potentially decrease workflow or patient safety concerns, and negative feelings during downtime. Materials, including procedures and downtime forms, must be accessible in the departments and on a schedule to be regularly reviewed.

LEADERSHIP AND MANAGEMENT IMPLICATIONS

Widespread adoption of meaningful EHRs in the US has been ongoing for over a decade. EHRs provide an opportunity for clinicians and leaders to learn about the care delivered in their organization in order to support real time decision-making and improve care outcomes. This is sometimes referred to as "Practice Based Evidence" (Linder et al., 2017) and "Learning Health Systems" (Friedman et al., 2015).

Data generated by nurses about their clinical decisions for patients, including identification of appropriate nursing diagnosis, selection of nursing interventions, and assessment of patients progress towards outcomes need to be an important part of learning health systems. Unfortunately, many organizations do not have systems for capturing nursing documentation data in a standardized manner. Fortunately, forward-thinking nurse leaders can advocate for the inclusion of standardized nursing terminologies as part of routine nursing documentation in order to capture important data about nursing care.

Standardized terminologies representing nursing diagnoses, interventions, and outcomes were developed by teams of nurse scientists with input from practicing nurses using rigorous research methods over four decades ago. For example, NIC (interventions) (Butcher et al., 2018) and NOC (outcomes) (Moorhead et al., 2018) were funded by the National Institute of Nursing Research. Standardized nursing terminologies have successfully been integrated into many EHRs and used by researchers to understand the impact of nursing care and predictive models (Macieira et al., 2019). Moorhead described ten ways to use NIC and NOC for practice-based evidence. These range from working with the EHR vendor to develop reports based on nursing documentation data and improving quality of care based on NIC and NOC data.

The constantly changing landscape of health information technologies' increasing use and regulatory issues have many implications for clinical nursing operations. In order to manage these changes, clinical nurse leaders need to leverage and sometimes improve their governance and organizational structures. Nurse leaders are also responsible for managing large- and small-scale implementation of technology.

Governance and Organizational Structure

Informatics processes touch every aspect of the health care system, from medication administration to mandatory health screening. It is essential to have not only interdisciplinary teams, but also ensure nursing leaders support informatics as project sponsors and operationalize the vision of the informatics team. Shared governance structures supported by nurse leaders and the prioritization of informatics work are imperative for new HIT initiatives and optimizing existing information systems. Nursing leaders and clinical informaticians collaborate on parallel committees with stakeholders such as IS, nursing councils, risk management, and accreditation departments to support a structured and sustainable clinical operation. Although there are many organizational structures for clinical informaticians, the role of the bedside nurse informs leadership of nursing work, where formalized informaticists positions serve to bridge the gap between IS and nurse end-users.

Some have found that EHR and other health information technology implementation is successful when (1) clinicians can define technology needs, (2) informatics goals are aligned with organizational strategy, (3) defined principles for EHR decision-making are aligned with strategy, (4) escalation protocols are well defined, (5) clinical informatics models are representative of shared governance models, and (6) clinical informatics are devoted full time to informatics positions with no patient care (Collins et al., 2015).

Managing Implementation of New Health Information Technologies

Not only must hospitals meet business objectives, but also external regulatory policy changes require leadership to work with interdisciplinary stakeholders to stay ahead and comply with new policies. Clinical nursing informaticians are in a unique position to create a structure of connectivity between top-level leadership, IS, and bedside nurses.

Organizational readiness projects should be assessed early to anticipate barriers to adoption and opportunities for engaging motivated stakeholders. Technology will not solve ineffective workflows, and failure to clearly implement a technology around the task needs of the nurse may potentially increase work/inefficiencies. Projects involving technology implementations are not technology projects, but people projects. Therefore prior assessments of culture, a clear understanding of the problem to be solved, analysis of the current state, and proposed future state must be defined. Creating effective teams and training, measuring key performance metrics, and sharing information with stakeholders early increases the chance of success.

Communications Plans

After assessing readiness to change, a communications plan and effective training strategy needs to be developed. New HIT changes come in many forms, from quarterly updates, to entire work processes that change how nurses perform daily tasks. Change is expected, and developing a standard communications plan will help users anticipate how to adjust smoothly. For example, quarterly updates should be in a standard template format and come from a leader who is invested in that change. A Vice President of Nursing Operations may send the message to the entire organization or the message may come directly from IS. Regardless of the sender, the communication needs to allow the user to reference current state with future state, and how the change will affect their work. Most importantly, how is the new state going to make the job easier and more efficient? Nurses need to know: what's in it for them?

Vetting the message with clinical nursing staff prior to delivery ensures it is congruent with the language nurses use to interpret the message's meaning. Nursing and IS may team up for traveling "road shows" and communicate changes in person or present at town hall meetings. Shift change reports and staff meetings are time-honored traditions for sharing new content. Whatever method, it is important to file the communications in a shared file where it may be referenced later.

Education Planning

Nurses expect change, whether it is a new piece of equipment or entire clinical process change and responsibilities. Any new HIT implementation should be coordinated with nursing leadership, frontline staff, and patients. The same holds true for education. Education should be done well before implementation, and the materials should relate to nursing work and contain expectations for what to do in case of failure. In-person education with protected time away from patients allows for focus and no interruptions. Asking a nurse to learn during patient care is distracting and unsafe. Training modules may be developed with nurses and subject matter experts to ensure alignment with clinical context and the environment of care.

Boilerplate education from IT vendors needs to be reviewed carefully or edited to match what is happening at the organization. Materials need to be available both electronically and via paper form during implementation. Relating any new technology or processes back to the previous one will help reinforce the existing mental model. What are the differences and similarities about how this process was done? What are the new tools needed, and how does the nurse get there? Nurses should know how to use any new tools and allow "hands on" testing before roll out. Technology documents from the manufacturer must be readily available and reviewed with nurses before implementations. When technical documents are not written in plain language or are cumbersome, shortened "quick tips" sheets written by nursing educators help the user when problems arise.

Creating Stakeholder Teams

Effective interdisciplinary teams ensure that the transition to a new technology is effective and efficient. The diffusion of new information technology innovations is dependent upon many factors, especially those most likely to be early adopters (Rogers, 2003). Nurses who welcome change and risk will be the "cheerleaders" for new HIT. Early adopters are respected leaders who communicate the message through social channels and influence others to do the same.

Frontline nurses should be part of the interdisciplinary team and inform leadership what happens at the bedside during new HIT implementations to eliminate unintended consequences like bottlenecks to workflow and nursing productivity at the bedside. If patients are part of the new change, they need to be part of the plan before it starts. For example, patients should be part of patient portal development and can guide usability and the way information is presented on the home screen. Nursing and patients can participate in usability testing months prior to roll out to ensure the right information is presented in a comprehensive, concise format.

CONCLUSION

In today's health care world of increasing reliance on technologies, all nurses need to have basic competencies in nursing informatics to provide safe and high-quality care. Nurse leaders can play a particularly important role in ensuring that the voice of nursing, as it relates to clinical technology use, is well represented in nursing governance structures and throughout every level of the organization. Clinical nursing informaticists play a key role in technology implementations, assessment, daily use, as well as the inclusion of nursing data in EHRs that fully represent nursing care. Their combined expertise in health care technologies and nursing work and workflow can save organizations money, prevent unintended consequences, and promote the success of technology implementations.

RESEARCH NOTE

Source

Mosier, S., Roberts, W.D., & Englebright, J. (2019). A systems-level method for developing nursing informatics solutions: The role of executive leadership. *Journal of Nursing Administration, 49*(11), 543–548.

Purpose

The challenge for nurse executive and nurse informaticists is how best to coordinate the efforts of experts from diverse fields to design, develop, and deploy solutions to complex systems problems. The purpose of this study was to describe the systems-level method and two successful applications of creating nursing informatics solutions to enhance patient care.

Discussion

The project was conducted within a large network of hospitals and facilities in the US and the UK. The Chief Nurse Executive developed a method to harmonize the work efforts of disparate groups of both clinical and informatics experts. The three guiding principles of the framework were clear lines of responsibility and authority, respect for each type of expertise needed, and clear commitment to the aims of the project. A visual model was displayed. Two large-scale nursing informatics solutions were discussed: one clinically focused (evidence-based clinical documentation for the flow of information in a patient-centric record), and one leadership focused (development of a nursing data portal with a common platform for sharing nursing performance data).

(*Continued*)

Application to Practice

Nurse executives advance the use of nursing knowledge by creating a data culture, developing data competencies, and establishing a data infrastructure. It takes specific leadership to guide a group of experts through idea development, design, development, data mapping, visualization, and subsequent application of the products that are developed. All of this goes through a technology and informatics life cycle. Clarity of roles was crucial. Leadership engagement stimulated ultimate adoption of the resulting solutions in two examples.

CASE STUDY

Clinical Decision Support System for Neonatal Hypoglycemia

Hypoglycemia is a very treatable condition with early intervention. A serious safety event was reported at a hospital where a neonate was not treated for hypoglycemia twelve hours after birth. Hypoglycemia is defined as low blood glucose concentration, is found in 5% to 15% of newborns, and is increasing in frequency. Hypoglycemia can lead to neurologic damage and abnormalities, such as seizures, and can result in learning disabilities (Wight et al., 2014).

A root cause analysis was completed by a team of clinicians, informatics nurses, and Information Technology Professionals (IT). It was determined there was a nursing educational gap, policies and procedures needed revision, hypoglycemia assessments were absent, and the system lacked alerts, reminders, or protocols. After the root cause analysis was performed, a project team was formed.

Stakeholders

Stakeholders for the project included Labor and Delivery and Special Care Nursery nurses, the Director and Manager of Women's and Children's Services, Quality Manager, Patient Safety Liaison, Project Manager, Informatics Nurse, Systems Analyst, Interface Engineer, analytics, and trainer.

Objectives

The objectives of the intervention were to improve adherence in testing neonates who are at risk for hypoglycemia or have signs and symptoms by obtaining blood glucose levels within the first hour of birth, to increase adherence to following hypoglycemic protocols in neonates who have abnormal glucose levels, and for an increase in staff satisfaction with the ERH related to functionality in the electronic health record to support clinical decision-making for the right patient at the right time in the workflow.

Interventions

The leadership team reviewed and updated the Hypoglycemia Policy and Procedure. Also, necessary documentation assessment points that were missing were added to the system. Finally, a hypoglycemic protocol was designed. There would be three Clinical Decision Support (CDS) interventions.

A clinical alert was designed by the project team and is based on the **Five Rights of CDS**. Table 25.4 summarizes each right and provides examples. The **Right information** will appear for the nurse when a newborn is at risk for hypoglycemia. The **Right person** is elicited from documented maternal risk factors during labor and delivery and neonatal assessment. The alert will appear for nurses who are caring for the mother and/or the neonate. The **Right format** is an active alert that requires input. The **Right channel** will be the Nursing Documentation System within the EHR. The format will contain a pop-up box with text suggesting the neonate is at risk for hypoglycemia and a link to hypoglycemia protocol. The **Right point in the workflow** is while the mother is in labor, during the newborn assessment, and when a point-of-care test result is entered into the system. The Five Rights of clinical decision support are mapped to an example in Table 25.4.

Workflow

Labor and Delivery

The first CDS intervention will occur while the mother is in labor. The patient must be admitted, be in labor, and have associated risk factors on the problem list or history. Upon opening up the record of a patient who meets the criteria, an active alert will appear. The nurse will be presented with the following information "this patient's newborn is at risk for hypoglycemia." The nurse is required to acknowledge the alert and has the option to review the policy and procedure: "select not applicable or remind me later." If the policy and procedure is not selected, the alert will continue to pop up every two hours. The purpose is to alert the nurse that the neonate may be at risk for hypoglycemia.

Neonatal

The second CDS intervention will occur after the neonate is born and will be directed toward the nurse who is

CASE STUDY cont'd

TABLE 25.4 Five Rights of Clinical Decision Support Mapped to Case Study

5 Rights[a]	Example
(What) Right information	A pop up alert for the nurse when a newborn is at risk for hypoglycemia: "This patient's newborn is at risk hypoglycemia." A pop-up alert for the nurse when the neonate is exhibiting signs and symptoms of hypoglycemia with a link to a suggested protocol to place orders.
(Who) Right person	The alert will appear for nurses caring for moms who are at risk for an infant with hypoglycemia or the infant that is exhibiting signs and symptoms. Based upon patient history and assessments documented in the EHR
(How) Right format	The alert will be active and display on the screen with the right information and will be required to acknowledge.
(Where) Right channel	The electronic health record
(When) Right point in the workflow	The alert will appear upon opening the laboring mom, newborns record, or when the point-of-care test is entered with an abnormal result.

[a] Adapted from Osheroff, J. A. (Ed.) (2012). *Improving outcomes with clinical decision support: an implementer's guide* (2nd ed.). Chicago, IL: HIMSS.

caring for the patient. The alert is based upon new documentation question selections added to the newborn admission history. The assessment will include maternal risk factors and signs and symptoms of hypoglycemia. When any of the choices are selected, the following information will appear in a pop-up box, "this patient is at risk for hypoglycemia, order the hypoglycemia protocol." The protocol will be based orders based and will require a response. After the order is placed a banner will appear in the electronic health record indicating the patient is at risk for hypoglycemia, nursing tasks will be added to the worklist related to feeding schedules and blood glucose levels. Nursing problems and goals will appear in the care plan.

Point-of-Care Testing

The third CDS intervention will be presented during the point-of-care testing. Blood glucose levels are interfaced from the point-of-care testing system. When the blood glucose is not within the parameters, the nurse is presented with the same alert in Intervention two. Also, graphical reports will display the glucose levels. Once the orders are placed, the active alert will cease.

Evaluation

Analytical reports were created for Nurse Managers to monitor patients who are at risk for neonates with hypoglycemia and neonates who have low blood glucose levels.

Staff Training

The project will include a training program that provides for baseline measurement of nurse's knowledge of hypoglycemia risk factors and interventions with a post quiz. Nurses needed to be trained on the new assessments, alerts, tasks, reports, and reminders.

The implementation of clinical decision support to alert nurses of mothers who may deliver a baby who is at risk or develop hypoglycemia will result in a higher quality of care and lead to improved outcomes. To achieve success multiple interventions at different points in the workflow needed to be implemented. Analytics were available to ensure clinical accuracy. The key to success in solving serious patient safety issues is to involve appropriate team members and engaging stakeholders. This will result in the right solution for the right person at the right time with the right information, at the right point in the workflow using the right channel.

CRITICAL THINKING EXERCISE

Nurses in all units of a large medical center are required to print and label patient point-of-care lab specimens that are automatically generated by physician orders in the EHR. Once an order is written and electronically "signed off" by the nurse, the label prints on a local printer designated for labs only.

Leaders from several nursing units have noticed an uptick in mislabeled specimens, and they need a way to improve compliance. Mislabeled specimens not only impede timely care, but can also potentially lead to the wrong care when specimens are labeled for the wrong patient. The nursing leadership team asked the Nursing Informatics department and Information Systems (IS) to help develop a solution to the problem by investigating the process by which labels are generated and applied to specimens.

The IS team decided to create a verification process where once the label is generated, a separate "task" of scanning the patient's ID band would need to be completed in the patient's room, whereby the label is linked to the patient. This "task" also shows up as a nursing task in a list in the EHR. After the band is scanned, the task will show as "completed" in the EHR and disappear from the list. Any labels that are not verified in the patient room showed up as unfinished tasks in the EHR. Leaders would then be able to monitor adherence via an unfinished task window in the EHR.

Prior to implementation, communications were sent out by IS to the nursing units on the process. There was no in-person training and during the implementation day, scanning tasks did not complete the nursing "task" in the list, and some patient labels did not scan. Nurses went back to the traditional method to print labels and send specimens. In some cases, nurses had to ask physicians to reorder labs just to generate lab labels. It was found later that during integration of the lab information system to the EHR, orders that were generated before the new process were not included in the new workflow. In addition, nurses had questions about how to scan multiple labels in one task, and how that would be captured in the EHR. IS could not answer whether that workflow was possible. Of note, IS was the only stakeholder to validate the process before go-live, and all testing occurred outside of the production environment.

1. Which stakeholders were missing in the development of this new process?
2. Where should the new process have been tested prior to implementation?
3. How should the process have been better tested?
4. What type of training would have been beneficial prior to the implementation?
5. What key performance metric would have been more effective in measuring outcomes besides task list completion? (Hint: number of mislabeled specimens after implementation)
6. What role do nursing leaders have in ensuring the success of any new HIT project?
7. How could education about the new process have been communicated better?
8. What types of communication channels are needed in HIT implementations such as this one?
9. What other unintended consequences and extra work came out of this new process?
10. What would you have done differently and why?

REFERENCES

Adler-Milstein, J., & Jha, A. K. (2017). HITECH Act drove large gains in hospital electronic health record adoption. *Health Affairs, 36*(8), 1416–1422.

Alexander, S., Frith, K. A., & Hoy, H. (2019). *Applied clinical informatics for nurses* (2nd ed.). Burlington, Mass: Jones and Bartlett Learning.

American Association of Colleges of Nursing (AACN). (2006). *DNP essentials*. https://www.aacnnursing.org/dnp/dnp-essentials.

American Association of Colleges of Nursing (AACN). (2008). *The essentials of baccalaureate education for professional nursing practice*. http://www.aacnnursing.org/portals/42/publications/baccessentials08.pdf.

American Association of Colleges of Nursing (AACN). (2011). *The essentials of master's education in nursing*. http://www.aacnnursing.org/portals/42/publications/mastersessentials11.pdf.

American Association of Colleges of Nursing. (2019). *AACN Essentials, DRAFT Domains and descriptors*. https://www.aacnnursing.org/Portals/42/Downloads/Essentials/Essentials-Revision-Domains-Descriptors.pdf.

American Medical Informatics Association. (2020). *What is informatics?* https://www.amia.org/fact-sheets/what-informatics.

Butcher, H. K., Bulechek, G. M., Dochterman, J. M. M., & Wagner, C. M. (2018). *Nursing interventions classification*

(NIC)-E-Book. Amsterdam, NL: Elsevier Health Sciences.

Clark, J., & Lang, N. (1992). Nursing's next advance: an internal classification for nursing practice. *International Nursing Review, 39*(4), 109–111 128.

Cohen, I. G., & Mello, M. M. (2018). HIPAA and protecting health information in the 21st century. *Journal of the American Medical Association, 320*(3), 231–232.

Coiera, E., Ash, J., & Berg, M. (2016). The unintended consequences of health information technology revisited. *Yearbook of Medical Informatics, 25*(01), 163–169.

Collins, S. A., Alexander, D., & Moss, J. (2015). Nursing domain of CI governance: recommendations for health IT adoption and optimization. *Journal of the American Medical Informatics Association, 22*(3), 697–706.

Dunn Lopez, K., & Fahey, L. (2018). Advocating for greater usability in clinical technologies: The role of the practicing nurse. *Critical Care Nursing Clinics, 30*(2), 247–257.

Friedman C., Rubin J., Brown J., Buntin M., Corn M., Etheredge L., et al. (2015). Toward a science of learning systems: a research agenda for the high-functioning Learning Health System. *Journal of the American Medical Informatics Association, 22*(1), 43–50.

Garcia, A., & Lovett, R. (2018). Use of nursing outcomes classification to measure patient acuity and optimize nurse staffing. In S. Moorhead, E. Swanson, M. Johnson, & M. Maas (Eds.), *Nursing Outcomes Classification*. Amsterdam, NL: Elsevier.

Hawkins, M., Messier, A., Myers, K., Nihsen, A., & Kniewel, M. (2019). Using an acuity tool that interfaces with the electronic health record to balance nursing workload. *Manager's Journal on Nursing, 9*(2), 36.

Kahn, M. J., & Baum, N. (2020). MIPS MACRA and Payment Models. In N. Baum, & M. J. Kahn (Eds.), *The Business Basics of Building and Managing a Health Care Practice* (pp. 75–79). New York, NY: Springer.

Linder, L. A., Gerdy, C., Abouzelof, R., & Wilson, A. (2017). Using practice-based evidence to improve supportive care practices to reduce central line–associated bloodstream infections in a pediatric oncology unit. *Journal of Pediatric Oncology Nursing, 34*(3), 185–195.

Lowry S., Quinn M., Ramaiah M., Schumacher R., Patterson E., North R., et al. (2012). *Technical evaluation, testing, and validation of the usability of electronic health records*. Gaithersburg, MD: National Institute of Standards and Technology. *NISTIR*(780).

Lye, C. T., Forman, H. P., Daniel, J. G., & Krumholz, H. M. (2018). The 21st Century Cures Act and electronic health records one year later: will patients see the benefits? *Journal of the American Medical Informatics Association, 25*(9), 1218–1220.

Macieira, T. G., Chianca, T. C., Smith, M. B., Yao, Y., Bian, J., Wilkie, D. J., et al. (2019). Secondary use of standardized nursing care data for advancing nursing science and practice: a systematic review. *Journal of the American Medical Informatics Association, 26*(11), 1401–1411.

Moorhead, S., Johnson, M., Maas, M. L., & Swanson, E. (2018). *Nursing Outcomes Classification (NOC)-E-Book: Measurement of Health Outcomes*. Elsevier Health Sciences.

Mosier, S., Roberts, W. D., & Englebright, J. (2019). A systems-level method for developing nursing informatics solutions: The role of executive leadership. *Journal of Nursing Administration, 49*(11), 543–548.

Nelson, R. (2019). Informatics: evolution of the nelson data, information, knowledge and wisdom model: part 1. *OJIN: The Online Journal of Issues in Nursing, 23*(3). https://ojin.nursingworld.org/MainMenuCategories/ANAMarketplace/ANAPeriodicals/OJIN/Columns/Informatics/Informatics-Evolution-of-Nelson-Model-Part-1.html.

O'Grady, E., Mason, D., Hopkins Outlaw, F., & Gardner, D. (2016). Frameworks for action in policy and politics. In D. Mason, D. Gardner, F. Hopkins Outlaw, & E. O'Grady (Eds.), *Policy politics in nursing in health care* (7th ed.). Philadelphia, PA: Saunders.

Osheroff, J. A. (2012). *Improving outcomes with clinical decision support: an implementer's guide* (2nd ed.). Chicago, IL: HIMSS.

Quality and Safety Education for Nursing (QSEN). (2020). *About QSEN*. https://qsen.org/about-qsen/.

Rogers, E. M. (2003). *Diffusion of innovations* (5th ed.). New York, NY: Free Press.

Staggers, N., & Thompson, C. B. (2002). The evolution of definitions for nursing informatics: A critical analysis and revised definition. *Journal of the American Medical Informatics Association, 9*(3), 255–261. https://doi-org.proxy.lib.uiowa.edu/10.1197/jamia.M0946.

Stossel, L. M., Segar, N., Gliatto, P., Fallar, R., & Karani, R. (2012). Readability of patient education materials available at the point of care. *Journal of General Internal Medicine, 27*(9), 1165–1170.

The Office of the National Coordinator for Health Information Technology. (2016). *Safety assurance factors for EHR resilience*. https://www.healthit.gov/sites/default/files/safer/guides/safer_high_priority_practices.pdf.

United States Department of Health and Human Services (USDHHS). (2020). *Strategy on reducing regulatory and administrative burden relating to the use of Health IT and EHRs*. https://www.healthit.gov/topic/usability-and-provider-burden/strategy-reducing-burden-relating-use-health-it-and-ehrs.

Wight, N., & Marinelli, K. A. (2014). ABM clinical protocol# 1: Guidelines for blood glucose monitoring and treatment of hypoglycemia in term and late-preterm neonates, Revised 2014. *Breastfeeding Medicine, 9*(4), 173–179.

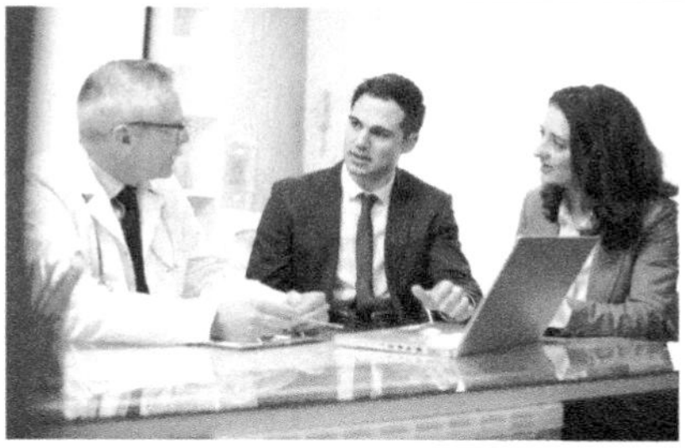

Marketing

Lyn Stankiewicz Losty

http://evolve.elsevier.com/Huber/leadership

Marketing is as old as civilization itself. In ancient Greece, the agora was the center of all aspects of economic life. Market stalls were set up and traders actively engaged in persuasive communications (Fig. 26.1). Marketing is also mentioned in the Bible, with references to marketplaces and the exchange of goods and services in both the Old and New Testament. Marketing is essential for any business to thrive as it helps to build and maintain an organization's goods and services while building the brand equity of the organization. Marketing also assists in building a relationship of trust and understanding with customers. Marketing also creates revenue opportunities for an organization. Since health care systems are businesses, they rely on promotion and advertising to attract patients; thus, marketing is paramount to health care.

Traditionally, nurses are educated to care for patients and their families. Nurse leaders and nurse managers are challenged to care not only for patients and families but also for organizations, especially in today's turbulent

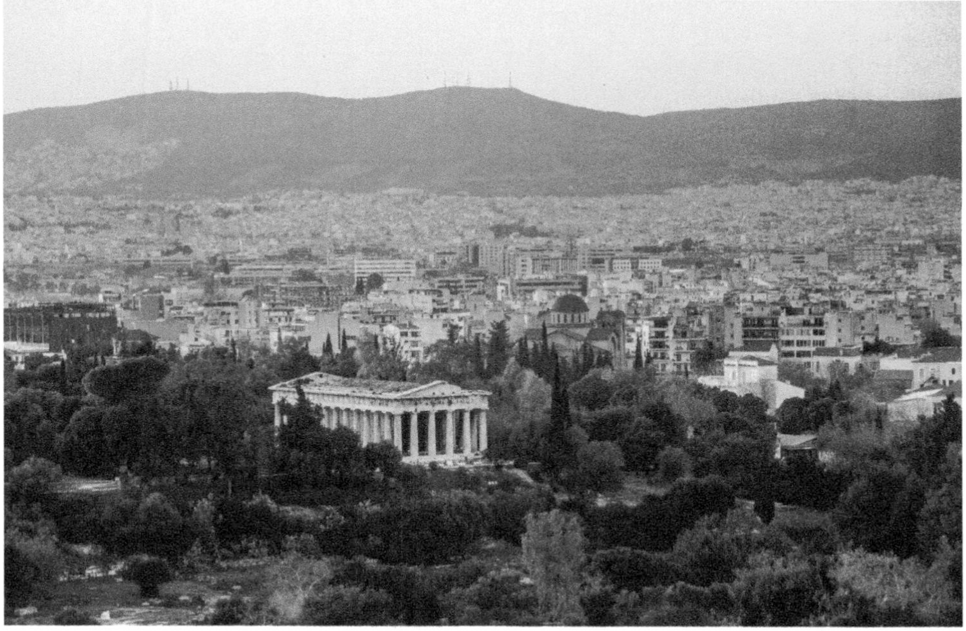

Fig. 26.1 Greece agora.

times. Nurse leaders and managers have a responsibility to foster collaborative relationships among all individuals within our health care organization in order to implement the mission and vision of the organization. They are responsible for recruiting, hiring, orienting new providers, evaluating performances, budgeting, setting policies and procedures, and most importantly, delivering safe and effective care to the patients served. All of these activities are included in the discipline of marketing. The purpose of this chapter is to present key marketing concepts and definitions, identify key current issues and trends of marketing in health care, and discuss implications for nurse leaders and nurse managers.

DEFINITIONS

Defining the Discipline of Marketing

Marketing seems relatively simple because it is about identifying and meeting human and social needs. However, similar to nursing, marketing is both an art and a science as it is achieved by careful planning and execution using state-of-the-art tools and techniques. To understand marketing, some definitions of the discipline of marketing are presented:

- **Armstrong and Kotler** (2017, p. 5) defined marketing as "engaging customers and managing profitable customer relationships."
- **Kotler and Keller** (2016, p. 5) articulated marketing as "the art and science of choosing target markets and getting, keeping, and growing customers through creating, delivering, and communicating superior customer value."
- The **American Marketing Association** (AMA, 2020) described marketing as "the activity, set of institutions, and processes for creating, communicating, delivering, and exchanging offerings that have value for customers, clients, partners, and society at large."
- **Peter Drucker**, a famous management theorist, described "the aim of marketing is to know and understand the customer so well that the product or service fits him and sells itself. Ideally, marketing should result in a customer who is ready to buy. All that should be needed then is to make the product or service available" (Kotler & Keller, 2016, p. 5).

From these definitions, it is apparent that much of what the average person understands about marketing focuses on the words such as "relationships," "customers," and "needs." Simply put, marketing is about meeting a need. **Marketing** is the art and science of identifying a private or social need and turning it into a profitable business opportunity. For example, when Google recognized that people needed to more effectively and efficiently access information on the internet, they created a powerful search engine that organized and prioritized information. When Apple saw that people wanted to carry one device that was a phone, music player, and organizer, they created the iPhone. Overall, there are ten different categories of entities that are marketed by organizations all over the world (Table 26.1).

TABLE 26.1 **Types of Marketed Entities**

Goods	Physical goods constitute the bulk of most countries' marketing efforts. Examples include furniture, cars, machines, sports equipment, etc.
Services	Services include the work of airlines, hotels, car rental firms, barbers and beauticians, maintenance and repair people, and accountants, bankers, lawyers, engineers, doctors, software programmers, and management consultants. Many market offerings mix goods and services, such as a fast-food meal.
Events	Marketers promote time-based events, such as major trade shows, artistic performances, and company anniversaries. Global sporting events such as the Olympics and the World Cup are promoted aggressively to companies and fans. Local events include craft fairs, bookstore readings, and farmer's markets.
Experiences	By orchestrating several services and goods, an organization can create, stage, and market experiences. Walt Disney World's Magic Kingdom lets customers visit a fairy kingdom, a pirate ship, or a haunted house.
Persons	Artists, musicians, CEOs, physicians, high-profile lawyers and professional athletes are examples of people who are marketed. For example, NFL quarterback Peyton Manning, talk show veteran Oprah Winfrey and rock-and-roll legend, Tom Petty are branded.

Continued

TABLE 26.1 Types of Marketed Entities—cont'd

Places	Cities, states, regions, and whole nations compete to attract tourists, residents, factories, and company headquarters. For example, Atlanta is the "hub" for Delta Airlines.
Properties	Property are intangible rights of ownership to either real property, real estate, or financial property such as stocks and bonds.
Organizations	Museums, art studios, corporations, and non-profits all use marketing to boost their public image and compete for audiences and funds.
Information	Information is essentially what books, schools, and universities produce, market, and distribute "this information" to consumers.
Ideas	Most products and services are platforms for some idea or benefit. Such ideas include "Friends Don't Let Friends Drive Drunk," "Just Say No," or "A Mind Is a Terrible Thing to Waste."

BACKGROUND

Marketing is not much different in health care, where the literature is replete with examples of the need for marketing. First, health care revenues were approximately $3.6 trillion in 2018, making it the single largest industry in the United States at 17.7% of GDP (Centers for Medicare & Medicaid Services [CMS], 2019a). Second, the industry faces many challenges, ranging from financial, regulatory, technological, and environmental that often create the need for radical, complex change. Continued consolidation among health care organizations has created a multi-faceted, convoluted, competitive environment. Overlying these challenges, health care leaders and managers need to balance concerns of quality of life and quality of care with "bottom line profits in a way that no other industry is challenged to do" (Kennett et al., 2005, p. 5). Thus, marketing skills are and will continue to be one of the key tools for nurse leaders and managers in the health care field.

Here is a scenario. A working mother with a family of four and an aging father to care for, may wonder if her father's unstable gait should be a concern or if it is part of the normal aging process. She commits to exploring possible solutions and Googles terms like "unstable walking" or "unstable gait in the elderly." She finds the webpage for the local hospital, which provides information about "change in gait for older adults" and sees that the hospital offers an evening program geared towards assisting adult children of aging parents. She calls the program and plans to attend as she has determined that her father's unstable gait is of concern and is committed to seeking a suitable solution. She attends the meeting, meets a geriatric nurse practitioner, and schedules an appointment for her father.

In this brief scenario, the individual becomes aware of an issue (an identified need), considers possible solutions, decides on the type of solution that works best, and commits to the solution. Before any of these events occurred, the marketing team at the local hospital recognized that assisting adult children of aging parents was a need for the community, thus became a priority for their organization. By understanding the customers' needs prior to "actual occurrence of the need," organizations are able to anticipate and meet the customer's need by marketing the solution prior to the need being identified. Thus, when a customer is ready to receive the information that he or she is looking for, an organization is "one step ahead" by advertising and marketing that good or service.

In health care, marketing is focused on establishing customer relationships and satisfying customer identified needs and wants. It is here that nurse leaders and managers are crucial members of the hospital marketing team. Nurse leaders and managers may provide input regarding the organization's marketing strategy; but more importantly, nurse leaders and managers also supervise the team that most directly affects the value that a customer (the patient and family) receives and, ultimately, may report in terms of outcomes. Every interaction between a patient and a nurse creates and communicates value—the very definition of marketing. Therefore, it is imperative that a health care environment which is to be built on patient satisfaction, is created and enhanced through the discipline of marketing.

Marketing Activities

Marketing activities within health care organizations occur at the organizational, departmental, and unit levels. Such activities are also classified as **internal or**

external, with each targeting a different audience or market. Target audiences can be patients and families, physicians, payers, and employees. Marketing departments within health care agencies take the lead in organizational-level, departmental-level, and unit-level activities to ensure that customer-driven marketing strategies and programs are in alignment with the organization's mission, vision, and strategic plan. The primary product that is offered and marketed by health care organizations is care delivery (a service), which includes the nurses who deliver most care in health care organizations. Patient satisfaction is a common and accepted indicator of the service, and a high level of satisfaction is imperative to viability in today's competitive marketplace (Kennedy et al., 2013). This is an example of an internal marketing strategy: marketing the quality of care to patients. For example, the nurse communication section of the Hospital Consumer Assessment of Healthcare Providers and Systems (HCAHPS) survey, which is a standardized survey of patients' perspectives about hospital care, has an important impact on patients' satisfaction with hospitalization. Thus, nurses and nurse leaders are important members of the marketing team because of their primary focus on providing patient care and managing patients' health care needs.

Not only are nurses at the center of health care delivery, but nurse leaders are also accountable for the workforce that provides this service. Marketing initiatives that focus on care delivery, customer satisfaction, and recruitment and retention of the nursing workforce are essential in hospitals. Nurse leaders who possess marketing acumen within their business skill set are invaluable to the development of more sensitive customer/patient service programs delivered by a competent, experienced nursing workforce. These initiatives may be internal (retention) or external (recruitment) or a blend of both.

Previous chapters in this text have addressed the challenges faced by top-level and frontline nurse leaders. These challenges include delivery of high-quality patient-centered care; recruitment and retention of a culturally diverse, competent workforce; promotion of a positive and inspiring image of nursing; design of a healthy work environment; and development of practices to satisfy patients and improve outcomes. Marketing initiatives can be designed and implemented to assist the nurse leader and nurse manager to successfully identify and meet these challenges.

KEY MARKETING CONCEPTS

The Market

Traditionally, a "market" was a physical place where buyers and sellers came together to buy and sell tangible goods. However, in today's environment, markets operate a bit differently. A market is a collection of buyers and sellers who interact over a particular product, product class or service, such as the housing market or the grain market. Manufacturers go to resource markets (raw material markets, labor markets, money markets), buy resources, turn them into goods and services, and sell finished products to intermediaries, who sell them to consumers. Consumers sell their labor and receive money with which they pay for goods and services. The government collects tax revenues to buy goods from resource, manufacturer, and intermediary markets and uses these goods and services to provide public services.

Each nation's economy consists of interacting sets of markets linked through exchange processes. Marketers view sellers as the industry and use the term "market" to describe customer groups. There are a variety of market types, such as need markets (the diet-seeking market), product markets (the shoe market), demographic markets (the "millennium" youth market), geographic markets (the Chinese market), voter markets, labor markets, and donor markets (Fig. 26.2). Sellers communicate to the market through ads and direct mail in the hope that the "market" or customer will purchase their goods and services, and, in return, the sellers receive money for the goods and services and information such as customer attitudes and sales data from the interaction. The inner loop shows an exchange of money for goods and services; the outer loop shows an exchange of information (Fig. 26.3).

Market Brand

A brand is a name, term, design, symbol, or any other feature that identifies a seller's good or service as distinct from those of other sellers. Brands are used in business, marketing, and advertising for recognition. Name brands are sometimes distinguished from generic or store brands. Interestingly, the practice of branding begun with the ancient Egyptians, who were known to have engaged in livestock branding as early as 2700 BCE. Branding was used to differentiate one person's cattle from another's by means of a distinctive symbol burned into the animal's skin with a hot branding

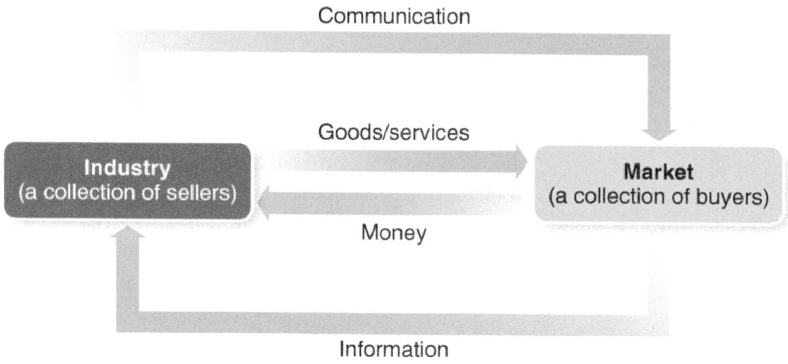

Fig. 26.2 A simple marketing system.

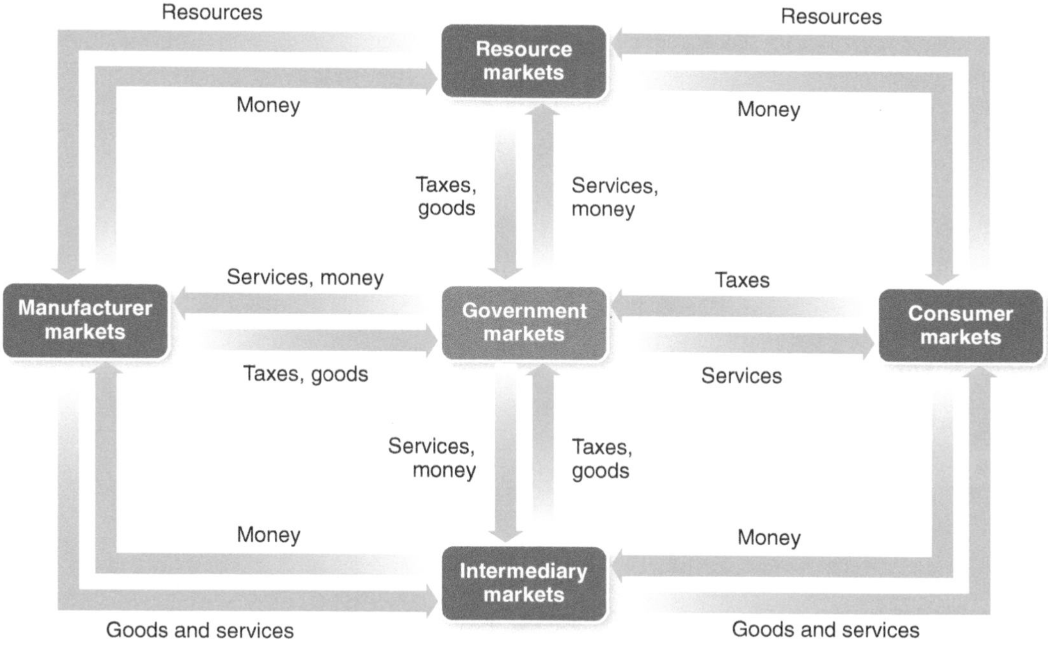

Fig. 26.3 Structure of flows in an exchange economy.

iron. If a person stole any of the cattle, anyone else who saw the symbol could deduce the actual owner. The term has been extended to mean a strategic personality for a product or company, so that "brand" now suggests the values and promises that a consumer may perceive and buy into. Over time the practice of branding objects extended to a broader range of packaging and goods offered for sale including oil, wine, cosmetics, and fish sauce. Branding in terms of painting a cow with symbols or colors at flea markets was considered to be one of the oldest forms of the practice.

In the modern era, the concept of branding has expanded to include the marketing and communication techniques that help to distinguish a company or products from competitors, aiming to create a lasting impression in the minds of customers. The key components that form a brand's toolbox include a brand's identity, brand communication (such as by logos and trademarks), brand awareness, brand loyalty, and various branding (brand management) strategies. Many companies believe that there is often little to differentiate between several types of products in the 21st century,

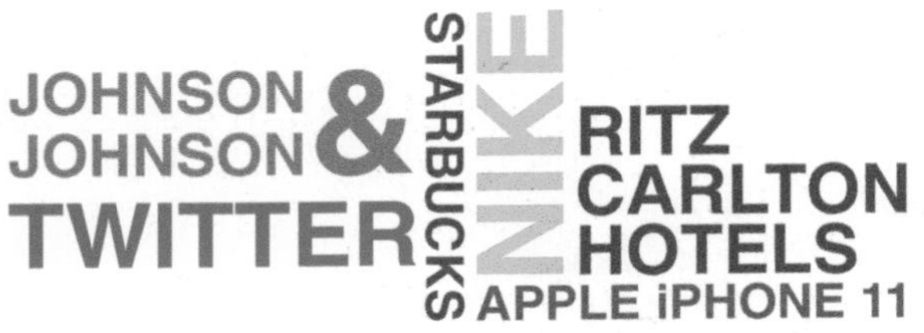

Fig. 26.4 Can you identify these popular brands by their logo?

hence branding is among a few remaining forms of product differentiation (Fig. 26.4).

Product Differentiation

Product differentiation is a marketing strategy that businesses use to distinguish a product from similar offerings on the market. The difference could be something concrete, like speed, power, performance, and better service. Or, it could be a more ephemeral quality, such as just being cooler or more stylish than your competitors. For small businesses, a product differentiation strategy may provide a competitive advantage in a market dominated by larger companies.

When an organization uses a differentiation strategy that focuses on the cost value of the product versus other similar products on the market, it creates a perceived value among consumers and potential customers. A strategy that focuses on value highlights the cost savings or durability of a product in comparison to other products. The cost savings can revolve around the initial selling price of the product, or focus on longer-term, life cycle costs. An energy-saving product, for example, might save consumers money in the long run, even if they pay a bit more at the front end.

Needs, Wants, and Demands

Needs. Needs are considered to be the basic human requirements such as for air, food, water, and shelter. The core of marketing starts with understanding the customer's needs. One of the most effective ways that nurses have accessed patients' needs is using Maslow's Hierarchy of Needs (Fig. 26.5). Maslow's Hierarchy of Needs is a motivational theory in psychology that depicts a classification system that reflects the universal needs of society as its base, then proceeds upward in the shape of a pyramid. Interestingly, marketing also uses

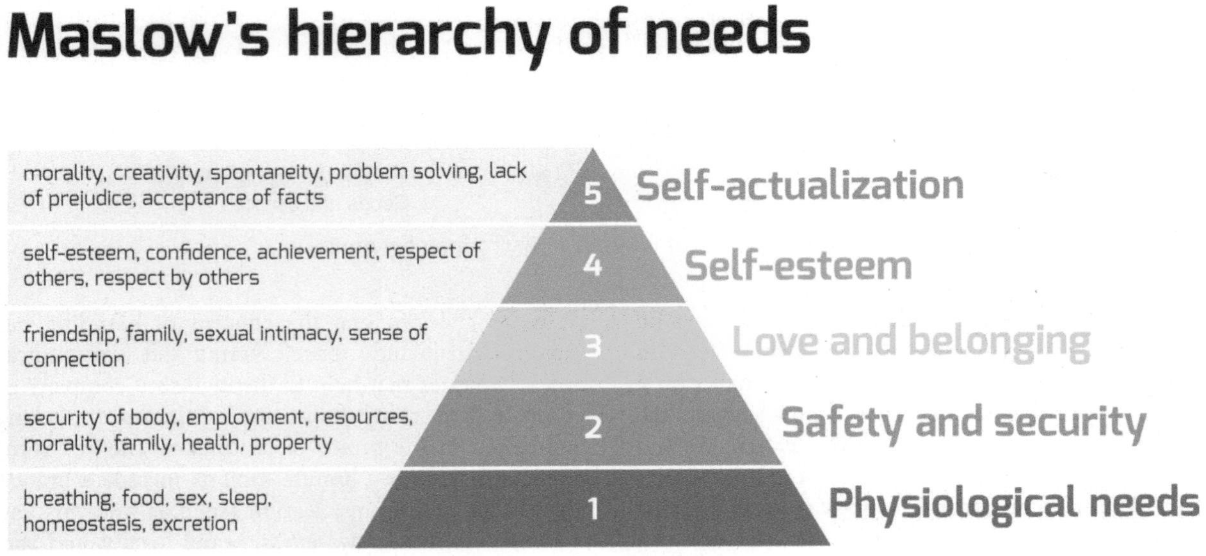

Fig. 26.5 Maslow's hierarchy of needs. *(©iStock.com (Credit:PytyCzech))*

Maslow's Hierarchy of Needs. The levels of the pyramid include:

- **Physiological:** Food, clothing, shelter, money, sleep, and homeostasis.
- **Safety:** Financial security, personal safety, health and wellness, and stability.
- **Love and Belonging:** Close bonds, recognition, compassion for others and affection.
- **Self-Esteem:** Respect, status, recognition, praise, confidence, and independence.
- **Self-Actualization:** Desire to become the most that one can be; full use and exploitation of talents, capabilities, and potentials.

Although the theory is generally portrayed as a fairly rigid hierarchy, Maslow noted that the order in which these needs are fulfilled does not always follow this standard progression. For example, he noted that for some individuals, the need for self-esteem is more important than the need for love. For others, the need for creative fulfillment may supersede even the most basic needs. Interestingly, some people consider health care to be a need while others see health care as a luxury, thus representing different levels on the hierarchy. When the Affordable Health Care Act (ACA) was passed in 2010, the law had three primary goals:

1. To make affordable health insurance available to more people with incomes between 100% and 400% of the federal poverty level,
2. Expand the Medicaid program to cover all adults with incomes below 138% of the federal poverty level, and
3. Support innovative medical care delivery methods designed to lower the costs of health care generally.

As a result of the ACA, individuals faced rigid fines for being without coverage. Despite this federal mandate, millions of working Americans remain uninsured because they are unable to afford the premiums, thus, unable to meet their need for health care.

Wants. Wants are a type of need when an individual is directed to a specific object that may satisfy a specific need. When deciding whether something is a need or a want, start with the basic definitions outlined in economics. A need is something necessary to survive. Without meeting a need, one would be in grave danger or even die as one's safety and health depend on it. If one can survive without something, then it's not a need. On the other hand, a want is simply something one desires but can live without.

Interestingly, research has determined that patients want safety more than savings when differentiating between various providers for necessary health care. In fact, 97% of the time, consumers will choose hospitals that are rated safer, regardless of cost (Byrnes, 2015). However, wants are not fixed. Wants change because both related factors and priorities can shift. For example, private insurance mitigates the impact of cost on patient choices. If the insurance environment changes, cost may become a more important factor in the choices patients make to meet their health care needs.

Demands. Demands are the "wants" for specific products backed by an ability to pay. In other words, demand refers to a buyer's desire to purchase goods and services at given price. For example, a person may want a diamond necklace; however, only a few individuals can actually buy one. We may want health care, but health care comes at a cost. Marketers spend a considerable amount of money to determine the amount of demand the public has for a good or a service. How much of their goods will they actually be able to sell at any given price? Incorrect estimations either result in money left on the table if demand is underestimated or losses if demand is overestimated. Demand is what helps fuel the economy, and without it, businesses would not produce anything.

Demand is closely related to supply. Consumers try to pay the lowest prices they can for goods and services, suppliers try to maximize profits. If suppliers charge too much, the quantity demanded drops and suppliers do not sell enough product to earn sufficient profits. If suppliers charge too little, the quantity demanded increases, but lower prices may not cover suppliers' costs or allow for profits. Some factors affecting demand include the appeal of a good or service, the availability of competing goods, the availability of financing, and the perceived availability of a good or service.

Supply and Demand

Supply and demand are perhaps one of the most fundamental concepts of economics, and it is the backbone of a market economy. Demand refers to how much (quantity) of a product or service is desired by buyers. The quantity demanded is the amount of a product people are willing to buy at a certain price; the relationship between price and quantity demanded is known as the demand relationship. Supply represents how much the market can offer. The quantity supplied refers to the amount of a certain good producers are willing to supply when receiving a certain price. The correlation between price and how much of a good or service is supplied to the market is known as the supply relationship. Price, therefore, reflects supply and demand.

Interestingly enough, there are only four basic laws that govern supply and demand. They include:

- If demand increases and supply remains unchanged, it leads to a higher price and higher quantities.
- If demand decreases and supply remains unchanged, it leads to a lower price and lower quantities.
- If supply increases and demand remains unchanged, it leads to a lower price and a higher quantity.
- If supply decreases and demand remains unchanged, it leads to a higher price and lower quantity.

So, exactly how does this work? Think about demand and the "want" for something. A new Apple watch or a reservation at the newest restaurant in New York are in high demand. As a result of the high demand, suppliers can charge a higher price, because there is a demand and the quantity of the goods will slowly increase to meet that demand. In health care there is a demand for services, however, the quantity is limited. For example, a hospital may have 350 available beds and 357 patients that need a bed (the demand is greater than the supply). An outpatient clinic may have five providers that can see 10 patients per day (50 appointments), but there are only 46 appointments (the supply is greater than the demand). This principle was in sharp focus during the 2020 COVID-19 pandemic.

Market Equilibrium

The point at which supply and demand meet represents the market clearing or market equilibrium price. An increase in demand shifts the demand curve to the right. The curves intersect at a higher price, and consumers pay more for the product. Equilibrium prices typically remain in a state of flux for most goods and services because factors affecting supply and demand are always changing. Free, competitive markets tend to push prices toward market equilibrium (Fig. 26.6).

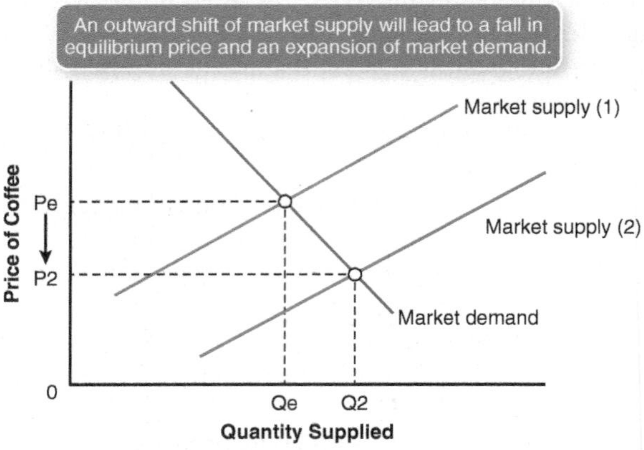

Fig. 26.6 Market equilibrium.

Market Demand Versus Aggregate Demand

The market for each good in an economy faces a different set of circumstances, which vary in type and degree. Aggregate demand in an economy is examined by macroeconomics. Aggregate demand refers to the total demand by all consumers for all good and services in an economy across all the markets for individual goods. Because aggregate includes all goods in an economy, it is not sensitive to competition or substitution between different goods or changes in consumer preferences between various goods in the same way that demand in individual good markets can be.

Utility

Utility is an abstract concept rather than a concrete, observable quantity. The units to which we assign an "amount" of utility, therefore, are arbitrary, representing a relative value. Total utility is the aggregate sum of satisfaction or benefit that an individual gain from consuming a given amount of goods or services in an economy. The amount of a person's total utility corresponds to the person's level of consumption. Usually, the more the person consumes, the larger their total utility will be. Marginal utility is the additional satisfaction, or amount of utility, gained from each extra unit of consumption.

Although total utility usually increases as more of a good is consumed, marginal utility usually decreases with each additional increase in the consumption of a good. This decrease demonstrates the law of diminishing marginal utility. Because there is a certain threshold of satisfaction, the consumer will no longer receive the same pleasure from consumption once that threshold is crossed. In other words, total utility will increase at a slower pace as an individual increases the quantity consumed.

Take, for example, a chocolate bar. Let us say that after eating one chocolate bar your sweet tooth has been satisfied. Your marginal utility (and total utility) after eating one chocolate bar will be quite high. But if you eat more chocolate bars, the pleasure of each additional chocolate bar will be less than the pleasure you received from eating the one before - probably because you are starting to feel full or you have had too many sweets for one day (Table 26.2).

TABLE 26.2 Chocolate Bars and Utility		
Chocolate Bars Eaten	**Marginal Utility**	**Total Chocolate Utility**
0	0	0
1	70	70
2	10	80
3	5	85
4	3	88

The Four Ps of Marketing

The four Ps of marketing are the four essential factors that come into play when a good or service are being marketed to the public (Fig. 26.7). Neil Borden popularized the idea of the Four Ps in the 1950s and E. Jerome McCarthy (1964) updated the Ps in 1960. The Four Ps include:

Product. Product refers to a good or service that a company offers to customers. Ideally, a product should fulfill a certain consumer demand or be so compelling that consumers believe they need to have it. To be successful, marketers need to understand the life cycle of a product, and business executives need to have a plan for dealing with products at every stage of their life cycles. The type of product also partially dictates how much businesses can charge for it, where they should place it, and how they should promote it in the marketplace.

Price. Price is what the consumer pays. Some industries garner only a small markup on price, while others have huge profit margins, because they are highly sought after. Price is affected by sales cycles, product life cycles, supply and demand. Business strategies might consider a cost leadership strategy by trying to beat the market with the lowest price, or a business strategy might choose to inflate the price, based on a luxury component or brand image.

Place. As a strategy, place has become a more significant component of marketing success. Place involves where the product is stored, perhaps even where it is manufactured. The internet has created a dramatic evolution of where products are sold and distributed, from small, local companies to global. This strategy also considers where the product is advertised and in which format, including radio, infomercials, magazines, online ads, and even in film product placements.

Promotion. This strategy component is tied directly to the other three Ps. The promotional strategy aims to show consumers why they need to buy this specific product over others. Timing heavily influences the amount of promotional marketing, and when. It may also adjust the location, such as commercials during football season games that target pizza delivery deals. It may try to entice consumers to try a product with an irresistible promotional or introductory offer. In today's digital age, the "place" and "promotion" factors are as much online as offline. Online considerations include where a product appears on a company's web page or social media, as well as which types of search functions trigger corresponding, targeted ads for the product.

An Important Fifth "P": PEOPLE

One of the most important Ps is the fifth P: people. Interestingly, a leader could have the best strategy in the world, but if the people are unable to execute the strategy

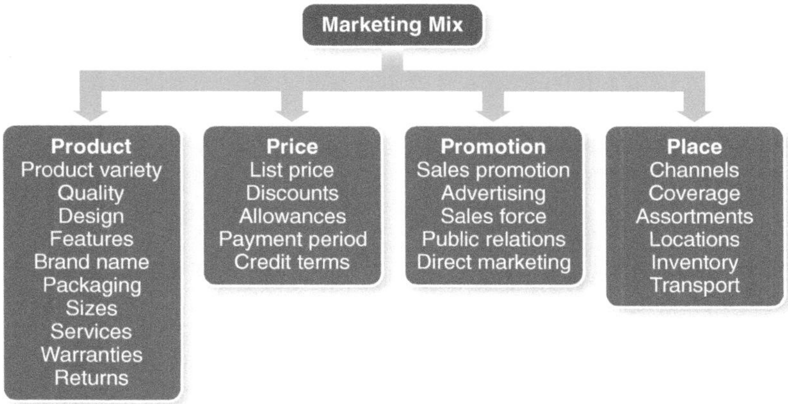
Marketing Mix
Product
Product variety
Quality
Design
Features
Brand name
Packaging
Sizes
Services
Warranties
Returns
Price
List price
Discounts
Allowances
Payment period
Credit terms
Promotion
Sales promotion
Advertising
Sales force
Public relations
Direct marketing
Place
Channels
Coverage
Assortments
Locations
Inventory
Transport

Fig. 26.7 Four Ps of marketing.

or closing sale, then there will not be a successful marketing campaign. For people to be positive factors in executing the strategy, the leader needs to take the time to properly hire, onboard, train, and monitor the team. Finding talent is one of the most difficult things any business leader must do. There is a great deal of competition for people who are looking for work, but there is a smaller pool of people who are a great fit for a company. Spend the time needed to review team positions and the team's exact needs. Understand what is required to make someone successful on the team.

When new hires are brought on board ("onboarding"), the leader needs to share their vision and the strategy for success. Having new employees buy into the company vision from day one sets the tone for success. Properly train people in the process of sales or service, whichever division they will be responsible for. Every person is a promotional face for the company, whether they know it or not. If your employee is leaving work and speaking negatively about their job, it is a reflection on the company.

The Four As of Marketing

In reviewing the Four Ps, it is evident that the Four Ps are completely company driven. The organization decides on the price, builds the product, decides where to distribute it and how to promote it. The missing piece is that it does not consider the customer. Sheth and Sisodai (2006) made the case that customer knowledge is more reliable. Thus, their framework emphasizes consumer value in terms of the Four As. This approach is organized around the values that matter most to the customers as it focuses on the four distinct roles that customers play in the market: acceptability, affordability, accessibility, and awareness.

Acceptability. The extent to which the organization's product or service meets and exceeds the customers' needs and expectations. The two dimensions of acceptability include:

Functional Acceptability: Indicated by the functionality of the product, performance attributes, ease of use, and reliability.

Psychological Acceptability: includes brand image, social and emotional value. Psychological acceptability is often associated with "luxury brands".

Affordability. The extent to which the targeted customers are economically and psychologically willing to pay the product or service's price. The two dimensions of affordability include:

Economic Affordability: The ability to pay for the product or service as determined by factors such as income, assets, financing, and fit within a budget. In other words, does the customer have sufficient economic resources to pay a product or service's price?

Psychological Affordability: The willingness to pay for a product or service determined by the perceived value for money, perceived price fairness, and price relative to other options.

Accessibility. The extent to which a customer is able to readily acquire and use the product or service. Accessibility has two dimensions:

Availability: As determined by factors such as supply and demand; the degree to which a product is kept in-stock and readily available to customers.

Convenience: Determined by the time and effort in acquiring the product, the ease in which the product can be found and accessed.

Awareness. The extent to which customers are informed regarding a product's characteristics and are in the process of making a decision that demonstrates they are "on board" with the product, ranging from the most obvious, a purchasing decision, to a surrogate, such as clicking on a coupon to print out. Awareness has two dimensions:

Product Knowledge – as demonstrated by interest or understanding

Brand Awareness – as demonstrated by brand recall or brand association.

In order for an organization to benefit from the four A's, Sheth and Sisodai (2006) posit that an organization be measured on each "A" on a 0 to 100 percent scale for a target market as each element is important. To succeed, an organization must do well on all four dimensions. However, an organization can fail simply by failing in one of the dimensions.

Marketing Mix

Previous sections of this chapter have focused on marketing at the organizational level to external markets. Familiarity with the marketing terminology and concepts that have been presented are imperative to building business skills and to applying the marketing mix. There are many complex marketing models that depict steps in the marketing process. Most begin with an appraisal and understanding of the environment and potential customers, include the design and delivery of a customer-driven marketing strategy, and end with customer loyalty and equity. A more in-depth understanding of such models is required as nurses advance in their career. At this point, understanding basic aspects of the marketing process is more meaningful. The marketing mix is the set of tactical tools used in the marketing process. The marketing mix was introduced almost 50 years ago (McCarthy, 1964) but remains a useful organizing framework for successful marketing programs. Nurse leaders at all levels can apply this framework in programs and initiatives designed to meet everyday challenges.

Although the Four Ps framework has been in existence for more than five decades, both frameworks are helpful in understanding how nurses can deliver health care effectively. The Four Ps framework is particularly well suited to a manufacturing and industrial economy and reflects a business-centric perspective. As the US economy has become more service-oriented, an alternative framework that assumes a customer-centric perspective might be more helpful in conceptualizing the ways in which a hospital's products are priced, placed, and promoted.

The Four As, therefore, describe a business environment in which the patient has far more influence over the marketing mix. This has been facilitated by the development of a digital marketplace, where services can be delivered without the more traditional boundaries established by brick and mortar buildings and regular business hours. The health care market is increasingly located in digital environments like electronic medical health records, computers and smartphones. In fact, Deloitte (2014) predicted that 75 million physician visits in North America annually would occur via some form of electronic technology.

Marketing Orientation

Organizations develop distinctive orientations or viewpoints that define their organizational culture. Hospital organizational cultures also have distinctive orientations. Orientation is usually presented in one of four ways:

- **Product orientation:** An organizational culture that assumes what the customer wants is the very best quality, regardless of cost.
- **Selling orientation:** An organizational culture that assumes the customers must be persuaded to buy the firm's products.
- **Marketing orientation:** An organizational culture that assumes the customer's needs and wants should determine the quality, price, and availability of the product.
- **Holistic orientation:** An organizational culture that focuses on the customer's needs and wants, as well as the societal impact of products that meet those needs and wants. Communication and promotion of the products involve both employees and potential customers.

Institutions that are committed to sustaining a relationship with their customers strive for a culture that can be labeled as a **marketing** or **holistic orientation**. Nurses can reflect on and evaluate these four orientations (product orientation, selling orientation, marketing orientation, and holistic orientation) and describe which of these most closely resembles their current workplace (or a prior workplace). What practices can be identified as evidence of the company's orientation? How does this company orientation affect the nurses' work? How are nurses' relationships with patients and colleagues affected by the culture that this orientation describes?

Segmentation → Targeting → Positioning

Segmentation. Segmentation is the process of dividing a market into distinct groups of buyers by identifying demographic, psychographic, and behavioral differences between them (Kotler & Keller, 2016). Segmentation has become particularly crucial as hospitals work to refine ways of predicting which patients are more or less likely to be hospitalized initially or readmitted after discharge. Identifying such segments of the population and creating relevant, effective interventions can save significant health care costs. Given this, there are many different approaches an organization can take when segmenting the target market. Generally speaking, there are four different types of market segmentation. These segmentation helps an organization to define a population into smaller "segments" so that each segment can be targeted. For example, in a health care organization, segmenting by lifestyle stage (infants, toddlers, adults, and geriatrics) can assist in identifying the specific needs of the group (Fig. 26.8).

Targeting. Targeting is the process through which an organization identifies users that they would like to reach and then advertises to them through various channels. For example, an organization may divide their population into segments by age and gender and then target specific groups, such as child-bearing women for their new maternity wing. By identifying which segment is most relevant presents the greatest opportunity for a given business (Kotler & Keller, 2016).

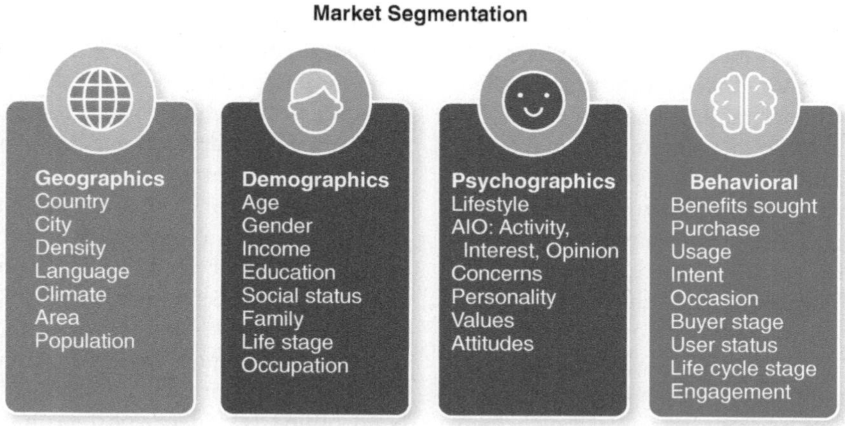

Fig. 26.8 Market segmentation.

Positioning. Positioning focuses on how the customer ultimately views the product or service in comparison to the competition. In other words, it is what a business should do to market its products and services. The more intense a positioning strategy, the more effective the market strategy is for an organization. In positioning, the marketing department creates an image for the product based on its intended audience. This is created through the use of promotion, price, place, and product.

Nurses are essential providers of the health care product and are engaged in marketing when delivering care. This is in part because interpersonal relationships are an important part of the therapeutic "product" of care. A health care organization dedicated to achieving excellence realizes this and works hard to inform all care providers and support staff about meeting customer needs. In excellence-driven organizations, particularly those with a holistic company orientation, marketing is more than a department; it is at the core of the organizational business framework. The American Organization for Nursing Leadership (AONL) has noted the identification of marketing opportunities and the development of marketing strategies as key business skills for nurse leaders in executive practice and for those with a career goal of leadership (AONL, 2015). Nurse leaders and aspiring nurse leaders who operate within a business framework benefit from understanding marketing concepts that underlie programs and initiatives in health care organizations.

Marketing Strategy

Strategic planning, a process discussed in Chapter 14, sets the overall direction for an organization. Defining the business, determining the mission, and developing long-term objectives form the basis of an organization's strategic plan. Marketing strategies and programs need to be aligned and guided by the organization-wide strategic plan (Kotler & Keller, 2016). This cannot be done effectively without investing adequate time and resources in evaluating the organization's competitive environment.

A market research approach is used for environmental scanning and is a critical step in both the strategic and marketing planning processes. During the environmental scanning, marketing departments explore and evaluate the internal and external environments to gain an understanding of demographic and societal trends, competition, and potential customers. Also, internal business performance indicators such as profits (or losses), customer and staff satisfaction, and quality indicators are evaluated. To be most effective, compilation, review, and analysis of environmental data should involve every functional area in an organization, including the nursing department. The results of the market research need to be shared across business units, and all key stakeholders need to participate in the subsequent planning process.

Marketing strategy is based on how target markets are defined. Markets are both broad and narrow. Mass marketing, which is broad, offers a product to an entire external market. Niche marketing represents a narrower view and focuses on capturing a small but important part of the market. Consider the difference between a full-service community hospital and a children's hospital. The former serves a broad market; the latter targets very specific customers: children and their families. Understanding the application of four critical concepts of segmentation, targeting, product differentiation, and positioning is essential to becoming fluent in the language of marketing.

By analyzing information about the competitive market, a hospital can determine key strategies to meet the unmet needs in its service area. A small rural community hospital in a market 200 miles from any other hospital will adopt strategies for defining and serving its market that are very different from the strategies of a large suburban hospital in a market with four other hospitals within a 25-mile radius. The rural hospital would likely position itself as a full-service facility capable of meeting the most frequently occurring needs of their target audience or the local community. For example, its profile of services is likely to include women's services, emergency care, diagnostic care, and general surgery. On the other hand, the large suburban hospital in a highly competitive market might seek to differentiate itself from competitors by creating a specialty center for heart disease or cancer. However, product or service lines are not the only way to differentiate.

In today's health care environment, differentiation is often based on quality measures and other distinctions that are prevalent today. Measures used to assess and compare the quality of health care organizations are classified one of three ways: structure, process, or outcome measures. This is known as the Donabedian model (1966).

Structure. Structure includes all of the factors that affect the context in which care is delivered. This includes the physical facility, equipment, and human resources, as well as organizational characteristics such as staff training and payment methods. These factors control how providers and patients in a health care system act and are measures of the average quality of care within a facility or system. Structure is often easy to observe and measure, and it may be the upstream cause of problems identified in process.

Process. Process is the sum of all actions that make up health care. These commonly include diagnosis, treatment, preventive care, and patient education but may be expanded to include actions taken by the patients or their families. Processes can be further classified as technical processes, how care is delivered, or interpersonal processes, which all encompass the manner in which care is delivered. According to Donabedian (1966), the measurement of process is nearly equivalent to the measurement of quality of care because process contains all acts of health care delivery. Information about process can be obtained from medical records, interviews with patients and practitioners, or direct observations of health care visits.

Outcome. Outcome contains all the effects of health care on patients or populations, including changes to health status, behavior, or knowledge as well as patient satisfaction and health-related quality of life. Outcomes are sometimes seen as the most important indicators of quality because improving patient health status is the primary goal of health care. However, accurately measuring outcomes that can be attributed exclusively to health care is very difficult. Drawing connections between process and outcomes often requires large sample populations, adjustments by case mix, and long-term follow ups as outcomes may take considerable time to become observable.

Although it is widely recognized and applied in many health care related fields, the Donabedian (1966) Model was developed to assess quality of care in clinical practice. The model does not have an implicit definition of quality care so that it can be applied to problems of broad or narrow scope. Donabedian noted that each of the three domains has advantages and disadvantages that necessitate researchers draw connections between them in order to create a chain of causation that is conceptually useful for understanding systems as well as designing experiments and interventions.

A handful of analytic frameworks for quality assessment have guided measure development initiatives in the public and private sectors. One of the most influential is the framework put forth by the Institute of Medicine (IOM, 2001), which includes the following six aims for the health care system:

Safe: Avoiding harm to patients from the care that is intended to help them.

Effective: Providing services based on scientific knowledge to all who could benefit and refraining from providing services to those not likely to benefit (avoiding underuse and misuse, respectively).

Patient-centered: Providing care that is respectful of and responsive to individual patient preferences, needs, and values and ensuring that patient values guide all clinical decisions.

Timely: Reducing waits and sometimes harmful delays for both those who receive and those who give care.

Efficient: Avoiding waste, including waste of equipment, supplies, ideas, and energy.

Equitable: Providing care that does not vary in quality because of personal characteristics such as gender, ethnicity, geographic location, and socioeconomic status.

Frameworks like the (IOM 2001) make it easier for consumers to grasp the meaning and relevance of quality measures. Studies have shown that providing consumers with a framework for understanding quality helps them value a broader range of quality indicators. For example, when consumers are given a brief, understandable explanation of safe, effective, and patient-centered care, they view all three categories as important. Further, when measures are grouped into user-friendly versions of those three IOM domains, consumers can see the meaning of the measures more clearly and understand how they relate to their own concerns about their care.

Setting marketing strategy is a shared responsibility within a health care organization. This critical activity needs to be guided by the strategic plan with input from every key stakeholder group, especially nursing, that is engaged in meeting customer needs during many and varied exchanges. Likewise, the organization's marketing team is engaged at the start when new services are planned. With multiple perspectives represented at the planning table, an organization will respond more effectively to the needs and challenges of its markets.

LEADERSHIP AND MANAGEMENT IMPLICATIONS

At a glance, nurses may consider that marketing is outside of the realm of nursing and care delivery. However, nurses (and nursing) are critical components to health care marketing. This is because marketing is about building relationships with customers so that needs and wants are satisfied and value is created. Marketing goals are incorporated in the organizational strategic plan. These goals focus on satisfying and creating value with respect to customers. They also may be focused on attracting new customers or increasing volume to enhance financial viability. Nursing is affected by such strategies and also can have an impact on goal achievement.

Health care marketing can be challenging in today's environment as health care marketing refers to marketing strategies that targets providers, insurers, suppliers, advocacy groups, patients, and families in order to increase awareness of their business and attract new patients. An understanding of the marketing framework as well as basic marketing concepts allows nurse leaders and managers to be knowledgeable contributors at the table where high-level goals are established and decisions about meeting goals are made. Nursing executive leadership generally would be involved in corporate strategic planning. Nurse leaders and managers then implement corporate strategies at the marketing management level by promoting the value nursing brings to the organization and managing the implementation of the marketing mix. Financial viability comes through the delivery of high-quality care product across varied settings and in a timely and efficient manner and price. Nurse leaders can challenge themselves and their colleagues to ask and answer questions such as:

- How do I create value for my organization?
- How do I help my organization become more patient centric?
- How do I help my organization recognize the centrality of nursing care in affecting the organization's reputation and brand?

The nurse's interactions with patients and their families are critical to patent satisfaction and good clinical outcomes. Nursing relationship management is a major component of the product/service element of the marketing mix. All employees need to focus on establishing and maintaining satisfactory customer relationships. In hospitals and other health care organizations, frontline nurses are critical in creating value for customers.

Advertising messages and promotion about nurses and nursing care can reinforce a positive image of nursing to internal and external markets. One opportunity for promotion of nursing to all markets is to have a nursing focus on the hospital's website. Nurse leaders can ensure the promotion of nursing and nursing roles in as many venues as possible to communicate the importance of nursing, nursing practice, or nursing care to potential target markets (Hoeve et al., 2013; Walker, 2014). This can be done by capturing stories of nurses who have been exemplars of compassionate and skilled care and featuring them on the hospital's intranet. These stories help define the profession and strengthen the organization's self-image as a place where branding tag lines such as "the skill to heal" and "the spirit to care" intersect with and exemplify the commitment to health and healing.

Kotler and Keller (2016) believed the future of marketing will be horizontal: consumer-to-consumer. They say that the economic downturn has not fostered trust in the marketplace and that customers now increasingly turn to one another for credible advice and information when selecting products (Kotler & Keller, 2016). In their book *Social Media for Nurses: Educating Practitioners and Patients in a Networked World*, Nelson and colleagues (2013, p. 2) noted that "Over the last several decades, the role of the patient has been evolving from passive recipients of health care to informed, empowered, and engaged patient/consumer." Digital marketplaces have empowered consumers to improve their own health literacy, research providers, and write reviews of health care services (Hotopf, 2013). Nurse managers can work with their colleagues to creatively imagine how social media (promotion) can be used to leverage this technology as well as this growing cultural trend of patient-to-patient trust to build patient loyalty and brand strength. Nurse leaders and managers are responsible for promoting the merits of nursing service internally and externally.

Finally, another marketing application for nurse leaders and managers relates to workforce characteristics. Nurses who are employed make up an internal market, and the pool of nurses who are potential new hires makes up an external market. In these instances, nurses are the customers. Nurse leaders can use marketing to increase "customer" retention and attraction. When considering nurse retention and recruitment, leaders consider what value proposition (product) the nursing department or unit offers to nurses. Highlighting department or unit characteristics deemed important, such as shared governance and professional development opportunities, provides details about the product. Leaders can give attention to the unit (place) where nurses provide service. Consideration of the physical layout and whether the unit design is conducive to an efficient and effective workflow is important. Nurse leaders can ensure that nurses' salaries are competitive and that nurses do not feel underpaid and undervalued (Evans, 2013). Market research in collaboration with the human resources department can analyze salaries (price) in the external market and adjust accordingly.

CURRENT ISSUES AND TRENDS

The hospital industry continues to evolve, streamlining and improving patient care, integrating big data and moving from a fee-for-service to a fee-for-outcome payment model. The hospitals of yesterday were quite different from the sprawling health care centers that are common in the United States today. Although the previous focus was on payment and legal changes that would be required to move health care forward, more recently the focus has been more about how the private sector has responded and shifted to answer new challenges. A brief environmental analysis of marketing in health care reveals an emphasis on issues of social media, cost and transparency, patient-centered care, the nursing shortage, geriatric workforce shortage, work–life balance, and data analytics.

A Dramatically Changed Marketplace

Overall, the first half of the 20th century began with childbirth, influenza, and everyday trauma inflicting high casualties. Medical education improved such that in 1911, the average patient seeing an average doctor for an average problem had better than a fifty-fifty chance of benefiting from the transaction. By the mid 1950s, progress in sanitation, immunizations, and antibiotics led to the eradication of polio and smallpox, the expectation of living to old age, and new wonder drugs. Knowledge, technologies, and entrepreneurism accelerated ever faster. Acute diseases have been replaced by new illnesses of body and psyche such as coronary heart disease, chronic fatigue syndrome, pain syndromes, arthritis, cancers, teenage suicide, and addictions of all varieties. Gauging the quality of health care systems is often difficult and restricted by the availability of data. One method for measuring quality is to look at mortality rates, which, though influenced by a myriad of factors, are in part affected by the quality of the health care system in addressing diseases for which mortality is amenable to health care.

Social Media

In this era of information and communication technology, every sector is taking advantage of social media, and the health care industry is no exception. In particular, social media can help engage patients, providers, and the public with relevant and timely information as well as communicate the value and credibility of health care organization. Research has demonstrated that posts with *links to more information* are the most preferred type of content on social media. In addition, 30% of consumers posited that social media is the primary way to receive information. Thus, any organization that desires to be in the public domain has to use social media.

Health care has now become patient-centered which makes patient engagement and satisfaction a top priority, hence the need to implement a social media strategy. Hospitals need social media experts, a new emerging opportunity, as well as a public relations department. Employing a social media expert has become one of the necessities for many health care organizations. For example, organizations can facilitate patient empowerment and patient education by enabling and engaging in patient forums and research networks online. For example, many organizations allow patients to manage their own health conditions by discussing treatment options with other patients who have similar conditions through social media. Moreover, organizations can use social media to physician alignment and collaboration.

Another example is *The Medical Directors Forum*, a social networking site for medical directors that provides a verified, secure, closed-loop environment for peer-to-peer interaction. The resources on this site include a comprehensive library, discussion groups, calendar postings, and alerts. The site also provides dedicated group pages for medical directors working in a wide range of sectors, including hospital, veterans' affairs, Medicare, group practice, employer, behavioral health, managed care, correctional facility, and long-term care.

It is important to understand that social media has the potential to be both beneficial and challenging to an organization. Health Insurance Portability and Accountability Act (HIPAA) compliance is one the biggest challenges of social media-facing organizations today.

Health care professionals are leery of entering into the social media fray for fear that they will compromise patient privacy, either through what they post or by exposing their networks to viruses or hacking. Although HIPAA offers specific guidelines on how to safely post information, comments, photos, or videos online without violating patient privacy laws, organizations must be diligent in their online security. Some of the guidelines include "de-identification" of patients by removing or omitting names, insurance or Social Security numbers, date of birth, photos, and eliminating specific details of rare medical issues, including the dates they occur. Health care providers can also obtain consent from patients to post their photos on social media sites.

When nurses post on social media sites such as Facebook, HIPAA and privacy violations may occur. A robust social media policy needs to exist and be enforced. Health care professionals worry that their presence on social media may label them as unprofessional with potential patients. Thus, it is important to consider the extent and reach of posts as a medical professional. Every post does offer more detail into you as a person, much less as a health care professional and care should be taken to post only content that is appropriate. The American College of Physicians and the Federation of State Medical Boards have been working on guidelines for health care professionals that can help physicians and providers make better choices regarding what is posted on social media. Overall, health care organizations have a duty to protect patients and providers by ensuring that the best possible information is made public to its customers through social media.

Cost and Transparency

Price transparency in health care is an important issue to watch for in health care. Prior to January 1, 2019, California was the only state that required hospitals to post their prices online for consumers to view. As of January 1, 2019, the CMS required all hospitals to post prices online (CMS, 2019b). However, prices don't provide the whole story as a patient's costs remain non-specific. For example, if a patient has a hip replacement surgery at an outpatient center versus in a hospital as an inpatient, the costs are going to vary considerably and include a wide range of variables. To aid consumers in understanding the billing process, the state of Maryland hosts a website where total cost is available for some procedures. The site shows the hospital costs and a potential total cost per condition, along with some quality metrics related to that condition for individual hospitals. This is a good example of how states can help improve transparency for consumers, enabling them to make informed choices about their health care.

An important consideration for nurses related to cost and value is that current payment models do not unbundle nursing care from room and board, thus making adjustments for nursing intensity in billing mechanisms impossible. Recommendations for incorporating a nursing intensity adjustment to existing inpatient billing could lead to determination of the economic value of nursing care. The marketing mix could more closely reflect the "price" of nursing care, which would contribute to the establishment of a value-based purchasing system for hospitals (Kavanagh et al., 2012).

There will be continued efforts and initiatives to address the costs of nursing care and subsequent reimbursement decisions in order to deliver and market cost-effective and efficient care. Nurses also need to stay informed about, and engaged in, evolving accountable payment models in order to create care delivery systems that prevent negative outcomes for which reimbursement will be withheld and/or to capture payment as an Advance Practice Provider. The shift away from fee-for-service models places an increasing emphasis on customer relationships and increasing pressure on nurses to manage such relationships and build value for the customer and the system (Healthcare Financial Management Association, 2015).

Patient-Centered Care

The focus on patient-centered care began in the 1970s, but implementation remains an issue for many health care organizations. Varied patient-centered models and frameworks exist. Attributes in patient-centeredness include patient satisfaction, the patient experience of care, patient engagement, and shared decision-making. Evidence supports the view that patient-centered care improves patient outcomes and is one approach to addressing racial, ethnic, and socioeconomic disparities in health care and health care outcomes (Long, 2012; Radwin et al., 2013).

Planetree is a designation that differentiates a hospital on the basis of excellence in patient- and person-centered care. The Planetree philosophy reveals a simple view of what it means to be patient-centered (Planetree, 2018). Components of the Planetree model that move an organization toward a culture of patient-centeredness can be found on their website. It is easy to determine the importance of patient-centeredness to marketing goals and ultimately to patient satisfaction, therefore models for delivery of patient-centered care will continue to evolve (Millenson & Macri, 2012).

Nursing Shortage

The US is projected to experience a shortage of registered nurses (RNs) that is expected to intensify as Baby Boomers age and the need for health care grows (American Association of Colleges of Nursing [AACN], 2020). According to the Bureau of Labor Statistics (BLS, 2015), RNs are listed among the top occupations in terms of job growth through 2026. Moreover, the Bureau projects the need for an additional 203,700 new RNs though 2026 to fill newly created positions and to replace retiring nurses. Buerhaus et al, (2017) estimated that one million RNs will retire by 2030 because according to a 2018 survey, nearly 51% of the RN workforce is aged 50 or older. Compounding this concern is that by 2050, the number of US residents aged 65 and over will almost double to 83.7 million. With this larger number of older adults, there will be an increased need for geriatric care, including care for individuals with chronic diseases and comorbidities.

Despite these needs, US nursing schools have turned away more than 75,000 qualified applicants from baccalaureate and graduate nursing programs in 2018 due to insufficient number of faculty, clinical sites, classroom space, and clinical preceptors, and budget constraints. The AACN (2020) projected a shortage of 260,000 nurses nationally by 2024 (Irish, 2014). This trend calls for internal marketing initiatives that address nurse turnover, job satisfaction, and occupational and organizational commitment. External marketing challenges will be encountered by hospitals seeking a more qualified nurse workforce (i.e., those with baccalaureate [BSN] degrees). This is supported by the American Nurses Credentialing Center's (ANCC) Magnet Recognition Program® (ANCC, 2016) as well as studies finding that higher percentages of RNs with BSN degrees in hospitals are linked to lower patient mortality rates (Aiken et al., 2014; Blegen et al., 2013; Kutney-Lee et al., 2013). This calls for competitive marketing strategies to recruit successfully from the target market of BSN-prepared nurses.

Geriatric Workforce Shortage

The baby boomer population as a whole will increase the demand for health care services over the next several decades (Irish, 2014). The combination of the aging of the baby boom population, increases in life expectancy, and decreases in the number of younger persons will mean that older adults make up a much larger percentage of the US population than ever before. As a result, the scarcity of workers specializing in the care of older adults, the eldercare workforce, will be even more pronounced (Bureau of Labor Statistics, 2015). This is an external marketing opportunity to recruit young people into nursing.

Work–Life Balance

About two-thirds of the close to 3 million nurses who live in the United States work in hospitals. Generally speaking, hospitals are high-stress environments. In one study, only 23% of female participants who worked in health care indicated that they were able to balance their personal and professional lives well (Delina & Raya, 2013). Research shows the importance of caring for oneself in order to provide outstanding patient care. Fatigue can lead to dangerous or costly mistakes, thereby affecting one's professional reputation and mental well-being (Steege & Pinekenstein, 2016). Nurse leaders need to advocate for policies that promote work–life balance in health care organizations and use this in internal marketing in order to improve retention of qualified nurses and increase the value of care provided to their customers.

Data and Analytics

The health care industry is at a point where core, foundational technology for the end user is almost fully digitized and automated. Structured data captured in data warehouse-centric models and electronic health records (EHRs) provides information that can be executed on in real time to improve patient care. Reducing the prevalence of hospital-acquired conditions (HACs) continues to be an output of new technology and tools combining with data and analytics. Early warning systems for sepsis that utilize continually updated EHR data, and subsequent treatment protocols, are helping organizations successfully lower sepsis rates nationwide. Algorithms for fall risk management, catheter-associated urinary tract infection (CAUTI) prevention, and diabetes management are now commonplace.

Avoiding costly and preventable readmissions is one area where health care has seen the valuable application of data and machine learning. Conservative estimates put the cost of readmissions at more than $41 billion annually for hospitals, and 30-day readmissions continue to be a quality measure for health care organizations. As hospital outcome data become more transparent, hospitals with excellent outcomes have a marketing advantage.

CONCLUSION

In a marketplace where patient needs and wants are the primary drivers of value, nurses are crucial participants in the marketing efforts of the health care organizations where they work. An understanding of the concepts and tools that are the foundation of modern marketing will enable nurses and nurse managers to advocate for their profession within health care organizations, recruit and retain high-quality peers, and build relationships with patients that facilitate meaningful exchange.

RESEARCH NOTE

Source: Elrod, J.K., & Fortenberry, J.L. (2018). Formulating productive marketing communications strategy: A major health system's experience. *BMC Health Services Research, 18*(1), 1–5.

Purpose

Health care organizations traditionally have selected marketing strategies from a standard marketing communications mix, including advertising (i.e., the paid use of mass media to deliver messages), personal selling (i.e., the use of sales agents to personally deliver messages), sales promotion (i.e., the use of incentives, such as contests and free giveaways, to encourage patronage), direct marketing (i.e., the delivery of messages via mail, the Internet, and similar routes directly to customers), and public relations (i.e., the use of publicity and other unpaid promotional methods to deliver messages). The purpose of this article is to describe one health system's expansion of marketing strategies.

Discussion

Willis-Knighton Health System decided to forge a new and different communications pathway, with this innovative course fostering its expansion initiatives and providing insights that influence its communications approach. The Willis-Knighton Health System was a small system desirous of growth. However, despite having a skill at identifying innovations emerging outside of the health care industry for use within that led to numerous product-related advancements that were driving growth, it also had to communicate effectively with target audiences. Submitting press releases to news media organizations and requesting these be placed with associated stories was not an effective strategy, so they experimented with and embraced advertising at a time when this was not common. Advertising required payment. They pursued two media types: newspaper advertising and billboard advertising. For example, the initial billboard advertisement provided a public service message promoting childhood immunizations. Advertising was well received by stakeholders. This evolved into a full communications strategy and formal marketing operation.

Application to Practice

Without effective communications as a centerpiece of the marketing strategy, current and prospective patients will remain unaware of available offerings. Health care organizations are a key community resource for improving health and wellness, yet this needs to be effectively communicated. Forging a new pathway created expertise in provider-patient engagement initiatives and leading to an enduring marketing communications approach. Being a trailblazer gave the organization an advantage over other competitors. As a result there was the opportunity to innovate, leading to communications prowess, informed audiences, and lasting mutual benefits resulting in growth.

CASE STUDY

Health System A is the only children's hospital in Soufriere for the last 75 years. This system has the entire market share for pediatric hospitalizations and many pediatric services. For the past five years, Health System B has conducted market research. This research required environmental scanning. Some actions included exploring and evaluating the internal and external environments, examining demographic and societal trends, examining competitors, and searching for potential customers. Findings revealed a need for children's services both inpatient and outpatient.

The results of the market research were shared across business units, and all key stakeholders had the opportunities to participate in the evaluation of the data and the planning process. Therefore, after 5 long years, the C-suite leadership in Health System B decided that it was time to build a children's hospital.

Mid-level leadership thought that continuing to provide supportive services for teenagers was sufficient and were not motivated with the future goal to penetrate the Children's space. Many thought that since Health System A was Magnet, it would be very difficult to penetrate.

You are a Nursing Director and the liaison for marketing. You noticed that one of the reasons Health System A is increasing their market share is because customers prefer to go to one system for all services. You communicate to marketing that ensuring customer knowledge will be the key in gaining market share. You started to brainstorm ways to build the new children's brand. Using the framework below how will you develop value for both current customers and new ones. Below here are the updated 4As with their prompts:

Acceptability: How will you ensure that this new service meets and exceeds the customers needs?

Affordability: Will old and new clientele have the resources to pay for an improved service within the community?

Accessibility: Will old and new clientele see this service as convenient?

Awareness: How will you ensure awareness in a market where Health Care System A, has had the market share for 75 years? What type of content will you need to differentiate your system?

CRITICAL THINKING EXERCISE

1. Review your organization's mission, vision, and values statement. How are these components marketed to individuals such as:
   a. The organization's employees?
   b. The organization's customers?
   c. The organization's stakeholders?
   d. The community at large?
2. Identify two to four service lines of your organization.
   a. What methods are used to market these service lines?
   b. Are these methods effective? What measures are used?
   c. How could the marketing efforts be enhanced?
3. Identify your organization's brand.
   a. What does your brand represent?
   b. How is your brand related to your organization?
   c. Does your organization's brand need to be updated? Why or why not?
4. In their book *Marketing Management,* Kotler and Keller (2016) suggested that marketing communications allow companies to link their brands to other people, places, events, experiences, feelings, and things.
   a. Identify three major organizations, their brand, and the target audience for their brand.
   b. Have these organizations changed their brand over time? If so, how?
   c. What factors may influence an organization to change its brand?
5. Often, such communications are understood in terms of advertisements or social media campaigns designed to promote a company's brand. In health care, however, the most important link between brands and experiences or feelings depends largely on communication between one patient and one nurse. Using your organization's website, how does your organization brand and market its nursing services? What strategies would you use to enhance the marketing of nursing services in your organization to:
   a. New nurses
   b. Current patients
   c. Potential patients
   d. Stakeholders
6. In 2015, Johnson & Johnson (J&J) pulled advertising from ABC's "The View" after controversial comments were made about nurses by the show's host. The company decided to "put some of the money we saved" by donating a dollar for every photo shared through the company's website to National Nurses Association.
   a. What potential harm, if any, did J&J avoid by pulling its ads?
   b. What does this say about the importance of marketing?
   c. What implications does this have for nursing as a profession?
7. Simon Sinek (2009), author of the national bestseller, *Start With Why,* posits that good marketing and good leadership begins with purpose, not product. View the TED talk: How Great Leaders Inspire Action found at https://www.ted.com/talks/simon_sinek_how_great_leaders_inspire_action?language=en
   a. What is your personal "why, how, and what"?
   b. What is your organization's ""why, how, and what"?
   c. What is the relationship between your own "why" and the "why" of your organization?
   d. As a nurse manager, how can you identify or screen for an individual's "why" in your recruitment and retention process?
8. At Good Hope Hospital, the HCAHPS scores for physician communication are consistently lower than those for nurses. Research has demonstrated that patients are more likely to accept the instructions of their physicians without question, despite having concerns about the instructions (Kennedy et al., 2013). Using this research as a basis, create a list of possible marketing campaigns to increase the physicians' HCAHPS scores at Good Hope Hospital.
9. Between Memorial Day and Labor Day, research has demonstrated that the risk of death and injury increasing significantly among teens aged 13 to 18. To raise awareness of these risks, the Arkansas Children's Hospital developed and marketed the "#100DeadliestDays" campaign. Search the web for examples of other marketing campaigns that are health related.
   a. How are these campaigns used?
   b. Are these campaigns successful?
   c. What strategies would you use to improve these campaigns?

10. Nurses must often manage patient care circumstances that require a complex balance between respecting individual autonomy, maintaining a high standard of care, and providing excellent customer service that is the basis for marketing. An indigenous patient is nearing the end of his life. As you discuss palliative care with the patient, who is now unable to leave his hospital bed, he makes a request. Because he subscribes to a deeply held set of religious beliefs, the patient asks that you facilitate adherence to end-of-life rituals involving ceremonies performed around an open fire.
    a. How would you respond to this request?
    b. What information and/or guidelines would you investigate and use to assist you in your response.
    c. What elements of this request would you be able to honor and in what way?
    d. How would this patient experience reflect your organization's mission and vision?
    e. How would this patient experience reflect your organization's marketing plan?

REFERENCES

Aiken, L. H., Sloane, D. M., Bruyneel L., Van den Heede, K., Griffiths, P., Busse, R., et al. (2014). Nurse staffing and education and hospital mortality in nine European countries: A retrospective observational study. *Lancet, 383*, 1824–1830.

American Association of Colleges of Nursing (AACN). (2020). *Nursing shortage*. https://www.aacnnursing.org/news-information/fact-sheets/nursing-shortage.

Americ Marketing Association. (2020). *Definition of marketing*. https://www.ama.org/the-definition-of-marketing-what-is-marketing/.

American Nurses Credentialing Center (2016). *Magnet Recognition Program®: Testimonials and case studies*. https://www.nursingworld.org/organizational-programs/pathway/overview/testimonials-and-case-studies/.

American Organization for Nursing Leadership (AONL). (2015). *Nurse executive competencies*. http://www.aone.org/resources/nurse-executive-competencies.pdf.

Armstrong, G., & Kotler, P. (2017). *Marketing: An introduction* (13th ed.). New York, NY: Pearson Education, Inc.

Blegen, M. A., Goode, C. J., & Park, S. H. (2013). Baccalaureate education in nursing and patient outcomes. *Journal of Nursing Administration, 43*(2), 89–94.

Buerhaus, P. I., Skinner, L. E., Auerbach, D. I., & Staiger, D. O. (2017). State of the registered nurse workforce as a new era of health reform emerges. *Nursing Economic, 35*(5), 229–237.

Bureau of Labor Statistics. (2015). *Employment projections – 2014-24* (BLS Publication No. USDL-15-2327). http://www.bls.gov/news.release/pdf/ecopro.pdf.

Byrnes, J. (2015). The value proposition in action. *Healthcare Financial Management, 69*(5), 106–107.

Centers for Medicare & Medicaid Services (CMS). (2019a). *Historical*. https://www.cms.gov/Research-Statistics-Data-and-Systems/Statistics-Trends-and-Reports/NationalHealthExpendData/NationalHealthAccountsHistorical.

Centers for Medicare & Medicaid Services (CMS). (2019b). *Trump administration announces historic price transparency requirements to increase competition and lower healthcare costs for all Americans*. https://www.cms.gov/newsroom/press-releases/trump-administration-announces-historic-price-transparency-requirements-increase-competition-and.

Delina, G., & Raya, R. P. (2013). A study on work-life balance in working women. *International Journal of Commerce, Business and Management, 2*(5), 274–282.

Deloitte. *eVisits: The 21st century housecall*. (2014). https://www2.deloitte.com/content/dam/Deloitte/au/Documents/technology-media-telecommunications/deloitte-au-tmt-evisits-011014.pdf.

Donabedian, A. (1966). Evaluating the quality of medical care. *Milbank Memorial Fund Quarterly, 44*(3), 166–206.

Elrod, J. K., & Fortenberry, J. L. (2018). Formulating productive marketing communications strategy: A major health system's experience. *BMC Health Services Research, 18*(1), 1–5.

Evans, J. D. (2013). Factors influencing recruitment and retention of nurse educators reported by current nurse faculty. *Journal of Professional Nursing, 29*(1), 11–20.

Healthcare Financial Management Association. (2015). Developing a blueprint for accountable care. *Healthcare Financial Management, 69*(11), 1–8.

Hoeve, Y., Jansen, G., & Roodbol, P. (2013). The nursing profession: Public image, self-concept, and professional identify. *Journal of Advanced Nursing, 70*(2), 295–309.

Hotopf, M. (2013). How patients' review sites will change health care. *Journal of Health Services Research and Policy, 18*(4), 251–254.

Institute of Medicine (IOM). (2001). *Crossing the quality chasm: A new health care system for the 21st century*. Washington, DC: National Academies Press.

Irish, K. (2014). Trends affecting the future of home healthcare. *Home Healthcare Nurse, 32*(9), 567–568.

Kavanagh, K. T., Cimiotti, J. P., Abusalem, S., & Coty, M. (2012). Moving healthcare quality forward with nursing-sensitive value-based purchasing. *Journal of Nursing Scholarship, 44*(4), 385–395.

Kennedy, B., Craig, J. B., Wetsel, M., Reimels, E., & Wright, J. (2013). Three nursing interventions' impact on HCAHPS scores. *Journal of Nursing Care Quality, 28*(4), 327–334.

Kennett, P. A., Henson, S. W., Crow, S. M., & Hartman, S. J. (2005). Key tasks in healthcare marketing: Assessing importance and current level of knowledge. *Journal of Health & Human Services Administration, 27*(4), 414–427.

Kotler, P., & Keller, K. L. (2016). *Marketing management* (15th ed.). New York, NY: Pearson.

Kutney-Lee, A., Sloane, D. M., & Aiken, L. H. (2013). An increase in the number of nurses with baccalaureate degrees is linked to lower rates of post-surgery mortality. *Health Affairs, 32*(3), 579–586.

Long, L. (2012). Impressing patients while improving HCAHPS. *Nursing Management, 43*(12), 32–37.

McCarthy, E. J. (1964). *Basic marketing: A managerial approach* (rev. ed.). New York, NY: McGraw-Hill.

Millenson, M. L., & Macri, J. (2012, March). Will the Affordable Care Act move patient-centeredness to center stage? Timely analysis of immediate health policy issues. *Urban Quick Strike Series*, 1–10. http://www.rwjf.org/en/library/research/2012/03/will-the-affordable-care-act-move-patient-centeredness-to-center.html?cid=XEM_A5765.

Nelson, R., Joos, I., & Wolf, D. M. (2013). *Social media for nurses: Educating practitioners and patients in a networked world.* New York, NY: Springer Publishing Company.

Planetree. (2018). *Person-centered care.* https://www.planetree.org/.

Radwin, L. E., Cabral, H. J., & Woodworth, T. S. (2013). Effects of race and language on patient-centered cancer nursing care and patient outcomes. *Journal of Health Care for the Poor and Underserved, 24*, 619–632.

Sheth, J. N., & Sisodia, R. (2006). *The 4 A's of marketing: Creating value for customer, company and society.* Milton Park, UK: Routledge.

Sinek, S. (2009). *Start with why: How great leaders inspire everyone to take action.* Westminster, MD:Penguin Group.

Steege, L. M., & Pinekenstein, B. (2016). Addressing occupational fatigue in nurses. *Journal of Nursing Administration, 46*(4), 193–200.

Walker, L. (2014). Promoting nursing's professionalism. *Nursing New Zealand, 20*(3), 2.

APPENDIX

Answers for Next-Generation NCLEX ® Case Studies and Item Types

CHAPTER 1: LEADERSHIP AND MANAGEMENT PRINCIPLES

Case Study

The medical/surgical units at St. Helens Community Hospital are busy with a complex mix of patient diagnoses and conditions and have a staff of 88 employees, with a few nurses of long tenure, but mostly new graduates and nurses with less than 2 years of experience. They have four very different leaders:

1. Nurse Manager Dan has 3 years of experience as a nurse manager. He prefers to tell the followers what to do and how to do it in order to get tasks done.
2. Nurse Manager Maria has 3 years of experience as a nurse manager. She prefers to use her outgoing personality and likability to achieve success, using positive motivation and team morale.
3. Nurse Manager Jorge has 3 years of experience as a nurse manager. He prefers to have a hands-off approach and let his employees assume responsibility in the decision-making process.
4. Nurse Manager Olivia has 3 years of experience as a nurse manager. Her unit is busy with a complex mix of patient diagnoses and conditions. She prefers to use her inspiring energy and personality to create a magnetic workplace by engaging with others, centering on followers' needs and goals, and thus raising each other to higher levels of motivation.

SLO/Objective: Analyze leadership styles for effectiveness
NGN Item Type: Matrix
Cognitive Skill: Analyze cues

Question

Use the numbered scenarios above, to indicate the best approach and priority area to lead the unit.

Nursing Situation	Best Approach
The entire facility has a power outage in a storm. Backup generators do not come on in the ICU.	#1
Nurses complain about being understaffed for Christmas vacation.	#4
Nurses have organized a shared governance committee.	#2
The bariatric unit does not have an adequate number of Hoyer lifts, and the NM is concerned about future back injuries.	#3

Answers/Rationales

1. The primary priority approach is #1. This situation will require an all-hands-on-deck approach, and a leader who does not operate in isolation, but one who requires cooperation and collaboration: specifically, one who will guide and motivate nurses to achieve the goal of patient safety during a power outage supported by effective followers.
2. The second priority approach is #2. In this situation the leader has empowered the nursing staff using a shared governance committee. In this case, she is acting as a servant leader. The leader is ensuring that other people's highest priorities are being addressed so that she promotes personal growth and helps others become freer and more autonomous.
3. The third priority approach is #3. In this situation, the leader is recognizing that the bariatric unit has increasing admissions and that there are not adequate resources to manage their care. This is a great example of clinical leadership using interpersonal understanding.

4. The fourth priority approach is #4. In this situation nurses are voicing a potential issue. This scenario is future-oriented and provides the leader with the opportunity to model an authentic leader approach. She can use self-awareness: How would I feel in this situation? She would use an internal moral perspective, determine what is relevant, and be open about the situation with subordinates.

Reference: Huber & Joseph (2021). Chapter 1.

CHAPTER 5: MANAGING TIME AND STRESS

Case Study

Caitlin has been working on 2 North for 6 months since graduating from nursing school. Every day seems stressful, and every new situation makes her feel like she does not have what it takes to be a nurse. She often feels overwhelmed. There are very few senior experienced nurses on the unit, and they are burned out from constantly orienting new nurses. Productivity and effectiveness are low. Caitlin is concerned about her own coping yet also wants to build a higher-functioning and more resilient team. There are lots of recommended stress reduction techniques. Key to success is choosing techniques that are practical and able to be accomplished by a busy nurse daily.

SLO/Objective: Determine highest priority actions
NGN Item Type: Cloze
Cognitive Skill: Take action

Choose the most likely options for the information missing from the question below by selecting from the list of options provided.

Question
Caitlin spent 2 days observing the employees on the unit and noticed that they were always busy, skipped breaks and lunch, drank lots of coffee, and never had down time, confirming her personal perceptions. The top three strategies an employee may use while at work to relieve stress are:
1. ___________ (Drink 8 glasses of water a day),
2. ___________ (Use your getaway place),
3. ___________ (Take scheduled lunches).

Options for Strategies
Getting a massage at the massage parlor 10 min from work
Eat French fries
Drink 8 glasses of water a day
Taking scheduled lunches
Taking a long walk in nature
Taking yoga classes in your neighborhood
Eat at your desk
Use your getaway place

Answers/Rationales
The only three correct anti-stress strategies that are feasible while at work include drinking water for hydration, taking scheduled breaks, and going to your getaway spot. The other choices will require that you leave work (massage parlor 10 min away, walk in nature, and yoga class in your neighborhood) and engage in activities that are not healthy (eat at desk and eat French fries).

Reference: Huber & Joseph (2021). Chapter 5.

CHAPTER 8: COMMUNICATION LEADERSHIP

Case study: Nurse Manager

Tyler has been in his job for 9 months in a busy academic medical center and is just beginning to settle in. He has noticed a spike in medication errors on the unit. It is difficult to manage health care providers' incoming orders as well as the confusion and complexity of multiple provider teams (e.g., neuro, cardiovascular, oncology) rounding independently and making medication and treatment changes that sometimes conflict. Tyler just got the latest data on his unit's quality and safety measures. The medication error rate has increased. He calls the Chair of the unit's Shared Governance Council (SGC) to help evaluate ideas to address communication breakdowns.

SLO/Objective: Apply knowledge of communication theory to determine effective actions
NGN Item Type: Extended multiple response
Cognitive Skill: Analyze cues

Question

Which communication strategies will Tyler, the nurse manager, use to support effective communication interventions? **Select all that apply.**

_______ **A.** Confrontive communication style
__X___**B.** AHRQ's CUS assertive statements.
_______ **C.** Incident reporting
__X___**D.** Crucial conversations
_______ **E.** Formal referral to immediate supervisor
__X__ **F.** TeamSTEPPS SBAR

Answers/Rationales

The correct responses (AHRQ's CUS assertive statements, crucial conversations, and TeamSTEPPS SBAR) are proactive communication tools or strategies to enable a constructive outcome. However, the incorrect responses (confrontive communication style, incident reporting, and referral to immediate supervisor) are all disciplinary in nature.

Reference: Huber & Joseph (2021). Chapter 8.

CHAPTER 13: DECENTRALIZATION AND GOVERNANCE

Case study

After 1 year of employment on 3 South, nurse Maria was invited to join the unit's Shared Governance Council Committee (SGCC). Maria has listened to her fellow nurses complain about not being listened to or valued, and the unit's nurse turnover rate is climbing. Morale is low. She is thrilled that this will be a venue to communicate ways to mitigate the increasing turnover and to communicate her peer's perceptions of being powerless and not having a voice. However, it is important that the SGCC operate as an effective structure. At the first meeting, Maria decided to observe and gain trust with the group versus voicing her concerns. After the meeting, Maria made an appointment with the chairperson (Elyssa) to discuss her observations about how the SGCC operates. Elyssa was open to her feedback.

SLO/Objective: Utilize competencies of shared governance
NGN Item Type: Extended multiple response
Cognitive Skill: Take action

Choose the most likely options to complete the question below.

Question

Which actions, observed while on the committee, indicate that the Shared Governance Council is demonstrating effectiveness? **Select all that apply.**

1. The council meetings are skillful.
2. The council enables leadership.
3. The information discussed is useful.
4. The committee goals are supported by management.
5. The council members are empowered to act.
6. The council is improving patient safety.
7. The council is improving nursing practice.

Answers/Rationales

All responses apply and define council effectiveness.

Reference: Huber & Joseph (2021). Chapter 13.

According to the General Effective Multilevel Theory for Shared Governance (GEMS), there are seven competencies that demonstrate council effectiveness, and these are all provided as the correct responses.

CHAPTER 21: NURSING WORKFORCE STAFFING AND MANAGEMENT

Case Study

Nurse Manager Dan's budget has been cut and is projected to have increasing cuts over the next 2 years due to COVID-19 implications. He made the decision to not hire new employees and use the existing employees to cover staffing needs. Employees on his unit are feeling overworked. Many employees are being asked to do mandatory overtime without adequate compensation. Dan's director was told by human resources that employees are feeling overwhelmed with the increasing staffing demands without adequate compensation. The director pulls Dan's non-salary YTD expense report to examine where opportunities may exist to reallocate funds toward staffing.

SLO/Objective: Evaluate solutions to reallocate funding for staffing management
NGN Item Type: Extended multiple response
Cognitive Skill: Take action

Question

Utilizing the non-salary expense report, the director makes the recommendation for Dan to redirect dollars from some itemized items in the budget. Dan decides to redirect budgetary dollars. Which options indicate an effective strategy to fund staffing?

Select all that apply.

1. Redirect dollars from food service to staffing.
2. Redirect dollars from equipment rental to staffing.
3. Redirect dollars from departmental supplies to staffing.
4. Redirect dollars from travel to staffing.
5. Redirect dollars from other expenses to staffing.

YTD Non-Salary Expense Report

Non-salary expense	Actual	Budget	Var %	Prior
Purchase professional	350	0	0.0%	0
Patient non-chargeable (e.g., Kleenex, bath wipes, deodorant)	100,655	60,656	(65.0%)	59,999
Drugs	0	178	100.0%	0
Food service	6,252	4,200	(48.0)%	4,736
Medical supplies	0	449	100.0%	0
Department supplies	8,668	8,546	(1.4)%	5, 429
Forms and access to databases	1,025	1,255	18.3%	1,204
Minor equipment (e.g., vital signs machine, IV vein finder)	0	1,080	100%	0
Equipment rental (e.g., wound VAC, low bed, bariatric bed)	6,148	6,800	9.5%	1,529
Publications	350	50	(600)%	44
Dues and Memberships	0	8	100%	0
Travel	567	1,058	46.4%	1,325
Other expenses (e.g., outside catering, holiday parties, recognition trophies)	0	8000	100%	3,000
Total non-salary expenses	124,015	92,280	34.3%	77,266

Answers/Rationales

- #4 Redirect dollars from travel for staffing and
- #5 Redirect dollars from Other Expenses

Answer #4: The itemized budget line for "travel" is $1,058, but only $540 has been utilized. Therefore, these funds may be redirected toward staffing and traveling can be put on hold.

Answer #5: The itemize budget line for "other expenses" is $8,000, and $0 has been utilized. Therefore, the $8,000 may be redirected to staffing fully or partially. To consider the redirection of partial budgeted funds, the manager must look at historical spending in that category. They may keep the same or reduce the amount previously allocated.

Reference: Huber & Joseph (2021). Chapter 21 and Chapter 22.

INDEX

Page numbers followed by *b*, *t*, and *f* indicate boxes, tables, and figures, respectively

B

G

H

J

N

O

S

PROFESSIONAL NURSING
CONCEPTS & CHALLENGES

TENTH EDITION

PROFESSIONAL NURSING

CONCEPTS & CHALLENGES

Beth Perry Black, PhD, RN, FAAN
Associate Professor Emeritus
University of North Carolina at Chapel Hill
School of Nursing
Chapel Hill, North Carolina

ELSEVIER

Elsevier
3251 Riverport Lane
St. Louis, Missouri 63043

PROFESSIONAL NURSING: CONCEPTS & CHALLENGES, TENTH EDITION ISBN: 978-0-323-77665-3

Senior Content Strategist: Sandra Clark
Content Development Manager: Danielle Frazier
Senior Content Development Specialist: Maria Broeker
Publishing Services Manager: Julie Eddy
Senior Project Manager: Rachel E. McMullen
Design Direction: Ryan Cook

Printed in the United States of America

Last digit is the print number: 9 8 7 6 5 4 3 2 1

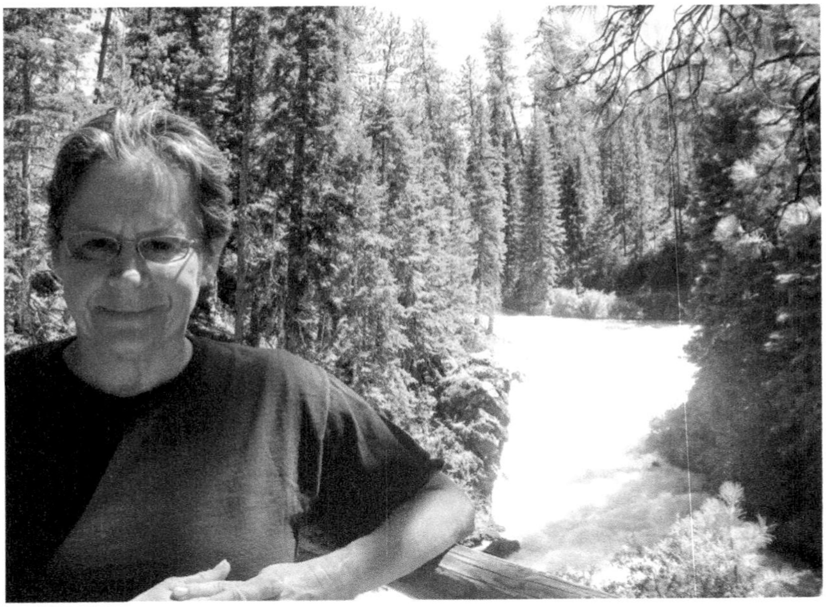

Photo courtesy Grant and Rebeckah Berry.

I dedicate this edition to the life and memory of Diane Berry, who graced our lives with her rare ability to make everyone in her sphere feel like her best friend; in her presence, you were the only person who mattered in the moment. An expert nurse and accomplished researcher, Diane was a gift—a kind, loving, loyal, courageous human unafraid to be herself. And she made us all kinder, more loving, more loyal, more courageous, and more human. That was her enduring gift to those of us—all her best friends—who miss "Mama Bear."

—BPB

PREFACE

As the largest group of health care providers in the U.S., nurses are well-positioned to be leaders in re-envisioning and reforming health care access and delivery. To be effective leaders, nurses must master knowledge about health and illness and human responses to each, think critically and creatively, participate in robust interprofessional education and collaborations, be both caring and professional, and grapple with complex ethical dilemmas that challenge providers in a time when health care resources are strained. As leaders, nurses should understand their history because the past informs the present; vision for the future builds on the lessons of today.

The tenth edition of *Professional Nursing: Concepts & Challenges* reflects my commitment to present current and relevant information. This edition is written while the COVID-19 global pandemic still rages. The stresses on the health care system are enormous, and the effects of the COVID-19 pandemic on the most vulnerable citizens in the U.S. provide irrefutable evidence of the consequences of severe, prevalent disparities related to access to both health and illness care. Ongoing legislative reluctance to address injustices related to climate change creates another barrier to optimal health and wellbeing among economically disadvantaged U.S. citizens, who tend to live in areas most affected by flooding and other sequelae of a changing climate. Nurses are learning that health care is not just what happens in hospitals and clinics but that it plays out in every aspect of daily life.

In this edition, the order of the chapters has remained the same as in the ninth edition, based on generous feedback from faculty that this order provides a cohesive view of nursing; its history, education, and conceptual and theoretical bases; and the place of nursing in the U.S. health care system. Faculty are encouraged, however, to use the chapters in any order that reflects their own pedagogic and theoretical approaches. This edition continues to address the effects of social media on nursing, especially with regard to the legal and ethical implications of their use by nurses and their role in professional socialization and communication. With the easy and free availability of health-related statistics from .gov and other websites, I am continuing with the format and content that was successful in the ninth edition: more narrative and fewer statistics. I have rarely met an engaged nurse who didn't start a story with, "I had a patient once who…" These narratives teach us about what is important in nursing.

Words matter. Throughout the book, I have been very careful to use inclusive language, to avoid heteronormative and ethnocentric words, to use examples that avoid stereotypes of all types, and to include photographs that capture the diversity of American nursing. You will notice that I use the gender-neutral "they" as a now-accepted singular pronoun, and its related possessive form "theirs," both avoiding the awkward "he and/or she" term and assigning a specific gender to a situation or person.

A note about references: older references refer to classic papers or texts. There are a few references that do not reach the level of "classic" texts, but the author turned a phrase in a clever or elegant way that needed to be cited. No manner of updated paper could replace these interesting comments or points of view. Research and clinical works are relevant and contemporary.

As with the last five editions, the tenth edition is written at a level appropriate for use in early courses in baccalaureate curricula, in RN-to-BSN and RN-to-MSN courses, and as a resource for practicing nurses and graduate students. An increasing number of students in nursing programs are seeking second undergraduate degrees, such as midlife adults seeking a career change and others who bring considerable experience to the learning situation. Accordingly, every effort has been made to present material that is comprehensive enough to challenge users at all levels without overwhelming beginning students. The text has been written to be engaging and interesting, and care has been taken to minimize jargon so prevalent in health care. A comprehensive glossary is provided to assist in developing and refining a professional vocabulary. As in previous editions, key terms are highlighted in the text itself. All terms in color print are in the Glossary. The Glossary also contains basic terms that are not necessarily used in the text but may be unfamiliar to students new to nursing.

I hope that the tenth edition continues to meet the high standards set forth by Kay Chitty, who edited the first four editions of this book. I hope that students and faculty will find this edition readable, informative, and thought provoking. More than anything, I hope that *Professional Nursing: Concepts & Challenges,* Tenth Edition, will contribute to the continuing evolution of the profession of nursing and, ultimately, to the excellent care of patients, their families, and their communities.

Beth Perry Black

ACKNOWLEDGMENTS

With each new edition of *Professional Nursing: Concepts & Challenges,* I find myself increasingly in awe of the intelligence, creativity, humility, and work ethic of the nurses who continue to inspire me.

I am grateful to the many people whose support and assistance have made this book possible, each in different ways:

- To nursing faculty who used earlier editions and shared their helpful suggestions to make this book better.
- To nursing students who sent e-mails, expressing their gratitude for an interesting and readable textbook while offering ideas for improvement.
- To the contributors from the ninth edition whose efforts on their chapters provided a solid foundation for my work on this edition.
- To my former colleagues in the School of Nursing at the University of North Carolina at Chapel Hill, and to our extraordinary nursing students and alumni, who make us proud.
- To Amanda Black, whose keen eye for detail was invaluable in preparing the final manuscript for submission. More important, however, was Amanda's sensitivity to the issues and language of gender, race, and diversity. Her incisive, exacting critique of the manuscript and her tireless work in searching out original sources and better references are an editor's dream! This text is better because of her work on it, and I am truly grateful.
- To Tarteel Suliman, who, as my mentee in her undergraduate honors course, demonstrated enviable wisdom and courage, and taught me much about what I do not know. I was privileged to be her teacher, and grateful for the opportunity. Remember her name.
- To Grant and Rebeckah Berry, who shared their photo of their beloved wife and mother Diane, and for sharing her with us in her all-too-short time on this earth.
- To my erstwhile pandemic companion, Abbey, my big goofy furball because, well, everyone who owns a dog knows why. She isn't much for conversation, but she looks at me with great interest while I talk, and her needs are pretty simple.
- To my grandson, Calvin, who as a two-year-old shows remarkable willingness to say "yes" instead of "no." That's a great lesson for all of us who are learning something new.

CONTENTS

Nursing in Today's Evolving Healthcare Environment

To enhance your understanding of this chapter, try the Student Exercises on the Evolve site at http://evolve.elsevier.com/Black/professional.

LEARNING OUTCOMES

After studying this chapter, students will be able to:

- Describe the demographic profile of registered nurses today.
- Recognize the wide range of settings and roles in which today's registered nurses practice.
- Identify evolving practice opportunities for nurses.
- Consider nursing roles in various practice settings.
- Explain the roles and education of advanced practice nurses.

Nurses comprise the largest segment of the healthcare workforce in the United States and have increasing opportunities to practice in a wide variety of settings. More than ever, the profession requires a well-trained, flexible, and knowledgeable workforce of nurses who can practice in today's evolving healthcare environment. Recent legislation, demands of patients as consumers of health care, and the need to control costs while optimizing outcomes have had a great influence on the way that health care is delivered in the United States. Nursing is evolving to meet these demands.

As this edition of *Professional Nursing: Concepts & Challenges* is being developed, the United States continues to face the significant challenges of the worldwide pandemic caused by SARS-CoV-2, more commonly known as *COVID-19.* The long-term health and socioeconomic effects of the pandemic are numerous and are not yet fully realized, although researchers, scientists, and healthcare providers are recognizing the presence of a phenomenon known as *long COVID* or *postacute COVID*, the symptoms of which do not appear to be related to the severity of the initial COVID infection (Centers for Disease Control and Prevention [CDC], 2021). As the numbers of newly diagnosed COVID infections and deaths related to acute COVID may be abating in the U.S. at the time of this writing, the array of new or ongoing symptoms of long COVID continues to widen. This poses a threat to a healthcare system already burdened by significant changes in care delivery required by this infectious, airborne virus, and the sometimes overwhelming numbers of patients with COVID infections requiring acute and critical care.

Furthermore, how to manage the spread of COVID became the source of much political and sociocultural debate. Topics of debate included whether and how to mandate wearing masks and vaccinations, the effectiveness of social distancing, and how to address the spread of disinformation related to COVID-19 transmission and the use of untested, unsupported, and even dangerous substances to prevent or cure infection. Importantly, the long-term effects of the pandemic and its overwhelming strain on the healthcare workforce, including registered nurses, continues to evolve, and will likely result in an acute shortage of nurses in the near future.

The issue of access to care and how to pay for it continues to challenge U.S. citizens, which has lagged behind other nations of comparable economic development in terms of accessibility of adequate health care, mortality rates, disease burden, and other key health metrics (Peterson-KFF, 2021). One of the most notable influences on today's healthcare environment is the Affordable Care Act (ACA), passed in 2010 by the

111th Congress and signed into law by President Barack Obama. The ACA is actually two laws: the Patient Protection and Affordable Care Act (PL 111–148) and the Health Care and Education Affordability Reconciliation Act (PL 111–152). These laws provide for incremental but progressive change to the way that Americans gain access to and pay for their health care. The ACA provided increased opportunities for nurses: the Committee on the Robert Wood Johnson Foundation (RWJF) Initiative on the Future of Nursing at the National Academy of Medicine (NAM) noted nursing's opportunities to act in partnership with other health professions in improving and reconfiguring the U.S. healthcare system and how care is delivered (National Academy of Medicine [NAM], 2010). The most recent study by NAM on the Future of Nursing 2020-2030 built on the findings from 2010-2020, noting the primacy of the health of its citizen to ensure that a nation will thrive, and that nurses as "trusted bridge builders" are catalysts for implementing changes in to the U.S. healthcare system to advance health equity by building on a stronger and more expert nursing workforce (NAM, 2021). The Future of Nursing 2020-2030 document and related resources can be found at https://nam.edu/publications/the-future-of-nursing-2020-2030/.

Writing about "nursing today" poses a challenge because what is current is likely to change by the time you read this. What does not change, however, is the commitment of nurses to what Rosenberg (1995) referred to as "the care of strangers": professional caring, learned through focused education and deliberate socialization (Storr, 2010). In other words, you will be taught to think like a nurse and to do well those things that nurses do. You will become a nurse. Importantly, some of you are already nurses and are returning to school to further your education. Thank you for your commitment to the profession and to your own professional development! You have experienced firsthand the sometimes quickly shifting needs of the profession in an evolving healthcare system in a changing world and are poised to move nursing forward with your knowledge from both your education and your wide variety of experiences.

In this chapter you will learn some basic information about today's nursing workforce: who nurses are, the settings where they practice, and the patients for whom they are providing care. You will also be introduced to some nurses who have had intriguing experiences and opportunities that you may not know are even possible. Your nursing education will provide you with a flexible set of skills and opens to you a wide variety of experiences that await you as you begin—or continue—your career as a professional registered nurse (RN).

NURSING IN THE UNITED STATES TODAY

A diverse nursing workforce is fundamental to meeting healthcare needs in the U.S., and to address health inequities, including access to care among historically underserved communities (American Association of Colleges of Nursing [AACN], 2020). To achieve this fundamental goal, schools of nursing must recruit and admit individuals from diverse backgrounds (AACN, 2020). Understanding the composition of the nursing workforce is necessary to identify underrepresented groups and to recognize workforce trends such as the age of nurses in practice and the percentage of licensed nurses holding jobs in nursing.

As an initial mechanism to respond to the need for understanding the nursing workforce, the U.S. Department of Health and Human Services conducted a comprehensive survey of the nursing workforce every 4 years, beginning in 1977. Known as the National Sample Survey of Registered Nurses (NSSRN), this effort gave policymakers, educators, and other nurse leaders data about the workforce, allowing them to make informed decisions about allocation of resources, development of programs, and recruitment of nurses. This important survey was discontinued, however, after its final report issued in 2010.

In response and the ongoing need to understand the nursing workforce, in 2013 the National Council of State Boards of Nursing (NCSBN) and the Forum of State Nursing Workforce Centers (FSNWC) combined efforts to conduct a comprehensive national survey of a randomized sample of 157,459 registered nurses and 39,765 licensed practical nurses/licensed vocational nurses (Smiley et al., 2021). In this chapter, data from the 2020 National Nursing Workforce Survey are presented to provide you with a thumbnail sketch of nursing, specifically focusing on the number of nurses in the workforce, and their gender, age, race, ethnicity, and educational levels. Any data retrieved from sources other than the 2020 National Nursing Workforce Survey are cited; otherwise, data are from this survey. For more comprehensive data, you can download the survey as a .pdf in its entirety for free at https://www.journalofnursingregulation.com/action/showPdf?pii=S2155-8256%2821%2900027-2.

Nurses in the Workforce

With more than 4.1 million active licenses, RNs are the largest group of healthcare providers in the United States, growing by 6.7% between 2017 to 2019 (note: "active" does not mean that a nurse is currently employed in nursing). A nursing license is issued by an entity or body such as a state board of nursing (BON) that assures the public that the person holding the license meets predetermined standards for safe practice (National Council State Boards of Nursing, 2011). You will learn more about this in Chapter 6. A significant number of RNs (84.1%) reported they are actively employed in nursing, with 64.9% reporting working full time, a slight decrease since the previous survey. Among nurses not currently in the workforce, 49.0% reported taking care of home and family as the reason for not being employed in nursing; interestingly, 14.6% reported difficulty in finding a nursing position, and 32.1% reported other, a nonspecific and undefined category. The 2020 survey asked an additional question regarding plans for retirement or leaving nursing in the next 5 years; 22.1% reported having these plans, an alarming statistic given the anticipated nursing shortage related to COVID-related stresses and other reasons for leaving nursing. In 2017, 13.9% of RNs reported working 2 positions and 2.8% working ≥ 3 positions; in 2020 these percentages decreased slightly to 13.7% and 2.4% respectively.

Gender

The RN workforce currently has 9.4% males, an increase of 0.3% since 2017 and 2.8% since 2013. In 2020, 0.1% identified as "other," a nonspecific, undefined term to capture responses of persons whose gender identity is not reflected in binary male/female signifiers previously used in the survey. In the AACN 2018–2019 report on baccalaureate and graduate programs in nursing, men comprised 12.9% of students in entry-level Bachelor of Science in Nursing (BSN) programs, 12.2% of students in masters programs, 13.4% in Doctor of Nursing Practice (DNP) programs, and 11.2% in research-focused doctoral programs, typically doctor of philosophy (PhD) programs (AACN, 2019).

Age

The future of any profession depends on the infusion of younger persons, and the steady increase in the age of the nursing workforce has been a concern. The median age—the point at which half of the nurses are older and half are younger—provides a more useful metric of the workforce than does calculating a mean age. Since 1988, when their median age was 38, the median age of nurses rose by 2 years between each national survey so that by 2004, the median age was 46, a worrisome figure that meant the nursing workforce was continuing to grow older. By 2020, 19.0% of nurses were ≥ 65 years old and an additional 12.2% were 60 to 64 years old, meaning that a combined 31.2%, or almost one-third, of the nursing workforce is ≥ 60 years old. The increasing number of nurses aged 60 and older who are still in the workforce may reflect economic conditions requiring older nurses to remain employed rather than retiring. The profession of nursing must continue to recruit, educate and retain younger nurses to prevent a severe nursing shortage as older nurses move toward retirement.

Race and Ethnicity

Racial and ethnic minorities comprise 39.9% of the U.S. population today but only 19% of the RN population, an underrepresentation by slightly more than 50% in 2020 (U.S. Census.gov, 2020; Smiley et al, 2021). This is a troublesome number, given the burgeoning emphasis on health equity and the need for a diverse nursing workforce. Detailed data from the 2020 National Nursing Workforce Survey showed that the largest disparity between the U.S. general population and the RN population is seen with Hispanics/Latinos of any race. Although this group forms about 18.5% of the U.S. population (U.S. Census Bureau, 2020), they make up only 5.6% of RNs. Black/African American, non-Hispanics also have a significant disparity; now constituting 13.4% of the U.S. population, this group makes up just 6.7% of RNs. The Asian population, comprising 5.9% of the general U.S. population, makes up 7.2% of the RN population, a moderate overrepresentation. Although many nurses identifying as Asian in practice in the U.S. were educated in Asia and immigrated to the U.S., this may not fully explain the overrepresentation of the population in nursing. Although the profession of nursing has a long way to go to reach proportional representation across racial/ethnic groups, there is evidence of some improvement. In 1995 fewer than 18% of students enrolled in a professional nursing program were from underrepresented racial or ethnic minority groups in contrast to more than 34.2% in 2019 (AACN, 2019).

Education

Entry level into practice is the term for one's basic education to become a nurse. Successful completion of your basic education, however, does not qualify you to become a nurse. Once you have graduated from a school of nursing approved by your state, you are qualified to take the National Council Licensure Examination for Registered Nurses, known as the NCLEX-RN®. After passing the NCLEX-RN®, you can be licensed as an RN if you meet other requirements by your state board of nursing, such as passing a background check.

Nursing has three mechanisms by which you can get basic nursing education to qualify to take the NCLEX-RN®: (1) a four-year education at a college or university conferring a BSN degree; (2) a two-year education at a community college or technical school conferring an associate degree in nursing (ADN); and (3) a diploma in nursing, awarded after the successful completion of a hospital-based program that typically takes three years to complete, including prerequisite courses that may be taken at another school.

Diploma programs educated only 3% to 4% of all new RNs in between 2003 and 2014 (NLN, 2014) as nursing education shifted to colleges and universities (AACN, 2011). Significantly, 41.8 % of nurses responding to the 2020 U.S. nursing workforce survey were graduates of BSN programs, while 37.7% were graduates of ADN programs. In comparison, in 2013, 36.0% reported having a BSN as their first degree or credential, while 38.7% reported having an ADN as their first degree or credential (Health Resources and Services Administration, 2013). In addition, in 2020, 3.6% of RNs reported receiving their MSN as their first nursing degree or credential, meaning that a combined 45.4% of respondents in the workforce survey received their entry level nursing education in a university setting. Between the years 2013 and 2020, ADN-prepared RNs decreased slightly from 38.7% to 37.7%, while the number of graduates from nursing schools offering a diploma decreased more significantly, from 17.6% to 11.1% (Smiley et al, 2021).

Many ADN-prepared RNs eventually return to school to complete a BSN degree. Between 2004 and 2012, the number of RNs enrolled in BSN programs almost tripled, from 35,000 to slightly fewer than 105,000 (RWJF, 2013). In December 2017, the state of New York implemented a law requiring nurses who graduate from ADN or diploma programs from that date forward must earn a BSN or higher degree within 10 years of graduation; students enrolled in ADN and diploma programs at the time the law was implemented had a grace period of 18 additional months to earn a BSN or higher (University of Buffalo, 2021). Importantly, many colleges and universities offer BSN programs, often online, to accommodate RNs in practice who want or are required to work toward a BSN degree as a supplement to their entry level ADN or diploma nursing education. Nursing education is discussed in greater detail in Chapter 4.

Globalization and the international migration of nurses have increased the number of internationally educated nurses (IENs) practicing in the United States by 40% between 2006 and 2015. In 2016, approximately 15% of all RNs in the United States were educated in other countries (World Education Service, 2018). The recruitment of IENs to the United States has been a strategy to expand the nursing workforce in response to nursing shortages. This strategy, however, may result in shortages in nurses' countries of origins. IENs may face challenges as they join the workforce in the United States, including English as a second language for some, and discrimination from co-workers who may not perceive them as knowledgeable (Thekdi et al., 2011). Cultural differences may further separate the IENs from their American peers. Thekdi and colleagues (2011) noted that IENs might have views of gender, authority, power, and age that vary from those of Americans, and which may affect their communication styles.

Practice Settings for Professional Nurses

As members of the largest healthcare profession in the United States, nurses practice in a wide variety of settings. The most common setting is the hospital, and many new nurses seek employment there to strengthen their clinical and assessment skills. Nurses practice in clinics, community-based facilities, medical offices, skilled nursing facilities (SNFs), and other long-term settings. Nurses also provide care in places where people spend much of their time: homes, schools, and workplaces. In communities, nurses work in the military, community and senior centers, children's camps, homeless shelters, and in clinics found in some pharmacies and other retail settings. Nurses also provide palliative care—symptom management to improve quality of life of persons with serious and/or chronic conditions—and end-of-life care, often in the homes of patients who are terminally ill or in inpatient hospice homes or facilities. Increasingly, nurses with advanced degrees, training, and certification are working in their own private practices or in partnership with physicians or other providers. This expansion of practice holds promise for nurses to widen their roles in health care, especially as the American healthcare system continues to evolve.

Noncritical inpatient care (29.6%) in hospital settings was the most common work setting for RNs, with 20.0% in general medical-surgical care units (U.S. Dept. of Health and Human Services [DHHS], Health Resources and Services Administration [HRSA], 2020). Ambulatory and primary care settings were the next most common places of RN employment. The HRSA report noted that fewer than 1% of RNs worked in pulmonary/respiratory or infectious/communicable disease settings, a statistic that held significant implications for the nursing workforce during the COVID-19 pandemic (DHHS HRSA, 2020). Other specialty areas of significance to the COVID-19 pandemic response were emergency care (8.1% of RNs), critical care (7.4%), and psychiatric/mental health (3.8%). The capacity of the RN workforce was challenged by the COVID-19 pandemic. HRSA (2020) noted that "understanding where nurses work provides valuable information for epidemic or pandemic responses regarding the mobilization and capacity of healthcare workers" (p. 8).

Ambulatory care settings, such as nurse-based practices, physician-based practices, and free-standing emergency and surgical centers, accounted for 13.1%, the second largest segment of the nurse workforce. Public and community health accounted for 7.8% of employed nurses, and an additional 6.4% worked in home health. Long-term care, skilled nursing (SNFs), or subacute care facilities employed 4.8% of nurses in the workforce. The remainder of employed RNs worked in settings or roles such as schools of nursing; healthcare management/administration; informatics, and school nursing, among others (U.S. DHHS HRSA, 2020).

Not all nurses provide direct patient care as their primary role. A small but important group of nurses spend the majority of their time conducting research, teaching undergraduate and graduate students in the classroom and in clinical settings, managing companies as chief executives, and consulting with healthcare organizations. Nurses with advanced levels of education, such as master's and doctoral degrees, are prepared to become researchers, educators, and administrators. Nurses can practice as advanced practice nurses (APNs), including a variety of types of nurse practitioners (NPs), clinical nurse specialists (CNSs), certified nurse-midwives (CNMs), and certified registered nurse anesthetists (CRNAs). These advanced practice roles are described later in this chapter.

Nurses have much to consider in deciding where to practice. Some settings will not be immediately open to new nurses because they require additional educational preparation or work experience. Importantly, nurses entering the workforce need to consider their special talents, likes, and dislikes; neither the nurse nor patients benefit when a nurse is working with a population for which they have little affinity. A nurse who enjoys working with children may not feel at ease in caring for older patients; on the other hand, a nurse who loves children may find that caring for sick children is emotionally stressful. A nurse with excellent communication skills may find that a postanesthesia care unit (PACU) does not allow the formation of professional relationships with patients that this nurse might appreciate in a psychiatric setting. Nursing school offers the chance to experience a variety of settings with diverse patient populations. At the end of your studies, you may be surprised by the skills you have developed and populations that appeal to you (Fig. 1.1).

With healthcare reform and the concomitant push to transform the healthcare system, and with full manifestation of the effects of COVID illness still to

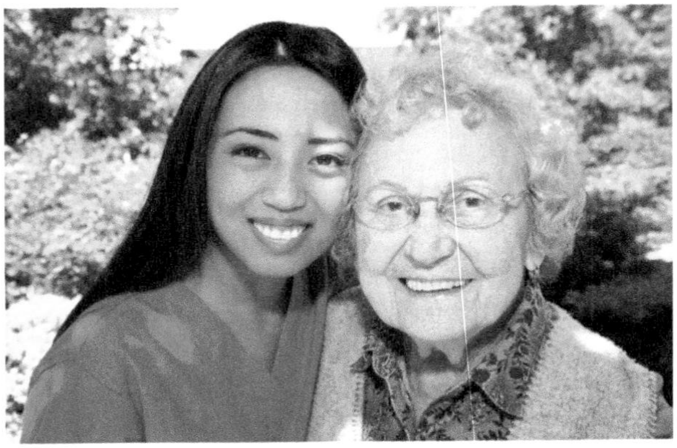

Fig. 1.1 Although most nurses work in hospitals, nurses in home health settings often enjoy long-term relationships with their patients. (Photo used with permission from iStockphoto.)

be determined, the profession of nursing continues to evolve. Numerous new opportunities and roles are being developed that use nurses' skills in innovative and exciting ways. In the following section, you will be introduced to a range of settings in which nurses practice. These areas are only a sample of the growing variety of opportunities available to nurses entering practice today.

Nursing in Hospitals

Nursing care originated and was practiced informally in home and community settings and moved into hospitals only within the past 150 years. Hospitals vary widely in size and services. Certain hospitals are referred to as medical centers and offer comprehensive specialty services, such as cancer centers, maternal-fetal medicine services, and heart centers. Medical centers are usually associated with university medical schools and have a complex array of providers. Medical centers can have 1000 or more beds and have a huge nursing workforce. Medical centers are often designated as level 1 trauma centers because they offer highly specialized surgical and supportive care for the most severely injured patients. The patients at community-based hospitals usually are less severely ill than those needing comprehensive care or trauma care at a medical center. However, if a patient becomes unstable or if the patient's condition warrants, he or she can be transported to a larger hospital or a medical center. Nurses play an important role in identifying very ill patients, assisting in stabilizing their conditions, and preparing them for transport.

In general, nurses in hospitals care for patients who have medical or surgical conditions (e.g., those with cancer or diabetes, those in need of postoperative care), children and their families on pediatric units, women giving birth and their newborns, and patients who have had severe trauma or burns. Specialty areas are referred to as *units*, such as operating suites or emergency departments, intensive care units (e.g., cardiac, neurology, medical), and step-down or progressive care units, among others. In addition to providing direct patient care, nurses are educators, managers, and administrators who teach or supervise others and establish the direction of nursing on a hospital-wide basis.

Various generalist and specialist certification opportunities are appropriate for hospital-based nurses, including medical-surgical nursing, pediatric nursing, pain management nursing, informatics nursing, genetics nursing–advanced, psychiatric–mental health nursing, nursing executive, nursing executive–advanced, hemostasis nursing, and cardiovascular nursing, among others. *Certification* means that nurses have demonstrated their expertise in a particular area of care and have passed rigorous credentialing testing offered by the American Nurses Credentialing Center (ANCC), one of three entities comprising the American Nurses Association (ANA) Enterprise. No other types of healthcare facilities offer the variety of opportunities for practice as hospitals offer.

The educational credentials required of RNs practicing in hospitals can range from associate degrees and diplomas to doctoral degrees. In general, entry-level positions require only RN licensure. Many hospitals require nurses to hold bachelor's degrees to advance on the clinical ladder or to assume management positions. A **clinical ladder** is a multiple-step program that begins with entry-level staff nurse positions. As nurses gain experience, participate in continuing education (CE), demonstrate clinical competence, pursue formal education, and become certified, they become eligible to move up the clinical ladder. There is no single model for clinical advancement for nurses across hospitals and other healthcare agencies. When exploring work settings, nurses as prospective employees should ask about the clinical ladder and opportunities for career advancement.

Most new nurses choose to work as staff nurses in hospitals initially to gain experience in organizing and delivering care to multiple patients. For many, staff nursing is extremely gratifying, and nurses continue in this role across their careers. Others pursue additional education, sometimes provided by the hospital, to work in specialty units such as neonatal intensive care or cardiac care. Although specialty units often require clinical experience and additional training, some hospitals allow new graduates to work in these units.

Some nurses find that management is their strength. **Nurse managers** are in charge of all activities on their units, including patient care, continuous quality improvement (CQI), personnel hiring and evaluation, and resource management, including the unit budget. Being a nurse manager in a hospital today requires business acumen and knowledge of business and financial principles to be most effective in this role. Nurse managers typically assume 24-hour accountability for the units they manage and are often required to have earned a master's degree.

Most nurses in hospitals provide direct patient care, sometimes referred to as bedside nursing. In the past, becoming administrators or managers was often necessary for nurses to be promoted or receive salary increases, which removed them from bedside care. Today, in hospitals with clinical ladder programs, nurses no longer must make that choice; clinical ladder programs allow nurses to progress professionally while staying in direct patient care roles.

At the top of most clinical ladders are **clinical nurse specialists** (CNSs), who are APNs with master's, post-master's, or doctoral degrees in specialized areas of nursing, such as oncology (cancer) or diabetes care. The CNS role varies but generally includes responsibility for serving as a clinical mentor and role model for other nurses and setting standards for nursing care on one or more particular units. The oncology clinical specialist, for example, works with the nurses on the oncology unit to help them stay informed regarding the latest research and skills useful in the care of patients with cancer. The clinical specialist is a resource person for the unit and may provide direct care to patients or families with particularly difficult or complex problems, establish nursing protocols, and ensure that nursing practice on the unit is evidence based. **Evidence-based practice (EBP)** refers to nursing care that is based on the best available research evidence, clinical expertise, and patient preference. More details about EBP are found in Chapter 10.

Salaries and responsibilities increase at the upper levels of the clinical ladder. The clinical ladder concept benefits nurses by allowing them to advance while still working directly with patients. Hospitals also benefit by retaining experienced clinical nurses in direct patient care, thus improving the quality of nursing care throughout the hospital. Research has demonstrated that patient outcomes are more positive for patients cared for by RNs with a bachelor's or higher degree. Linda Aiken, PhD, RN, FAAN, is a leader in nursing who has conducted important research documenting the positive impact of adequate RN staffing on patient outcomes. Two decades ago, Aiken and colleagues (2003) published a groundbreaking study in which they found that patients on surgical units with more BSN-prepared nurses had fewer complications than patients on units with fewer BSN nurses. Aiken has published widely on nurse staffing and safety since publishing this landmark study. In 2010 Aiken and colleagues reported on a comparison of nurse and patient outcomes among hospitals in California, which has state-mandated nurse-to-patient ratios, and in Pennsylvania and New Jersey, neither of which has state-mandated nurse-to-patient ratios. Furthermore, concern about patient quality and safety is an international issue. In 2012 Aiken and colleagues led a very large team in examining nurse and patient satisfaction, hospital environments, quality of care, and patient safety across 12 European countries and the United States (Aiken et al, 2012). Again in 2014, Aiken and her team conducted a retrospective observational study of nine European countries analyzing 422,730 patient records (Aiken et al, 2014). They found the proportion of nurses with a baccalaureate education is associated with significantly fewer deaths after surgery: every 10% increase in baccalaureate-prepared nurses is associated with a 7% reduction in mortality.

The World Alliance of Patient Safety was formed by the World Health Organization (WHO) after the alarming results of the U.S. Institute of Medicine (now National Academy of Medicine [NAM]) study published in 1999 demonstrated the high incidence of patient harm associated with healthcare delivery across the world. At the University of Pennsylvania, USA, the Center for Health Outcomes and Policy Research initiated an international research program known colloquially as RN4CAST. In 2018 Aiken and colleagues published a summary of key findings from RN4CAST and described the work in progress from Chile on patient safety. A key finding was that "higher nurse resourced hospitals" (p.324), with higher labor costs, had better patient outcomes, with 40% fewer expensive intensive care unit (ICU) admissions and shorter patient lengths of stay than hospitals who did not invest in hiring more professional nurses. This means that the costs of providing care by a larger workforce of professional nurses were offset by fewer expensive patient complications that required ICU admission and longer hospital stays (Aiken, Cerón, Simonetti, et al, 2018). See Evidence-Based Practice Box 1.1 for a description of these landmark studies.

Rigid work scheduling was one of the greatest drawbacks to hospital nursing in the past. These schedules usually included evenings, nights, weekends, and holidays. Although hospital units must be staffed around the clock, **flexible staffing** is more common now, a process by which nurses on a particular unit negotiate with one another and establish their own schedules to meet personal and family responsibilities while ensuring that appropriate staffing for high-quality patient care is provided. Staffing needs may be predictable, such as in the emergency department or surgical units when times of

EVIDENCE-BASED PRACTICE BOX 1.1

The Evidence: Better Professional Nurse Staffing Improves Quality and Safety of Patient Care

Linda Aiken, PhD, RN, FAAN, Professor of Nursing and Professor of Sociology at the University of Pennsylvania School of Nursing and director of the Center for Health Outcomes and Policy Research, is noted for her work spanning her career examining issues of health care outcomes and the nursing workforce. She is an authority on causes, consequences, and solutions for nursing shortages both in the United States and worldwide, and has published extensively. Twenty years ago, Dr. Aiken and her colleagues noted growing evidence suggesting "that nurse staffing affects the quality of care in hospitals, but little is known about whether the educational composition of registered nurses (RNs) in hospitals is related to patient outcomes" (Aiken et al., 2003). They wondered whether the proportion of a hospital's staff of bachelor's or higher degree–prepared RNs contributed to improved patient outcomes. To answer this question, they undertook a large analysis of outcome data for 232,342 general, orthopedic, and vascular surgery patients discharged from 168 Pennsylvania hospitals over a 19-month period. They used statistical methods to control for risk factors such as age, gender, emergency or routine surgeries, type of surgery, preexisting conditions, surgeon qualifications, size of hospital, and other factors. Their findings were very important:

To our knowledge, this study provides the first empirical evidence that hospitals' employment of nurses with BSN and higher degrees is associated with improved patient outcomes. Our findings indicate that surgical patients cared for in hospitals in which higher proportions of direct-care RNs held bachelor's degrees experienced a substantial survival advantage over those treated in hospitals in which fewer staff nurses had BSN [bachelor of science in nursing] or higher degrees. Similarly, surgical patients experiencing serious complications during hospitalization were significantly more likely to survive in hospitals with a higher proportion of nurses with baccalaureate education (p. 1621).

Noting that fewer than half of all hospital staff nurses nationally are prepared at the bachelor's or higher level, and citing a shortage of nurses as a complicating factor, this group of researchers recommended "placing greater emphasis in national nurse workforce planning on policies to alter the educational composition of the future nurse workforce toward a greater proportion with bachelor's or higher education and ensuring the adequacy of the overall supply" (p. 1623). They concluded that improved public financing of nursing education and increased employers' efforts to recruit and retain highly prepared bedside nurses could lead to substantial improvements in quality of care.

More recently, California became the first state to enforce state-mandated minimum nurse-to-patient ratios. Much commentary about the pros and cons of these types of mandates has been generated. To determine whether nurse and patient outcomes were different in California than in two states without mandated staffing, Aiken and colleagues (2010) analyzed survey data from 22,336 hospital staff nurses in California, Pennsylvania, and New Jersey, and state hospital discharge databases. From this highly complex analysis they determined the following:

When we use the predicted probabilities of dying from our adjusted models to estimate how many fewer deaths would have occurred in New Jersey and Pennsylvania hospitals if the average patient-to-nurse ratios in those hospitals had been equivalent to the average ratio across the California hospitals, we get 13.9% (222/1598) fewer surgical deaths in New Jersey and 10.6% (264/2479) fewer surgical deaths in Pennsylvania (p. 917).

In addition, the nurses in California experienced lower levels of burnout (a condition associated with intense and prolonged stress in work settings) and were less likely to report being dissatisfied with their jobs. These important findings can inform ongoing debates in other states regarding legislation regulating nurse-patient ratio or mandatory reporting of nurse staffing. Aiken and colleagues (2010) concluded, "Improved nurse staffing, however it is achieved, is associated with better outcomes for nurses and patients" (p. 918).

Quality and safety of patient care are of international concern. In 2012 Aiken and a team of researchers from the U.S. and Europe published findings from a very large, cross-sectional study of 488 general acute care hospitals in 12 European countries and 617 similar hospitals in the United States. Despite deficits in the quality of care present in all countries, Aiken and colleagues found that hospitals providing good work environments and better staffing by professional nurses had nurses and patients who were more satisfied with care. Furthermore, their findings suggested that good work environments and better professional nurse staffing resulted in improving quality and safety of care. The implication of these findings is that improvement of hospital work environments could be an affordable strategy to improve both patient outcomes and retention of professional nurses who provide high-quality care.

EVIDENCE-BASED PRACTICE BOX 1.1—cont'd

The Evidence: Better Professional Nurse Staffing Improves Quality and Safety of Patient Care

In 2014 Aiken et al. published foundational research assessing the impact of nursing patient ratios and educational qualifications in 300 hospitals in nine European countries. They reviewed more than 422,730 patient records of patients who underwent common surgeries and surveyed 26,516 nurses practicing in the study hospitals to gather data on nurse staffing and education. The researchers found that an increase of 10% of nurses holding a baccalaureate degree in the hospital setting is associated with a 7% reduction in mortality. Also, an increase of a nurse's patient load by one patient increased the likelihood of an inpatient dying within 30 days of admission by 7%. In other words, cutting nurse staff to reduce the nursing budget may adversely affect patient outcomes. Also, increasing the number of baccalaureate-prepared nurses may prevent hospital deaths.

In 2018 New York became the first state to require that new RNs obtain their baccalaureate degree within 10 years of graduation. Much of the evidence presented to back this legislative bill came from the pivotal work done by Aiken and colleagues. Furthermore, in 2018, Aiken et al. reported on the business case for improved nurse staffing, noting the continuing accumulation of compelling evidence from around the world demonstrating the same phenomenon: investing in improved nurse staffing simply makes hospitalization safer for patients and less expensive for the institutions. Despite the tendency for policy-makers and executives to try to minimize the expense of nurse staffing, allocation of additional resources to professional nurse staffing pays off in better health and financial outcomes.

Resources

Aiken LH, Cerón C, Simonetti M, Lake ET, Galiano A, Garbarini A, Soto P, Bravo D, Smith HL: Hospital nurse staffing and patient outcomes, *Revista Médica Clínica Las Condes* 29(3):322-327, 2018.

Aiken LH, Clarke SP, Cheung RB, Sloane D, Silber JH: Educational levels of hospital nurses and surgical patient mortality, *Journal of the American Medical Association* 290(12):1617–1623, 2003.

Aiken LH, Sermeus W, Van den Heede K, Sloane DM, Busse R, McKee M, Kutney-Lee A: Patient safety, satisfaction, and quality of hospital care: cross sectional survey of nurses and patients in 12 countries in Europe and the United States, *British Medical Journal* 344:1717, 2012.

Aiken LH, Sloane DM, Bruyneel L, Van den Heede K, Griffiths P, Busse R, Sermeu W: Nurse staffing and education and the hospital mortality in nine European countries: a retrospective observational study, *Lancet* 383(9931):1824–1830, 2014.

Aiken LH, Sloane DM, Cimiotti JP, Clarke SP, Flynn L, Seago JA, Spetz J, Smith HK: Implications of the California nurse staffing mandate for other states, *Health Services Research* 45(4):904–921, 2010.

high use can be anticipated. Accordingly, some units may decrease staffing over major holidays because numbers of admissions are known to be low during certain days of the year when elective procedures are not routinely scheduled.

Each hospital nursing role has its own unique characteristics. In the following profile, an RN discusses his role as a nurse in a neonatal intensive care unit (NICU):

> *Many people are surprised when I tell them that I work in a NICU. They don't seem to expect that a man might enjoy working with the tiniest patients in the hospital. But I appreciate the technical challenges of providing care for an infant born very prematurely or who has a serious congenital condition. The biggest challenge for me though is working with a full-term baby that had some kind of unexpected trauma during labor and birth. These babies can be very, very sick, and their families need a lot of support and information. I take care of my little patients the same way I would want someone to take care of my own child. I can only imagine how terrifying it is for the parents for their baby to be so sick. I know that some of the procedures that I have to do are painful, so I make sure that I talk to the baby while I am doing a procedure and try to provide comfort the best I can. Sometimes, when things are quiet in the unit, I'll wrap a blanket around a baby whose family can't visit often and rock him or her for a while. The only thing better than that is the day the family takes the baby home.*

When the "fit" between nurses and their role requirements is good, being a nurse is particularly gratifying, as an oncology nurse demonstrates in discussing her role:

Being an oncology nurse and working with people with cancer that may shorten their lives brings you close to patients and their families. The family room for our patients and their families is much like someone's home. Families bring in food and have dinner with their loved one right here. Working with terminally ill patients is a tall order. I look for ways to help families determine what they hope for as their loved one nears the end of life. It varies. Sometimes they hope for a peaceful death, or hope to make amends with an estranged family member or friend or hope to go to a favorite place one more time. The diagnosis of cancer can be traumatic, and patients may struggle to cope, especially if their cancer is advanced or untreatable. I love getting to know my patients and their families and feel that I can be helpful to them as they face death, sometimes by simply being with them. They cry, I cry—it is part of nursing for me, and I would have it no other way.

These are only two of the many possible roles nurses in hospital settings may choose. Although brief, these descriptions convey an idea of the responsibility, complexity, and fulfillment to be found in hospital-based nursing (Fig. 1.2).

Nursing in Communities

Lillian Wald (1867–1940) initiated public health/community health nursing when she established the Henry Street Settlement in New York City in 1895, provided care to families living in poverty, and was an early proponent of nurses in public schools. In 2013 the American Public Health Association (APHA) published a statement defining and describing the practice of public health nursing: "...the practice of promoting and protecting the health of populations using knowledge from nursing, social, and public health sciences" (American Public Health Association [APHA], 2013). The writers of this comprehensive statement noted that the terms *public health nursing* and *community health nursing* are often used interchangeably and did not make a distinction between the two. Some make a distinction in that public health nursing is a broader concept and focuses on population-based health concerns, while community health nursing focuses on individuals, families and community-based health concerns. For purposes of this chapter, the term public health nursing, as defined by the APHA, is used.

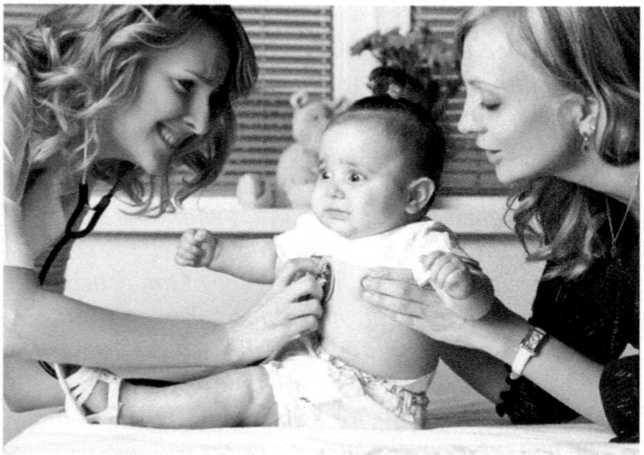

Fig. 1.2 Hospital staff nurses work closely with the families of patients, as well as with the patients themselves. (Photo used with permission from Photos.com.)

The COVID-19 pandemic put issues of public health front and center in American life and beyond. As the world grappled with how to prevent and then manage the transmission of this highly contagious airborne virus, public health efforts also had to address and counter widespread disinformation and confusion about the virus, how it is spread, testing for contact tracing, masking, and vaccine administration. Much media and public attention was placed on nurses and other healthcare providers in in-patient settings, particularly ICUs, because these units faced a burgeoning number of extremely ill patients requiring ventilatory and other extensive support to survive the effects of the viral infection. Early in the pandemic, these nurses were deemed "heroes." At the same time, other nurses faced challenges in communities to prevent the spread of the virus among particularly vulnerable populations. One of these efforts occurred in Alaska, where the Alaska Native Tribal Health Consortium (ANTHC), the largest and most comprehensive tribal health organization in the United States, works to address the needs of Alaska Native and American Indian people, both populations at high risk for COVID-19 (CDC Foundation, 2021). Evidence-Based Practice Box 1.2 features the efforts of three nurses—Elizabeth Aarons, MS, RN; Elizabeth Arteaga, DNP, RN; and Tracy Frost, CMSRN—who led an impressive effort to provide testing for a geographically dispersed population in Alaska for whom intensive care may be delayed if not impossible. You will learn in Chapter 10 that evidence-based

EVIDENCE-BASED PRACTICE BOX 1.2

Nurses Taking Care Into Their Community: Covid-19 Testing Among the Resilient Alaskan Native People

Elizabeth Aarons, MS, RN

I am Inupiaq, from the Native Village of Unalakleet. I come from a lineage of healers. Before the time when pregnancy, labor, and birth became medicalized in Western health care, my great-great-grandmother on my mom's side was one of the local midwives in my home village. On my dad's side, my great-grandfather was a doctor trained in Western Medicine. The duality of their practices has given me perspective and respect for where knowledge originally came from: Indigenous healers.

Before attending nursing school, I earned my bachelor's degree in Anthropology from the University of Colorado, Boulder. I was an intern in the Epidemiology Dept at ANTHC. I created fact sheets for data dissemination related to Alaska Native health disparities and outcomes, using the Behavioral Risk Factor Surveillance System. I also assisted in facilitating focus groups to develop the Getting Together safety card for Alaskan teens in both rural and urban settings. I received a MS in Public Health Nursing from the University of California at San Francisco (UCSF). At UCSF, I worked as a Research Assistant at Larkin Street Youth Services, and I helped develop an evidenced-based evaluation tool and collected data among HIV-positive homeless youth for an intervention that addressed substance use and mental illness.

My interest in public health nursing stemmed from a class I took in undergraduate studies on the intersection between race, class, gender. This sparked my interest in health intersectionality. I chose a career in public health because I am passionate about health literacy, and its role in primary prevention. I chose to work at Alaska Native Tribal Health Consortium (ANTHC) because I wanted to serve my people. As a nurse, I am in a position to improve health literacy among Alaska Native People; this empowers patients to be advocates for themselves or family members, which allows people to make informed and ethical decisions in critical situations. I moved back to Alaska and cared for critically ill patients in the ICU, at Alaska Native Medical Center.

When the pandemic hit, I was still able to work with my fellow Alaska Native People at ANTHC through my position at the CDC Foundation. Here I was able to do Program Management and Program/Team Development at ANMC Testing Site, and Contact Tracing. Each tribal community has specific COVID-19 restrictions. We have had to help community members navigate airline and regional restrictions, while testing them within a timeframe where they can get a negative result that allows them to go home. Resource availability was a variable that affected this greatly and was a great challenge. We were able to work with our lab to determine prioritization, so our patients could travel home safely.

Alaska Native People are experts at survival and have lived off the land for tens of thousands of years. We nurture and use the land, animals, plants, and weather to survive. Although colonization-related trauma has resulted in health problems among Alaska Native People, we are resilient. Despite adversity, we continue to live off the land, while participating in the global economy.

Tracy Frost, CMSRN

I am Yupik Eskimo, born and raised in rural Alaska where there isn't a hospital or doctors and nurses, but only a village clinic run by health aides. I marveled at their ability to help others who were in need of health care. I decided to become a nurse to help others in their health and wellness journey. I decided to work for ANTHC specifically because I want to help my fellow Alaskan Natives become the healthiest people in the world, which is ANTHC's vision. I also love ANTHC's mission statement: "Providing the highest quality health services in partnership with our people and the Alaska Tribal Health System." The Alaska Native people have so many strengths, most of which they are not fully aware. They are resilient and they love and respect the land. We gather and live off the land, and this in turn, keeps us a healthy people. Alaska has so many delicious and very nutritious wild foods and Alaska Natives use this valuable asset to great extent.

I graduated from nursing school in 2014. After becoming a registered nurse, I immediately came to work for ANTHC and have been employed here since. I am a certified medical surgical RN and worked mainly in the oncology and medical surgical inpatient unit. I also worked as a 'swat nurse' where I would assist in many of the other inpatient departments. I dabbled in school nursing for a few years with the Anchorage School District as a second job, which was a rewarding experience. In partnership with the CDC Foundation and ANTHC, I now help manage the Alaska Native Medical Center COVID Testing Site, because the need for widespread testing is imperative to mitigate or stop the pandemic.

Our testing site staff are an amazing group of healthcare providers who are willing to work through the elements in Alaska. The pandemic started in the middle of winter, so setting up testing sites while maintaining safety and social distancing was a challenge. We worked outdoors through subfreezing temperatures, high windstorms, and other inclement weather that our beautiful state has to offer. The rewarding part of this was to know that we were there for our patients, who were quite anxious because of the pandemic,

Continued

EVIDENCE-BASED PRACTICE BOX 1.2—cont'd

Nurses Taking Care Into Their Community: Covid-19 Testing Among the Resilient Alaskan Native People

and despite these challenges, we helped stop the spread of COVID-19 through widespread testing. Being there to lend them a helping hand, sharing an encouraging word, or giving a smile beneath your mask is important to public health, because mental well-being plays a role in optimal health.

Elizabeth Arteaga, DNP, RN

It was always a dream of mine to work for the Native community. My father's family is from the Yukon-Kuskokwim Delta region of Alaska, and he helped build the Native hospital. He would continually express gratitude and yearning to give back to the community.

I decided to become a nurse, and first earned an ADN in 2008. Three years later, I graduated with a BSN from Jacksonville State University. In 2019 I earned an MSN and then graduated in 2020 from Chatham University with my Doctor of Nursing Practice (DNP), with a focus on executive leadership and management. My nursing career began working as a Registered Nurse in a Progressive Care Unit, then Surgical Intensive Care Unit, and Post-Anesthesia Care Unit. Afterward, I worked as a travel nurse at various locations through the United States before seeking employment at ANTHC. I worked in the PACU and comprehensive pain management at ANTHC before the pandemic. I began working as the Director of COVID-19 Testing and Resulting Operations in April of 2020.

In remote Alaskan village settings, prevention is absolutely imperative because resources—including health care—are limited. As news of the pandemic swept across the globe, I could only envision the impact the virus would have on the vulnerable population of the Alaska Native communities. I had a fortunate opportunity to work with a phenomenal team to build the COVID-19 Testing and Resulting department where our focus was just that – to offer widespread testing to identify positive cases to mitigate community spread.

Early in the pandemic, we quickly outlined priorities and how best to use the resources we had available. We set up operations quickly, but the volume was not as high as we had expected. We learned we needed to bring these testing opportunities to those who needed it most. We planned and initiated Mobile Testing Units and brought testing to many different Native corporations, businesses, and congregate settings such as homeless shelters, etc. We will continuously grow and adapt to meet the needs of this resilient population we serve. We continually focus on adapting what we do to meet the needs of our people.

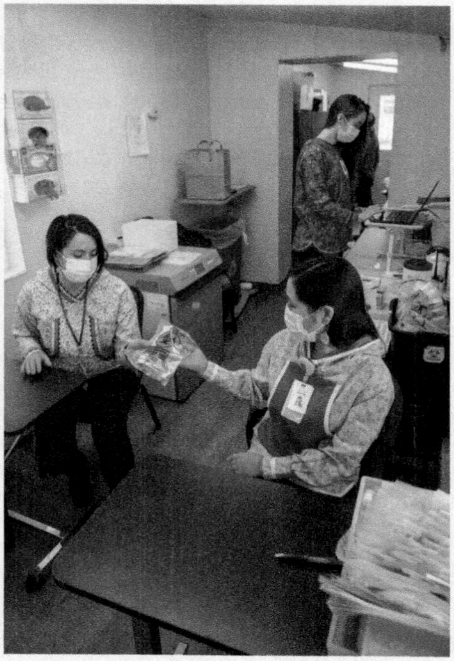

Elizabeth Aarons, RN, MS; Tracy Frost, CMSRN; Elizabeth Arteaga, DNP, RN

Tribal Nation Testing and Resulting Statewide Services Director and Coordinators

Alaska Native Tribal Health Consortium

Acknowledgment: The CDC Foundation is an independent nonprofit organization created by the U.S. Congress to mobilize philanthropic and private-sector resources in support of the work of the Centers for Disease Control and Prevention to protect the health, safety and security of the United States and the world. The CDC Foundation featured the work of Nurses Aarons, Frost, and Arteaga on the foundation website, aptly describing them as battling "COVID and the elements" in their work to mitigate the spread of COVID in Native Alaska communities. I am grateful for the CDC Foundation's public recognition of the work of these nurses and other nurses who became part of the massive-scale efforts to "crush COVID." I encourage students and faculty to take a long look at the CDC Foundation's website www.cdcfoundation.org; you will be both inspired and humbled by the incredible work your nurse colleagues and other healthcare providers have done and are continuing to do. –BPB

Courtesy Elizabeth Aarons, MS, RN; Tracy Frost, CMSRN; Elizabeth Arteaga, DNP, RN; CDC Foundation

practice consists of the integration of findings from research studies, clinician expertise and patient preference. The work of the ANTHC nurses is a good example of how expertise and patient preference, in addition to the research used to create and test vaccines to prevent or mitigate COVID-19, makes for a powerful way to get health care to the where communities need it most. You will learn in Chapter 2 that the ANTHC nurses follow in the footsteps of important pioneers in public health nursing such as Lillian Wald and Jessie Sleet Scales, who were instrumental in identifying problems and improving health in their communities in New York City over a century ago.

Public health nurses may work for either the government or private agencies. Those working for public health departments provide care in clinics, schools, retirement communities, and other community settings. They focus on improving the overall health of communities by planning and implementing health programs, as well as delivering care for individuals with chronic health problems. Public health nurses provide educational programs in health maintenance, disease prevention, nutrition, and child care, among others. They conduct immunization clinics and health screenings and work with teachers, parents, physicians, and community leaders toward a healthier community.

Many health departments also have a home health component. Over the past several decades an increasing number of public and private agencies provides home health services, a form of community health nursing. In fact, home health care is a growing segment of the healthcare industry.

Home health care is a natural fit for nurses. Home health nurses across the United States provide quality care in the most cost-effective and, for patients, most comfortable setting possible. Patients cared for at home may face significant health challenges from significant chronic illnesses requiring management or early hospital discharges in efforts to control costs. As a result, technological devices such as ventilators and intravenous pumps, and significant interventions such as administration of chemotherapy and total parenteral nutrition are encountered in home health care. Wound care is another domain of home health nursing. Wounds managed in the patient's home can be extensive, and home health nurses who provide wound care can assess the patient's home environment for factors that help or hinder healing.

Home health nurses must possess up-to-date nursing knowledge and be secure in their own nursing skills because, unlike in an in-patient setting, they may not have the expertise of more experienced nurses quickly available. Strong assessment and communication skills are essential in home health nursing, and effective home health nurses recognize the importance of respect for person's cultural and social practices in the home that may differ from their own. These nurses must make independent judgments and be able to recognize patients' and families' learning needs. Home health nurses must also recognize the limits of their education and experience and seek help when the patient's needs are beyond the scope of their abilities. An RN working in home health care relates her experience:

> *I have always found home care to be very rewarding. I get to know patients in a way I could never have if I had continued to work in a hospital. One of my favorite success stories involved a man in his late 30's with a long history of osteomyelitis—an infection in the bone—resulting from a car wreck 18 years earlier. He had a new central line and was going to receive three types of antibiotics for six months. If this treatment didn't work, he would require an above-the-knee amputation. I taught his wife how to assess the central line dressing and site, how to change the dressing, and how to do the infusions twice per day. I noted on my initial visit that the patient was obese with a BMI of 38, and he smoked at least one pack of cigarettes each day. At my once-a-week visits to draw blood, I got to know the patient and his wife well and began to feel comfortable that I could talk to him about his weight and smoking and how they both can interfere with healing. He lost 80 pounds, quit smoking completely, and at the end of six months, he had no signs of infection. He described himself as "a new man." I was so happy for him and his wife. Holistic nursing care in his own home made a huge difference for the rest of his life.*

In your clinical rotations in nursing school, you might encounter nurses who are ANCC-certified as community health or home health nurses. The examinations for these two specialties have now been retired, but previously certified nurses can have their credentials renewed. The demand for nurses to work in a variety of community settings is expected to continue to increase as care moves from hospitals to homes and other community sites.

Nursing in Medical Offices

Nurses who are employed in medical office settings work in collaboration with physicians, NPs, and their patients. Office-based nursing activities include performing health assessments, reviewing medications, drawing blood, giving immunizations, administering medications, and providing health teaching. Nurses in office settings also act as liaisons between patients and physicians or NPs. They expand on and clarify recommendations for patients, as well as provide emotional support to anxious patients. They may visit hospitalized patients, and some assist in surgery. Often, RNs in office practices supervise other care providers, such as licensed practical/vocational nurses, nurse aides, and, depending on the size of the practice, other employees of the practice such as assistants who schedule patient appointments and manage patient records.

An RN who works for a nephrology practice with three nephrologists describes a typical day:

> *I first make rounds independently on patients in the dialysis center, making sure they are tolerating the dialysis procedure and answering questions about their treatments and diets. I then make rounds with one of the physicians in the hospital as she visits patients and prescribes new treatments. The afternoon is spent in the office assessing patients when they come for their physician's visit. I might draw blood for a diagnostic test on one patient and do patient teaching regarding diet with another. No two days are alike, and that is what I love about this position. I have a sense of independence but still have daily patient contact.*

RNs considering employment in office settings need good communication skills because many of their responsibilities involve communicating with patients, families, employers, pharmacists, and hospital admissions offices. Nurses should be careful to ask prospective employers the specifics of the position because nursing roles in office practices can range from routine tasks to challenging responsibilities requiring expertise in a particular practice setting, such as that described by the nurse in the nephrology practice. Educational requirements, hours of work, and specific responsibilities vary, depending on the preferences of the employer. Some nurses find a predictable daily schedule with weekends and holidays off to be an advantage in working in an office practice. An important advantage of employment in an office setting is that over time, nurses get to know their patients well, including several members of a family, depending on the type of practice.

Nursing in the Workplace

Many companies today employ **occupational and environmental health nurses** to provide health and safety education, including the prevention of injury, basic healthcare services, screenings, and emergency treatment to employees in the workplace. Corporate executives have long known that good employee health reduces absenteeism, insurance costs, and worker errors, thereby improving company profitability. Occupational health nurses (OHNs) represent an important investment by companies in the health and safety of their employees. They are often asked to serve as consultants on health matters within the company. OHNs may participate in health-related decisions, such as policies affecting health insurance benefits, family leaves, and acquisition and placement of automatic external defibrillators. Depending on the size of the company, the OHN may be the only health professional employed in a company and therefore may have a good deal of autonomy.

Being licensed is generally the minimum requirement for nurses in occupational health roles. The American Association of Occupational Health Nurses (AAOHN) recommends that OHNs have a bachelor's degree. OHNs must possess knowledge and skills that enable them to perform routine physical assessments (e.g., vision and hearing screenings), first aid and basic life support. Good interpersonal skills to provide counseling and referrals for lifestyle problems, such as stress or substance abuse, are needed in this setting, as is the ability to do counseling and crisis intervention for employees. OHNs also need to know laws and regulations related to health and safety in their setting, such as those of the Occupational Safety and Health Administration (OSHA), and to understand how to maintain legal and regulatory compliance. If employed in a heavy industrial setting where the risk of burns or trauma is present, OHNs must have special training to manage those types of medical emergencies.

OHNs also have responsibilities for identifying health risks in the entire work environment. They must be able to assess the environment for potential safety hazards and work with management to eliminate or reduce them. They may instruct new workers in the effective use of protective devices such as safety glasses and noise-canceling earphones. OHNs also understand workers' compensation regulations and coordinate the care of injured workers with the facilities and providers who provide care for an employee with a work-related injury. Some injuries may be life threatening; others may be chronic but clearly related to work, such as musculoskeletal injuries from repetitive motion or poorly designed workspaces. Recently OHN, like many nurses, faced significant issues related to the COVID-19 pandemic in doing testing, contact tracing, implementing safe distancing, masking regulations and vaccine requirements of the company, in addition to assisting employees in dealing with disinformation and confusion about the virus and its spread, vaccinations and vaccine hesitancy, and recognizing the onset of symptoms of COVID in employees.

Nurses in occupational settings have to be confident in their nursing skills, effective communicators with both employees and managers, able to motivate employees to adopt healthier habits, and be able to function independently in providing care. The AAOHN is the professional organization for OHNs. The AAOHN provides conferences, webcasts, a newsletter, a journal, and other resources to help OHNs stay up-to-date (website: www.aaohn.org). Certification for OHNs is available through the American Board for Occupational Health Nurses (ABOHN), and experienced nurses may take the more advanced specialist OHN certification exam.

Nursing in the Armed Services

Nurses practice in both peacetime and wartime settings in the armed services. Nurses serving in the military ("military nurses") may serve on active duty or in military reserve units, which means that they will be called to duty in the case of an emergency. They serve as staff nurses and supervisors in all major medical specialties. Both general and advanced practice opportunities are available in military nursing, and the settings in which these nurses practice use state-of-the-art technology.

Military nurses often find themselves with broader responsibilities and scope of practice than do civilian nurses because of the demands of nursing in the field, on aircraft, or onboard ship. Previous critical care, surgery, or trauma care experience is desirable but not required. Military nurses are required to have a BSN degree for active duty. They enter active duty as officers and must be between the ages of 21 and 46½ years when they begin active duty. Professional Profile Box 1.1 is a profile of the work of Lt. Joseph Biddix, NC, USN, whose work as a Navy nurse has given him a wide variety of experiences and opportunities in his development as an RN.

A major benefit of military nursing is the opportunity for advanced education. Military nurses are encouraged to seek advanced degrees, and support is provided during schooling. The U.S. Department of Defense pays for tuition, books, moving expenses, and even salary for nurses obtaining advanced degrees. This allows students to focus on their studies. Nurses with advanced degrees are eligible for promotion in rank at an accelerated pace.

Travel and change are integral to military nursing, so these nurses must be flexible. Military nurses in the reserves must be committed to readiness; they must be ready to go at a moment's notice. All military nurses may be called on for active wartime duty anywhere in the world.

In 2011 Lieutenant General (Lt. Gen.) Patricia Horoho was nominated and confirmed to become the Army Surgeon General, the first nurse and the first woman to serve in this capacity. Horoho had previously commanded the Walter Reed Health Care System and was serving in the Pentagon on September 11, 2001, where she cared for wounded persons after terrorists crashed a plane into the building. Lt. Gen. Horoho is an experienced clinical trauma nurse (Brewin, 2011).

Nursing in Schools

School nursing is an interesting, specialized practice of professional nursing, and is a specific role for public/community health nurses. The National Association of School Nurses (NASN) defines school nursing as "a specialized practice of nursing [that] protects and promotes student health, facilitates optimal development, and advances academic success. School nurses, grounded in ethical and evidence-based practice, are the leaders who bridge health care and education, provide care coordination, advocate for quality student-centered care, and collaborate to design systems that allow individuals and communities to develop their full potential" (NASN, 2021). To that end, school nurses facilitate positive student responses to normal development; promote health and safety, including a healthy environment; intervene with

PROFESSIONAL PROFILE BOX 1.1

Military Nurse

My nursing path was untraditional. I graduated from college in 2005 with an Arts degree in Media Studies and Production and immediately began an internship with the entertainment industry in Los Angeles. I eventually worked for a top talent management firm, yet after 4 successful years in the business, something was missing. I kept asking myself, "Why doesn't this feel more rewarding?"

I began exploring other options in search of professional gratification, and the idea of military service kept popping into my head. I questioned what the military would do with a film major whose only job experience was working in Hollywood. While deciding options, a close friend told me that he was planning to return to school for a second-degree nursing program. It didn't sound like a bad idea and this would be a perfect career for the military. My internal wheels were spinning, so I called my mom for advice about what I should do, because she was a nurse of 30 years. She said, "I've always thought you would make an excellent nurse, but I never wanted to push it. I figured I would let you find your path on your own."

That was all the encouragement I needed. Once accepted into a nursing program, I contacted the local Navy recruiter. After a rigorous application process, I was accepted into a program to become a Nurse Corps Officer, and on graduation, I was commissioned as an ensign in the United States Navy.

Nearly 9 years later, I have found military nursing to be a phenomenal experience. I have the opportunity to provide nursing care to active duty and retired service members and their families. I also deployed aboard the USNS Comfort (T-AH 20) for six months in 2015 providing humanitarian assistance alongside partner nation and civilian experts to patients in 11 countries in Central and South America and the Caribbean.

One of the primary responsibilities of Navy nurses is training our hospital corpsmen who regularly care for our forward deployed sailors and marines. These young men and women carry a heavy responsibility to provide first responder care to our warfighters. As a Navy nurse, I have a direct role in mentoring them. There is no greater reward than training newly enlisted corpsmen and seeing their faces light up when they "get it." Whether we're discussing the physiology of hypertension or how to treat for shock after a blast injury, you know when the light bulb turns on and the sailor has added another layer to their knowledge base.

Military nursing also requires flexibility and the ability to adapt to new situations quickly. COVID-19 has tested the durability of the global healthcare system, and military nurses and medical professionals have answered the call to aid in the fight against this pandemic. I would guess that many active duty nurses never thought they would deploy *within* the United States, but when state and local health systems declared states of emergency, military medicine answered the call. Active duty and reserve medical professionals from all branches and disciplines including providers, nurses, corpsmen and medics have deployed nationwide to support the COVID-19 response and our national vaccination drive. As a Navy nurse, you have to be prepared, whether it is to deploy abroad to provide medical to support to warfighters, provide needed humanitarian assistance to a region hit by a natural disaster, or shore up the capabilities of our fellow Americans whose health systems have been strained by a pandemic. While the nature of the need is ever changing, Navy nurses will always answer the call.

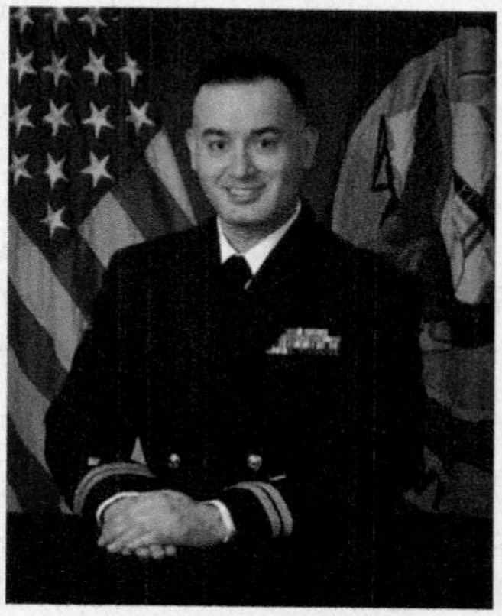

Lt. Joseph Biddix, NC, USN
Navy Medicine Readiness & Training Command – Bethesda

Note: The views expressed in this article are those of the author and do not necessarily reflect the official policy or position of the Department of the Navy, the Department of Defense, or the United States government.
Courtesy Lt. Joseph Biddix

actual and potential health problems; provide case management services; and actively collaborate with others to build student and family capacity for adaptation, self-management, self-advocacy, and learning.

During the COVID-19 pandemic, school nurses face significant challenges in maintaining the safety of children in school. Routinely, school nurses evaluate students for COVID symptoms or possible exposures. Moreover, they provide guidance to school administrators and teachers on prevention strategies, contact tracing, school-based testing strategies, and assist in the support of students, families and school staff as they face their own challenges related to the pandemic and its accompanying concerns, anxieties and losses. The CDC provided guidance to school nurses in addressing the wide variety of challenges they faced during the uncertainty and frequently changing recommendations based on a quickly evolving science related to the virus and its transmission.

School nurses are in short supply. Very few states achieve the federally recommended ratio of 1:750 (a recommended minimum number of 1 school nurse for every 750 students). In 2016 only 8 states had set a nurse-to-student ratio; however, these ratios were not necessarily consistent with the guidelines set by the CDC and NASN. For instance, Pennsylvania's ratio was set at 1 nurse per 1500 students, twice the prescribed ratio (Camera, 2016). This poses a serious problem for children with disabilities, for those with chronic illnesses in need of occasional management at school, and for children who become ill or are injured at school. With higher than recommended ratios of students per RN, children may lack the substantial health benefits of having a school nurse available to them during the school day. In a position statement revised in 2020, NASN stated, "All students need access to a school nurse every day" (NASN, 2020).

School nursing has the potential to be a significant source of communities' health care. In medically underserved areas and with the number of uninsured families increasing, the role of school nurse is sometimes expanded to include members of the student's immediate family. This requires many more school nurses, requiring willingness of state and local school boards to hire them. Without adequate qualified staffing, the nation's children cannot receive the full benefits of school nurse programs.

Most school systems require nurses to have a minimum of a bachelor's degree in nursing, whereas some school districts have higher educational requirements. Prior experience working with children is also usually required. School health has become a specialty in its own right, and in states where school health is a priority, graduate programs in school health nursing have been established. The National Board for Certification of School Nurses (NBCSN) is the official certifying body for school nurses.

School nurses need a working knowledge of human growth and development to detect developmental problems early and refer children to appropriate therapists. Counseling skills are important because many students turn to the school nurse as a counselor. School nurses keep records of children's required immunizations and are responsible for ensuring that immunizations are current. When an outbreak of a childhood communicable illness occurs, school nurses educate parents, teachers, and students about treatment and prevention of transmission. For children with special needs, school nurses must work closely with families, teachers, and the students' primary providers to care for these children while at school—and these needs can be significant. Management of the health of children with diabetes and serious allergies is important in the daily life of school nurses.

School nurses also work with teachers to incorporate health concepts into the curriculum. They endorse the teaching of basic health practices, such as handwashing and caring for teeth. School nurses encourage the inclusion of age-appropriate nutritional information in school curricula and work with children to make healthful food choices in the cafeteria and when choosing snacks. They conduct vision and hearing screenings and make referrals to physicians or other healthcare providers when routine screenings identify problems outside the nurses' scopes of practice.

School nurses must be prepared to handle both routine illnesses of children and adolescents and emergencies. One of their major concerns is safety. Accidents are a leading cause of death in children of all ages, yet some accidents are preventable. Prevention includes both protection from obvious hazards and education of teachers, parents, and students about how to avoid accidents. School nurses work with teachers, school bus drivers, cafeteria workers, and other school employees to provide the safest possible environment. When accidents occur, first aid for minor injuries and emergency care for more severe ones are additional skills school nurses use (Fig. 1.3). Detection of evidence of child neglect and abuse is a sensitive but essential aspect of school nursing. School violence or bullying can also result in injury, absenteeism, and anxiety. In the wake of school violence involving guns and the possibility of experiencing

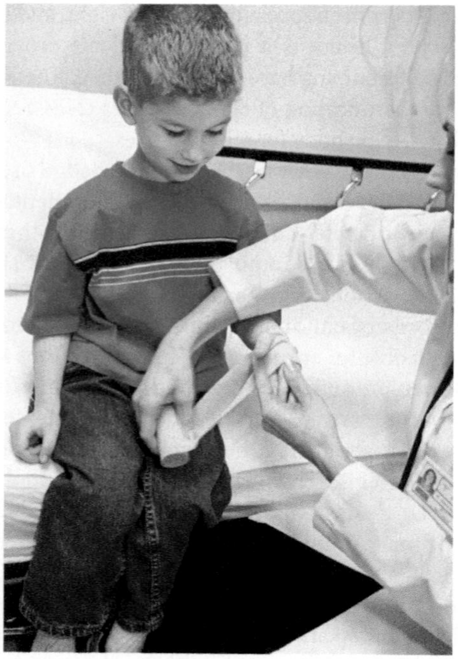

Fig. 1.3 School nurses manage a variety of students' health problems, from playground injuries to chronic illnesses such as asthma and diabetes. (Photo used with permission from iStockphoto.)

a natural disaster, the NASN has made disaster preparedness a priority.

The mission of NASN is "advancing school nurse practice to keep students healthy, safe, and ready to learn" (www.nasn.org). This underscores their commitment to both the health and education of schoolchildren across the United States. The NASN 2013-2014 annual report noted that sensitivity to the cultural needs of students is important in assisting with a child's health and to that end created a section on their website focusing on cultural competence (NASN, 2014). The 2019-2020 Annual Report was notable for its announcement on page 4—just after the introduction to the document—of its position brief "Eliminate Racism to Optimize Student Health and Learning," their unequivocal position being that "systematic racism must be eliminated from the United States" (NASN, 2020).

Nursing in Palliative Care and Hospice Settings

Palliative care and hospice nursing is a nursing specialty dedicated to improving the quality of life of patients who are seriously or terminally ill and their families. The World Health Organization (WHO) defines *palliative care* as "an approach that improves the quality of life of patients (adults and children) and their families facing the problem associated with life-threatening illness. It prevents and relieves suffering through the early identification, correct assessment and treatment of pain and other problems, whether physical, psychosocial or spiritual" (WHO, 2020). Hospice care is "the model for quality, compassionate care at the end-of-life, hospice involves a team-oriented approach to expert medical care, pain management, and emotional and spiritual support expressly tailored to the patient's needs and wishes. Support is extended to the patient's loved ones, as well" (National Hospice and Palliative Care Organization, 2021).

In 1986 the Hospice and Palliative Nurses Association (HPNA) was established, and it is now the largest and oldest professional nursing organization dedicated to the practice of palliative care and end-of-life care. The HPNA journal, *JHPN—Journal of Hospice and Palliative Nursing*, is a peer-reviewed publication promoting excellence in palliative and end-of-life care, is published six times each year, and can be followed on Twitter at @JHPN_online. HPNA's website is https://advancingexpertcare.org/ and can be followed on Twitter at @HPNAinfo. In addition to HPNA, two other organizations are central to supporting this domain of nursing: the Hospice and Palliative Nurses Foundation (HPNF) and the Hospice and Palliative Credentialing Center (HPCC). In 2014, HPNA, HPNF, and HPCC adopted shared mission and vision statements, in addition to pillars of excellence held in common. The shared mission is "to advance expert care in serious illness" and the shared vision is "to transform the care and culture of serious illness." The pillars of excellence on which these organizations base their work are education, competence, advocacy, leadership, and research (HPNA, 2021).

Because nursing curricula traditionally have not included extensive content to prepare nurses to deal effectively with dying patients and their families, the AACN developed *CARES: Competencies and Recommendations for Educating Undergraduate Nursing Students Preparing Nurses to Care for the Seriously Ill and Their Families.* This document provides palliative care competencies for undergraduate nursing students and may be viewed online at http://www.aacnnursing.org/Portals/42/ELNEC/PDF/New-Palliative-Care-Competencies.pdf.

In 2000, the End-of-Life Nursing Education Consortium (ELNEC) was funded by the Robert Wood Johnson Foundation, and it has since received additional funding by a variety of organizations. The foundation for the ELNEC project reflects the core areas identified by the AACN in the *CARES* document. In 2020 the AACN announced 39.915 individuals had participated in the ELNEC train-the-trainer course, and in turn, these trainers had provided state-of-the-art palliative care education to 1,256,000 nurses and other professionals worldwide (AACN, 2020). Currently there are seven available curricula: core, pediatric palliative care, critical care, geriatric, advance practice registered nurse, international, and veterans (AACN, 2018). To expand the reach of *CARES* and ELNEC, AACN launched six interactive online modules for undergraduate students and new graduates. The online ELNEC modules had more than 200 schools and more than 7000 users enrolled in its first year. For more information see http://elnec.academy.reliaslearning.com.

Hospice and palliative care nurses work in a variety of settings, including inpatient palliative and hospice units, free-standing residential hospices, community-based or home hospice programs, ambulatory palliative care programs, teams of consultants in palliative care, and long-term care facilities. Both generalists and APNs work in palliative care. In Professional Profile Box 1.2 you will meet Lily Gillmor, RN, a nurse who works in a large community-based pediatric palliative care program, who describes her career path and passion for her work with children with serious illness and their families.

PROFESSIONAL PROFILE BOX 1.2

Pediatric Palliative Care Nurse

I graduated from college with a Bachelor of Arts in Psychology and a minor in Health Care Studies. Convinced I was destined for a career in public health, I immediately enrolled in a Master of Public Health (MPH) program. Almost as immediately, I realized I had made a terrible mistake: an MPH was not the right fit for me. A physician classmate also recognized this was not the right fit for me, and I decided to go to nursing school. A year and a half and a lot of prerequisites later, I enrolled in UNC at Chapel Hill's accelerated BSN program. And from day one, I knew I had found the right fit.

My first job after nursing school was in inpatient pediatrics, before hospitals had pediatric palliative care teams. One particular situation bothered me: the medical team proceeded with an organ transplant knowing the child would likely not survive, and there was no discussion with the family of the likelihood of a poor outcome. When I questioned why we were not discussing all options with the child's parents, I was told, "We don't want them to think we have given up. We need to give them hope." I was struck by this response and knew that I did not see an honest discussion with the family as giving up or taking away hope, and I worried perhaps nursing was not the right fit after all.

A few years later I was fortunate enough to fall into the world of hospice and palliative care. It was there that I realized nursing itself was not the problem, but that I just had not yet found my people! I was suddenly immersed in a world where honest conversations were the foundation of my work and walking with patients and families through these conversations was the expectation, not the exception. I learned the fundamentals of palliative care, focusing on managing the symptoms of a disease rather than the disease itself, providing discussions around goals of care and quality of life, and supporting patients and families through the complexities of serious illness. Having found my right fit I have continued in this field my entire career, and I currently work in a community-based organization that provides palliative and hospice services to both adults and children. Our organization is unique in that all pediatric services are provided by a dedicated pediatric program, which includes perinatal, palliative, hospice, and bereavement care to children and families.

I often get asked how and why I work in the field of pediatric palliative care; my answer is always "the kids and their families." *They* are the foundation of our work. Families of children with chronic or life-limiting illnesses, are, quite simply, rock stars. They are immersed in a world of juggling, balancing, and coordinating provider appointments, supplies, medications, schooling, nursing, and more, while also trying to work full time jobs and keep up with the regular household needs such as grocery shopping and paying bills. Their work requires an extraordinary amount of time, patience, planning, and a good sense of humor. Every family's journey is different, with a unique set of experiences throughout their child's illness. Having the privilege to witness these journeys, and support kids and families throughout is the how and why I work in the field of pediatric palliative care.

Continued

PROFESSIONAL PROFILE BOX 1.2—cont'd

Pediatric Palliative Care Nurse

The moment I tell someone I work in hospice and palliative care—specifically pediatrics—I can feel the air get sucked out of the room as silence descends, followed by the statement, "Wow. I don't know how you do that; it's just too sad for me." This has always been an intriguing statement to me, the implication being that because I work in this area, it is not sad for me. It is sad. The work we do is sad for every single team member. It is heavy work that challenges us daily. Children aren't supposed to get seriously ill and die so there is not a lot of discussion about it. Our team gives patients and families a safe place for their questions and concerns, often giving them the opportunity to discuss difficult things for the first time. Holding this space for families can be taxing, and an important part of our roles as pediatric palliative care specialists is to take time to care for ourselves. Our pediatric team builds self-care into daily practice, treating it with same importance as the care we provide our patients. The team is accountable to each other, and we have the support and resources necessary to keep the team healthy.

What people don't often think about with this work though is the happy: the chance to work with kids and families to make the most of whatever time there is, focusing on what is most meaningful and important to them. Just because a child has an illness does not mean they stop being a kid. There is a level of joy and fun that we get to see in our work that you don't get to see anywhere else. Visits with kids may include a serious discussion of goals of care, but they also may break into a nerf gun battle or splatter paint bonanza. We also get to witness a depth of love between a child and their family that cannot easily be described. No one gets to decide how much time they have on this earth, and for some, it may not be very long. As a palliative care nurse, I get to help people fill that time however they would like, focusing on what is important to them and their families and making the most out of it. There is no career more difficult, no career more rewarding, and no other career I can imagine having.

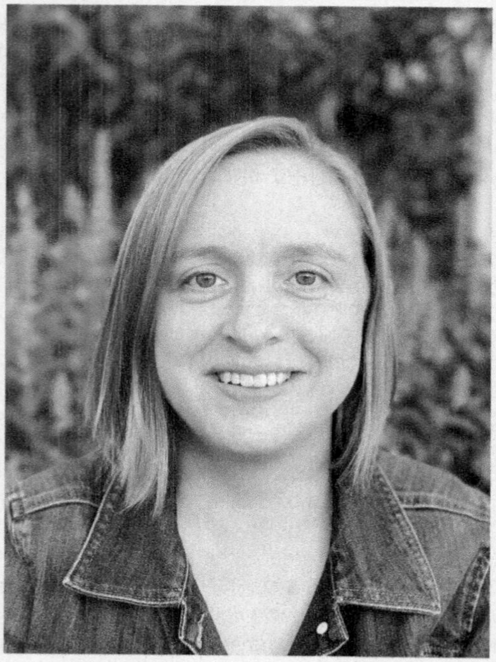

Lily Gillmor, RN
BSN, University of North Carolina at Chapel Hill, 2006

Courtesy Lily Gillmor, RN

Information Technologies in Nursing: Telehealth and Informatics

Telehealth is the delivery of healthcare services and related healthcare activities through telecommunication technologies. **Telehealth nursing** is not a separate nursing specialty, because few nurses use telehealth systems exclusively in their practices. Rather, it is most often found as a part of other nursing roles. Current technology includes bedside computers, interactive audio and video links, teleconferencing, real-time (synchronous) transmission of patients' diagnostic and clinical data, and more. The fastest growing applications of these technologies are phone triage, remote monitoring, and home care. Some aspects of patient health can be monitored from a distance via remote patient monitoring (RPM) and include physiologic data (e.g., blood pressure, blood glucose, oxygen levels) (healthit.gov, 2017). The use of telehealth devices expands access to health care for underserved populations and individuals in both urban and rural areas. Telehealth can also reduce the sense of professional isolation experienced by those who work in such areas and may assist in attracting and retaining healthcare professionals in remote areas.

Technologies available for telehealth nurses include remote access to laboratory reports and digitalized imaging; counseling patients on medications, diet, activity, or other therapy on mobile phones or by voice-over-Internet (VOI) protocol services; or participating in interactive video sessions, such as an interdisciplinary team consultation about a complex patient issue. Although the fundamentals of basic nursing practice do not change because of the nurse's use of telehealth technologies, their use may require adaptation or modification of usual procedures. In addition, telehealth nurses must develop competence in the use of each new type of telehealth technology, which changes rapidly.

Numerous legal and regulatory issues surround nursing care delivered through telehealth technologies; for instance, care of patients across state lines may require licensing in the state not only where the nurse is employed but also where the patients reside. You can learn more about telehealth, an area of growing interest in nursing and other health professions, as well as some controversy, from the American Telemedicine Association (www.americantelemed.org), and from the American Academy of Ambulatory Care Nursing (www.aaacn.org). A lesson from the COVID-19 pandemic is the burgeoning need for expertise in delivery of telehealth. In addition, access to telehealth services needs to be increased by widening the availability of broadband Internet across the U.S., so that persons in remote areas or those for whom in-person visits mean unacceptable risk for exposure to COVID can receive adequate health care from a distance.

Nursing informatics (NI) is a rapidly evolving specialty area defined by the Nursing Informatics Nursing Group as "the science and practice [integrating] nursing, its information and knowledge, with management of information and communication technologies to promote the health of people, families, and communities worldwide" (American Medical Informatics Association, 2021). Informatics nurses (also known as *nurse informaticians*) were well positioned to assist in the implementation of the 2009 American Recovery and Reinvestment Act and the Health Information Technology Act. This legislation contained federal incentives for the adoption of electronic health records (EHRs) with criteria known as meaningful use. To qualify for Centers for Medicare and Medicaid Services (CMS) incentive payments, healthcare organizations had to select, implement, enhance, and/or measure the impact of EHRs on patient care. Meaningful Use (MU) focused on the use of technology to improve patient outcomes through the engagement of patients and families, improved care coordination, and increased privacy and security of patient information. MU is now included as part of the Medicare Access and Chip Reauthorization Act, which focuses on merit-based incentives and the use of EHR technology for multiple purposes, including quality care (HealthIT.gov, 2017).

Because they are nurses themselves, nurse informaticians are best able to understand the needs of nurses who use the systems and can customize or design them with the needs, skills, and time constraints of those nurses in mind. In contrast to computer science systems analysts, nurse informaticians must clearly understand the information they handle and how other nurses will use it. According to the 2017 Healthcare Information and Management Systems Society Nursing Informatics Work Survey, nurses in this field were overall satisfied with their work. Their two main job responsibilities included systems implementation and utilization/optimization, suggesting that their role is imperative in the effective use of electronic medical and health records (EMR/EHR) (2017).

As healthcare organizations continue to adopt and implement EHRs, nurse informaticians will be in increasing demand. At a minimum, nurses specializing in informatics should have a BSN and additional knowledge and experience in the field of informatics. An increasing number of nurse informaticians have advanced degrees, including doctorates. Certification as an informatics nurse is available through the ANCC. The American Medical Informatics Association (AMIA; www.amia.org) and the Health Information and Management Systems Society (HIMSS; www.himss.org) sponsor the Alliance for Nursing Informatics (ANI), whose mission is to "advance nursing informatics practice, education, policy and research through a unified voice of nursing informatics organizations" (ANI, 2021). The ANI website is www.allianceni.org.

Nursing in a Faith Community

Interest in spirituality and how it is related to wellness and healing in recent years prompted the development of the rapidly growing practice specialty of faith community nursing (FCN), previously known as *parish nursing*. "FCN is a nursing practice specialty that focuses on the intentional care of the spirit, promotion of an integrative model of health, and prevention and minimization of illness within the context of a faith community" (ANA, 2017). FCN takes a holistic approach to healing that involves partnerships among congregations, their pastoral staffs, and healthcare providers. Since its development in the Chicago area in the 1980s by a hospital chaplain, Dr. Granger E. Westberg, FCN has spread rapidly and now includes more than 15,000 nurses in paid and volunteer positions in a variety of religious faiths, cultures, and countries.

The FCN reclaims the historical custom of health and healing found in many faith traditions. The spiritual dimension is central to FCN practice with a focus on the intentional care of the spirit while assisting individuals and faith-based communities to regain wholeness in body, mind, and spirit (Westberg Institute for Faith Community Nursing, 2018). FCNs are instrumental in connecting individuals disconnected from the healthcare system with preventative services and local healthcare resources, can clarify provider orders, and identify and recommend needed medical care (Schroepfer, 2016). Research with small FCN projects and partnerships demonstrates the benefits of the combined health and spiritual ministry; however, follow-up research that can more broadly address the impact of the FCN is needed (Schroepfer, 2016).

Since 1997 the ANA (2017) has recognized FCM as a specialty nursing practice within diverse faith communities. The Health Ministries Association Inc. and the ANA in their third edition of *Faith Community Nursing: Scope and Standards of Practice* collaboratively define six standards of practice for FCN and 11 standards of professional performance (ANA, 2017). Faith community nurses serve as members of the pastoral team in a faith community. The practice of FCN is governed by the nurse's state nurse practice act, *Nursing: Scopes and Standards of Practice* (ANA, 2015a), *Faith Community Nursing: Scope and Standards* (ANA, 2017), and the *Code of Ethics for Nurses with Interpretive Statements* (ANA, 2015b). FCNs work as health educators and counselors, advocates for health services, referral agents, and coordinators of volunteer health ministers. Faith community nurses often sponsor health screenings and facilitate support groups while integrating the concepts of health and spirituality.

Many FCNs work independently and benefit from networking with other FCNs. Throughout the U.S., many local and regional FCN organizations support FCN networking and collaboration, providing grant opportunities and even specialized training in the ministry of FCN practice. Nurses interested in FCN may pursue specialized training with a local or regional FCN organization. According to NurseJournal (2021), citing the U.S. Bureau of Labor Statistics, there is a growing job market for RNs at a projected 7%, increase between 2019 and 2029, which presumably should translate into similar growth for faith community nursing. The salary for FCNs tends to be somewhat lower than the median for RNs (NurseJournal, 2021).

NURSING OPPORTUNITIES REQUIRING ADVANCED DEGREES

Many RNs choose to pursue careers that require a master's degree, doctoral degree, or specialized education in a specific area. These roles include clinical nurse leaders, nurse managers, nurse executives in hospital settings, nurse educators (whether in clinical or academic settings), nurse anesthetists, nurse-midwives, clinical nurse specialists, and advanced practice nursing in a variety of settings. Some of these careers are described next.

Nurse Educators

Nurse educators teach across all levels of nursing education. Nurse educators in accredited schools of nursing offering a bachelor's or higher degree must hold a minimum of a master's degree in nursing. Nurse educators such as those teaching basic (prelicensure) nursing education typically have expertise in the clinical area in which they teach students and can be excellent mentors for nursing students. Being a nurse educator requires being highly organized, having good communication skills, possess the ability to help learners feel comfortable in clinical settings, and having the ability to evaluate student performance fairly. A primary responsibility of nurse educators in clinical settings is to maintain safety for both students and patients, a significant aspect of the role. For this reason, state boards of nursing set firm limits on the ratio of faculty to prelicensure students in clinical settings.

In September 2021, the AACN released a survey indicating a vacancy rate for faculty positions at 8%, up from 6.5% in 2020. Additionally, the survey showed that U.S. schools of nursing turned away more than 80,000 qualified applicants, generally because of the lack of adequate numbers of faculty. At a time when demand for nurses continues to grow, the lack of adequate numbers of nursing faculty limits the number of new nurses entering the workforce (NC Health News, 2021). In response, several states have implemented initiatives to improve salaries of nurse educators, usually in the form of tax credits for clinical preceptors, in order to improve the bottleneck that occurs in the nursing workforce due to inadequate numbers of educators (campaignforaction.org, 2018). Preceptors are clinicians working on-site who provide clinical education. Concerns about a critical shortage of nursing faculty in the future continue.

Clinical Nurse Leaders

The credential clinical nurse leader (CNL) is a designation intended to give master's-prepared nurses opportunity to oversee and manage care at the point of care in various settings, with the goal of improving patient outcomes. CNLs are clinical experts who focus on several aspects of patient care. The AACN (2021) notes seven key elements of the CNL's clinical focus: case coordination, outcomes measurement, transitions of care, interprofessional communication and team leadership, risk assessment, implementation of best practices based on evidence, and quality improvement.

The role of CNL was not without controversy and objections from Clinical Nurse Specialists (CNSs), advanced practice nurses (APNs) who see the CNL role as duplicating and potentially disenfranchising CNSs. Currently, the AACN lists 155 schools offering CNL programs (AACN, 2021).

Advanced Practice Nursing

Advanced practice nurse is a general term applied to an RN who has met educational and clinical practice requirements beyond the 2 to 4 years of basic nursing education required of all RNs. Advanced practice nursing has grown since it evolved more than 40 years ago. The U.S. Bureau of Labor Statistics reported that 271,900 APNs work in advanced practice roles in 2020, and the projected demand for these roles will increase 45% by 2030 (U.S. Bureau of Labor, 2021). Heightened demand for efficient and cost-effective treatment mean that advanced practice poses excellent career opportunities for nurses.

The implementation of the Affordable Care Act (ACA) stimulated even greater interest and growth in the numbers of APNs. In a discussion paper containing a comprehensive review of pertinent literature, and updated four times since its original publication in 2007, the American Association of Nurse Practitioners (2020) found that NPs provide safe, effective, patient centered, efficient, equitable and evidenced based care, comparable in quality to that of physician colleagues, and that under the care of NPs, patients have fewer unnecessary hospital readmissions, fewer potentially preventable hospitalizations, higher patient satisfaction and fewer unnecessary emergency room visits than patients under the care of physicians.

There are four categories of APNs: nurse practitioner, clinical nurse specialist, certified nurse-midwife, and certified registered nurse anesthetist. The following section provides a short overview of each of these roles.

Nurse Practitioner

Opportunities for nurses in expanded roles in health care have created a demand in nurse practitioner (NP) education. These programs grant master's degrees or postmaster's certificates and prepare nurses to sit for national certification examinations as NPs. The length of the programs varies, depending on the student's prior education. Programs of study leading to the doctor of nursing practice (DNP) degree have been implemented in schools of nursing across the country in response to the AACN member institution's endorsement of a clinical doctorate for advanced practice. The DNP is consistent with other health professions that offer practice doctorates, including medicine (MD), dentistry (DDS), pharmacy (PharmD), physical therapy (DPT), and psychology (PsyD), among others. As of the end of 2020, 357 DNP programs were actively enrolling students across all 50 states, and another 136 programs in the planning stages, which demonstrates the rapid growth of this degree path (AACN, 2020).

States vary in the level of practice autonomy accorded to NPs. NPs beginning practice in a new state should check the status of the advanced practice laws in that state before making firm commitments, because some states still place limitations on NP independence. The scope of practice across states can vary, which has implications for practice opportunities, and reimbursement (payor) policies may be linked to state practice regulations.

NPs work in clinics, nursing homes, their own offices, or physicians' offices. Others work for hospitals, health maintenance organizations, or private industry. Most NPs choose a specialty area such as adult–gerontology, psychiatric–mental health, family, or pediatric care. They are qualified to handle a wide range of health problems in primary or acute care settings. Nurse practitioners can perform physical examinations, take medical histories, diagnose and treat common acute and chronic illnesses and injuries, order and interpret laboratory tests and x-ray films, and counsel and educate patients. Despite the restrictions on practice in some states, in other states NPs are independent practitioners with full prescriptive authority and can be directly reimbursed by Medicare, Medicaid, and military and private insurers for their work.

During the COVID-19 pandemic, the need for an all-hands-on-deck approach to the delivery of prompt, safe health care was unprecedented, thus presumably opening the doors for nurse practitioners for more unrestricted practice. In a national survey to which almost 7500 APNs responded (86.8% of which were nurse practitioners), researchers found that despite the acute need for health care across the U.S., 84.8% of APN respondents identified that practice restrictions posed barriers to their ability to provide care during the pandemic (Kleinpell, Myers, Schorn & Likes, 2021).

The American Association of Nurse Practitioners is the professional organization for NPs. If you would like more information about the NP role, their website is www.aanp.org.

Clinical Nurse Specialist

Clinical nurse specialists (CNSs) are APNs who work in a variety of settings, including hospitals, clinics, nursing homes, their own offices, industry, home care, and health maintenance organizations. These nurses hold master's or doctoral degrees and are qualified to handle a wide range of physical and mental health problems. They are experts in a particular field of clinical practice, such as mental health, gerontology, cardiac care, cancer care, community health, or neonatal health, and they perform health assessments, make diagnoses, deliver treatment, and develop quality control methods. In addition, CNSs work in consultation, research, education, and administration. Direct reimbursement to some CNSs is possible through Medicare, Medicaid, and military and private insurers.

The National Association of Clinical Nurse Specialists (NACNS) is the professional organization for CNSs. If you are interested in additional information about the CNS role, the NACNS website is www.nacns.org.

Certified Nurse-Midwife

Certified nurse-midwives (CNMs) provide well-woman care and attend or assist in childbirth in various settings, including hospitals, birthing centers, private practice, and home birthing services. By 2010 all CNM training programs were required to award a Master of Science in Nursing (MSN) degree. CNM programs require an average of 1.5 years of specialized education beyond basic nursing education and must be accredited by the Accreditation Commission for Midwifery Education (ACME).

CNMs are licensed, independent healthcare providers who can prescribe medications in all 50 states, the District of Columbia, and most U.S. territories. Federal law designates CNMs as primary care providers. More than half of CNMs identify reproductive care as their main responsibility rather than attending births. According to the CDC, CNMs attended 387,297 births in 2018, representing 9.4% of the total births in the United States in 2018 (CDC, 2019). Historically, births attended by CNMs have had half the national average rates for cesarean sections and higher rates of successful vaginal births after a previous cesarean, both considered measures of high-quality obstetric care. The American College of Nurse-Midwives (ACNM) is the professional organization representing CNMs and certified midwives (CMs) and sets education and practice standards. If you are interested in additional information about the profession, the ACNM website is www.midwife.org. Karen Sheffield-Abdullah, PhD, CNM is an experienced CNM and describes her work in Professional Profile Box 1.3.

Certified Registered Nurse Anesthetist

In 2021, there were approximately 66,300 certified registered nurse anesthetists (CRNAs) and CRNA students in the United States, 89% of whom were members of the American Association of Nurse Anesthetists (AANA), the professional organization for CRNAs (AANA, 2021). Nurse anesthetists administer more than 50 million anesthetics each year and are the only anesthesia providers in more than 80% of U.S. counties (AANA, 2021). Collaborating with physician anesthesiologists or working independently, CRNAs are found in a variety of settings, including operating suites; obstetric delivery rooms; the offices of dentists, podiatrists, ophthalmologists, and plastic surgeons; ambulatory surgical facilities; and military and governmental health services (AANA, 2021).

To become a CRNA, nurses must complete 2 to 3 years of specialized education beyond the required

PROFESSIONAL PROFILE BOX 1.3

Certified Nurse-Midwife

Being a nurse-midwife is at the core of who I am, not just what I do. I decided to become a nurse-midwife after working as a chemist for many years and recognizing that my true passion resided in all aspects of women's health care. After the birth of two of my children, one by a physician and one by a nurse-midwife, I realized that I was "called" to the profession of nurse-midwifery and the philosophy of care that nurse-midwives provide. Providing comprehensive, holistic wellness care to women across their life span is one of the most rewarding and inspirational aspects of my profession. I feel privileged and honored to share in the important and often life-changing decisions that women make during the many transitions between puberty and menopause and beyond.

I have a Bachelor of Arts in physics from Connecticut College, an MSN from Yale University in 2005 with a specialty in nurse-midwifery, and a PhD in Nursing from the UNC at Chapel Hill School of Nursing. Additionally, I am certified in nurse-midwifery by the American Midwifery Certification Board (AMCB). Certification by the AMCB is the gold standard in midwifery and is recognized in all 50 states. As a nurse-midwife, I must also complete the requirements of the Certification Maintenance Program through AMCB by completing continuing education units every 5-year certification cycle. Maintaining competence in evidence-based, up-to-date management and treatment for women's health is critical to being an effective clinician.

Although the professional work environment for nurse-midwives varies, a typical day as a nurse-midwife with a full scope of practice involves providing gynecologic, antepartum, intrapartum, and postpartum care, including hospital rounds on women who have given birth and seeing patients in the office. Evidence-based care in the office setting includes contraceptive management, family planning, primary care, gynecologic care, and sick visits, among others. In addition to gynecologic care, nurse-midwives provide obstetric care that is grounded in our belief that childbirth is a normal, healthy human event. We are, however, educated in how and when to collaborate with physician colleagues for emergent care that necessitates a physician's specific expertise.

I strongly believe that my role as a nurse-midwife is to be "with a woman" and to honor her journey toward health and wellness and respecting her wishes for her birth within the limits of safety. When I reflect on my journey as a nurse-midwife over the past decade, I know that I am truly carrying out my purpose in providing holistic women's health care to the highest standard of excellence.

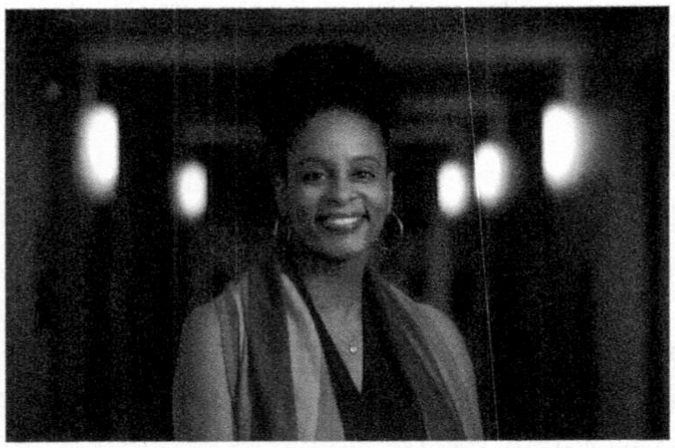

Karen Sheffield-Abdullah, PhD, RN CNM
PhD, University of North Carolina at Chapel Hill, 2019

Courtesy Karen Sheffield-Abdullah, PhD, RN, CNM

bachelor's degree; in mid-2021, 128 nurse anesthesia programs operated in the U.S. and Puerto Rico, and 113 programs are approved to award doctoral degrees for entry into CRNA practice. Importantly, as of January 1, 2022, all CRNA students matriculating into an accredited program must be enrolled in a doctoral program (AANA, 2021). Nurse anesthetists must also meet national certification and recertification requirements. The safety of care delivered by CRNAs is well established, and numerous outcome studies have demonstrated that there is "no difference in the quality of care provided by CRNAs and their physician counterparts" (AANA, 2021).

The COVID-19 pandemic resulted in the supervision requirements for CRNAs by the Centers of Medicare and Medicaid Administration (CMS) and in several states, additional barriers to their practice were lifted. This was to increase the capacity of the healthcare delivery system in the COVID crisis, and CRNAs were among the top 20 specialties providing non-telehealth care during the height of the pandemic in mid-2020 (AANA, 2021). The website for the AANA is www.aana.com.

Issues in Advanced Practice Nursing

Each year in January, *The Nurse Practitioner: The American Journal of Primary Health Care* publishes an update on legislation affecting advanced practice nursing. Over the years, advances have been made toward removing the barriers to autonomous practice for APNs in many, but not all, states.

In the past, substantial barriers to APN autonomy existed because of the overlap between traditional medical and nursing functions. A decade ago, the picture was considerably less optimistic than it is now. The issue of APNs practicing autonomously was a politically charged arena, with organized medicine positioned firmly against all efforts of nurses to be recognized as independent healthcare providers receiving direct reimbursement for their services. Organized nursing, however, persevered. Nurses, through their professional associations, continued their efforts to change laws that limit the scope of nursing practice. Their efforts were aided by the fact that numerous published studies validated the safety, cost efficiency, and high patient acceptance of advanced practice nursing care.

Both the public and legislators at state and national levels have begun to appreciate the role that APNs have played in increasing the efficiency and availability of primary healthcare delivery while reducing costs; however, opposition to APN autonomy persists. Roadblocks to full practice autonomy continue, primarily because of the resistance of organized physician groups despite data indicating positive patient outcomes. Despite progress, there remains the need for APNs to continue to work with their professional organizations to promote legislation mandating full autonomy.

EMPLOYMENT OUTLOOK IN NURSING

The Bureau of Labor Statistics is confident about nursing's overall employment prospects in the near and distant future. According to the bureau (U.S. Department of Labor, 2021), nurses can expect their employment opportunities to grow at 9%, which is approximately average for all occupations. The bureau estimates that, during this time, 276,800 new RN jobs will be created to meet growing patient needs and to replace retiring nurses (U.S. Department of Labor, 2021). Several factors are fueling this growth, including technological advances and the increasing emphasis on primary care. The aging of the nation's population also has a significant impact because older people are more likely to require medical care. As aging nurses retire, many additional job openings will result. Notably, these statistics did not take into account the alarming attrition to the healthcare workforce, including nurses, as a result of the COVID-19 pandemic. The need for nurses will become increasingly intense over the next several years as the pandemic lingers and the long-term effects of COVID infections become clearer.

An additional factor influencing employment patterns for RNs is the tendency for sophisticated medical procedures to be performed in physicians' offices, clinics, ambulatory surgical centers, and other outpatient settings. RNs' expertise will be needed to care for patients undergoing procedures formerly performed only in hospital settings. APNs can also expect to be in higher demand for the foreseeable future. The evolution of integrated healthcare networks focusing on primary care and health maintenance and pressure for cost-effective care are ideal conditions for advanced practice nursing.

Salaries in the nursing profession vary widely according to practice setting, level of preparation, credentials, experience, and region of the country. According to the U.S. Board of Labor Statistics, in 2020, median annual salary for nurses was $75,300 (as a comparison, the median salary for all workers was $41,950). Salaries were the highest with government and hospital employers and lowest in educational services. About 21% of RNs are members of unions or are covered by union contracts. Interestingly, California has the highest nursing salaries in the United States and has a vigorous union in the California Nurses Association/National Nurses United. Salaries in nursing vary by region, as do salaries in other professions and occupations.

APNs have higher salaries than do staff nurses; CRNAs average the highest salary of any advanced practice specialty group. In nursing as in most other professions, additional preparation and responsibility increase earning potential.

Most of the wage growth for nurses occurs early in their careers and tapers off as nurses near the top of the salary scale. This leads to a flattening of salaries for more experienced nurses in a phenomenon known as *wage compression*. Wage compression may account for nurses leaving patient care for additional education or other careers in nursing or outside the profession, an issue that must be addressed to improve retention of the most experienced nurses in the profession.

RECOGNIZING AN EXEMPLARY NURSE AND HIS CAREER

Some of this chapter has been, in all honesty, a sobering look at lingering issues and new ones that challenge our profession. Throughout this text you will be introduced to other challenges facing the nursing workforce as the healthcare system in the United States and throughout the world adapts to postpandemic realities that are yet to be fully manifested. Across the history of nursing, however, are stories of nurses and their careers that are inspirational and aspirational. Ernest Grant, PhD, RN is one of those nurses. Now the past president of the American Nurses Association, Dr. Grant describes his career trajectory as an African American man who understood that, albeit unfairly, he had to "be better" than other nurses in order to lead the profession, an acknowledgment that shaped his educational and career path. Dr. Grant was the first African American man to earn a PhD at the University of North Carolina-Greensboro School of Nursing. It is an honor to share Dr. Grant's story, found in Professional Profile Box 1.4.

PROFESSIONAL PROFILE BOX 1.4

Recognizing an Exemplary Nurse and His Career

My work life started when I was in high school, in the deli-bakery department of a local grocery store chain during my junior and senior years. I managed that department in the evening and weekends, and I recall being the one of the first persons hired there and remained until I graduated from nursing school. Although nursing was not my first job, it was my first professional career.

I had wanted to be an anesthesiologist ...and drive a 1968 lime green Mercury Cougar with a red leather interior. Being the youngest of seven children whose mom was widowed, I knew in high school that there was probably no money available for me to go to college, let alone to medical school. My high school guidance counselor told me I definitely had the grades (I graduated #13 of 197 students), so I could probably get some scholarships for undergraduate school, but perhaps not for medical school. He suggested that I look at nursing as a career. I could become a CRNA and if I still wanted to go to medical school and become an anesthesiologist, at least I could work my way through med school as a CRNA making more money than I would as a staff nurse. Then he suggested that I might not like nursing, so he suggested that I first take a one-year LPN course at local community college, and if I liked nursing, I could then apply to the college's associate degree in nursing (ADN) program to become an RN. About three months into the LPN course, I totally forgot about medical school. I realized that nursing was my calling, and a BSN would give me the opportunity to do more for my patients than I could as an LPN. I enjoyed being an LPN, but mostly in that role I was doing patient care and being the unit's medication nurse. I wanted to be an advocate for the patients that I took care of.

After completing the LPN course, I immediately started taking college courses toward my BSN, graduating from North Carolina Central University (Durham, NC) in 1985. After five years, I realized I could advocate more on behalf of the profession and my patients by earning my MSN, which I completed in 1993, and 25 busy years later, I completed my PhD at the University of North Carolina - Greensboro. During the interval between my MSN and PhD, I was doing what I loved... advocating for patients and the profession. I also got very busy as a member of the North Carolina Nurses Association (NCNA) and ANA, serving on several committees and boards.

The first two years of my career as an LPN, I worked on a med-surg floor at a community-based hospital in the NC mountains. I began to float to the adult ICU due to staffing shortages and eventually transferred to that unit because I loved the challenge of caring for trauma, stroke and post open-heart patients. As an LPN, I had extensive ICU training and had taken board of nursing-approved critical care courses that allowed me to run a balloon pump and care for patients after open-heart surgery and other critically ill persons. When I moved to the Triangle (Raleigh, Durham, Chapel Hill) area in central NC, I found out that, compared with the NC mountain area where BSN-prepared RNs were still a rarity, they were a dime a dozen here. ICUs were fully staffed with RNs; the only exceptions were

Continued

PROFESSIONAL PROFILE BOX 1.4—cont'd

Recognizing an Exemplary Nurse and His Career

the North Carolina Jaycee Burn Center at UNC, and an special oncology floor at a local regional hospital. I didn't think I could do oncology nursing. Coincidentally, I was a member of the Black Mountain-Swannanoa chapter of the North Carolina Jaycees, the organization that had built and still supports the burn center. One of major fundraisers for the Jaycees is the annual jelly sale, and as a Jaycee I had actually chaired three of these projects. Based on my relationship as a member of the Jaycees, I joined the staff of the Burn Center. My intention was to only work there until I graduated from NCCU with my BSN, and then I would head back to the mountains where my family lived.

About three months into working at the Burn Center, I guess you could say that I was convinced this was my calling. I really felt that I was able to make a difference in the lives of the patients and families that I cared for. This was an era during which we used wire scratch brushes to debride the wounds and administered very little pain medication. Wound care was done three times a day, so that if you worked day shift, you did dressing changes first thing in the morning, and around 5:00 p.m. Night nurses would change dressings between 9:00 p.m. and 11:00 p.m. Some dressing changes would take up to 3 hours to complete, and the room temperature was set at 85 degrees to prevent the patients from becoming hypothermic. It was not unusual to step out of the room and have to change scrubs because they were soaked through with sweat. My plan to work there only until I completed my BSN turned into 36.5 years!

I grew to love my work at the burn center and welcomed the challenge, as I quickly realized that I was able to use everything I learned in nursing school in that setting—and I do mean EVERYTHING—including OB! Our burn center admitted pediatric, geriatric and all persons in between, so I had to remain very well versed in the care of all patient populations and their cultures. I found myself applying knowledge of anatomy and physiology, nutrition, pediatric and adult care, med-surg, orthopedic, neuro ... the list goes on and on. Many of our patients had mental health problems either before or after entering the burn center, especially if they had burns to their face or hands which could not be covered up. This work required all my skills to help the patients and their families, even if it was as the patient transitioned from this life to the next, or helping them get through their hospital stay and beyond.

A couple of issues triggered my desire to seek further education, specifically an MSN degree. First, as I mentioned earlier, in the Triangle area, RNs with BSN degrees common. To advance up the career ladder and into leadership roles, you needed the MSN or higher degree to even be considered for a career beyond the bedside. Significantly, I knew as an African American male, I had to be better than those that I may be competing against for those leadership positions. In hospital administration at that time, maybe one or two BIPOC (Black, Indigenous, People of Color) persons held leadership positions. Second, I realized a graduate degree had some weight in giving nurses a voice. Two years after completing my BSN, I had become the Education Clinician for the Burn Outreach program. I knew that in order to go to other hospitals and teach physicians and other providers how to care for and prepare patients who would be transferred to our unit, I needed a graduate degree to be seen as credible. The same principle applied when going to the NC General Assembly to seek passage of legislation containing measures to make our homes safer by having a working smoke alarm, or decreasing the hot water heater temperature, among others.

Shortly after completing my MSN, I realized I wanted to obtain my PhD; however, work and my professional career path got in the way for about 25 years! I became very active in NCNA, ANA and the Burn community. Even though I was making great strides at advocating for my patients and the profession, I could not yet find the time it would take to study for my PhD. After completing my term as the President of the NCNA, I realized that I did not have anything else to do – so it was a good time to start working on my PhD. Also driving me was my desire to run for President of the ANA, although I was concerned that by not having a degree beyond an MSN, I might not be seen as well qualified as others running for this office. I knew that because I would be working with leaders in the federal government and other organizations, having a PhD would give me additional leverage to be taken seriously and to have my voice heard. I used my work experience as the basis for my PhD research, focusing on prevention of burns in elderly persons, and I'm considered a geriatric burn expert with a concentration of critical care as well. My dissertation was a qualitative study that examined whether older Black and White men changed their habits after sustaining a burn injury. It yielded some very interesting results!

I became involved in NCNA during nursing school. My instructors instilled into their students the need to belong to their professional associations. They would assign extra

PROFESSIONAL PROFILE BOX 1.4—cont'd

Recognizing an Exemplary Nurse and His Career

credit for students to attend our local chapter meetings and the state meeting. They not only walked-the-walk, but talked-the talk: they attended those meetings. They were *active* participants on committees, asking questions at the microphones after presentations, or debating an issue. They showed us how it was to be done. About 2 weeks after graduating from NCCU in 1985, I became a member of NCNA, and shortly afterward, began serving on a committee. The next thing I knew, I was chairing committees and being asked to serve on the Board of Directors.

I think unconsciously, I was preparing myself for the next role in my career: that of becoming the president of the ANA. I knew that somewhere deep down, I would be involved in helping the nursing profession to advance to have its voice heard and to advocate for mankind on every level, whether well, sick or somewhere in between with chronic illnesses, nurses needed to be at the table advocating for health and healthcare!

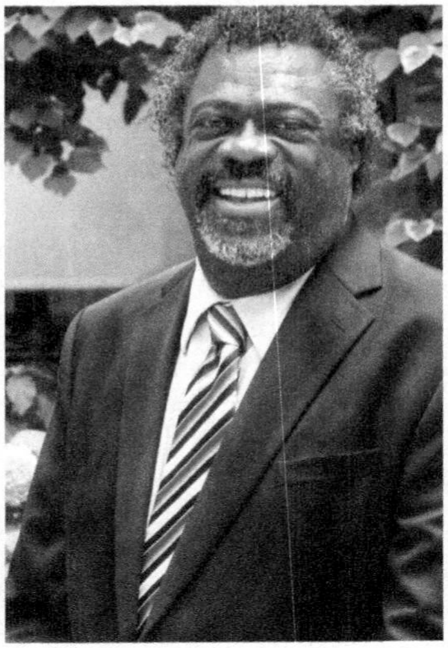

Ernest Grant, PhD, RN
PhD, University of North Carolina – Greensboro, 2015

Courtesy Ernest Grant, PhD, RN

CONCEPTS AND CHALLENGES

- ***Concept:*** Nursing is the largest workforce in health care in the United States.
  Challenge: The effects of the COVID-19 pandemic on the healthcare workforce, including nursing, and its effects on long-term health of survivors of COVID infection are yet undetermined.
- ***Concept:*** More than half of working nurses are employed in hospitals, a traditional setting for nursing practice.
  Challenge: As health care becomes increasingly based in the community, more nurses will be working outside of the hospital. Nursing must consider the effects of the migration from hospital to community.
- ***Concept:*** The Affordable Care Act and other changes in healthcare delivery and payment will create more opportunities for practice for nurses. Increased use of APNs as providers of primary care may be part of the solution to the American healthcare crisis as the population ages, the number of older persons increases, and the need for healthcare cost containment becomes critical.
  Challenge: APNs deliver high-quality and cost-effective care; however, educating adequate numbers of APNs is essential to meet the demands on the healthcare system.
- ***Concept:*** Nursing will continue to be a profession in high demand.
  Challenge: Nursing faculty shortages at all levels of nursing education pose an ongoing challenge to educate enough professional nurses to meet the health needs of the population.

IDEAS FOR FURTHER EXPLORATION

1. Think of the areas of nursing that interest you most. How do your personal interests and nursing education compare with the characteristics needed in the roles presented in this chapter?
2. As you continue your nursing education, ask questions of nurses in various practice settings to learn how they prepared for their positions, what their work life is like, and what they find most challenging and rewarding about their work.
3. Call the nurse recruiter or personnel office of a nearby hospital to inquire about education, experience, and salaries and other benefits for entry-level and advanced practice nursing. Is there a clinical ladder program? How does it work?
4. Ask an APN in your community about their practice. What are the advantages and major barriers to practice that they encounter?
5. Look up the COVID-19 statistics in your state/region/county/town. Ask an RN in your community what effects the pandemic had on them personally and professionally.

REFERENCES

Aiken LH, Cerón C, Simonetti M, Lake ET, Galiano A, Garbarini A, Soto P, Bravo D, Smith HL. Hospital nurse staffing and patient outcomes. *Revista Médica Clínica Las Condes*. 2018;29(3):322–327.

Aiken LH, Clarke SP, Cheung RB, et al. Educational levels of hospital nurses and surgical patient mortality. *JAMA*. 2003;290(12):1617–1623.

Aiken LH, Sermeus W, Van den Heede K, et al. Patient safety, satisfaction, and quality of hospital care: cross sectional survey of nurses and patients in 12 countries in Europe and the United States. *BMJ*. 2012;344:1717.

Aiken LH, Sloane DM, Bruyneel L, et al. Nurse staffing and education and the hospital mortality in nine European countries: a retrospective observational study. *Lancet*. 2014;383(9931):1824–1830.

Aiken LH, Sloane DM, Cimiotti JP, et al. Implications of the California nurse staffing mandate for other states. *Health Serv Res*. 2010;45(4):904–921.

Alliance for Nursing Informatics (ANI): *Our mission*, 2021. (website). Available at: www.allianceni.org.

American Association of Colleges of Nursing (AACN): *White paper: promising practices in holistic admissions review*, 2020. (website). Available at: https://www.aacnnursing.org/Portals/42/News/White-Papers/AACN-White-Paper-Promising-Practices-in-Holistic-Admissions-Review-December-2020.pdf.

American Association of Colleges of Nursing (AACN): Fact Sheet, The impact of education on nursing practice, 2019. (website). Available at: https://www.aacnnursing.org/Portals/42/News/Factsheets/Education-Impact-Fact-Sheet.pdf.

American Association of Colleges of Nursing (AACN): *Clinical nurse leader (CNL)*, 2021. (website). Available at: https://www.aacnnursing.org/CNL.

American Association of Colleges of Nursing (AACN): DNP fact sheet, 2020. (website). Available at: http://www.aacnnursing.org/DNP/Fact-Sheet.

American Association of Colleges of Nursing (AACN): Fact sheet: enhancing diversity in the nursing workforce, 2019. (website). Available at: https://www.aacnnursing.org/Portals/42/News/Factsheets/Enhancing-Diversity-Factsheet.pdf.

American Association of Colleges of Nursing (AACN): *ELNEC project reaches historic milestone with one million nurses trained*, 2020. (website). Available at: https://www.aacnnursing.org/News-Information/Press-Releases/View/ArticleId/24730/ELNEC-Historic-2020-Milestone.

American Association of Nurse Anesthetists (AANA): *Certified registered nurse anesthetists fact sheet*, 2021. (website). Available at: https://www.aana.com/membership/become-a-crna/crna-fact-sheet.

American Association of Nurse Practitioners (AAPN): *Discussion paper: quality of nurse practitioner practice*, 2020. (website). Available at: https://storage.aanp.org/www/documents/advocacy/position-papers/Quality-of-NP-Practice-Bib_11.2020.pdf.

American Nurses Association. *Nursing: scope and standards of practice*. Silver Spring, MD: American Nurses Association; 2015a.

American Nurses Association. *Code of ethics for nurses with interpretive statements*. Silver Spring, MD: American Nurses Association; 2015b.

American Nurses Association. *Faith community nursing, scope and standards of practice*, 3rd ed, Silver Spring, MD, 2017, Nursing Knowledge Center.

American Medical Informatics Association: Nursing informatics, 2021. (website). Available at: https://amia.org/communities/nursing-informatics.

American Public Health Association: *The definition and practice of public health nursing*, 2013 (website). Available at:

https://www.apha.org/~/media/files/pdf/membergroups/phn/nursingdefinition.ashx, 2013.

Brewin, B: *First nurse nominated as Army Surgeon General*, Government Executive, 2011. (website). Available at: https://www.govexec.com/federal-news/2011/05/first-nurse-nominated-as-army-surgeon-general/33918/.

Camera L: *Many school districts don't have enough school nurses,*2016. (website). Available at: https://www.usnews.com/news/articles/2016-03-23/the-school-nurse-scourge.

CDC.gov: Centers for Disease Control and Prevention: *Post-COVID* conditions, 2021. (website). Available at https://www.cdc.gov/coronavirus/2019-ncov/long-term-effects/index.html.

CDC.gov: *National Vital Statistics Reports: Table 1-4, Birth, by attendant*, 2019. (website). 2019. Available at: https://www.cdc.gov/nchs/data/nvsr/nvsr68/nvsr68_13_tables-508.pdf.

CDC Foundation: *Alaska Native Nurses Battle COVID and the Elements*, 2021. Available at: https://www.cdcfoundation.org/stories/alaska-native-nurses-battle-covid-and-elements, 2021.

Healthcare Information and Management Systems Society Nursing Informatics: 2017 *Nursing informatics work survey,* 2017. (website). Available at: https://www.himss.org/sites/hde/files/d7/FileDownloads/2017_HIMSS_Leadership_Workforce_Survey_Executive_Summary_Final.pdf.

healthIT.gov: *Meaningful use and the shift to merit-based incentive payment system,* 2017. (website). Available at: https://www.healthit.gov/topic/federal-incentive-programs/meaningful-use.

healthIT.gov: *Telemedicine and telehealth*, 2017. (website). Available at: https://www.healthit.gov/topic/health-it-initiatives/telemedicine-and-telehealth

Health Resources and Services Administration: *National center for health workforce analysis: The U.S. nursing workforce: trends in supply and education,* 2013. (website). Washington, DC. Available at: https://www.ruralhealthinfo.org/assets/1206-4974/nursing-workforce-nchwa-report-april-2013.pdf.

Hospice and Palliative Nurses Association (HPNA): *Mission, vision and pillars of excellence*, 2021. (website). Available at: https://advancingexpertcare.org/HPNA/About/Mission_Strategic_Plan/HPNA/About_Us/About.aspx?hkey=63b4511d-eba6-4c88-b732-4685a5988b6d.

Kleinpell R, Myers CR, Schorn MN. Likes W: Impact of COVID-19 pandemic on APRN practice: results from a national survey. *Nurs Outlook*. 2021;69:783–792.

National Academy of Medicine. *The future of nursing 2010-2020: leading change*. Washington, DC: National Academy of Sciences; 2010.

National Academy of Medicine. *The future of nursing 2020-2030: charting a path to achieve health equity*. Washington, DC: National Academy of Sciences; 2021.

National Association of School Nurses (NASN). *Transforming school health*; 2014. (website). Available at. www.joomag.com/magazine/annual-report-2013-2014/0147811001426704218?short.

National Association of School Nurses (NASN). *FAQ: about school nursing: the definition of school nursing*; 2021. (website). Available at. https://www.nasn.org/faq.

National Association of School Nurses (NASN): *School nurse workload: staffing for safe care*, 2020. (website). Available at: https://www.nasn.org/advocacy/professional-practice-documents/position-statements/ps-workload.

National Association of School Nurses (NASN): *School nurses: leading the way, 2019-2020 annual report,* 2020. (website). Available at: https://higherlogicdownload.s3.amazonaws.com/NASN/3870c72d-fff9-4ed7-833f-215de278d256/UploadedImages/About/2019-2020-NASN-Annual-Report.pdf.

National Council of State Boards of Nursing: *What you need to know about nursing licensure and boards of nursing,* 2011. (website). Available at: https://www.ncsbn.org/Nursing_Licensure.pdf. 2011

National Hospice and Palliative Care Organization: *Hospice care: a consumer's guide to selecting a hospice program*, 2021. (website). Available at: www.nhpco.org.

National League for Nursing: *Percentage of basic RN programs by program type*, 2014. (website). Available at: http://www.nln.org/docs/default-source/newsroom/nursing-education-statistics/percentage-of-basic-rn-programs-by-program-type-1994-to-1995-and-2003-to-2012-and-2014-%28pdf%29.pdf?sfvrsn=0.

NC Health News: *COVID-19 didn't help the North Carolina nursing shortage*, 2021. (website). Available at: https://www.northcarolinahealthnews.org/2021/10/05/covid-19-didnt-help-the-north-carolina-nursing-shortage/.

NurseJournal: *Faith community nurse career overview*, 2021. (website). Available at: https://nursejournal.org/careers/parish-nurse/.

Peterson-KFF Health System Tracker: *How does the quality of the U.S. health system compare to other countries?* 2021. (website). Available at: https://www.healthsystemtracker.org/chart-collection/quality-u-s-healthcare-system-compare-countries/#item-start.

Robert Wood Johnson Foundation: *Charting nursing's future: the case for academic progression*, 2013. (website). Available at: www.rwjf.org/content/dam/farm/reports/issue_briefs/2013/rwjf407597.

Rosenberg CE. *The care of strangers: the rise of America's hospital system*. Baltimore, MD: Johns Hopkins University Press; 1995.

Schroepfer E. A renewed look at faith community nursing. *MEDSURGNursing*. 2016;25(1):62–66.

Smiley RA, Ruttinger C, Oliviera CM, et al. The 2020 national nursing workforce survey. *J Nurs Regulation*. 2021;12(supplement):S1–96.

Storr GB. Learning how to effectively connect with patients through low-tech simulation scenarios. *Int J Hum Caring.* 2010;14(2):36–40.

Thekdi P, Wilson BL, Xu Y. Understanding post-hire transitional challenges of foreign-educated nurses. *Nurs Manage.* 2011;42(9):8–14.

University of Buffalo: *New York's BSN in 10 law: what you need to know,* 2021. (website). Available at: http://nursing.buffalo.edu/news-events/nurses-report.host.html/content/shared/nursing/articles/nurses-report/posts/bsn-in-10.detail.html.

U.S. Census: *Quick facts, United States,* 2020. (website). Available at: https://www.census.gov/quickfacts/fact/table/US/PST045219.

U.S. Department of Health and Human Services, Health Resources and Services Administration: National Center for Health Workforce Analysis: *Characteristics of the U.S. nursing workforce with patient care responsibilities: resources for epidemic and pandemic response,* Rockville, MD, 2020. (website). Available at: https://bhw.hrsa.gov/sites/default/files/bureau-health-workforce/data-research/nssrn-pandemic-response-report.pdf.

U.S. Department of Labor Bureau of Labor Statistics: Occupational outlook handbook, 2021. (website). Available at: https://www.bls.gov/ooh/healthcare/nurse-anesthetists-nurse-midwives-and-nurse-practitioners.htm#tab-3.

Westberg Institute for Faith Community Nurses: *What is faith community nursing?* 2018. (website). Available at: https://westberginstitute.org/faith-community-nursing/.

World Education Service: *How Well Do Foreign-Educated Nurses Integrate into the U.S. and Canada?,*2018. (website). Available at: https://wenr.wes.org/2018/03/how-well-do-foreign-educated-nurses-integrate-into-the-u-s-and-canada#_edn6

World Health Organization: *Fact sheet: palliative care,* 2020. (website). Available at: https://www.who.int/news-room/fact-sheets/detail/palliative-care.

2

The History and Social Context of Nursing

ⓔ To enhance your understanding of this chapter, try the Student Exercises on the Evolve site at http://evolve.elsevier.com/Black/professional.

LEARNING OUTCOMES

After studying this chapter, students will be able to:

- Identify the social, political, and economic factors and trends that influenced the development of professional nursing in the United States.
- Explain the significance of early nurse leaders to the development of modern nursing.
- Describe the development of schools of nursing.
- Explain the role that the military and wars have had on the development of the nursing profession.
- Describe how issues of gender and race/ethnicity have influenced the development of the profession of nursing.
- Describe nursing's efforts to manage and improve its image in the media.
- Evaluate the implications for nursing in a technologically driven era.
- Describe how nursing has reacted to nursing shortages.
- Explain how nursing shortages affect patient outcomes.

HISTORICAL CONTEXT OF NURSING

From the work of Florence Nightingale and Mary Seacole in the Crimea and beyond in the mid-1800s to the present-day efforts of nurses to address the onslaught of demands on the healthcare system by the COVID-19 pandemic, the profession of nursing has been influenced by and reacted to the social, political, and economic climate of the times, as well as by advances in science and technology. This chapter presents an overview of some of the highlights of nursing's history and its early leaders, and a discussion of current and past social forces that have shaped the profession's course of development.

Mid–19th-Century Nursing in England

Nursing's most recognized early figure, Florence Nightingale, was born into the aristocratic social sphere of Victorian England in 1820. As a young woman, Nightingale (Fig. 2.1) often felt stifled by her privileged and protected social position. As was customary, aristocratic women visited sick and poor persons to deliver, food, render care, and provide religious and spiritual support. When she was young, Nightingale often accompanied her mother on these visits; however, her parents were surprised by and opposed her decision when, at age 30, she entered the 3-year nurse training program at Kaiserswerth, Germany, where she learned basic nursing care under the guidance of Protestant deaconesses. Later, Nightingale continued her nursing education when she studied with the Sisters of Charity in Paris. Care of persons with illness was often in the purview of women and men in religious orders, within both Roman Catholic and Protestant religious traditions.

Having secured her education and training in nursing practice, Nightingale sought the means to communicate her emerging ideas about health and illness. On hearing of the terrible conditions suffered by sick

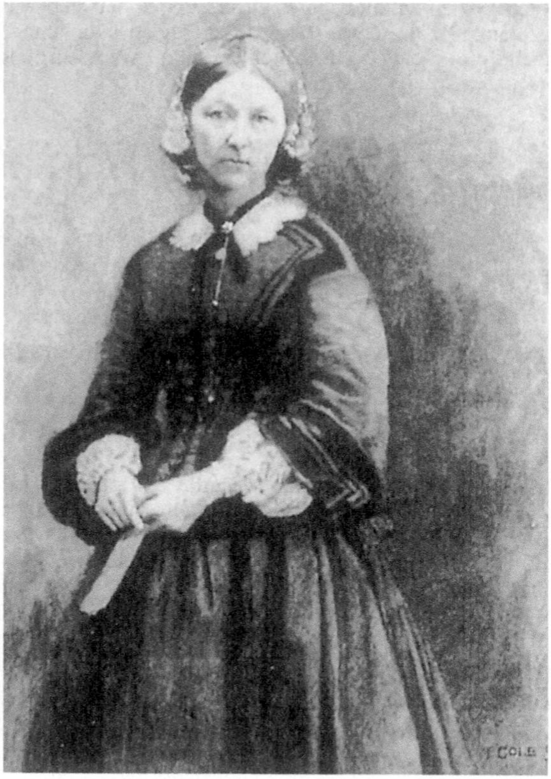

Fig. 2.1 Florence Nightingale (1820–1910), founder of modern nursing. (T. Cole, wood engraving, National Library of Medicine, Bethesda, MD.)

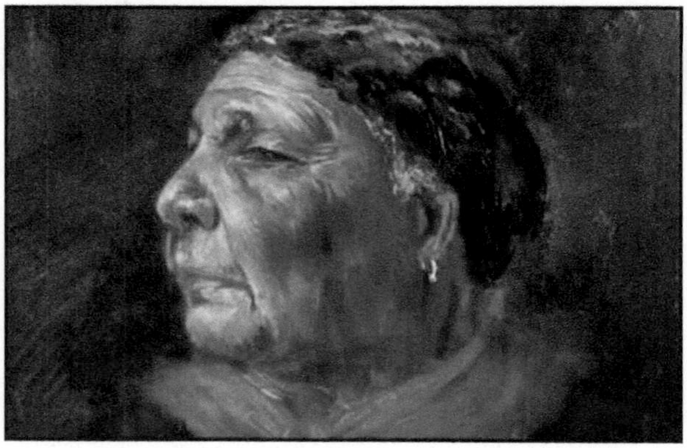

Fig. 2.2 Mary Seacole (1805–1881). Seacole's contributions in the Crimea and elsewhere are often overlooked. A beloved figure, in 2003 she was voted as the "Greatest Black Briton" in history. (Albert Charles Challen, oil on panel, National Portrait Gallery, London.)

and wounded British soldiers in Turkey during the Crimean War (1853–1856), Nightingale lobbied British decision makers to support her travel and interventions to aid the soldiers needing care. Nightingale took 38 nurses to the British hospital in Scutari, Turkey. Despite the opposition of military officers, Nightingale and the other nurses organized and cleaned the hospital and provided care to the wounded soldiers. Armed with an excellent education in statistics, Nightingale collected detailed data on morbidity and mortality of the soldiers in Scutari. Using this dramatic supporting evidence, she effectively argued the case for reform of the entire British Army medical system. Gill and Gill (2005) claimed that "Nightingale's influence today extends beyond her undeniable impact on the field of modern nursing to the areas of infection control, hospital epidemiology, and hospice care" (p. 1799).

On her return to England after the Crimean War, in 1860 Nightingale founded the first English training school for nurses at St. Thomas' Hospital in London, which became the model for nursing education in the United States. Among her publications, Nightingale's most famous was *Notes on Nursing: What It Is and What It Is Not* (1859). In this document, Nightingale stated for the first time that mastering a unique body of knowledge was required of those wishing to practice professional nursing (Nightingale, 1859). Her writings, dedication to hospital reform, commitment to upgrading conditions for the sick and wounded in the military, and establishment of nurse training schools influenced the development of nursing in the United States, especially after the American Civil War, as well as in England.

Mary Seacole (1805–1881; Fig. 2.2) made significant contributions to the health of soldiers in the Crimean War. Described as a Jamaican nurse and businesswoman, Seacole was voted as "the greatest Black Briton" in history in a 2003 poll and campaign to raise the profile of contributions of persons of African heritage to Britain over the past 1000 years (100 Great Black Britons, 2015). Although historical accounts of Seacole's life and contributions refer to her as a nurse, Seacole did not refer to herself as a nurse despite her initial desire to be part of Nightingale's team of nurses going to the Crimea, a request that was denied.

An independent woman with some wealth, Seacole funded her own travel to the Crimea, where her offer to be of service at the British hospital run by Nightingale was again refused. Seacole later reflected in her 1857 autobiography, *Wonderful Adventures of Mrs. Seacole*, "Once again I tried, and had an interview this time with one of Miss Nightingale's companions. She gave me the same reply, and I read in her face the fact that, had there been a vacancy, I should not have been chosen to fill it… Was it possible that American prejudices against colour had some root here? Did these ladies shrink from accepting my aid because my blood flowed beneath a somewhat duskier skin than theirs?" (Seacole, 1857, p. 80). Not only did Seacole encounter racism when she sought to join Nightingale in her work, but she also faced discrimination directed toward "colonials," residents of the widely dispersed countries of the British Empire, which included Seacole's home of Jamaica.

Undeterred, Seacole gathered resources to establish what she referred to as a "hotel," where injured soldiers received care. Seacole visited the battlefield to tend to injured and sick soldiers and brought many to her hotel. Seacole had much experience in the management of cholera because an outbreak occurred in Panama while she was there visiting her brother; cholera and other infectious diseases were the cause of a significant percentage of deaths of soldiers in the Crimea. In her autobiography, Seacole described performing an autopsy on a small child who had died of cholera in Panama, the results of which she did not make public but shaped her understanding of the effects of cholera and how it should be managed. British soldiers called her "Mother Seacole," and news accounts of the day described her as a heroine, compassionate, fearless, and determined (maryseacoletrust.org, 2021). When Seacole filed for bankruptcy soon after her return to England, 80,000 persons attended a 4-day fundraising event organized in her honor.

1861–1873: The American Civil War: An Impetus for Training for Nursing

At the onset of the American Civil War 5 years after the end of the Crimean War, no professional nurses were available to care for wounded soldiers, and no organized system of medical care existed for either the Union or the Confederate soldiers. Conditions on the battlefield and in military hospitals were unimaginable, with wounded and dying men lying in squalor. Military leadership made appeals for nurses, and the women of both the North and the South responded. Most significant perhaps was the response by the Roman Catholic orders, particularly the Sisters of Charity, the Sisters of Mercy, and the Sisters of the Holy Cross, who had a long history of providing care for the sick (Wall, 1995). Likely the most skilled and devoted of the women who provided nursing care in the Civil War, the Catholic sisters were disciplined, organized, and efficient.

A number of leaders emerged among the women responding to appeals for nurses, including Dorothea L. Dix, a longtime advocate for persons with mental illnesses in prewar years. She was appointed Superintendent of Women Nurses by the Union Army. In that position she was instrumental in creating a month-long training program at two New York hospitals for women who wanted to serve. Thousands of women volunteered and gained nursing skills that made them employable in the postwar era. Dix's efforts saved the lives of countless Union soldiers.

Black women who provided care for injured Union soldiers included abolitionists Sojourner Truth and Harriet Tubman, a formerly enslaved person who established the Underground Railroad and led others to freedom in the North. Susie King Taylor, also once enslaved, first worked doing laundry but was called on to assist as a nurse. Significantly, she taught soldiers how to read and write. She herself was taught to read and write in schools kept secret by Black women in Georgia. After being led to freedom by her uncle at age 14, she became a refugee behind Union army lines on the coast of South Carolina, where she aligned herself with the First South Carolina Volunteers, the first black regiment of the US Army.

Mary Ann ("Mother") Bickerdyke, who attended Oberlin College in Ohio, was a widow who moved to Illinois and worked as an herbalist, creating alternative treatments with plants and herbs. An active member of the Congregationalist Church, she learned of the squalid conditions in battlefield hospitals through a letter sent to the church by her friend, a surgeon with the 22nd Illinois infantry. She was selected by her congregation to deliver supplies to troops on the Western Front and to investigate the situation in the hospital camp at Cairo, Illinois, where she found that conditions were as bad as described. Although she had no official authority and was opposed by the camp surgeons, Bickerdyke was undeterred in her efforts to bring cleanliness and order to the chaotic conditions. She set up field hospitals as she accompanied Ulysses S. Grant and his troops down the Mississippi River, making cleanliness a priority, and hired formerly enslaved persons to work with her. Even though she was not trained formally as a nurse, she provided vital nursing care.

A nursing pioneer from Massachusetts, Clara Barton was copyist in the US Patent Office who initiated an independent campaign to provide relief for the soldiers. Appealing to the nation for supplies of woolen shirts, blankets, towels, lanterns, camp kettles, and other necessities (Barton, 1862), she established her own system of distribution, and chose not to enlist in the military nurse corps headed by Dorothea Dix (Oates, 1994). Barton took a leave of absence from her copyist work and traveled to Culpeper, Virginia, a strategically important site of many battles, including Cedar Mountain, Kelly's Ford, and Brandy Station, the largest cavalry battle in the Western Hemisphere, with more than 20,000 soldiers in combat. Barton set up a makeshift field hospital and cared for the wounded and dying, gaining the nickname "Angel of the Battlefield." In 1881, Barton founded the American Red Cross, an organization whose name continues to be synonymous with compassionate service.

In the South, women responded to support for Confederate soldiers. Until late 1861 and early 1862, women volunteers and wounded soldiers staffed Confederate hospitals. When the Confederate government assumed control, several women were appointed as superintendents of hospitals. Superintendent Sallie Thompkins, who had earlier established a private hospital in Richmond, Virginia, was commissioned a "captain of Cavalry, unassigned" by Confederate President Jefferson Davis and was the only woman in the Confederacy to hold military rank. Women living near battlefields in both the North and South brought men wounded in battle into their homes to care for them.

Although thousands of women supported the war effort, only a few were appointed as hospital matrons. One of the earliest was Phoebe Pember, whose initial assignment in 1862 to Chimborazo Hospital in Richmond, Virginia, put her in charge of a sprawling government-run institution crowded with "sick or wounded men, convalescing and placed in that position, however ignorant they might be until strong enough for field duty" (Pember, 1959, p. 18).

The Civil War set the stage to advance professional nursing practice because women providing care as nurses, although largely untrained, had achieved dramatic improvements in conditions during the conflict. The successful reforms in military hospitals served as models for reform of civilian hospitals nationwide.

After the Civil War: Moving toward Education and Licensure Under the Challenges of Segregation

The move toward formal education and training for nurses grew after the Civil War. Support was garnered from physicians and the US Sanitary Commission, a private relief agency created by the federal government in 1861 to provide and coordinate care of sick and wounded soldiers during the Civil War. After the war, the Sanitary Commission raised the equivalent of an estimated $385 million in today's dollars to fund their efforts. At the 1869 American Medical Association meeting, Dr. Samuel Gross, Chair of the Committee on the Training of Nurses, presented three proposals, the most significant of which was the recommendation that large hospitals begin the process of developing nurse training schools. At the same time, the influential US Sanitary Commission, who had seen the effectiveness of nursing care during the Civil War, also lobbied for the creation of nursing schools (Donahue, 1996). Support for their efforts gained momentum as advocates of social reform reported the shockingly inadequate conditions that existed in many hospitals.

The First Training Schools for Nurses

In 1872, the New England Hospital expanded its "nursing course" into "the first general training school for nurses in America" (Kalisch and Kalisch, 2004, p. 65–66). Linda Richards, who earned its first diploma, is considered America's first professionally trained nurse.

Three American training schools were based on Nightingale's St. Thomas Hospital model: Bellevue (New York) Training School for Nurses, Connecticut Training School for Nurses (New Haven), and Boston Training School for Nurses at Massachusetts General Hospital. Opened in 1873, these American schools were called *Nightingale Schools*.

The Victorian belief that White women were innately sensitive and moral led to the early requirement that applicants to these programs be women because program leaders thought that these qualities were important in nurses. Conversely, men were generally prevented from entering the profession, except among Roman Catholic orders, such as the Alexian Brothers. The number of training schools increased steadily during the last decades of the 19th century. By 1900 these schools provided hospitals with a steady supply of nursing students who worked

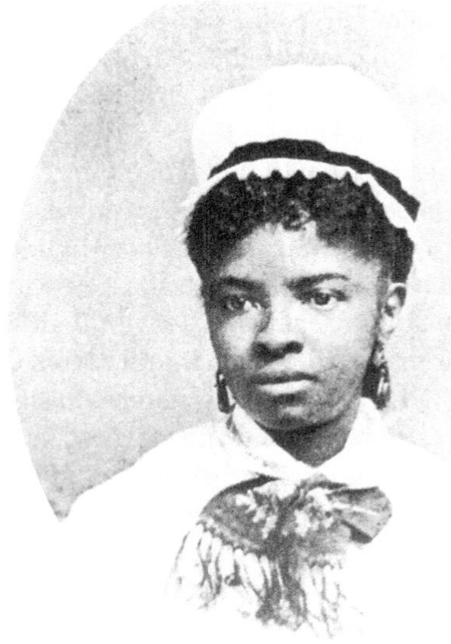

Fig. 2.3 Mary Eliza Mahoney (1845–1926), the first trained Black nurse in the United States.

HISTORICAL NOTE 2.1

Mary Eliza Mahoney (1845–1926) was the first professionally trained Black nurse (Miller, 1986). She began her nursing training at the New England Hospital for Women and Children at age 33. The course of study was rigorous, and admission was highly competitive. When Ms. Mahoney applied, there were 40 applicants; 18 were accepted for a probationary period; nine were kept after probation, and only three earned the diploma—Mahoney being one of those three. As was common in her day, her practice mainly consisted of private duty nursing with families in the Boston area. To celebrate her accomplishments and her status as the first Black professional nurse, the Mary Mahoney Award was established by the NACGN in 1935, with the first award given in 1936. This organization was later combined with the ANA.

Miller HS: *America's first black professional nurse,* Atlanta, 1986, Wright Publishing.

fundamentally as poorly or unpaid trainees learning on the job: hospitals were staffed primarily by students.

Some Northern schools admitted a small number of Black women to their programs. The training school at the New England Hospital for Women and Children in Boston agreed to admit one Jewish and one Black student in each of their classes if they met all entrance qualifications. Mary Eliza Mahoney (Fig. 2.3), the first Black professionally educated nurse, received her training there. Historical Note 2.1 gives some details about Mahoney.

The development of separate schools for Black and White nursing students reflected the segregated American society. Black and White persons received care at separate hospitals, and nurses at those institutions reflected the race of patients of the hospitals. The first program exclusively for training Black women in nursing was established at the Atlanta Baptist Female Seminary (later Spelman Seminary, now Spelman College) in Atlanta, Georgia, in 1886. Training lasted two years and led to a diploma in nursing. Spelman closed its nursing program in 1928 after graduating 117 nurses (Carnegie, 1995).

In the early years post–Civil War, Washington, D.C. had become a destination for persons who had been freed from enslavement in the South. Their often poor physical and psychological health necessitated the establishment in 1865 of the Freedmen's Bureau of Relief of Freed Men and Refugees by the US War Department. Known as the Freedmen's Bureau, Major General O.O. Howard, for whom Howard University was named, was appointed by President Andrew Jackson as bureau commissioner. Over the following decades, Freedmen's Hospital became one of the most prominent schools in training Black nurses and physicians, at one point training more than 50% of Black physicians in the U.S. In 1894 Freedmen's Hospital opened its School of Nursing, and by the time it closed in 1973, almost 1700 Black nurses had earned diplomas in nursing there. The Howard University School of Nursing opened its BSN program in 1969, and in 1973 graduated its first class at the same time the Freedmen's Hospital diploma program ended its mission after 79 years (Howard University, 2021). The first graduating class from Freedmen's Hospital School of Nursing is shown in Fig. 2.4. More details about this important piece of nursing history is available at the Howard University digital history website: https://dh.howard.edu/cgi/viewcontent.cgi?article=1001&context=fhsn_pub.

The earliest school established exclusively for the training of men in nursing was the School for Male Nurses at the New York City Training School, established in 1886. The Mills College of Nursing at Bellevue Hospital was the second school for men, founded in 1888. In 1898 the Alexian Brothers Hospital in Chicago established a nursing school to train men. They opened a second school in 1928 in St. Louis, Missouri.

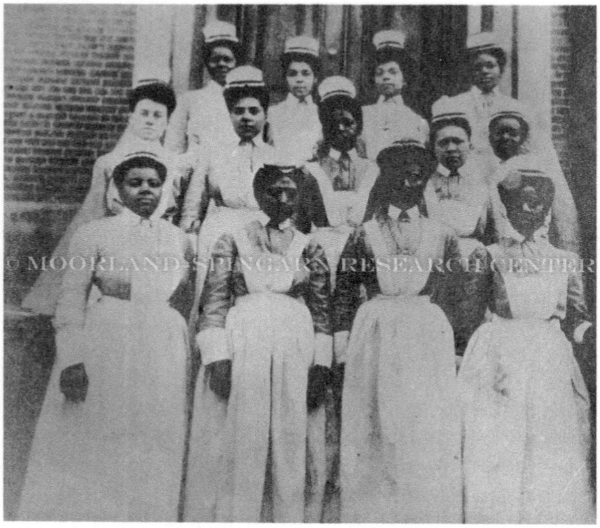

Fig. 2.4 The first graduating class of the Freedmen's Hospital School of Nursing in Washington, D.C., circa 1894. (Printed with permission from Moorland-Spingarn Research Center, Howard University, Washington, DC. ©Moorland-Spingarn Research Center.)

The Alexian Brothers ministry dates back to the Middle Ages in Europe, where they tended to the sick and hungry and, in the mid-1300s, cared for victims of the Black Plague that devastated the continent. The Alexian Brothers Health System still exists today.

Professionalization Through Organization

The 1893 Chicago World's Fair was an unlikely setting for a turning point in nursing's history. Several influential nursing leaders of the century, including Isabel Hampton Robb, Lavinia Lloyd Dock, and Bedford Fenwick of Great Britain, gathered to share ideas and discuss issues pertaining to nursing education. Isabel Hampton Robb presented a paper in which she protested the lack of uniformity across nursing schools, which led to inadequate curriculum development and nursing education. A paper by Florence Nightingale on the need for scientific training of nurses was presented at this same meeting. Also at this event the precursor to the National League for Nursing, the American Society of Superintendents of Training Schools for Nurses, was formed to address issues in nursing education. The society changed its name in 1912 to the National League of Nursing Education (NLNE), and in 1952 it became the National League for Nursing (NLN). This event held during the Chicago World's Fair became a pivotal point in nursing history.

Three years later, in 1896, Isabel Hampton Robb founded the group that eventually became the American Nurses Association (ANA) in 1911. Originally known as the Nurses' Associated Alumnae of the United States and Canada, the initial mission of this group was to enhance collaboration among practicing nurses and educators.

At the close of the century, in 1899, this same group of visionary American nursing leaders, along with nursing leaders from abroad, collaborated with Bedford Fenwick of Great Britain to found the International Council of Nurses (ICN). The ICN is dedicated to uniting nursing organizations of all nations; fittingly, its first meeting was held in 1901 at the Pan American Exposition in Buffalo, New York. At that meeting, state registration of nurses was a major topic of discussion, and an issue that would dramatically change the practice of nursing.

Early nursing professional organizations reflected the segregation that characterized post–Civil War America. Initially nurses from minority populations were excluded from the ANA. After 1916, Black nurses were admitted to membership, but only through their constituent or state associations. In the parts of the United States that remained segregated, including southern states and the District of Columbia, Black nurses lacked a pathway to membership.

In response, Black nurses recognized the need for their own professional organization to represent and manage their specific challenges. Martha Franklin sent 1500 letters to Black nurses and nursing schools across the country to gather support for this idea (Carnegie, 1995). In response, the National Association of Colored Graduate Nurses (NACGN) was formed in 1908 in New York with the objectives of achieving higher professional standards, breaking down discriminatory practices faced by Black students in schools of nursing and nursing organizations, and developing leadership among Black nurses. Believing they had met their objectives, and with declining funding for the NACGN, in 1949 the group accepted a proposed merger with the ANA, which was finalized in 1951.The ANA had by that time committed full support to minority populations and abolishment of discrimination in all aspects of the profession.

Nursing's Focus on Social Justice: The Henry Street Settlement

From the late 1800s into the 20th century, the young profession of nursing addressed the serious health conditions

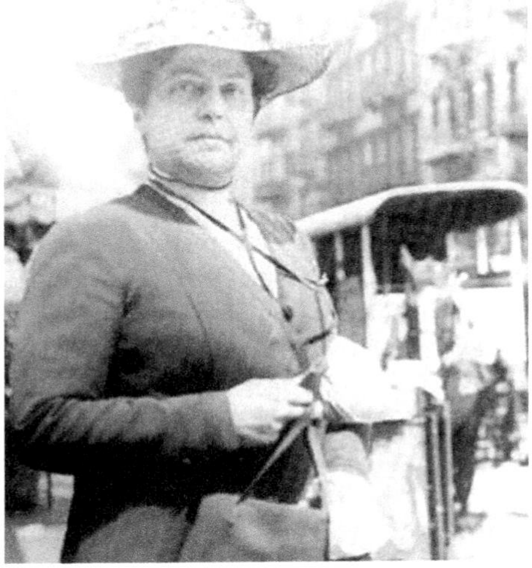

Fig. 2.5 Lillian Wald (1867–1940), nurse and social activist. Wald founded the Henry Street Settlement, which is still in operation today, and was one of the founders of the National Association for the Advancement of Colored People (NAACP).

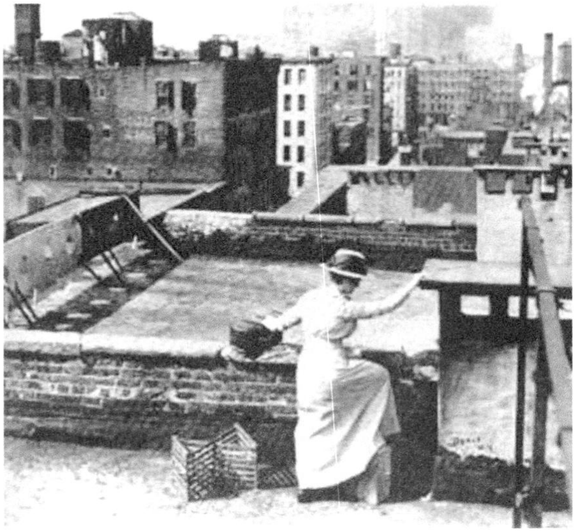

Fig. 2.6 The Henry Street Settlement nurses were undeterred from their daily visits to their patients in New York's Lower East Side.

related to the arrival of persons who had immigrated from Europe and sought work in the urban and rural factories of the northeastern U.S. Infectious diseases were easily spread in the overcrowded conditions in which newly immigrated persons often lived. In response to the difficult living conditions and the lack of sufficient healthcare services, the Henry Street Settlement was established on New York's Lower East Side in 1893. Its founders, Lillian Wald (Fig. 2.5) and her colleague Mary Brewster, obtained financial assistance from local philanthropists and began the first formalized public health nursing practice established in a settlement house. The Henry Street Settlement continues to serve its immediate community in the 21st century. Social activist and reformer Lavinia Dock and others worked with Wald to provide services through visiting nurse home visits and clinic services that cared for well babies, treated minor illnesses, prevented disease transmission, and provided health education to the neighborhood. Through the Henry Street Settlement, in 1902 Lina Rogers became the first school nurse in the United States. The public health nurses of the Henry Street Settlement were relentless in establishing and achieving broad goals to improve the health of persons who had immigrated to the U.S. (Fig. 2.6). Margaret Sanger, a nurse concerned by the plight of women living in poverty on the Lower East Side (Kennedy, 1970), became a champion for safe contraception and family planning for women. Her controversial work was sometimes dangerous, yet she persisted in her efforts to ensure reproductive and contraceptive rights for women. It is necessary and important to note that although Sanger founded the Planned Parenthood Federation of America, she endorsed the inherently racist and ableist ideology of eugenics, a stance that Planned Parenthood (2021) denounced in a detailed public statement found at https://www.plannedparenthood.org/uploads/filer_public/cc/2e/cc2e84f2-126f-41a5-a24b-43e093c47b2c/210414-sanger-opposition-claims-p01.pdf. The Henry Street Settlement still addresses urban poverty in New York's Lower East Side, providing care to persons of all ages with a variety of health and social services; it also has a robust arts program. A more comprehensive view of the remarkable history and work of the Henry Street Settlement is available at www.henrystreet.org.

A Common Cause, but Still Segregated

Tuberculosis was a major health problem in crowded industrial cities in the U.S. Dr. Edward T. Devine, president of the Charity Organization Society, noted the high incidence of tuberculosis among New York City's Black population. Aware of racial barriers to receiving health

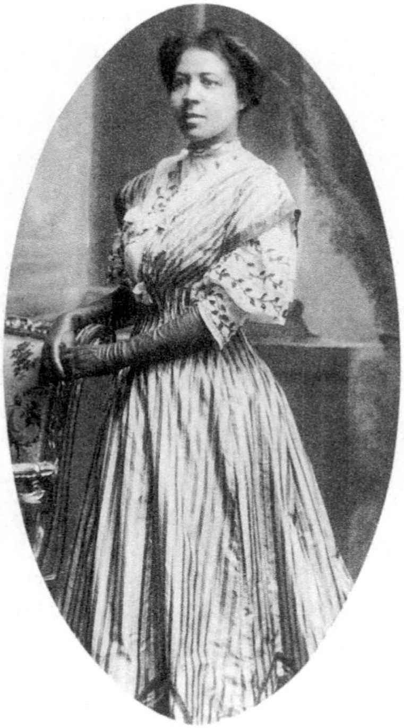

Fig. 2.7 Jessie Sleet Scales was a visionary nurse and was among the first to bring community health nursing to persons living in poverty in New York City around 1900. (Courtesy Hampton University Archives.)

care and the related cultural resistance to seeking medical care, Dr. Devine determined that a Black district nurse should be hired to conduct outreach into the Black community to persuade local residents to accept health services, screen for tuberculosis, and provide treatment if needed. Jessie Sleet Scales (Fig. 2.7), a Canadian-born Black nurse, trained in nursing at Providence Hospital in Chicago, and after a six-month course of study at Freedman's Hospital in Washington, D.C., was hired as a district nurse and soon earned a permanent position. Her report to New York's Charity Organization Society, published in the *American Journal of Nursing* in 1901, was titled "A Successful Experiment":

> *I beg to render to you a report of the work done by me as a district nurse among the colored people of New York City during the months of October and November. I have visited forty-one families and made 156 calls in connection with these families, caring for nine cases of consumption, four cases of peritonitis, two cases of chickenpox, two cases of cancer, one case of diphtheria, two cases of heart disease, two cases of tumor, one case of gastric catarrh, two cases of pneumonia, four cases of rheumatism, and two cases of scalp wound. I have given baths, applied poultices, dressed wounds, washed and dressed newborn babies, cared for mothers.*
>
> **(Sleet, 1901, p. 729)**

Jessie Sleet Scales later recommended to Lillian Wald that Elizabeth Tyler, a graduate of Freedmen's Hospital Training School for Nurses, work with Black patients through the Henry Street Settlement. Working within the confines of segregation, Scales and Tyler established the Stillman House, a branch of the Henry Street Settlement that served Black persons in a small store on New York's West 61st Street. For community health nursing, the addition of these pioneer Black nurses to the ranks of the Henry Street Settlement signified activism, expansion, and growth. Despite the persistent barriers related to race, Scales and Tyler succeeded in providing effective nursing care to underserved families living in poverty with burgeoning but manageable health problems.

War Again Creates the Need for Nurses: The Spanish-American War

In 1898 the US Congress declared war on Spain, and once again nursing had a major role in the care of those soldiers sick and injured in war. Anita M. McGee, MD was appointed head of the Hospital Corps, a group formed to recruit nurses. Encouraged by Isabel Hampton Robb and the fledgling Nurses' Associated Alumnae of the United States and Canada, McGee initially wanted only graduates of nurse training schools in the Hospital Corps (Wall, 1995); however, it soon became clear that this requirement could not be met because of a typhoid fever epidemic. Untrained nurses immune to typhoid fever because they had previously contracted the illness were accepted for service, as were Sisters of the Holy Cross, whose order had served during the Civil War and (Wall, 1995). Namahyoke Curtis was employed as a contract nurse by the War Department during the Spanish-American War, making her the first trained Black nurse in this capacity. Despite having to use untrained persons to care for sick and injured soldiers during the Spanish-American War, McGee's and Robb's efforts set the stage for the development of a permanent Army Nurse Corps (1901) and Navy Nurse Corps (1908) (Fig. 2.8).

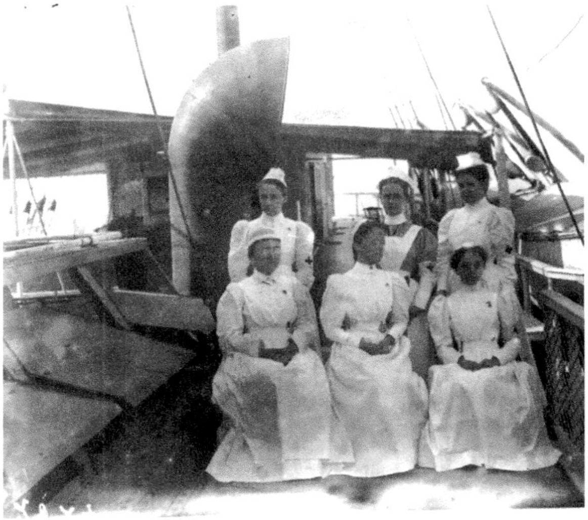

Fig. 2.8 Red Cross nursing in the Spanish-American War, circa 1898. Nurses on deck of the hospital ship Relief near Cuba. (National Library of Medicine, Bethesda, MD.)

Professionalization and Standardization of Nursing through Licensure

State licensure for nurses was a significant milestone for nursing in the early 20th century, despite lack of widespread support for it. After an educational campaign, the ICN passed a resolution asking each nation and US state to license nurses. As a result, state legislatures in New Jersey, New York, North Carolina, and Virginia passed what were known as permissive licensure laws for nursing in 1903, meaning that although nurses did not have to be registered to work, the title registered nurse (RN) was limited to nurses who were licensed. By 1923, all states required examinations for permissive licensure, however examinations were not standardized. Although in the 1930's, New York became the first state to require licensure, it was not fully mandated until 1947. In 1950 the NLN assumed responsibility for administering the first nationwide State Board Test Pool Examination, meaning all candidates for nursing licensure took the same examination.

The first edition of the *American Journal of Nursing*, published in October 1900, was a key event of this decade. Nurse leaders Isabel Hampton Robb, Mary Adelaide Nutting, Lavinia L. Dock, Sophia Palmer, and Mary E. Davis were heavily involved in the development of the journal. Sophia Palmer, director of nursing at Rochester City Hospital, New York, was appointed as the first editor, with the goal of presenting "month by month the most useful facts, the most progressive thought and the latest news that the profession has to offer in the most attractive form that can be secured" (Palmer, 1900, p. 64).

1917–1935: Challenges of World War I, the 1918 1919 Influenza Pandemic, and the 1930s Depression Era

The years 1917–1918 posed significant challenges to nursing. As the United States entered World War I, the utility of trained female nurses in caring for soldiers during warfare had been demonstrated successfully in previous military campaigns and wars. In early April 1917, the National Committee on Nursing was formed (Dock and Stewart, 1920) and chaired by Mary Adelaide Nutting, professor of Nursing and Health at Columbia University. Charged with supplying an adequate number of trained nurses to US Army hospitals abroad, the National Committee on Nursing initiated a national publicity campaign to enhance recruitment of young women to enter nurse training (Fig. 2.9),

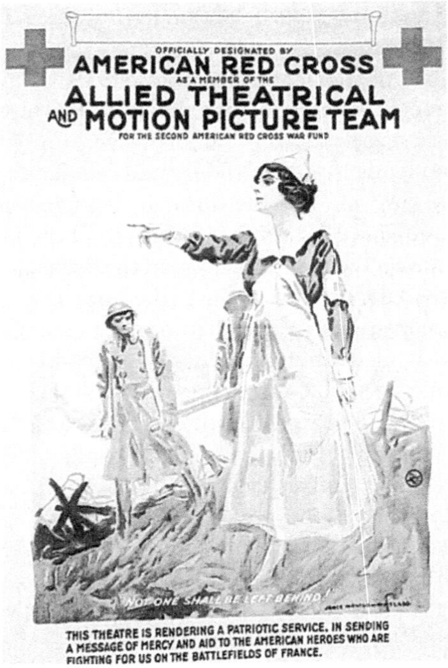
OFFICIALLY DESIGNATED BY
AMERICAN RED CROSS
AS A MEMBER OF THE
ALLIED THEATRICAL
AND MOTION PICTURE TEAM
FOR THE SECOND AMERICAN RED CROSS WAR FUND
NOT ONE SHALL BE LEFT BEHIND!
THIS THEATRE IS RENDERING A PATRIOTIC SERVICE. IN SENDING A MESSAGE OF MERCY AND AID TO THE AMERICAN HEROES WHO ARE FIGHTING FOR US ON THE BATTLEFIELDS OF FRANCE.

Fig. 2.9 A World War I Red Cross nursing poster, 1918. "Not one shall be left behind!" by James Montgomery Flagg is typical of World War I recruitment posters. Nurses responded in record numbers. (Collection of the Library of Congress.)

HISTORICAL NOTE 2.2

The influenza pandemic of 1918 to 1919 increased the public's awareness of the necessity of public health nursing. A pandemic is an epidemic over a very large geographic area—a continent or even the world, crossing international boundaries—and simultaneously affects a large proportion of the population. Across the United States, the Public Health Service, American Red Cross, and local Visiting Nurse and Public Health Nursing agencies mobilized to provide care for the millions of Americans who contracted influenza, known as "La Grippe" or "Spanish flu." [Note: "Spanish flu" is a misnomer: this virulent strain of influenza originated in the United States and was spread widely when troops deployed for combat in World War I. Because Spain was not involved in WWI, the Spanish press reported heavily on the pandemic, hence the incorrect assumption of the origins of virus and its spread.] One-third of the world's population (approximately 500,000,000 persons) contracted the illness, and in the U.S., 28% of Americans became infected, leading to the deaths of an estimated 675,000 citizens. The influenza was most deadly to persons 20 to 40 years of age. This age group is typically least susceptible to death by infectious disease, whereas infants, children, and the elderly are usually most affected—but this was no ordinary seasonal influenza. Approximately half of the fatalities among soldiers in Europe were caused by influenza, not war injuries, and in total, an estimated 43,000 servicemen mobilized during World War I died of influenza. In spring 1919, the second wave of the flu pandemic struck the East Coast and swept across the country. Although not as lethal as the first wave, second wave resulted in closed businesses, schools, and churches. The demand for nursing services increased across these two waves of influenza.

established the Army School of Nursing with Annie Goodrich as its dean, and introduced college women to nursing through participation in the Vassar Training Camp for Nurses.

From September 1918 to August 1919, an influenza pandemic first swept across the U.S., and eventually infected a staggering one-third of the world's population. The pandemic spurred widespread public education in home care and hygiene through Red Cross nursing. Historical Note 2.2 describes the effects of the influenza pandemic on the United States and the profession.

By the end of World War I, the nursing profession had demonstrated its ability to provide care to injured soldiers while responding effectively to the influenza pandemic. In 1920 Congress passed a bill that provided nurses with military rank (Dock and Stewart, 1920). The 1920s were notable in that use of hospitals increased, and the public began to accept the scientific basis of medicine.

Two other noteworthy events of the 1920s included the publication of the 1923 Goldmark Report, a study of nursing education (discussed further in Chapter 4) that advocated for the establishment of schools of nursing associated with colleges and universities, as opposed to hospital-based diploma programs. The Report encouraged the establishment of rural programs in midwifery, and in 1925 the Frontier Nursing Service (FNS) was established by Mary Breckinridge, a nurse and midwife. Originally established as the Kentucky Committee for Mothers and Babies, this service provided the first organized nurse-midwifery program in the U.S. Nurses of the FNS worked in isolated rural areas in the Appalachian Mountains, traveling by horseback to serve the health needs of the persons living in poverty (Fig. 2.10). FNS nurses assisted women during labor and birth, provided prenatal and postnatal care, educated women and their

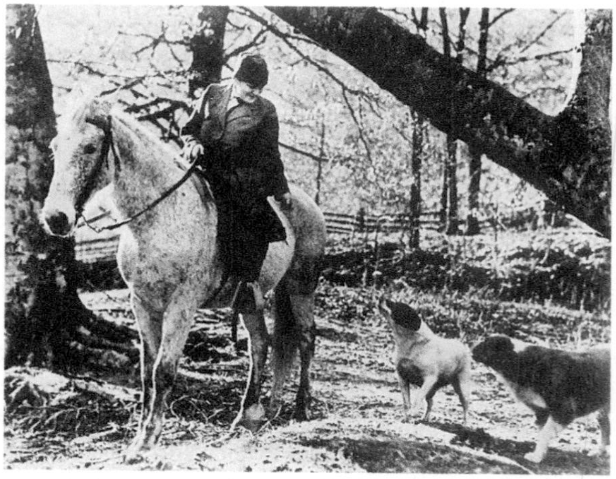

Fig. 2.10 Mary Breckinridge, founder of the FNS, rode on horseback to visit patients in rural Kentucky. (Used with permission of the Frontier Nursing Service, Wendover, KY.)

families about nutrition and hygiene, and cared for the sick. Through this rural midwifery service, Breckinridge demonstrated that nurses could play a significant role in providing primary rural health care.

1931–1945: Challenges of the Great Depression and World War II

With hospitals largely staffed by nursing students, most nurses who had completed their training worked as private duty nurses in patients' homes. The Great Depression, however, meant that many families could no longer afford private duty nurses, forcing them into unemployment. In 1933 President Franklin D. Roosevelt established the Civil Works Administration (CWA) in which nurses participated by providing rural and school health services. They also took part in specific projects such as conducting health surveys on communicable disease and nutrition of children. Many hospitals, facing significant economic hardships as result of the Depression, closed their schools of nursing, which resulted in the loss of a reliable, inexpensive student workforce. At the same time, the number of patients needing charity care increased. The solution soon became apparent: unemployed graduate nurses, willing to work for minimum pay, were recruited to work in the hospitals rather than doing private duty for wealthy families. This had a lasting effect on the staffing of hospitals.

The Social Security Act (SSA) of 1935, a significant part of President Roosevelt's plans to bring the U.S. out of the Depression, enhanced the practice of public health nursing. A purpose of the SSA was to strengthen public health services, including public health nursing, which then provided health care for mothers needing assistance and their children, children with disabilities and blind persons.

World War II: Challenges and Opportunities for Nursing

During World War II, the nation's military once again needed nurses, and in response Congress enacted legislation to provide substantial financial support for nursing education. The Cadet Nurse Corps was an alliance between the military and college schools of nursing to train nurses. Students received tuition, books, a stipend, and a uniform in return for a commitment to serve as nurses for the duration of the war in either civilian or military hospitals, the Indian Health Service, or public health facilities. Between 1943 and 1948, about 179,000 women ages 17–25 volunteered, and of these 124,000 graduated and were certified for military services in the Army and Navy Nurse Corps. As a result of lobbying by US Congresswoman Frances Payne Bolton, First Lady Eleanor Roosevelt, and the National Association of Colored Graduate Nurses (NACGN), for the first time in US history, Black nurses were permitted to provide nursing services to injured soldiers overseas. Despite ongoing racial segregation, HBCUs (Historically Black Colleges and Universities) and NACGN participated in preparing nurses for the Cadet Nurse Corps.

Historical Note 2.3 describes the experience of nurses in the Philippines at Corregidor and Bataan during World War II, who were held in an internment camp for 3 years.

1945–1960: The Rise of Hospitals: Bureaucracy, Science, and Shortages

In 1947, 2 years after the end of World War II, military nurses were awarded full commissioned officer status in both the Army and the Navy Nurse Corps, and Black and White nurses were no longer segregated. Julie O. Flikke was the first nurse to be promoted to the rank of colonel in the US Army. In 1954 men were allowed to enter the military nursing corps.

In 1946, US President Harry S. Truman signed into law the Hospital Survey and Construction Act. Often called the *Hill-Burton Act*, this legislation provided funds to construct hospitals, which led to a surge in the growth of new facilities. The rapid expansion in the number of hospital beds resulted in an acute shortage of nurses and increasingly difficult working conditions. Long hours, inadequate salaries, and increasing patient loads made many nurses unhappy with their jobs, and threats of strikes and collective bargaining followed.

In response to the shortages, the concept of "team nursing" was introduced. Team nursing involved the provision of care to a group of patients by a group of care providers. Although efficient, the method fragmented patient care and removed the RN from the bedside. Another response to the shortage was the institution of the associate degree in nursing (ADN), discussed in more detail in Chapter 4. As nursing leaders continued to search for a clear identity for the profession, they focused on the scientific basis for nursing practice, and in 1952, the *Journal of Nursing Research* was first published.

HISTORICAL NOTE 2.3

Hours after Pearl Harbor was attacked on December 7, 1941, a successful surprise attack on US installations in the Philippines crippled the air force in the South Pacific. At that time, more than 100 nurses were enlisted with the US Army and Navy units in the Philippines. Some of the most dramatic stories in nursing's history played out over the next weeks and months during the takeover by Japan of the Bataan peninsula, a large land mass at the northern tip of the Philippines, and then Corregidor, a small island (about 6 square miles) in a strategically advantageous location at the opening on the Manila Bay. Nurses proved their ingenuity, commitment, courage, and intelligence during the first months of 1942 as they were forced to provide care under the most extreme conditions. The two field hospitals, built to handle 1000 patients each, had 11,000 sick and wounded patients by the end of March 1942; one month later there were 24,000. The field hospitals themselves were bombed twice. With the imminent fall of the Bataan to Japanese control, the nurses were evacuated to Corregidor.

Corregidor contained a huge bomb-proof tunnel system, a complex of a main tunnel (the Malinta Tunnel, 1400 feet long and 30 feet wide) and numerous lateral tunnels with electricity and ventilation, and a hospital. At first, the conditions deep in the tunnel were a stark contrast to the horrors of Bataan, until conditions deteriorated over the next few weeks as Corregidor continued to be under relentless air attack by Japan. The number of wounded soldiers increased, until finally 1000 young men were being cared for by the nurses in a space where power outages, poor ventilation, oppressive heat, and vermin were common.

Although many nurses were evacuated from Corregidor before the final takeover of the island fortress by the Japanese military, about 85 American and Filipino nurses remained in the tunnel hospital to attend to the wounded. On May 4, 1942, the American forces on Corregidor surrendered. The nurses remaining on Corregidor were confined to the tunnel hospital, were not allowed to go outside for fresh air, and were given only two small meals a day, and yet they continued to provide nursing care for 1000 sick and injured soldiers. After six weeks, they were moved to the old hospital site outside the tunnel. One week later, they were bound for Manila, not knowing they were headed to an internment camp, where they would be held for the next 33 months. On February 3, 1945, U.S. troops liberated the internment camp.

For more details of the nurses' work during their ordeal at Bataan, Corregidor, and the internment camp, consult these excellent resources:

1. Kalisch PA, Kalisch BJ: Nurses under fire: the World War II experiences of nurses on Bataan and Corregidor, *Nurs Res* 44(5):260–271, 1995.
2. Norman E: *We band of angels: the untold story of American nurses trapped on Bataan by the Japanese,* New York, 1999, Random House.

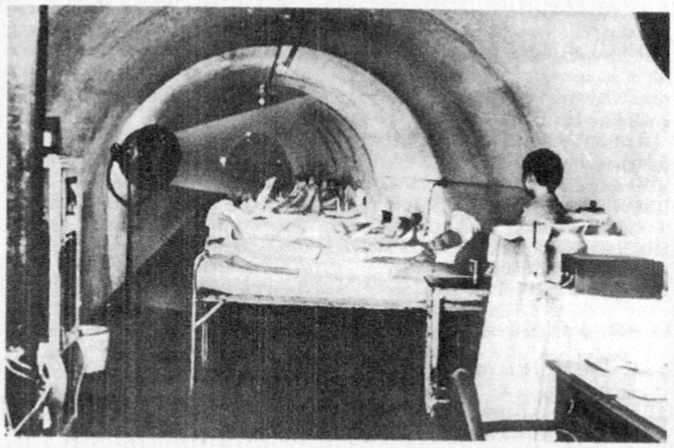

1961–1982: The Great Society, the Vietnam War, and Women's Social Movements

Two 1965 amendments to the Social Security Act, designed to ensure access to health care for elderly, poor, and disabled Americans, resulted in the establishment of Medicare and Medicaid. Soon after, hospitals began to rely heavily on reimbursements from Medicare and Medicaid. Care for sick persons shifted from homes to hospitals, and accordingly hospitals became the preferred place of employment for nurses, with new opportunities and roles.

The 1960s were the era of specialty care and clinical specialization for nurses. The successful development of the clinical specialist role in psychiatric nursing—combined with the proliferation of intensive care units and technological advances of the period—fostered the growth of clinical specialization, including cardiac-thoracic surgery and coronary care. During this era, the role of nurse practitioners (NP) in providing primary care emerged. Two factors influenced the rise in NPs. First, with the increase in medical specialization, fewer physicians provided primary care. Second, the public demanded improved access to health care as a result of President Lyndon B. Johnson's "Great Society" reforms. In 1971 Idaho became the first state to recognize diagnosis and treatment as part of the legal scope of practice for NPs.

The Vietnam War served to stretch the boundaries of the nursing, because the much of the combat occurred in jungle and remote areas difficult to access by rescue workers or medics. There were often no clearly drawn lines of combat. When mobile hospital units were set up in inaccessible areas, nurses often worked without the direct supervision of physicians as they fought to save the lives of wounded soldiers. Nurses performed advanced emergency procedures such as tracheotomies and chest tube insertions, never before executed by nurses. They also had to deal with the lack of support at home, where the Vietnam War was controversial, unpopular, and widely protested. The trauma of the battlefield was intensified by the lack of support in the U.S., and many nurses suffered posttraumatic stress disorder (PTSD), as did the returning soldiers. In 1993 the Vietnam Women's Memorial statue was dedicated in Washington, D.C., and features two nurses tending to the prostrate figure of an injured soldier. Most American women who served in Vietnam were nurses. This memorial captured the difficult and crucial role of nurses in the Vietnam War, and its purposeful feature of a Black nurse and a White nurse is a sharp contrast to the days of segregation among nurses in the military just a few decades earlier.

1983–2000: Challenges for Nursing: HIV/AIDS and Life Support Technologies

The early 1980s was marked by the recognition of the rapid spread of a retrovirus that later became known as the human immunodeficiency virus (HIV). This virus was isolated from a person with acquired immunodeficiency syndrome (AIDS) and ultimately resulted in a change in health care globally. First believed to be confined to the gay community, in 1983 HIV was found in persons with hemophilia as a result of HIV-contaminated blood products, thus making it clear that all persons were susceptible to HIV. Although much is known about HIV and its transmission now, 40 years ago the questions that surrounded HIV were frightening and resulted in significant changes to the daily routines in health care, including the implementation of universal precautions. The development of antiretroviral treatments proved to be useful in prolonging the time from infection with HIV to the development of AIDS, and the use of antiretroviral drugs during pregnancy reduced the incidence of maternal-fetal transmission from 30% to 3%. Very quickly, the HIV/AIDS epidemic changed the landscape of health care, affecting everything from materials such as needles, intravenous catheters, and gloves to global AIDS initiatives in impoverished nations, particularly on the African continent.

The 1980s and 1990s were also marked by an enormous increase in the use of medical technologies, including the wide use of life support. Notable ethical questions were raised during these years regarding the use of life support technologies and when they are appropriate. A prominent case involved the decision of the parents of Karen Ann Quinlan to discontinue ventilatory support after she lapsed into a drug- and alcohol-induced coma in 1975. The phrase "persistent vegetative state" became well known, if not entirely understood, by the public. Ms. Quinlan lived for a decade after the discontinuation of the ventilator, never regaining consciousness. Another case involving a young woman, Nancy Cruzan, raised questions of "right to die" and what the patient would have wanted. Ms. Cruzan was in a persistent vegetative state, and her parents asked for her feeding tube to be removed, eventually taking their fight to the U.S. Supreme Court, which upheld a ruling by the Missouri court that prevented them from discontinuing her nutritional support. They eventually won a court order under the Due Process Clause that supports a person's right to refuse medical treatment. The Cruzans provided evidence that their daughter would have wanted her life support terminated, and they were allowed to have nutritional support discontinued. These prominent cases moved forward support for advance directives to provide evidence of a patient's wishes while still competent.

2001–2020: The Post–9/11 Era, Natural Disasters, and Health Care Reform

The United States underwent a sudden and cataclysmic social and cultural shift in the aftermath of the September 11, 2001, attacks on the World Trade Center towers in New York City and on the Pentagon in Washington, D.C., plus the crash of a hijacked airliner in rural Pennsylvania. Almost all areas of American life were touched by the events of that day, including nursing. Disaster management became a focus of nursing efforts to be better prepared for mass casualties, and disaster drills have become part of the routine in hospitals to ensure that nurses and other personnel can respond effectively and efficiently, with a focus on saving as many lives as possible during a wide-scale disaster.

In 2005 Hurricane Katrina created a disaster along the Gulf Coast of Louisiana, Mississippi, and beyond. Parts of the city of New Orleans were underwater, and the images of people sitting on housetops and propped in wheelchairs along the walls of the Superdome became part of the story of Katrina. In hospitals filled with floodwaters in their lower floors, nurses, physicians, and other providers sought to protect and comfort patients under intolerable conditions. In 2006 in response to the arrest of two nurses for administering lethal doses of morphine and midazolam to four terminally ill patients in the aftermath of Hurricane Katrina, the ANA published comments on nursing care during disasters, citing the "unfamiliar and unusual conditions with the health care environment that may necessitate adaptations to recognized standards of nursing practice"; the comments, however, did not address the specific details of these nurses' situations. The ANA comments can be found at https://www.nursingworld.org/~4af058/globalassets/docs/ana/ethics/who-will-be-there_disaster-preparedness_2017. What was clear from both the September 11th attacks and the aftermath of Hurricane Katrina is that nurses were called on to act in conditions that had been previously unimaginable and unaddressed. Nursing as a profession has responded by increasing preparedness for human catastrophes and natural disasters that are certain to occur in the future.

Another marker of the current social context of nursing was the passage of the Affordable Care Act (ACA), signed into law by President Barack Obama in March 2010. This legislation was and continues to be debated vigorously. This legislation was often referred to as "health care reform." The ANA supported the passage of this Act and in 2011 affirmed its continuing support for the Act in the face of efforts by subsequent sessions of Congress to repeal it. Provisions of the ACA were implemented over time. Early provisions banned lifetime limits on insurance coverage by insurers so that patients with extreme medical costs can be assured of continuing benefits over the course of their illness and lifetime. Young adults up to age 26 were allowed coverage on their parents' insurance plan unless they had insurance coverage at work. The ACA also prevented insurance companies from denying coverage to children and teens younger than age 19 because of a preexisting condition. An estimated 162,000 children benefitted from these two provisions. Later provisions included coverage of recommended preventive services with no out-of-pocket expenses for insurance holders, the right to appeal coverage decisions, and having a choice of primary care providers. By 2019, 8.5 million persons signed up for a health care plan under the ACA, with a total of 23 million people insured, and in 2017, 73.8 million persons were enrolled in the ACA-based Medicaid insurance program (policyadvice.net, 2021). The Congressional Budget Office, a nonpartisan department of the federal government, estimated a cost savings of more than $1.7 trillion over two decades. Interestingly, the ACA improved patient safety and prevented an estimated 50,000 deaths between 2010 and 2013 from health care–related harm. An important provision of the ACA was that persons with a preexisting health condition could not be denied health insurance coverage. This provision affected 129 million Americans.

Another major development in the health care field that affects the nursing profession has been the rapid development of informational and medical technologies. Electronic health records have become common as the U.S. healthcare system is moving toward becoming paperless. Digitalized health records allow for access across disciplines and across distance, with the goal to improve continuity of health care no matter where a person may require medical treatment. In many institutions, nurses enter patient data into computers at the bedside. Life-sustaining medical technologies have created new ethical challenges for nurses, who continue to be the first line of defense on behalf of their vulnerable patients. This role has never changed for nurses, even though technologies have altered the terrain of health care over time.

2021 and Beyond: SARS-CoV-2, the COVID Pandemic, and Its Aftermath

In late 2019, news media began reporting on a new viral pneumonia known as COVID-19, caused by the SARS-CoV-2 (severe acute respiratory syndrome coronavirus 2), occurring in Wuhan, Hubei Province, China. In a matter of months, the world was in the throes of a severe public health crisis, and by the end of the third quarter of 2021, 246,000,000 cases had been reported worldwide, and an estimated 5,000,000 persons had died, although experts believe the number is actually much higher. In late 2020, vaccines became available and were approved in the United States for progressively younger populations. (At the time of this writing, a vaccine for children under age 5 had been approved.) In the interval between the first reports of the new viral pneumonia and the widespread availability of vaccines in the U.S., the world changed in ways that have yet to be fully realized.

Many persons who survived a COVID-19 infection have reported symptoms of "long COVID"—ongoing health problems and symptoms months after the initial infection. Although hospitalization and death rates plummeted among vaccinated persons, those individuals could contract the virus, although typically their symptoms were mild. The pandemic exposed—again—the huge disparities in health, standards of health care and access to health care across various communities, such that persons of color, persons living in poverty and who are uninsured suffered tremendous negative effects attributed to the pandemic. Not only was physical health negatively affected in vulnerable populations, but also emotional, psychological and economic health.

Moreover, healthcare providers themselves experienced tremendous stresses during the pandemic. Many nurses and other providers died from COVID-19 infections and complications; those who survived an infection may suffer with symptoms of long COVID, thus limiting their availability in the workforce. With large numbers of nurses needing to leave the workforce as a result of burnout and competing priorities with their families related to the pandemic, there is likely to be a further eroding of the adequacy of health care across the U.S. healthcare system. The solutions to these many serious problems are yet to be determined, even as more problems emerge over time.

SOCIAL CONTEXT OF NURSING

No endeavor functions separately from its social and historical context, and nursing is no exception. The influences on nursing in several contexts are identified and discussed in the remaining pages of this chapter. The social context also influences who chooses nursing as a career.

As you read this section, think about what drew you into the profession of nursing. What is the story of your own journey into nursing? One nurse's story is found in Thinking Critically Box 2.1. As you read his story, identify the factors that influenced his career choice and the challenges that he faced as he became a nurse. Then think of your own story and identify the social forces that may have influenced your career choice.

Several social factors that have influenced the development of professional nursing will be explored in this section, including the following:

- Gender
- The image of nursing
- National population trends
- Technology
- The shortage of nurses

THINKING CRITICALLY BOX 2.1

Challenging Gender Norms: One Nurse's Journey Into Nursing

Analyze the following story, and determine some of the factors that influenced this nurse's choice of a career. What assumptions did he make about the profession before entering it? Were his assumptions accurate? How would his assumptions hold up today?

"I never wanted to be anything but a nurse. As a child, I loved to bandage my sister's dolls and stuffed animals, and later as a teen, I volunteered at the animal shelter and took care of sick and injured animals. As soon as I was old enough, I volunteered at a local skilled nursing facility taking care of elderly persons, helping feed them and reading to them, and sometimes writing letters for them. When I was 18, I was hired as an 'orderly' (a male assistant) at a small hospital and provided care to male patients who were being prepared for surgery. One of the doctors there asked me if I was going to go to medical school, and I told him that I was saving my money to go to nursing school. He told me, 'What a waste. You have a great mind. And how is a man going to provide for a family on a nurse's salary?' Needless to say, I was upset by his response, and didn't feel like I could defend my career choice very well at the time. I have now completed my bachelor of science in nursing (BSN) and am working as an RN in a large, busy emergency department, and am planning to return to graduate school. I sometimes think about that conversation with that doctor, and wish that I could go back in time and answer him better than I did then."

Gender

Gender is a social construction of behaviors, roles, beliefs, and values that are specific to women, girls, boys, and men. Gender is not the same as sex, which is a biologic entity. A fundamental example has to do with asking a pregnant woman whether she is having a girl or a boy. This is a question of biology: is the fetus a female (XX) or a male (XY)? If the woman responds, "It's a girl. She's so graceful, she just moves so gently, and we can see in her ultrasound that she has long legs and arms. I can tell that she is going to be a ballerina someday!" she has assigned a gender role to the biologic entity of a female fetus. Because the fetus moves gently and has long limbs, the pregnant woman has interpreted these attributes in light of the fetus's sex: she is going to be a ballerina.

Assignment of gender roles starts early (even before birth in some cases) and is part of *socialization*, the process through which values and expectations are transmitted from generation to generation. Parents and others in a child's sphere of influence teach lessons about gender roles and behavior, both intentionally and unintentionally. A consequence of this is that gender-role stereotyping occurs. Stereotypes are also social constructions that portray how men and women "should" behave in society or within their cultural group. Gender-role stereotyping is often subtle and begins early with cues as commonplace as pink clothing exclusively for baby girls and blue for boys; dolls for girls and trucks for boys; and comments such as "big boys don't cry" and "girls shouldn't get dirty when they play."

Gender-specific stereotypes have affected nursing for 170 years. When nursing as a modern profession began in the mid-1800s, the most common roles assumed by women were those associated with care of their families, maintaining a household, and taking care of their husbands and children. Women often did not work outside the home for money but rather relied on their husbands or families for support. The first formal schools of nursing in the U.S. were developed to attract "respectable" women into nursing, a criterion that was designed to increase the value society put on nursing. Stereotyping of women also included the notion that women were intellectually inferior to men and hence women were not called on to make decisions or think for themselves. This type of stereotyping shaped the type of training that nurses received, which was fundamentally task oriented, and this form of instruction persisted for decades.

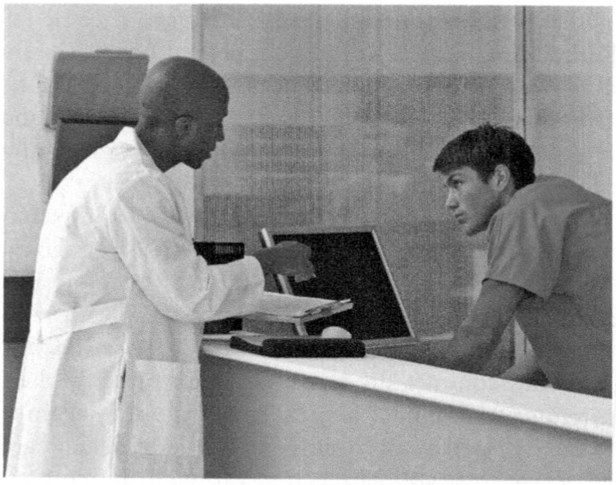

Fig. 2.11 Bringing men into nursing continues to be a priority for the profession. (Photo used with permission from Photos.com.)

Men are not new to the profession of nursing. During the 11th, 12th, and 13th centuries in Europe, men provided much of the nursing care, often under the authority of military or religious orders. Florence Nightingale worked hard to establish nursing as a career path for women and largely ignored the historical contributions of men. In her estimation, the role of men was confined to supplying physical strength, such as lifting, moving, or controlling patients when needed. Early schools of nursing in the U.S. did not admit men, establishing an early tradition of discrimination in the profession. An exception was psychiatric nursing, which often required physical stamina and strength and was therefore considered an appropriate setting for men in nursing. Now women and men in nursing have the same choices of settings available to them (Fig. 2.11).

Today about 11% of students enrolled in undergraduate programs are men. Men in nursing, compared with women in nursing, are likely to be younger, to be employed full time in nursing, to have more nonnursing education, and to have chosen nursing as a second career. Their motivations for entering nursing, however, are similar to those of women. The top three reasons identified by men for becoming nurses are (1) a desire to help people, (2) the perception that nursing is a growth profession with many career paths, and (3) the desire for a stable career. Professional Profile Box 2.1 contains the story of Eugene Farrug, DNP, FNP-BC, who was introduced to nursing by his mother who was an RN, and how his career and educational paths have developed.

PROFESSIONAL PROFILE BOX 2.1

Shaped by Family, He Became a Nurse

Nursing was introduced to me by my mother, Virginia Farrug, labor and delivery registered nurse, and my father, Joseph Farrug, rehabilitation counselor and disabled air force veteran. I grew up the youngest of four children in Detroit Michigan. We were raised between hospital work and rehabilitation work within our community. I was a cheerful, helpful, caring child, and my family encouraged me to help support our grandmother, Bridget, who had bipolar disorder. She liked me and I listened. At an early age she confided to me she preferred to go by Mary. She felt her name sounded guttural and proclaimed, "Mary was the mother of Jesus, and a good Irish woman should honor our Lord." Known then as Mary, she lived with us for most of my childhood. She tested my understanding of the art and science of nursing persons with mental illness well into college. From an early age, my family provided color and meaning to my nursing career.

I often had to help my parents with Mary. Her outfits, outrageous behavior, and interesting opinions were common discussions among the neighborhood children or nosy neighbors. In this spirit, I started working with persons with mental illness, veterans, and convalescent patients as a teenager as a certified nursing assistant (CNA) and later as an EMT. When I was 20, I entered a BSN program at Western Michigan University, and later, after moving to North Carolina, enrolled in an MSN program at UNC at Chapel Hill, where I trained to become a Family Nurse Practitioner (FNP). During my training, I fondly remembered my grandmother Mary—she solidified my lessons on patience and caring from my mother, and respect and tolerance from my father.

My patients also played a tremendous role in my nursing education. For example, in the 1990's I worked as an EMT in a Michigan Level 1 Trauma and Emergency room, during the time when HIV and precautions were being instituted. I had an unfortunate accident: while I was suturing an injury in a 5-year-old child, blood splashed into my eye. During follow-up HIV testing, some of my lab values were irregular, and the hospital's infectious disease department was unsure if my test was negative.

Fortunately, an Infectious Disease NP counseled me, did retesting, and was my advocate until everything was cleared. This experience cemented my desire to become an RN. I then became an NP to provide treatment and education to people before they became severely ill, treat them when they were ill, and provide holistic care along the way. And now, preventing and treating HIV and COVID-19 are big parts of my practice.

In 2016, I completed my Doctor of Nursing Practice (DNP) at East Carolina University with a specialty in biometric screening. Our biometric screening program included HIV screening for employees. Working with a large health insurance company., we developed a more cost effective biometric screening and referral program. This served as the basis of my DNP project, and now work with biometric screening data, equipment, and patients has become foundational to my clinical practice.

As an NP, my typical day now consists of working with patients and mentoring UNC NP students in two primary care practices, in Hillsborough and Mebane, NC, where I have witnessed the ravages of the COVID-19 pandemic. Days are long, challenging, and full of testing, assessing, managing, and treating patients. Primary care, COVID-19, and opioid recovery patients have all become part of my practice over the last few years. The COVID-19 pandemic has co-occurred with the opioid epidemic in a politically charged and polarized community. We now have a mental health crisis due to the far reaching nature of the pandemic.

COVID-19 has created a huge crater in the healthcare community, and we will be digging out for years. In terms of scale, the COVID-19 pandemic is bigger than the HIV epidemic and the opioid crisis combined. Biometric screening, testing, measuring biochemical values, and avoiding infections will continue to be regular activities for all of us working in healthcare. My goal is to continue working with UNC colleagues to provide patients with exceptional care, and students with innovative experiences. The pandemic has given me the chance to provide leadership, education, and treatment. I firmly believe nurses have shined throughout this time, and we can be proud of our service to the state, the U.S., and the world.

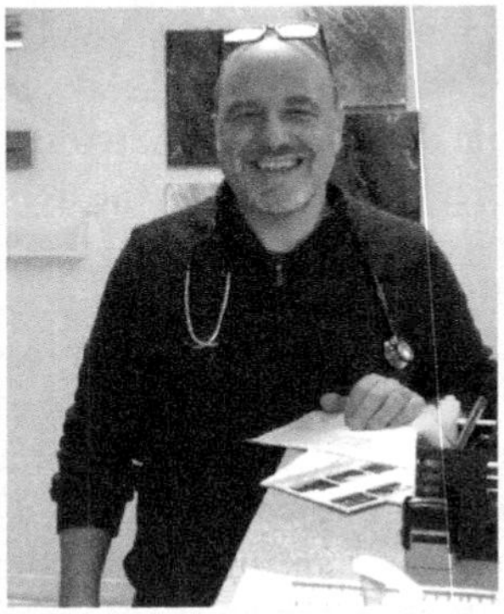

Eugene Farrug, DNP, FNP-BC
UNC Primary Care at Mebane.

Courtesy Eugene Farrug.

In 1974 the American Association for Men in Nursing (AAMN) was organized to address, discuss, and influence factors affecting men in nursing. Open to men and women, this national organization has local chapters. The goals for AAMN organization are as follows:

- Encourage men of all ages to become nurses and join together with all nurses in strengthening and humanizing health care to Americans.
- Encourage men who are nurses to grow professionally and demonstrate to each other and to society the increasing contributions being made by men in the nursing profession.
- Support members' full participation in the nursing profession and its organizations, and use this Assembly for the limited objectives stated earlier (AAMN, 2021).

Social change in the 1960s had a profound effect on society, and thus affected the nursing profession. Women began to recognize that they had career opportunities beyond the traditional and stereotypical "female" ones, such as teaching and nursing. Gifted women who might have otherwise become nurses pursued careers in a variety of other fields. This meant that nursing faced more competition for students than it once did because of the heightened interest in other careers by young women. Women took opportunities offering higher salaries, better working conditions, and schedules more accommodating of family life.

An interesting recent phenomenon occurred, however. Across the U.S., nursing programs began to see an increasing number of applicants who have degrees in other areas or who have had careers in other disciplines. The appeal of nursing seemed to be related to economic and employment security. Furthermore, a reason for this trend is that, in spite of the wide array of career choices, nursing's appeal is strong to individuals who seek a vocation with a positive effect on the lives of others.

The women's movement of the 1960s and 1970s benefited nursing in numerous ways. First, economic inequities and poor working conditions for women were exposed. The movement provoked a conscious awareness that equality and autonomy for women were inherent rights, not privileges, and stimulated the passage of legislation to ensure those rights. Unfortunately, however, a significant gender pay gap in nursing persists: in 2020, men reported earning $7300 more than women as RNs, and is even more pronounced among BIPOC women. Overall, women who are RNs earn 91% of what men who are RNs earn, and the pay disparity is most pronounced among nurses in pediatric settings (nursejournal.org, 2021).

Nursing also benefited from the women's movement in more subtle ways. As nursing students were increasingly educated in colleges and universities, they were exposed to campus activism, protests, and organizations committed to improving the status of women. Learning informal lessons about influence and power and how to foster change had a positive effect on students, who later used this knowledge to improve the status of nursing. With the firm commitment of all of its practitioners, the profession of nursing can give voice to all its members and ultimately contribute to the advancement of society at large.

Image of Nursing

A recent search of images available on a popular search engine using the word "nurse" recently resulted in 15 million results. Of the first 25 images returned in the search, all 25 were stock photos (professional copyrighted photographs for purchase) of young women and men, most wearing scrubs with their stethoscopes around their necks, and only one that appeared to show a nurse with a patient. This search—in contrast to those reported on in previous editions of this text—is remarkably representative of nursing now, with the exception of the youthfulness of those posing as nurses in the photos. The photos show ethnic diversity and a slight overrepresentation of men in nursing. Nurses older than 30 years are not well-represented, despite the "graying" problem of the profession as many highly experienced nurses are nearing retirement. Importantly, the highly sexualized images that have plagued the representation of nursing were notably absent among the first 300 images. In an earlier edition of this text, published in 2015, the same search returned two cartoon images of White females wearing nurse's caps and white dresses among the first 25 images, and further down the page was a photo of a tired, distressed woman with her hand to her forehead, eyes closed, with the words "nursing crisis" and "JOB" in large capital letters superimposed on her image. One image was of a young Asian woman in a highly sexualized image, wearing a very short, white, fake nursing uniform, complete with a plunging neckline and a large red cross on her chest; the same red cross was on her nursing cap. One was a photo of a nurse in a 1950s-era uniform and cap with a large syringe, smiling into the camera; her words in a text balloon are, "I have no idea what I'm injecting into your child." The author noted: "Finally, gratefully, there is an image of a nurse who appears to be talking to an elderly man in his hospital bed. If this was a representative sample of nursing, it is no wonder that we have a shortage. If this is a representative sample of the public's image of nursing, we have an image problem." The difference between results of the 2015 search and the 2022 search are encouraging in the lack of attention to sexist stereotypes and cartoonish images of nurses and, importantly, the increased attention to diversity and the seriousness of the profession. This is progress; however, these images leave the impression that nurses spend a significant proportion of their time conversing with each other while holding a clipboard or standing together with their arms folded. One image, among the first 100, has a banner superimposed that asks the question: "What does a Registered Nurse do?" The answer is certainly not found among this collection of photos.

Images are powerful. They surround us, and we become saturated by images. The images of nurses in advertisements and on television may be the first and lasting impression that people have of nursing. These impressions based on media images affect public attitudes toward the profession. Although the public's view of nursing has changed over time, most people still do not appreciate the complexity and range of the work of today's professional nurses.

Nurses are not so identifiable in health care settings as they once were. Once worn by nurses everywhere, caps were for decades a symbol of the profession. In the U.S., each school had a unique cap that was instantly recognizable. Nursing schools held capping ceremonies during which they presented caps to students as a symbol of their progress toward graduation. The cap saw its demise by the late 1970s; many, if not most, nurses were glad to forgo wearing a cap, believing it was part of the stereotypical image of nursing. With many different providers involved in the care of patients, there is often no distinct way of determining who is an RN. Identification badges carry titles but may be difficult to read. Interestingly, in the interest of safety, some personnel on certain units, such as urban emergency departments, are no longer including last names on ID badges or have them in a font so small as to be unreadable in usual emergency department lighting. Some medical centers and hospitals have recently made some movement toward reestablishing identifiable dress norms across health care disciplines. This is often accomplished by having staff of various professions wear attire or scrubs that are distinct in color or style. Others identify registered nurses by "RN" printed in large red letters on ID badges.

The manner in which health professionals address one another is a matter of image. Nurses in most agencies refer to themselves by first name, for example: "Good morning, my name is David, and I'm going to be your nurse for this shift." Physicians usually introduce themselves by title and last name, for example: "I am Dr. Roberts." Nurses rarely refer to each other by last name such as "Ms. Kyle" or "Mr. Pierce," and it is even rarer to hear them refer to each other as "Nurse Kyle" or "Nurse Pierce." Moreover, physicians often refer to nurses by their first names, whereas nurses typically refer to physicians by their title and last name. Nurses have reported being uncomfortable introducing themselves by last name, thinking that it establishes a formality that could interfere with the nurse-patient relationship. One of the most damaging and lingering images of nursing was the portrayal by Louise Fletcher of a cold, sadistic, and controlling psychiatric nurse in the 1975 movie *One Flew Over the Cuckoo's Nest*. Fletcher won an Academy Award for her role as Nurse Ratched, a name that has become synonymous for a cold, uncaring nurse. In fall 2020, Netflix, the popular streaming service, released Season 1 of the series Ratched, in which the history of the title character predating "Cuckoo's Nest" is presented, presumably to explain what shaped the older Mildred Ratched. A second season is expected to be released, but at the time of this writing, the date is unknown.

In spite of the challenges facing the nursing profession, nurses are well respected by the public and enjoy a generally positive image. In a report released by Gallup in late 2019, for the 18th consecutive year and in 20 of the past 21 years, nurses were rated the highest among a number of professions and occupations on honesty and ethics. Nursing ranked second to firefighters in the wake of the September 11 attacks, at a time when a great deal of positive media coverage focused on firefighters (news.gallup.com, 2020).

Foundations and corporations, as well as nursing groups, have undertaken initiatives to analyze and/or improve nursing's image. Three major initiatives are discussed here.

The Woodhull Study on Nursing and the Media

The Woodhull Study on Nursing and the Media was a comprehensive study of nursing in the print media conducted in September 1997 by 17 students and 3 faculty coordinators from the University of Rochester (New York) School of Nursing (URSN). In this study, sponsored by Sigma Theta Tau International (STTI) and URSN, students examined approximately 20,000 articles from 16 newspapers, magazines, and trade publications. The study was named in memory of Nancy Woodhull, a founding editor of *USA Today*. Woodhull became an advocate of nursing after her diagnosis of lung cancer, when she was impressed with the comprehensive nursing care she received. She suggested the study and assisted in the design of the survey after she became concerned about the absence of media attention to nurses and nursing.

In December 1997 the students presented their findings and recommendations to a mixed audience of nurses and national media representatives at the STTI Biennial Convention. The key finding was that "Nurses and the nursing profession are essentially invisible to the media and, consequently, to the American public" (STTI, 1998, p. 8). The purpose of the Woodhull Study, its major findings, and strategies to guide the nursing profession's collective response are found in Box 2.1.

The Johnson & Johnson Campaign

Johnson & Johnson, the giant health care corporation, began a multimillion-dollar campaign, the Campaign for Nursing's Future, in 2002, "to enhance the image of the nursing profession, recruit new nurses and educators, and to retain nurses currently in the system" (Donelan et al., 2005). This campaign included initiatives in print media, television advertising, student scholarships, fundraising, and research.

Johnson & Johnson now describes their work as "proudly advocating for, elevating and empowering nurses to drive transformative health change" on their popular website https://nursing.jnj.com. The site has an easy access to a variety of resources for nurses and prospective nurses, including support for nursing innovation and accompanying podcast, nursing school resources, career guidance and information on nursing specialties (nursing.jnj.com, 2021). This landmark effort by a major American corporation provides an example to the nursing profession of the potential for effective corporate partnership.

BOX 2.1 The Woodhull Study at a Glance

Purpose, Findings, and Recommendations

Purpose of the Study

The Woodhull Study was designed to survey and analyze the portrayal of health care and nursing in U.S. newspapers, news magazines, and healthcare industry trade publications.

Key Study Findings

1. Nurses and the nursing profession are essentially invisible in media coverage of health care and, consequently, to the American public.
2. Nurses were cited only 4% of the time in the more than 2000 health-related articles gathered from 16 major news publications.
3. The few references to nurses or nursing that did occur were simply mentioned in passing.
4. In many of the stories, nurses and nursing would have been sources more germane to the story subject matter than the references selected.
5. Healthcare industry publications were no more likely to take advantage of nursing expertise, focusing more attention on bottom-line issues such as business or policy.

Key Study Recommendations

1. Both media and nursing should take more proactive roles in establishing an ongoing dialogue.
2. The often-repeated advice in media articles and advertisements to "consult your doctor" ignores the role of nurses in health care and needs to be changed to "consult your primary healthcare provider."
3. Journalists should distinguish researchers with doctoral degrees from medical doctors to add clarity to healthcare coverage.
4. To provide comprehensive coverage of health care, the media should include information by and about nurses.
5. It is essential to distinguish health care from medicine as subject matter in the media.

Modified from Sigma Theta Tau International: *The Woodhull Study on nursing and the media: health care's invisible partner*, Indianapolis, 1998, Sigma Theta Tau International–Center Nursing Press.

The Truth about Nursing

The Truth about Nursing is a nonprofit organization with the mission to "increase public understanding of the central, front-line role nurses play in modern health care," with the ultimate goal of "[fostering] growth in the size and diversity of the nursing profession at a time of critical shortage, strengthen nursing practice, teaching and research, and improve the health care system." Its focus is to "promote more accurate, balanced and frequent media portrayals of nurses and increase the media's use of nurses as expert sources" (Truth about Nursing, 2021). Currently there are local chapters of The Truth about Nursing in many states and numerous nations around the world. Founded in 2001 by Sandy Summers, RN, and a group of seven graduate students at Johns Hopkins University School of Nursing, The Truth about Nursing uses a variety of social media, including Facebook, Twitter, and LinkedIn, among others, to shape the public's image of nursing. Some of their efforts have included convincing a number of major corporations to change their advertising when they have portrayed nurses in a sexualized or otherwise trivialized manner.

Ultimately all nurses hold the professional responsibility to reinforce positive images of nursing and, equally important, to speak out against negative ones. The nursing profession has the major responsibility for improving its own image. The major avenue for changing the image of nursing occurs one nurse-patient encounter at a time, where nurses demonstrate what nurses do and how to look and behave professionally. In addition, organizations such as the ANA can enhance nursing's image by offering services as consultants to media and setting professional standards.

One way in which nursing can take responsibility for its public image is for nurses to become sensitive to portrayals of nurses and nursing in the media. Box 2.2 contains a checklist for monitoring media images of nurses

BOX 2.2 Checklist for Monitoring Images of Nurses and Nursing in the Media

Prominence in the Plot

1. Are nurse characters seen in leading or supportive roles?
2. Are nurse characters shown taking an active part in the scene, or are they shown primarily in the background (e.g., handing instruments, carrying trays, pushing wheelchairs)?
3. To what extent are nurse characters shown in professional roles, engaged in nursing practice?
4. Do nurse characters or other characters provide the actual nursing care?
5. In scenes with other healthcare providers, who does most of the talking?

Demographic Characteristics

1. Does the portrayal show persons of all gender identities as nurses?
2. Are nurse characters of varying ages and ethnicities?

Personality Traits

1. Are nurse characters portrayed as:
   a. Intelligent?
   b. Trustworthy?
   c. Confident?
   d. Problem solvers?
   e. Assertive?
   f. Powerful?
   g. Nurturing?
   h. Compassionate?
   i. Kind?
2. If other healthcare providers are included in the show, how does their portrayal compare with that of nurse characters?
3. When nurse characters exhibit personality traits listed earlier, are they shown as positive traits?

Primary Values

1. Do nurse characters demonstrate value in:
   a. Service to others?
   b. Scholarship, achievement?
2. How do the values portrayed in nurse characters compare to those portrayed in other health professions?
3. When nurse characters exhibit the primary values of scholarship and achievement, do such portrayals show them to be an aberration in the expected values of nurses?

Sexual Objectification of Nurses

1. Are nurse characters portrayed in a sexualized manner?
2. Are nurse characters referred to in sexually demeaning terms?
3. Are nurse characters presented as appealing because of their physical attractiveness as opposed to their intellectual capacity, professional commitment, or skill?

Role of the Nurse

1. Is the profession of nursing shown to be a fulfilling long-term career?
2. Is the work of the nurse characters shown to be creative?

Continued

BOX 10.2 Checklist for Monitoring Images of Nurses and Nursing in the Media—cont'd

Career Orientation

1. How important is the career of nursing to the nurse character portrayed?
2. How does this compare with other healthcare professionals depicted in the show?

Professional Competence

1. Do nurse characters exhibit autonomous professional judgment?
2. Does the program send a message that a nurse's role in health care is a supportive rather than central one?
3. Do nurse characters positively influence patient/family welfare?
4. Are nurse characters shown harming or acting to the detriment of patients?
5. How does the professional competence of nurse characters compare with the professional competence of other healthcare providers?

Education

1. In shows that include nursing students, who actually teaches the nursing students?
2. Is there evidence that the practice of nursing requires special knowledge and skills?
3. What is actually taught to nursing students?

Nursing Administration

1. Are any roles filled by nurse administrators or managers, or are all nurse characters shown as staff nurses or students?
2. Is there evidence of a responsible administrative hierarchy in nursing, or are nurses shown answering to physicians or hospital administrators?
3. Overall, is this a positive or negative portrayal of nursing? Support your response.

Adapted from Kalisch P, Kalisch B: *The changing image of the nurse,* Menlo Park, CA, 1987, Addison-Wesley, Health Sciences Division.

and nursing on TV and in movies; however, you should keep this checklist in mind as you visit websites, read blogs, books, and other media, and notice commercials and advertisements. Then take action:

1. Contact those responsible for negative nursing images on television and in movies.
2. Contact the companies that sponsor television programs with negative images of nurses.
3. Contact the editors of publications that present nursing in a negative manner.
4. Boycott shows, films, and products that promote negative images of nurses and nursing.
5. Importantly, contact those responsible for accurate portrayals of nurses and the profession of nursing, letting them know that you have noticed and appreciate their efforts.

Of note, during the early weeks and months of the COVID-19 pandemic, nurses were often referred to "heroic" and their work as "self-sacrificing," among many other descriptors. Nurses soon chafed at this representation of their work, however, because it appeared to overlook their professionalism, and difficult and caring efforts of their day-to-day work in more ordinary times. Their point is well-taken. A pandemic should not be required for the key role of nurses and nursing care to become public knowledge.

National Population Trends

Over the course of American nursing history, nurses have responded as individuals and as a profession to wars, poverty, epidemics, pandemics, and various social movements. Contemporary nursing also seeks to respond as a profession to social changes that shape our nation and the world. Two in particular will be examined here: the aging population and increasing diversity.

Aging of America

People in the United States are living longer than they have in the past. The median age of the population in 2020 was 38.1 years (meaning that half the population is older than this) and ~16.5% are ages 65 older (U.S. Bureau of the Census, 2020). Life expectancy in the United States is currently 78.8 years for people born today: 76.2 for males and 81.2 for females (Centers for Disease Control and Prevention [CDC], 2020). This means that the people who have lived to 65 years of age are expected to live into their early to middle 80s. The very old (older than 85 years) represent the fastest-growing segment of the total population. In contrast, the number of 35- to 44-year-old Americans is expected to decline. This phenomenon is sometimes referred to as the "graying of America." The CDC website (www.cdc.gov) lists a tremendous number of age and health statistics.

Persons older than 75 years are more likely than younger persons to be widowed, female, and live alone and in poverty, and are more likely to have chronic conditions such as arthritis, hypertension, and heart disease. As a consequence of these and other factors, this age group uses a disproportionately higher share of health services than other age groups. The leading causes of death in people 65 years of age and older are heart disease, cancer, and chronic lower respiratory disease (CDC, 2020). (The full effect of COVID-19 and deaths in older persons, known to be the age group most likely to succumb to an infection, is as yet unknown at the time of this writing.) A significant percentage of older men and women have obesity and hypertension, and 22.2% of noninstitutionalized (i.e., not living in skilled nursing facilities, etc.) report having only fair or good health (CDC, 2020). The oldest "baby boomers"—those Americans born between 1946 and 1964—are well into their retirement years, and the younger baby boomers are in their 50s. This group of citizens will create an increase in the aging population between 2010 and 2030. As these postwar babies enter their 70s, their large numbers are expected to create an additional strain on the healthcare system. For the first time in U.S. history, the number of elderly people is increasing as the number of adults in early midlife is decreasing. The projected change in proportion over the next 2 decades may create stress on the U.S. economic and social systems. The "graying of America" plus the long term effects on the profession from the COVID pandemic is likely to have a profound effect on the healthcare system and nursing, stretching an already challenged capacity to provide adequate medical and nursing care.

Diversity

Historically and currently, the United States is widely diverse racially, ethnically, and culturally. The circumstances under which people immigrate to the United States range considerably; however, regardless of the period of history, the healthcare system has always been affected by the change in demographic characteristics of its population. In earlier U.S. history, immigrants were most often from European and Asian countries and often were located within major cities. For example, Washington, D.C.; Brooklyn, New York; and San Francisco, California (among many others), are cities with large enclaves of persons who immigrated from China in districts known as Chinatown. As described earlier in this chapter, persons who had immigrated often came through Ellis Island and subsequently lived New York City's Lower East Side. Lillian Wald and other nurses responded to their needs by starting what was to become the first visiting nurse association in the United States and had a significant positive effect on the health of residents of the Lower East Side.

Enslavement of the people of Africa by Americans and persons of other typically White nations is deeply shameful, and this tragic history continues to affect the lives of Black persons today. Deep distrust of a healthcare system that exploited Black persons continues. Two notable but certainly not the only examples of exploitation are the U.S. Public Health Service Syphilis Study at Tuskegee, and the unrestricted use without permission of cell lines of Henrietta Lacks, a Black woman who died at age 31 of an aggressive adenocarcinoma of the cervix; both are examples of exploitation that continue to foment distrust. The COVID-19 pandemic disproportionately affected the Black population in the U.S., a function of medical mistrust based not simply on the exploitation at Tuskegee and that of Lacks, but of higher infant and maternal mortality, disparate cancer care and HIV care, and care of those with substance abuse disorders (The Commonwealth Fund, 2021).

In 2018, 44.8 million persons—13.7% of the U.S. population—were foreign born (Pew Research Center, 2020). The first decade of the 21st century in the United States was characterized by significant immigration, and by 2017, ~18% of the total US population was Hispanic, a population with a diverse heritage (Pew Research Center, 2020). People immigrating from other nations bring a wealth of values, health beliefs, and practices, and may find assimilation into U.S. culture daunting. Some persons who immigrate prefer to preserve their own cultural heritage while living in the U.S.

The exact number of persons in the various racial/ethnic groups is difficult to pinpoint. Identifying by race or ethnicity does not necessarily capture a complete picture of the many different cultures represented by persons who immigrate to the United States. The concept of race and ethnicity as used by the U.S. Census Bureau depends on "self-identification by respondents; that is, the individual's perception of his/her racial identity" (U.S. Bureau of the Census, 2021). The U.S. Census Bureau is required to adhere to the Office of

Management and Budget's (OMB's) 1997 regulations in classifying race (U.S. Bureau of the Census, 2021). The minimum number of categories allowable by the OMB are White, Black or African American, American Indian or Alaska Native, Asian, and Native Hawaiian or Other Pacific Islander. People who identify themselves as Hispanic, Latino, or Spanish may be of any race, according to the U.S. Census Bureau (U.S. Bureau of the Census, 2020). People may report being of more than one race. Information on race and ethnicity is critical in policy decision making, including congressional redistricting, civil rights legislation, and promotion of equal employment opportunities. Particularly important to health care is the ability to assess health disparities and environmental risk (CDC, 2020). The next census in 2030 will likely show significant shifts in race and ethnicity statistics in the United States.

Projections indicate that the White population will become a minority by the middle of the 21st century. This represents a significant change in the historical demographics and attitudes of the nation, with important implications. Nursing must also change to meet the requirements of persons of varying ethnicities and cultural responses to health and illness. Certain illnesses and health conditions occur disparately across race, ethnicity, and sex. The changing demographic profile of the U.S. population will continue to pose a significant challenge to nursing in order to ensure a diverse workforce that is responsive to the differing needs across communities and populations.

Diversity in the Profession

To meet the challenge of an increasingly diverse population entering the healthcare system, nurses need to be educated to be aware and respectful of cultural differences between themselves and their patients and among their patients. The language of cultural education has varied over time, from "cultural competence" to "cultural sensitivity" to a more recent phrase, "cultural humility." This is the view that one understands that they cannot be competent in another's culture, but can take a posture of willingness to learn about practices and preferences of other cultures from those who are of the culture. Nurses are, compared with the general population, disproportionately White. (This is presented in detail in Chapter 1.) This represents an opportunity for schools of nursing to recruit and educate nurses of a wide variety of cultural backgrounds. Attention to the development of nurses who are attuned to culture and cultural differences has become an integral part of progressive nursing education programs. Issues of culture are discussed in detail in Chapter 13.

Technological Developments

The word *technology* seems to be everywhere today and has a place in many domains in health care. For purposes of this basic introduction, four types of technological developments will be presented: genetic, biomedical, information, and knowledge.

Genetics, *genomics*, and *epigenetics* are three important words that have shaped and will continue to shape health care for the foreseeable future. Genetics is the science of heredity, and genomics is the study of genomes: DNA sequences. Epigenetics is an important field of study: the examination of the causes of changes in phenotypes or gene expressions not explained by the underlying DNA sequence. The Human Genome Project was a study funded by the National Institutes of Health in which the 20,000 to 25,000 genes on the human genome were mapped out. This took 13 years. The data from the Human Genome Project will continue to have a significant effect on our understanding of health and illness, and on predicting who is likely to develop certain conditions, and when.

Pharmacogenetics will have a significant effect on nursing practice eventually, in which the mechanisms and actions of medications can be determined by their genetic structures. This will mean that medications can be prescribed that will be more effective than those that are given generically. For example, advances are being made in chemotherapy for certain cancers, such as leukemias and lymphomas, in which methylation that occurs at the gene level causes the expression of the genes to be aberrant—that is, to go wrong—leading to the development of malignant cell growth. Certain drugs used to treat these cancers are "hypomethylating" agents that reverse the increased ("hyper") methylation occurring in the cells' genetic material.

Biomedical technology involves complex machines or implantable devices used in patient care settings for a variety of reasons; for example, pacemakers, internal automated defibrillators, insulin pumps, artificial organs, and various invasive monitoring systems such as those used to measure intracranial pressure. This form of technology affects nursing practice because nurses assume responsibility for monitoring data generated from these machines and for assessing the safety and effectiveness of implantable equipment in relation to patient well-being. Nurses are as a matter of safe practice required to react to data being generated and respond accordingly. An important consideration in nursing when working in a high-tech environment: there is a "human in there" under all of the lines and monitors. The human touch and a word of reassurance are comforting to your patient, and no technology can replace you. Family members usually need help distinguishing monitoring equipment from those technologies supporting the patient's basic functions, such as a ventilator. Showing them what you are reading and seeing can be reassuring to them at a time when families are in a great deal of distress. During the pandemic, this was taken to a level previously not seen in wide use: nurses used video technologies in ICUs to help family members unable to visit their sick loved ones because of COVID restrictions. Sometimes these video calls meant that family members and friends were saying their goodbyes to a dying person at a time when they would otherwise have gathered at the bedside as their loved one died. Nurses proved over and over again to be conduits of human caring for families at these raw and tender moments that were never what anyone would have wanted at the point of their dying.

IT refers to a variety of computer-based applications used to communicate, store, manage, retrieve, and process information. Nurses assumed much of the responsibility for entry and retrieval of data with the development of this technology. Computers are common on nursing units and at the bedside, and with the Centers for Medicare and Medicaid Services' "meaningful use" initiative, most hospitals have moved to electronic health records, as described in Chapter 1. One goal in healthcare reform included going "paperless"; that is, that all medical prescriptions, patient records, and other documents will be digitally stored and available for convenient transmittal across various record systems and healthcare facilities. Any other care provider can access data at any time, as opposed to the single hard copy chart that only one person can view or use at a time.

In some healthcare organizations, nursing information systems are handheld, allowing nurses to enter and access data about the patient directly from the patient's side, whether in an inpatient, outpatient, or home setting. This type of technology allows for more timely documentation of care, and because documentation is done at the time of care, the information is likely to be more accurate. This convenience can come at the expense of patient privacy, and the privacy and confidentiality of patient information are critical ethical and legal issues. The Health Insurance Portability and Accountability Act (HIPAA) of 1996 is legislation designed to protect patients' healthcare information from misuse. A more complete discussion of HIPAA's provisions is found in Chapter 6.

Knowledge technology is described as "technology of the mind." It involves the use of computer systems to transform information into knowledge and to generate new knowledge. Through the creation of expert systems, this form of technology assists nurses with clinical judgments about patient management problems. An example of knowledge technology includes medication administration systems that prompt the nurse for data before giving a particular medication. Nurse clinicians and nurse leaders should have a significant role in developing these mechanisms to maximize their effectiveness in improving nursing care and patient outcomes.

In addition, sophisticated human simulation mannequins are gaining popularity in schools of nursing (Fig. 2.12). They make it possible to simulate a

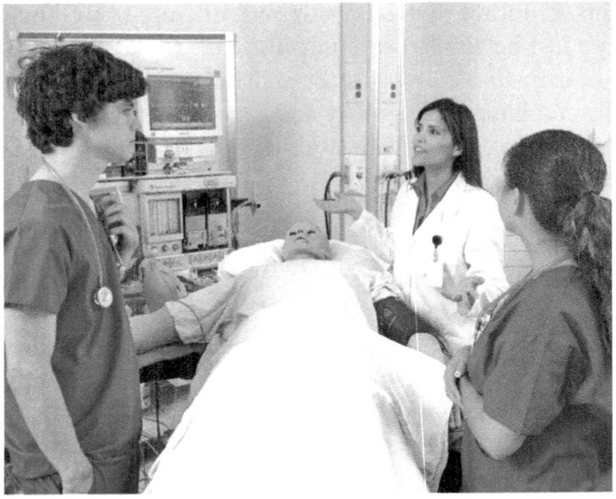

Fig. 2.12 Advances in simulation technology have enhanced clinical decision making. Here students use a human simulator in a laboratory setting to refine their skills. (Photo courtesy the UNC at Chapel Hill School of Nursing.)

clinical event such as cardiac arrest, pneumothorax, or childbirth, allowing the student to practice clinical assessment and intervention skills. One of the benefits of computerized expert systems is that they can provide practice in decision making for novice nurses and nurses who may be working outside their area of expertise without increased risk to a patient. Simulation training is common in other professions such as aviation where the stakes are very high in the event of a mistake. Learning to manage crises in simulated situations allows a person to become confident in his or her skills and accustomed to working under pressure without the risk of harm.

As technology becomes more pervasive, nurses must be very intentional in providing compassionate, personalized care for patients. Technological advances such as telehealth allow nurses to interact with and assess their patients remotely. Without even seeing the patient in person, nurses can gather large amounts of data and make nursing decisions based on that information. As nurses rely more on technology, they may actually spend less time with the patient, with the possibility of creating dissatisfaction for patients and families. Although being able to monitor one's patient on a telemetry unit from the nurses' station is convenient and practical, continuous monitoring of a contraction pattern and fetal heart rate from the nurses' station in a labor and birth suite diminishes the nurse's role to one of labor and fetal surveillance rather than labor support. The use of technology must be applied carefully and never take the place of human-to-human contact and interaction. Successfully combining technology and caring requires specific attention to patients' physical, emotional, and spiritual needs.

Nursing Shortages

Periodic imbalances are not uncommon between the numbers of nurses working and the number of available nursing positions. Over many decades, there have been rare, brief periods of oversupply of nurses and more frequent and longer-lasting nursing shortages. By far the more common concern is an inadequate supply of RNs to meet the healthcare needs of the nation.

The term *nursing shortage* can be misleading because actual shortages are usually confined to institutional settings such as hospitals and nursing homes. Causes of shortages may be seen as either external or internal. Internal causes include inadequate pay, long hours, increased responsibility for unlicensed workers, and significant responsibility with little authority. External causes include changes in demand for nursing services, the increasing age of the American population, greater acuity (degree of illness) of hospitalized individuals, and the public perceptions of nursing as a profession.

A key aspect of recent nursing shortages is the shortage of nursing faculty. Qualified applicants are often denied admission to U.S. schools of nursing because of insufficient numbers of faculty, clinical sites, and classroom space. Faculty shortages are attributed to several factors. First, doctorally prepared and master's degree–prepared faculty are now, on average, more than 50 years of age, foreshadowing a large number of retirements in the next decade. Second, nurses with advanced degrees who are otherwise eligible for faculty appointments are being hired into more lucrative private sector or clinical positions. Third, not enough doctorate- and master's-level graduates are being produced to meet the demands of nursing education. The American Association of Colleges of Nursing (AACN) continues to search for remedies for this situation (AACN, 2021).

In the past, when a shortage of RNs became serious, two solutions were attempted: (1) increase the supply of nurses, and (2) create a role requiring less training to supplement the number of nurses. Practical nursing programs that are completed in 1 year were created to meet civilian and military needs of the United States during World War II. The nursing shortage of the 1950s gave rise to 2-year associate degree (ADN) programs. In the 1960s, shortages led to the creation of the position of unit manager; this manager was expected to take over certain tasks to relieve nurses, who could then concentrate on providing patient care. The 1970s produced other new positions, such as emergency medical technicians, respiratory therapists, and others who took on various aspects of patient care formerly performed by nurses. The shortage of nurses in the late 1980s resulted in a proposal by the American Medical Association to create yet another "nurse extender" called the *registered care technician*. However, this initiative was short-lived when nurses responded quickly and negatively, with nurse leaders stating that nurses could not be responsible for direct caregivers that nurses had not trained.

Another method of increasing the supply of nurses is to encourage immigration from other English-speaking countries. Nurses from the United Kingdom, Australia, New Zealand, certain Caribbean islands, South Africa, and the Philippines have been targeted for recruitment. Companies have been established to prepare them to take the National Council Licensure Examination for Registered Nurses (NCLEX-RN®) successfully to practice in this country. The ethics of this solution are addressed in Chapter 7.

Shortages are often limited to certain geographic areas or specialties. In those cases, redistributing RNs who are already licensed may be seen as a solution, and many hospitals use agencies to provide nurses for short-term assignments. These nurses often called *traveling nurses* or *travelers*. In fact, the acute nursing shortage wrought by the overwhelming number of patients during the COVID pandemic required some hospitals to lean heavily on this solution. Travel nursing can provide individual nurses with opportunities to live in and experience different parts of the country and world, but little incentive exists for traveling nurses to work toward long-term goals on the units where they are, for all practical purposes, filling in until a nurse can be hired permanently.

Explaining why there is a shortage is complex. Like many issues in nursing, there is no simple explanation. What is known is that the shortage exists and is more crucial in traditional settings such as hospitals and long-term care facilities. A significant reason for shortages of nurses is that there is a shortage of nursing faculty, as mentioned earlier, because nurses with advanced degrees may find more lucrative positions in the private sector or in clinical settings. Schools of nursing report turning away thousands of otherwise qualifying candidates each year because of constraints on the number of students per faculty member in clinical settings, and even the availability of adequate numbers of clinical settings for a large number of students.

Additionally, nurses are in increased demand because of the growth in total population, especially an aging population with extensive healthcare needs. The shortage is also compounded by the fact that the nursing workforce is aging, and the number of new entrants to the profession may not keep pace with the numbers who are exiting.

Initiatives to Provide a Stable Workforce of Registered Nurses

Recognizing that dramatic swings in the supply of and demand for RNs harm the profession, jeopardize patient care, and are costly to nurses and their employers, organizations inside and outside of nursing have called for mechanisms to ensure more even distribution of the workforce. Here are four major initiatives that made or are making an impact on the nursing workforce:

1. The American Recovery and Reinvestment Act of 2009, the goal of which was to stimulate the U.S. economy, had a provision for $500 million to strengthen the U.S. healthcare workforce. This included the training and education of the next generation of nurses and physicians.
2. The Robert Wood Johnson Foundation (RWJF), a private foundation that funds innovative healthcare initiatives, committed tens of millions of dollars to pursuing programs that help nursing schools, hospitals, and other healthcare agencies create regional workforce development systems. This initiative was named Colleagues in Caring.
3. Corporate support of nursing was mentioned earlier. For example, Johnson & Johnson is working in partnership with the National Student Nurses Association (NSNA), the NLN, the ANA, the Association of Nurse Executives (AONE), and the STTI Honor Society of Nursing.
4. The ANCC Magnet Recognition Program is a model for employers to earn the designation "employer of choice" by implementing a model program designed to attract and retain nurses in acute hospital settings.

Nursing faces numerous challenges related to today's social context. Yet in the history of nursing, nurses have risen to the challenges they face, improving the terrible conditions in war, developing public health initiatives, and becoming proactive in shaping their public image. The challenges to the upcoming generation of nurses may be completely unforeseen, such as the HIV epidemic that challenged nurses in the 1980s, and the COVID-19 pandemic of the 2020s. Nurses have confronted the challenges of yesterday and today with ingenuity and intelligence and have set the stage for the next generation to continue this legacy.

CONCEPTS AND CHALLENGES

- ***Concept:*** In 1860 Florence Nightingale founded a school for nurses at St. Thomas' Hospital, London, which became the model for nursing education in the United States. Formal nursing education programs were established in the United States in 1873.
  Challenge: Nursing must continue to evolve in response to its social context. This means that nursing education must continue to evolve.
- ***Concept:*** The period between the 1893 World's Fair and 1908 marked a time of organizing for nurses, including the formation of forerunners of the NLN and the ANA.
  Challenge: The evolution of the profession depends on visionary nurses taking leadership roles now and in the future.
- ***Concept:*** The initiation of state licensure in 1903 meant that nursing education programs would be standardized. Until then, nursing education varied widely.
  Challenge: With the rapid evolution of nursing practice opportunities, consistent, thorough education is particularly important.
- ***Concept:*** The establishment of the Henry Street Settlement and the rise of community health nursing played a major role in the widespread public acceptance of nurses.
  Challenge: Remembering that nursing has led significant social changes in the past, we can draw inspiration and guidance from the work of nurses such as Lillian Wald, who faced tremendous challenges to care for persons who had immigrated, those who were living in poverty, had substandard living conditions, and whose health was poor, with little access to health care.
- ***Concept:*** Nursing has responded to wars, epidemics/pandemics, and economic disasters that created a high demand for nursing care. Hospital expansion, technological advances, and social changes have created new and progressively autonomous roles for nurses, especially advanced practice nurses.
  Challenge: The profession of nursing must remain vigilant for new, promising spheres of practice.
- ***Concept:*** The nursing shortage is projected to increase again.
  Challenge: Identifying and responding to the cause of shortages, such as the shortage of nursing faculty, will require the attention of nurse leaders.
- ***Concept:*** New data suggest that men in nursing earn more than $7,300 more per year than do women, regardless of setting, specialty, or position.
  Challenge: Nurse leaders and employers must act to correct the injustice of pay inequity.
- ***Concept:*** Nurses have been stereotyped in the media, which has resulted in misperceptions and lack of clarity by the public about what nurses do and their importance in health care.
  Challenge: Individual nurses must act when nursing is presented in an unfavorable light in the media. Responsibility for the image of the profession belongs to all nurses.

IDEAS FOR FURTHER EXPLORATION

1. Florence Nightingale is often credited with being the first nurse researcher. What were her contributions to the science of nursing?
2. Consider the significance of the events that occurred during the Chicago World's Fair, 1893, to the advancement of the nursing profession. What would nurse leaders address today if they were to hold a leadership summit across all domains of the profession?
3. Think about the role the military had in opening the profession of nursing for Black persons and other minority populations, including men. Why did nursing require military conflicts to expand entry into the profession to persons other than White women?
4. How has being a profession in which most practitioners are women influenced the development of nursing?
5. What do you think accounts for the documented pay inequity between women and men in nursing? What challenges do you think nursing leaders and employers should take to correct pay inequity?
6. Describe your idea of the "perfect" nurse. What stereotypes does your description reveal? Does your image of the perfect nurse include a particular gender, race, ethnic group, or generation?
7. Think about social factors that have the potential to stimulate or stifle interest in nursing as a profession. What effects—positive and negative—could these factors have on nursing? What recommendations do you have for the profession to address these factors?

REFERENCES

American Association of Colleges of Nursing (AACN): *Data spotlight: insights on the nursing faculty shortage*, 2021 (website). Available at: https://www.aacnnursing.org/News-Information/News/View/ArticleId/25043/data-spotlight-august-2021-Nursing-Faculty-Shortage.

American Association for Men in Nursing (AAMN): *Purpose and objectives*, 2021. (website). Available at: www.aamn.org.

Barton C: *Diary: The papers of Clara Barton (1812–1912)*, Washington, DC, 1862, Library of Congress Manuscript Division.

Carnegie ME: *The path we tread: Blacks in nursing*, Philadelphia, 1995, JB Lippincott, pp 1854–1994.

Centers for Disease Control and Prevention: (website). In National vital statistics reports, 2020. Available at https://www.cdc.gov/nchs/data/nvsr/nvsr69/nvsr69-12-508.pdf.

Dock LL, Stewart IM: *A Short History of Nursing*, New York, 1920, Putnam.

Donahue MP: *Nursing: the finest art: an illustrated history*, ed 2, Philadelphia, 1996, Mosby.

Donelan K, Buerhaus PI, Ulrich BT, et al.: Awareness and perceptions of the Johnson & Johnson Campaign for Nursing's Future: Views from nursing students, RNs, and CNOs, *Nurs Econ* 23(4):150–156, 2005.

Gill CJ, Gill GC: Nightingale in Scutari: her legacy reexamined, *Clin Infect Dis* 40(12):1799–1805, 2005.

Howard University: *History of the Freedmen's Hospital School of Nursing, 1974*, 2021 (website). Available at https://dh.howard.edu/cgi/viewcontent.cgi?article=1001&context=fhsn_pub.

Johnson & Johnson: *Johnson & Johnson Nursing*, 2021 (website). Available at: nursing.jnj.com.

Kalisch PA, Kalisch BJ: *American nursing : a history*, ed 4, Philadelphia, PA, 2004, Lippincott Williams & Wilkins.

Kennedy D: *Birth control in America: the career of Margaret Sanger*, New Haven, CT, 1970, Yale University Press.

Mary Seacole Trust: *Read Mary's Story*, 2021 (website). Available at: https://www.maryseacoletrust.org.uk/learn-about-mary/#.

Miller HS: *America's first Black professional nurse*, Atlanta, 1986, Wright Publishing.

news.gallup.com: *Nurses continue to rate highest in honest, ethics*, 2020 (website). Available at: https://news.gallup.com/poll/274673/nurses-continue-rate-highest-honesty-ethics.aspx.

Nightingale F: *Notes on nursing: what it is and what it is not*, London, 1859, Harrison and Sons. Reprinted e-book #17366, Project Gutenberg, 2005 (website). Available at: https://www.gutenberg.org/cache/epub/17366/pg17366-images.html.

nursejournal.org: *The gender pay gap in nursing 2021*, 2021. Available at: https://nursejournal.org/resources/the-gender-pay-gap-in-nursing/.

Oates SB: *A woman of valor*, New York, 1994, The Free Press.

100 Great Black Britons: *100 Great Black Britons*, 2015 (website). Available at: www.100greatblackbritons.com.

Palmer S: The editor, *Am J Nurs* 1(1):64, 1900.

Pember PY: *A southern woman's story*, Atlanta, 1959, Bill Wiley.

Pew Research Center: *Facts on U.S. immigrants, 2018*, 2020 (website). Available at https://www.pewresearch.org/hispanic/2020/08/20/facts-on-u-s-immigrants/.

Planned Parenthood: *Opposition claims about Margaret Sanger*, 2021 (website). Available at: https://www.plannedparenthood.org/uploads/filer_public/cc/2e/cc2e84f2-126f-41a5-a24b-43e093c47b2c/210414-sanger-opposition-claims-p01.pdf.

policyadvice.net: *27+ Affordable Care Act statistics and facts*, 2021 (website). Available at: https://policyadvice.net/insurance/insights/affordable-care-act-statistics/.

Seacole M: *Wonderful Adventures of Mrs. Seacole in Many Lands*, London, 1857, W.J.S. Reprinted e-book #23031, Project Gutenberg, 2007 (website). Available at: https://www.gutenberg.org/cache/epub/23031/pg23031-images.html.

Sigma Theta Tau International (STTI): *The Woodhull study on nursing and the media: health care's invisible partner*, Indianapolis, 1998, Sigma Theta Tau International–Center Nursing Press.

Sleet J: A successful experiment, *Am J Nurs*, 1901 2(729).

The Commonwealth Fund: *Understanding and ameliorating medical mistrust among Black Americans*, 2021 (website). Available at: https://www.commonwealthfund.org/publications/newsletter-article/2021/jan/medical-mistrust-among-black-americans.

Truth about nursing: *Mission statement*, 2018 (website). Available at www.truthaboutnursing.org.

U.S. Bureau of the Census: *Race*, 2021 (website). Available at https://www.census.gov/topics/population/race/about.html.

U.S. Bureau of the Census: *2020 Census Results*, 2020 (website). Available at https://www.census.gov/programs-surveys/decennial-census/decade/2020/2020-census-results.html.

Wall BM: Courage to care: the Sisters of the Holy Cross in the Spanish-American War, *Nurs Hist Rev* 3:55–77, 1995.

3

Nursing's Pathway to Professionalism

ⓔ To enhance your understanding of this chapter, try the Student Exercises on the Evolve site at http://evolve.elsevier.com/Black/professional.

LEARNING OUTCOMES

After studying this chapter, students will be able to:

- Identify the characteristics of a profession.
- Distinguish between the characteristics of professions and occupations.
- Describe how professions evolve.
- Identify barriers to nursing's development as a profession.
- Explain the elements of nursing's contract with society.
- Recognize characteristic behaviors that exemplify professional nurses.
- Assess themselves in the development of professional conduct.

The word *professional* shows up in everyday conversation and in the media. A professional athlete is one who is paid and is no longer considered an amateur. A professional stunt actor is one whose dangerous activities should not be "tried at home," according to warning messages at the bottom of your monitor or TV screen. Job seekers are encouraged to "look professional" when applying for a position. Services such as dry cleaning, lawn care, and plumbing are often referred to as "professional" when they are rendered by someone with specific expertise or tools of their trade.

Historically, physic (medicine), law, and divinity (clergy) were considered "learned professions." Over time, however, the meaning of *profession* has expanded to include other domains of work and career, including nursing. You will learn in this chapter various characteristics of a profession and how nursing fits those characteristics. Furthermore, you will learn what **professionalism** means generally and what professionalism in nursing means specifically.

CHARACTERISTICS OF A PROFESSION

For nearly a century, scholars have grappled with the meaning of **profession**. They have generally agreed that a profession is an occupational group with a set of attitudes or behaviors, or both. In the early 1900s the Carnegie Foundation issued a series of papers about professional schools. In 1910 Abraham Flexner, a sociologist, published what became groundbreaking work for reform in medical education, calling on medical schools to implement high standards for admission and graduation and to follow long-accepted tenets of science in teaching and research (Flexner, 1910). Five years after his initial report, Flexner published a list of criteria that he believed were characteristic of all true professions (Flexner, 1915). These criteria stipulate that a profession:

1. Is basically intellectual (as opposed to physical) and is accompanied by a high degree of individual responsibility.

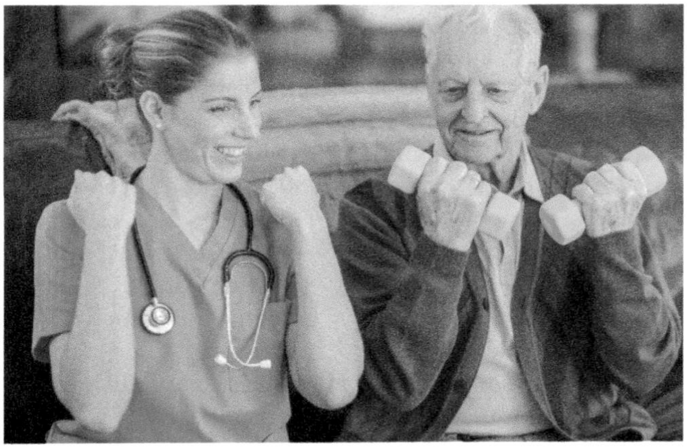

Fig. 3.1 According to experts, professionals are motivated by *altruism,* a desire to help others. (Photo used with permission from iStockphoto.)

2. Is based on a body of knowledge that can be learned and is developed and refined through research.
3. Is both practical and theoretical.
4. Can be taught through a process of highly specialized professional education.
5. Has a strong internal organization of members and a well-developed group consciousness.
6. Has practitioners who are motivated by altruism (the desire to help others) and who are responsive to public interests (Fig. 3.1).

Since the 1910 report was published, Flexner's criteria have been widely used as the benchmark for determining the professional status of various occupations and have had a profound influence on professional education in several disciplines, including nursing. In 1968 R. H. Hall, a sociologist, published his work on professionalism. Similar to Flexner's criteria, Hall (1968) described a professional model with five attributes of professions:

1. Use of a professional organization as a primary point of reference
2. Belief in the value of public service
3. Belief in self-regulation
4. Commitment to a profession that goes beyond economic incentives
5. A sense of autonomy in practice

Recognizing the uniqueness of disciplines, Hall (1968) recommended each profession develop its own methods of measuring professionalism. In recent years, individuals and groups have continued to identify what professionals believe, think, and do. In the 1990s a pharmacy profession task force spent 5 years studying and promoting pharmacy student professionalism (Task Force on Professionalism, 2000). This task force, in examining the history of professional development in a broad sense, reviewed the work of numerous scholars. From this review, they found that members of a profession share the following 10 characteristics:

1. Prolonged specialized training in a body of abstract knowledge
2. A service orientation
3. An ideology based on the original faith professed by members
4. An ethic that is binding on the practitioners
5. A body of knowledge unique to the members
6. A set of skills that forms the technique of the profession
7. A guild of those entitled to practice the profession
8. Authority granted by society in the form of licensure or certification
9. A recognized setting in which the profession is practiced
10. A theory of societal benefits derived from the ideology

Although scholars have not always agreed on the number of criteria and the types of behaviors and characteristics of professions, three criteria consistently appear: service/altruism, specialized knowledge, and autonomy/ethics (Carr-Saunders and Wilson, 1933; Flexner, 1915; Hall, 1968, 1982; Huber, 2000).

FROM OCCUPATION TO PROFESSION

The distinction between an occupation and a profession is not always clear. The term occupation is often used to mean "profession"; for example, the Collins English Dictionary (2021) defines *occupation* as "[one's] job or profession," inferring that occupation is a more encompassing term than profession. In this discussion, Huber's (2000) definition of *profession* is used to make the distinction between an occupation and a profession: "a calling, vocation, or form of employment that provides a needed service to society and possesses characteristics of expertise, autonomy, long academic preparation, commitment, and responsibility" (p. 34).

Professions usually evolved from occupations that originally consisted of tasks but developed more specialized educational pathways and publicly legitimized status. The earliest recognized "learned" professions (law, medicine, and divinity) generally followed a sequential development. First, practitioners of these professions performed full-time work in the discipline. They then determined work standards, identified a body of knowledge, and established educational programs in institutions of higher learning. Next, they promoted organization into effective occupational associations and then worked to establish legal protection that limited practice of their unique skills by outsiders. Finally, they established codes of ethics (Carr-Saunders and Wilson, 1933). This is the process known as professionalization.

The evolution from occupation to profession was further analyzed by Houle (1980), who identified a number of characteristics that indicate that an occupational group is moving along the continuum toward professional status. Defining the group's mission and foundations of practice is the first step, followed by mastery of theoretical knowledge, development of the capacity to solve problems, use of practical knowledge, and self-enhancement (continued learning and development). Finally, Houle described the necessity of the development of a collective identity as an occupation evolves into a profession. Signs of a developing collective identity, and hence a profession, include formal training, credentialing, creation of a subculture, legal right to practice, public acceptance, ethical practice, discipline of incompetent/unethical practitioners, relationship to other practitioners, and formalization of the relationship of practitioners of the profession to users of the practitioners' services.

In an analysis of the concept of professionalism in nursing, Ghadirian and colleagues (2014) determined three attributes of professionalism. First, through nursing education, nurses develop a cognitive framework to understand the profession of nursing, including how and why to conduct oneself in a professional manner, with the goal of learning to prioritize and make decisions correctly in practice. This suggests that nursing education should be consistent across formal settings for entry to practice education. Second, nurses acquire professional values (beliefs and ideals) that are consistent across individuals and groups and continue to develop these values through experiences shaping one's professional identity. Third, standards of practice and psychomotor competencies are requirements of professionalism in nursing. Common descriptors of professional behavior were *safety* and *competency*.

Professional Preparation

A profession is different from an occupation in at least two major ways—preparation and commitment (Table 3.1). Professional preparation, typically taking place in a college or university, requires instruction in the specialized body of knowledge and techniques of the profession. In addition to knowledge and skills, professional preparation includes orientation to the beliefs, values, attitudes expected of the members of the profession, as well as the standards of practice and ethical considerations. These components of professional education are part of the process of socialization into a profession and are discussed in more detail in Chapter 5. This intense preparation enables professional practitioners to act in a logical, rational manner using scientific knowledge and prescribed ways of thinking through problems rather than relying on simple problem solving, custom, intuition, or trial and error. The nursing process, described in detail in Chapter 11, is an example of how the profession of nursing uses scientific knowledge and prescribed ways of thinking through patient problems amenable to nursing care.

Professional Commitment

Professionals are usually highly committed to their work, deriving much of their personal identification from it, and consider it an integral part of their lives; some people even refer to their profession as their "calling" (Fig. 3.2). Historically, professionals' commitment to their profession has transcended their expectation of material reward. The

TABLE 3.1 Comparing Occupations and Professions

Occupation	Profession
Training may occur on the job.	Education takes place in a college or university.
Length of training varies.	Education is prolonged.
Work is largely manual.	Work involves mental creativity.
Decision making is guided largely by experience or by trial and error.	Decision making is based largely on science or theoretical constructs (evidence-based practice).
Values, beliefs, and ethics are not prominent features of preparation.	Values, beliefs, and ethics are an integral part of preparation.
Commitment and personal identification vary.	Commitment and personal identification are strong.
Workers are supervised.	Workers are autonomous.
People often change jobs.	People are unlikely to change professions.
Material reward is main motivation.	Commitment transcends material reward.
Accountability rests primarily with employer.	Accountability rests with individual.

strong identity that professionals develop means that it is less common for them to change careers compared with persons involved in occupations, which may not involve such a strong commitment and identity.

Interprofessionality

Educators across health care professions have recognized the importance of the development of core competencies for their students (and future practitioners) in response to initiatives calling for more teamwork across disciplines and team-based care. *Interprofessionality* is a "process by which professionals reflect on and develop ways of practicing that provides an integrated and cohesive answer to the needs of the client/family/population … [involving] continuous interaction and knowledge sharing between professionals" (D'Amour and Oandasan, 2005, p. 9). The World Health Organization (WHO) noted that in the current global climate, "it is no longer enough for health workers to be professional …. [They] also need to be interprofessional" (World Health Organization, 2010, p. 36). A report by the Interprofessional Education Collaborative Expert Panel (2011) identified four domains of interprofessional collaborative practice competency:

1. Values/ethics for interprofessional practice
2. Roles/responsibilities
3. Interprofessional communication
4. Teams and teamwork

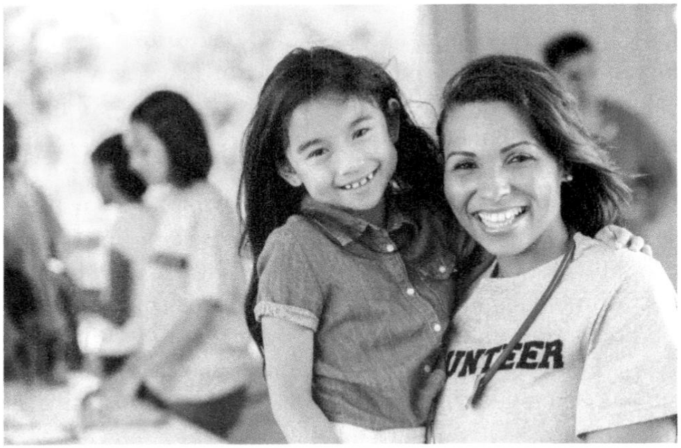

Fig. 3.2 Nurses often put their skills to use as volunteers as part of their strong commitment to their profession and to helping others. (Photo used with permission from iStockphoto.)

The National Academy of Medicine (2015), in a robust effort to ensure optimal patient outcomes, challenged American healthcare educators and providers to expand the traditional view of separate professional foci and to consider alternate ways of shaping education and models of care. Interprofessional education (IPE) across disciplines such as nursing, medicine, social work, pharmacy, and others has gained significant momentum. Although IPE is receiving increasing emphasis in health educational settings, there is a current gap in practice that will depend on the development of a workforce for which IPE has provided with skills and knowledge to address the health needs of individuals and communities (Derouin et al., 2018).

NURSING'S PATHWAY TO PROFESSIONALISM

The question of whether nursing is a profession was debated for decades. In the mid-20th century, Roy Bixler and Genevieve Bixler examined nursing's status as a profession. Bixler and Bixler, neither of whom were nurses but both of whom were advocates and supporters of nursing, used seven criteria that are similar to those listed earlier in this chapter. In 1959 they reappraised nursing, noting progress in nursing's professional development (Bixler and Bixler, 1959). More recently, nurse leaders, rather than those outside of nursing, have explored the professionalization of nursing.

Kelly's Criteria

Lucie Kelly, PhD, RN, FAAN, is an accomplished nurse writer, teacher, and influential leader. Now retired from Columbia University, Kelly was editor of the journal *Nursing Outlook* and president of Sigma Theta Tau International, among many career highlights. Dr. Kelly spent much of her nursing career exploring the dimensions of professional nursing. Although she compiled the following set of eight characteristics of a profession many years ago, contemporary nursing still embodies these characteristics (Kelly, 1981, p. 157):

1. The services provided are vital to humanity and the welfare of society.
2. There is a special body of knowledge that is continually enlarged through research.
3. The services involve intellectual activities; individual responsibility (accountability) is a strong feature.
4. Practitioners are educated in institutions of higher learning.
5. Practitioners are relatively independent and control their own policies and activities (autonomy).
6. Practitioners are motivated by service (altruism) and consider their work an important component of their lives.
7. There is a code of ethics to guide the decisions and conduct of practitioners.
8. There is an organization (association) that encourages and supports high standards of practice.

Services Vital to Humanity and the Welfare of Society

If you ask nursing students why they want to become nurses, the most likely answer would be "to help people." You yourself may have included a statement like this in your application to nursing school. Nursing provides services that are essential to the well-being of people and to society as a whole. The word *services*, however, minimizes the essence of nursing; caring is the core of professional nursing, shaping the way that nurses interact with and intervene on behalf of their patients. Nursing interventions in the most general sense are the "services" nurses provide. Nursing is essential in today's world, providing vital care to humanity and the welfare of society.

Special Body of Knowledge Enlarging through Research

Nursing has an increasingly well-developed body of knowledge. Nursing has its own doctor of philosophy (PhD), a research degree earned by nurses at the highest levels of education. Through research, the specialized body of knowledge for nursing is developed. In the past, nurse researchers often had PhDs from other academic disciplines, and nursing science was based on principles borrowed from the physical and social sciences. As opposed to practice based in problem-solving earlier in our history, the basis for current nursing practice is theory and research. One of the key principles of evidence-based practice is the use of research evidence. You will learn more about theory, research, and evidence-based practice in later chapters.

Services Involve Intellectual Activities and Feature Individual Responsibility (Accountability)

Nursing is a cognitive (mental) activity that requires both critical and creative thinking and serves as the basis for providing nursing care. Nursing developed and refined its own unique approach to practice, called the *nursing process.* (You will learn more about the nursing process in Chapter 11.)

Individual accountability in nursing has become a hallmark of practice. Accountability, according to the American Nurses Association's (ANA's) *Code of Ethics for Nurses*, is being answerable to someone for something one has done. Provision 4 of the Code states, "The nurse has authority, accountability, and responsibility for nursing practice. Makes decisions; and takes action consistent with the obligation to promote health and to provide optimal care" (ANA, 2015, p. 15). Furthermore, accountability is firmly rooted in the ethical principles of "fidelity (faithfulness), loyalty, veracity, beneficence, and respect for the dignity, worth, and self-determination of patients" (p. 15).

Education Occurs in Institutions of Higher Learning

The first university-based nursing program began in 1909 at the University of Minnesota. Three decades later, Esther Lucille Brown (1948) wrote *Nursing for the Future,* calling for nursing education to be based in universities and colleges. In 1965 the ANA published a significant position paper, taking the official position that all nursing education should take place in institutions of higher education (ANA, 1965).

The debate about entry level into practice continues. Despite the ANA's long-held position, only recently has the number of graduates of Bachelor of Science in Nursing (BSN) programs been greater than those of associate's degree in nursing (ADN) programs, and increasing numbers of registered nurses (RNs) with ADN degrees are returning to colleges and universities to earn their BSN degree. (Chapter 1 introduced you to recent legislation signed into law in New York requiring RNs to earn a BSN in the next 10 years). In addition, the number of nurses prepared at the master's and doctoral levels continues to increase, although that number is small compared with other health professions.

Practitioners Are Relatively Independent and Control Their Own Policies and Activities (Autonomy)

Licensure by state boards of nursing means that nurses are autonomous practitioners who are responsible for their own practice. *Autonomy* means that one has control over one's practice. Although nursing actions are independent, most RNs are employed in settings in which nurses carry out prescriptions for care or medical regimens by physicians, nurse practitioners, or physician assistants (PAs). Recently nurses who understand that language matters have criticized the use of the phrase "doctor's orders": the word *orders* connotes obedience and thus has outlived its usefulness (Reuter and Fitzsimons, 2013). Although nursing practice acts in many states establish and acknowledge nurses' independent practice, nurses occasionally face constraints on practice in settings in which their scope of practice can be narrowed (but never expanded) by their employer or a supervising physician.

Three groups have historically attempted to control nursing practice: organized nursing, organized medicine, and health service administration. *Organized* in this context refers to the collective professional bodies that are the voice speaking for the interests of their respective professions, specifically the ANA and the American Medical Association (AMA), although other organizations have vested interests in these professions too. The interests of these groups are often expressed through lobbying efforts at the state and federal levels to influence legislative decisions that benefit their constituencies. Organizations such as National Nurses United (NNU) and its affiliates use collective bargaining and other strategies to protect the interests of nurses and patients. Although the discussion of nursing unionization is beyond the scope of this chapter, you will find the NNU website (www.nationalnursesunited.org) to be highly informative regarding organized nursing's efforts to keep the best interests of nursing, and therefore patients, front and center in the evolution of health care in the U.S. today.

Both the medical profession and health service administration have attempted to limit the autonomy of nursing to hinder financial competition for patients by nurses in independent practice. Medicine and health service administration are well organized, well-funded and have powerful lobbies at state and national levels, posing a major challenge to full autonomy for nurses. Conversely, organized nursing does not yet have available economic resources to compete effectively against these influential forces seeking to minimize nursing autonomy.

The Magnet Recognition Program® is an initiative of the American Nurses Credentialing Center (ANCC), the updated 2020 mission statement of which states: "The Magnet Recognition Program will continually elevate patient care around the world in an environment where nurses, in collaboration with the interprofessional team, flourish by setting the standard for excellence through leadership, scientific discovery and dissemination and implementation of new knowledge." (nursingworld.org, 2020).

In 2021, 549 hospitals had achieved Magnet designation, or fewer than 10% of the more than 5000 hospitals in the U.S. (Campaign for Action, 2021). The Magnet credential was established to recognize hospitals that attract and retain nurses, acknowledging that this achieves better patient outcomes. Nursing autonomy and control over practice were identified in 1983 as crucial characteristics of these hospitals. Significantly, the COVID-19 pandemic beginning in 2021 exacerbated the shortage of nurses, and the final effects of this public health disaster on the healthcare system, including nursing, has yet to be determined.

Motivated by Service (Altruism), Practitioners' Work Is Important in Their Lives

As a group, nurses are dedicated to the ideal of service to others, also known as *altruism*. The desire to "help people" is foundational to altruism. Moreover, many, if not most, nurses consider nursing to be a key part of their identity and recognize that their work is important. The ideal of service has sometimes become intertwined with economic issues and historically has been exploited by employers of nurses. Although no one questions the rights of other professionals to charge reasonable fees for the services they render, nurses' altruism is sometimes questioned when they demand higher compensation and better working conditions. The COVID-19 pandemic exacerbated this phenomenon. Early in the pandemic, nurses were widely hailed in the public and media as "heroes," doing exceptional work in exceptional times (and, sadly, underscoring the invisibility of the work of nursing in "ordinary" times). In a 2021 survey of more than 6000 critical care nurses administered by the American Association of Critical-Care Nurses, 66% of the respondents reported that their experiences during the pandemic have caused them to consider leaving nursing, an alarming statistic in and of itself; moreover, 92% agreed that the pandemic had depleted the nursing staff at their institution, and that their careers will be shorter (Medscape.com, 2021). The pandemic and its prolonged strain on the health care system exposed the fallacy of altruism being enough to sustain a profession. Nursing's value must be acknowledged by adequate compensation because a sense of altruism erodes when working conditions are unsatisfactory and pay is inadequate.

Commitment to the profession is not a value equally shared by all nurses. Some nurses regard nursing as simply a job with schedule flexibility to meet needs of their families, and to ensure a regular income. This point of view, although appealing to many nurses and conducive to management of family responsibilities, may inadvertently delay the development of professional attitudes and behaviors for the profession as a whole.

Code of Ethics to Guide the Decisions and Conduct of Practitioners

A code of ethics provides professional standards and a framework for moral decision making; however, a code does not stipulate how an individual should act in a specific situation. The trust placed in the nursing profession by the public requires that nurses act with integrity. Both the International Council of Nurses and the ANA, among others, have established codes of nursing ethics articulating standards of ethical practice.

In 1893, long before these codes were written, "The Florence Nightingale Pledge" (Box 3.1) was created by a committee headed by Lystra Eggert Gretter and presented to the Farrand Training School for Nurses located at Harper Hospital in Detroit, Michigan (Dock and Stewart, 1920). The Nightingale Pledge functioned

BOX 3.1 The Florence Nightingale Pledge

I solemnly pledge myself before God and in the presence of this assembly to pass my life in purity and to practice my profession faithfully.

I will abstain from whatever is deleterious and mischievous, and will not take or knowingly administer any harmful drug. I will do all in my power to maintain and elevate the standard of my profession, and will hold in confidence all personal matters committed to my keeping and all family affairs coming to my knowledge in the practice of my calling.

With loyalty will I endeavor to aid the physician in his work and devote myself to the welfare of those committed to my care.

From Dock LL, Stewart MM: *A short history of nursing*, New York, 1920, Putnam.

as nursing's first code of ethics; although its language and some of its ideals are archaic, it has historical value, and it established the roots for our current code.

An Association Encouraging and Supporting High Standards of Practice

The ANA is the official voice of nursing and therefore is the primary advocate for nursing interests in general. The ANA is a federation of state nurses associations that all RNs are eligible to join. Membership in a state nurses association automatically conveys membership in the ANA. According to its bylaws, the ANA has four purposes: (1) work for the improvement of health standards and the availability of healthcare services for all people; (2) foster high standards of nursing; (3) advocate for workplace standards that foster safe patient care and support the profession; and (4) to stimulate and promote the professional development of nurses and advance their welfare (ANA, 2021). The ANA continues to be limited by the relatively low percentage of nurses (fewer than 20%) who belong to the ANA and their constituent state nurses associations. This represents significant unrealized political influence for the profession.

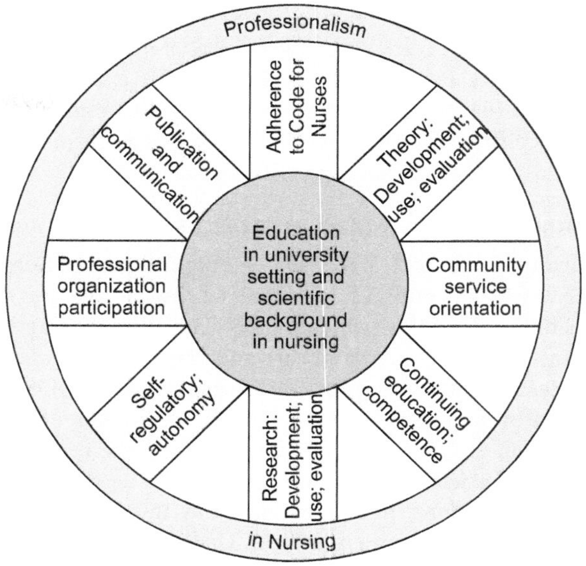

Fig. 3.3 The Wheel of Professionalism in nursing. (Copyright 1984 Barbara Kemp Miller.)

Miller's Wheel of Professionalism in Nursing

Miller (1985; Adams and Miller, 2001) created a model, the Wheel of Professionalism, based on common themes she identified in the work of sociologists and nursing leaders, as well as statements from *Nursing's Social Policy Statement* and *Code of Ethics for Nurses*. The wheel's center represents the essential foundation of nursing education in an institution of higher learning (Fig. 3.3). According to Adams and associates (1996):

> *Each of the eight spokes represents other behaviors deemed necessary in maintaining or increasing nurses' professionalism. They are competence and continuing education; adherence to the code of ethics; participation in the primary and referent professional organization, i.e., ANA and state constituent member association; publication and communication; orientation toward community services; theory and research development and utilization; and self-regulation and autonomy.* (p. 79)

Standards Established by the Profession Itself

Three major documents guide all nurses in their professional commitments: Nursing's Social Policy Statement: The Essence of the Profession (ANA, 2010), Nursing: Scope and Standards of Practice, 4th edition (ANA, 2021), and the Code of Ethics for Nurses with Interpretive Statements (ANA, 2015).

Nursing's Social Policy Statement: The Essence of the Profession

A Contract With Society

Although criteria for professions vary, all professions have one criterion in common: an obligation to the recipients of their services. Nursing therefore has an obligation to those who receive nursing care. The nature of the social contract between the members of the nursing profession and society is summarized in the latest version of *Nursing's Social Policy Statement: The Essence of the Profession*, revised in 2010 (ANA, 2010). This edition was the result of several years of work by many nurses from a variety of settings and holding an assortment of educational degrees and credentials, collectively known as the Congress on Nursing Practice and Economics. The Social Policy Statement serves as a framework for understanding professional nursing's relationship with society and nursing's obligation to those who receive professional nursing care. This statement also includes the ANA's contemporary definition of nursing and pertinent discussions related to the knowledge base of nursing, specialty and advanced practice, and professional regulation. A careful reading of this 45-page document will provide the reader with the essence of nursing's professionalism. It is available online without appendices as a PDF document at https://essentialguidetonursing-practice.files.wordpress.com/2012/07/pages-from-essential-guide-to-nursing-practice-chapter-1.pdf.

Nursing: Scope and Standards of Practice

Nursing: Scope and Standards of Practice, 4th edition (ANA, 2021), outlines the expectations of the professional role within which all RNs must practice and delineates the standards of care and associated competencies for professional nursing. The goal of establishing standards is to improve the health and well-being of all recipients of nursing care and to establish the responsibilities for which nurses are accountable. Several editions of *Standards* have been issued by the ANA since the first one was written in 1973. Under the leadership of the ANA, each edition has been carefully revised with input from a large number of nurses.

The current document (ANA, 2021) itemizes a combined 18 Standards of Practice and Standards of Professional Performance. For each standard, there are numerous competencies by which practice for that standard can be assessed, and additional competencies for graduate-level prepared RNs, including APNs. Although all the standards are important to the practice of nursing, the Standards of Professional Performance are particularly germane to this chapter's emphasis on professionalism. The depth and scope of this document are impressive; you should consider adding this book, available as a downloadable ebook, to your professional library.

The Code of Ethics for Nurses

The ANA designated 2015 as the Year of Ethics and published a revision of the 2001 code. The *Code of Ethics,* like the Social Policy Statement, was revised by a committee of nurses from a variety of roles and settings across the United States. As you recall, most of the early scholars attempting to define *profession* mentioned ethical behavior as a hallmark of a profession. In fact, a code of ethics is generally considered a tool that guides a group toward professional self-definition and provides evidence of professional legitimacy. The healthcare environment often presents situations that pose ethical problems for nurses. The Code exists to strengthen and guide nurses' decision making as they navigate the ethical dilemmas frequently faced in many practice settings today. The Code empowers nurses to maintain their focus on the patient as the center of health care.

A **code of ethics** is a written public document that reminds practitioners and the public they serve of the specific responsibilities and obligations accepted by the profession's practitioners. Ever since education was formalized for nurses, the practice of nursing has been guided by ethical standards promoted first by Florence Nightingale and thereafter by nursing groups and organizations. The *Code of Ethics for Nurses* has been modified over the years as nursing and its social context have evolved. It is intended to guide the practice of RNs in all practice settings, with all types of patients, families, groups, and communities receiving care. The *Code of Ethics* serves three distinct purposes: (1) it is a statement of the "ethical values, obligations, duties, and professional ideals of nurses individually and collectively"; (2) it is nursing's "nonnegotiable ethical standard"; and (3) it expresses "nursing's own understanding of its commitment to society" (ANA, 2015, p. 10).

There are nine provisions in the 2015 Code, each of which is accompanied by interpretive statements intended to clarify the provision. The first three provisions describe "the fundamental values and commitments of the nurse; the next three address boundaries of duty and loyalty; and the last three address aspects of duties beyond individual patient encounters" (p. 16). The entire document, including interpretive statements, can be found here: www.nursingworld.org/MainMenu-Categories/EthicsStandards/CodeofEthicsforNurses/Code-of-Ethics-For-Nurses.html.

COLLEGIALITY IN PROFESSIONAL NURSING

A sometimes overlooked but increasingly important aspect of professionalism in nursing is collegiality. The promotion of a supportive and healthy work environment, cooperation, and recognition of interdependence among members of the nursing profession is the essence of **collegiality**. Professional nurses demonstrate collegiality by sharing with, supporting, assisting, and counseling other nurses and nursing students. These behaviors can be seen when nurses, for example, share knowledge with colleagues and students, take part in professional organizations, mentor less experienced nurses, serve as role models for nursing students, welcome learners and their instructors in the practice setting, assist researchers

BOX 3.2 To Be a Professional

Be respectful. You do not have to like or agree with a person to be civil. Treat him or her as you would want to be treated.
Be ethical. Understand that in professional settings, professional ethics are mandatory.
Be honest. Be trustworthy; do not participate in gossip and rumor.
Be the best. Strive to be better than just good enough.
Be consistent. Behavior should be consistent with professional values and beliefs.
Be a communicator. Invite ideas, opinions, and feedback from patients and colleagues.
Be accountable. Do what you say you will do. Take responsibility for your own actions.
Be collaborative. Collaborations benefit your patients.
Be forgiving. Everyone makes mistakes—including yourself.
Be current. Keep knowledge and skills up-to-date.
Be involved. Be active at local, state, and national levels in professional organizations.
Be a model nurse. What a person says and does reflects on his or her profession.
Be responsible for your own learning. Be assertive in making your learning needs known to teachers and mentors.
Be prepared. Do assignments for classes, and prepare for labs and clinical shifts in advance, making sure that you have a good foundation for your practice.

Modified from Bruhn JG: Being good and doing good: the culture of professionalism in the health professions, *Health Care Manag* 19(4):47–58, 2001; and Cheyne D: Take responsibility for your learning needs, *Nurs Standard* 20(7):88, 2005.

with data gathering, publish in professional literature, and support peer-assistance programs for impaired nurses.

Box 3.2, "To Be a Professional," contains 14 characteristics of professional nurses. Several serve as reminders of the value of collegiality. You may find this list helpful in considering where you are in your development as a professional nurse.

BARRIERS TO PROFESSIONALISM IN NURSING

Nurses own the profession of nursing and thus own the struggle for recognition as a profession. To reduce the barriers to professionalization, the first step is to identify those barriers, several of which are discussed here.

Varying Levels of Education for Entry into Practice

The most obvious barrier to nursing's achievement of professional status is the variability of educational backgrounds for entry into practice: the BSN, the ADN, and the diploma in nursing. Other healthcare professions—for example, medicine, dentistry, and physical therapy—require postgraduate preparation for professional practice. Because professional status and power increase with education, a legitimate question is, "How can nursing establish itself as a profession, and nurses be recognized as professional peers with other healthcare providers, when a significant percentage of nurses currently in practice do not hold a bachelor's degree?"

In 2000, David described this "never-ending fracas" (p. 87) over the varying credentials for entry into practice as contributing to the continuing subordination of nursing in the healthcare arena. Almost two decades later, this "fracas" continues. Nursing's lack of a standardized requirement for a minimum of a BSN, and preferably a master's degree, stands in sharp contrast with other healthcare professions requiring more education to practice (David, 2000). Nurses prepared in the three different types of basic educational programs have thus far failed to develop a unified identity that would allow the continuing professionalization of nursing. Lack of resolution of these differences threatens to undermine nursing's continued steady development as a profession. This remains a difficult issue for nurses, creating division and defensiveness. A solution would be for nurses to move beyond personal feelings and opinions to look objectively at how nursing compares with other professions with whom we collaborate.

Gender Issues

Although gender was not identified as a criterion by any of the scholars of professionalism, it continues to play a role in the perceived value of professions dominated by women such as teaching, social work, and nursing. Although the number of men in nursing has increased, a gender balance remains elusive (Fig. 3.4). The persistent devaluing of women's work in our society has created an ongoing struggle for members of professions such as nursing and teaching to increase their status, increase their compensation, and improve their working conditions. Referenced previously, David (2000) provided an incisive critique of nursing and the detrimental and continuing effects of gender politics on nursing's professional development.

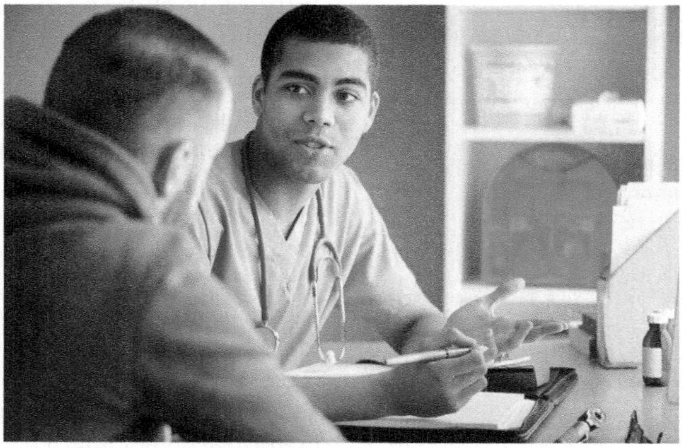

Fig. 3.4 The number of men in nursing is slowly increasing.

Historical Influences

Nursing's historical connections with religious orders and the military continue to have influence, both positive and negative, today. Aspects that have become liabilities with the passage of time include deference to other professionals, which runs counter to the professional values of autonomy and self-determination, and altruism, which prevents nurses from demanding the fair economic valuation of the work of nursing. Deference to management, physicians, and other stakeholders in the workplace stifles creative and critical thinking required for professional practice. Furthermore, nurses must resist pressure to defend their expectation to be compensated fairly for their complex and demanding work.

Florence Nightingale, the historical figure most strongly associated with the development of modern-day nursing, died in 1910. That same year, Isabelle Hampton Robb died suddenly. As you read in Chapter 2, Robb was a central figure in the women's movement of the late 19th century, and in nursing specifically. Professional Profile Box 3.1 contains a tribute to Robb published in 2011 examining the challenges to nursing Robb faced and the challenges of reenvisioning of the profession today, more than a century later.

External Conflicts

As nurses have become more highly educated and as advanced practice nurses increasingly assume responsibilities for patient care once considered in the domain of medicine, tensions between nursing and medicine continue. The influence and resources of organized nursing and professional associations have gone toward lobbying efforts in state legislatures to ensure that the legal scope of nursing practice is protected and appropriately reflects current training and expertise of professional nurses.

Internal Conflicts

Professional nursing's power and influence are fragmented by subgroups and dissension. Tensions among diploma-educated, associate degree–educated, and bachelor's degree–educated nurses reduce the vitality of the profession. The proliferation of nursing organizations and competition among them for members may diminish rather than increase nursing's influence in the healthcare arena by diluting concentrations of interested stakeholders across many organizations. Fewer than 20% of the more than 4.1 million RNs in the U.S. are members of the ANA. The fact that most nurses are not members of any professional organization hampers nursing's ability to govern itself, set standards, and use its collective power to lobby effectively. These are major challenges for nursing if it is to realize its potential collective professional power and autonomy.

Nursing Image and Professionalism: Are These Related?

In Thinking Critically Box 3.1, you will first read the results of a study completed by a senior honors student of nursing, Lindy Beyer, who has now graduated and is an RN. Ms. Beyer did a systematic review and analysis of nurse-authored blogs, where she found a forum where nurses describe what it means to be a nurse. Once you have read these results, consider these questions:

PROFESSIONAL PROFILE BOX 3.1

Repaving the Path to Professionalism in Nursing Education

In Remembrance of Isabel Hampton Robb

Celebrated as the international year of the nurse, 2010 marked the centennial remembrance of the death of Florence Nightingale in 1910. For nurse educators, it was also a time to remember the contributions of Isabel Hampton Robb, a younger contemporary of Nightingale, who died an untimely death the same year. Like many nurses of her day, Robb was an immigrant to the United States who began her second career as a nurse after attending New York Training School for Nurses attached to Bellevue Hospital. After practice abroad, she was recruited into nursing education administration, first in Illinois and then as principal of the Training School and as superintendent at Johns Hopkins Hospital. A politically astute young woman, Robb helped build a path to professionalism for nursing education, drawing on professional and political connections to advance nursing and the quality of patient care. In 1893 she chaired the first major meeting of nursing leaders in Chicago at the Columbian Exhibition and World's Fair, where she presented a paper sent by Nightingale titled "Educational Standards for Nurses." Acknowledging the importance of collaboration in advancing the quality of nursing education and practice, she was a primary founder and first leader of the Association of Nursing Superintendents, the precursor to the National League for Nursing. Her work to unite trained nurses resulted in the Association of Nursing Alumni, which preceded the ANA. Robb set the bar high for nursing education in an era of hospital growth and proliferation of nursing schools. With nursing education highly disorganized, she advocated for admission standards and a formalized curriculum. A scholar of nursing, she took on the task to disseminate teaching materials nationally and wrote reports, articles, and textbooks to provide a sound basis for practice. She addressed the clinical practices of her day, the ethics of nursing, and standards for nursing education. In an era when travel was slow, Robb traveled nationally and internationally and maintained an active correspondence in support of her vision for nursing education. Some 100 years after Robb's death, nursing is again faced with the challenge of reenvisioning standards for the future. The focus now is on the transformation of nursing education to better support the expected changes in a remodeled healthcare system. Walking along a path initially laid by Robb and her coterie of nursing leaders, a collaboration of nursing and nonnursing leaders set out a call for action in the 2010 Institute of Medicine (IOM) report, *The Future of Nursing: Leading Change, Advancing Health.* This effort to set a national course for nursing education and practice balances optimism for the potential of nursing and pragmatism grounded in the recognition of barriers to change. In their report, commissioned by the Carnegie Foundation for the Advancement of Teaching, Benner, Sutphen, Leonard, and Day (2010) address the perceived disconnect between the classroom and clinical education. They urge nurse educators to attend to the methods of education and to teach with greater emphasis on clinical reasoning and clinical salience. Noting the challenges that nurses face in practice, from the diversity of patients to the need to manage multiple chronic diseases to the complex and too often fragmented healthcare system, they underscore the importance of developing in nursing students the ability to readily access and integrate knowledge and skills and transcend discrete classes and clinical experiences. Both the IOM and Carnegie reports reflect the belief, long espoused by nursing leaders, that nurses must be prepared as agents of change. Both reports call for strengthening and empowering nursing leadership. Echoing a call first launched by Robb, the Carnegie report highlights the importance of attending to the socialization, roles, and ethics of nursing graduates as they develop their foundational values, attitudes, and behaviors for leadership. Throughout nursing's history, leaders such as Robb have taken risks to strategically develop, articulate, and promote not simply standards for nursing education but rather a vision of what nursing education and nursing practice offer society. Today, as we reenvision nursing's future and engage in repaving the road of nursing's professionalism, it is fitting to mark the centennial of Isabel Hampton Robb's death and her contributions to nursing education.

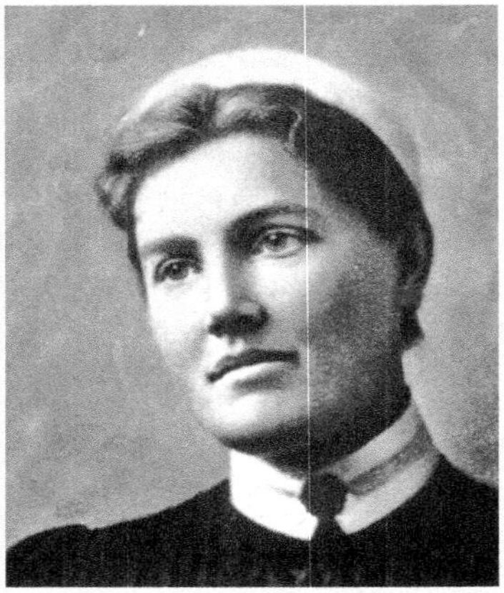

Isabel Hampton Robb

From Wolf KA: End note: Repaving the path to professionalism in nursing education: in remembrance of Isabel Hampton Robb, *Nurs Educ Perspec* 32(2):138, 2011.

THINKING CRITICALLY BOX 3.1

Rethinking the Professional Image of Nursing: A Content Analysis of Nurse-Authored Blogs

Nursing has suffered from a poor image since the 1800s, which has been perpetuated by the media, physician influence, and societal stereotypes. In much of the literature, image problems have been implicated in contributing to the nursing shortage. The image of nursing has the potential to be influenced by Internet representation. Americans occupying the 18- to 29-year-old age group cite the Internet as their primary source of information because it is convenient and it provides more in-depth and varied viewpoints than does traditional media. The Internet is the number one source of healthcare information, with more than 12.5 million health-related searches conducted daily, including nurse-authored blogs.

Blogs are a useful adjunct to traditional media as a source of information. Through blogs, nurses are able to describe their life and experiences—what it means to be a nurse—directly to an audience without many filters or external editing processes. How nurses choose to represent themselves in the media has yet to be described. In this study I systematically reviewed and analyzed blogs written by nurses, examining the authors' portrayal of the profession of nursing with respect to image to yield insight on how nurses represent their profession via Internet blogs and whether these insights support or refute the view that nursing has a poor image.

A sample of 101 blog posts containing information about the professional life of the nurse-author revealed that nurses rarely blogged about the image of nursing (24.85%), with few examples related to actual experience (6.45%). Three themes—"Variety in professional settings," "Nursing as physically/mentally demanding," and "Detailed descriptions of duties/priorities"—accounted for 12.8% of the coding decisions in the analysis. Importantly, 54.5% of coded content fit within the category "Positive or neutral descriptors of nursing," indicating that nurse-authored blogs do not contribute to the poor image of nursing. Furthermore, the experiences nurses blog about do not reinforce the idea that nursing has a poor image.

Beginning with Nightingale's assertion that nursing is a scientific profession with a distinct body of knowledge requiring training, several efforts have transformed the modern landscape of professional nursing: educational requirements have evolved; professional improvement campaigns are progressively being adopted at the institutional level; and image-enhancing advocacy groups work toward correcting misperceptions and stereotypes in the public eye. Considering that the theoretical bases for the poor image argument were formed 20 to 30 years ago when nursing was a very different profession, this study indicates a need to reevaluate the idea that modern nursing has a poor image.

Lindy Beyer, BSN, RN

1. What positive effect does blogging in the public domain have on the profession of nursing?
2. What are possible negative effects that these accounts could have on the profession?
3. Find an example of two nursing blogs, one that promotes a positive view of the nursing profession and another that promotes a negative view of nursing. What are the characteristics of each of these examples?
4. What are your responsibilities as a member of the profession of nursing in responding to the posts on these blogs?
5. What is the relationship of the image of nursing and the professionalization of nursing?

FINAL COMMENTS

The World Health Organization/ Assembly designated the year 2020 as the "Year of the Nurse and the Midwife," with no idea that the year would be characterized by a world health crisis during which nurses had a key role in caring for the overwhelming number of seriously ill and dying persons. Health care, its delivery and its priorities changed in a matter of weeks and months, and the full impact of this health disaster is yet to be manifested. Debates regarding whether nursing is a profession may need to take a back seat to more pressing issues that were made clear by the pandemic and its effects on nurses and nursing, especially the need to improve workplace conditions and compensation. Nursing has made progress in the past few decades in developing its science and improving its image. Although considerable barriers remain, healthcare reform in the United States and improvement of healthcare delivery mean that nurses can establish themselves as primary stakeholders in this debate and move forward.

To summarize this discussion of professionalism in nursing, read Thinking Critically Box 3.2, and identify the professional behaviors exhibited in the case study presented.

THINKING CRITICALLY BOX 3.2

The Challenge to be a Professional Nurse: Identifying Professional Nursing Behaviors

Instructions: If being a professional nurse is different from practicing the occupation of nursing, there must be certain behaviors that differentiate the two. Read the following (fictionalized) case study; then, using various criteria for professions presented in this chapter and the Code of Ethics for Nurses, identify professional behaviors exhibited by Joan. For each behavior you identify, state which source or document, such as the Code or Social Policy Statement, promotes that behavior.

Joan is a 32-year-old married mother of two. She graduated from River City College of Nursing at the age of 26 years and has been practicing as an RN since her graduation. Her first position was as a staff nurse at Providence Hospital, a 300-bed private hospital. Nursing administration at Providence encourages nurses to provide individualized nursing care while protecting the dignity and autonomy of each patient and family. She chose Providence because the hospital's philosophy of nursing paralleled her own. Another reason Joan selected this hospital was that she wanted to practice oncology (cancer) nursing, and there is an oncology unit at Providence.

Each day Joan arrives promptly on her nursing unit. Her neat grooming and positive attitude convey pride in herself and her profession. She uses the nursing process in caring for her patients and in dealing with their families. That means she assesses their condition, plans and implements their care, and evaluates the care she has given. Then she documents what she has done in each patient's database in the accepted format. She communicates clearly to the other members of the nursing staff and collaborates with other healthcare professionals involved in the care of the patients on her unit but is careful not to discuss her patients with others not involved in their direct care.

After 2 years as a staff nurse, Joan accepted a position as a team leader. This means that now she takes responsibility not only for her own practice but also for that of licensed practical/vocational nurses and nursing assistants on her team. To do this effectively, she stays abreast of changes in her state's nurse practice act and Providence Hospital's policies and procedures. In addition, she updates her knowledge by reading current journals and research periodicals to base her practice on evidence rather than intuition. She makes it a policy to attend at least two nursing conferences each year to stay on top of trends. She belongs to her professional organization and participates as an active member. She finds that this is another source of the latest information on professional issues.

Joan looks forward to working with the nursing students at Providence Hospital. She remembers when she was a student and how a word from a practicing nurse could make or break her day. Of course, students do mean extra work, but she sees this as a part of her role and patiently provides the guidance they need, even when she is busy.

In the course of her daily work, Joan sometimes has questions. She is not embarrassed to seek help from more experienced nurses, from textbooks, professional websites or from other healthcare providers. Sometimes she offers suggestions to the nurse manager and the oncology clinical nurse specialist about possible research questions and participates in gathering data when the unit is participating in a research study.

Providence Hospital uses a shared governance model, which means nurses serve on committees that develop and interpret nursing policies and procedures. Joan serves on two committees and chairs another. Because the hospital is preparing a self-study for upcoming accreditation, meetings are frequent. Instead of complaining about the meetings, Joan prepares and organizes her responsibilities for the meeting so it will run efficiently. While attending meetings, she delegates her patient care responsibilities to others, and because she has taken time to understand her colleagues' skills, she knows her patients are safe and asks for a full report when she returns to her unit.

In her evenings at home, Joan occasionally gets a call from a friend with a health-related question or a request from a neighbor to give an allergy injection. Although she is tired, she understands that in the eyes of others she represents the nursing profession and is proud to be trusted and respected for her knowledge and skills. Helping others through nursing care is something Joan has wanted to do since she was a child, and she finds it very fulfilling.

Lately Joan has recognized in herself some troubling signs: she has been irritable and impatient with family and co-workers and generally "not herself." She has gained weight and is exercising less than usual, and because she rotates 12 hour shifts equally between days and nights, she is not sleeping well. She wonders if working with terminally ill patients and their families is the source of her stress, and acknowledges that her work life and personal life are out of balance. Joan's husband has suggested

Continued

THINKING CRITICALLY BOX 3.2—cont'd

The Challenge to be a Professional Nurse: Identifying Professional Nursing Behaviors

that she take a break from nursing and stay home with their children, but after talking it over with her nurse manager, she decides to transfer to a different nursing unit for a while. Although she will miss her colleagues and patients on the oncology unit, Joan knows that she needs to be her own advocate and take care of herself. She will work 10-hour day shifts four days each week in an outpatient surgery unit where the emotional intensity will be lower. Joan hopes to return eventually to oncology nursing—her first love—but for now, she understands she cannot take care of her patients well if she is not taking care of herself.

CONCEPTS AND CHALLENGES

- ***Concept:*** Commitment to a profession is different from having a job or an occupation.
  Challenge: Commitment to nursing as a profession may be challenged by ongoing problems with workplace conditions and compensation.
- ***Concept:*** A body of knowledge, specialized education, service to society, accountability, autonomy, and ethical standards, among others, are hallmarks of professions.
  Challenge: Nursing is still troubled by lack of autonomy, varying educational preparation, and long-term commitment to practice that function as barriers to professionalism.
- ***Concept:*** Nursing has a social contract with society to serve the public safely, competently, and ethically.
  Challenge: Many nurses in practice are not familiar with *Nursing's Social Policy Statement: The Essence of the Profession,* which describes nursing's contract with society, and the *Code of Ethics with Interpretive Statements,* which is the nonnegotiable ethical standard for professional nursing.

IDEAS FOR FURTHER EXPLORATION

1. Determine where nursing currently stands on each of Kelly's criteria for professions.
2. Describe at least five characteristic behaviors of professional nurses.
3. Discuss the Nightingale Pledge (see Box 3.1) as a historical document, as an ethical statement, and as a reflection of Florence Nightingale's social and cultural environment. What value does this document have for today's nurse?
4. Using Miller's Wheel of Professionalism, identify specific activities that fit under each of the "spokes." How might a beginning nurse's behaviors in relation to each spoke differ from those of an experienced nurse? Where does evidence-based practice fit into this model?
5. How might nursing be different today if all nurses viewed it as their profession rather than a job?

REFERENCES

Adams D, Miller BK: Professionalism in nursing behaviors of nurse practitioners, *J Prof Nurs* 17(4):203–210, 2001.

Adams D, Miller BK, Beck L: Professionalism behaviors of hospital nurse executives and middle managers in 10 western states, *West J Nurs Res* 18(1):77–88, 1996.

American Nurses Association (ANA): *Educational preparation for nurse practitioners and assistants to nurses: a position paper*, Kansas City, MO, 1965, The Association.

American Nurses Association (ANA): *Bylaws of the American Nurses Association as amended March 23, 2021*, 2021, The Association. (website). Available at https://www.nursingworld.org/~4965b2/globalassets/ana/leadership-governance/ana-bylaws.pdf.

American Nurses Association (ANA): *Code of ethics for nurses with interpretive statements*, Washington, DC, 2015, The Association.

American Nurses Association (ANA): *Nursing: scope and standards of practice*, ed 4, Washington, DC, 2021, The Association.

American Nurses Association (ANA): *Nursing's social policy statement: the essence of the profession*, ed 2010, Washington, DC, 2010, The Association.
Bixler GK, Bixler RW: The professional status of nursing, *Am J Nurs* 59(8):1142–1147, 1959.
Brown EL: *Nursing for the future*, New York, 1948, Russell Sage Foundation.
Carr-Saunders AM, Wilson PA: *The professions*, Oxford, 1933, Clarendon Press.
Campaign for Action: *Number of hospitals in the United States with Magnet status*, 2021. (website). Available at: https://campaignforaction.org/resource/number-hospitals-united-states-magnet-status/.
Collins English Dictionary: *Occupation*, 2021. (website). Available at: https://www.collinsdictionary.com/dictionary/english/occupation.
D'Amour D, Oandasan I: Interprofessionality as the field of interprofessional practice and interprofessional education: an emerging concept, *J Interprof Care* 19(Suppl 1):8–20, 2005.
David BA: Nursing's gender politics: reformulating the footnotes, *Adv Nurs Sci* 23(1):83–93, 2000.
Derouin A, Holtscheider ME, McDaniel KE, Sanders KA, McNeill DB: Let's work together: interprofessional training of health professionals in North Carolina, *NC Med J* 79(4):223–225, 2018.
Dock LL, Stewart IM: *A short history of nursing*, New York, 1920, Putnam.
Flexner A: *Medical education in the United States and Canada: a report to the Carnegie Foundation for the Advancement of Teaching*, Bethesda, MD, 1910, Science & Health Publications.
Flexner A: Is social work a profession? *School Soc* 1(26):901, 1915.
Ghadirian F, Salsali M, Cheraghi MA: Nursing professionalism: an evolutionary process, *Iran J Nurs Midwifery Res* 19(1):1–10, 2014.
Hall RH: Professionalization and bureaucratization, *Am Sociol Rev* 33:92–104, 1968.
Hall RH: *The professionals, employed professionals, and the professional association. professionalism and the empowerment of nursing*, Kansas City, MO, 1982, American Nurses Association.
Houle C: *Continuing learning in the professions*, San Francisco, 1980, Jossey-Bass.
Huber D: *Leadership and nursing care management*, Philadelphia, 2000, Saunders.
Interprofessional Education Collaborative Expert Panel: *Core competencies for interpersonal collaborative practice: report of an expert panel*, Washington, DC, 2011, Interprofessional Education Collaborative.
Kelly L: *Dimensions of professional nursing*, ed 4, New York, 1981, Macmillan.
Medscape.com: *Nurses 'at the breaking point', consider quitting due to COVID issue: survey*, 2021. (website). Available at https://www.medscape.com/viewarticle/959043.
Miller BK: Just what is a professional? *Nurs Success Today* 2(4):21–27, 1985.
National Academy of Medicine (Institute of Medicine): *Measuring the impact of interprofessional education on collaborative practice and patient outcomes*, Washington, DC, 2015, National Academies Press.
nursingworld.org: *About Magnet: new 2020 Magnet mission and vision statement*, 2020, ANCC. (website). Available at: https://www.nursingworld.org/organizational-programs/magnet/about-magnet/.
Reuter C, Fitzsimons V: Viewpoint: physician orders, *Am J Nurs* 113(8):8–11, 2013.
Task Force on Professionalism: White paper on pharmacy student professionalism, *J Am Pharm Assoc* 40(1):96–100, 2000.
Wolf KA: End note: Repaving the path to professionalism in nursing education: in remembrance of Isabel Hampton Robb, *Nurs Educ Perspec* 32(2):138, 2011.
World Health Organization (WHO): *Framework for action on interprofessional education and collaborative practice*, Geneva, 2010, World Health Organization. (website). Available at https://www.who.int/publications/i/item/framework-for-action-on-interprofessional-education-collaborative-practice.

4

Nursing Education in an Evolving Healthcare Environment

To enhance your understanding of this chapter, try the Student Exercises on the Evolve site at http://evolve.elsevier.com/Black/professional.

LEARNING OUTCOMES

After studying this chapter, students will be able to:

- Trace the development of basic and graduate education in nursing.
- Discuss the influence of early nursing studies on nursing education.
- Describe traditional and alternative ways of becoming a registered nurse.
- Discuss program options for registered nurses and students with nonnursing bachelor's degrees.
- Differentiate between licensed practical/vocational nurses and registered nurses.
- Differentiate between associate degree and bachelor's degree nursing education.
- Explain the difference between licensure and certification.
- Define *accreditation*, and analyze its influence on the quality and effectiveness of nursing education programs.
- Discuss recommendations of the Institute of Medicine and major nursing organizations regarding transforming nursing education.
- List Quality and Safety Education in Nursing (QSEN) competencies.
- Define *Interprofessional Education* (IPE), and describe its importance in health care today.

Produced more than three decades ago, *Sentimental Women Need Not Apply: A History of the American Nurse* is a classic documentary featuring a comprehensive view of the history of nursing in the United States. In this film, nursing is shown to be both shaped by and shaping of its sociocultural and historical contexts. A century ago, nursing education was often exploitative, with students staffing hospital wards as part of their training, only to be unemployed at the end of their training. Nursing education was typically hospital based, and students lived together in tightly controlled environments. The film's narrator made the wry observation of mid–20th-century nursing education: "Schools of nursing took women and turned them into girls." Nursing education, although becoming formalized at the time, did not serve nursing's—or society's—best interests.

Leaders in nursing education today continue to work to evolve nursing education in response to the changing landscape of healthcare delivery in the United States. Furthermore, nursing education must honor nursing's social contract with the public, recognizing that education of nurses plays a critical role in their ability to achieve optimal outcomes for their patients and to practice safely. In 2009 Patricia Benner, PhD, RN, FAAN, and her team at the Carnegie Foundation for the Advancement of Teaching published a landmark study, *Educating Nurses: A Call for Radical Transformation*. In addition to calling for a bachelor of science in nursing (BSN) as the entry level for registered nurse (RN) practice, this team recommended that all RNs be required to earn a master of science in nursing (MSN) within 10 years of licensure. Over ten years ago, they found nurses to be undereducated to meet the demands of current practice. Their recommendations called for a significant shift in basic nursing education, but they made a compelling argument for extending the education of nurses entering the workforce (Benner et al., 2009).

Within a year of the publication of the Carnegie Foundation study, in October 2010 the Institute of Medicine (IOM; now the National Academy of Medicine) published a report, *The Future of Nursing: Leading Change, Advancing Health* (IOM, 2011). This report was compiled as the result of a 2-year initiative by the Robert Wood Johnson Foundation and the IOM to address the need to transform the profession of nursing. Four key messages were at the center of the 2010 *Future of Nursing* report:

1. Nurses must practice to the fullest extent of their education and training.
2. Nurses should attain higher education levels through a system of improved education with seamless progression across degrees.
3. As health care in the United States is being transformed, nurses should be full partners with other healthcare professionals in this effort.
4. Improved data collection and information infrastructure can result in more effective workforce planning and policy development.

In 2016, a follow-up report was published that noted progress in nursing since the 2010 Future of Nursing report but also noted the lack of awareness of nurses' ability for being full participants in professional education, collaboration and leadership (IOM, 2016). In the newest version of the Future of Nursing report, *The Future of Nursing 2020-2030: Charting a Path to Achieve Health Equity*, Chapter 7 lays out a broad appeal for schools of nursing to look past preparation for the NCLEX®, which focuses heavily on acute care nursing, and to educate nurses to understand the complex influences on the health of populations including social determinants, and the need for health equity (NASEM, 2021). This will require a significant shift in nursing education, but will in turn produce a generation of nurses well-equipped for recognizing and acting on the profound challenges to population health in the U.S. *The Future of Nursing 2020–2030* is available as a free .pdf download at https://nam.edu/publications/the-future-of-nursing-2020-2030/.

A decade ago, nursing education was challenged to address a different set of needs. The National Council of State Boards of Nursing (NCSBN) indicated that nursing responded to challenges to increase the sophistication and innovation in nursing education (Spector and Odom, 2012). These innovations, some of which are likely embedded in your nursing school curriculum now, included increased use of simulation, integration of Quality and Safety Education for Nurses (QSEN) principles, development of practice partnerships, and the development of dedicated education units (DEUs), among others. Also, more attention is being paid to ways to manage an ongoing shortage of nursing faculty, which has a direct effect on the number of students that can be educated and added to the nursing workforce.

In addition to the Carnegie and IOM reports, two other important sources called for advancement in nursing education. Linda Aiken, PhD, RN, FAAN, and her colleagues called for increased federal support for the preparation of nurses at the BSN level and higher (Aiken et al., 2009). They suggested policy changes to address the growing need for nursing faculty and in the preparation of advanced practice nurses (APNs) to serve in primary care. In 2010 the Tri-Council for Nursing (an alliance of the American Nurses Association [ANA], American Association of Colleges of Nursing [AACN], American Organization of Nurse Executives, and National League for Nursing [NLN]) released a policy statement that included the following:

> *Current healthcare reform initiatives call for a nursing workforce that integrates evidence-based clinical knowledge and research with effective communication and leadership skills. These competencies require increased education at all levels. At this tipping point for the nursing profession, action is needed now to put in place strategies to build a stronger nursing workforce. Without a more educated nursing workforce, the nation's health will be further at risk (Tri-Council for Nursing, 2010).*

The ANA continues to support funding for the Title VIII Nursing Workforce Development Programs as contained in the Public Health Service Act, which are administered by the Health Resources and Services Administration (HRSA). (At the time of this writing, the Title VIII Nursing Workforce programs were operating without authorization, and there was an effort by nurse leaders to pressure the U.S. Congress to pass the Title VIII Nursing Workforce Reauthorization Act, which would be in force through 2024.)

Two of the major program areas of HRSA related to nursing are Advanced Education Nursing, grants to schools of nursing to enhance advanced nursing education, including nurse practitioners (NPs), certified nurse-midwives (CNMs), certified registered nurse anesthetists (CRNAs), nurse educators, and others; and Workforce Diversity Grants that increase opportunities for persons from disadvantaged backgrounds and who are underrepresented in the nursing workforce (HRSA.gov, 2021).

The contemporaneous release of the IOM report, the Carnegie Foundation report, the Aiken findings, the Tri-Council statement, and the HRSA Title VIII initiatives represented a substantial change in nursing education. Their strong language with regard to the educational basis for nursing required for today's healthcare environment, combined with the increase in funding for education at a time of serious economic constraints, make it necessary for even the staunchest critic of requirements for higher education for nurses to reconsider.

You are entering nursing at a challenging and nearly unprecedented time. The remainder of this chapter will focus on nursing education of today and its current structures and requirements. This includes the history behind educational programs, descriptions of the various programs, and trends and future issues.

DEVELOPMENT OF NURSING EDUCATION IN THE UNITED STATES

Florence Nightingale (Fig. 4.1) is credited with founding modern nursing and creating the first educational system for nurses. After hospitals came into existence in Western Europe, and before the influence of Florence Nightingale, nurses had no formal preparation in giving care because there were no organized programs to educate nurses until the late 1800s. Before this, nursing care was administered by either the patient's relatives, individuals affiliated with religious or military nursing orders, or self-trained persons who were often held in low regard by society.

Nightingale revolutionized and professionalized nursing by arguing that nursing was not a domestic, charitable service but a respected occupation requiring advanced education. In 1860 she opened a school of nursing at St. Thomas' Hospital in London and established the following principles, which were considered highly innovative at the time (Notter and Spalding, 1976):

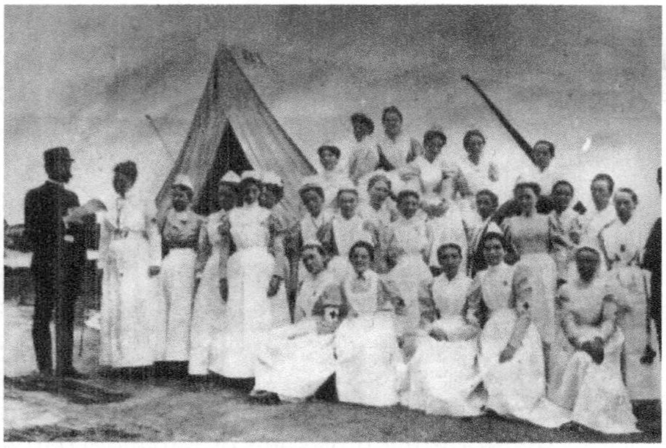

Fig. 4.1 Florence Nightingale's nurses in Scutari, Turkey, during the Crimean War. Nightingale's vision for formalized nursing education transformed nursing.

1. The nurse should be trained in an educational institution supported by public funds and associated with a medical school.
2. The nursing school should be affiliated with a teaching hospital but also should be independent of it.
3. The curriculum should include both theory and practical experience.
4. Professional nurses should be in charge of administration and instruction and should be paid for their instruction.
5. Students should be carefully selected and should reside in "nurses' houses" that form discipline and character. (Nightingale envisioned nursing as a profession only for women.)
6. Students should be required to attend lectures, take quizzes, write papers, and keep diaries. Student records should be maintained.

Nightingale also believed that nursing schools should be financially and administratively separate from the hospitals in which the students trained. This was not the case, however, when nursing schools were first established in the United States.

The first training schools for nurses in the United States were established in 1872. Located at Bellevue Hospital in New York; the New England Hospital for Women and Children in New Haven, Connecticut; and Massachusetts General Hospital in Boston, the programs of study were 1 year long. These schools became known as the "famous trio" of nursing schools. In October 1873, Melinda Anne "Linda" Richards became the first "trained nurse" educated in the United States. By 1879, there were 11 U.S. nursing training schools. Other schools rapidly developed, and by 1900 there were 432 hospital-owned and hospital-operated programs in the United States (Donahue, 1985). These early training programs differed in length from 6 months to 2 years, and each school set its own standards and requirements. On graduation from these programs, students were awarded a diploma. The term *diploma program* was, and still is, used to identify hospital-based nursing education programs. The primary reason for the schools' existence was to staff the hospitals that operated them; therefore high-quality education of student nurses was not always the primary concern of these hospitals.

Early Studies of the Quality of Nursing Education

Nursing leaders of the early 1900s were concerned about the poor quality of many of the recently formed nurse training programs. They initiated studies about nursing and nursing education to prompt changes. October 1899 marked the culmination of approximately 4 years of work by the American Society of Superintendents of Training Schools for Nurses. Isabel Hampton Robb chaired a Society-selected committee to investigate ways to prepare nurses better for leadership in schools of nursing. Teachers College, which had opened in New York 10 years earlier for the training of teachers, seemed the logical location for the leadership training of nurses. A program, originally designed to prepare administrators of nursing service and nursing education, began as an 8-month course in hospital economics (Donahue, 1985).

Mary Adelaide Nutting came to Teachers College in 1907 as the first nursing professor in history and became a pioneer in nursing education. The school at Teachers College became known as the "Mother House" of collegiate education because it fostered the initial movements toward undergraduate and graduate degrees for nurses (Donahue, 1985). In 1912 Nutting conducted a nationwide investigation of nursing education, *The Educational Status of Nursing*, that focused on students' living conditions, nursing education curricula, and teaching methods (Christy, 1969).

Another major and important study of nursing education was published in 1923. Titled *The Study of Nursing and Nursing Education in the United States* and referred to as the Goldmark Report, the study focused on the clinical learning experiences of students, hospital control of the schools, the desirability of establishing university schools of nursing, the lack of funds specifically for nursing education, and the lack of prepared teachers (Kalisch and Kalisch, 1995). It is notable that some of the findings of the Goldmark Report in terms of funding and faculty shortages remain applicable to nursing today.

The year 1924 marked another first in nursing education: Yale University opened its School of Nursing, the first nursing school to be established as a separate university department with an independent budget and its own dean, Annie W. Goodrich. The school demonstrated its effectiveness so well that in 1929 the Rockefeller Foundation ensured the permanency of the school by awarding it an endowment of $1 million (Kalisch and Kalisch, 1995). This was an enormous endowment, equivalent to $13.7 million in 2015, and even more astounding given that in 1929 the stock market crash accelerated the collapse of the global economy that spiraled into the Great Depression.

In 1934 a study titled *Nursing Schools Today and Tomorrow* reported the number of schools in existence, gave detailed descriptions of the schools, described their curricula, and made recommendations for professional collegiate education (National League for Nursing Education, 1934). In 1937 *A Curriculum Guide for Schools of Nursing* was published, outlining a 3-year curriculum and influencing the structure of diploma schools for decades after its publication (National League of Nursing Education, 1937).

Although published over a 30-year period and undertaken by different groups, these early studies consistently made five similar recommendations:

- Nursing education programs should be established within the system of higher education.
- Nurses should be highly educated.
- Students should not be used to staff hospitals.
- Standards should be established for nursing practice.
- All students should meet certain minimum qualifications on graduation.

These studies set the stage for the development of the educational programs that exist today.

EDUCATIONAL PATHS TO BECOME A REGISTERED NURSE

Today, preparation for a career as an RN usually begins in one of three ways: in a hospital-based diploma program, a BSN program, or an associate degree in nursing

(ADN) program. These basic programs vary in the courses offered, length of study, and cost. After the completion of a basic program for RNs, graduates are eligible to take the National Council Licensure Examination for Registered Nurses (NCLEX-RN®). On successful completion of the licensing examination, graduates may legally practice as RNs and use the RN credential.

Having three different educational routes to achieve RN licensure is confusing to the public and even to many nurses themselves. In the following sections, each type of basic program is described, along with its history, unique characteristics, and special issues. These basic programs are discussed in the chronologic order in which they were developed.

Diploma Programs

The hospital-based diploma program was the earliest form of nursing education in the United States. At the peak of diploma education in the 1920s and 1930s, approximately 2000 programs existed, with numerous programs in almost every state. Since their numbers peaked in the first third of the 20th century, the number of diploma programs has decreased, with a dramatic decline since the mid-1960s, when nursing education moved rapidly into collegiate settings. Over the past 50 years, the number of these programs has declined from more than 800 to fewer than 60. This decline in the number of diploma programs is attributable to several factors: the growth of ADN and BSN programs, which moved the education of nurses into the mainstream of higher education; the inability of hospitals to continue to finance nursing education; accreditation standards that have made it difficult for diploma programs to attract qualified faculty; and the increasing complexity of health care, which has required nurses to have greater academic preparation.

Despite the significant decrease in the number of diploma programs, many outstanding nurses practicing today received their basic nursing education in these programs. In the early days of formal nurses' "training" in this country—that is, during the late 1800s and early 1900s—diploma programs provided one of the few avenues for women to obtain formal education and jobs. Most of the early programs followed a modified apprenticeship model. Physicians gave lectures, and students' clinical training was supervised by head nurses and nursing directors. Nursing courses paralleled medical areas and included surgery, obstetrics, pediatrics, operating room experience, and, somewhat later, psychiatry. Students were sometimes sent to affiliated institutions where they could obtain experiences that were not available at the home hospital.

The schedule was demanding, with classes being held after patient care assignments were completed. Critics charged that students were used as inexpensive labor to staff the hospitals and that education was given a lower priority. The truth of those charges varied, depending on which hospital was scrutinized, but there is no question that early nursing students virtually ran the hospitals. Programs lasted 3 years, and, at graduation, students were awarded diplomas in nursing. Today most diploma programs are about 24 months in duration.

A problem that many diploma program graduates faced was that hospitals were not part of the higher education system in the United States. Therefore most colleges and universities did not recognize the nursing diploma as an academic credential and often refused to give college credit for courses taken in diploma programs, regardless of the quality of the courses, students, and faculty. Most diploma programs today have established agreements with colleges and universities that allow students to earn college credit in courses such as English, psychology, and the sciences, thereby enabling them to attain advanced standing in a bachelor's degree program on completion of the diploma program.

Baccalaureate Programs

Informed by early studies of nursing education, nursing leaders have continued to push for nursing education to move into the mainstream of higher education—that is, into colleges and universities where other professionals were educated. There is increasing understanding that nurses need a bachelor's degree, the BSN, to qualify nursing as a recognized profession and to provide leadership in administration, teaching, and public health.

By the time the first BSN program was established in 1909 at the University of Minnesota, diploma programs were numerous and firmly entrenched as the system for educating nurses. This first BSN program was part of the university's School of Medicine and followed the 3-year diploma program structure. Despite its many limitations, it was the start of the movement to bring nursing education into the recognized system of higher education.

Seven other BSN programs were established by 1919 (Conley, 1973). Most of the early BSN programs were 5 years in duration. This structure provided for 3 years of nursing education and 2 years of liberal arts. The growth in the numbers of these programs was slow both because of the reluctance of universities to accept nursing as an academic discipline and because of the power of the hospital-based diploma programs. The theoretical, scientific orientation of the BSN program was in sharp contrast to the "hands-on" skill and service orientation that was the hallmark of hospital-based diploma education.

Influences on the Growth of Baccalaureate Education

National studies of nursing and nursing education have reiterated the need for nursing education and practice to be based on knowledge from the sciences and humanities. A forward-looking study was conducted by Esther Lucille Brown, who in 1948 published *Nursing for the Future*, more commonly known as the Brown Report. The Brown Report recommended that basic schools of nursing be placed in universities and colleges, with efforts made to recruit men and minorities into nursing education programs (Brown, 1948). This report, sponsored by the Carnegie Foundation, was widely reviewed, discussed, and debated.

In 1965 the ANA published a position paper titled *Educational Preparation for Nurse Practitioners and Assistants to Nurses* (American Nurses Association, 1965). Although not all nursing historians agree, this paper, which subsequently created conflict and division within nursing, had a significant influence on the growth of baccalaureate education in nursing. In preparing the position paper, the ANA studied nursing education, nursing practice, and trends in health care, although the ANA did not refer to a critical, groundbreaking change in American health care that occurred in 1965: the implementation of Medicare and Medicaid. The ANA concluded that baccalaureate education should become the foundation for professional practice. Major recommendations included the following:

- Education for all those who are licensed to practice nursing should take place in institutions of higher learning.
- Minimum preparation for entering professional nursing practice should be the baccalaureate degree in nursing.
- Education for assistants in health service occupations should consist of short, intensive preservice programs in vocational education institutions rather than on-the-job training programs.

Despite tremendous opposition from proponents of diploma and ADN programs, in 1979 the ANA further strengthened its stance by proposing three additional positions (ANA, 1979):

- By 1985 the minimum preparation for entry into professional nursing practice should be the BSN.
- Two levels of nursing practice should be identified (professional and technical) and a mechanism to devise competencies for the two categories established by 1980.
- There should be increased accessibility to high-quality career mobility programs that use flexible approaches for individuals seeking academic degrees in nursing.

The controversy created by the 1965 ANA position paper and the 1979 additions continued for many years. Practicing nurses across the United States, who were mainly diploma program graduates, as well as hospitals supporting diploma programs, vehemently protested the recommendations.

In 1970 the National Commission for the Study of Nursing and Nursing Education published a report titled *An Abstract for Action* (Lysaught, 1970). Also known as the Lysaught Report, it made recommendations concerning the supply and demand for nurses, nursing roles and functions, and nursing education. Among the priorities identified by this study were (1) the need for increased research into both the practice and the education of nurses and (2) enhanced educational systems and curricula.

In the mid-1980s, the National Commission on Nursing suggested that the major block to the advancement of nursing was the ongoing conflict within the profession about educational preparation for nurses. The Commission recommended establishing a clear system of nursing education, including pathways for educational mobility and development of additional graduate education programs (De Back, 1991).

The National League for Nursing (NLN) is another major national nursing group supporting the BSN as the entry credential. The organization's membership consists of nurses, faculty, healthcare agencies, all types of nursing programs, and nonnursing citizens who are supportive of nursing. After much debate, in 1982 the

NLN board of directors approved the *Position Statement on Nursing Roles: Scope and Preparation*, which affirmed the BSN as the minimum educational level for professional nursing practice and the ADN or diploma as the preparation for technical nursing practice (NLN, 1982).

In 1996 the AACN board approved a position statement, *The Baccalaureate Degree in Nursing as Minimal Preparation for Professional Practice*. This document supports, among other things, articulated programs, which enable associate degree nurses to attain the BSN (AACN, 2000). This document was last updated in 2000 and still reflects the AACN's current position. It can be found online at https://www.aacnnursing.org/news-information/position-statements-white-papers/bacc-degree-prep.

The latest recommendations by influential nursing groups demonstrate a renewed interest in moving toward a BSN as a minimum degree for entry into practice. These recommendations were used to introduce this chapter, which will now focus on the current state of nursing education in the United States.

Today's Baccalaureate Education

Today, baccalaureate programs provide education for students getting a college degrees in preparation for licensure, and for diploma- or ADN-prepared RNs enrolling in colleges and universities to earn a BSN. This section focuses on the program characteristics of prelicensure baccalaureate education. Baccalaureate programs for RNs are discussed later in this chapter.

Basic BSN programs combine nursing courses with general education courses in a 4-year curriculum in a college or university. Students may be admitted to the nursing program as entering freshmen or after completing certain liberal arts and science courses. Students meet the same admission requirements to the university as other students and often must meet even more stringent requirements to be admitted to the school of nursing with a major in nursing. (Some universities have departments or colleges of nursing rather than schools of nursing.) Courses in the nursing major focus on nursing science, communication, decision making, leadership, and care to persons of all ages in a wide variety of settings (Fig. 4.2).

Faculty in BSN programs are typically required to have a minimum of a master's degree for clinical faculty and a doctorate in nursing or a related field for permanent, tenure-track faculty. This can vary by size and location of an institution, however. Some colleges and universities now require that all faculty, whether tenure track or clinical track, have an earned doctorate. The requirement of a doctorate ensures that nursing faculty members are able to meet the teaching, research, and service requirements expected of all faculty in universities.

Nursing faculty work leads to many interesting possibilities for collaboration in unexpected places and in distant countries. For example, the author of this text spent two and a half memorable weeks in Malawi, a small

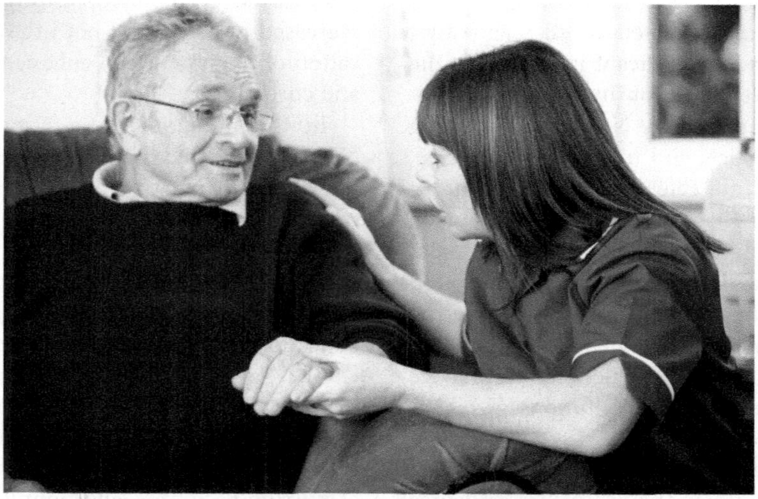

Fig. 4.2 Clinical experience is a vitally important aspect of every basic nursing program. This student is working with her elderly patient in a hospice setting. (Photo used with permission from iStockPhoto.)

country in eastern Africa affected by HIV and malaria, teaching Malawian nurses how to manage two research protocols related to HIV transmission. With three colleagues from other universities, the author spent two weeks in Russia helping nurses there plan their first nursing research projects and, as a result of a visiting professorship at a school of nursing in China, became the mentor for a graduate student in Guangzhou who is now working toward her PhD in Europe. Caring for the health of populations takes many different forms across nations. Nursing and the skills you develop provide you with opportunities to experience firsthand how citizens of other countries care for persons across the continuum of ages, development, and health. The long-term mentoring relationships that can develop between faculty members and students are a reward of working in a school of nursing. (The author's opportunity to teach in Malawi was a direct result of her relationship from a long-time mentor from graduate school.) Professional Profile Box 4.1 contains the first half of a story of how an encounter in a clinical setting was the unexpected start of an important mentor/mentee relationship based on a difficult, shared experience, albeit from different perspectives. Nancy Jo Thompson, DNP, RN, a faculty member, shares her side of the story first in "Room to Zoom."

PROFESSIONAL PROFILE BOX 4.1

From "Room to Zoom": A Nurse's Move From the ICU Bedside to Teaching Online, and an Important Lesson About Inspiration

In August 2020, I was working part-time as a critical care nurse in a large tertiary center in a metropolitan area. Simultaneously, I was excited to be embarking on a new career path teaching in one of the nation's top nursing programs. Anxiety, fears, and uncertainty of abandoning my fellow critical nurses were in full force as I fulfilled my career goals to transition from the patient room to the classroom during an unprecedented pandemic. My first day jitters were intensified by virtual learning platforms, a hundred new faces in tiny Zoom boxes, and fear of failure, all of which were completely forgotten when Danielle, a student in the class, sent me a message in the Zoom chat asking if I could meet via Zoom for a few minutes after class.

The class came to an end and Danielle was the only student left in the Zoom classroom. We exchanged pleasantries and Danielle shared her journey to nursing school after witnessing the inspirational nursing care her sister-in-law Carolyn received in the ICU at a tertiary hospital in a metropolitan area four years earlier. Danielle shared a memory of the nurse at her sister-in-law's bedside immediately after a brief interaction with the neurologist who had told the family that Carolyn was brain dead. Danielle recalled the primary nurse sobbing at the bedside as her family received the news. I was crying when I said, "It was me that day, I was that nurse." Danielle said, "Yes you were!" and she continued, "I remember watching you say to her mom as you leaned in to hug her, 'may I hug you?' Not as a nurse, but as a mom." Danielle went on to say, "Everything changed for me that day, I knew that I had to be a critical care nurse!" Danielle added, "My inspiration for changing my career path and going back to school was you and now you are my professor in my first nursing class." I was speechless, honored, humbled, and moved as the memories of being Carolyn's nurse came flooding back. As we both wept, I shared my perspective of being that bedside nurse who provided care for her dying loved one.

All critical care nurses have patients, families, and dynamic scenarios that will forever affect their practice and life. Carolyn's story was one of those for me. She was admitted and diagnosed with acute respiratory distress syndrome (ARDS) after a suffering an acute asthma attack. I vividly remember the beautiful artwork covering Carolyn's tiny body as she was fighting for every breath. She was in a corner room of the MSICU. The prognosis was grim. I recall Carolyn's siblings and parents sitting by her side and grieving for days. Even in their grief and sadness, they were kind, respectful, and took time to get to know the ICU care team. I could tell that Carolyn was loved by many and their hearts would be broken. Critical care nurses frequently know when the prognosis is bad. My heart ached for my Carolyn's family because I knew their time with her was limited. Sadly, Carolyn did not recover. Her family made the decision to donate life—her organs—on her behalf.

In the days after Caroline's death, I received an award from the hospital in response to a letter submitted by her father. He thanked several of my colleagues and me for the outstanding care we provided his daughter during her illness. I immediately attached the award, a small pewter acorn, to my nurse ID badge and wore it with honor from that day forward. The beautiful letter and receiving of the award provided a gentle reminder of why nurses

Continued

PROFESSIONAL PROFILE BOX 4.1—cont'd

From "Room to Zoom": A Nurse's Move From the ICU Bedside to Teaching Online, and an Important Lesson About Inspiration

chose the profession. Four years have passed since this remarkable patient and her family impacted my practice in a profound way. Although, I did not keep in touch with Carolyn's family, I continue to carry the memories of her last days in my heart.

Critical care nurses provide care for patients and their families during what many describe as the worst days of their lives, a sad and sometimes disheartening description often felt by the nurse, patient, and family. The critical care environment is sterile, cold, and intimidating. The sounds are strange, frequent, and anxiety-inducing. Conversations are deliberate, heartfelt, challenging, and extremely difficult. As nurses working in such an environment, we risk becoming numb to the experiences we encounter during a 12-hour shift. Critical care nurses find themselves in numerous roles at the bedside, now more than ever. The COVID-19 pandemic has increased critical care nurse responsibilities immensely. Responsibilities are compounded by fear and loneliness for both nurse and patient. The increase in emotional and physical workload has been immeasurable in critical care units across the globe since March 2020. The increased workload has decreased nurses' resiliency and led to some nurses questioning their ability to remain working in the critical care specialty.

I will admit, I was one of the critical care nurses asking myself how long I could stay.

I can remember the ICU conversations, questions, hugs, life-altering decisions, and family arguments about their loved ones. The impact of our patient's illness and their loved one's pain is powerful, unrelenting, and we rarely experience closure—the sense of feeling like we know the "rest of the story." Reconnecting with Danielle and hearing her story of inspiration after family tragedy represents the first time I have experienced a sense of closure as a critical care nurse who cared for a dying patient. Critical care nurses are expected to set aside so many feelings into compartments to ensure they maintain the ability to support patients and their families during some of the most difficult times in their lives. COVID has made this worse.

Critical care nurses are strong, resilient, and dedicated persons who learn to compartmentalize their feelings to support the heavy-hearted emotion existing in their patient rooms. This is how we survive and practice effectively in the face of adversity. Conversely, these journeys of patients and families also stick with us. Danielle's story of inspiration to become a critical nurse after witnessing nursing care provided to her sister-in-law demonstrates the power of extraordinary nursing care. I had no idea I was inspiring a future nurse. Danielle will go on to provide care for many critically ill patients and their families, recalling how she was inspired to join the greatest profession on Earth!

Full circle moments rarely come along in a lifetime. I feel blessed to have experienced a beautiful full circle moment reminding me of the importance of inspiration even during times of adversity. As Danielle and I wrapped up our Zoom meeting, I held my nursing badge up the screen pointing out the pewter acorn pin I have proudly worn for the last four years. As we smiled, laughed, and cried together in the last moments of our conversation, we both knew we would be forever changed by our full circle moment, from the room in the ICU to her online class on Zoom.

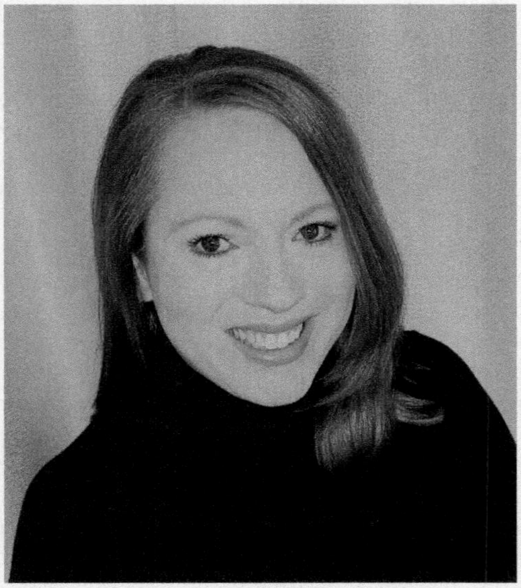

Nancy Jo Thompson, DNP, RN
University of North Carolina at Chapel Hill

Acknowledgment: Carolyn's family was generous in sharing her story and theirs with future nurses who read this and its companion "Zoom to Room" in Chapter 16. Her name and diagnosis are real. Her family honors Carolyn's life by sharing it with all of us, and I am grateful.—BPB

BSN graduates are prepared to take the NCLEX-RN® and, after licensure, enter practice and eventually can become leaders in numerous healthcare settings, including hospitals, community agencies, schools, clinics, and homes. Graduates with BSN degrees are also prepared to move into graduate programs in nursing and advanced practice certification programs. Programs granting a BSN are the most costly of the basic programs in terms of time and money, but the investment can result in long-term professional advancement. Today, with a great demand for BSN graduates, these nurses have the greatest career mobility among all basic program graduates in nursing.

According to *The Essentials of Baccalaureate Education for Professional Nursing Practice* (AACN, 2008), nurses who graduate from BSN programs are prepared "to practice within complex healthcare systems and assume the following roles: provider of care; designer/manager/coordinator of care; and member of a profession" (p. 3). The AACN document also stressed the concepts of patient-centered care, interprofessional teams, evidence-based practice, quality improvement, patient safety, informatics, clinical reasoning/critical thinking, genetics and genomics, cultural sensitivity, professionalism, and practice across the life span in an increasingly complex healthcare environment (p. 3).

The challenge to enhance opportunities for students to pursue a career in nursing has been met in an innovative, significant way by visionary nurse educators in Rhode Island, who 10 years ago opened the Rhode Island Nurses Institute Middle College Charter School (RINI) in Providence. This school is for students who have completed 8th grade and who are interested in a career in nursing. Students continue at RINI through their first year of college. The curriculum focuses on science and math skills necessary to be successful in nursing school and then in practice. The mission of the school is "to prepare a diverse group of students to become the highly educated and professional nursing workforce of the future" (Rhode Island Nurses Institute Middle College, 2021).

Associate Degree Programs

ADN (associate degree in nursing) education was initiated in 1952 to address the post–World War II nursing shortage. Based on a model developed by Mildred Montag, EdD, during her doctoral studies, and fueled by interest in community college education after World War II, associate degree programs became the most common type of basic nursing education program in the U.S. and until recently graduated the most RN candidates of all the basic programs.

The popularity of ADN programs can be attributed to several features: accessibility of community colleges, low tuition costs, part-time and evening study opportunities, shorter duration of programs, and graduates' eligibility to take the licensure examination for RNs.

When first envisioned by Dr. Montag, ADN programs were proposed as a solution to a nursing shortage. She suggested a shorter program designed to prepare nurse technicians who would function under the supervision of professional nurses. ADN nurses were to work at the bedside, performing routine nursing skills for patients in acute and long-term care settings. The original ADN program, as outlined by Montag (1951), offered general education courses in the first year and nursing courses in the second year. Montag originally viewed the ADN as a final, end-point degree, not an incremental step to the BSN.

In practice, Montag's original conceptions of ADN programs have been greatly modified. ADN curricula now offer more nursing credits than she suggested. They also include content on leadership and clinical decision making, abilities that Montag did not anticipate as needed in technical nurses. Because of additions to the curriculum, students may need to enroll for more than 2 years to complete the program of study. ADN graduates are employed in a variety of settings and function autonomously with BSN and diploma graduates. In the educational system of nursing today, the ADN can be a step in the progression to the BSN or master's degree.

Since 1990, the NLN Council of Associate Degree Programs has sought to differentiate the competencies of the ADN nurse from those of the BSN nurse. The original document, first written in 1990 (NLN, 1990), was revised in 2000 in response to a changing healthcare delivery system. Titled *Educational Competencies for Graduates of Associate Degree Nursing Programs*, the revised document identified eight core competencies of ADN education: professional behaviors, communication, assessment, clinical decision making, caring interventions, teaching and learning, collaboration, and managing care (NLN, 2000). The most current version, *Outcomes and Competencies for Graduates of Practice/Vocational, Diploma, Associate Degree, Baccalaureate, Master's Practice, and Research Doctorate Programs in*

Nursing (2012), addresses four core competencies across all educational levels—human flourishing, nursing judgment, professional identity, and spirit of inquiry (NLN, 2012). Landmarks in the history of nursing education are listed in Table 4.1.

External Degree Programs

External degree programs in nursing are different from traditional basic nursing education in that students attend no classes. Learning is independent and is assessed through highly standardized and validated competency-based outcomes assessments, leading to the description "virtual university." Students are responsible for arranging their own clinical experiences in accordance with established standards.

Excelsior College, formerly known as the New York Regents External Degree Nursing Program, is a well-recognized external degree model. Beginning in 1970 with an ADN program, Excelsior College now offers ADN, BSN, and MSN degrees, all of which are accredited by the National League for Nursing Accreditation Commission (NLNAC). The Excelsior College School of Nursing was designated by the NLN as a Center of Excellence in Nursing Education, 2016–2021. Since 1981, the California State University Consortium has offered a statewide external BSN program. The California program is for RNs already holding current licenses to practice in the state. Numerous external degree programs are in existence today, many of which are marketed online and by direct mail. Prospective students must exercise caution when deciding on which type of entry-level program to attend. Program accreditation ensures prospective students that the curriculum and faculty meet external requirements for nursing education.

Articulated Programs

In response to the demand for educational mobility, articulation (mobility) among programs has become much more common in today's nursing education system. The purpose of articulation is to facilitate opportunities for nurses to increase their education. An example of a fully articulated system is the LPN/LVN/ADN/BSN/MSN program in which students spend the first year preparing to be an LPN/LVN and the second year completing the ADN. Depending on the program, students can leave at the end of the first year, take the licensure examination for LPN/LVN, and return to complete the ADN program later. These students may continue study in the program after the initial 2 years to earn a BSN degree and even continue for a master's or doctorate.

TABLE 4.1 Landmarks in the History of Nursing Education

1860	Florence Nightingale founded the first organized program to educate nurses at St. Thomas' Hospital in London.
1872	The "famous trio," the first year-long training schools for nurses, was established in the United States, founded at Bellevue Hospital, the New England Hospital for Women and Children, and Massachusetts General Hospital.
1873	Melinda Anne "Linda" Richards became the first "trained nurse" to graduate in the United States.
1899	Teachers College, Columbia University, offered the first postgraduate course in hospital economics for nurses.
1907	Mary Adelaide Nutting became the first nursing professor at Teachers College, Columbia University.
1909	The first BSN program was established at the University of Minnesota.
1923	The Goldmark Report was published, the first such report focusing on hospital control of schools of nursing and lack of proper teacher preparation.
1924	Yale University established the first nursing school as a separate university department with its own dean, Annie W. Goodrich.
1932	The first EdD in nursing was granted by Teachers College.
1934	The first PhD program in nursing was initiated by New York University.
1948	Esther Lucille Brown's report Nursing for the Future was published, recommending that basic nursing programs be situated in colleges and universities rather than in hospitals.
1952	The first ADN program, based on Dr. Mildred Montag's model, was established to prepare nurse technicians.
1954	The University of Pittsburgh started the first PhD program in clinical nursing.
1965	The ANA issued a position paper advocating the BSN degree as the minimum educational preparation for entry into nursing practice.
2004	The AACN passed a resolution to create the DNP degree.

Multiple-entry, multiple-exit programs are difficult to develop. A tremendous amount of joint institutional planning is needed to create equivalent courses and to keep the programs congruent across institutions. A change in one curriculum dictates changes in all the others. These challenges explain why fully articulated programs have been slow to develop. In increasing numbers, however, articulation agreements between BSN and ADN programs and between ADN and LPN/LVN programs are being established that facilitate student movement among programs and accept transfer credit among institutions. These requirements may result in acceleration or advanced placement within the higher-degree school.

Despite the difficulties in developing articulated programs, several state legislatures have mandated their public institutions to create these programs to facilitate upward educational mobility for nurses. Other states have statewide voluntary articulation plans, and still others have individual school-to-school agreements in place.

RN-TO-BSN, ACCELERATED BSN, DISTANCE LEARNING: ALTERNATE PATHS IN NURSING EDUCATION

In addition to the basic programs leading to entry-level nursing practice, alternative programs exist.

Baccalaureate Programs for Registered Nurses

After nursing organizations of the 1960s and 1970s publicly advocated for the BSN degree to be the minimum education level for professional practice, the demand for the BSN degree increased. Employers of nurses recognized that nurses with broad education matched well with the complexities of health care. As a result, many supported the BSN as a requirement for career mobility. Diploma and ADN graduates returned to school in increasing numbers. Today, many students enter ADN programs with plans to earn a BSN eventually. Baccalaureate programs for RNs allow these nurses, as well as diploma nurses, to accomplish this goal.

Historically, RNs with diplomas and associate degrees did not always find a place in BSN programs. In the early years of baccalaureate education for RNs, many schools required these students to take courses in areas the students had already mastered, constituting barriers for these nurses to complete their BSN degrees. Now, however, BSN programs recognize the importance of RN-to-BSN education and have developed alternative tracks to accommodate the unique learning needs of the RN student.

Baccalaureate programs for RNs are most often offered by universities that also offer basic nursing education in baccalaureate programs. The RN students may be integrated with the traditional BSN students, or they may be enrolled in a separate or partially separate sequence. Some baccalaureate programs for RNs are freestanding; that is, they are offered by colleges that do not have a basic BSN program or are in single-purpose institutions. Many of these programs are now offered online.

Most 4-year colleges and universities allow the transfer of general education credits from ADN programs. With increasing frequency, transfer credit is given for nursing courses as well, or there is the option of receiving credit for previous nursing courses through a variety of advanced placement methods such as examinations, demonstrations, and portfolios.

For diploma graduates, transfer credit is usually given for previous college courses, such as English, if they were included as part of the diploma program and taught by college faculty. Options for advanced placement of diploma graduates into BSN programs vary widely, and prospective RN students should seek detailed information to select a program that fits individual needs and goals.

The demand for the BSN degree by large numbers of ADN and diploma graduates continues to be strong. More nurses are returning to school to prepare for the wider opportunities offered by the BSN degree. With broad preparation in clinical, scientific, community health, and patient education skills, the baccalaureate nurse is well positioned to move across community-based settings such as home health care, outpatient centers, and neighborhood clinics, where opportunities are fast expanding.

Programs for Second-Degree Students

A noteworthy trend is the significant increase in the number of students with bachelor's degrees in other fields making a career change to nursing. The educational system in nursing has responded to this group of students by offering options to the traditional basic baccalaureate education. Increasingly, baccalaureate programs offer these students an accelerated or fast-track sequence, awarding either a second bachelor's degree or, in some cases, an MSN. Accelerated MSN programs for individuals with bachelor's degrees in another field are known as generic master's degree programs. They usually require about 3 years to complete, depending on the number of prerequisite courses needed. Graduates take the RN licensure examination (NCLEX-RN®) after completing the generic master's program.

Online and Distance-Learning Programs

The majority of nursing programs, particularly entry-level programs, are still offered in the traditional way with in-person course work. Technological advances, however, have made it possible for students to take courses online, and a significant percentage of colleges and universities are now offering some or all of their courses online as distance learning (DL). Originally intended to improve educational access for nurses from rural areas, students enrolled in web-based courses today might live in the same town as the educational institution but have significant demands on their time and prefer the flexibility of online offerings.

Master's and doctoral programs in nursing have been at the forefront in the development of online programs, with up to 30% of MSN programs and up to 50% of doctor of nursing practice (DNP) programs now offering half or more of their courses online. According to the AACN, relatively few entry-level BSN programs offer half or more of their courses online, and the majority offer few if any online courses, although this number is increasing. In contrast, RN-to-BSN programs are often offered online.

As more schools of nursing offer coursework and entire degrees through DL, the issue of adequate and properly supervised clinical experience arises. Technology may again provide at least a partial answer to this dilemma through use of virtual environments. DL students validate their clinical competence in a number of traditional ways, including preceptorships, clinical examinations, demonstrations, and clinical portfolios. When the programs are properly structured, well monitored, and offered to carefully selected students, the achievement levels of DL students are comparable with those of traditional students.

Some fraudulent online programs exist in which students are charged very large fees. Other programs may be appealing at the outset, but sometimes enrolled students find serious flaws in how content is delivered online and how their learning is evaluated. Students contemplating enrolling in online programs should be educated consumers and consider several factors when evaluating options, such as the reputation of the college or university offering the courses and access to faculty and student support services such as academic advisement or disability services. Before committing to an online degree program, you should answer these important questions:

- Do you have the self-discipline needed to keep up with assignments outside a traditional classroom setting?
- Do you learn best when you can interact with other students and faculty, or do you prefer working alone?

ACCREDITATION: ENSURING QUALITY EDUCATION

Accreditation of educational programs in nursing is crucial. Although all nursing programs must be approved by their respective state boards of nursing for graduates to take the licensure examination, nursing programs may also seek accreditation, which goes beyond minimum state approval. Accreditation refers to a voluntary review process of educational programs by a professional organization known as an accrediting agency, which compares the educational quality of the program with established standards and criteria. Accrediting agencies derive their authority from the U.S. Department of Education. Two agencies, the Accreditation Commission for Education in Nursing (ACEN) and the Commission on Collegiate Nursing Education (CCNE), are responsible for accrediting nursing educational programs today.

Accreditation of nursing schools grew out of concerns by leaders of the profession about the lack of quality and standards for nursing education. An accredited program voluntarily adheres to standards that protect the quality of education, safety, and the profession itself; in other words, maintains nursing's social contract with the public. Accreditation provides both a mechanism and a stimulus for programs to initiate periodic self-examination and self-improvement. This process assures students that their educational program is accountable for offering quality education.

Accrediting bodies establish standards by which a program's effectiveness is measured. Programs under review prepare self-study reports that show how the school meets each standard. The self-study report is reviewed by a volunteer team composed of nursing educators from the type of program being reviewed, and an on-site program review is conducted by the same team. After the site visit, the visitors' report and the program's self-study are reviewed by the accrediting organization, and a decision is made about the accreditation status of each nursing program.

Prospective nursing students should inquire about the accreditation status of any nursing program they are considering. Qualifying for certain scholarships, loans, and military service typically requires an accredited program. Acceptance into a graduate program in nursing will likely depend on graduation from an accredited BSN program. Employers of nurses are usually interested in hiring only nurses who are graduates of accredited programs.

Once a program is accredited and in good standing, continuing accreditation reviews take place every 8 to 10 years. Programs not meeting standards may receive a warning or be placed on probation and given a specific time limit to correct deficiencies. Accreditation can be withdrawn if deficiencies are not corrected within the specified time.

In 1996 the AACN organized the CCNE, which is recognized by the U.S. Department of Education as the national accrediting body for BSN and higher degree nursing programs. CCNE began operation in 1998 and has subsequently established an organizational structure, policies and procedures, and accreditation standards and criteria. In December 1999 CCNE received a recommendation from the National Advisory Committee on Institutional Quality and Integrity, a panel of the U.S. Department of Education, that the Secretary of Education grant initial recognition of CCNE as a national agency for the accreditation of bachelor's and graduate nursing education programs. This status was renewed in 2002. The establishment of a second national accrediting body for nursing education represented a significant development in the evolution of the nursing profession. Originally commissioned as the National League for Nursing Accrediting Commission (NLNAC), the ACEN is the accreditation agency for LPN/LVN programs, diploma programs, and ADN programs. Bachelor's and higher degree programs may choose which of the two accrediting bodies they wish to use.

TAKING THE NEXT STEPS: ADVANCED DEGREES IN NURSING

A variety of economic, educational, and professional trends are fueling the demand for RNs with advanced degrees (master's or doctorate). The evolving healthcare system requires nurses to possess increasing knowledge, clinical competency, greater independence, and autonomy in clinical judgments. Trends in community-based nursing centers, case management, complexity of home care, sophisticated technologies, and society's orientation to health and self-care are rapidly causing the educational needs of nurses to expand, thereby requiring graduate education. Reforms in health care are expected to increase the demand for nurses with master's and doctoral degrees.

Nurses who have advanced education can become researchers, NPs, clinical specialists, educators, and administrators. Some of the opportunities available to nurses with advanced degrees are described in Chapter 1. Having a workforce of highly educated nurses strengthens the profession.

Master's Education

The purpose of master's education is to prepare people with advanced nursing knowledge and clinical practice skills in a specialized area of practice. Teachers College, Columbia University, is credited with initiating graduate education in nursing. As mentioned, beginning in 1899, the college offered a postgraduate course in hospital economics, which prepared nurses for positions in teaching and hospital administration. From this beginning, there has been consistent growth in the number of master's nursing programs in the United States.

Most nurses in the 1950s and 1960s viewed the master's degree in nursing as the terminal degree—that is, the highest degree in a profession or academic discipline. The master's degree was considered the highest degree nurses would ever need. Early master's programs were longer and more demanding than master's programs in other disciplines. Master's programs in the 1950s and 1960s prepared students for careers in nursing administration and nursing education.

With the rapid development of doctoral programs for nurses during the 1970s, however, the master's degree was no longer considered nursing's terminal degree. Programs were shortened and advanced practice through clinical specialization became the emphasis.

Master's programs in nursing are most often found in colleges and universities that have basic BSN programs. These programs may also seek voluntary accreditation from either ANEC or CCNE.

Entrance requirements to master's programs in nursing typically include the following: a BSN degree from an accredited program, licensure as an RN, completion of the Graduate Record Examination or other standard aptitude test, a minimum undergraduate grade point average of 3.0, recent work experience as an RN in an area related to the desired area of specialization, and specific goals for graduate study. These entry requirements vary among colleges and universities, so prospective students need to be aware of specific requirements for the master's programs to which they are applying.

The average traditional program length is 18 to 24 months of full-time study, although part-time study and accelerated curricula are far more common today than in the past. The Master of Science (MS) and the MSN are the two most common graduate degrees offered. The curriculum includes theory, research, clinical practice, and courses in other disciplines. Master's students generally select both an area of clinical specialization, such as adult health or gerontology, and an area of role preparation, such as informatics, administration, or teaching. Students may be required to write a comprehensive examination and/or to complete a thesis or research project.

Major areas of role preparation include administration, case management, informatics, health policy/healthcare systems, teacher education, clinical nurse specialist, NP, nurse-midwifery, nurse anesthesia, and other clinical and nonclinical areas of study. With the increasing demand for NPs, master's programs have expanded their practitioner tracks.

Another option in master's education is the RN/MSN track, which allows RNs who are prepared at the associate degree or diploma level and who meet graduate admission requirements to enter a program leading to a master's degree rather than a bachelor's degree. Other recent graduate program options are combined degrees such as the master of science in nursing/master of business administration (MSN/MBA) for nurse administrators or the master of science in nursing/juris doctor (MSN/JD) for nurse attorneys. Clearly diversity in nursing education extends to the graduate as well as the basic level.

Doctoral Education

Doctoral programs in nursing prepare nurses to become faculty members in universities, administrators in schools of nursing or large medical centers, researchers, theorists, and advanced practitioners. Doctoral programs in nursing offer several degree titles. These can be divided into two categories: a research-focused degree (PhD) and a practice-focused degree (DNP).

History of Doctoral Education in Nursing

Formal doctoral education for nurses began at Columbia University's Teachers College in 1910 with the creation of the Department of Nursing and Health. The first student completed work for the Doctor of Education (EdD) in nursing education and was awarded the doctorate in 1932. In 2016 the Teachers College of Columbia University began offering an online program leading to an EdD in nursing education.

In 1934 New York University initiated the first PhD program for nurses. The programs at Teachers College and New York University provided many of the profession's early leaders, who worked over the years for improvements in nursing education. From 1934 through 1953, no new nursing doctoral programs were opened. In 1954 the University of Pittsburgh opened the first PhD program in clinical nursing and clinical research in the United States. By the end of the 1950s, only 36 doctoral degrees had been awarded in nursing (Parietti, 1990).

Because of the limited number of nursing doctoral programs, most nurses in the 1950s and 1960s earned doctorates in nonnursing fields, such as education, sociology, and physiology. Doctoral education for nurses moved into a new phase when the federal government initiated nurse scientist programs in 1962, which awarded the doctor of nursing science (DNS, DNSc, DSN) degrees. These programs were created to increase the research skills of nurses and provide faculty for the development of doctoral programs in nursing. The nurse scientist programs were discontinued in 1975 after more universities began offering doctoral programs in nursing. Some universities converted these degrees retroactively to PhD degrees (Ponte and Nicholas, 2015).

Current Status of Doctoral Education in Nursing

The research-focused doctorate for students with prior degrees in nursing is the PhD. The PhD is an academic degree and prepares nurse scholars for research and the development of theory. Nurses with PhDs focus their work on the development of the science of nursing. Some nurses hold the DNS degree. It is an academic research degree that has generally been phased out in the United States but is recognized to be the equivalent of a PhD. Other countries award the DNS as the terminal degree (highest academic degree) in nursing. In the U.S., the PhD is the terminal degree.

In October 2004, members of the AACN debated and passed a resolution calling for a new doctorate, the DNP (AACN, 2004). Designed to replace the master's degree, the DNP would be required to be completed by nurses who wish to practice in advanced roles, such as NP or nurse-midwife. Proponents of this change suggested that it would put nursing on an even footing with other healthcare disciplines that require a clinical doctorate. Detractors argued that the proposed change could increase confusion within and outside the profession about the qualifications of nurses prepared at the doctoral level; it could also discourage nurses from seeking the PhD in nursing and thereby further deepen the shortage of nurse faculty prepared in the manner of other professors on college and university campuses (Dracup and Bryan-Brown, 2005). Despite early concerns, the degree has proven to be popular, and increasing numbers of universities are offering the DNP. The number of programs and graduates has grown rapidly.

Enrollment trends indicate that there is continued demand for all types of doctoral education in nursing. The number of programs, as well as the number of requests for admission to these programs, continues to increase. This trend has partially stemmed from the requirement of a doctorate for academic advancement and tenure for university nursing faculty. A research doctorate is typically required to become a well-trained researcher who can compete for grants and develop nursing science; PhD-prepared nurses can assist DNP nurses in the development of sound research. DNP-prepared nurses move research into practice. This advances the profession as a whole. Large numbers of nurses with doctorates will continue to be needed in the future as positions requiring this degree expand in universities and throughout the healthcare system. In Professional Profile Box 4.2, you can read about Tom Bush, DNP, FNP-BC, FAANP, a nurse practitioner who decided to complete his DNP after several years of advanced practice as a family nurse practitioner in an orthopedic clinic in an academic medical center.

PROFESSIONAL PROFILE BOX 4.2

FNP Earning His Doctor of Nursing Practice Degree

Neither of my parents nor extended family attended college so I am the first in my family to earn a college degree. To fund my education, I worked part time while earning an associate's degree in nursing from a local community college in the mountains of eastern Kentucky. I chose nursing because of an interest in biologic and social science and could never have imagined the opportunities gained by choosing a career in nursing.

While working as a registered nurse, I soon realized the many rewards and challenges of the nursing profession. I was able to gain valuable on-the-job experience and work toward an advanced degree while earning a living. I quickly enrolled in an innovative bridge program that led to a master's degree in nursing.

My nursing career has included primary care, critical care, and specialty services. For 10 years I split my time between teaching nurse practitioner students at the University of North Carolina at Chapel Hill School of Nursing and clinical practice in the Department of Orthopedics at the University of North Carolina at Chapel Hill School of Medicine. The dual roles of clinician and educator positioned me to help others realize the vast opportunities that are the future of nursing.

The landmark report by the Robert Wood Johnson Foundation and the Institute of Medicine, *The Future of Nursing: Leading Change, Advancing Health*, recommends that nurses achieve higher levels of education and training through an education system that promotes seamless academic progression. I have lived this experience, and after two decades of practice I chose to return to school for a doctor of nursing practice degree at East Carolina University in Greenville, North Carolina.

The skills gained from additional education enable me to participate more fully in interprofessional teams to meet the healthcare needs of individuals and populations in North Carolina and throughout the United States. As our nation moves toward a redesigned healthcare system, it is imperative that nurses are well positioned to lead the way. Nursing addresses the pathophysiology of disease *and* the human response to illness. This perspective

Continued

PROFESSIONAL PROFILE BOX 4.2—cont'd

FNP Earning His Doctor of Nursing Practice Degree

helps inform my leadership role in interprofessional education among nurse practitioner students and physician residents. Experience as a clinician and educator allows me to share clinical expertise to improve patient outcomes. Demonstrating nursing leadership among multiple healthcare disciplines has a valuable impact on the next generation of clinicians.

Doctoral nursing education enabled me to apply analytical methodologies for the evaluation of education models for NP transition to practice. Postgraduate NP education (fellowships and residencies) is gaining popularity and is funded primarily by employers interested in recruiting and retaining qualified healthcare professionals. My DNP project produced the first evidence demonstrating that postgraduate education positively affects NP job satisfaction. Knowledge of factors that influence job satisfaction is valuable to NPs and employers considering formal postgraduate education programs.

It is an excellent time to be a nurse. Together we can improve our nation's health by building on the strengths of all health disciplines, celebrating the differences, and pointing to models of collaboration that serve our citizens well.

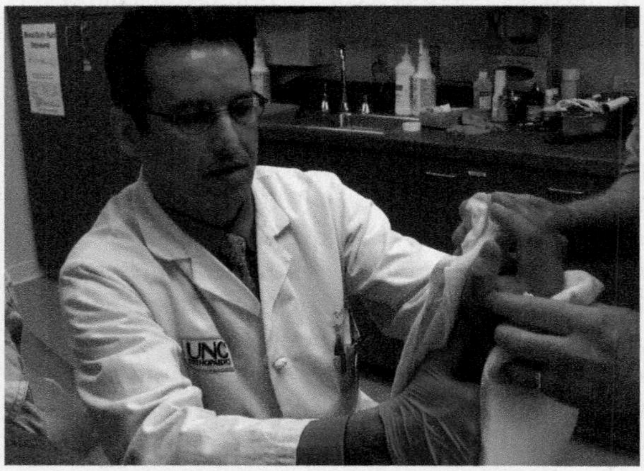

Tom Bush, DNP, FNP-BC, FAANP
East Carolina University, 2015

Courtesy North Carolina Health News.

BECOMING CERTIFIED: VALIDATING KNOWLEDGE AND PROFICIENCY

Licensure and certification are both forms of credentialing of nurses. Licensure refers to state regulation of the practice of nursing. Licensure is required of individuals at the entry point to practice and must be renewed periodically. It is a legal designation that ensures public safety by assessing basic and continuing competence. You will learn more about licensure in Chapter 6. Certification goes beyond licensure by validating a high level of knowledge and proficiency in a particular practice area. Certification has professional but not legal status.

Certification means that a certificate is awarded by a certifying body as validation of specific qualifications demonstrated by an RN in a defined area of practice. A comprehensive examination is required to become certified, as well as documentation of experience, letters of reference, and other documents. You can find a great deal of information about specialty certification at https://www.nursingworld.org/our-certifications.

Certified nurses may have greater earning potential, wider employment opportunities, a broader scope of practice, validation of their skills, knowledge, and abilities, public recognition, a sense of personal satisfaction, and prestige that sets them apart from noncertified nurses. Requirements for admission to certification programs vary, with some requiring only RN licensure and others requiring either a bachelor's or a master's degree. The ANCC, affiliated with the ANA, is the largest of the certification bodies, providing many certification programs for RNs at the associate degree, bachelor's degree, and advanced practice levels. APNs certified by the ANCC must have master's degrees and demonstrate successful completion of a certification examination based on nationally recognized standards of nursing practice and designed to test their special knowledge and skills. For most specialties, candidates also must show evidence of specified clinical practice experience. Once granted, certification is valid for 3 to 5 years, whereupon the individual must apply for recertification by retesting or by demonstrating continuing education (CE) credits and evidence of ongoing clinical practice.

Nurses holding certification may use the initials RNC (registered nurse certified) after their names. Board certified nurses are entitled to use RN, BC. Those certified as clinical specialists use APRN, BC (advanced practice registered nurse, board certified). The educational and practice requirements for board certification can be stringent, but becoming board certified identifies a nurse as having a high level of expertise in the field in which they are working.

Many in the nursing profession believe that nurses should be certified in a standardized manner by nationally recognized certifying boards only and that having multiple standards of certification is confusing and disadvantageous to the profession. The AACN has been particularly vocal in this regard and issued position statements in 1994, 1998, and 2008. The 2008 Consensus Model emphasized standardization goals focusing on APRNs. This could become a model for nursing certifications at all levels, thereby unifying certification processes and rendering them more understandable by both employers and the public and thereby benefiting nursing. The Consensus Model document can be found on the National Council of State Boards of Nursing website at https://www.ncsbn.org/Consensus_Model_Report.pdf.

MAINTAINING EXPERTISE AND STAYING CURRENT THROUGH CONTINUING EDUCATION

Continuing education (CE), also known as *lifelong learning*, is a term used to describe ways in which nurses maintain expertise during their professional careers. CE differs from staff development, which refers to how an agency or institution assists its employees in maintaining competence. CE opportunities are those pursued by individual nurses themselves and take place in a variety of settings: colleges, universities, hospitals, community agencies, professional organizations, and professional meetings. CE is available in many formats, such as workshops, institutes, conferences, short courses, evening courses, DL, and instructional modules offered in professional journals and by professional organizations online.

The ANCC is responsible for standards of CE, accreditation of programs offering CE, transferability of CE credit from state to state, and development of guidelines for recognition systems within states. The contact hour is the measure of CE credit. In general, nurses receive 1 contact hour of CE credit for each 50 or 60 minutes they spend in a CE course.

Most states require some evidence of CE for license renewal; the requirements, however, vary from state to state. Once you become licensed, you will need to be aware of the CE requirements for your state to maintain your license. Before renewing their licenses in states and territories with mandatory CE, nurses must provide evidence that they have met contact hour requirements. The requirement for mandatory continuing education is the mechanism through which a regulatory agency (e.g., state board of nursing) ensures that nurses remain current in their profession. CE is required in most professions, including medicine, law, pharmacy, and accounting, among others.

CHALLENGES: FACULTY SHORTAGES AND QUALITY AND SAFETY EDUCATION IN TODAY'S COMPLEX HEALTHCARE ENVIRONMENT

A number of challenges face nursing education. Two major challenges are discussed in this section: (1) faculty and other resource shortages resulting in the inability of nursing programs to produce enough nurses to meet society's needs, and (2) the need to transform nursing education to meet the need for quality and safety in the complex healthcare environment.

Faculty and Other Resource Shortages Resulting in Lack of Nurses

Despite the fact that enrollments in entry-level nursing programs across the nation have increased in recent years, the number of employed nurses still falls short of current needs and will fall further behind in the wake of the COVID-19 pandemic and as the population ages. The lack of capacity in nursing schools is a significant problem in educating sufficient numbers of nurses. Capacity to educate nurses includes size and preparation of faculty, classroom and lab facilities, and number and types of clinical sites. Several schools of nursing may compete for clinical sites when there are fewer adequate sites compared with the number of students needing clinical placements.

As the general population ages, so does the nurse faculty population. The latest available AACN data indicated that the average age of full professors in schools of nursing was 62 years and the average age of associate professors was 58 years (AACN, 2017;

http://www.aacnnursing.org/Portals/42/News/Factsheets/Faculty-Shortage-Factsheet-2017.pdf). This trend will result in increasing numbers of faculty retirements in the next decade. Faculty shortages are severe and seriously affect the nation's supply of RNs. Interest in nursing careers is strong, but access to professional nursing programs is increasingly difficult and is expected to become even more so for the foreseeable future. This represents a formidable challenge for the profession.

Continuing the Evolution of Nursing Education: Quality and Safety Education for Nurses

In response to the challenges of preparing future nurses adequately to "continuously improve the quality and safety of the healthcare systems," the QSEN project was funded by the Robert Wood Johnson Foundation. In phases 1 and 2 of the QSEN project, Drs. Linda Cronenwett and Gwen Sherwood of the University of North Carolina at Chapel Hill School of Nursing and their team developed and pilot-tested approaches to curricula that would ensure that future nursing graduates had competencies in patient-centered care, teamwork and collaboration, evidence-based practice, quality improvement, and informatics (QSEN, 2012).

In phase 3, which ended in 2012, Dr. Cronenwett and the AACN focused on three goals: (1) promote continuing innovation in the QSEN competencies and dissemination of these innovations; (2) develop faculty expertise required for students to achieve quality and safety competencies; and (3) create mechanisms to sustain the will to change among nursing programs through nursing textbooks, accreditation and certification standards, licensure examinations, and continued competence requirements. In Professional Profile Box 4.3, Linda Cronenwett, PhD, RN, FAAN, describes how the increasing complexity of health care has demanded new ways of thinking about quality and safety in nursing.

Some experts believe that education of all health professions is in need of systemic change. A notable example is the 2003 report of the IOM, *Health Professions Education: A Bridge to Quality*. This report built on the 2001 IOM report, *Crossing the Quality Chasm: A New Health System for the 21st Century*, which recommended a complete restructuring of clinical

PROFESSIONAL PROFILE BOX 4.3

Changing Meanings of Quality and Safety in Nursing Education

During most of the 20th century, patients were cared for by relatively few people. Even in the hospital, it was often one physician, one nurse per shift (working 5 days a week), and a head nurse who knew everything about each patient's condition. A nurse could know every medication she gave, and disruptions during medication rounds were few.

The sole purpose of nursing education was to prepare nurses to care for individual patients. Quality and safety were considered dependent on the knowledge and skills of individual professionals. A nurse could say, "I'm the best nurse on this unit. If your mother were sick, you'd want me caring for her. But don't bother me with committees or performance improvement teams or being a better team player. That's not the work I care to do." No one challenged that nurse's definition of what it meant to be a good nurse.

Today, health care is a complex enterprise. Multiple physicians and other healthcare professionals are involved in a hospitalized patient's care. Patients and families rarely have the same nurse 2 days in a row, and much nursing care is delivered by various types of assistants and technicians. There are thousands of pieces of medical equipment, multiple procedures and medications, and complex systems for documenting care. If you had to identify which professionals were responsible for the quality and safety of a patient's care, it would be hard to know who to hold accountable. In fact, quality and safety are more likely to be related to the way a healthcare microsystem (unit, clinic, or community-based setting) is designed to work than to the traits and skills of individual professionals. The reliability of the system is what meets or fails to meet patient needs, and although system reliability includes, it is not limited to, the quality of care any one professional gives any one patient.

With the 2003 IOM Report, *Health Professions Education: A Bridge to Quality*, all educators were challenged to alter the process of professional development so that health professionals, including nurses, would graduate understanding and accepting that their jobs consisted of both caring for individual patients and continuously improving the quality, safety, and reliability of the

PROFESSIONAL PROFILE BOX 4.3—cont'd

Changing Meanings of Quality and Safety in Nursing Education

healthcare systems within which they worked. The development of specific competencies related to patient-centered care, interprofessional teamwork and collaboration, evidence-based practice, safety sciences, quality improvement methods, and informatics was considered an essential element of future curricula. I served as the principal investigator of the Quality and Safety Education for Nurses (QSEN) project, an initiative funded by the Robert Wood Johnson Foundation to support faculty development to accomplish this paradigm shift in nursing education.

To be a good health professional into the future will mean knowing what constitutes good care (as it has in the past), but it will also mean knowing something about how the actual care delivered in one's unit or clinic compares to expected or best practices in the world at large. Furthermore, if there is a gap between good care and the results of care in one's own system, being a good healthcare professional will mean knowing what one can do to close that gap.

Gradually, nursing curricula are changing to meet these new expectations. We want you to be good nurses in this new world, ones who know what quality of care is all about.

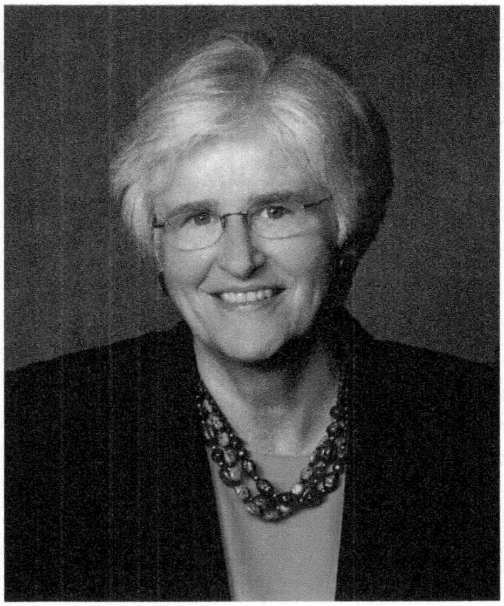

Linda R. Cronenwett, PhD, RN, FAAN
Dean Emeritus and Professor Emeritus, School of Nursing, University of North Carolina at Chapel Hill

Courtesy Linda R. Cronenwett.

education across all health professions (IOM, 2001). As a follow-up to the initial report, a multidisciplinary summit of health profession leaders met in 2002; this high-level panel composed of 150 participants recommended the goal of "an outcome-based education system that better prepares clinicians to meet both the needs of patients and the requirements of a changing health system" (IOM, 2003). Five major problems were identified in professional health education across disciplines (IOM, 2003):

- Students are not being educated to care for the increasingly diverse, elderly, and chronically ill patient populations.
- Students are not being prepared to work in teams, but once in practice, they are usually expected to work in interdisciplinary teams.
- Students are not consistently educated in how to find, evaluate, and use the rapidly expanding scientific evidence on which practice should be based.
- There is little opportunity to learn how to identify, analyze, and eliminate the root causes of errors and other quality problems in healthcare delivery systems.
- Students often are not provided basic informatics training to enable them to access information and use computerized order entry systems.

In 2005 the NLN issued a position statement titled *Transforming Nursing Education.* This statement promoted evidence-based education; that is, educational practices based on research into best educational practices rather than "tradition, past practices, and good intentions" (NLN, 2005, p. 1). The NLN statement of a decade ago shaped the view of the faculties of schools of nursing in terms of designing and implementing educational practices in which the focus is on developing professional nursing practice that is evidence based. There is an increased emphasis on evidence-based practice across all disciplines in today's evolving healthcare environment.

COLLABORATION IN HEALTHCARE EDUCATION: INTERPROFESSIONAL EDUCATION

Interprofessional education (IPE) is a highly significant development in the training and education of nurses, physicians, social workers, pharmacists, and other healthcare professionals, in which students in these disciplines take courses and have clinical experiences together. IPE involves structural changes in healthcare education to think beyond the traditional model in which healthcare professionals are educated separately, often without understanding the focus and expertise of practitioners in other disciplines. IPE enhances the development of respect across disciplines, increased understanding of the roles of other disciplines, and better communication among practitioners. Health care is more effective when delivered collaborative. Interprofessional teamwork and collaboration has the potential to increase patient satisfaction, decrease errors and improve safety, and be more cost effective (Derouin et al., 2018). In 2011 the IOM encouraged the healthcare professions to think differently about education, given the increasingly obvious need for collaboration among the professions to provide optimal health care and improve outcomes (IOM, 2015). Early adopters of IPE have begun to publish their experiences, with one noting that "IPE and practice are crucial to the development of future healthcare professionals" (Derouin et al., 2018, p. 225).

Nursing students should understand that nursing organizations and leaders are continually recognizing, analyzing, and responding to changes in the healthcare system and working to set standards by which high-quality education nursing programs can be designed, implemented, and evaluated. The complexity of healthcare delivery systems, variations in health across populations, faculty shortages, financial constraints and other limitations on resources make this a challenging task. Despite formidable challenges, nursing education will continue to evolve in response to significant changes in today's healthcare environment.

CONCEPTS AND CHALLENGES

- ***Concept:*** First provided in hospitals, entry-level nursing education has evolved into three major types of basic programs, diploma, ADN, and BSN, each of which has a range of features.
  Challenge: Differing levels of education for entry into practice pose a problem for nursing that has yet to be resolved, although an increasing number of employers are requiring a BSN as minimum education.
- ***Concept:*** Alternatives such as bachelor's degree programs for RNs, external degree programs, accelerated options for postbaccalaureate students, and online programs contribute the complex educational picture for RNs.
  Challenge: Standardization of nursing education across the various programs becomes a challenge across these various educational offerings.
- ***Concept:*** Voluntary accreditation is designed to ensure the quality of nursing education programs.
  Challenge: Students are often not aware of their program's accreditation status. Graduate programs require that applicants be graduates of accredited schools of nursing.
- ***Concept:*** Schools have found it necessary to restrict enrollments because of faculty shortages, lack of clinical sites, and budget constraints.
  Challenge: Nursing leaders must prioritize making nurse faculty positions attractive in terms of compensation and work environment. At a time of economic volatility, this is a particularly difficult challenge for nursing.
- ***Concept:*** Lifelong learning through CE is considered essential for all professionals, particularly in practice-based disciplines such as nursing.
  Challenge: States vary on their requirements for CE for license renewal. Even if your state does not require CE, your professional responsibility is to stay current in practice by engaging in CE opportunities.
- ***Concept:*** The problem of reduced resources in nursing education may soon reach crisis proportions and poses a threat to smaller schools and universities.
  Challenge: The underfunding of higher education in general and, in particular, diminishing sources of federal and state funding for schools of nursing require the attention of nurse leaders to ensure

an adequate workforce of well-educated nurses to manage today's complex healthcare problems.

- ***Concept:*** QSEN was developed to meet the challenge of ensuring competencies of nursing graduates in patient-centered care, teamwork and collaboration, evidence-based practice, quality improvement, and informatics.
  Challenge: QSEN and other initiatives required a change in thinking about nursing education and the way nurses practice to ensure the best possible patient outcomes in a healthcare environment where resources are strained.
- ***Concept:*** IPE is a newer model of education for healthcare providers across disciplines in response to the increasing need for professional collaboration to optimize patients' health outcomes.
  Challenge: Nursing stands to benefit from IPE through its potential to elevate communication, create shared goals, and increase mutual respect across healthcare disciplines.

IDEAS FOR FURTHER EXPLORATION

1. Watch *Sentimental Women Need Not Apply* (available on DVD). How does your experience of nursing school compare with that of students a century ago? What challenges to nursing have remained the same over time?
2. How did you determine which type of basic nursing program you entered? Knowing what you know now, what changes, if any, would you make in your choice? How would you advise a high school student interested in nursing to select a program?
3. Consider the challenge that states face in determining whether a BSN should be the educational degree for entry into practice. Discuss the pros and cons of requiring a BSN to take the NCLEX-RN®. In what ways would the unification of nursing education strengthen the profession? What are the drawbacks to this approach?
4. If you could create a curriculum for nursing school, what would you include? What courses have surprised you by being included in your nursing education?
5. What unique contributions to nursing are possible by nurses with master's-level education? With doctorates?
6. Find out if your school has implemented QSEN competencies. How prepared are you in each of the competencies?
7. Find out if your school offers any interprofessional courses or experiences with other healthcare disciplines. If so, consider enrolling in one or more to enhance your education and understanding of the focus and values of other health professionals.

REFERENCES

Aiken LH, Cheung RB, Olds DM: Education policy initiatives to address the nurse shortage in the United States, *Health Affairs Web Exclusive*, 2009. (website). Available at https://www.healthaffairs.org/doi/abs/10.1377/hlthaff.28.4.w646.

American Association of Colleges of Nursing (AACN): *Position statement: certification and regulation of advanced practice nurses*, Washington, DC, 1994, The Association (revised 1998).

American Association of Colleges of Nursing (AACN): *Position statement: the baccalaureate degree in nursing as minimal preparation for professional practice*, Washington, DC, 2000, The Association.

American Association of Colleges of Nursing (AACN): *Position statement: the practice doctorate in nursing*, Washington, DC, 2004, The Association.

American Association of Colleges of Nursing (AACN): *The Essentials of baccalaureate education for professional nursing practice*, Washington, DC, 2008, The Association. (website). Available at https://www.aacnnursing.org/portals/42/publications/baccessentials08.pdf.

American Association of Colleges of Nursing (AACN): *Nursing faculty shortage fact sheet*, Washington, DC, 2017, The Association. (website). Available at http://www.aacnnursing.org/Portals/42/News/Factsheets/Faculty-Shortage-Factsheet-2017.pdf.

American Nurses Association (ANA): *Position paper: educational preparation for nurse practitioners and assistants to nurses*, Kansas City, MO, 1965, The Association.

American Nurses Association (ANA): *A case for baccalaureate preparation in nursing*, Kansas City, MO, 1979, The Association.

Benner P, Sutphen M, Leonard V, et al.: *Educating nurses: a call for radical transformation*, San Francisco, 2009, Jossey-Bass.

Brown EL: *Nursing for the future*, New York, 1948, Russell Sage Foundation.
Christy T: Portrait of a leader: M. Adelaide nutting, *Nurs Outlook* 17(1):20–24, 1969.
Conley V Curriculum and instruction in nursing, *Boston*, 1973 Little, Brown.
De Back V: The National commission on nursing implementation project, *Nurs Outlook* 39(3):124–127, 1991.
Derouin A, Holtschneider ME, McDaniel KE, Sanders KA, McNeill DB: Let's work together: interprofessional training of health professionals in North Carolina, *NC Med J* 79(4):223–225, 2018.
Donahue MP: Nursing: the finest art: an illustrated history, St. Louis, 1985, Mosby.
Dracup K, Bryan-Brown CW: Doctor of nursing practice: MRI or total body scan, *Am J Crit Care* 14(4):278–281, 2005.
Health Resources and Services Administration (HRSA): Apply for a grant,2021. (website). Available at: https://bhw.hrsa.gov/grants/nursing.
Institute of Medicine (IOM): *Crossing the quality chasm: a new health system for the 21st century*, Washington, DC, 2001, National Academies Press.
Institute of Medicine (IOM): *Health professions education: a bridge to quality*, Washington, DC, 2003, National Academies Press.
Institute of Medicine (IOM): *The future of nursing: leading change, advancing health*, Washington, DC, 2011, National Academies Press.
Institute of Medicine (IOM): *Measuring the impact of interprofessional education on collaborative practice and patient outcomes*, Washington, DC, 2015, National Academies Press.
Institute of Medicine (IOM): *Assessing progress on the Institute of Medicine Report The Future of Nursing*, Washington, DC, 2016, National Academies Press.
Kalisch P, Kalisch B: *The advance of American nursing*, ed 3, Boston, 1995, Little, Brown.
Lysaught J: *An abstract for action*, New York, 1970, McGraw-Hill.
Montag M: *The education of nursing technicians,* New York, 1951, Putnam.
National Academy of Sciences, Engineering, and Medicine: *The future of nursing 2020-2030: charting a path to achieve health equity*, Washington, DC, 2021, National Academies Press, 2021.
National League for Nursing Education: *Nursing schools today and tomorrow*, New York, 1934, The League.
National League of Nursing Education: *A curriculum guide for schools of nursing*, New York, 1937, The League.
National League for Nursing (NLN): *Position statement on nursing roles: scope and preparation*, New York, 1982, The League.
National League for Nursing (NLN): *Council of associate degree programs: educational outcomes of associate degree nursing programs: roles and competencies*, New York, 1990, The League.
National League for Nursing (NLN): *Educational competencies for graduates of associate degree nursing programs*, New York, 2000, The League.
National League for Nursing (NLN): *Transforming nursing education*, 2005. (website). Available at www.nln.org/aboutnln/PositionStatements/index.htm.
National League for Nursing (NLN): *Competencies for graduates of nursing programs,* 2012. (website). Available at https://www.nln.org/education/nursing-education-competencies/competencies-for-graduates-of-nursing-programs.
National League for Nursing (NLN): Preparing the next generation of nurses to practice in a technology-rich environment: an informatics agenda, 2008. (website). Available at www.nln.org/aboutnln/PositionStatements/index.htm.
Notter L, Spalding E: *Professional nursing: foundations, perspectives and relationships*, ed 9, Philadelphia, 1976, JB Lippincott.
Parietti E: The development of doctoral education in nursing: a historical overview. In Allen J, editor: *Consumer's guide to doctoral degree programs in nursing*, New York, 1990, National League for Nursing, pp 1532.
Ponte RP, Nicholas PK: Addressing the confusion related to DNS, DNSc, and DSN degrees, with lessons for the nursing profession, *J Nurs Scholarsh* 42(4):347–353, 2015.
QSEN: Quality and safety education for nurses,2012. (website). Available at: www.qsen.org.
Rhode Island Nurses Institute Middle College: Mission and vision, 2021. (website). Available at: www.rinimc.org.
Spector N, Odom S: The initiative to advance innovations in nursing education: three years later, *J Nurs Regul* 3(2):40–44, 2012.
Tri-Council for Nursing: Tri-Council for Nursing issues new consensus policy statement on educational advancement of registered nurses, 2010. (website). Available at: www.nln.org/newsroom/news-releases/news-release/2010/05/14/tri-council-for-nursing-issues-new-consensus-policy-statement-on-the-educational-advancement-of-registered-nurses.

5

Becoming a Professional Nurse: Defining Nursing and Socialization In Practice

ⓔ To enhance your understanding of this chapter, try the Student Exercises on the Evolve site at http://evolve.elsevier.com/Black/professional.

LEARNING OUTCOMES

After studying this chapter, students will be able to:

- Describe the benefits of defining nursing and how this is related to professional socialization.
- Compare early definitions of nursing with contemporary ones.
- Recognize the impact of historical, social, economic, and political events on evolving definitions of nursing.
- Identify commonalities in existing definitions of nursing.
- Understand how students' initial images of nursing are transformed through professional education and experiences.
- Differentiate between formal and informal socialization.
- Identify factors that influence an individual's professional socialization.
- Describe two developmental models of professional socialization, and explain how they are used.
- Describe strategies to ease the transition from student to professional nurse.

Suppose you were to ask someone, "What do nurses do?" Then think about how you as a nursing student would answer the same question. You might be tempted to respond with a list of psychomotor skills such as injections, medication administration, and physical assessments you have been practicing in your clinical setting. You might use some of your communication skills to turn the question back on the person: "You are wondering about nurses. What is it that *you* think nurses do?" This might be your best means of buying some time until you come up with an answer; describing the work of nursing is not always easy.

This chapter will help you answer this question. Definitions of nursing and nursing's scope of practice delineate who nurses are and what they do. Definitions provide answers to these questions: "What is nursing?", "What is the role of the nurse?", "What is unique about nursing?", and "What are the boundaries of nursing practice?" Although the answers to these questions seem simple, agreement on a single definition of nursing has been elusive; however, the careful crafting of definitions of nursing by noteworthy nursing organizations has resulted in definitions that are increasingly similar and specific about what nursing is.

In this chapter, definitions of nursing are explored to determine how they have evolved over time. Once you have a clear understanding of definitions of nursing, you will learn how to make the move from student to nursing student and then from nursing student to professional nurse. This developmental trajectory from student to professional nurse involves a process known as *socialization*, which occurs over time but ultimately guides you in developing a safe and informed professional nursing practice. Defining nursing is an important first step in socialization. Having a clearer understanding of what nursing is (and, as Nightingale said, "What it is not") helps you move closer to incorporating the values of professional practice.

DEFINING NURSING: HARDER THAN IT SEEMS

You may be surprised to learn that finding a universally acceptable definition of nursing has been difficult historically. Common responses to your question "What do nurses do?" might be "They take care of people in the hospital" and "They help doctors." Few people outside of the healthcare setting understand who nurses are and what they do.

Even nurses themselves have been unable to agree on one definition. For more than 150 years, individuals and organizations around the world such as the International Council of Nurses (ICN), the United Kingdom's Royal College of Nursing (RCN), and the American Nurses Association (ANA) have attempted to achieve a consensus on a definition of nursing. In 1859 Florence Nightingale wrote a famous text, *Notes on Nursing: What It Is and What It Is Not*, an early attempt to define who and what nurses are and do. Some efforts have been more successful than others.

The definitions reviewed in this chapter have become increasingly aligned over time. Considering the variations in knowledge and technology during the different points in history when these definitions were written, the similarities are remarkable. All the definitions are rooted in history and were affected by significant political, economic, and social events that shaped nursing.

Why Define Nursing?

Having an accepted definition of nursing provides a framework for nursing practice. A definition establishes the parameters (or boundaries) of the profession and delineates the purposes and functions of the work of nursing. In addition, a definition guides the educational preparation of aspiring practitioners and guides nursing research and theory development. Importantly, a clear definition makes the work of nursing visible and valuable to the public and to policy makers who determine when, where, and how nurses can practice. Norma Lang, Professor and Dean Emerita at the University of Pennsylvania, described the need for definition succinctly: "If we cannot name it, we cannot control it, finance it, research it, teach it, or put it into public policy. It's just that blunt!" (Styles, 1991).

Definitions Clarify Purposes and Functions

Nursing is a complex enterprise that is often confusing to its own practitioners as well as to the public. Defining nursing assists people to grasp its nuances, many of which are not readily observable. The profession of nursing benefits when the public, other healthcare providers, policy makers, insurers, and journalists, among others, understand who nurses are and what they do.

Definitions Differentiate Nursing from Other Health Occupations

Five million allied healthcare providers in more than 80 different occupations represent approximately 60% of all providers (Explore Health Careers, 2021). Advances in technology require providers who need to be educated, hired, and oriented to their specific work setting and who are paid with limited healthcare dollars. These resulting costs figured greatly into the redesign of the healthcare system over the past decade and required the redefining of roles within the system. Defining nursing amid these new providers became even more important to avoid losing the core identity of nursing. Nurses have had to name and claim for their own what it is that nurses do.

Furthermore, with the implementation of healthcare reforms, nursing must be clearly defined and its importance within the healthcare system made unmistakable. Nurses understand that they have the skills and expertise to address a wide variety of health issues; keeping nurses in key positions of influence as the healthcare system continues to take shape in the next few years is crucial to fulfilling nursing's social contract with the public, which you read about in previous chapters. The ANA's *Nursing's Social Policy Statement: The Essence of the Profession* explicates this contract.

Definitions Influence Health Policy at Local, State, and National Levels

Policy makers such as legislators and regulators need a clear understanding of the role and scope of nursing. Without that understanding, they cannot institute good healthcare policy that maximizes use of nurses' particular skills to protect and improve the health of the public.

A key reason to define nursing is that nursing practice is regulated at the state level. Nursing practice acts of each state need to reflect the widening expertise and autonomy of nurses. When the roles of professional registered nurses (RNs), advanced practice nurses, licensed practical/vocational nurses, and nursing assistants are well defined, legislators can pass progressive laws regulating and expanding nursing practice. Otherwise, nursing practice acts that are legislated by state governing bodies may restrict nursing practice and inhibit professional growth.

Definitions Focus Educational Curricula and Research Agendas

When nursing faculty plan the curriculum of a school of nursing, one of the major determinants of the design is their definition of nursing. A definition of nursing provides a good starting point for curriculum development. Without the foundation of a clear definition, deciding what to include in a nursing curriculum and how to prioritize educational needs would be very difficult and unwieldy. In much the same way, nurse researchers cannot easily determine phenomena of interest for nursing unless they are clear about the boundaries and purposes of nursing actions that a definition of nursing sets in place.

Evolution of Definitions of Nursing

While nursing was progressing as a more formal academic discipline and practice profession over the past 150 years, a number of attempts were made to define nursing that reflect the profession's evolution over the years.

Nightingale Defines Nursing

Florence Nightingale was the first person to recognize the complexities of nursing that led to difficulty in defining it. Considering how relatively undeveloped nursing was during her time, Nightingale's definitions contain what today we recognize as contemporary concepts. Remember that during Nightingale's day, formal education in nursing was just beginning. In *Notes on Nursing: What It Is and What It Is Not* (originally published in 1859), she became the first person to attempt a written definition of nursing, stating, "And what nursing has to do … is put the patient in the best condition for nature to act upon him" (Nightingale, 1946, p. 75). She also wrote:

> *I use the word nursing for want of a better. It has been limited to signify little more than the administration of medicines and the application of poultices. It ought to signify the proper use of fresh air, light, warmth, cleanliness, quiet, and the proper selection and administration of diet—all at the least expense of vital power to the patient.*
>
> ***(Nightingale, 1946, p. 6)***

Although Nightingale lived in a time when little was known about disease processes and effective treatments were extremely limited, these definitions foreshadowed contemporary nursing's focus on the therapeutic environment as well as the modern emphasis on health promotion and health maintenance. Observation has always been integral to processes of nursing. Nightingale noted that, although simply possessing observational skills does not make someone a good nurse, without these skills a nurse is ineffective. She was also the first person to differentiate between nursing provided by a professional nurse using a unique body of knowledge and physical care provided by a layperson such as a mother caring for a sick child.

Early 20th-Century Definitions

Fifty years after Nightingale wrote *Notes on Nursing*, the search for a definition began in earnest. Following the English model, many schools of nursing had been established in the United States, and many nurses with formal education were practicing. These nurses sought to develop a professional identity for their rapidly expanding discipline. Shaw's *Textbook of Nursing* (1907) defined nursing as an art: "It properly includes, as well as the execution of specific orders, the administration of food and medicine, the personal care of the patient" (pp. 1–2). Harmer's *Textbook of the Principles and Practice of Nursing* (1922) elaborated on Shaw's bare-bones definition: "The object of nursing is not only to cure the sick … but to bring health and ease, rest and comfort to mind and body. Its object is to prevent disease and to preserve health" (p. 3). The fourth edition of the Harmer text, which showed the influence of coauthor and visionary Virginia Henderson, redefined nursing: "Nursing may be defined as that service to an individual that helps him to attain or maintain a healthy state of mind or body" (Harmer and Henderson, 1939, p. 2). Henderson's perceptions represented the emergence of contemporary nursing and were so inclusive that they remained useful over a long time. We will encounter her influence again in the next section.

Post–World War II Definitions

World War II helped advance the technologies available to treat people, which, in turn, influenced nursing. The war also made nurses aware of the influential role emotions play in health, illness, and nursing care. Hildegard Peplau (1952), widely regarded as a pioneer among contemporary nursing theorists and herself a psychiatric nurse, defined nursing in interpersonal terms: "Nursing is a significant, therapeutic, interpersonal process. Nursing is an educative instrument that aims to promote forward movement of personality in the direction of creative, constructive, productive, personal, and community living" (p. 16). Peplau reinforced the idea of the patient as an active collaborator in his or her own care. Recently Peplau's notion of patient participation and collaboration in their health and healthcare has reemerged and is referred to as active patient engagement. Patient engagement, or when patients take purposeful action in improving their health, is a crucial factor in helping transform the current healthcare paradigm. During the late 1950s and early 1960s, the number of master's programs in nursing rapidly increased. As more nurses were educated at the graduate level and learned about the research process, they were eager to test new ideas about nursing. Nursing theory was born. (See Chapter 9 for an in-depth discussion of nursing theory.)

Dorothea Orem was a significant nursing theorist who began work during this early period of theory development. Her 1959 definition captures the flavor of her later, more completely elaborated self-care theory of nursing: "Nursing is perhaps best described as the giving of direct assistance to a person, as required, because of the person's specific inabilities in self-care resulting from a situation of personal health" (Orem, 1959, p. 5). Orem's belief that nurses should do for a person only those things the person cannot do without assistance emphasized the patient's active role.

By 1960, Henderson's earlier definition had evolved into a statement with such universal appeal it was adopted by the ICN:

> *The unique function of the nurse is to assist the individual, sick or well, in the performance of those activities contributing to health or its recovery (or to a peaceful death) that he would perform unaided if he had the necessary strength, will or knowledge. And to do this in such a way as to help him gain independence as rapidly as possible.*
>
> **(Henderson, 1960, p. 3)**

This definition of nursing was widely accepted both in the United States and across the world. Many believe it is still the most comprehensive and appropriate definition of nursing in existence.

Another pioneer nursing theorist, Martha Rogers, included the concept of the nursing process in her definition: "Nursing aims to assist people in achieving their maximum health potential. Maintenance and promotion of health, prevention of disease, nursing diagnosis, intervention, and rehabilitation encompass the scope of nursing's goals" (Rogers, 1961, p. 86).

Professional Association Definitions

Nursing organizations worldwide have worked to define nursing, developing and revising them over time. Definitions reviewed here include those of the ANA, the RCN, and the ICN. As you study these definitions, notice that some new concepts and terms are introduced in the more recent American definitions. In the United States nursing has defined itself as the health discipline that "cares," although recent discussion suggests that limiting nursing to "caring" only overlooks the significant role that nurses have in the curative processes of health care (Gordon, 2005).

American Nurses Association. The ANA has published several definitions of nursing over the years. In 2021 the ANA published its revised definition of nursing:

> *Nursing integrates the art and science of caring and focuses on the protection, promotion and optimization of health and human functioning; prevention of illness and injury; facilitation of healing; and alleviation of suffering compassionate presence. Nursing is the diagnosis and treatment of human response; and advocacy in the care of individuals, families, groups, communities and populations in recognition of the connection of all humanity"*
>
> **(ANA, 2021, p.20).**

Nursing: Scope and Standards of Practice, 4th Edition reflects on the "who," "what," "where," "when," "why," and "how" of the practice of nursing, an intentional format that sets flexible boundaries on the scope of practice because "changes in scope of practice and overlapping responsibilities are inevitable in our current and future health care system." (ANA, 2021).

Nursing's Social Policy Statement: The Essence of the Profession defined contemporary nursing practice in terms of six essential features of (ANA, 2010):

1. Provision of a caring relationship that facilitates health and healing
2. Attention to the range of human experiences and responses to health and illness within the physical and social environments
3. Integration of objective data with knowledge gained from an appreciation of the patient or group's subjective experience
4. Application of scientific knowledge to the processes of diagnosis and treatment through the use of judgment and critical thinking
5. Advancement of professional nursing knowledge through scholarly inquiry
6. Influence on social and public policy to promote social justice

The wide focus of the practice of nursing is described in the preface to the *Code of Ethics for Nurses* (ANA, 2015): "Nursing encompasses the prevention of illness, the alleviation of suffering, and the protection, promotion, and restoration of health in the care of individuals, families, groups, and communities" (p. vii). The definition of nursing and the ethics to which nurses are bound are intertwined.

Royal College of Nursing. The RCN is the United Kingdom's voice of nursing and is the largest professional union of nurses in the world. This organization embarked on an 18-month-long initiative to define nursing, culminating in the April 2003 publication of the document titled *Defining Nursing* (RCN, 2021). In 2014 the RCN's Nursing Policy and Practice Committee upheld and affirmed the continuing appropriateness of the 2003 definition because it described nursing to persons who do not understand nursing; it clarified the role of nurses in multidisciplinary teams and identified areas of research that nursing needs to strengthen its science (RCN, 2021).

The RCN definition of nursing has a core statement supported by six defining characteristics:

> *Nursing is the use of clinical judgment in the provision of care to enable people to improve, maintain, or recover health, to cope with health problems, and to achieve the best possible quality of life, whatever their disease or disability, until death.*

The six defining characteristics are delineated by statements of the "particulars of nursing": purpose, mode of intervention, domain, focus, value base, and commitment to partnership. The particulars are explicated on page 3 of the Definition of Nursing document (RCN, 2021).

International Council of Nurses. The ICN is a federation of national nurses associations founded in 1899, and represents more than 27 million nurses in more than 130 countries worldwide. Although ICN's membership is diverse, its definition of nursing is similar to that of single-nation organizations such as the ANA and RCN. The ICN still uses a definition of nursing the Council created in 2002, the short version of which is as follows:

> *Nursing encompasses autonomous and collaborative care of individuals of all ages, families, groups and communities, sick or well and in all settings. Nursing includes the promotion of health, prevention of illness, and the care of ill, disabled and dying people. Advocacy, promotion of a safe environment, research, participation in shaping health policy and in patient and health systems management, and education are also key nursing roles.*
>
> ***(ICN, 2021)***

You can learn more about the ICN online at www.icn.ch, which includes an expanded version of the short definition.

Definitions Developed by State Legislatures

One of the most significant definitions of nursing is contained in the nursing practice act of the state in which a nurse practices. Regardless of how restrictive or permissive it may be, the definition contained in a nursing practice act constitutes the legal definition of nursing in a particular state. Professional nurses must maintain familiarity with the latest version of the act. North Carolina's Nursing Practice Act, most recently revised in

2009, contains particularly specific language defining nursing (North Carolina Board of Nursing, 2009):

> *"Nursing" is a dynamic discipline which includes the assessing, caring, counseling, teaching, referring and implementing of prescribed treatment in the maintenance of health, prevention and management of illness, injury, disability or the achievement of a dignified death. It is ministering to, assisting, and sustained, vigilant, and continuous care of those acutely or chronically ill; supervising patients during convalescence and rehabilitation; the supportive and restorative care given to maintain the optimum health level of individuals, groups, and communities; the supervision, teaching, and evaluation of those who perform or are preparing to perform these functions; and the administration of nursing programs and nursing services.*

Furthermore, the North Carolina Board of Nursing describes nursing as a dynamic discipline, described as both a science and an art:

> *The practice of nursing is a scientific process founded on a professional body of knowledge. It is a learned profession based on an understanding of the human condition across the life span and the relationship of a client with others and within the environment. The practice of nursing is an art dedicated to caring and to assisting clients by providing sustained, vigilant, and continuous care to those acutely or chronically ill. Nurses assist clients to attain or maintain optimal health, implementing a strategy of care to accomplish defined goals within the context of a client centered health care plan. Nursing is a dynamic discipline that increasingly involves more sophisticated knowledge, technologies and client care activities.*
>
> ***(North Carolina Board of Nursing, 2020)***

The language in this nursing practice act sounds like familiar nursing language. State nurses associations and boards of nursing actively assist legislators in drafting laws that reflect the nature and scope of nursing accurately. The current nursing practice act in each state and U.S. territory can be obtained online.

Before moving on to the next discussion on socialization, take time to look at the question posed in Thinking Critically Box 5.1. What would you do?

? THINKING CRITICALLY BOX 5.1

What Would You Do?

Imagine you are dining out and are seated next to a table where a young person who appears to be in their late teens tells their parents they want to be a nurse. The parents' reaction is one of disdain. They reply, "Are you serious? You want to be a nurse? You want to clean up messes and sling bedpans for the rest of your life? Why don't you become a doctor—it pays much better and is more respectable." The young person, visibly upset, leaves the table. The parents notice that you are eavesdropping and ask you, "Why would anyone want to be a nurse?"

What would you say to these parents? Using your thoughts and experience, as well as elements of definitions from this chapter, how would you explain and define nursing to them? You may want to save your response and refer to it after you graduate from nursing school. As you become more socialized into nursing, your explanation to these parents would likely evolve.

BECOMING A NURSE: SHAPING YOUR PROFESSIONAL IDENTITY

Defining nursing means identifying the essential elements of being a nurse: what a nurse is and what a nurse does. When you first decided to become a nurse, you had certain preconceived notions about what nursing was and how you saw yourself as a nurse. Your desire to be a nurse may have been shaped by an illness experience of your own or of a family member. Becoming a nurse may simply be something that you have always wanted to do without a specific event that spurred this desire. Or you may be pragmatic in your career choice by selecting a profession in which demand is high, the risk for unemployment is low, and the compensation is adequate. Whatever the reason(s) you decided pursue a career in nursing, your view of nursing and what it entails is almost certainly going to be challenged while in nursing school. How you think about the profession of nursing should evolve and mature over the course of your education and career.

Although many nursing students enter the profession with the worthy goal of "taking care of people," how this goal is translated into practice remains something of a mystery until you begin your education as a nursing student. Being a student of nursing is the first of many steps in socializing you into professional practice: the goal of socialization is the development of professionalism. The goal of your nursing education is not simply teaching you the tasks of nursing, although they are important elements of safe practice. Good quality nursing education teaches you to think like a nurse, to think critically, to develop a broad sense of the meaning of health care and its delivery, and to respond to your educational and clinical experiences with the development of professionalism.

This process requires that students internalize, or take in, new knowledge, skills, attitudes, behaviors, values, and ethical standards and make these a part of their own professional identity. For the RN returning to school for a bachelor of science in nursing (BSN) degree, a modification of an already formed professional identity occurs. This process of internalization and development or modification of an occupational identity are known as *professional socialization*; it begins during the period when students are in formal nursing programs and continues as they practice in the "real world."

Two conditions—structural and cultural—are part of professional socialization in nursing (Lai and Lim, 2012). Structural conditions are those in which one's professional role is shaped by rules (e.g., job descriptions, workplace policies, carrying out prescriptions for care by physicians and other providers). Cultural conditions are those in which traditions, symbols, language, and other idea systems in a society are at work in shaping how one becomes a fully socialized professional nurse. The goal, then, of socialization as a professional nurse is the development of a professional identity such that the attributes of nursing become "part of a nurse's personal and professional self-image and behavior" (p. 32).

From Student to Nurse: Facilitating the Transition

Nursing faculty are concerned with creating educational experiences that encourage and facilitate the transition from student to professional nurse. You may wonder how this transition occurs, especially when you are faced with the challenges of simply figuring out what is going on in your classes, labs, and clinical sites.

Learning any new role is derived from a mixture of formal and informal socialization. We have all been socialized into a variety of roles over the course of our lives. One that is so familiar to you now is the role of student in a generic sense. You learned in kindergarten that there are particular ways to behave in class, times to sit quietly and times to play, ways to get the teacher's attention, and ways that you did not want to get the teacher's attention. You learned the unwritten rules of being a student, and, unless you were particularly incorrigible, you learned your role as a student early and well.

In nursing, formal socialization includes lectures, online activities, assignments, and clinical experiences, such as planning nursing care, writing a paper on professional ethics, learning steps of a physical examination of a healthy child, starting an intravenous line, practicing communication skills with a person with mental illness, or spending time with a mentor (Fig. 5.1). A faculty

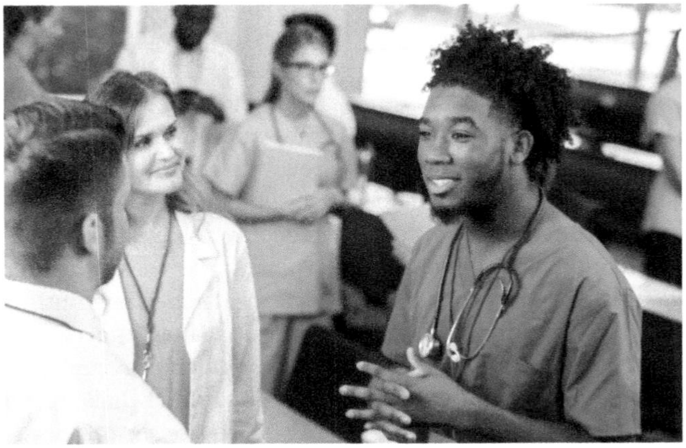

Fig. 5.1 During formal socialization, students internalize the knowledge, skills, and beliefs of nursing in planned educational experiences and interactions with faculty and other nurses. (Photo used with permission from iStockphoto.)

member may serve as your first nursing mentor. Formal socialization proceeds in an orderly, building-block fashion, such that new information is based on previous information. For that reason, more advanced nursing students are often encouraged to manage a larger number of patients than they did as novice students, when their skills were fewer and less tested.

Informal socialization includes lessons that occur incidentally, such as the unplanned observation of a nurse teaching a young mother how to care for her premature infant, participating in a student nurse association, or hearing nurses discuss patient care in the nurses' lounge. Part of professional socialization is simply absorbing the culture of nursing—that is, the rites, rituals, and valued behaviors of the profession. This requires that students spend enough time with nurses in work settings for adequate exposure to the nursing culture to occur. Most nurses agree that informal socialization experiences were often more powerful and memorable than formal socialization in their own development.

Learning a new vocabulary is also part of professional socialization. Each profession has its own jargon that is generally not well understood by outsiders. Professional students in any field usually enjoy acquiring the new vocabulary and practicing it among themselves. Although the vocabulary of any profession can be confusing and complex, students quickly become fluent as a function of both formal and informal socialization. Students should be aware, however, that certain informal vocabulary overheard on nursing units is not always appropriate in professional settings and may actually be denigrating to patients or their families. Deciding early to forgo these sorts of negative characterizations is a step toward maturity in your professional socialization.

Learning any new role creates some degree of anxiety. You likely remember your nervousness and anxiety as you started college or a new job. New students may find themselves particularly anxious as clinical experiences begin; the uncertainty of the situation, the unfamiliar language, the presence of patients with serious medical diagnoses, and a keen sense of the importance of the work of nursing can all contribute to this anxiety. Once the initial anxiety and excitement of entering nursing school have worn off, students may find themselves dealing with disappointment and frustration when their learning expectations come into conflict with educational realities. Students' ideas of what they need to learn, when they need to learn it, and what might be the best way to learn it may differ from how their education actually unfolds. Students sometimes become disillusioned when they observe nurses behaving in ways that conflict with an image they may hold of how nurses "should" behave. Knowing in advance that frustration and even disillusionment can occur can help students accurately assess the sources of their discomfort and manage it more effectively.

Factors Influencing Socialization

As students progress through nursing programs, a variety of factors challenge their customary ways of thinking. These include personal feelings and beliefs, some of which may conflict with professional values. For example, if students have strong religious beliefs, they may be uncomfortable working with patients who have no such belief or whose beliefs are different from their own. Provision 1 in the *Code of Ethics for Nurses* (ANA, 2015, p.v) states that "the nurse practices with compassion and respect for the inherent dignity, worth, and unique attributes of every person." This can be a difficult aspect of nursing to master. If you have a strong moral objection to a particular belief system of a patient or a negative reaction to a patient based on some characteristic of the patient, you should seek out your clinical faculty or other professional mentor to discuss your reaction and determine how to handle your conflicted feelings in an appropriate and professional way. This is not an uncommon response in nursing students as their sphere of contact with others different from themselves grows.

When children are growing up, they are first influenced by the values, beliefs, and behaviors of their adult caretakers. Later, peers become a significant influence. These influences also shape ideas about health, health care, and nursing. A common issue in nursing practice revolves around negative health behaviors of patients. If a nurse's family valued fitness, for example, that nurse may have difficulty empathizing with a patient with heart disease who refuses to exercise despite the clear health benefits. In this example, a personal value (fitness) comes into conflict with a professional value (nonjudgmental acceptance of patients). Students may encounter other challenges to their personal values, such substance abuse, self-destructive behaviors, abortion, issues related to sexuality, sexual orientation, expression of gender identity, fertility treatments, and care at the end of life.

All people have biases; however, unexamined biases are more likely to influence behavior than examined ones. Nurses need to be aware of their biases and discuss them with peers, faculty, and professional role models or mentors. Failure to address one's biases may adversely affect the nursing care provided to certain patients. Professional nurses should make every effort to avoid imposing their personal beliefs on others. (See Chapter 12 for further discussion of self-awareness and nonjudgmental acceptance as necessary attributes of professional nurses.) Becoming a professional nurse requires learning how to deal with conflicts in values while respecting patients' differing viewpoints. Having a systematic way to examine and think about your actions and responses to patient situations is a tenet of reflective practice (Sherwood and Horton-Deutsch, 2012). Reflective practice can help nurses cope with their role in a complex, emotionally charged healthcare system and concurrently help them develop their knowledge and nursing practice (Sherwood and Zomorodi, 2014). The key point is that you should begin to identify and reflect on those "hot button" issues that seem to affect you negatively so that you anticipate when you might encounter these issues, understand your own responses, and—importantly—know how to set them aside while still providing excellent care of your patients.

As seen from this brief overview, socialization is much more than the transmission of knowledge and skills. Socialization serves to develop a common nursing consciousness and is the key to keeping the profession vital and dynamic while preserving its fundamental focus on human responses in health and illness.

A New Factor Influencing Socialization: Distance Learning

The COVID-19 pandemic affected all aspects of the healthcare system, and the education of healthcare providers was not spared its effects. Classes moved abruptly from classrooms to online/videoconferencing, and clinical experiences were interrupted. Moreover, nurses in practice were faced with unprecedented working situations including uncertainty about the nature of viral transmission early in the pandemic, working while wearing personal protective equipment (PPE) that was uncomfortable and unwieldy, and managing tremendous changes in routines. Furthermore, like others, nurses were under stress about their own families' well-being, including their physical, psychological, and economic health and safety. Nursing students in those moments had little experience to draw from and the positive aspects of the profession sometimes seemed a fading ideal. As students were necessarily moved from clinical and classroom settings, their faculty faced the significant challenges of not simply teaching content but assisting students in understanding nursing roles and professionalism in context of a public health emergency.

Even before the pandemic, distance learning in nursing had become more common. Increasing numbers of nursing schools are using various media to deliver education to students who do not have access to traditional on-campus programs. Initially, single courses or continuing education short courses were offered by distance education. Today, entire nursing curricula are offered via video teleconferencing and online courses, with limited time spent on campus. This trend is expected to continue as demand increases. Even in traditional nursing curricula, some content is taught online combined with occasional classroom sessions (also known as "hybrid" courses).

Students have found some aspects of distance education to be useful; those born in the late 1990s and early 2000s use technology easily and would like to see faculty develop courses that appeal to their comfort with technology and distance learning (Fichten et al., 2015). Questions, however, arise about whether professional attitudes and values—in other words, professional socialization—can be effectively achieved through distance education. In a compelling large-sample study from Canada related to distance learning and socialization published by Loisier in 2014 (tonybates.ca, 2015), researchers found that, despite the support of the idea of collaborative learning and socialization via distance education, socialization does not occur automatically online in collaborative work and in fact it may conflict with distance students' desire for flexible and individual learning. This finding is somewhat at odds with Peddle, Bearman, and Nestel's integrative review (2016), suggesting that at least with regard to undergraduate health professional education, distance learning, including the use of virtual patients and environments, may be used successfully and with adequate socialization.

"JUST GOING THROUGH A STAGE": MODELS OF SOCIALIZATION

The transition from student to nurse is a topic of importance to nurse researchers interested in creating effective means of professional socialization. During the 1970s and 1980s, a number of models of professional socialization of basic and RN students were developed. Cohen (1981) and Hinshaw (1976) described developmental models appropriate for beginning nursing students. Bandura (1977) described a type of socialization he called *modeling*, which is useful when learning any new behavior. Benner (1984) identified five stages nurses pass through in the transition from novice to expert. Cohen's and Benner's models are explained in more detail below. Although these models were developed in the early 1980s, they serve to describe processes of transition and socialization that many faculty have come to recognize as almost universal among nursing students.

Cohen's Model of Basic Student Socialization

Cohen (1981) proposed a model of professional socialization consisting of four stages. Basing her work on developmental theories and studies of beginning students' attitudes toward nursing, she asserted, "Students must experience each stage in sequence to feel comfortable in the professional role" (p. 16). She believed that a positive outcome in all four stages is necessary for satisfactory socialization to occur. You may find yourself determining where you and your classmates stand amid these four stages. A reminder: this model is interesting and potentially useful; however it has not been subjected to rigorous testing or scientific validation. It does appear, thought, to fit the behaviors that experienced faculty note in the development of students' socialization into professional practice.

Cohen identified the first stage in her model, stage I, as unilateral dependence. Because they are inexperienced and lack knowledge, students at this stage rely on external limits and controls established by authority figures such as teachers. During stage I, students are unlikely to question or analyze critically the concepts teachers present, because they lack the necessary background to do so. An example of a student operating in a unilateral dependent stage would be the student who takes a clinical assignment without questioning the clinical faculty's thinking about the appropriateness of the assignment or what the student may gain from the assignment. The student absorbs the faculty's direction and discussion about the patient without yet making linkages of their own in thinking about the patient's condition. Fundamentally, students at this stage do as they are told because they lack the experience and knowledge to question.

In stage II (negativity/independence), students' critical thinking abilities and knowledge bases expand. They begin to question authority figures. Cohen called this occurrence *cognitive rebellion*. Students at this level begin to free themselves from external controls and to rely more on their own judgment. They think critically about what they are being taught. This is a stage when students begin to question, "Why do I have to learn about this? What does this have to do with nursing?" or complain, "I will never learn to give an injection to a patient if I have to sit here reading about the nursing process!" This can be a stage where a student's fledgling independence may cause some lack of judgment in the clinical setting; at this stage, students might not consult with their clinical faculty before attempting a new procedure because they do not appreciate the safety net clinical faculty provide in a patient care situation. In addition, students at this stage may begin to demand to care for additional or more complex patients, resisting their faculty's (more informed) judgment that the student is not yet ready.

Stage III (dependence/mutuality) is characterized by what Cohen described as students' more reasoned evaluation of others' ideas. They develop an increasingly realistic appraisal process and learn to test concepts, facts, ideas, and models objectively. Students at this stage are more impartial; they accept some ideas and reject others. This is a time when students begin to appreciate the usefulness of the nursing process in organizing care and begin to use more sophisticated critical thinking skills.

In stage IV (interdependence), students' needs for both independence and mutuality (sharing jointly with others) come together. Students develop the capacity to make decisions in collaboration with others. The successfully socialized student completes stage IV with a self-concept that includes a professional role identity that is personally and professionally acceptable and compatible with other life roles. Faculty appreciate the maturity and trustworthiness that students exhibit when they reach this stage in their professional development. These students are often highly self-directed, seeking out learning experiences to maximize their knowledge before the completion of their formal education. Table 5.1 summarizes the key behaviors associated with each of Cohen's stages.

TABLE 5.1 Cohen's Model of Basic Student Socialization

Stage	Key Behaviors
I: Unilateral dependence	Reliant on external authority; limited questioning or critical analysis
II: Negativity/ independence	Cognitive rebellion; diminished reliance on external authority
III: Dependence/ mutuality	Reasoned appraisal; begins integration of facts and opinions after objective testing
IV: Interdependence	Collaborative decision making; commitment to professional role; self-concept now includes professional role identity

Data from Cohen HA: *The nurse's quest for professional identity,* Menlo Park, CA, 1981, Addison-Wesley.

Benner's Stages of Nursing Proficiency (Basic Student Socialization)

Patricia Benner, a nurse, was curious about how nurses made the transition from inexpert beginners to highly expert practitioners. She described a process consisting of five stages of nursing practice, on which she based her 1984 book, *From Novice to Expert*. The stages Benner described are "novice," "advanced beginner," "competent practitioner," "proficient practitioner," and "expert practitioner." Advancing from stage to stage occurs gradually as nurses gain more experience in patient care. Clinical judgment is stimulated when the nurse's "preconceived notions and expectations" (p. 3) collide with, or are confirmed by, the realities of everyday practice.

Since its generation and publication in 1984, Benner's model has continued to receive significant attention from researchers testing how learning theories apply to adult skill acquisition (e.g., reflective thinking, clinical decision-making skills). Researchers have tested and confirmed that Benner's model is valid and suggested that her stages and theory can be used for all adult learning situations associated with nursing care (Oshvandi et al., 2016).

Benner's novice stage, or stage I, begins when students first enroll in nursing school. Because they generally have little background on which to base their clinical behavior, they must depend rather rigidly on rules and expectations established for them. Their practical skills are limited. For example, a novice nurse is faced with the request of a man who is terminally ill and wants to see and pet his beloved dog—a faithful companion—just one more time. The novice is very uncomfortable with the request because it is against institutional rules. The novice denies the request, citing these rules. Because the student is concerned about preserving the man's energy and does not want him to feel even more sad about missing his pet, they do not offer any alternative to an in-person visit, despite the availability of technology to make this happen.

By the time learners enter the advanced beginner period, or stage II, they have discerned that a particular order exists in clinical settings (Benner et al., 1996). Their performance is marginally competent. They can base their actions on both theory and principles but tend to experience difficulty in establishing priorities, viewing many nursing actions as equally important. When faced with the same situation as the novice nurse and the man approaching death who wants to cuddle and pet his dog one last time, the advanced beginner nurse also has an understanding of the needs of the man to continue his familiar ritual, bringing him the comfort and companionship he had at home with his dog, even if he soon tires. The advanced beginner suggests that the family take pictures and videos, or even arrange a video call (using FaceTime, WhatsApp, WeChat, etc.) so the man can see and even talk to his dog and reflect and reminisce about the good times and friendship they had together.

Competent practitioners, or stage III learners, usually have 2 to 3 years' experience in a setting. As a result, they feel competent, organized, and efficient most of the time. These feelings of mastery are a result of planning and goal-setting skills and the ability to think abstractly and analytically. These learners can coordinate several complex demands simultaneously. For example, the competent nurse spends a few moments at the start of their shift examining the needs of each patient and planning fundamental care. At this stage, the competent nurse understands that situations change quickly and that planning is the best way to ensure that care gets implemented even when emergencies or unexpected events arise. This nurse may or may not allow the beloved dog in the patient's room; however, they will examine the needs of everyone carefully and try to anticipate the contingencies involved before making a final decision.

Proficient practitioners (stage IV) have typically been in practice 3 to 5 years. These nurses see patient situations holistically rather than in parts, to recognize and interpret subtleties of meaning, and to easily recognize priorities for care. They can focus on long-term goals and desired outcomes. These experienced nurses are likely to be leaders on their units, having a wealth of experience and commitment to nursing. Concerned with patient outcomes rather than institutional rules, the proficient nurse would likely understand in a holistic way the needs of the man whose life is nearing its end and his desire to continue a cherished ritual of petting and cuddling with his dog. This nurse is likely to allow the "rules" to be broken in deference to the needs of the man.

Expert practitioner, or stage V, status is reached only after extensive practice experience. These nurses perform intuitively, without conscious thought, automatically grasping the significance of the patient's complete experience. They move fluidly through nursing interventions, acting on the basis of their feeling of rightness of nursing action. Their responses to a situation are so integrated that they may find it difficult to express verbally why they selected certain actions. To observers, their expertise seems to come naturally. Expert nurses on occasion have difficulty deconstructing their work, that is, being able to describe what they experience clinically, because it comes so naturally to them. The expert nurse might even initiate a suggestion to the family that they bring the dog to the man's bedside, because the expert recognizes and understands that this ritual that brings comfort and peace is even more important to honor as death approaches.

TABLE 5.2 Benner's Stages of Nursing Proficiency (Basic Student Socialization)

Stage	Nurse Behaviors
I: Novice	Has little background and limited practical skills; relies on rules and expectations of others for direction
II: Advanced beginner	Has marginally competent skills; uses theory and principles much of the time; experiences difficulty establishing priorities
III: Competent practitioner	Feels competent, organized; plans and sets goals; thinks abstractly and analytically; coordinates several tasks simultaneously
IV: Proficient practitioner	Views patients holistically; recognizes subtle changes; sets priorities with ease; focuses on long-term goals
V: Expert practitioner	Performs fluidly; grasps patient needs automatically; responses are integrated; expertise comes naturally

Data from Benner P: *From novice to expert: excellence and power in clinical nursing practice*, Menlo Park, CA, 1984, Addison-Wesley.

Table 5.2 summarizes Benner's stages from novice to expert. Professional Profile Box 5.1 contains a description of an experience in the first semester of undergraduate nursing school of this text's author that demonstrated the clear difference between novice and expert nursing; Professional Profile Box 5.2 contains the description of a memorable night shift early in the career of Maureen Baker, PhD, CNL, RN, who as an advanced beginner faced an onslaught of patient complications on a postoperative step-down unit.

PROFESSIONAL PROFILE BOX 5.1

From Novice to Expert: "How Did She Know That?"

The difference between a novice and an expert nurse was demonstrated to me in a stark way when I was in my first semester of nursing school. I was assigned to a surgical unit with other junior students. Our clinical instructor, Janie, had 8 years of surgical intensive care unit (SICU) experience as an RN and had been a faculty member for several years. The fact that she was 7 months pregnant never slowed her down. Janie just always seemed to know when we needed her, even when we did not know we needed her.

I had finished morning care for my patient, a kind elderly man who was going to be transferred to a long-term care facility later that morning. Because I had some extra time, I asked one of the other students if she needed any help. Her patient's situation was complex, having been transferred from the SICU the night before. He had a deep sacral decubitus ulcer ("bedsore") that needed to be assessed, in addition to poor perfusion resulting in gangrene in his lower extremities. She asked me to help turn him so she could assess his sacral area.

PROFESSIONAL PROFILE BOX 5.1—cont'd

From Novice to Expert: "How Did She Know That?"

Using our best communication skills, we told the patient exactly what we were going to do—turn him on his side and check his wound—and assured him that we were not going to hurt him.

Being the two novices that we were, we were fascinated by the size and depth of the ulcer and spent what seemed like several minutes staring at it. The patient never complained about the position we were holding him in. We continued talk about what to do about this pressure ulcer. I finally took a look at his face and began to reassure him that we were almost done. Then I realized that he was not responding. My novice assessment to the other student: "He looks funny" ("funny" in an odd way, not in a humorous way).

Thank goodness Janie, the expert nurse and clinical faculty member, was walking past the patient's door. She heard my novice assessment and immediately understood the severity of "looking funny" to a new student. In my memory she became airborne as she dashed into the room; in reality she simply walked in, made an immediate and correct assessment of the patient, and called a code. He was in full cardiac arrest. My classmate and I stood cowering in the corner as the room quickly filled with persons responding to the emergency. I wondered aloud, *"How did she know that?"*; with so little effort, on intuition, and with incredible calm, Janie took in the disastrous situation. I found myself envying her expertise in the resuscitation effort, the placement of a pacemaker, and coordination of his transfer back to the SICU.

My novice assessment: "He looks funny." Her expert assessment: "New students, odd assessment, complex patient. Risk for variety of complications caused by prolonged bed rest and postop infection; unresponsive, cyanotic, eyes open, not breathing, no heart rate. Call code, lower head of bed, start CPR, make sure IV is patent, make sure oxygen is available, etc."

Wisely, Janie took my classmate and me to lunch that day, encouraging us to discuss what had happened and reassuring us that nothing we did caused him to have an arrest. She allowed us to work through our own considerable distress (reflective practice). And I knew that I wanted to be "just like her" when I first became an RN and later when I became a nursing faculty member. I will always be grateful for her example of expert nursing and compassionate mentoring.

Beth Perry Black, PhD, RN, FAAN

School of Nursing, University of North Carolina at Chapel Hill

PROFESSIONAL PROFILE BOX 5.2

From Advanced Beginner to Expert: "Why Didn't I Think of That?"

I was only 6 months out of new nurse orientation and received report on the four patients I would be caring for that evening in the postoperative unit. The unit, often referred to as *the pit*, had a history of accommodating "heavy"—labor-intensive—and complex patients. As I listened to the day nurse give me report, my to-do list for each patient was growing by the second.

1. A nurse for 6 months with four complex postop patients. Four patients.
2. In bed 1, a large man, 1 day after coronary artery bypass surgery, had two chest tubes, a Foley catheter, and an external pacemaker. In bed 2, an elderly man with an active gastrointestinal (GI) bleed needed to be prepped for his bowel surgery tomorrow. His GoLytely® regimen to clean out his bowel was to begin at 6 p.m. (GoLytely® ... anything but...!). In bed 3, a fragile woman with a history of pulmonary disease was recovering from abdominal surgery. And one empty bed—I was awaiting an admission from the postanesthesia care unit (PACU).

"I got this!," I thought as I gazed over my to-do list, set my priorities, and got to work. But as the sun began to set on New York City that evening, the atmosphere in "the pit" began to change.

The man in bed 1, still calm and cooperative, asked if we were underwater: the bubbling of his chest tubes confused him. I quickly reassured him that we weren't underwater and adjusted the suction strength on the chest tube units.

I began to focus my efforts on the woman, who was now having dyspnea (difficulty breathing). I sat her up in bed, listened to her lungs, adjusted her oxygen, assessed urine output, and gave her her scheduled dose of furosemide, a strong diuretic. At that time, Barbara, a gruff woman and my nursing leadership (supervisor) for the evening, strode into the room with the pace and manner

Continued

PROFESSIONAL PROFILE BOX 5.2—cont'd

From Advanced Beginner to Expert: "Why Didn't I Think of That?"

of a drill sergeant and asked me for the unit's "bullet," a quick rundown of what is happening on the unit.

I implemented SBAR (*S*ituation *B*ackground *A*ssessment *R*ecommendation) on each patient and expressed concern for my dyspneic patient. Barbara listened as I methodically went through my nursing interventions as she looked over the unit, then she abruptly handed me her clipboard. Barbara immediately walked over to bed 3 and, with a calm, confident, yet tender voice, introduced herself. She gently assisted the woman, who was breathing rapidly, to a sitting position with her legs dangling at the side of the bed. In a reassuring tone, Barbara told the patient that gravity works on the excess fluid in her lungs when she sits up and dangles, making it easier to breathe. I sensed such relief from the woman while her breathing improved and anxiety dissipated. And I thought to myself, *"Why didn't I think of that?"*

Just then, the man with the GI bleed and GI prep began to have explosive bloody diarrhea, over and over again, and was moaning in discomfort. His daughter at the bedside was distraught. The lovely man in bed 1—the same man who was calling me "sweetheart" earlier in my shift—became more confused. Imagine a 250-pound man with multiple tubes and wires calling for the cops. He said he was leaving and would not be held prisoner. He was going to have me arrested and began to spit at me as he attempted to pull at his chest tubes and hurdle the bed rails. The phone was ringing because the PACU was getting "slammed" with postop patients, and the nurse wanted to give me the report for the patient who was on his way up to the empty bed in my unit.

I became paralyzed with fear and doubt, not knowing what to do first. I was not in control of this unit, but rather the unit was in control of me. Karen, a resource nurse, floated in with calmness amid the chaos. Karen enlisted a nursing assistant to help her with the man with the GI bleed while I tried to calm down and attend to the confused patient in bed 1.

Somehow that night, we restored order. I looked at my "to-do" list, which barely had a dent in it because all of my time and energy was spent on gaining control in a frenzied evening shift. Karen saw I was overwhelmed and exhausted at that point. She quietly reassured me and reminded me that nursing is a 24-hour/7-day-a-week profession, and if I could not get to every last thing on my list, the next nurse would. What was important that night was that we took care of our patients, not our "to-do" lists. Again, I thought to myself, *"Why didn't I think of that?"*

This is the difference between an expert and advanced beginner nurse. The advanced beginner—me—defaulted to task-oriented behavior in an attempt to gain some semblance of control. The expert nurses—Barbara and Karen—used prior experience, knowledge, and intuition amid what I thought was chaos to deliver effective, professional care.

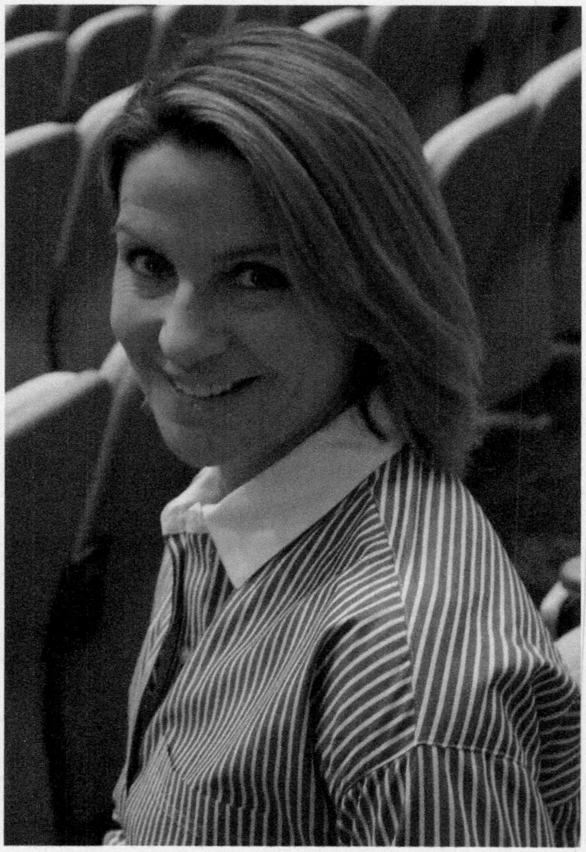

Maureen J. Baker, PhD, CNL, RN
Molloy College 1995, Rockville Centre, New York

Actively Participating in One's Own Professional Socialization

Many schools of nursing have programs for RNs with associate degrees or diplomas to complete their BSN degree. These students have special socialization needs as they return to the classroom, sometimes after years of nursing practice. Comfortable with their identities as nurses, becoming a student again can challenge adults returning to school. Students in RN to BSN or RN to MSN programs (and in prelicensure education) may find that they can reframe their own thinking about pursuing a BSN or MSN:

1. Keep your goal for returning to school front and center. Your stress is temporary, but your efforts will get you where you want to go professionally (e.g., certification, promotion, personal growth, or graduate education later).
2. Be an advocate for yourself in your studies, including being proactive on your own behalf in approaching your faculty for assistance and clarification.
3. Try to keep the opinions of others from concerning you. Colleagues may appear critical of your decision to return to school but creating your own path for professional and personal development is courageous and noteworthy.
4. Advanced education requires that you learn to think conceptually. Not all content that you encounter is immediately applicable to the clinical setting, but it is important nonetheless.
5. Become an excellent time manager, and be disciplined about how you spend your study time.
6. A mentor—another nurse, a more advanced student, or a faculty member—is an invaluable source of support.
7. Trust your faculty to help you, but remember that despite all appearances, they cannot read your mind. Ask for their help and guidance.

For other ideas about how to become an active participant in your own socialization process, use the checklist in Box 5.1.

BOX 5.1 A Do-It-Yourself Guide to Professional Socialization

The following are 18 behaviors demonstrated by students who take responsibility for their own professional socialization. Place a check next to the behaviors you regularly exhibit. Be honest with yourself.

1. I interact with other students in and out of class.
2. I participate in class by asking well-thought out questions and occasionally initiate discussion.
3. I have formed or joined a study group.
4. I use the library and librarians, labs, and teachers as resources.
5. I organize my work so that I can meet deadlines.
6. If I have a conflict with another student or a teacher, I take the initiative to resolve it.
7. I do not let minor personality problems distract me from my goals.
8. I seek out new learning experiences and sometimes volunteer to demonstrate new skills to others.
9. I have chosen professional role models and mentors.
10. I am realistic about my performance.
11. I work to accept constructive criticism because it helps me grow as a nurse.
12. I recognize that trying to do good work is not the same as doing good work.
13. I recognize that each faculty member has different expectations, and it is my responsibility to learn what is expected by each.
14. I demonstrate respect for my faculty members' time by making appointments or seeing them during office hours whenever possible.
15. I demonstrate respect for my classmates, patients, and teachers by coming to class and clinical prepared in advance.
16. I recognize my responsibility to help create an interactive learning environment and am not satisfied to be simply a spectator.
17. I participate in the student nurse association and encourage others to do the same.
18. One of my goals is to become a self-directed, lifelong learner.

Scoring

1. *1–9 checks:* You need to examine your behavior and think about taking more responsibility for your own socialization.
2. *11–14 checks:* You are active on your own behalf; try to begin using some of the remaining behaviors on the list, or come up with your own.
3. *More than 14 checks:* You are a role model of positive action in your own professional socialization process.

FROM STUDENT TO EMPLOYED NURSE: SOCIALIZATION SPECIFIC TO THE WORK SETTING

When nurses graduate, professional socialization is not over. In fact, the intensity of their socialization is likely to increase as their exposure to nursing and the culture of nursing increases. Just about the time that students become well socialized to the culture of the educational setting, they graduate and face socialization to a work setting. Most new nursing graduates feel somewhat unprepared and overwhelmed with the responsibilities of their first positions. Although settings that hire new graduates realize that the orientation period will take time, graduates may have unrealistic expectations of themselves and others.

During the early days of practice, most graduate nurses quickly realize that the ideals taught in school are difficult to achieve in everyday practice. This is largely a result of time constraints and can result in feelings of conflict and even guilt. In school, students are taught to spend time with patients and to consider their emotional as well as physical needs, and nursing students are likely to have a lighter patient assignment than they will have once they are licensed RNs in practice. Once in practice, however, new nurses may find that much emphasis seems to be placed on tasks and on documentation. Talking with patients, engaging in patient teaching, or counseling family members might not be considered central to care on a busy nursing unit. Early in professional practice, having time to do comprehensive, individualized nursing care planning, a staple of life for nursing students, may seem like an unrealistic luxury.

Optimal transitions for graduate nurses to professional practice often occur within the context of a positive and supportive working environment (Rush et al., 2013). Supportive relationships between nurses, demonstrating both recognition and acknowledgment of the learning and support needs of new nurses, can have a long-lasting impact on effectiveness in the work setting (Laschinger et al., 2016, p. 83). Recent research suggested that use of an organization's social media helps with rapid socialization of new employees into the organization, and intense use of social media has significant positive effects on performance proficiency and interpersonal relationships (Cai, Jiu, Zhao, Li, 2020). Social media then can provide a professional space for nurses to build supportive professional relationships, help develop nursing expertise and knowledge, and serve as an outlet for reflective practice in the forms of blogging or journaling. However, when using social media, nurses need to be extremely mindful of their ethical and legal responsibilities both as employees and as professional licensed nurses in keeping patient information private and confidential (National Council of State Boards of Nursing, 2018).

An interesting suggestion offered by Kopp (2008) is to "listen to gossip," a strategy that may help you determine who is integral to the culture of the unit and help you gain insight into the idiosyncratic behaviors or responses of co-workers. Participating in malicious gossip is unprofessional and hurtful to others but being aware of comments that provide insight into your new colleagues can help you understand the culture of the unit more quickly. For instance, you may overhear two co-workers discussing a third: "Alan is in the middle of everything. He manages to get appointed to every task force in the hospital, it seems." Now you know that Alan is a key person on the unit; however, if your co-workers had been speculating about the cause of Alan's recent breakup with his partner, you need to remove yourself from the conversation because it is unprofessional and no one's business except Alan's.

Speed of functioning is another area in which new nurses vary widely. Time management is a skill that is closely related to speed of functioning. Managing your time well means managing yourself well and requires self-discipline. The ability to organize and prioritize nursing care for a group of patients is the key to good time management. Box 5.2 and Fig. 5.2 provide guidance in determining and then improving your time management skills while you are a student. Once you have established the habit of good time management skills on a daily as a student, this habit will carry over to your practice setting both as a student in clinical and in professional practice.

New nurses also must adapt to working with other care personnel, such as unlicensed assistive personnel (UAP; e.g., nursing assistants, patient care technicians) and other unlicensed persons whose help is important in caring for patients. Some nurses may find working with UAPs uncomfortable when they are unaccustomed to delegating, are unsure or unaware of the abilities of others, or believe only they themselves can provide quality care.

BOX 5.2 Time Management Self-Assessment

Effective time management is a skill that can be developed. Listed are principles reflecting good time management. For each of the statements 1–10, circle the answer that most closely characterizes how you manage your time.

1. I spend some time each day planning how to accomplish school and other responsibilities.
   1. Rarely
   2. Sometimes
   3. Frequently
2. I set specific goals and dates for accomplishing tasks.
   1. Rarely
   2. Sometimes
   3. Frequently
3. Each day I make a "to-do" list and prioritize it, completing high priority tasks first.
   1. Rarely
   2. Sometimes
   3. Frequently
4. I plan time in my schedule for unexpected problems and unanticipated delays.
   1. Rarely
   2. Sometimes
   3. Frequently
5. I ask others for help when possible.
   1. Rarely
   2. Sometimes
   3. Frequently
6. I make time for short but regular breaks to refresh myself and stay alert.
   1. Rarely
   2. Sometimes
   3. Frequently
7. When I really need to concentrate, I work in a specific area that is free from distractions and interruptions.
   1. Rarely
   2. Sometimes
   3. Frequently
8. When I am working, I refuse other persons' nonurgent requests (even if they sound like fun!) that interfere with completing my priority tasks.
   1. Rarely
   2. Sometimes
   3. Frequently
9. During a clinical shift, I avoid unproductive and prolonged socializing with fellow students or employees.
   1. Rarely
   2. Sometimes
   3. Frequently
10. I keep a calendar of important meetings, dates, and deadlines.
    1. Rarely
    2. Sometimes
    3. Frequently

Scoring

Give yourself 2 points for each "Frequently," 1 point for each "Sometimes," and 0 points for each "Rarely."

1. *0–10 points:* You need to improve your time management skills.
2. *11–15 points:* You are doing fine but can still improve.
3. *16–18 points:* You have very good time management skills.
4. *19–20 points:* Your time management skills are excellent.

An overlooked aspect of stress in new graduates is the sheer physical fatigue caused by 8- to 12-hour shifts accompanied by the standing, walking, lifting, bending, and squatting that patient care requires. Some new prelicensure graduates will have never spent an entire shift on a unit while in school, and few have worked day after day on a nursing unit. Moreover, shift work, especially night shift, contributes its own significant physical demands in terms of quality and quantity of sleep. When physical fatigue is combined with the mental and emotional stress of decision making, efforts to become integrated into a peer group, uncertainty about policies or procedures, and lack of role clarity, sensory overload is almost certain to occur.

With all of this content about fatigue, gossip, demands of the job, and mental and emotional stress of decision making, it may have become evident to you that sometimes nursing units are difficult places to maintain one's good humor, much less create a culture of civility (Regan et al., 2017). Ariza-Montes and colleagues (2013) described the issues facing nurses in terms of incivility, including bullying, and noted that organizational structures that are hierarchical, are downsizing, or whose employees do not feel empowered contribute to incivility. This conduct is a form of workplace violence that most often occurs with new nurses, particularly inexperienced ones. The ANA defines incivility as "one or more rude, discourteous, or disrespectful actions that

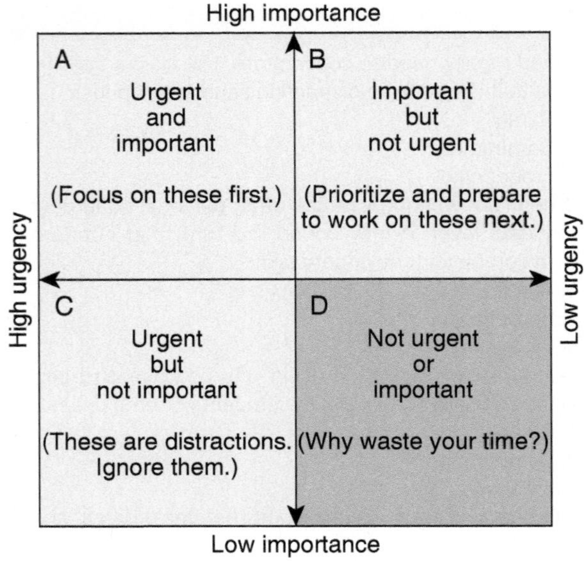

Fig. 5.2 Setting priorities is an important aspect of time management. Use this grid to determine whether a task should go to the top, middle, or bottom of your daily "to-do" list—or if it belongs on the list at all.

may or may not have a negative intent behind them." (nursingcenter.com, 2020). In 2015 the ANA published a position statement that nurses must make "a commitment to—and accept responsibility for—establishing and promoting healthy interpersonal relationships with one another" (nursingcenter.com, 2020).

A culture of civility involves respecting one another, honoring differences, listening and seeking common ground, and engaging in social discourse (Clark and Carnosso, 2008). Although the culture in many hospital units may be characterized by some degree of incivility, there are ways to turn the culture into one of civility. This starts with recognizing that incivility needs to be addressed, developing a framework at the institutional level setting and operationalizing behavioral standards, and being patient but persistent in creating a civil culture from one that is toxic. Nurses have the responsibility to intervene on behalf of their colleagues who are being harassed or bullied; silence from the other nurses is a form of acquiescence to bullying (Houck and Colbert, 2017). Similarly, not enforcing mandates for civility in the workplace implies that bullies in fact have permission to harass (Hébert, 2017). Bullying or allowing others to bully is antithetical to caring, the core value of nursing.

"Reality Shock": When Ideals and Reality Collide

A reality of nursing today is that nurses are expected to provide care in a complex healthcare system with an aging population and more persons living with chronic illness. Working conditions are sometimes very difficult, especially when acuity (severity of illness) of the patients is high and staffing is low. Despite the rewards of a career spent in nursing, nursing can be difficult at times. A current challenge in nursing is retention: keeping nurses in nursing. Replacing nurses who leave is extremely expensive for hospitals and other healthcare facilities. Many of the difficulties faced by nurses now are not very different from other times of shortage when the needs of the healthcare system were greater than the profession of nursing could address. This section is intended to leave you in a more powerful position to understand some of the negative feelings you may experience as you make the transition into professional nursing. Because "forewarned is forearmed," discussion is included of not only how to recognize these feelings but also how to manage them so that you will remain an involved, well-prepared, and productive professional nurse.

"Reality shock" (Kramer, 1974) was a term used to describe the feelings of powerlessness and ineffectiveness experienced by new graduates, a term that is still relevant more than four decades later. Psychological stresses generated by reality shock decrease the ability of individuals to cope effectively with the demands of the new role. Causes of reality shock include the following:

1. Absence of positive reinforcement (such as one gets from clinical faculty) and lack of frequent communication
2. Lack of support, such as the availability of faculty that students have
3. The gap between the ideals taught in school and the actual work setting
4. The inability to provide nursing care effectively because of circumstances such as a heavy case load or time constraints

Unfortunately, some new nurses "drop out" at this point, rather than taking steps to resolve reality shock. Kramer (1974) identified several ways nurses may drop out:

1. Disengaging mentally and emotionally
2. Driving oneself and others to the breaking point by trying to do it all

3. "Job hopping"—looking for the perfect, nonstressful job that is completely compatible with professional values
4. Prematurely returning to school (seeking the routine and known expectations of a student)
5. Burning out—a condition of unresolved reality shock with subsequent emotional exhaustion
6. Leaving the nursing profession entirely, which neither nursing nor society can afford

Much can be done to reduce reality shock in the transition from student to professional. Students must recognize that schools cannot provide enough clinical experience to make graduates comfortable on their first day as new nurses. They can take responsibility for obtaining as much practical experience as possible outside of school. Working in a healthcare setting during summers, on school breaks, and on weekends may be helpful. The current difficult economy requires some students to work in addition to going to school. To the extent possible, they should avoid work during the school week or keep it to a minimum because academic responsibilities take priority during that time, and exhausted students make poor learners. Also, exhausted students are at risk for making clinical errors. If you are a student who must work in addition to going to school, consider letting your faculty know. They may be helpful to you in helping you balance your study and work time.

An increasing number of schools of nursing offer programs in which students are paired with practicing nurses (preceptors) and work closely with them to experience life as an RN. Sometimes called *shadowing* programs, these opportunities are highly useful because preceptors are selected for both their clinical expertise and commitment to teaching students in their own work setting. If your school offers such a program, take advantage of it. If not, seek out information about similar programs at area hospitals. Many agencies, including hospitals and the military, are now providing excellent opportunities for students nearing graduation to function in expanded roles.

Nursing residency programs are 1-year programs that offer the new nurse graduate clinical and educational activities to facilitate transition into professional practice and to enhance competence, confidence, and professional development. Nursing residency programs can help bridge the gap between academic preparation and competency development in the clinical setting (Letourneau and Fater, 2015). The structured programs often focus on specific institutional policies, procedures, and standards of care to help new nurses assimilate, develop, and transition into their professional nursing role and practice. Nurses receive education and training in technical skills, critical thinking, organizational skills, prioritization skills, professionalism, and interprofessional communication, helping to ease the "reality shock" and transition from the role of nursing student to professional nurse.

Talking with other new graduates about your feelings is one of the best ways to combat reality shock. Take the initiative to form a group for mutual support; others need it too. Another interpersonal strategy is to seek a professional mentor, an experienced nurse who is committed to nursing and to sharing knowledge with less experienced nurses to help advance their careers. A mentor can be a great source of all types of knowledge, as well as another source of support. Having a mentor is different from having a preceptor. Mentoring involves the formation of a long-term relationship through which ideas, experiences, and successful behavior patterns are shared.

Ask a nurse whose work you wish to emulate to be your mentor, and identify what he or she can offer. Some inexperienced nurses are fearful of approaching potential mentors with this request. They should remember that this process is not a one-way street; it benefits both persons because it complements and validates the mentor's knowledge and experience, as well as provides important information and support to the nurse (the mentee) being mentored. To get the most from a mentoring relationship, first understand your professional and personal needs and select a mentor who seems to share your values and beliefs. Set up specific times to meet, and be willing to communicate openly with your mentor. A mentoring relationship is a powerful tool by which a new nurse can benefit from the experience, wisdom, and feedback from someone who has "been there" and who understands your experience because they have experienced the same transition.

The Internet provides opportunities for nursing students to learn more about the profession of nursing and to assist with socialization into practice. As noted in Chapter 3, nurses often blog about work and work issues. You may find that these serve as a good outlet for you, both to read and to contribute to. Writing serves as a means of organizing one's thoughts and helps you make sense of them; writing can also help you manage uncomfortable feelings and distress.

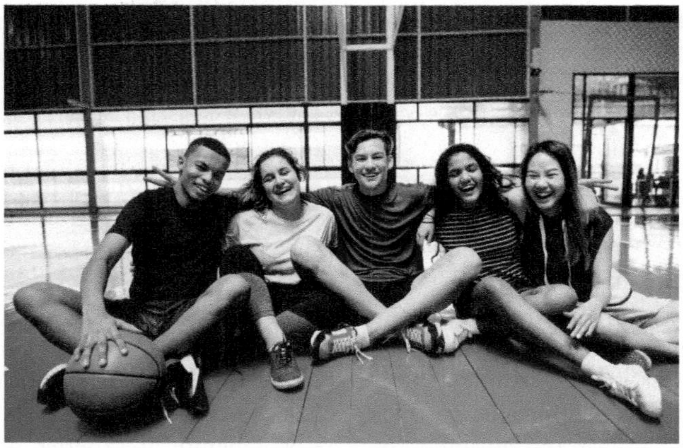

Fig. 5.3 Self-care, including time with friends, is an important aspect of managing the stress of a new career. (Photo used with permission from iStockphoto.)

Care of self is an important activity as you begin your career in the care of others. Recall that when you are traveling by plane, flight attendants instruct you to put on your oxygen mask first in the case of an emergency. You are then prepared to help those around you. The same principle applies here. You will provide better care to others if you care for yourself first, such as eating well, exercising regularly, avoiding tobacco and excessive alcohol use, seeking spiritual support if that is important to you, and having friends outside of work, all of those things that you know are enhance all aspects of your life. The stronger and healthier you are physically, psychologically, and spiritually, the better prepared you are to face the demands of your transition into the important work of nursing (Fig. 5.3).

In the final analysis, you—and only you—are responsible for your own lifelong professional socialization. Those nurses who maintain a good balance between their work and personal lives and who have reasonable expectations of the work of nursing without sacrificing their own values and ideals hold great potential to be effective nurses over a long career.

CONCEPTS AND CHALLENGES

- ***Concept:*** Although nursing has been difficult to define, definitions assist in distinguishing nursing from other healthcare professions.

  Challenge: Although the definitions of nursing in this chapter have much in common, the fluid nature and complexity of nursing, society, and health care may prevent the development of one standard definition of nursing.
- ***Concept:*** Nurses move across a trajectory from novice to expert, progressing from an orientation toward rules and procedures to a patient-centered approach to care that is intuitive.

  Challenge: Novices and advanced beginners should be alert to situations in which they need help from more experienced nurses in setting priorities and addressing patient needs.
- ***Concept:*** Socialization is a critical process through which novices become well-functioning professional nurses, and occurs in both school and the workplace.

  Challenge: Individuals have the responsibility to participate actively in their own professional socialization by seeking out experiences that enhance socialization.
- ***Concept:*** Reality shock occurs during a stressful period that new nurses may encounter when entering nursing practice.

  Challenge: By identifying and understanding reality shock, new graduates can move more easily through the transition from nursing student to practicing nurse.
- ***Concept:*** Mentors can be valuable resources in enhancing and enriching the professional socialization experience.

  Challenge: Identify an experienced nurse, colleague, or faculty member to help you through the transition to practice. Then be available to mentor new nurses as you gain experience and move along the trajectory from novice to expert.

IDEAS FOR FURTHER EXPLORATION

1. Examine your state's nursing practice act for its definition of nursing. How is it similar to or different from definitions in this chapter?
2. From among the definitions of nursing in this chapter, determine the one you think fits most closely with your understanding of nursing, and explain your choice.
3. How might new technologies, economic factors, social trends, and evolving practice options for nurses affect future definitions of nursing? How might these factors affect the scope of nursing?
4. If you are already a practicing nurse, how has your personal definition of nursing changed over time? How have you seen the scope of nursing change since you entered practice?
5. Describe how both formal and informal socialization experiences in school are affecting your understanding and image of nursing.
6. Examine one of the two models of socialization discussed in this chapter, and determine at which stage you are in your development as a student and nurse. Give your rationale for that placement. If none of the models or stages fits your experience, create your own model (or stage).
7. Talk to an experienced nurse about their experience with reality shock. How did this nurse handle the transition from student to practicing nurse? What can you learn from their experience?
8. Identify several personal and professional areas in which you think you could use mentoring and support. Select a potential mentor, and ask if you can have an honest conversation about how they can be helpful to you in your personal and professional development.

REFERENCES

American Nurses Association (ANA): *Code of ethics for nurses with interpretive statements* (website), 2015. Available at: https://www.nursingworld.org/coe-view-only.

American Nurses Association (ANA): *Nursing: scope and standards of practice*, 4th edition, Silver Spring, MD, 2021.

American Nurses Association (ANA): *Nursing's social policy statement: the essence of the profession*, Silver Spring, MD, 2010.

Ariza-Montes A, Muniz NM, Montero-Simó MMJ, Araque-Padilla RA: Workplace bullying among healthcare workers, *Intern J Environ Res and Pub Health* 10(8):3121–3139, 2013 http://doi.org/10.3390/ijerph10083121.

Bandura A: *Social Learning Theory*, Englewood Cliffs, NJ, 1977, Prentice-Hall.

Benner P: *From novice to expert: excellence and power in clinical nursing practice*, Menlo Park, CA, 1984, Addison-Wesley.

Benner P, Tanner CA, Chesla CA: *Expertise in nursing practice: caring, clinical judgment, and ethics*, New York, 1996, Springer.

Cai D, Liu J, Zhao H, Mingyu L: Could social media help in newcomers' socialization? The moderating effect of newcomers' utilitarian motivation. *Comput in Human Behav* 107:106273. 2020. http://doi.org.10.1016/j.chb.2020.106273.

Clark CM, Carnosso J: Civility: a concept analysis, *J Theory Constr & Testing* 12(1):11, 2008.

Cohen HA: *The nurse's quest for professional identity*, Menlo Park, CA, 1981, Addison-Wesley.

Explore Health Careers: *Allied health professions overview*, 2021. (website). Available at: https://explorehealthcareers.org/field/allied-health-professions/.

Fichten CCS, King L, Jorgensen M, et al.: What do college students really want when it comes to their instructors' use of information and communication technologies (ICTs) in their teaching? *International Journal of Learning, Teaching and Educational Research* 14(2):173–191, 2015.

Gordon S: *Nursing against the odds: how health care cost cuts, media stereotypes, and medical hubris undermine nurses and patient care*, Ithaca, NY, 2005, Cornell University Press.

Harmer B: *Textbook of the principles and practice of nursing*, New York, 1922, Macmillan.

Harmer B, Henderson V: *Textbook of the principles and practice of nursing*, ed 4, New York, 1939, Macmillan.

Hébert LLC: Protections from workplace bullying and psychological harassment in the United States: a problem in search of a cause of action. In *Psychosocial risks in labour and social security law*, Cham, 2017, Springer Press, pp 269–287.

Henderson V: *Basic principles of nursing care*, London, 1960, International Council of Nurses (ICN).

Hinshaw AS: *Socialization and resocialization of nurses for professional nursing practice*, New York, 1976, National League for Nursing.

Houck NM, Colbert AM: Patient safety and workplace bullying: an integrative review, *J Nurs Care Qual* 32(2):164–171, 2017.

International Council of Nurses (ICN): *The ICN definition of nursing*, 2021. (website). Available at: www.icn.ch/definition.htm.

Kopp G: How to fit in fast at your new job, *Am Nurse Today* 3(1):40–41, 2008.

Kramer M: *Reality shock: why nurses leave nursing*, St. Louis, 1974, Mosby.

Lai PK, Lim PH: Concept of professional socialization in nursing, *Int e-J Sci Med Educ* 6(1):31–35, 2012.

Laschinger HKS, Cummings G, Leiter M, et al.: Starting out: a time-lagged study of new graduate nurses' transition to practice, *Internat J Nursing Studies* 57:82–95, 2016.

Letourneau RM, Fater KH: Nurse residency programs: an integrative review of the literature, *Nurs Educ Perspect* 36(2):96–101, 2015.

National Council of State Boards of Nursing: *A nurse's guide to the use of social media*, 2018. (website). Available at: https://www.ncsbn.org/NCSBN_SocialMedia.pdf.

Nightingale F: *Notes on nursing: what it is and what it is not*, Philadelphia, 1946, JB Lippincott Reprint [originally published in 1859].

North Carolina Board of Nursing: *Nursing practice act, Article 9a*, 2009. [website]. Available at https://www.ncleg.net/enactedlegislation/statutes/html/byarticle/chapter_90/article_9a.html.

North Carolina Board of Nursing: *Practice/Overview*, 2020. (website). Available at: https://www.ncbon.com/practice-overview.

nursingcenter.com: *Lippincott Nursing Center: Workplace Incivility*, 2020. (website). Available at: https://www.nursingcenter.com/getattachment/Clinical-Resources/nursing-pocket-cards/Workplace-Incivility/Pocket-Card_Workplace-Incivility_March-2020.pdf.aspx.

Orem D: *Guidelines for developing curricula for the education of practical nurses*, Washington, DC, 1959, U.S. Government Printing Office.

Oshvandi K, Sadeghi Moghadam A, Khatiban M, Cheraghi F, Borzu R, Moradi Y: On the application of novice to expert theory in nursing: a systematic review, *J Chem Pharm Sciences* 9(4):3014–3020, 2016.

Peddle M, Bearman M, Nestel D: Virtual patients and nontechnical skills in undergraduate health professional education: an integrative review, *Clin Simul Nurs* 12(9):400–410, 2016.

Peplau H: *Interpersonal relations in nursing: a conceptual frame of reference for psychodynamic nursing*, New York, 1952, GP Putnam's Sons.

Regan S, Wong C, Laschinger HK, et al.: Starting out: qualitative perspectives of new graduate nurses and nurse leaders on transition to practice, *J Nurs Manag* 25(4):246–255, 2017.

Rogers M: *Educational revolution in nursing*, New York, 1961, Macmillan.

Royal College of Nursing (RCN): Defining nursing,2021. (website). Available at: http://anaesthesiaconference.kiev.ua/downloads/defining%20nursing_2003.pdf.

Rush KL, Adamack M, Gordon J, Lilly M, Janke R: Best practices of formal new graduate nurse transition programs: an integrative review, *International J Nurs Stud* 50(3):345–356, 2013.

Shaw CW: *Textbook of nursing*, ed 3, New York, 1907, Appleton.

Sherwood G, Horton-Deutsch S: *Turning vision into action: reflection to build a spirit of inquiry. Reflective practice: transforming education and improving outcomes, Sigma Theta Tau International*:3–19, 2012.

Sherwood G, Zomorodi M: A new mindset for quality and safety: the QSEN competencies redefine nurses' roles in practice, *Nephrology Nurs J* 41(1):15, 2014.

Styles MM: Bridging the gap between competence and excellence, *ANNA J* 18(4):353–366, 1991.

tonybates.ca: *Does distance education socialize students? A study from Québec*, 2015. (website). Available at: www.tonybates.ca/2014/04/04/does-distance-education-socialize-students-a-study-from-quebec/.

6

Nursing as a Regulated Practice: Legal Issues

To enhance your understanding of this chapter, try the Student Exercises on the Evolve site at http://evolve.elsevier.com/Black/professional.

LEARNING OUTCOMES

After studying this chapter, students will be able to:

- Describe the components of a model nursing practice act.
- Discuss the authority of state boards of nursing.
- Explain the conditions that must be present for malpractice to occur.
- Identify nursing responsibilities related to delegation, informed consent, and confidentiality.
- Explain the legal responsibilities of nurses to enforce professional boundaries, including the use of social media.
- Describe strategies nurses can use to protect their patients, thereby protecting themselves from legal actions.

Few aspects of professional nursing practice seem more daunting than those related to laws, rules, and regulations. Laws, rules, and regulations that shape any professional practice serve to protect the public from practitioners who are unsafe or otherwise unqualified. Sometimes you may feel like the "nursing police" are looking over your shoulder and a malpractice attorney is waiting around every corner. In this chapter, the goal is to clarify some of the basic legal issues related to nursing practice so you can understand their importance while not feeling overwhelmed. In fact, understanding nursing as a regulated profession can give you confidence by understanding the purpose of boards of nursing responsible for setting limits on practice, knowing the scope of your practice, and knowing how to protect your career by practicing within accepted standards of care.

Maintaining basic knowledge of the law as it relates to professional nursing practice is especially important now in this time of change in health care with expansion of nursing roles and practice settings. This chapter will give you a foundation of knowledge about the various ways that nursing practice is shaped and regulated by legislation and regulations. Nurses, especially early in their careers, are sometimes concerned about "breaking the law" regarding nursing practice or misinterpret the meaning and purposes of laws. Laws and regulations serve to protect both nurses and the patients for whom they are providing care.

AMERICAN LEGAL SYSTEM

The U.S. Constitution is the framework on which governance in the U.S. is built. The purpose of the law in the United States is found in the Preamble to the Constitution: to ensure order, protect the individual person, resolve disputes, and promote the general welfare. To achieve these broad objectives, the law concerns itself with the legal relationships between persons and the government. All U.S. law flows from the Constitution and must conform to its principles. This means that, although states themselves have the power to set laws for their citizens, no state or municipality can make laws that are not in accordance with the intentions of the

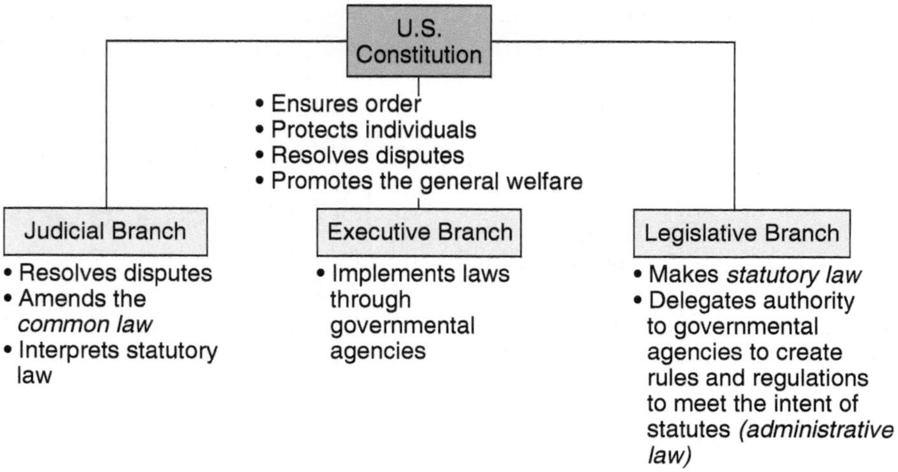

Fig. 6.1 Branches of the U.S. federal government were established by the Constitution to provide for a balance of power.

framers of the Constitution. These intentions are subject to interpretation; hence the constitutionality of a particular law or ruling is argued in the court system.

The Constitution established a government in which the balance of power was divided among three separate but equal branches: (1) the executive branch, charged to implement law and which includes the office of the president at its highest level and the Department of Justice; (2) the legislative branch, charged to create law and which includes the U.S. Congress and other regulatory agencies that set law; and (3) the judicial branch, charged to interpret law and which includes the Supreme Court and federal court system (Fig. 6.1). The separate but equal branches constitute a form of government with a built-in system of checks and balances to keep one body from claiming authority not recognized in the Constitution.

Laws are rules of conduct that are authored and enforced by formal authorities and hold people accountable for compliance. Three major types of laws govern American society: common law, statutory law, and administrative law. Common law is decisional, meaning that judges' rulings become law. U.S. law has its foundation in centuries-old English common law. Every time a judge makes a legal decision, the body of common law expands.

Statutory laws (statutes) are those established through formal legislative processes. Every time the U.S. Congress or a state legislature or assembly passes legislation, the body of statutory law expands.

Administrative laws are created when the legislative branch of a government delegates authority to governmental agencies to create laws that meet the intent of a statute. Both federal and state administrative laws have the force and effect of statutory law.

Laws are further categorized as either civil or criminal. Civil law recognizes and enforces the rights of individuals in disputes over legal rights or duties of individuals in relation to one another. In civil cases the party judged responsible for the harm may be required to pay compensation to the injured party. In contrast, criminal law involves public concerns regarding an individual's unlawful behavior that threatens society, such as murder, robbery, kidnapping, or domestic violence. The criminal court system both defines what constitutes a crime and also may mandate specific punishments, within limits set by legislative bodies and the Constitution. Individuals convicted of criminal charges are punished, usually through the loss of some degree of their freedom, ranging from probation to imprisonment. They may also be required to pay fines.

Administrative cases result when a person violates the regulations and rules established by administrative law. In nursing, examples of administrative cases would be when a nurse practices without a valid license or beyond the scope of nursing practice. These cases are reviewed by state boards of nursing, which administer laws related to nursing practice and determine the appropriate sanctions for the infraction. This is discussed in more detail later in this chapter.

STATE BOARDS OF NURSING, NURSING PRACTICE ACTS, AND LICENSURE

The boundaries of the practice of nursing, medicine, dentistry, law, and many others are established and regulated at the state level. This means that the legislative body in each state sets practice law and then assigns authority to implement the law to appropriate regulatory agencies and boards. These laws are in the form of professional practice acts, which set the licensing standards for various professions.

The purpose of licensing certain professions is to protect the public health, safety, and welfare. The statute that defines and controls nursing is called a *nursing practice act*. All 50 states, the District of Columbia, and several U.S. territories have nursing practice acts passed by their legislatures. State boards of nursing (SBNs) are the regulatory bodies by which nursing practice acts are administered and enforced. Ultimately, SBNs regulate nursing to protect the public from harm by unprepared or incompetent practitioners (Russell, 2017).

Statutory Authority of State Nursing Practice Acts

Nurses, as healthcare providers, have certain rights, responsibilities, and recognitions through various state laws, or statutes. The nursing practice act in each state accomplishes the following objectives (Russell, 2017):

1. Defines the standards and scope of professional nursing
2. Describes the authority, power, and composition of the board of nursing
3. Defines educational program standards
4. Sets the minimum educational qualifications and other requirements for licensure
5. Determines and protects the legal titles and abbreviations nurses may use
6. Provides for disciplinary action of licensees for certain causes

In many states, nursing practice acts also define the responsibilities and authorities of the SBN; thus the nursing practice act of the state in which nurses practice is statutory law affecting nursing practice within that state. For example, a registered nurse (RN) who is employed as a nurse in Virginia practices under the nursing practice act of Virginia, although the nurse's home address may be in Maryland. Maryland's state board of nursing has no jurisdiction over the nurse's practice as long as the nurse is working in Virginia.

Once the law regarding nursing practice is established or amended by the legislature, the legislative branch delegates authority to enforce the law to an executive agency, usually the SBN. SBNs are responsible for enforcing the nursing practice acts in the various states. The SBN publicizes rules and regulations that expand the law. The statutory law plus the rules and regulations propagated by the SBN give full meaning to the nursing practice act in each state. The board of nursing in each state has a comprehensive website containing crucial information for nurses practicing in that state. You should familiarize yourself with your SBN's website, which will include details of how you apply for and maintain your nursing license once you have passed the licensing examination. In addition, the nursing practice act for your state will be featured on the website so that you can be informed as to the specific rules and regulations under which you will practice and the "scope of practice," which defines your care (Ballard et al., 2016; National Council of State Boards of Nursing [NCSBN], 2016). Nursing practice acts are revised periodically to keep up with new developments in health care and changes in nursing practice. State nurses associations are usually instrumental in lobbying their state legislators for appropriate updating of nursing practice acts.

Because of the importance of practice acts to professional nurses, the American Nurses Association (ANA) and the NCSBN have collaborated to develop suggested language for the content of state nursing practice acts. Discussions over the past two decades at the national level, facilitated by both the NCSBN and ANA, have brought a national perspective on nursing regulation to the state level, fostered dialogue and the development of more consistent standards across state lines, and provided increased protection for the public. The current NCSBN's Model Nursing Practice Act (2014) is a comprehensive document developed to guide individual states' development and revisions of their nursing practice acts. The NCSBN describes the current model as both a standard toward which states may strive and a reflection of the current and changing regulatory and healthcare system environments.

Executive Authority of State Boards of Nursing

At both the federal and state government levels, the executive branch administers and implements law. The governor, who holds the state's highest executive office, generally delegates the responsibility for administering the nursing practice act to the SBN, the agency charged with executing (carrying out) laws. In most states, the SBN consists of RNs representing different areas of practice and education, licensed practical/vocational nurses (LPNs/LVNs), and consumers (members of the general public). In a few states, nurses elect members of the SBN; otherwise, they are appointed by the governor, who can also appoint consumers to the board.

The SBN's authority is limited. It can adopt rules that clarify general provisions of the nursing practice act, but it does not have the authority to enlarge the law. The law is set by the state governing body (legislature or assembly), and legislation is usually proposed by the SBNs, often in collaboration with state professional organizations. Within these confines, SBNs have three functions similar to those of the federal and state governments:

1. Executive, with the authority to administer the nursing practice act
2. Legislative, with authority to adopt rules necessary to implement the act (note that rules are different from laws, which are made by the state's legislative body)
3. Judicial, with authority to deny, suspend, or revoke a license or to otherwise discipline a licensee or to deny an application for licensure

Each of these functions is as broad or as limited as the state legislature specifies in the nursing practice act and related laws.

SBNs can be independent agencies in the executive branch of state government or part of a department or bureau such as a department of licensure and regulation. Some state boards have authority to carry out the nursing practice act without review of their actions by other state officials. Others must recommend action to another department or bureau and receive approval of the recommendation before the decision is finalized.

Licensing Powers

Because nursing is a regulated practice, nurses must hold a valid license to practice. Being granted a license to practice nursing takes several years of hard work, and keeping one's license active and in good standing is a professional priority. Each state determines who is qualified to receive a license to practice nursing, as well as the limits on the license. Licensure laws in general may be either mandatory or permissive. A mandatory law requires any person who practices a particular profession or occupation to be licensed. A permissive law on the other hand protects and limits the use of the title granted in the law but does not prohibit persons from practicing the profession or occupation if they do not use the title. All states now have a mandatory licensure law for the practice of nursing to safeguard the public. This means that only licensed nurses—RNs or LPN/LVNs—can practice nursing and call themselves nurses. Unlicensed assistive personnel (UAP) such as certified nursing assistants (CNAs) may not refer to themselves as nurses. Patients often mistake the roles of various practitioners who are providing care; however, the CNAs and other UAP must clarify with patients that they are not nurses when patients refer to them as such.

In most states, SBNs have the authority to set and enforce minimum criteria for nursing education programs. The practice act usually stipulates that an applicant for licensure must graduate from a state-approved nursing education program as a prerequisite to being admitted to the licensure examination. This means that schools of nursing must have state approval to operate. State approval requirements are generally less stringent than are national accreditation standards. Schools may voluntarily seek national accreditation to demonstrate that they meet higher than minimum standards. Although many other professions and occupations require graduation from a nationally accredited educational program as a prerequisite of licensure, only state approval is currently required in nursing. Some states are currently undertaking rule changes to require that nursing programs have national accreditation to achieve state approval.

Not only does the state, through the SBN, grant licenses, but it also has the power to sanction a nurse for performing professional functions in a manner that is dangerous to patients or the general public. Sanctions range from probation (i.e., predetermined period during which the nurse may not have any further complaints made against them); suspension of the nursing license for a specific period, after which the nurse may resume practice; or revocation of the license if the infraction is especially egregious or the nurse shows a pattern of unsafe practice. The most common reason nurses are disciplined by SBNs is for practicing while under the influence of alcohol or other substance, often a narcotic taken ("diverted") from the workplace.

Historically the nursing profession has demonstrated a commitment to the rehabilitation of nurses whose practice is impaired by mental health issues or substance abuse. The ANA first published a recommendation that a Nursing Disciplinary Diversion Act be implemented by states through their boards of nursing. Nurses are estimated to misuse drugs and alcohol at approximately the same rate—10% to 15%—as the general population; however, only a small percentage of nurses are disciplined each year for substance abuse. The goal of SBNs is to return to safe practice those nurses who have been identified as having a problem with drugs and/or alcohol use. This is accomplished through interventions that have shown evidence of effectiveness. Bettinardi-Angres and colleagues (2012) published a comprehensive description of alternative-to-discipline programs in the U.S., which explains efforts to help nurses return to safe practice.

Licensure Examinations

Individuals who have successfully completed their basic nursing education from a state-approved school of nursing are eligible to take the licensing examination. The nurse licensure examination for RNs is the National Council Licensure Examination for Registered Nurses (NCLEX-RN®). The NCLEX-RN®, which is updated regularly, tests critical thinking and nursing competence in all phases of the nursing process. The current test plan can be downloaded from the NCSBN website (www.ncbsn.org). Search for "test plan" on the website to find a list of the most recent and up-to-date test plans; they are updated every 3 years. Through the NCSBN, each state participates in the licensing process through test plan and item development, periodic validation of the examination content with current practice, and adoption of a minimum passing score.

The NCLEX-RN® is administered by computerized adaptive testing (CAT) at various testing centers across each state at a time scheduled by the test taker. CAT means that computer software will determine the level of difficulty of the next question based on whether you answered the previous question correctly. This purpose of this form of testing is to create an examination process that is as objective as possible. The minimum number of questions is 75; the maximum is 265. Each person taking the examination has 6 hours to complete it, including breaks. You will likely hear much speculation about the NCLEX-RN® from classmates. If testing stops at 75 questions, it is not an indication that you passed or failed. What it does indicate is that you either clearly passed with the minimum number of questions or clearly failed. Because around 88% of first-time test takers educated in the U.S. pass the examination, the "75 questions" benchmark has no predictive value for any one individual.

Test takers who do not pass the NCLEX-RN® may retake the examination after paying the examination fees and waiting a required 45 days after the previous attempt. Passing rates for graduates of different nursing schools are published online on SBNs' websites. Passing rates for first-time test takers reflect the quality of the education that specific programs are providing. Schools with consistently high scores among their first-time test takers are providing excellent education and preparation for professional nursing practice. Most if not all states include the first-time pass rate for each nursing school in their respective states. You can likely find your own school's first-time pass rate on your SBN's website.

Mobility of Nurses: Licensure by Endorsement

Since 1944, most SBNs have participated in a cooperative effort to assist in the interstate mobility of nurses. The NCLEX-RN® is a national examination; therefore all states recognize the licensure awarded in other states because all nurses have passed the same exam. This is called *licensure by endorsement*. Endorsement means that RNs may practice in different states without having to take another licensing examination. To receive a license in a different state, nurses submit proof of licensure in another state, pay a licensure fee and meet any other requirements imposed by the state, and they receive a license in the new state by endorsement. Licensure by endorsement is not available in all practice disciplines. Nursing's plan serves as a national model for other licensed professions and occupations.

Enhanced Nurse Licensure Compact (eNLC)

Because the United States has a mobile society, a regulatory approach known as a Nurse Licensure Compact (NLC)—a mutual recognition model of licensure—was developed by the NCSBN in 2000. In 2015 an extensive revision of the NLC was undertaken, and the enhanced

NLC (eNLC) was implemented in 2018 (Puente, 2017). The NLC and then the eNLC were developed to improve mobility of nurses while still protecting the public health, safety, and welfare. Mobility occurs in travel nursing, in crossing state lines from one's home to one's workplace, in the telehealth practices (being physically present in one state while providing nursing care to a patient in another state through digital technology), and in simply moving to another state for personal or career purposes. Having a mobile nursing workforce able to respond to regional and national disasters is an advantage for states in the compact.

The eNLC allows RNs to have one license (in the state of residency) yet practice in other compact member states without an additional license in the state of employment. Importantly, nurses are subject to the nursing practice act in the state where they practice, not to that of the state of licensure. A single license for each nurse and the concomitant reduction of state barriers provide better protection for the public through improved tracking of nurses for disciplinary purposes and information sharing.

Each state wanting to participate in the compact must pass legislation enabling the board of nursing to enter into the interstate NLC. Nurses licensed in any state that has implemented the compact can practice in their own states, as well as in any other compact state without applying for licensure by endorsement before beginning work. A nurse who has changed permanent residence from one compact state to another may practice under the license from their former state of residence for up to 90 days, which starts on the nurse's first day of work. The license in the new state of residence will be granted under endorsement rules if the nurse is in good standing with the SBN of the state from which the nurse is moving. This means that a nurse moving between compact states does not have to delay working as a nurse until a new license is granted. Updated information about states participating in or seeking legislation to participate can be found on the NCSBN website. Based on a demand from nurses educated abroad, the NCSBN began administering the NCLEX-RN® internationally to otherwise qualified nurses applying for U.S. licensure in January 2005. Testing sites are available abroad and are published at https://www.ncsbn.org/testing-locations.htm. Performance scores on the NCLEX-RN® for United States and abroad are published annually by the NCSBN at https://www.ncsbn.org/12171.htm.

LEGAL RISKS IN PROFESSIONAL NURSING PRACTICE

Nurses make decisions daily affecting the well-being of their patients. Because they have access to personal information about patients and interact with them during stressful times, they are in positions of responsibility and trust. Several areas of nursing practice—delegation, informed consent, and confidentiality—are particularly important in terms of risk. Furthermore, nurses may also be charged with malpractice or assault and battery. Being fully informed, however, will help you minimize risks related to these areas.

Malpractice

Malpractice is the primary legal concern of healthcare professionals. Nurses are accountable for their own practice and can be named in a malpractice suit, just as any practitioner can be named. Malpractice suits are very complex. This discussion will give you basic information about malpractice and, importantly, how to protect yourself from practices that make you susceptible to claims of malpractice.

Negligence is the central issue in malpractice. Negligence is the failure to act as a reasonably prudent person would have acted in the same circumstances. For example, a person parks a car on a steep hill and does not engage the parking brake. The car then rolls down the hill and into the porch of a nearby house. The homeowner may seek damages in a civil suit on charges of negligence. Because a reasonably prudent person would have set the parking brake, the result—the damage to the porch—can be shown to be a direct result of the failure to act reasonably.

Malpractice is negligence applied to the acts of a professional. In other words, malpractice occurs when a professional—for example, a nurse or a physician—fails to act as a reasonably prudent professional would have acted under the same circumstances. Malpractice does not have to be intentional; that is, the professional did not mean to act in a negligent manner. Malpractice may occur in two ways: (1) by commission (doing something that that should not have been done) and (2) by omission (failing to do things that should have been done) (Box 6.1).

A patient or someone acting on behalf of the patient who brings a claim of malpractice against a nurse (or other professional) is known in the legal system as the

BOX 6.1 Malpractice: Professional Negligence

Malpractice is not limited to what a nurse *does* (commission); it also refers to what a nurse *fails to do* (omission) in a nursing care situation. The following is an example in which an RN is negligent in both ways.

A patient had surgery one morning for an abdominal mass. He was given morphine 8 mg intravenously (IV) at 5 p.m. At 5:20 p.m., he was very drowsy, but when the nurse woke him and asked about his pain, he complained that his "stomach still hurts some." She gave him a second dose of morphine 8 mg IV. When the nurse went back to check on him an hour later, he was in respiratory arrest. After aggressive resuscitation, the patient was placed on a ventilator and admitted to the intensive care unit, where he stayed for 4 days after showing signs of new-onset neurologic impairments.

The nurse was negligent by commission when she gave the patient a second dose of morphine because (1) the nurse had to awaken the patient to ask him about his pain, and (2) the patient's complaint of "some pain" likely did not warrant a second dose of intravenous morphine so soon after the first dose. A reasonably prudent nurse in the same situation would not have given a relatively large dose of morphine so soon after the first, especially given that the patient was drowsy and had to be awakened to assess his pain.

The nurse was negligent by omission because she did not check on her patient for 1 hour after giving a second substantial dose of morphine. The first dose made him very drowsy after 20 minutes; this would indicate that he had a significant response to the first dose. The nurse also failed provide evidence that they assessed the patient for causes of his continuing pain, such as examining his abdomen and checking his vital signs for evidence of a surgical complication.

plaintiff. Malpractice suits are civil, not criminal, cases. The nurse (or other professional) becomes the defendant. Advancing a malpractice case to the point of being argued in front of a judge and jury is a long process and is actually unlikely to get this far. Often, malpractice cases are settled out of court, meaning that the outcome is negotiated between attorneys for the plaintiffs and defendant(s) (Thinking Critically Box 6.1).

The central question in any charge of malpractice is, "Was the prevailing standard of care met?" The nursing standard of care is what a reasonably prudent nurse, under similar circumstances, would have done. Standard of care reflects a basic minimum level of prudent care based on the ethical principle of nonmaleficence ("do no harm"). Nurses, not practitioners from other disciplines, determine whether standard of care is met. For instance, a physician cannot testify what the standards of care are for nurses. Nurse expert witnesses are hired by both the plaintiff and the defendant and will testify as to whether the nurse met the prevailing standard of care.

"Prevailing" is an important qualifier. As practice changes and develops, standards of care change accordingly. The issue in malpractice cases is the standard of care that prevailed—or was in effect—at the time the negligent act occurred. What may be considered negligent now may not have been considered negligent at the time. The standard of care prevailing at the time is key and is ascertained through expert witness testimony; documents, including national standards of nursing practice; the patient record; and other pertinent evidence, such as the direct testimony of the patient, the nurse, and others. Box 6.2 illustrates the presumed failure of an RN to meet the prevailing standard of care.

THINKING CRITICALLY BOX 6.1

What or Who Needs the Most Attention: The EHR or Your Patients?

You hear nursing colleagues discussing prevention of malpractice, and you notice that some nurses are spending more time attending to patients' EHRs than they are in providing care to patients. Think about how this emphasis on "defensive practice"—that is, making sure that your patient's medical record is perfect—may actually impede the delivery of safe care. As you think about this issue, consider what the purpose of documentation is. How can you use the medical record to enhance the care of your patients? How might excessive documentation harm you in a malpractice suit?

EHR, Electronic health record.

BOX 6.2 Standards of Care: A Case Example

An 8-month-old infant was brought by his parents to the emergency department (ED) with significant fever and dehydration. The family with the infant was Spanish-speaking and included a family member trained in nursing in her country of origin.

Intravenous (IV) fluids were ordered for rehydration. Because of the need for the infant to be able to move from bed to the arms of his caregivers, the IV line was set up before IV catheter insertion with both regular- and extension-length tubing. The ED RN, in her second year in the ED, failed to flush the line to clear air from the extension tubing and then inserted the catheter and began the infusion. This was noted by the family, and an unsuccessful attempt was made to alert the nursing and medical staff. The infant subsequently died of a significant air embolus. The family engaged an attorney, who eventually filed a malpractice suit against the hospital and the nurse. The following standards of care were considered in this case.

1. Hospital policy indicated that an interpreter should have been called for communication with family.
2. Hospital policies and orientation competency guidelines, completed by this nurse, indicated that flushing of an IV line was a required step in the process.
3. Local schools of nursing indicated that flushing of an IV line was part of basic skills training, and current textbooks about fundamentals of nursing confirmed this content.
4. Other nurses in local EDs were interviewed, and all reported that flushing of an IV line before infusion was standard practice.
5. The company manufacturing the IV tubing had visual and written instructions on the box indicating proper use of the product, including flushing of the line.

There are two requirements of a malpractice action. First, the defendant (nurse) has specialized knowledge and skills, and second, through the practice of that specialized knowledge the defendant causes the plaintiff's (patient's) injury. All four elements of a cause of action for negligence must be proven. These elements are the same for any professional accused of malpractice:

1. The professional (nurse) has assumed the duty of care (responsibility for the patient's care).
2. The professional (nurse) breached the duty of care by failing to meet the standard of care.
3. The failure of the professional (nurse) to meet the standard of care was the proximate cause of the injury.
4. The injury is proved.

A high degree of proof is needed in each of these four elements. Monetary damages are awarded when a plaintiff prevails. These awards are based on proved economic losses, such as time missed from work, out-of-pocket healthcare costs, and future costs of care, and on remuneration for pain and suffering caused by the injury. In the case of a death, the next of kin can become the plaintiff on behalf of the deceased patient. In a clinical setting, you may occasionally hear a nurse or other provider complain about a patient's care as being "malpractice." This term is often misused and applied to what may be bad practice, but remember that to be sued for malpractice, an injury must have occurred that is directly and demonstrably caused by the act.

In the past, only some malpractice lawsuits involved nurses, but the physician or hospital defendants were typically sued for damages even when nurses provided the substandard care. In these instances, physicians were implicated through the "captain of the ship" doctrine. This archaic doctrine implied that the physician is ultimately in charge of all patient care and thus should be responsible financially. Hospitals were implicated through the legal theory of *respondeat superior* (from Latin, meaning "let the master answer"), which attributes the acts of employees to their employer. However, as nurses have obtained more credentials and their expertise, autonomy, and authority for nursing practice have increased, direct liability for nursing care has risen correspondingly.

In a paper that is still widely cited, Croke (2003) conducted a review of more than 350 trial, appellate, and supreme court case summaries from a variety of legal research sources and analyzed 253 cases that met the following criteria: a nurse was engaged in the practice of nursing as defined by his or her state's nursing practice act; a nurse was a defendant in a civil lawsuit as the result of an unintentional action (no criminal cases were considered); and a trial was held between 1995 and 2001. Sixty percent of the cases occurred in acute care hospitals. Six major categories of negligence resulted in malpractice lawsuits against nurses: failure to follow standards of care, failure to use equipment in a responsible manner, failure to communicate, failure to document, failure to assess and monitor, and failure to act as a patient advocate. More details of Croke's analysis are presented in Box 6.3. The findings from this review paper remain relevant today.

BOX 6.3 Six Major Categories of Negligence That Result in Malpractice Lawsuits

1. Failure to follow standards of care, including failure to
   - Perform a complete admission assessment or design a plan of care
   - Adhere to standardized protocols or institutional policies and procedures (for example, using an improper injection site)
   - Follow a physician's verbal or written orders
2. Failure to use equipment in a responsible manner, including failure to
   - Follow the manufacturer's recommendations for operating equipment
   - Check equipment for safety before use
   - Place equipment properly during treatment
   - Learn how equipment functions
3. Failure to communicate, including failure to
   - Notify a physician in a timely manner when conditions warrant it
   - Listen to a patient's complaints and act on them
   - Communicate effectively with a patient (for example, inadequate or ineffective communication of discharge instructions)
   - Seek higher medical authorization for a treatment
4. Failure to document, including failure to note in the patient's medical record
   - A patient's progress and response to treatment
   - A patient's injurise
     - Pertinent nursing assessment information (for example, drug allergies)
     - A physician's medical orders
     - Information about telephone conversations with physicians, including time, content of communication between nurse and physician, and actions taken
5. Failure to assess and monitor, including failure to
   - Complete a shift assessment
   - Implement a plan of care
   - Observe a patient's ongoing progress
   - Interpret a patient's signs and symptoms
6. Failure to act as a patient advocate, including failure to
   - Question discharge orders when a patient's condition warrants it
   - Question incomplete or illegible medical orders
   - Provide a safe environment

Reprinted with permission from Croke EM: Nurses, negligence, and malpractice: An analysis based on more than 250 cases against nurses, *Am J Nurs* 103(9):54–63, 2003.

The key point is that professional nurses must consider carefully the legal implications of practice and be willing to and capable of conforming to prevailing professional standards and all legal expectations. Among factors leading to the increase in the number of malpractice cases against nurses is delegation.

Delegation

Delegation—giving someone authority to act for another—is an issue that carries great legal and safety implications in nursing practice. The ability to delegate has generally been reserved for professionals because they hold licenses that sanction the entire scope of practice for a particular profession. RNs, for example, may delegate independent nursing activities (as well as medical functions that have been delegated to them) to other nursing personnel. State nursing practice acts do not give LPNs or LVNs the authority to delegate.

Professional RNs retain accountability for acts delegated to another person. This means that the RN is responsible for determining that the delegated person (delegatee) is competent to perform the delegated act. Likewise, the delegatee is responsible for carrying out the delegated act safely. The professional nurse remains legally liable, however, for the nursing acts delegated to others unless the delegatee is also a licensed professional whose scope includes the assigned act. For example, an RN can assign an LPN who has been properly trained to take vital signs of all the patients under the RN's care. The LPN cannot, however, reassign this responsibility to another person. The RN remains accountable for the data that the LPN collects, because it is not the LPN's responsibility, nor is it within their training and scope of practice to interpret those data. However, if the RN asks another RN to take the vital signs of a patient, and the second RN agrees, the second RN then becomes responsible for carrying this out, interpreting the data, and acting on them accordingly. The video in this link describes a case of nursing malpractice that involved delegation of care by an RN to an LPN, and the ensuing death of a previously stable patient in a postanesthesia care unit: https://www.nso.com/Learning/Videos/Failure-to-Assess-and-Monitor.

Delegation must also be considered in terms of ethical implications. The ANA's Code of Ethics for Nurses, Provision 4.4, Delegation of Nurse Activities (2015), states,

> *The nurse must make reasonable efforts to assess individual competence when assigning selected components of nursing care to other healthcare workers. This assessment involves evaluating the knowledge, skills, and experience of the individual to whom the care is assigned, the complexity of the assigned tasks, and the health status of the patient. ... Nurses may not delegate responsibilities such as assessment and evaluation; they may delegate tasks. ... Employer policies or directives do not relieve the nurse of responsibility for making judgments about the delegation and assignment of nursing care tasks. (p. 2)*

Importantly, the Code of Ethics is clear that workplace policies or directives do not supersede the ethical standards described in the Code.

Delegation is an important liability and one not fully appreciated by many practicing nurses. The professional nurse's primary legal and ethical consideration must be the patient's right to safe, effective nursing care. Box 6.4 contains a list of "five rights" to ensure safe delegation of tasks to nursing assistants and other UAP. With the present nursing shortage, the use of UAP has expanded, further increasing the RN's liability related to delegation. Additional information on delegation can be found on the NCSBN website at www.ncsbn.org.

In an attempt to further clarify issues of delegation, the ANA (2015) also defined the responsibilities of the nurse when delegating to nursing assistive personnel. They reinforce the stance that the RN may delegate elements of care but cannot delegate the nursing process itself. Furthermore, they reaffirm that the judgment of the nurse is primary in determining the patients, environments, and care situations for safe delegation and that the nurse remains responsible for evaluating the outcomes of nursing care.

Significantly, the ANA and the NCSBN published a joint statement on delegation (NCSBN, 2015), noting that there is more to do for patients than there are nurses to do the work, and the increasingly complex therapies have created a demand for nursing care. Therefore delegating, assigning, and supervising assistive personnel are "critical competencies for the 21st century nurse" (p. 1, introduction). The importance of this principle became a key feature of the work of nurses on ICUs during the COVID-19 epidemic, when nurses where overwhelmed by the numbers of patients and acuity of care required by these very ill persons, many of whom died in the ICUs without benefit of their families' presence. As the work required of nurses becomes more chaotic, errors are more likely to occur, including inadequate supervision of UAPs. The pandemic underscored two separate but related issues: the high volume of patients per nurse, and the vulnerability of nurses and other healthcare providers to burnout and other stress responses, in addition to threats to their own health and that of their families.

BOX 6.4 Five Rights to Ensure Safe Delegation

The following are standards that delineate responsibility for the RN who is delegating responsibility to unlicensed personnel such as nursing assistants.

1. *Right task:* Is the task appropriate for delegation in a specific care situation?
2. *Right circumstances:* Is delegation appropriate in this case? Consider the patient's health status, care delivery setting, complexity of the activity and delegate's competency, and available resources, and determine any other relevant factors.
3. *Right person:* Can the nurse verify that the person delegated to do the task is competent to complete this task?
4. *Right direction/communication:* Has the RN given clear, specific instructions? These include identifying the patient clearly, goals of care, time frames, and expected results.
5. *Right supervision/evaluation:* Can the RN or other licensed nurse provide supervision and evaluation of the patient and the performance of the task?

Data from National Council of State Boards of Nursing: The Five Rights of Delegation, approved August 1997 by the Delegate Assembly. Retrieved from www.ncsbn.org.

Informed Consent

All patients or their guardians (e.g., parents of minor children) must be given an opportunity to grant informed consent before treatment unless there is a life-threatening emergency. The following are the three major conditions of informed consent:

1. Consent must be given voluntarily.
2. Consent must be given by an individual with the capacity and competence to understand.

3. The patient must be given enough information so that the locus of the decisions lies with the patient and not the provider; in other words, the provider cannot influence the patient unduly by giving incomplete information or obscuring data that the patient should have to make a truly informed decision.

Informed consent, then, is the full, knowing authorization by the patient for care, treatment, and procedures and must include information about the risks, benefits, side effects, costs, and alternatives. Consumers of health care need a great deal of information and should be told everything they would consider significant in making a treatment decision. This is a long-standing element of healthcare law (*Canterbury v. Spence*, 464 F2 772, 1972).

For informed consent to be legally valid, elements of completeness, competency, and voluntariness are evaluated. *Completeness* refers to the quality of the information provided. *Competency* takes into account the capability of a particular patient to understand the information given and make a choice. *Voluntariness* refers to the freedom the patient has to accept or reject alternatives. *Autonomy* is the key ethical principle that supports voluntariness as foundational to informed consent. When patients are minors, are under the effects of drugs or alcohol (including preoperative medications), or otherwise have cognitive impairments, their competency to consent is in question. In these situations, consent needs to be granted by the patient's spouse, next of kin, or court-ordered guardian or healthcare proxy.

The role of nurses in informed consent, unless they are themselves primary providers, is to collaborate with the primary provider, most often a physician. A nurse may witness a patient's signing of informed consent documents but is not responsible for explaining the proposed treatment (Fig. 6.2). The nurse is not responsible for evaluating whether the physician has fully explained the significant risks, benefits, and alternative treatments; however, professional nurses are responsible for determining that the elements for valid consent are in place, providing feedback if the patient wishes to withdraw consent or grant consent previously withheld, and communicating the patient's need for further information to the primary provider. Advocacy is a key nursing responsibility when the nurse is not certain that a patient is fully informed or understands what he or she has signed.

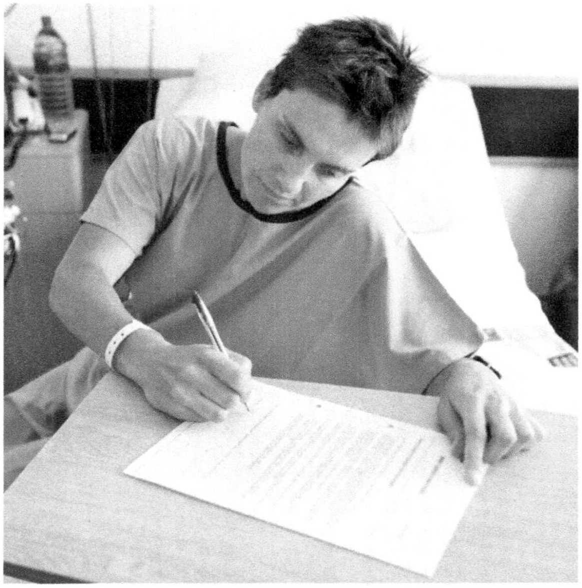

Fig. 6.2 Professional nurses may be called on to witness a patient's signing of informed consent documents. The primary provider, however, is responsible for providing necessary information to the patient or legal guardian. (Photo used with permission from iStockPhoto.)

CONFIDENTIALITY: THE CHALLENGE TO PROTECT PRIVACY

Confidentiality is both a legal and an ethical concern in nursing practice. Confidentiality is the protection of private information gathered about a patient during the provision of healthcare services. The Code of Ethics for Nurses Provision 3.1 states that "the nurse has a duty to maintain confidentiality of all patient information, both personal and clinical in the work setting and off duty in all venues, including social media and any other means of communication. Nurses are responsible for providing accurate, relevant data to members of the health care team and others who have a need to know" (ANA, 2015).

The Code acknowledges exceptions to the obligation of confidentiality. These include discussing the care of patients with others involved in their direct care, quality assurance activities, legally mandated disclosure to public health authorities, and information required by third-party payers (ANA, 2015). The Code also recognizes the need to disclose information without the patient's consent when the safety of innocent parties is

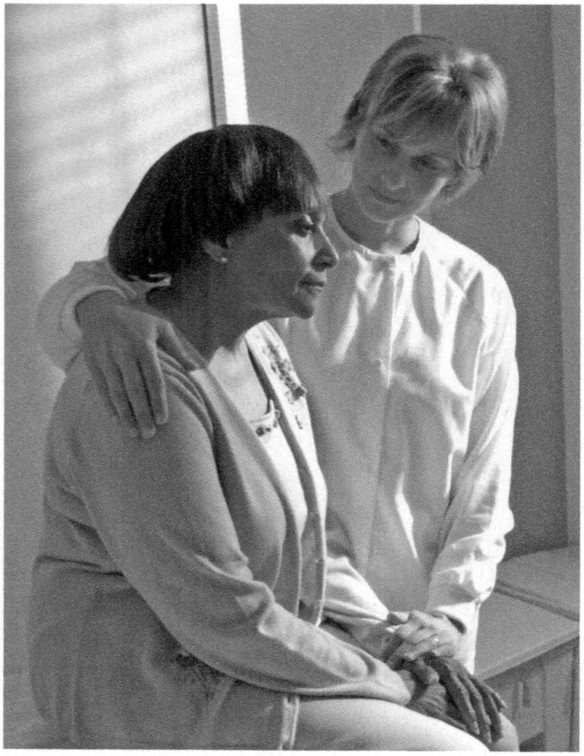

Fig. 6.3 Nurses have an obligation for confidentiality but are not protected by privileged communication statutes. In some cases, nurses are required to report what a patient has told them. (Photo used with permission from Photos.com.)

in question (*Tarasoff v. Board of Regents of the University of California,* 551 P2 334, 1976).

The principle of confidentiality is protected by state and federal statutes, but there are exceptions and limitations. Although some professions have privileged communication protected by statutes (e.g., attorneys, priests) nurses are usually not included in such statutes (Fig. 6.3). Nurses then may be ordered by a court to share information without the patient's consent. The professional nurse must understand these legal limitations to confidentiality.

Based on common, state, or municipal law, nurses have the duty to report or disclose certain information such as suspected abuse or neglect of a child (or adults, in some states), gunshot wounds, certain communicable diseases, and threats toward third parties. These laws vary by state and may be the responsibility of institutions providing healthcare services and not of an individual practitioner. Nurses should be aware of these requirements, however, and if uncertain of what to do in a particular situation, make sure their nurse manager or other supervisor or hospital administrator on duty.

The Health Insurance Portability and Accountability Act of 1996

The Health Insurance Portability and Accountability Act (HIPAA) of 1996 is the first federal privacy standard governing protection of patients' medical records. The privacy provisions in the act began as a 337-word guideline, but as the final regulations were written, the provisions expanded to 101,000 words. HIPAA was designed, in part, to reinforce the protection of patient information as it is transmitted electronically, but the final act goes far beyond that goal. The regulations protect medical records and other individually identifiable health information, whether on paper, electronically, or communicated orally.

HIPAA requires all healthcare providers, including physicians, hospitals, health plans, pharmacies, public health authorities, insurance companies, billing agencies, information systems sales and service providers, and others, to ensure the privacy and confidentiality of patients. Although passed in 1996, the confidentiality regulations were not implemented until April 2003 to give providers time to prepare the necessary safeguards and documents and to train workers in their use.

HIPAA regulations require several major patient protections:

- Patients can see and obtain copies of their medical records, generally within 30 days of their request, and to request corrections if they detect errors. Providers may charge patients for the cost of copying and mailing the records.
- Providers must give patients written notice describing the provider's information practices and explaining patients' rights. Patients must be asked to agree to these practices by signing or initialing the notice.
- Limitations are placed on the length of time records can be retrieved, what information can be shared, where it can be shared, and who can be present when it is shared.

A number of other protections are provided in this comprehensive federal legislation. A current guide to the complicated HIPAA regulations can be found online at the Department of Health and Human Services (2018). The increasingly widespread use of electronic health records and digital transmission of health information has necessitated the development of comprehensive guidelines ("Guide to Privacy and Security of Electronic Health Information") to help with the implementation of the Meaningful Use programs while still protecting the privacy and security of patient information (U.S. Department of Health and Human Services, 2015). The integration of HIPAA into clinical practice was not easy because it necessitated changing many aspects of day-to-day care on nursing units, such as having patients' names on whiteboards at nursing stations with detailed information about their diagnoses, care teams, and plans. HIPAA regulations, however, served to remind nurses and other practitioners of the importance of determining what and how much information on patients to share, and who actually needed to know information. For many nurses, then, HIPAA affirmed nursing's long-standing responsibility to our patients.

Social Media: Maintaining Confidentiality and HIPAA Standards

The NCSBN has published a white paper, "A Nurse's Guide to the Use of Social Media," in response to the burgeoning social media outlets, such as social networking sites, blogs and microblogs (e.g., Twitter), photo and video sites (e.g., YouTube, Instagram, Snapchat), and other online forums, including sites specifically for nurses and nursing students (NCSBN, 2018). Healthcare settings now generally have policies in place to govern the use of social media from workplace settings, as do many non–health-related employers. However, the use of social media outside of nursing school or the workplace can cause tremendous consequences if used in ways that interfere with the privacy of patients, even if the nurse's or student's intentions are not malicious. *The ethical principle of confidentiality and HIPAA regulations place significant limitations on the content of nurses' social media activities and comments.* Violations of patient privacy by posting photos or identifiable information on social networking sites are offenses reportable to the board of nursing in the state where the nurse is in practice. Violating HIPAA regulations means that the nurse has broken federal law and may have also broken state laws in the process.

NCSBN identified six common myths and misunderstandings regarding social media. You should be aware of these and structure your online communication accordingly. It is a professional obligation with important ethical and legal ramifications. The following is a list of these pervasive myths and misunderstandings (you can find the full white paper at the NCSBN website for details):

- *Myth 1:* Posts and photos are private and accessible only to the intended recipient.
  - Fact: They can be reposted, "retweeted," copied, and otherwise disseminated in ways completely beyond your control.
- *Myth 2:* Once content has been deleted, it is no longer accessible.
  - *Fact:* There is no "erasing" digital content. Cached versions and screenshots of posts and photos are available. Even sites such as Snapchat in which content quickly "disappears" retain digital evidence of the content.
- *Myth 3:* No harm is done if patient information is disclosed only to the intended recipient.
  - *Fact:* This is still a breach of confidentiality, just as if you used spoken words to share private information about patients. As soon as you write or tell something, you have lost control of the message. You cannot control what happens to the information you have passed along.
- *Myth 4:* It is acceptable to refer to a patient by a nickname, room number, or diagnosis/condition.
  - *Fact:* This still remains a breach of confidentiality and is disrespectful to the patient.
- *Myth 5:* If your patient is posting about their health condition, you may also post about it.
  - *Fact:* Patients can say or write anything about their own health; however, this does not in any way release you from the obligations of confidentiality and HIPAA regulations.
- *Myth 6:* Social media blurs the distinction between one's professional and personal lives.
  - *Fact:* This is an illusion. Professional boundaries are still firmly in place, although social media may cause you to believe that they are not.

The use of social media makes it tempting to respond to online social contact with patients and former patients. For instance, you may get a "friend" request from a former patient that you liked very much. As difficult as this is to do, you should ignore that request or decline it for the sake of your professional boundaries. Establishing an online relationship will interfere with your ability to provide care for that patient if and when you encounter that person in the healthcare setting in the future.

Furthermore, the quick availability of mobile phone cameras makes it easy to take photos of patients of whom you are fond, or of their new baby, or of milestones in the patient's recovery. Your employer or school of nursing is likely to have a policy in place prohibiting the use of cameras in the clinical setting. Although there are certain times in which photography in the clinical setting is appropriate, it is in very circumscribed situations and will involve the use of the institution's camera, not your personal smartphone. Box 6.5 contains an example of a situation in which a mobile phone photo taken by a nursing student in a clinical setting led to unforeseen problems.

BOX 6.5 A Cautionary Tale: The Far-Reaching Effect of Digital Technology

During her rotation in the maternity unit, a nursing student really enjoyed taking care of the infants in the newborn nursery. One evening, a baby with a rare and distinctive facial defect was admitted to the nursery. The baby's parents had come from another state so the mother could give birth at this institution because of its known expertise in the management of craniofacial defects. The defect was severe, and the student was curious about it. She took a photo of the baby in his bassinet with her phone, wanting to use the photo in a presentation she was preparing on genetic defects for another class.

She consequently downloaded the photo onto her computer and included it in her PowerPoint presentation, which was posted online for her classmates. A few weeks later, she was called to the office of the director of her nursing program. A complaint had been filed against her and her school by the infant's parents, who had neither known about nor consented to having their baby photographed. They found the photo while using a search engine's "image" function as they were seeking more information about their infant's genetic condition. The photo was embedded in the student's PowerPoint presentation, which was available online, with the student's name, school, and course number on the title slide. It was not difficult for them to figure out where and when the photo was made. Tracing their identity would not be difficult, and their privacy was compromised.

The student was dismissed from her nursing program because there was a policy in place at both the school and the clinical institution forbidding use of phone photography. Although she tried to defend herself that the baby's name band was obscured, the presence of the rare facial defect served as enough of an identifier to compromise the family's privacy. She was reminded that even without the clear policy forbidding photography, she had committed an egregious ethical violation by not protecting the family's privacy. One seemingly simple photograph created a career-threatening situation for this student who failed to understand the far-reaching effects of digital technologies.

Assault and Battery

Assault and battery is occasionally the basis for legal action against a nurse defendant. Assault is a threat or an attempt to make bodily contact with another person without the person's consent. Assault precedes battery; it causes the person to fear that battery is about to occur. Battery is the assault carried out: the impermissible, unprivileged touching of one person by another. Actual harm may or may not occur as a result of assault and battery.

If, for example, a nurse threatens a patient with a vitamin injection if the patient does not eat, the patient may charge assault. Actually giving the patient a vitamin injection against their will leaves the nurse open to charges of battery, even if there is a physician's prescription for this treatment. Patients have the right to refuse treatment, even if the treatment would be in their best interest. This is both a legal and an ethical principle (autonomy). Both by common law and by statute, informed consent is required in the healthcare context as a defense to battery (42 U.S.C. 1395 cc., 1990).

EVOLVING LEGAL ISSUES AFFECTING NURSING

As the healthcare system and the profession of nursing evolve, legal issues affecting nursing practice are also evolving. Specific legal issues illustrating the changing nature of nursing practice are related to role changes, supervision of UAP, payment mechanisms, and issues associated with the implementation of the Patient Self-Determination Act (PSDA). Each of these issues is discussed briefly in the following sections.

Role Changes in Health Care

Just as a nurse's knowledge base and the nurse's accountability for nursing practice have increased over time, so too has the need to expand the legal authority for nursing practice. Professional nurses realize the importance of states' nursing practice acts to reflect nursing practice accurately and to keep up with changes in healthcare delivery as they occur. In other words, states' nursing practice acts must be responsive to changes in practice. Advanced practice nurses set the pace for evolving nursing practice, and the nursing practice act must support their ability to offer nursing services to consumers in various settings. Otherwise, the legal basis for nursing practice is unclear and nurses are vulnerable to litigation.

Nurses face legal exposure and are vulnerable when their state's nursing practice act is not updated periodically to support explicitly an expanded scope of practice. Collaboration between the constituent member (state nurses) association and the SBN to expand the evolving scope of nursing practice ensures the growth of the profession and increases the number of primary care providers needed by the public. Professional nurses should support their professional associations and SBN, which guide the development of legislation that accurately reflects current nursing practice at all levels. Your practice is directly affected by the work of professional organizations at the legislative levels.

An interesting role for nurses has been developed over the past 30 years—legal nurse consulting. The American Association of Legal Nurse Consultants, founded in 1989, is a nonprofit organization dedicated to the professional enhancement of RNs who practice as consultants in the legal field. Box 6.6 contains more information about legal nurse consulting and the interesting work legal nurse consultants do.

Prescriptive Authority

An important role expansion for advanced practice nurses is prescriptive authority. *Prescriptive authority* is defined as the legal acknowledgment of prescription writing as an appropriate act of nursing practice. The ANA, the American Academy of Nurse Practitioners, and others support prescriptive authority for advanced practice nurses, as distinguished from generalist RNs.

By 2006, advanced practice nurses had some type of prescriptive authority in all 50 states. This authority ranged from completely independent authority with no collaborative requirements to a limited authority in which nurse practitioners can prescribe (excluding controlled substances) with some degree of physician involvement or delegation of prescription writing. In other states, nurse practitioners can prescribe (including controlled substances) with some degree of physician involvement or delegation of prescription writing). This is an evolving area of practice, and advanced practice nurses must be aware of the boundaries on prescriptive authority given to them in the state where they are practicing. Your state's board of nursing website will give you the most up-to-date information regarding prescriptive authority for advanced practice nurses in your state. The ultimate goal is a uniform consensus practice model across all states. Progress toward this goal may be viewed online at https://www.ncsbn.org/5397.htm.

BOX 6.6 What Is a Legal Nurse Consultant?

A legal nurse consultant (LNC) is an experienced nurse who brings expertise from their professional nursing education and clinical experience to the evaluation of standard of care, causation, damages, and other medically related issues in medicolegal cases or claims. For instance, if a nurse is named in a malpractice suit, the attorneys for both the plaintiffs (the person/persons who filed the suit) and the defendants (the persons being sued) will seek the expertise of nurses who can evaluate if the nurse met the standard of care and other important aspects of the case. LNCs have additional education and experience regarding applicable legal standards and/or strategy to the evaluation of medicolegal cases or claims. LNCs know how to analyze healthcare records and medical literature critically, as well as other relevant legal documents and other information to the case or claim on which they are consulting.

LNCs practice in a variety of settings, such as law firms, governmental agencies, healthcare facilities, forensic environments, and LNC consulting firms, among others. Some LNCs are self-employed in their own practices. In addition to medical malpractice, LNCs practice in a variety of areas such as personal injury, long-term care litigation/elder law, product liability, workers' compensation, life care planning, and forensic/criminal settings. Among their many activities, LNCs serve as expert witnesses; they interview clients, evaluate the strengths and weaknesses of cases, and locate or prepare evidence for trial.

LNCs can become board certified through the Legal Nurse Consultant Certified program, which allows them to use the LNCC credential. This certification demonstrates that the nurse has met the experience and education requirements and has passed the certification examination. For more information about this very interesting and challenging career, you can contact the American Association of Legal Nurse Consultants (AALNC) at info@aalnc.org or visit their website at www.aalnc.org. You can also find them on Facebook and LinkedIn (AALNC, 2021).

Both RNs and advanced practice nurses (APRNs) must understand prescriptive authority of advanced practice in their states. RNs must know from whom they can accept medication prescriptions, and APRNs must stay within their legal scope of practice.

Supervision of Unlicensed Assistive Personnel

Another evolving legal issue is the continued role expansion of UAP or limited licensed (LPN/LVN) personnel by healthcare institutions. Nursing assistants (i.e., UAP) are increasingly being substituted for nurses, thus creating greater risks to patients and increasing the liability of RNs, who supervise their work. indicate that lack of professional nurse supervision and the educational level of nurses themselves significantly affect patients, institutions, and nurses alike. (See Chapter 1: Evidence-Based Practice Box 1.1 for details.) Convening expert panels of educators, researchers, and practitioners to develop standards for delegation, the NCSBN published a comprehensive National Guidelines for Nursing Delegation NCSBN, (2016) to provide guidance for the complex process of delegation and patient care assignment across both licensed and unlicensed personnel.

The licensure or state approval of unlicensed personnel is a complex issue that has relevance for RNs because professional nurses are legally responsible for the tasks delegated to unlicensed persons. Nationally standardized education and training for these workers would assure nurses that their co-workers have a minimum level of competence. The NCSBN has developed the National Nurse Aide Assessment Program (NNAAP) examination, a test of both cognitive and skill performance to certify nurse aide competency. The Medication Aide Certification Examination (MACE) also administered by the NCSBN, certifies competency in administration of simple medications by UAP. Regardless of certifications by UAP, it remains the responsibility of professional nurses to know the limitations of the particular assistive personnel under their supervision.

Payment Mechanisms for Nurses

Nurses may practice in nontraditional roles and settings. Many professional nurses are both capable of and interested in offering nursing services as private practitioners, but payment mechanisms may limit such activities. Nurses are concerned about offering services for which consumers are unable to obtain reimbursement from their insurance carriers, and third-party reimbursement has traditionally been limited to care provided by physicians.

Over time, nurses and nursing professional associations have supported state and federal legislation to provide direct and indirect payments to nurses for nursing services rendered. Advanced practice nurses and their advocates scored a major legislative victory with the passage of the 1997 Balanced Budget Act after an 8-year fight to obtain direct reimbursement. The resistance to advanced practice nurse reimbursement was significant and protracted. This legislation authorized nurse practitioners and clinical specialists, beginning in January 1998, to bill the Medicare program directly for nursing services furnished in any setting. Even now, it remains a regulatory challenge to devise a fair and equitable payment system for advanced practice nurses, whose scopes of practice vary from state to state. Nurses are concerned that these changes are often not implemented or that advanced practice nurses are paid less for services similar to those provided by other healthcare professionals who are paid at a higher rate.

Laws are passed that are sometimes not implemented. This occurs when the group affected by the law (for example, the insurance industry) is unwilling to implement the changes and no "watchdog" agency is created to ensure that changes occur. For example, federal legislation was enacted requiring state Medicaid agencies to pay certain nurses (nurse practitioners, nurse-midwives, and nurse anesthetists) directly for services provided to Medicaid recipients. As with the laws affecting private insurers, these requirements were not implemented in every state. Nurses may need to seek legal remedies to require implementation of policies mandated by federal law (*Nurse Midwifery Associates v. Hibbett,* 918 Fed 2 605, 1990).

The Patient Protection and Affordable Care Act (ACA) was passed in 2010 and enacted with a number of initiatives implemented incrementally. This law reformed health care and health insurance industries in the United States, with the goal of increasing quality, availability, and affordability of health insurance. In 2008 President Barack Obama campaigned on a platform of health insurance for all Americans. The debate about health care in general over the course of the debate over the ACA in particular brought healthcare inequities, high costs, and poor access to preventive care into the spotlight. As a result of the new spotlight on these issues of great concern to the profession of nursing, the ANA and constituent member (state) associations are working to ensure that nurses are included in discussions and roundtables addressing the management of healthcare reform in the United States. The ACA faced two significant challenges before the U.S. Supreme Court (*National Federation of Independent Business v. Sebelius*, 2011–2012; *King et al. v. Burwell*, 2014–2-15). In each case the court ruled to uphold key provisions of the ACA. Further challenges to the ACA are expected, and currently many provisions of the ACA remain vulnerable to repeal, including coverage for persons with preexisting medical conditions, among others.

Patient Self-Determination Act

Although the PSDA became effective in 1991, many problems in its implementation remain. Nurses are in a position to help patients and families understand this law and how it can assist them to have the end-of-life care they prefer. The PSDA applies to acute care and long-term care facilities receiving Medicare and Medicaid funds. It encourages patients to consider which life-prolonging treatment options they desire and to document their preferences in the event they become incapable of participating in the decision-making process. Written instructions recognized by state law describing an individual's preferences in regard to medical intervention should the individual become incapacitated are called an *advance directive*. Additional details about the PSDA are included in Chapter 7.

This Act was passed partly in response to the U.S. Supreme Court's decision in *Cruzan v. Director Missouri Department of Health* (110 Supreme Court 2841, 1990), which was viewed as limiting an individual's ability to direct health care when unable to do so. The Cruzan case is explained in more detail in Chapter 2. The PSDA requires the healthcare facility to document whether the patient has completed an advance directive.

The PSDA's basic assumption is that each person has legal and moral rights to informed consent about medical treatments with a focus on the person's right to choose (the ethical principle of autonomy). The Act does not create any new rights, and no patient is required to execute an advance directive.

According to the PSDA, acute care (hospitals) and long-term care facilities must do the following:

1. Provide written information to all adult patients about their rights under state law.
2. Ensure institutional compliance with state laws on advance directives.
3. Provide for education of staff and the community on advance directives.
4. Document in the medical record whether the patient has an advance directive.

The Agency for Healthcare Research and Quality (AHRQ) reported that even when patients had advance directives in place, the directives were not guiding end-of-life care as legislators and advocates had anticipated. This was attributable to several factors: patients were not considered ill enough to implement their advance directives; family members were not available, were too overwhelmed to implement the patient's wishes, or disagreed with the patient's wishes; and the advance directive itself was not specific enough or did not cover pertinent clinical issues. A model for advanced directives developed by the American Association of Retired Persons, the American Bar Association, and the American Medical Association seeks to address these issues and can be accessed at the American Bar Association website (American Bar Association, 2012). Documentation of the existence of advance directives and use of them in planning care is an important patient advocacy role for nurses and is a legal requirement that needs careful implementation in clinical settings.

PROTECTING YOURSELF FROM LEGAL PROBLEMS

Although the discussion about legal issues related to nursing practice has covered many topics, it is important that new nurses realize that the vast majority of nurses never encounter a legal problem during their professional careers. This is because there are a number of effective strategies that professional nurses can use to limit the possibility of legal action (Butler and Lostritto, 2015).

Practice in a Safe Setting

To be truly safe, facilities in which nurses work must be committed to safe patient care. The safest situation is one in which the agency does the following:

1. Employs an appropriate number personnel with a variety of skills to care adequately for the number of agency patients at all levels of acuity

2. Has policies, procedures, and personnel practices promoting quality and safety (Smith, 2018)
3. Keeps equipment in good working order
4. Provides comprehensive orientation to new employees, supervises all levels of employees, and provides opportunities for employees to learn new procedures consistent with the level of health care services provided by the agency (note that a comprehensive orientation is not "on-the-job training") (Paradiso, 2018)

Risk management is a key part of an active quality and safety program. Risk management seeks to identify and eliminate potential safety hazards, thereby reducing patient and staff injuries. Common areas of risk include a wide range generally and specifically involving failure to ensure patient safety: medication errors, failure to monitor or respond to a patient, patient falls, failure to follow workplace procedures, and failure to supervise when delegating, among others.

In a desire to promote improvements in patient safety, The Joint Commission on Accreditation of Healthcare Organizations (i.e., The Joint Commission) adopted patient safety goals in 2005 that were revisited in 2012 and again in 2015. A summary of these goals is online (The Joint Commission, 2018). These goals identify significant ways in which patient safety can be enhanced through environmental, educational, practice, and policy changes. They are far-reaching and affect patients at almost every level and setting of care, from hospitals to office-based surgery to laboratory services.

Communicate With Other Health Professionals, Patients, and Families

RNs must have open and clear communication with other nurses, physicians, and other healthcare professionals. Nurses who practice safely trust their own assessments, inform physicians, APRNs, physician assistants, and others of changes in patients' conditions, and question unclear or inaccurate physicians' prescriptions or treatment plans. A key aspect of communication essential in preventing legal problems is keeping good patient records. This written form of communication is called *documentation*.

The medical record (often referred to as the *electronic health record* [EHR]), particularly the nurse's notes, provides the core of evidence about each patient's nursing care. No matter how good the nursing care, if the nurse fails to document it in the medical record, from the perspective of the law the care did not take place. (You may hear nurses remind each other, "Not documented—not done.") Be sure to document accurately, in a timely manner, and concisely. Know the documentation policies of your agency and your unit, particularly the acceptable abbreviations.

Current and descriptive documentation of patient care is essential, not only to provide quality care but also to protect the nurse. Assessments, plans, interventions, and evaluation of the patient's progress must be reflected in the patient's medical record in case malpractice is alleged. Nurses must also document phone conversations with patients, family members, physicians, and other healthcare providers.

If a patient is angry, not adhering to their treatment plan, or complaining, nurses should be even more careful to document thoroughly. Professional nurses recognize that establishing and maintaining good communication and rapport with patients and their families not only is an aspect of best practice but also is a means of protection from lawsuits. If you encounter a negative patient or family situation that you sense is escalating, seek the advice and guidance of a nurse manager or other person in a position of authority in your organization. You do not have to settle problems with patients and families by yourself, and in fact it is wise to involve those in leadership situations to help deescalate difficult situations.

Accountability for accurate documentation has increased in recent years because of the advent of electronic documentation and multiple uses of recorded data, such as reimbursement, research, and quality assurance audits. The importance of the patient record as the basis for safe practice remains. You will learn how to document correctly as you advance through nursing school. Common problems in documentation include gaps in data or entries, subjectivity or bias, and deviating from policies and procedures established by your place of employment.

Meet the Standard of Care

The most important protective strategy for the nurse is to be a knowledgeable and safe practitioner and to meet the standard of care with all patients (Strong, 2016). Meeting the standard of care involves being technically competent, keeping up to date with healthcare innovations, being aware of peer expectations, and participating as an equal on the healthcare team.

Nurses must familiarize themselves with the policies and procedures of the agency in which they work, and if policies deviate from the current standard of care, they must take steps through organizational processes to bring institutional practices in line with standards and law. They must know how to use equipment properly and know when it is malfunctioning. Nurses must keep up with the current evidence to guide their practice by reading the professional literature and attending continuing education conferences and workshops. Professional nurses must use national standards of practice, care planning, and care evaluation. The ANA has developed generic and specialty standards of nursing practice and published these in the document *Nursing: Scope and Standards of Practice*, described in more detail elsewhere in this text. These national standards can be used by quality improvement programs in individual hospitals in establishing their own specific standards of nursing care appropriate for the setting.

Continued competence is an issue the nursing profession has not uniformly addressed (Strong, 2016). At this time, different states have differing requirements for continuing education as a prerequisite for license renewal. Professional nurses recognize that continuing education and maintaining competence are essential to safe practice, regardless of state requirements.

In the final analysis, the best protection a nurse can have is to know the limits of their own education and expertise and the provisions of the state's nursing practice act. Staying within those limits may sometimes require nurses to enlist assistance from more experienced nurses to be able to meet the standard of care. This should be viewed as a learning opportunity and an indication of maturity rather than as a failure or evidence of incompetence. Box 6.7 contains information about documents that all professional nurses should own, read, and understand to ensure that they meet the standard of care.

BOX 6.7 Four Documents You Should Own

Professional nurses are accountable for practicing within their scope of practice. To stay current with changes that may affect the scope of nursing practice, you should always have the latest revision of the following four documents. You must read and understand them and be mindful of their provisions as you practice.

1. A copy of the nursing practice act of the state in which you practice. These are generally available for downloading from states' board of nursing websites. Familiarity with the law in your state is a key safeguard against inadvertently overstepping your limits of practice while understanding the full set of responsibilities that your state requires you to fulfill as a professional RN.
2. *Nursing's Social Policy Statement: The Essence of the Profession.* Available from the ANA (www.nursingworld.org), this short but important document lays out in concise language the most current definition of nursing; the knowledge base for nursing, including specialization and advanced practice roles; and the regulation of practice. It represents "an expression of the social contract between society and professional nursing" (p. v) in the United States. The ANA has taken the position that the scope of nursing practice should flow from the definition of nursing that is contained in this document. It therefore has considerable impact on the national scope of practice.
3. *Nursing: Scope and Standards of Practice.* Also published by the ANA, this document expands on the *Social Policy Statement.* It focuses on defining and delimiting clinical practice and its safe implementation. *Scope and Standards'* statements, in conjunction with other documents, are widely used in legal cases to determine whether a nurse has met the "standard of care" in a particular case. In addition to this general document, the ANA has published standards for numerous specialized areas of practice, such as hospice and palliative care and gerontologic, pediatric, neuroscience, vascular, and psychiatric–mental health nursing, among others.
4. ANA's *Code of Ethics for Nurses with Interpretive Statements.* This document is available for viewing only (http://www.nursingworld.org/MainMenuCategories/EthicsStandards/CodeofEthicsforNurses) and may be purchased even if you are not yet a member of the ANA. It describes the ethical provisions that cover all aspects of nursing practice. In addition, it adds a number of interpretive (clarifying) statements for each provision. Knowledge of your professional organization's code of ethics is an important protection for you as you begin or continue your nursing practice.

The three ANA documents are available on the ANA website, www.nursingworld.org.

Carry and Understand Professional Liability Insurance

Despite the efforts of dedicated professionals, sometimes they make mistakes and patients are injured. It is essential for nurses to carry professional liability insurance to protect their assets and income in case they are required to pay monetary compensation to an injured patient (Pohlman, 2015). Nursing students should also carry insurance, and most nursing education programs require that they do so. In addition to carrying the insurance, nurses must read and understand the provisions of their malpractice coverage.

Professional liability insurance policies vary. The amount of coverage varies by insurance carrier, so you must become familiar with your policy and coverage. The amount of coverage depends on the nurse's specialty. Certified nurse-midwives, for example, pay higher liability insurance premiums than do psychiatric nurses because a nurse-midwife's potential for being named as a defendant in a malpractice suit is greater. Look for a policy that has portable coverage, and make sure that it covers court judgments, out-of-court settlements, legal fees, and court costs (Watson, 2014). Furthermore, a good policy covers incidents occurring any time, as long as the incident took place while the policy was in force, even if you no longer carry the insurance (occurrence policy).

Professional liability insurance is available through most state nurses associations, nursing students associations, and private insurers. Group policies, such as those available through professional associations, are usually less expensive than individual policies and are an important benefit of association membership. Box 6.8 provides information about the two main types of professional liability policies.

BOX 6.8 Basic Types of Professional Liability Insurance Policies

Occurrence Policies

Cover injuries that occur during the period covered by the policy, whether or not the policy is still in effect at the time the suit is brought.

Claims-Made Policies

Cover injuries only if the injury occurs within the policy period and the claim is reported to the insurance company during the policy period or during the "tail." A tail is an uninterrupted extension of the policy period and is also known as the extending reporting endorsement.

Promote Positive Interpersonal Relationships

Even in the face of untoward outcomes from a healthcare provider, it is usually only the disgruntled patient who sues. Therefore the best strategy for the professional nurse is prevention of legal actions through positive interpersonal relationships.

Prevention includes giving personalized, concerned care; including the patient and the family in planning and implementing care; and promoting positive, open interpersonal relationships that communicate caring and compassion. When confronted with angry patients or family members, you must avoid criticizing or blaming other healthcare providers and maintain a concerned and nondefensive manner.

The professional nurse who is clinically competent and caring, and communicates openly with patients is likely to prevent most legal problems. Box 6.9 summarizes the important steps nurses can take to avoid legal problems in professional practice. When or if you commit an error, follow your agency's reporting requirements, learn from the experience, and then begin the process of self-compassion, "being warm and understanding toward yourself when you make a mistake, rather than punishing yourself with self-criticism" (Curtin, 2017, p. 64).

BOX 6.9 Guidelines for Preventing Legal Problems in Nursing Practice

- Practice safely in a safe setting.
- Communicate with other health professionals, patients, and—with the patient's permission—family members. Document fully, carefully, and in a timely manner.
- Delegate wisely, remembering the "five rights" of delegation.
- Meet or exceed the standard of care by staying on top of new developments and skills.
- Carry professional liability insurance and know the specifics of the policy.
- Promote positive interpersonal relationships and a nondefensive manner while practicing caring, compassionate, holistic nursing care.

CONCEPTS AND CHALLENGES

- ***Concept:*** Law is a system of rules that governs conduct and attaches consequences to certain behavior. These consequences include civil or criminal action or both.
  Challenge: Nursing is subject to and its boundaries set by the definition of practice in the state nursing practice act and the qualifications for licensure to practice nursing in that state. Become familiar with your state's nursing practice act.
- ***Concept:*** The law is dynamic and must be responsive to society's needs.
  Challenge: Being responsive has broadened the scope of nursing practice and increased the possibility for legal actions involving nurses.
- ***Concept:*** Technological advances have increased concern about informed consent and patients' rights to direct the care they choose to receive or refuse.
  Challenge: The use of social media may blur the lines between personal and professional boundaries; however, the nurse needs to maintain firm professional boundaries with current and former patients when using social media.

IDEAS FOR FURTHER EXPLORATION

1. Using your state's nursing practice act, describe the scope of practice of the RN. When was the last time the law was modified? Does it accurately reflect current nursing practice?
2. Read the section of the nursing practice act relating to advanced practice. What are differences between the scope of practice of RNs and that of APRNs?
3. If a physician, nurse practitioner, or physician's assistant writes a prescription for an unusually high dose of a medication, what steps should the RN take to ensure patient safety?
4. What are the liability issues for a nurse who fails to raise the side rails on a postoperative patient's bed if the patient is injured in a fall?
5. Do you have an advance directive in place? Think about what you would want if you become incapacitated. Write your wishes down, and then consider taking whatever steps your state requires to create an official advance directives document. Be willing to have that "hard conversation" about end-of-life wishes with your family or close friends.
6. It will not be long before you will be interviewing for your first nursing position. What questions should you ask to determine whether employer provides a legally safe setting in which to practice?
7. Discuss ways that social media have complicated how you determine where your professional and personal boundaries are.

REFERENCES

American Association of Legal Nurse Consultants: *What is an LNC?*, 2021. (website). Available at: http://www.aalnc.org/page/what-is-an-lnc.

American Bar Association: *Law for older Americans: health care advance directives,* 2012. (website). Available at: https://www.americanbar.org/groups/public_education/resources/law_issues_for_consumers/directive_whatis.html.

American Nurses Association (ANA): *Code of Ethics for Nurses, Provision 4.4 Delegation of Nurse Activities,* 2015. (website). Available at: https://www.nursingworld.org/practice-policy/nursing-excellence/ethics/code-of-ethics-for-nurses/coe-view-only/.

Ballard K, Haagenson D, Christiansen L, et al. Scope of nursing practice decision-making framework, *J Nurs Adm* 7(3):19–21, 2016.

Butler KA, Lostritto MD: Malpractice 101:strategies for defending your practice, *J Radiol Nurs* 34(1):13–24, 2015.

Bettinardi-Angres K, Pickett J, Patrick D: Substance use disorders and accessing alternative-to-discipline programs, *J Nurs Regul* 3(2):17–23, 2012.

Croke EM: Nurses, negligence and malpractice: an analysis based on more than 250 cases against nurses, *Am J Nurs* 103(9):54–63, 2003.

Curtin L: Self-compassion, mistakes and moral behavior, *Am Nurse Today* 12(3):64, 2017.

The Joint Commission: *National Patient Safety Goals,* 2018. (website). Available at: https://www.jointcommission.org/assets/1/6/2018_HAP_NPSG_goals_final.pdf.

National Council of State Boards of Nursing: *Scope of Nursing Practice Decision-Making Framework,* 2016. (website). Available at: https://www.ncsbn.org/decision-making-framework.htm.

National Council of State Boards of Nursing (NCSBN): *A nurses guide to the use of social media,* 2018. Available at: https://www.ncsbn.org/NCSBN_SocialMedia.pdf.

National Council of State Boards of Nursing (NCSBN): *Model Nursing Practice Acts,* 2014. Available at:
https://www.ncsbn.org/model-acts.htm#:~:text=The%20APRN%20Model%20Act%20defines,(APRNs)%20in%20every%20state.

National Council of State Boards of Nursing (NCSBN): National guidelines for nursing delegation, *J Nurs Regul* 7(1):5–14, 2016.

Paradiso L: Everyone is responsible for a culture of safety, *Am Nurse Today* 13(3):33–34, 2018.

Pohlman KJ: Why you need your own malpractice insurance, *Am Nurse Today* 10(11):28–30, 2015.

Puente J: The enhanced nurse licensure compact, *Am Nurse Today* 12(10):50–53, 2017.

Russell KA: Nurse practice acts guide and govern, *J Nurs Regulation* 8(3):18–25, 2017.

Smith CA: Promoting high reliability on the front-line, *Am Nurse Today* 13(3):30–34, 2018.

Strong M: Maintaining clinical competency is your responsibility, *Am Nurse Today* 11(7):46–47, 2016.

U.S. Department of Health and Human Services.: *Privacy and Security Guide,* 2018. (website). Available at: https://www.healthit.gov/sites/default/files/pdf/privacy/privacy-and-security-guide.pdf.

Watson E: Nursing malpractice: costs, trends, and issues, *J Leg Nurse Consulting* 25(1):26–31, 2014.

7

Ethics: Basic Concepts for Professional Nursing Practice

To enhance your understanding of this chapter, try the Student Exercises on the Evolve site at http://evolve.elsevier.com/Black/professional.

LEARNING OUTCOMES

After studying this chapter, students will be able to:

- Differentiate between values, morals, ethics, and bioethics.
- Explain the difference between Kohlberg's and Gilligan's approaches to moral reasoning.
- Compare and contrast the three normative ethical theories.
- Identify and define basic ethical principles.
- Discuss the concept of justice as an ethical principle in healthcare delivery.
- Discuss the relevance of a code of ethics for the profession of nursing.
- Understand how professional ethics override personal ethics in professional settings.
- Describe ethical dilemmas resulting from conflicts between patients, healthcare professionals, family members, and institutions.
- Identify a model for ethical decision making, and discuss the steps of the model.
- Recognize sociocultural challenges to professional ethical behavior, including social media and substance abuse.
- Understand the important ethical issues related to immigration, migration, and health care.
- Recognize moral distress, and describe the individual and organizational issues resulting from unaddressed moral distress.
- Describe the process of using moral courage with the CODE Moral Courage Model.

In our everyday, nonwork lives, the "rightness" or "wrongness" of a situation or how to act can seem obvious. We sometimes refer to these clearly and sharply delineated acts or decisions as being "black or white." Often in health care, nurses face an uncertain space known as the "gray area": the rightness or wrongness of acts are not clear or sharply delineated. You have learned that nursing focuses on human responses, so as with all endeavors that deal with humans and responses, nurses face the messiness—the gray area—inherent in individuals' lives and actions. Understanding ethical principles, frameworks, nursing's code of ethics, and your values and beliefs can help you face the many complex ethical issues that nurses confront. You will learn to act in accord with nursing's code of ethics, which will give you a firm foundation on which to practice nursing ethically.

Scholars have devoted their entire careers to the study of *ethics,* the examination of questions of right and wrong, how values are determined, and how ethics are applied in specific situations. Ethics are also known as moral philosophy. There are three general types of ethics: (1) *metaethics*, which focus on universal truths, and where and how ethical principles are developed; (2) *normative ethics*, which focus on the moral standards that regulate behaviors; and (3) *applied ethics*, which focus on specific issues such as allowing a natural death, capital punishment, abortion, and health disparities. In a practice profession such as nursing, ethical issues often arise, created by the very nature of the work of nursing.

The purpose of this chapter is to give you a basic introduction to the complex issues of ethics so that you will be better prepared to recognize and work through situations with ethical implications.

Common situations with ethical implications for nurses include making decisions about the allocation of time and resources, what and how much information to share with patients and their families, how to manage and deal with colleagues professionally, and how to resolve problems when the desires and needs of patients and families conflict with institutional policies or the values of those providing the care. More dramatic ethical issues for nurses include assisting families making end-of-life decisions, allocating care in emergency situations (triage), managing pain near the end of life with large doses of narcotics, and advocating for a patient even when the nurse does not agree with the patient. To manage the complex ethical issues they face, nurses need an understanding of the theoretical basis for ethical decision making.

Throughout their education and practice, nurses must exercise judgment when making clinical decisions. However, when nurses encounter ethical dilemmas, they need both an ethical decision-making model to apply to the situation and one that works for individual nurses in the context of his or her value system. Box 7.1, "To Be Guardians of the Ethical Treatment of Patients," describes the importance of the role of nurses and nursing faculty in achieving high standards of integrity to provide ethical care for our vulnerable patients.

DEFINITIONS OF BASIC CONCEPTS IN ETHICS

Defining *values*, *morals*, *ethics*, and *bioethics* is useful as a first step in understanding ethics and their relationship to health care. **Values** are attitudes, ideals, or

BOX 7.1 To Be Guardians of the Ethical Treatment of Patients

Anne Bavier (2009), PhD, RN, FAAN, Dean of the University of Texas at Arlington College of Nursing and President-elect of the National League for Nursing, wrote to nursing students and their faculty in an editorial about the high standards of integrity for themselves and for all who serve patients:

To become the guardians of patients' well-being and of the nursing profession, nurses must learn more than technical skills, even more than just critical thinking or ethical criteria.... The topic is timely: If recent headlines are any indication, professional ethics are in critical condition. We are all familiar with reports of financial dishonesty that have contributed to a contracted global economy, and we have seen recent surveys about student cheating and plagiarism. It seems that a chronic ailment, human frailty, is the underlying disorder.

For nurses and nurse faculty, the outcomes of dishonesty are, without hyperbole, a matter of life and death. When a math student or an English student cheats without learning, society is impaired, to be sure. However, if a nursing student cheats without learning, patients may sicken or die.... When the (National League for Nursing [NLN]) adopted its core values, it included integrity, "evident when organizational principles of communication, ethical decision making, and humility are encouraged, expected, and demonstrated consistently." The NLN states that "not only is doing the right thing simply how we do business, but our actions reveal our commitment to truth-telling and to how we always see ourselves from the perspective of others in a larger community" (http://www.nln.org/about/core-values). *Most schools and universities have similar codes of conduct that stress the greater good of individual actions and the pursuit of truth.*

Nurses and nurse faculty must be the guardians of the ethical treatment of patients. Aristotle's deceptively simple rationale for living well and doing good seems exquisitely suited to nursing education: "Every art and every inquiry, and similarly every action and choice, is thought to aim at some good; and for this reason the good has rightly been declared to be that at which all things aim." Nursing, as both art and inquiry, action and choice, must always reflect on its aims. That is what Aristotle called phronesis, practical wisdom, change for good by planning an effective route to a desirable goal. Thus a nurse educator (whether in classroom or clinic) is not just a master of skills conveyed to the student but also a teacher of practical wisdom: ethical action.

Deeply mentored by nurse faculty, they must become confident, autonomous healthcare professionals who have high standards of integrity for themselves and for all who serve patients.

beliefs that an individual or a group holds and uses to guide behavior. Values are usually expressed in terms of right and wrong, hierarchies of importance, or how one should behave. Values are freely chosen and indicate what the individual considers important, such as honesty and hard work. Values are assimilated from and influenced by personal and professional experiences and are deeply rooted in an individual's culture. Attitudes are integrated with values and can shape nurses' judgments and actions. Attitudes may, however, result in nurse bias if the nurse is not cognizant of how the beliefs may affect the nurse's judgment. The terms *morals* and *ethics* are often used interchangeably, but for the purposes of this chapter, a distinction is made. Philosophers and scholars have conflicting views on how to define these terms. **Morals** provide standards of behavior that guide the actions of an individual or social group and are established rules of conduct to be used in situations where a decision about right and wrong must be made. Morals typically focus on behaviors and actions of what to do (good) and what to avoid (harm). An example of a moral standard is "One should not lie." Morals are learned over time and are influenced by life experiences and culture.

Ethics is a term used to reflect what actions an individual should take and maybe "codified," as in the ethical code of a profession. "Ethics" is derived from the Greek word "ethos," which means habits or customs. Ethics are process oriented and involve a critical analysis of actions. If ethicists (persons who study ethics) reflected on the moral statement "One should not lie," they would clarify definitions of lying and explore whether there are circumstances under which lying might be acceptable.

Bioethics are the application of ethical theories and principles to moral issues or problems in health care. Bioethics (also referred to as *biomedical ethics*) as an area of ethical inquiry came into existence around 1970, when healthcare providers began to embrace a holistic view of the patient and the rights of patients, in addition to treating and curing disease. Bioethics are concerned with determining what should be done in a specific situation by applying ethical principles. For instance, discussions about genetic testing often have a strong bioethical component surrounding use of knowledge from this type of testing. The website www.bioethics.net is a source of comprehensive and up-to-date information about issues related to bioethics that you may find interesting.

Advances in science and medical technologies have allowed healthcare providers to sustain lives under circumstances that once would have caused a patient's death. On the one hand, these technologies are excellent tools in the management of some problems—for example, in assisting with ventilation until a patient can breathe without assistance, as sometimes happens in the case of a life-threatening but reversible condition (e.g., severe pneumonia, moderately severe head injury). Conversely, these advances sometimes create ethical dilemmas for healthcare providers. For example, a patient may be "kept alive" even when there is no discernible brain activity or hope for the return of spontaneous respiration. Nurses struggle with situations such as these, asking whether a patient should be sustained ("kept alive") under these circumstances. These situations sometimes raise serious questions for nurses about the meaning of life and what constitutes being "alive."

A critical attribute of providing care in a professional setting is that professional ethics override personal morals and values. The American Nurses Association (ANA) published a position statement in 1983 that remains in effect today and that contains this statement: "The ANA believes the Code [of Ethics] for Nurses is nonnegotiable and that each nurse has an obligation to uphold and adhere to the code of ethics" (ANA, 1994). Holding all nurses accountable to the same ethical code is a means of protecting patients by establishing a clear standard by which nurses make ethical decisions and carry out their duties. Provision 2 of the Code of Ethics describes the nurse's primary commitment to the patient; provision 5 describes the responsibility of nurses to maintain their own integrity. These two provisions are not in conflict, but they do underscore the importance of understanding nursing's primary ethical obligations to the care of patients.

Nurses, then, must think carefully about personal values and morals. Being clear on where one stands personally on a situation will help the nurse make careful choices about their work environment and the types of patients with whom he or she would like to work. For instance, if a nurse's personal moral belief is that abortion is wrong under any circumstances, they would find untenable the requirements of a work setting in which pregnancy terminations are performed for genetic disorders. Similarly, if a nurse believes that drug addiction represents a moral shortcoming, seeking employment on an infectious disease unit or mental health setting where

PROFESSIONAL PROFILE BOX 7.1

Nurses' Ethical Reasoning Skills Model

A dynamic, ethically based reasoning process became apparent to me over a period of years as I worked with patients and families as a registered nurse (RN) in the emergency department and in hospice/palliative care. This dynamic is proposed to involve the interplay of several important internal cognitive processes, as depicted in the nurses' ethical reasoning skills (NERS) model (Fairchild, 2010). With this theory, I propose that when faced with an ethical dilemma, the professional nurse's cognitive processes include reflection, reasoning, and a review of competing values, ultimately leading to purposeful *action* on behalf of patients and families in the nurse's care.

I developed this model during my doctoral studies at Indiana University, based on my work experiences as an RN, and also based on current evidence in ethical decision making, and in nursing and health systems theory and research (Fairchild, 2010). During my studies, a diverse mix of coursework in ethics and theory seemed to coalesce, allowing me to visualize the complexity of patient care decision-making processes as a unique and ongoing cycle for nurses, akin to a phenomenon called *systems thinking* (Pesut and Herman, 1999). In systems thinking, we continually take experiences in and reflect on them from a holistic, values-based, knowledge-driven stance. Thus what nurses and other healthcare providers strive to accomplish every day in emergent and/or crisis situations needs to be represented and supported by a fluid, interactive thought dynamic that promotes sound ethical decision making at the "sharp end" (Cook and Woods, 1994) of care.

As challenges in patient care are managed on a daily basis in practice, I believe that practical ethical decision-making skills need to be pushed to the forefront of healthcare delivery, based on ever-changing characteristics of today's complex healthcare systems. In addition, as nurses, our experiences teach us that *context* is of utmost importance as we strive to follow basic tenets of our profession; that is, to do good, and above all, to do no harm (Gilligan, 1987) on behalf of patients and families. Nurses' unique commitment and calling to apply both higher level knowledge and humanistic, holistic caring are what set us apart from the medically based disease model of care. Knowing and cooperatively manifesting our uniqueness allow us to act wholeheartedly and in good faith with other members of the healthcare team, because we are consciously realizing the complexity, as well as the fragility, of the human caring work we engage in each day.

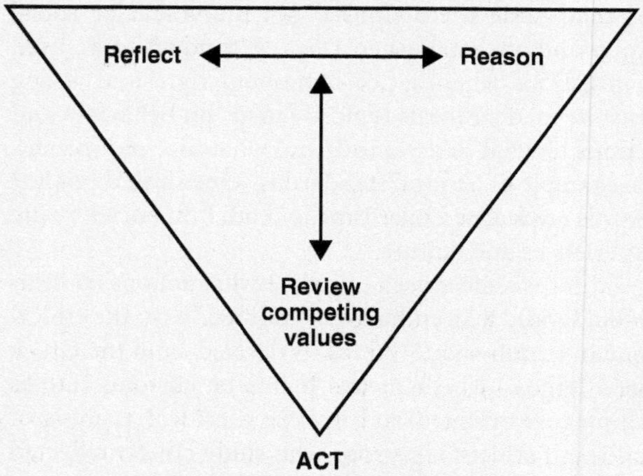

Theoretical model of nurses' ethical reasoning skills.

Roseanne M. Fairchild, PhD, RN, CNE, NE-BC
Indiana State University, Clayton, IN

many patients have addiction problems would be a poor choice. By understanding their personal values, nurses can anticipate situations in which their personal morals and professional ethics may be in conflict. A thoughtful nurse who is aware of deep personal values and moral standards will make decisions regarding practice setting so that the nurse's own personal integrity remains intact, while putting patients and their needs first.

Moral reflection—critical analysis of one's morals, beliefs, and actions—is a process through which a person develops and maintains moral integrity. Moral integrity in a professional setting is a goal in which one's professional beliefs and actions are assessed and analyzed (reflected on) so that professional ethics continue to mature and respond to changes in practice (Hardingham, 2004). In any complex ethical situation, nurses should analyze their own actions so that they can reduce inner conflicts between their personal values and morals and their professional ethics. A model of nurses' ethical reasoning developed by Roseanne Fairchild, PhD, RN, CNE, NE-BC, is featured in Professional Profile Box 7.1.

Moral distress is a phenomenon of spiritual, emotional, and behavioral anguish (Burston and Tuckett, 2013). Moral distress may arise when one knows the morally correct action to take but is unable to act as a result of internal constraints (such as lack of moral courage) or external constraints, including power differentials (Saureland et al., 2014). Moral distress may also occur when a nurse's moral action is ineffective in ensuring the moral outcome, often because of constraints beyond the nurse's control (Rushton et al., 2016).

Repercussions of moral distress affect not only the nurse but also the broader healthcare context, including risk to healthcare quality and patient outcomes, job satisfaction, and retention, as well as the physical, spiritual, and emotional wellness of the nurse (Burston and Tuckett, 2013). Unaddressed moral distress can lead to nurse behaviors that exacerbate an integrity-compromising situation, including nurse apathy, indifference, avoidance, disengagement in patient care situations, feelings of powerlessness, and loss of moral sensitivity (McCarthy and Gastmans, 2015).

The following scenario and the one later in this chapter have several important ethical implications that cause a moral dilemma for the healthcare team and the family. Examine the scenarios for various ethical issues, and think about what parts of this situation might pose a moral dilemma or moral distress for you.

Scenario 1: What are the implications of "doing everything"? A newborn infant was admitted to the neonatal intensive care unit (NICU). She was born very prematurely and weighs only 520 grams (about 1 pound). The parents want "everything done" for the infant to ensure her survival; the infant, however, has multiple setbacks including serious infections; feeding problems; and then a grade IV intraventricular hemorrhage, which is severe bleeding into the ventricles of the brain. The neonatologists are convinced that the infant will have profound physical, cognitive, and developmental problems if she even survives and ask for a meeting with the parents to discuss discontinuing the infant's life support. The parents want life support to be continued and for the infant to be a "full code," meaning that all efforts will be made to resuscitate her in case her heart stops. The infant's primary care nurse understands the parents' deep desire to give their child every chance to live; however, he also understands the severe physical and neurologic complications of extreme prematurity. He is concerned about the pain and suffering the infant may be experiencing because of her numerous treatments and extensive supportive technology. He thinks about the resources in terms of time and money that continuing support of this infant requires, and although he does not like thinking about patient care in those terms, he recognizes the tension he feels about the effort the infant is requiring. The nurse realizes that he dreads going in to work every day to take care of this infant and finds himself dwelling on the situation when he is not at work. After a long shift one night, he goes home and blurts out to his wife, "This just isn't right, and I don't know what to do about it."

This example demonstrates numerous aspects of moral dilemmas and resulting moral distress. The nurse experienced moral distress, a sense of being unable to act in a way that he believes is moral in this situation. The nurse recognized the parents' desire for their child to live; the possibility of pain and suffering of the infant; the real possibility of severe, long-term problems if she survives; the expense in terms of time and resources; the emotional toll of care of the infant; and his own discomfort and sense of helplessness. This nurse also demonstrated that he was reflecting on his own practice and beliefs, which will help maintain his moral integrity. He will also use the lessons from this patient situation as he matures as a nurse, so that similar situations in the future may not be so distressful for him. Thinking Critically Box 7.1 refers to this patient situation; once you have studied the remainder of this chapter, you will have additional knowledge, tools, and perspective with which to consider the complexities of this scenario.

THINKING CRITICALLY BOX 7.1

Addressing Distressful Ethical Situations

Reflect on the clinical example of the nurse's moral distress related to the infant born extremely prematurely in the NICU. Now that you have some basic knowledge about ethics, consider these questions:

1. What would a deontologist's position be with regard to the sustaining of the infant's life?
2. What would a utilitarian's position be in this case?
3. What virtues of the nurse do you see at work in this case?
4. What basic ethical principles do you think the nurse may be using in analyzing this moral dilemma?
5. What are your own personal beliefs and values regarding the sustaining of an infant born extremely prematurely on extensive life support?
6. What are alternative ethical viewpoints that someone else may hold regarding this situation?
7. Who holds the primary responsibility for determining what should happen in this case—the parents or healthcare providers? Explain your response from an ethical perspective.
8. What is the state's (government's) role in intervening in this type of situation?

To function effectively in today's complex healthcare arena, nurses need to understand approaches to moral reasoning, theories of ethics, basic ethical principles, and ethical decision-making models. A significant advance in the professionalization of a traditional occupation such as nursing is the adoption of a formal code of ethics (Baker, 2009). Professional ethical codes such as that of the ANA provide substantial guidance in determining how to respond and act in practice settings when faced with an ethical dilemma. The remainder of this chapter will provide a basic orientation to these complex topics.

APPROACHES TO MORAL REASONING

Similar to other forms of human development, moral reasoning is a process in which maturation occurs over time as persons become more abstract in their thinking and understanding of the world. Moral development describes how a person learns to handle moral dilemmas from childhood through adulthood. Two important theorists in moral development and reasoning are Lawrence Kohlberg and Carol Gilligan.

Kohlberg's Stages of Moral Reasoning

Kohlberg (1976, 1986) proposed three levels of moral reasoning as a function of cognitive development: (1) preconventional, (2) conventional, and (3) postconventional. Each of these three levels is then considered in terms of stages. In the preconventional level, the individual is inattentive to the norms of society when responding to moral problems. Instead, the individual's perspective is self-centered. At this level, what the individual wants or needs takes precedence over right or wrong. A person in stage 1 of the preconventional level responds to punishment. In stage 2, the person responds to the prospect of personal reward. Kohlberg observed the preconventional level of moral development in children younger than 9 years of age, as well as in some adolescents and adult criminal offenders. A more typical example, however, is that of a toddler for whom the word *no* has yet to have meaning as he or she persists in reaching for a breakable object on a table.

The conventional level is characterized by moral decisions that conform to the expectations of one's family, group, or society. The person making moral choices based on what is pleasing to others characterizes stage 3 within this level. An individual in stage 4 of the conventional level makes moral choices based on a larger notion of what is desired by society. When confronted with a moral choice, people functioning at the conventional level follow family or cultural group norms. According to Kohlberg, most adolescents and adults generally function at this level. "Because it's the law" is a common explanation of persons operating at a conventional level of moral reasoning.

The postconventional level consists of stage 5 and stage 6 and involves more independent modes of thinking than previous stages. The individual has developed the ability to define his or her own moral values. Individuals who apply moral reasoning at the postconventional level may ignore both self-interest and group norms in making moral choices. Part of their moral reasoning and behavior is based on a socially agreed-on standard of human rights (Haynes et al., 2004). In this highest level of moral development, people create their own morality, which may differ from society's norms. Kohlberg believed that only a minority of adults achieve this level.

Progression through Kohlberg's levels and their corresponding stages occur over varying lengths of time for different individuals. The stages are sequential, they build on each other, and each stage is characterized by a higher capacity for moral reasoning than the preceding stage. Kohlberg (1976) suggested that certain conditions might stimulate higher levels of moral development. Intellectual development is one necessary characteristic. Individuals at higher levels intellectually generally operate at a higher stage of moral reasoning than those with lower levels of intellect. An environment that offers people opportunities for group participation, shared decision-making processes, and responsibility for the consequences of their actions also promotes higher levels of moral reasoning. Moral development is stimulated by the creation of conflict in settings in which the individual recognizes the limitations of present modes of thinking. For example, students have been stimulated to higher levels of moral reasoning through participating in courses on moral discussion and ethics (Kohlberg, 1973).

Gilligan's Stages of Moral Reasoning

Gilligan (1982) was concerned that Kohlberg did not adequately recognize women's experiences in the development of moral reasoning. She noted that Kohlberg's theories had largely been generated from research with men and boys, and when women were tested by using Kohlberg's stages of moral reasoning, they scored lower than men. Gilligan believed that women's and girls' relational orientation to the world shaped their moral reasoning differently from that of men and boys. Women do not have inadequate moral development but different development because of their gender. Kohlberg's inattention to gender differences meant that his theory was inadequate in explaining women's moral development.

Gilligan described a moral development perspective focused on care. In Gilligan's view, the moral person is one who responds to need and demonstrates consideration of care and responsibility in relationships. This perspective differed from the orientation toward justice described by Kohlberg (1973, 1976). In Gilligan's research on moral reasoning, women most often exhibited a focus on care, whereas men more often exhibited a focus on justice. Gilligan described the differences between women's and men's moral reasoning not as a matter of better or worse, or mature or immature, but simply as a matter of having "a different voice" in moral reasoning.

Gilligan (1982) suggested that women view moral dilemmas in terms of conflicting responsibilities. She described women's development of moral reasoning as a sequence of three levels and two transitions, with each level representing a more complex understanding of the relationship between self and others. Each transition resulted in a critical reevaluation of the conflict between selfishness and responsibility. Gilligan's levels of moral development are (1) orientation to individual survival; (2) a focus on goodness with recognition of self-sacrifice; and (3) the morality of caring and being responsible for others, as well as oneself. The focus of nursing on care as a moral attribute is congruent with Gilligan's assertion that the dynamics of human relationships are "central to moral understanding, joining the heart and the eye in an ethic that ties the activity of thought to the activity of care" (p. 149). Critical thinking within a caring professional relationship is a sound basis for nursing practice.

Nurses at times combine the care/justice perspective when forced to make ethical decisions. Nurses have shifted from the moral perspective of care to a justice orientation where universal rules and principles are used in moral decision making (Zickmund, 2004). Furthermore, as economics and scarcity of resources shape the delivery of health care, nurses may find themselves less able to use critical thinking, reflection, and higher stages of moral reasoning in their practice setting.

The nature of the practice of nursing has deeply ethical implications. Some implications are clear, such as those described in the case of the NICU earlier in this chapter. The ethical implications of day-to-day practice and decisions are often obscured by more dramatic scenarios. In scenario 2, a nurse organizes her day and addresses her patients' needs by a cynical strategy she calls "time management."

Scenario 2: At the beginning of her shift on an orthopedic trauma unit, Michelle, a registered nurse with 3 years' experience, identified and prioritized several tasks that she needed to complete during her shift, listing times for scheduled medications, three complex dressing changes, helping a patient on postoperative day 1 to get out of bed, and discharge teaching for her patient Mr. Thomas, who was going home after a long hospitalization for the treatment of a severe compound fracture of his lower leg. Michelle knew that there was another patient in the emergency department (ED) waiting for admission to the unit, but there were no empty beds; the only bed that was going to be available was the one Mr. Thomas now occupied. Michelle anticipated a busy shift.

Also, Michelle's patient Mr. Dillard complained of pain in his abdomen and asked for medication frequently. After assessing each of her six patients, Michelle collected the discharge papers for Mr. Thomas and started her teaching with him and his wife, who was going to continue care of the large wound in Mr. Thomas' leg at home. Mrs. Thomas had numerous questions and what seemed to be a routine discharge became more complicated when she asked Michelle for a home health referral so a nurse could help them manage Mr. Thomas' wound at home. Soon, Mr. Dillard rang his call light and asked for pain medication; a nurse colleague stepped into the room to tell Michelle, "Your frequent flyer in Room 312 rang again." Several minutes later, the ED charge nurse called to ask when a bed was going to be ready. The patient in the ED had been there since 10 p.m. the previous evening. Michelle began to feel a bit of stress but decided to reprioritize her day.

As she stood at the med cart and reviewed Mr. Dillard's pain med use, she noted to her colleague, "He has got to be drug seeking. That is the only explanation." She decided that she could forgo temporarily calling the social worker to initiate a home health referral for Mr. Thomas; she understood that until he went home, she would not have to do the long admission process for the new patient coming from the ED. When Mr. Dillard

THINKING CRITICALLY BOX 7.2

Day-to-Day Ethical Considerations

Reread Scenario 2 carefully, and then consider the perspectives from various persons described in it.

1. You are the new nurse in orientation. Describe the scenario from your perspective, and identify what you understand as elements of the scenario with ethical implications.
2. You are Michelle. Describe the scenario from your perspective as a competent nurse with a busy day ahead.
3. You are Mr. Dillard. Your pain in your abdomen was not part of your original admission diagnosis. You are hospitalized for treatment for injuries after an automobile accident in which the air bag deployed. You ask Michelle to call your doctor because you are not getting pain relief. Michelle tells you that you are to get pain medication every 4 to 6 hours, and it has only been 3.5 hours. Consider the ethical implications of pain management. What did Michelle mean in referring to Mr. Dillard as "drug seeking"? What does "being ethical" mean for a nurse in this situation? Was Michelle being ethical?
4. You are Mrs. Thomas, and as you walk away you hear Michelle's "time management" comment. You return to the desk to ask Michelle if she had even called a social worker yet. From an ethical perspective, how should Michelle respond?

asked for pain medication a second time, Michelle rolled her eyes and continued to check the morning laboratory reports; when Mrs. Thomas came to the nurses' station to ask if Michelle had started the home health referral, Michelle told her, "I called the social worker to come up to see you, but she is busy and can't get here until midafternoon." Mrs. Thomas thanked Michelle and walked away, at which point Michelle turned to a new nurse in orientation and told her, "And that's the time management skill they don't teach you in nursing school" and high-fived another colleague.

In Thinking Critically Box 7.2, you will be considering this scenario and how day-to-day nursing acts have ethical implications.

The article described in this chapter's Evidence-Based Practice Box 7.1 demonstrates that nurses often fall short of established ethical standards to complete their daily work. This problem is not exclusive to American nurses: the problem exists across nursing internationally.

THEORIES OF ETHICS

Theories of ethics, like all theories, are conceptual descriptions of phenomena. In ethics, the phenomena described are understandings of behaviors in terms of their moral implications. Theories are broad descriptions, and no single ethical theory can be applied universally in healthcare situations. As previously introduced, there are three general types of ethics: (1) *metaethics*, which focuses on universal truths, and where and how ethical principles are developed; (2) *normative ethics*, which focuses on the moral standards that regulate behaviors; and (3) *applied ethics*, which focuses on specific difficult issues such as euthanasia, capital punishment, abortion, and health disparities. In this section, selected ethical theories useful to nurses are introduced with emphasis on the normative ethical theories (virtue ethics, deontological ethics, and utilitarian ethics), and principlism ethics. Table 7.1 provides the highlights and contrasts among the three normative ethical theories, and Table 7.2 summarizes principlism ethics.

Deontology

The term *deontology* has its origins from the Greek word *deon,* which means "obligation" or "duty." German philosopher Immanuel Kant (1724–1804) was a preeminent deontologist. He believed that an act was moral if its motives or intentions were good, regardless of the outcome. An ethical action consists of doing one's duty or honoring one's obligations to human beings: to do one's duty was right; to not do one's duty was wrong. The deontological perspective does not look primarily at the consequences of actions or outcomes; rather, it focuses on the intent of the act. For example, Charlotte, a nursing student, was providing care to Mr. Wallace, an older man who was dying and who had been estranged from his son for many years. From his wallet, Mr. Wallace pulled out a tattered piece of paper with a phone number on it. Handing it to Charlotte, he asked her to promise him that she would call his son and ask him to come for a final visit. She promised.

Although she was filled with dread, Charlotte recognized her obligation to her patient to honor her promise to him. With trembling hands, she called the number. The man who answered listened to her for a few moments; then he said, "I wouldn't go to see him if you paid me. Tell him I am glad he's dying." And then he hung up on her. Charlotte

EVIDENCE-BASED PRACTICE BOX 7.1

Nurses' Ethical Decision Making: Conformist Practice

A growing concern exists regarding nurses' ethical competence. Barriers to ethical practice compromise nurses' ability to care for patients in a manner that they consider to be moral. De Casterlé and colleagues (2009), an international team of nurse researchers, conducted a meta-analysis using data from nine different studies in four countries to determine how nurses became involved in ethical decision making and action in their daily practice. A meta-analysis is a means of using similar data from different studies that address similar hypotheses and research questions to get results from a larger sample. By combining data, these researchers were able to pool the responses of 1592 RNs who completed the Ethical Behavior Test, which is based on an adaptation of Kohlberg's theory of moral development.

De Casterlé and colleagues first reviewed the existing literature about nurses' ethical decision making in practice. They found in their review that nurses typically were often poorly prepared to address ethical dilemmas and that nurses do not use critical thinking in making ethical decisions. Nurses were also found to experience conflicts between their personal values and professional ethics, and few nurses were able to express ethical problems to the healthcare team. In addition, nurses found that their work environment hindered their ability to practice nursing in a manner that they believed was ethical. Heavy workloads, time and financial constraints, and staffing problems all interfered with nurses' ability to make ethical decision making a priority.

Among the 1592 RNs included in the sample of this meta-analysis, 58 nurses were recruited specifically because they were known to demonstrate high-level ethical reasoning and practice. These nurses constituted the "expert group." This strategy is known as "purposeful sampling," to include in a study a very specific group of participants as a comparison group.

The expert group exhibited a significantly higher likelihood to make ethical decisions from a postconventional level of moral reasoning, usually at Kohlberg's sixth stage. The nonexpert group (the other 1534 nurses) generally preferred moral decisions that corresponded to Kohlberg's fourth stage, the conventional level of moral reasoning. The nonexpert nurses were significantly more likely than expert nurses to prefer moral decisions from the preconventional level, at Kohlberg's second stage.

The findings suggested that nurses typically make ethical decisions at a conventional level and that this is an international phenomenon among nurses. The researchers referred to this as "conformist practice" that "excludes a critical and creative search for the best caring answer" (p. 547) to ethical dilemmas. The conventions of practice—medical prescriptions, rules of the nursing unit, and policies and procedures—serve as a framework for practice but should not preclude individualized patient care. The findings of this study confirmed much of what the researchers had seen from their review of the literature: that nurses often face ethical challenges, that workplace conditions hinder nurses from ethical practice, and that there is a growing concern about nurses' ability to practice ethically. In addition, de Casterlé and colleagues found that nurses tend to conform to workplace rules and norms rather than using creativity and reflecting critically on their practice. The researchers suggest that, to provide the best care possible for patients, nurses must develop maturity in their moral reasoning, especially at a time when economic values tend to predominate in shaping workplace decisions.

Data from de Casterlé BD, Izumi S, Godfrey NS, et al.: Nurses' responses to ethical dilemmas in nursing practice: meta-analysis, *J Adv Nurs* 63(6):540–549, 2009.

was horrified and upset about what to tell Mr. Wallace. From a deontological perspective, Charlotte acted ethically, because she had a duty to respond to her patient's request and to keep her promise, despite the outcome.

Deontology can be further divided into act deontology and rule deontology. Act deontologists determine the right thing to do by gathering all the facts and then making a decision. Much time and energy are needed to judge each situation carefully. Once a decision is made, there is a commitment to universalizing it. In other words, if one makes a moral judgment in one situation, the same judgment will be made in any similar situation. Rule deontologists, on the other hand, emphasize that principles guide our actions. Examples of rules might be "Always keep a promise" or "Never tell a lie." In all situations, the rule is to be followed. Deontologists are not concerned with the consequences of adhering to certain rules or actions. If one's guiding principle is "Always keep a promise," a deontologist

TABLE 7.1 **Highlights and Contrasts Among the Three Normative Ethical Theories**

Framework	Virtue	Consequentialist	Duty
Deliberative Process	What kind of person should I be (or try to be), and what will my actions show about my character?	What kinds of outcomes should I produce (or try to produce)?	What are my obligations in this situation, and what are the things I should never do?
Focus	Person: Attempts to discern character traits (virtues and vices) that are, or could be, motivating the people involved in the situation.	Outcome: Directs attention to the future effects of an action, for all people who will be directly or indirectly affected by the action.	Duty: Directs attention to the duties that exist before the situation and determines obligations.
Definition of Ethical Conduct	Ethical conduct is whatever a fully virtuous person would do in the circumstances.	Ethical conduct is the action that will achieve the best consequences.	Ethical conduct involves always doing the right thing: never failing to do one's duty.
Motivation	Aim is to develop one's character.	Aim is to produce the most good.	Aim is to perform the right action.
Limitations	Assumes everyone has moral motives and strives to develop virtues. Requires a case-by-case approach without a defined decision-making process.	In interest of benefiting the majority, the interests of the minority are overlooked. Impossible to calculate all consequences.	Assumes humans make moral judgments. Life situations vary, and rules for all circumstances are unrealistic. Disregard for consequences of actions.

Adapted by Brown University, 2017.

Acknowledgement: This framework for thinking ethically is the product of dialogue and debate in the seminar Making Choices: Ethical Decisions at the Frontier of Global Science held at Brown University in the spring semester 2011. It relies on the Ethical Framework developed at the Markkula Center for Applied Ethics at Santa Clara University (http://www.scu.edu/ethics/practicing/decision/) and the Ethical Framework developed by the Center for Ethical Deliberation at the University of Northern Colorado as well as the Ethical Frameworks for Academic Decision-Making on the Faculty Focus website (https://www.facultyfocus.com/articles/faculty-development/ethical-frameworks-for-academic-decision-making/), which in turn relies on Understanding Ethical Frameworks for E-Learning Decision-Making, December 1, 2008, Distance Education Report. Primary contributors include Sheila Bonde and Paul Firenze, with critical input from James Green, Margot Grinberg, Josephine Korijn, Emily Levoy, Alysha Naik, Laura Ucik, and Liza Weisberg. It was last revised in May 2013.

will keep promises, even if circumstances have changed. For Charlotte, the nursing student in the previous example, by judging that making a call under these circumstances was ethical, she set for herself a precedent—that she would act the same way in each circumstance like this one. Similarly, if she acted on the principle to never tell a lie, she would find a caring way to tell her patient not to expect his son to visit when he asked.

A limitation of this duty-based theory is there is an assumption that humans will all make moral judgments. Additionally, life situations vary, and a guide (rules of duty) for all circumstances is unrealistic. Last, a significant theory limitation of deontology is the disregard of consequences of actions.

Utilitarianism

Utilitarianism is based on a fundamental belief that the moral rightness of an action is determined solely by its consequence. Utilitarianism was first described by David Hume (1711–1776) and was developed further by many notable philosophers, including Jeremy Bentham (1748–1832) and John Stuart Mill (1806–1873). Mill had a significant influence on utilitarian ethics as it is known today.

Those who subscribe to utilitarian ethics believe that "what makes an action right or wrong is its utility, with useful actions bringing about the greatest good for the greatest number of people" (Guido, 2006, p. 4). In other words, maximizing the greatest good for the benefit,

TABLE 7.2 Summary of Principlism Theory

Ethical Principle	Moral Basis	Overemphasis/ Downside	Challenges in Health Care
Autonomy (includes confidentiality)	Respect for individuals	Lack of caring, not interfering with decision making	Some patients defer autonomy to their provider. Who is granted the autonomy with incompetent or unconscious patients, minors, and those with cultural power differentials? Autonomy as a principle is typically weighted highest in health care.
Beneficence (includes patient advocacy)	Do good	Paternalism—inflicting own values	Context of patient's life and situation must be considered. Beneficence may conflict with informed refusal.
Nonmaleficence	Do no harm	Lack of action, questionable treatments not offered	Therapeutic interventions may cause harm. Often conflicts with autonomy. Rule of double effect used to justify actions that may cause harm.
Justice	Be fair; provide care appropriate to needs	With lack of resources impossible to be fair or individualize	Is health care a right or a privilege? Should nonadherent patients continue to receive health care resources? Health disparities highlight the lack of health care justice.
Fidelity (includes confidentiality and synergistic with veracity)	Loyalty and truthfulness	Confidentiality may impede efficiency and quality of care	No absolute duty to keep promises; in each situation, the harmful consequences of the promised action must be weighed against the benefits of promise keeping.
Veracity	Truth telling or not lying	Truth may cause harm	Cultural variances existing regarding truth telling with healthcare information. Sometimes a desire to justify why deceit is best in situations occurs.

happiness, or pleasure of the greatest number of people is moral. Utilitarianism assumes that it is possible to balance good and evil with a goal that most people experience good rather than evil. Professional healthcare providers use utilitarian theory in many situations. Consider, for example, the concept of *triage*, in which sick or injured persons are classified by the severity of their condition to determine the priority of treatment. Imagine that there is a plane crash in a remote area in which many of the survivors are severely burned. The local healthcare facility cannot manage all of the patients, and although air transport is available from a large medical facility 3 hours away, only those with the possibility of surviving can be transported. Those with less serious burns can be managed at a smaller hospital. This means that someone must decide who will and will not be treated. The most gravely injured will not be treated until those with a reasonable chance of survival are taken care of, although this means that some of the more severely injured will die while waiting for care. As a function of utilitarianism, triage is accepted worldwide as an ethical basis for determining treatment.

Often, utilitarianism is the basis for deciding how healthcare dollars should be spent. For example, money is more likely to be spent on research for diseases that affect large numbers of people than for research on diseases that affect relatively few. Some healthcare systems, such as the National Health Service in the United Kingdom, depend on utilitarian ethics as one determinant of who receives treatment. For example, inexpensive procedures that benefit large numbers of people, such as cataract surgeries, are easier to access than expensive ones, such as organ transplantations, that benefit a few. A difficulty inherent in utilitarianism is that in the interests of benefiting the majority, the interests of the individual or minority, who also deserve help, may be overlooked. Another limitation of utilitarianism is that it is impossible to calculate all consequences of an action.

Virtue Ethics

Virtue ethics was first noted in the works of Plato, Aristotle, and early Christians. According to Aristotle, virtues are tendencies to act, feel, and judge that develop through appropriate training but come from natural tendencies. This suggests that individuals' actions are built from a degree of inborn moral virtue (Burkhardt and Nathaniel, 2002).

More recently, bioethics literature has emphasized the character of the decision maker. *Virtues* are specific character traits, including truth telling, honesty, courage, kindness, respectfulness, compassion, fairness, and integrity, among others. These virtues become obvious through one's actions and are expressions of specific ethical principles. Truthfulness, for example, embodies the principle of veracity, which will be discussed in the next section of this chapter. When virtuous people are faced with ethical dilemmas, they will instinctively choose to do the right thing because they have developed character through life experiences (Butts and Rich, 2005).

Descriptions of character in terms of virtues portray an individual's way of being, rather than the process of decision making. One's actions in both personal and professional domains extend from this way of being. This does not guarantee right behavior, but it may predispose an individual to right behavior. Similarly, the development of a profession's code of ethics provides a framework of virtues and qualities of character that shape the behaviors of persons engaged in that profession; however, there is no guarantee that members of the profession will act ethically. In other words, a limitation of virtue ethics is the assumption everyone has moral motives and strives to develop their virtues.

The ability to respond to ethical dilemmas or situations in the healthcare arena is dependent on the nurse's own integrity, honesty, courage, or other personal attributes. Practicing ethically requires a decision to act within the ethical code of the profession, demanding commitment, personal investment, and the intention and motivation to become a good nurse. Nurses' ways of being and acting are essential to the integrity of nursing practice and patient care. Nurses often practice in challenging circumstances in which they must rely on their own integrity to ensure that care is given conscientiously and consistently. Another limitation of virtue ethics is that it requires a case-by-case approach without a defined decision-making process.

Principlism

In 1976 the Belmont Report formalized principlism as a moral decision-making approach to assess the ethics of research with human subjects in response to the horrific history of biomedical research, including the thalidomide case and the Tuskegee syphilis study (Bulger, 2007). Ethical principles, rather than theories, are emphasized in the Belmont Report. Application of ethical principles is a practical approach to ethical decision making that brings together the best elements of each ethical theory while aligning with most societal and religious belief systems.

Principlism uses key ethical principles of beneficence (do good), nonmaleficence (do no harm), autonomy (respect for the person's ability to act in his or her own best interests), and justice in the resolution of ethical conflicts or dilemmas. Fidelity (faithfulness) and veracity (truth telling) are also important ethical principles that may be at work in managing ethical dilemmas. Nurses are often more knowledgeable about ethical principles than theories and are more likely to use a combination of these principles when critically analyzing ethical dilemmas. Although judging ethical dilemmas with ethical principles is useful, principlism does have limitations when applied to healthcare ethical dilemmas. Principlism provides no guidance on which ethical principle is prioritized when two or more ethical principles are in conflict. In other words, principlism does not provide a clear process for arriving at a decision; rather, it allows the principles to guide a decision.

SIX ETHICAL PRINCIPLES BASED ON HUMAN DIGNITY AND RESPECT

Respect for humans as a function of human dignity is the primary ethical responsibility for nurses in practice. The *Code of Ethics for Nurses* states that "the nurse practices with compassion and respect for the inherent dignity, worth, and uniqueness of every individual, unrestricted by consideration of social or economic status, personal attributes, or the nature of health problems" (ANA, 2015). Respect for persons requires that each person be valued as a unique individual equal to all others and that every aspect of a person's life is valued. This can be difficult, because it is sometimes hard to value those parts of human lives that differ from our own. Human dignity and respect for persons are the foundation of the six ethical principles discussed in this section: autonomy, beneficence, nonmaleficence, justice, fidelity, and veracity. Table 7.2 summarizes the moral basis for each principle, the downside of overemphasis of each principle, and the potential challenges with each ethical principle within the healthcare context.

Autonomy

The principle of *autonomy* asserts that individuals have the right to determine their own actions and the freedom to make their own decisions. Respect for the individual is the cornerstone of this principle. Autonomous decisions are based on (1) individuals' values, (2) adequate information, (3) freedom from coercion, and (4) reason and deliberation. Autonomous decisions lead to independent, autonomous actions. Autonomous actions by a patient include deciding to refuse treatment; giving consent for treatment or procedures; and obtaining information regarding results of diagnostic tests, diagnosis, and treatment options.

Autonomy, however, is sometimes overlooked in the healthcare system. Healthcare providers sometimes take actions that affect patients' lives without adequate consultation with the patients themselves. Some healthcare providers, including physicians and nurses, may operate inadvertently in a paternalistic way that assumes the providers are better equipped than patients to make healthcare decisions for patients. Some patients, however, prefer to have decisions made for them, possibly because of a lack of information, fear of making a poor choice, or trusting that a provider will make the right decision for them.

Incorporating the principle of autonomy in all healthcare situations can be difficult. Autonomy poses a problem for healthcare providers when the patient is unable to make decisions because of physical condition, psychological or mental status, or developmental age. Examples of those unable to participate in decisions include infants or small children, persons with serious cognitive or psychological conditions, and unconscious patients. Other patients may be unable to participate in decision making because of external constraints, such as inadequate information, or cultural norms. Nevertheless, the principle of autonomy is an increasingly important principle in health care and nursing. In fact when two or more principles are in conflict, autonomy is likely to take priority.

Beneficence

Beneficence is "the doing of good" and is one of the critical ethical principles in health care. In determining what is "good," nurses should always consider one's actions in the context of the patient's life and situation. Although this sounds simple, healthcare providers are challenged daily when what constitutes "good" for a patient may also cause them harm or is in conflict with what the patient wants. Suppose, for example, that an older hospitalized patient has become confused, especially at night, and is at high risk for falls. She has fallen at home twice. Now that she has confusion at night and is an unfamiliar setting, she is at even more risk for a fall, especially because confusion can become worse at night in older persons. The healthcare team decides that the patient needs a sitter to stay with her in her room all night. The patient objects stridently, because she is very dignified and proud, and values her privacy. She complains that she "doesn't need a babysitter" and cries for a long time. The patient is prevented from falling but experiences emotional distress because, by arranging for a sitter, her healthcare providers have put limitations on her independence, freedom, privacy, and dignity.

Virtually everyone would agree that promoting good and avoiding harm are important to all human beings, and certainly to healthcare providers. It may seem surprising, therefore, how often conflicts occur surrounding the principle of beneficence. A beneficent act may conflict with other ethical principles, most often autonomy. Even though a nurse or physician may understand that a particular treatment has a benefit for the patient, the patient may decide to forgo that treatment (autonomy) for a variety of reasons. In this instance healthcare providers should avoid acting paternalistically, recognizing the autonomy of the patient, even if the providers themselves would choose differently for themselves.

Nonmaleficence

Nonmaleficence is defined as the duty to do no harm. This principle is the foundation of the medical profession's

Hippocratic Oath; it is likewise critical to the nursing profession. Inherent in the *Code of Ethics for Nurses* (ANA, 2015), the nurse must not act in a manner that would intentionally harm the patient. Although this point appears straightforward, the nature of health care dictates that some therapeutic interventions carry risks of harm for the patient, but the treatment will eventually produce good for the patient. Classic examples of this are chemotherapy and bone marrow or stem cell transplantation procedures. Both interventions can make patients sicker for a time, posing a risk for complications such as opportunistic infections, but the possibility of achieving a cure or remission of disease may justify the temporary harm. The concept that justifies risking harm is referred to as the rule of "double effect."

Double effect considers the intended foreseen effects of actions by the professional nurse. The doctrine states that as moral agents we may not intentionally produce harm. It is ethically permissible, however, to do what may produce a distressful or undesirable temporary situation if the intent is to produce an overall good effect (Beauchamp and Childress, 2001).

The rule of double effect justifies that an individual may rightfully perform an act that produces a good and bad effect provided the following four conditions are met at one and the same time (Buckley et al., 2012):

1. The action must be good or at least morally indifferent (neutral).
2. The healthcare provider must intend only the good effect, and the bad effect is unintended.
3. The good effect is not achieved by means of the bad effect.
4. There is a favorable balance between the desirable and undesirable effects (the good outweighs the bad).

Justice

The principle of *justice* is that equals should be treated the same and that unequals should be treated differently. In other words, patients with the same diagnosis and healthcare needs should receive the same care, and those with greater or lesser needs should receive care that is appropriate to their needs.

Basic to the principle of justice are questions of who receives health care and whether health is a right or a privilege. These questions have been central to discussions surrounding healthcare reform in the United States in the past several years. Such questions involve the allocation of resources: how much of our national resources should be appropriated to health care; what healthcare problems should receive the most financial resources; what persons should have access to healthcare services?

Numerous models have been developed for distributing healthcare resources. These models include the following (Jameton, 1984):

- To each equally
- To each according to merit (this may include past or future contributions to society)
- To each according to what can be acquired in the marketplace
- To each according to need

You may disagree with each or all of these models of resource distribution; certainly, no single one is adequate in ensuring a just model for the distribution of healthcare resources. In an ideal world, all people would receive all available treatment and resources for their health needs, including those targeting disease prevention and health promotion. Unfortunately, this is not possible because of costs and limited resources. When people with wealth have advantageous access to the best quality health care available, which may include lifesaving medical devices or innovations, how does one apply the concept of justice? Conversely, how does the issue of justice apply when access to care known to be cost effective and simple, such as prenatal care, is difficult or impossible for women who must be at work during clinic hours?

Health disparities among ethnic minorities with regard to types of treatments and services that are available represent a difficult problem in terms of an ethic of justice. Research has demonstrated that allocation of resources in the healthcare system is not equitable across all race/ethic groups and that "racial disparity exists in health care access, treatment options and outcomes" (Harrison and Falco, 2005, p. 252). Thinking Critically Box 7.3 describes lessons learned by nursing students who participate in international learning experiences and how to continue one's growth of social consciousness and sense of justice.

Furthermore, how does one decide what is just when a natural disaster strikes, crippling healthcare facilities, and providers are left with critically ill patients in dire circumstances? The situation of Memorial Medical Center (now Oschner Baptist Medical Center) in New Orleans, Louisiana, in the aftermath of the devastating Hurricane Katrina in 2005 brought these questions of justice and ethical decision making in a disaster to the

THINKING CRITICALLY BOX 7.3

To Keep the Vision of Social Justice

Nursing students often have a great deal of interest in and energy for international learning experiences. These experiences expose students to the huge gap in healthcare practices and availability between developed and undeveloped nations. In an article by Kirkham and colleagues (2009), they describe the challenge of "keeping the vision" for nursing students and their faculty as they return home—sustaining the social consciousness that is raised during these international experiences.

Kirkham and colleagues (2009) defined social consciousness in terms of "personal awareness of social injustice," borrowed from Giddings (2005, p. 224). Specifically, they described social injustice as unfairness in the burdens and rewards of a society in which there is inequitable access to healthcare services. Social injustice is the foundation of health disparities, a serious ethical issue that challenges the human right to health and health care.

In their study of student learning that took place in international settings and the long-term benefits and effects of these experiences, Kirkham and colleagues sought to describe students' experiences but also to find ways to integrate and maintain the students' learning once they returned home (in this case, Canada).

Students had many experiences that opened their eyes to the healthcare practices and accessibility of care in Guatemala). Students related the realization that "statistics … became faces of people I know" (p. 6) and that "people are the same everywhere" (p. 6). They also recognized the significant prosperity and power gradients that exist between North and Central America. From these realizations, the students began to have a deep sense of social injustice and the consequences of short-term international efforts that are not sustained. These insights challenged the students' worldview.

Despite the immense learning and intense reflection that resulted from these experiences, "keeping the vision" became hard as students returned home. Kirkham and colleagues (p. 9) suggested four strategies that may help students in translating their learning and sustaining their new vision for social justice. Individually, students can write journals of their reflections and insights, read journals, and maintain contact with their host families. In formal groups, students can mentor new students who will go through the same experiences, participate in forums and focus groups, and become involved in other humanitarian projects. In informal groups, students can reflect on and share their experiences with other students and faculty who participated in the international experience. And last, nursing school curricula can be shaped to integrate themes of social justice.

Data from Kirkham SR, Van Hofwegen L, Pankratz D: Keeping the vision: sustaining social consciousness with nursing students following international learning experiences, *Int J Nurs Educ Scholarsh (online)* *6*(1):article 3, 2009.

general public in a way that was unprecedented in modern American history. Desperate healthcare providers were in a dire situation with no electricity, rising water, unbearable heat, and no reasonable hope of rescue for their many patients, many of whom were critically ill even before the hurricane struck. An investigation later found that nurses and physicians had administered lethal doses of morphine and midazolam to more than 20 patients whom the providers determined were unlikely to survive the disaster. A physician and two nurses were eventually charged with second-degree murder. The charges were dropped against the nurses, and a grand jury did not indict the physician. Other questions were raised related to whom nurses had primary ethical responsibilities during the storm: their patients or their own families?

In 2015, the ANA sponsored an ethics symposium that featured an interactive address with Sheri Fink, MD, PhD, who won the Pulitzer Prize for her book *Five Days at Memorial*, an investigation of the patients' deaths after Katrina. Dr. Fink noted that thinking about situations in disasters in advance is a way to prepare for distressing ethical situations that arise under conditions that are barely imaginable under normal circumstances (ANA, 2015).

Justice as a principle often leaves us with more questions than answers. Thinking through questions of justice can be helpful in recognizing unjust situations and in shaping just resolutions, but applying the principle of justice does not determine what the answer should be. A single ethical principle cannot typically be used to resolve complex ethical dilemmas such as those encountered in healthcare settings.

Fidelity

The principle of *fidelity* refers to faithfulness or honoring one's commitments or promises. For nurses, this specifically refers to fidelity to patients. Through the process of licensure, nurses are granted the privilege to practice. The licensure process is intended to ensure that only a qualified nurse, appropriately trained and educated, and passing a standardized national examination, can practice nursing. When nurses are licensed and become a part of the profession, they accept certain responsibilities as part of the contract with society. Nurses must be faithful in keeping their promises of respecting all individuals, upholding the *Code of Ethics for Nurses* (ANA, 2015), practicing within the scope of nursing practice, keeping nursing skills current, abiding by an employer's policies, and keeping promises to patients. Fidelity entails meeting reasonable expectations in all these areas. Fidelity is a key foundation for the nurse-patient relationship. When nurses receive patient assignments and accept hand-off reports, they are committed to and required to provide care to those patients assigned to them. Failure to carry out the prescribed care is unethical (provided that the prescribed care is safe and consistent with good practice) and may constitute patient abandonment or neglect. This is a serious charge that would likely require a state board of nursing review of the specific details of the case to determine whether the nurse failed to carry out this responsibility ethically.

Fidelity suggests that one is faithful to the promises, agreements, and commitments made. This faithfulness creates the trust that is essential to any relationship. Most ethicists believe there is no absolute duty to keep promises, however. In every situation the harmful consequences of the promised action must be weighed against the benefits of promise keeping (Burkhardt and Nathaniel, 2002). This is an ethical posture that may explain decisions by some nurses during Hurricane Katrina, described earlier, to stay at home with their families rather than going to the hospitals for their shifts.

Veracity

Veracity is defined as telling the truth, or not lying. Truth-telling is fundamental to the development and continuance of trust among persons and is an expected behavior. Truthfulness is necessary to basic communication, and societal relationships are built on an individual's right to know the truth, or not to be deceived. Inherent in nurse-patient relationships is the understanding that nurses will be honest with their patients. However, in some (rare) instances nurses are constrained in some healthcare systems that place limits on what a nurse can tell a patient. These situations, however, can pose an ethical dilemma for nurses who believe that it is unethical to withhold information from patients, especially when patients ask for information about their condition or diagnosis. A nurse can still remain truthful by telling the patient, "Dr. Roberts always prefers to discuss her findings with her patients directly. I will call her and ask when you can expect her to make rounds tonight to talk to you." Intentional deception, however, is considered morally wrong. (Consider the situation again of Michelle, the nurse who was asked by Mrs. Thomas, her patient's wife, whether she had called a social worker yet: caught in a lie, what was the best thing Michelle could do?)

Some healthcare providers attempt to justify deceiving their patients. For the most part, these justifications are related to the idea that patients would be better off not knowing certain information or that they are not capable of understanding the information. This reflects a posture toward patients known as "paternalism," in which someone believes that they know what is best for another person who is competent to make their own autonomous judgments about a course of action. Some justify not being truthful with a patient if they perceive that the patient might refuse medical treatment if they knew the "complete" truth. However, if both patient and healthcare provider are respectful of each other as individuals, it is difficult to accept that deception is ever justified. Two exceptions exist, however. If a patient asks not to be told the truth, the nurse can, under the ethical principles of beneficence and nonmaleficence, withhold the truth. This does not mean that the nurse must lie but that the nurse is released from the obligation to report to the patient what they may know. Furthermore, if a patient is mentally incompetent, autonomy and the capacity for self-determination are diminished, thereby justifying the withholding of healthcare information.

Cultural humility is a posture that requires clinicians to make every effort to understand their patients' beliefs and how their patients want themselves and their illness to be treated. Hines (2008) observed that true cultural humility is tied to respecting patient preferences for information and treatment. Although Hines was writing about care in an oncology setting, her observation that "goals of care can be established, refined, or refocused at any point in the trajectory of care, whether truth-telling or not telling is occurring" (p. 415) holds true for any practice setting for nurses.

CODES OF ETHICS FOR NURSING

A code of ethics is a hallmark of mature professions and a social contract through which the profession informs society of the principles and rules by which it functions. Ethical codes shape professional self-regulation, serving as guidelines to the members of the profession, who then meet their responsibility as trustworthy, qualified, and accountable caregivers. Codes of ethics, however, are useful only to the extent that they are known and upheld by the members of the profession in practice.

American Nurses Association's Code of Ethics for Nurses

Ethical practice has been a priority for nurses in America since the late 19th century. In 1893 the Nightingale Pledge (Box 7.2) became the first public evidence of an ethical code in nursing. In 1896 the Nurses' Associated Alumnae of the United States and Canada, which later became the ANA, was organized with the purpose to establish and maintain a code of ethics. A suggested code was developed in 1926 and published in the *American Journal of Nursing (AJN)* but was never formally adopted. Similarly, a "tentative" code was published in the *AJN* in 1940, but this version also was never formally adopted. Finally, in 1950, with the addition of 17 provisions, the 1940 version was formally adopted as the Code of Ethics for Nurses. Between 1950 and 1985, the Code was revised and refined six times; the ANA's House of Delegates adopted a complete revision of the Code in 2001.

BOX 7.2 The Florence Nightingale Pledge

The Florence Nightingale Pledge was written in 1893 by Lystra Gretter at the Farrand Training School in Detroit, Michigan. It was modeled after the Hippocratic Oath taken by physicians as they begin their medical careers. The pledge is dated in its wording and gender references; however, key ethical principles discussed in this chapter and elsewhere in this text are present in this early statement intended to hold nurses to a high standard of professional ethical behavior. These principles are noted parenthetically in ***bold italics***.

I solemnly pledge myself before God and presence of this assembly; to pass my life in purity and to practice my profession faithfully ***(fidelity)***.

I will abstain from whatever is deleterious and mischievous and will not take or knowingly administer any harmful drug ***(nonmaleficence)***.

I will do all in my power to maintain and elevate the standard of my profession ***(beneficence)*** and will hold in confidence all personal matters committed to my keeping and family affairs coming to my knowledge in the practice of my calling ***(confidentiality)***.

With loyalty will I endeavor to aid the physician in his work ***(fidelity)***, and devote myself to the welfare of those committed to my care ***(justice)***.

The *Code of Ethics for Nurses with Interpretive Statements* is the nursing profession's expression of its ethical values and duties to the public (ANA, 2015). The Code has undergone no fewer than eight revisions, each clarifying meanings, defining terms, and making the Code more relevant to nursing practice at the time. Codes through the years have also reflected trends in social awareness issues, such as women's and patients' rights. The consequences of breaking the Code have become more specific with later versions.

In 2015 the ANA published the latest version of the *Code of Ethics for Nurses with Interpretive Statements*. A view-only version is available at https://www.nursingworld.org/coe-view-only. The ANA is responsible for the periodic review of the code to ensure that it reflects the contemporary issues of this dynamic profession and is consistent with the ethical standards of the society in which we live.

The ANA's *Nursing: Scope and Standards of Practice* (4th edition) is another very important document for professional nurses. It defines standards of practice and standards of professional performance. The standards describe the minimal expectations and duties a registered nurse should perform competently regardless of role or population served. The current version of the *Nursing: Scope and Standards of Practice* was published in 2021. Standard 7: Ethics emphasizes that an ethical practice spans across all roles and settings and is integral to nursing professionalism (ANA, 2021). Standard 7 also incorporates the ANA *Code of Ethics for Nurses* recognizing its moral foundation for nursing practice. Chapter 6 contains more detailed information on the Scope and Standards of Practice.

International Council of Nurses Code of Ethics for Nurses

The International Council of Nurses (ICN) also has published a code of ethics for the profession (ICN, 2012). This document discusses the rights and responsibilities

BOX 7.3 International Council of Nurses Code of Ethics for Nurses: Preamble

Nurses have four fundamental responsibilities: to promote health, to prevent illness, to restore health, and to alleviate suffering. The need for nursing is universal.

Inherent in nursing is respect for human rights, including cultural rights, the right to life and choice, to dignity, and to be treated with respect. Nursing care is respectful of and unrestricted by considerations of age, color, creed, culture, disability or illness, gender, sexual orientation, nationality, politics, race, or social status.

Nurses render health services to the individual, the family, and the community and coordinate their services with those of related groups.

of nurses related to people, practice, society, co-workers, and the profession. The ICN first adopted a code of ethics in 1953. Its last revision, adopted in 2012, represents an agreement by more than 80 national nursing associations that participate in the international association. The preamble of *The ICN Code of Ethics for Nurses* (Box 7.3) is unchanged from the previous version and details the four fundamental responsibilities for nurses and describes the ethical foundations of nursing practice. In 2020 the ICN initiated a consultation to update the code of ethics, but at the time of this writing the update was not yet available.

NAVIGATING THE GRAY AREAS: ETHICAL DECISION MAKING

The "gray area" in nursing practice entails addressing ethical dilemmas. An ethical dilemma is a moral conflict in which the decision maker experiences indecision because the available choices or alternatives result in conflicting values or ethical principles. When facing an ethical dilemma, there is no one good decision; however, two or more decisions may be deemed as right (also known as a right versus right dilemma). Table 7.3 illustrates the complexity of an ethical dilemma and the clarity of a "black and white" decision when an issue is not a dilemma.

Nurses encounter situations daily that require them to make and act on professional judgments. The judgments (decisions) are usually made in collaboration with other persons involved in the situation: patients, families, and/or other healthcare professionals. Ethical decision-making requires that the nurse make judgments or decisions when the values between two or more of the other persons are incongruent with the nurse's values. When an ethical decision is made, respect and valuing of the perspectives

TABLE 7.3 The Gray Area of an Ethical Dilemma

No Ethical Dilemma = Wrong Versus Right	Ethical Dilemma = Gray Area With Right Versus Right	No Ethical Dilemma = Right Versus Wrong
	• Includes a conflict of two or more ethical principles and possible conflict of values/ beliefs. • Two or more equally unfavorable choices to resolve the dilemma.	
It is clear after morally and ethically analyzing the situation there is clearly one or more wrong choices that should not be pursued and one right choice.	Ethical decision making requires a contextual factor analysis: • Ethical principles at stake/in conflict • Beliefs and values of the stakeholders • Legal mandates, organizational policy • Professional Codes of Ethics Note: most professional codes of ethics allow for conscientious objection to participate in care against individual values/beliefs as long as the patient has competent professionals to care for him or her.	It is clear after morally and ethically analyzing the situation there is only one or more clear "right" action(s) to take, and the other action(s) are wrong and should not be pursued.

TABLE 7.4 Comparison of the Nursing Process, Ethical Decision-Making Model, and CODE Moral Courage Model

Nursing Process	Ethical Decision-Making Model	CODE Moral Courage Model (Lachman, 2010)
Assess	Clarify the dilemma, gather additional data	Courage: Critically evaluate does action need to be taken to address the situation?
Analyze/ diagnose	Identify options	Obligation to honor: Analyze/reflect—what is the right thing to do? Consider what is at risk with the ANA Code of Ethics for Nurses, stakeholder beliefs and values, and ethical principles.
Plan	Make a decision	Danger management: What do I need to do to handle my fear?
Evaluate	Evaluate	(Should reflect on situation and outcome.)

held by others, even when all do not agree on the resolution, is important professional behavior. Through respectful collaboration, the best decision can be reached in even the most difficult dilemma. Note that the "best decision" will be made in response to an ethical dilemma.

Ethical Decision-Making Model

Whether involved in a collective or individual decision, nurses need to be knowledgeable about suggested steps in ethical decision making. Table 7.4 demonstrates the similarity in the processes required in ethical decision making and the nursing process, both of which are based on sound critical thinking. A variety of ethical decision-making models are available in published literature across many disciplines and share more similarities than differences. The steps are not always necessarily sequential, nor are they intended to be rigid processes. Instead, ethical decision making is a process that guides exploration of the dilemma and examination of options to determine the best solution to a difficult situation.

The following steps can be used in ethical decision making:

1. What is the specific issue in question? Who should actually make the decision? Who is affected by the dilemma? Determine the ethical principle or theory related to the dilemma. Are there value conflicts? What is the timeframe for the decision?
2. After the ethical dilemma is clarified, in most instances more information needs to be collected. Clarity is enhanced when you have as many facts as possible about the situation. Make sure you are up-to-date on any legal cases or precedents related to the situation, because ethical and legal issues often overlap.
3. Most ethical dilemmas have several solutions, some of which are more feasible than others. Identifying more options increases the likelihood an acceptable solution will be identified. Brainstorm with others, and consider every possible alternative.
4. To make a decision, think through the identified options, and determine the impact of each option. Ethical principles and theories, as well as universal basic human values, may help determine the significance of each option. When a nurse is confronted with an ethical dilemma, they should when possible make an active decision, as opposed to refusing to make a decision (being passive). Passivity is a form of decision-making; it is a decision not to act, which may be professionally irresponsible.
5. Once a course of action has been determined, the decision must be implemented, which usually involves working collaboratively with others.
6. Unexpected outcomes are common in crisis situations that result in ethical dilemmas. Decision makers should consider the effect an immediate decision may have on future ones. Reflecting on a decision and action can help determine whether a different course of action might have resulted in a better outcome. If the action accomplished its purpose, the ethical dilemma should be resolved. If the dilemma has not been resolved, engage in additional deliberation, and reexamine alternative options. Consider the six suggested ethical decision-making steps in the context of Case Study 7.1 of Daniel, who is terminally ill and who wants you—his nurse—to help him end his life.

(1). *Clarify the ethical dilemma.* The specific issue is the patient's right to autonomy versus the nurse's professional ethics and personal morals.

(2). *Gather additional data.* Is Daniel responding to something that happened before you even got to

CASE STUDY 7.1

Your Hospice Patient Wants to Die ... and He Wants You to Help Him

Daniel is a 55-year-old gay man with advanced lung cancer and is positive for human immunodeficiency virus (HIV). He has a longtime partner, Juan, with whom he has lived for more than 20 years. Daniel is miserable, with profuse secretions from his lungs; every breath is a struggle. Despite his weakened physical condition, he is still very alert. He is getting oxygen via nasal cannula. He is very image-conscious, and part of each of your visits is spent helping him groom himself and put on fresh designer pajamas. His mother is staying with him and Juan, and she has never been told that Daniel is gay or that he has HIV. He confides to you that trying to maintain the secret that he has kept from his mother is exhausting and is becoming burdensome. In the middle of your visit, he asks for a mirror to see what he looks like. You hand him a small mirror, and he is shocked at what he sees—a gray, shrunken, emaciated image looking back at him. He sets the mirror down carefully on the bedside table, looks at you evenly, and with great seriousness says, "I am ready to die, and I want you to help me."

As a new nurse, you are not ready for this. You know that in his bedside drawer there is enough oral morphine to stop his breathing. You know that his death is still probably days away, and you are very sad for him in his misery. When you say, "I can't do that, Daniel," he starts crying and says, "I trusted you to help me...."

What should you do in response to this situation? What does the ANA say about assisted suicide and euthanasia? What is your personal moral code in this situation?

his home today, such as an argument or a confrontation? Is he becoming depressed?

(3). *Identify options.* Options may include the following:
 (a). Simply tell Daniel you will not help him die.
 (b). Respond to his dire request with compassion, and try to determine what is behind his sudden sense that he wants to die.
 (c). Determine whether there is better symptom management that you can implement to make him more comfortable.
 (d). With Daniel and his partner's support, enlist the assistance of other hospice agency that might have services such as pastoral care to help him ease his spiritual distress. (*Note:* There are many choices available here. These are just some suggestions.)

(4). *Make a decision.* Make sure that everyone, especially Daniel, agrees with the plan.

(5). *Act.* This may include a number of interventions, both physical and psychoemotional.

(6). *Evaluate.* Does Daniel continue to express his desire to die now? Is he more comfortable? Is his distress less troublesome? Is he at some level of peace with his partner, his mother, and his life? Did your actions enhance the nurse-patient relationship with mutual trust and caring?

EXPLORING ETHICAL DILEMMAS IN NURSING

Many ethical dilemmas arise in nursing because of conflicts among patients, their families, healthcare professionals, and institutions. The following section will explore the major issues involved in these conflicts: (1) personal value systems, (2) peers' and other professionals' behaviors, (3) patients' rights, (4) institutional and societal issues, and (5) patient data access issues.

Dilemmas Resulting From Personal Value Systems

Values are important preferences that influence the behavior of individuals. Values are learned beliefs that help people choose among difficult alternatives, even when there may not be a good choice.

Each person has a set of values that was shaped in part by the beliefs, purposes, attitudes, and qualities of a child's early caregivers. In time, individuals develop their own value systems that are grounded in their culture and life experiences. Variations in value systems become highly significant when dealing with critical issues such as health and illness or life and death. Value systems enable people to resolve conflicts and decide on a course of action based on a priority of importance.

Professions have a "built-in" value system known as a code of ethics, discussed earlier in this chapter. A very difficult issue for nursing students to come to terms with on occasion is when their personal values conflict with their professional values, or, more specifically, when they are faced with a professional situation that has some elements that are not in keeping with the nurse's personal moral code or values. The overriding principle

BOX 7.4 Childhood Value Messages

By the time we are about 10 years old, most of our values have already been "programmed." Values are taught to us by family members and friends, through the media, in churches and schools, and by watching other people. What are the value messages you learned as a child?

Recall as many values as you can remember hearing as a child, and write them in the blanks provided below. Here are a few examples to get you thinking:

"Be nice."

"You can do anything you want to if you try hard enough."

"Clean your plate; there are starving children in ______!"

"Making money is the number one goal in life."

"You always have to tell the truth, no matter what."

"Crying is a sign of weakness. You have to be strong."

Now it is your turn to write some of your childhood values. How many of these values still influence the way you think and act today? Which ones influence you professionally? If you want to further explore your values, you may do the following:

1. Next to each value on your list, write the person's name who taught or modeled that value.
2. Put a star next to those messages that are still your values today.
3. Put a check mark next to those messages that you need to alter.
4. How are some of these values still influencing you today? Is this a positive or negative influence?

Reprinted with permission of Uustal DB: *Clinical ethics and values: issues and insights in a changing healthcare environment,* East Greenwich, RI, 1993, Educational Resources in Healthcare.

in this situation is that *professional ethics outweigh personal ethics in a professional setting*. It is incumbent on the nurse to find a work situation in which their personal ethics are not routinely challenged by situations that occur with patients.

Nurses must have a good sense of their own values and be able to identify clearly what they believe to be good or right. We each develop our own value systems based on a variety of messages that we received in our formative years from our parents, siblings, relatives, friends, teachers, and religious training. The "childhood value messages" exercise (Box 7.4) can help you identify values learned as a child that may still influence you today.

To understand how personal and professional values can conflict in nursing practice, consider the following situation: Marta had been a nurse on a postpartum unit for a number of years. Over time, an increasing number of pregnant women (antepartum) with serious pregnancy-related problems were admitted to the unit where Marta worked. Although Marta preferred to work with new mothers and their infants, she occasionally took care of antepartum patients. One day in report, she learned that a newly admitted patient, Mrs. Anderson, was 11 weeks pregnant with triplets. Mrs. Anderson had a history of serious heart disease, but her condition was thought to be stable. Marta agreed to take care of her, having very little information about her.

Shortly after receiving her hand-off report, Marta went into Mrs. Anderson's room to do her usual assessment, only to find Mrs. Anderson crying, being comforted by her husband, who was also crying. Mrs. Anderson related to Marta that the maternal-fetal medicine specialist and her cardiologist had recommended that they do what is known as a selective reduction (also known as multifetal pregnancy reduction [MFPR]), a form of pregnancy termination in which a multiple pregnancy (meaning more than one embryo or fetus) is reduced to one or two remaining embryos. Even though still in the first trimester of pregnancy, Mrs. Anderson was already having signs of cardiac decompensation, evidenced by her increasing difficulty breathing, necessitating her sitting straight up all the time. Already it was clear that Mrs. Anderson was not going to be able to tolerate the demands on her heart of a multiple pregnancy. Remaining pregnant at all would put her health at great risk. She and her husband, although sad, understood that the selective reduction was their only chance of having a child at all and that without it her own life was in serious danger.

Marta was very upset with this news. As a practicing Catholic, she had a very strong moral stance against abortion, and as a nurse, she had worked specifically with mothers and their new infants to avoid issues related to pregnancy termination. The procedure was going to be performed in Mrs. Anderson's room under ultrasound guidance within the next few minutes. Marta faced a serious moral dilemma in determining what to do. She sought the advice and counsel of a colleague whose wisdom she admired and trusted. In a few moments, Marta decided that her responsibility was to her patient and that, although she was present during the termination, she was not participating in performing it in any way. She understood her patient's deep distress and sadness.

Before reentering the room, Marta took a moment to calm herself to be in a better state of mind to provide care for her patient. After taking a deep breath, she went into Mrs. Anderson's room and encouraged Mr. Anderson to sit near his wife where they could see each other; then she took Mrs. Anderson's hand, saying "I will be with you through this." Mrs. Anderson whispered, "Thank you."

Marta had set aside her personal values to take excellent care of her patient as a trained and caring professional nurse.

Dilemmas Involving Peers' and Other Professionals' Behavior

All practicing nurses participate as members of the healthcare team, which involves cooperation and collaboration with other providers. As is true in all situations involving human beings, conflicts can easily develop, particularly in stressful circumstances. These conflicts may be between two nurses, nurse and physician, nurse and agency policies, or nurse and other healthcare professional (Professional Profile Box 7.2).

As noted earlier, conflicts can evolve because of differing value systems, cultures, education levels, or a variety of other factors. Like Marta in the previous example, a nurse may believe that abortions are wrong under any circumstances, whereas the institution in which they are employed routinely performs them. This creates a conflict between the nurse's value system and the institution's practices, which can be the source of distress. Conflicts relevant to human rights often center around one of the ethical principles discussed earlier: autonomy, beneficence, nonmaleficence, veracity, or justice.

Sociocultural Influences Posing Ethical Challenges: Social Media and Substance Abuse

Nurses face two serious ethical challenges in today's sociocultural context: (1) the use of social media and (2) substance misuse. Substance misuse by healthcare providers is not new but still poses a tremendous dilemma for nurses who may suspect that a colleague is impaired at work or has developed a substance abuse problem. More recently, social media has changed the landscape of communication; ethical problems have arisen in nursing related to the use of social media.

The widespread use of social media, such as TikTok, Twitter, and blogs, has created two distinct problems: (1) the transmission of potentially identifiable patient information and (2) the blurring of professional and personal boundaries. Moreover, nurses who are posting on social media may fail to realize that, depending on their privacy settings, their content is widely available to professional and personal contacts, including their employers and colleagues. In response to the ethical challenges posed by social networking, the ANA and the National Council of State Boards of Nursing (NCSBN) have both issued guidelines for maintaining professional boundaries within social networking.

The ANA has developed a page on its website explaining best practices regarding social media (https://www.nursingworld.org/social/). The NCSBN website has an informative video Social Media Guidelines for Nurses (https://www.ncsbn.org/347.htm) detailing the challenges related to ethical use of social media. The ANA and NCSBN mutually endorsed their positions regarding nurses' professional use of social media. It is important to realize that the principles foundational to the protection of patients regarding social media do not change, even as digital media continue to grow and thrive. In other words, what is not appropriate for posting on TikTok is also not appropriate for Instagram or any other forms of digital communication yet to be developed. Box 7.5 contains five basic principles related to the ethical use of social media.

Consider the following situation, and think about the ethical considerations related to the use of social media. You and your colleague who works on the same nursing unit enjoy sports and share a passion for the local university's football program. You are both members of a sports website that features a message board, and you know each other's screen names under which you post anonymous comments. One of the team's star athletes sustained a serious neck injury during a game and was admitted to the trauma center where you work, although not on your unit. The following day, you see a comment posted by your colleague under his screen name that details the injured player's condition. You realize that your colleague has obtained information about the player from the hospital's electronic health record (EHR) system and has posted it on the website.

What is your responsibility in this situation? What do you do next?

The second sociocultural problem is the number of nurses and other healthcare professionals impaired by

PROFESSIONAL PROFILE BOX 7.2

Distress in an Expert Labor and Delivery Nurse

This is a true account of a moral dilemma and moral distress in a labor and delivery nurse, Mary Tilghman, RN, who had been in practice for 6 years at the time of this event. She asked to use a pseudonym in recounting this story, because she does not want anyone to identify her situation or the location where this event happened. But the story itself is true and illustrates the very difficult ethical situations that nurses find themselves in and the lingering distress that these situations can cause. Here is her story:

I was working on a slow evening in a labor and delivery unit. We got a call from our dispatcher that emergency medical services (EMS) was bringing in a patient who was 25 weeks pregnant and having some vaginal bleeding. This is not really unusual, but it can be serious. I notified the resident physician and another nurse, and I set about getting a labor room ready. In about 10 minutes, EMS arrived with a young woman who was extremely pale and sobbing loudly. Her young husband was with her.

When we moved her to the labor bed, it was obvious that "some bleeding" was an understatement. She was bleeding from everywhere—even her gums, nose, and a small crack in her lip were bleeding. I listened for fetal heart tones, and when I could not hear them, I asked her when the last time was that she had felt the baby move. I suspected that she had DIC—disseminated intravascular coagulation—a rare but severe problem that can occur when a fetus has died but labor does not begin. She said it had been "2, maybe 3 weeks." Her husband was shocked, because she had not told him that she had not been feeling the baby move. I called for the doctor right away, and then I paged the anesthesiologist to come to labor and delivery STAT. This was a severe emergency. I started a large-gauge intravenous (IV) line so that we could give her blood and fluids, and sent some blood samples for laboratory testing, including a type and crossmatch.

The physician confirmed the fetal death by doing a quick ultrasound examination, and then he explained to the woman that this was an emergency and had her sign a consent form. We hurried the patient to the operating room (OR) on our unit for an emergency dilation and evacuation (D&E). At the time, I had seen a lot as an obstetric nurse in a high-risk unit, but I was horrified at her huge and rapid blood loss. The anesthesiologist ordered as many units of O-negative blood (universal donor) as we could get until donor blood could be matched to hers in the blood bank. Weakly, but as firmly as she could, the woman declared, "No blood. No blood. I am a Jehovah's Witness. Please no blood. If I die, I will be all right. No blood. Please." Everyone in the OR heard her. The anesthesiologist patted her shoulder and told her that she would "be okay."

Everybody there could tell that the woman was bleeding to death. The anesthesiologist prepared to give her medications to increase her blood pressure and perfusion. By then the senior resident physician and the attending physician were working quickly to perform the D&E. The junior obstetric resident was very concerned by the situation. He left the room in a hurry and found the woman's husband, who was pacing outside in the hallway. The resident asked him, "Were you planning to be with your wife when she gave birth to your baby?" The husband said yes. The resident then told him, "Your wife is going to die. I think that you might want to be with her as she dies."

He gave the husband some scrubs to put on over his clothes and started toward the OR. By then, the woman's blood had begun to run out from under the OR door and into the hallway. When the husband saw it, he threw up his hands, saying, "Just give her the blood. Give her the blood...." The resident patted him on the back and told him it was a good decision. The husband left the OR, and the anesthesiologist began infusing unit after unit of blood and blood products into the woman. I reminded them of her plea not to give her blood, but the physicians agreed that her husband's verbal consent was enough for them. The junior resident said, "I just don't think they [Jehovah's Witnesses] understand what it means to bleed to death. I thought he'd change his mind if I showed him."

The patient went to intensive care for many days but recovered. I never saw her again. But I was very distressed over what I interpreted coercion on the part of the resident physician, showing the husband his wife's blood, and overriding the woman's clear and unmistakable pleas for no blood products. Also, the resident had made assumptions and judgments about what Jehovah's Witnesses "really" understood. The woman was willing to die rather than break her deep religious conviction. No matter what I believed about her religious views, my role was to advocate on her behalf—to be her voice. This situation is still distressful to me many years after it happened. I was so relieved that she lived, but I also felt like I was part of something that she had made clear she didn't want. Sometimes ethical dilemmas in nursing are unforgettable. For me, this is the one that stands out most clearly, the one that still haunts me. I hope she made peace with what happened to her, or maybe she never even knew. I hope she has had a good life.

BOX 7.5 Ethical Use of Social Media

The use of social media has created professional and personal opportunities, yet it can pose significant ethical challenges. Keep these principles in mind when you engage in blogging, including microblogs, or communicating via social networking sites.

1. You must not post or otherwise transmit digitally anything about your patients that may violate their rights to privacy and confidentiality. Their privacy is not ensured by your use of privacy settings. This is both an ethical and a legal obligation.
2. Never post images of patients. Even though it is tempting to take a photo of a favorite patient, a cute baby, or some curiosity you encounter in the clinical setting, you must not. And even if you pixelate (blur) some identifying features on the photo, its metadata is still available. Metadata provides digital information as to who made the photo and exactly where and when it was made, in addition to other technical info.
3. Online contact with patients blurs professional and personal boundaries. Although it is difficult to turn down a patient's (or former patient's) request that you follow or "friend" them on social media, you are obligated to enforce the professional boundary that separates you.
4. You are ethically obligated to report any breach in confidentiality or privacy that you encounter online.
5. Remember that posting anything leaves a permanent digital footprint. Even deleting a post, tweet or photo leaves evidence behind, sometimes in the form of a screenshot that is no longer in your control. If you have the slightest question as to the appropriateness of a blog entry or update, err on the side of extreme caution.

From National Council of State Boards of Nursing (NCSBN): White paper: a nurse's guide to the use of social media, 2012. Retrieved from www.nursingworld.org/FunctionalMenuCategories/AboutANA/Social-Media/Social-Networking-Principles-Toolkit.aspx.

drug dependence, alcohol abuse, or other addictions. Deciding how and when to confront a colleague who is impaired may constitute an ethical dilemma. When a colleague appears to be under the influence of some type of substance (e.g., exhibiting slurred speech, unsteady gait, combativeness, the smell of alcohol on their breath), the decision to report is usually easy, even if personally painful. Be aware, however, that certain acute medical conditions may be responsible for changes in behavior or gait; your colleague may be experiencing a medical emergency. It is crucial that you engage the assistance of a nurse manager or supervisor before confronting your colleague if you suspect your colleague is impaired in some way.

When a colleague is showing a pattern of behavior that may indicate a substance abuse problem (e.g., frequent tardiness, excuse making, excessive absences, leaving the work setting frequently, increasingly poor clinical judgment), the dilemma can be overwhelming. Nurses agonize over whether to report suspected instances of unethical conduct or incompetent care, including an impairment caused by alcohol or drugs. Fortunately, some employers and state boards of nursing have developed plans to assist impaired nurses in getting the help they need and make provisions for them to return to the profession once they are far enough along in their recovery. The board of nursing in each state, as well as each state nurses association, can provide information on specific programs for impaired nurses in the state. However, the process must begin with a colleague who follows the ANA ethical standard that obligates professional nurses to report colleagues who "pose a threat or danger to patients, self or others" (ANA, 2015, p. 13).

To understand how the suspicion of substance abuse can be triggered, consider the following situation: Gloria is an RN who works on a surgical floor. She has just assisted in the transfer of Mr. Hudson to his room from the postanesthesia care unit (PACU) after surgery and heard the PACU nurse report that Mr. Hudson had received morphine 6 mg intravenously before transfer, and he is resting comfortably. Gloria sees another nurse drawing up morphine, a narcotic, in a syringe and then leaving the medications room. Ten minutes later, she returns with an empty syringe. Gloria asks, "Who needed pain medication?" The other nurse replies, "Mr. Hudson. He was in pain after surgery." Confused, Gloria checks Mr. Hudson's room and learns from his wife that he has neither asked for nor received pain medication since arriving on the surgical floor.

What should Gloria do now? What are her options, and how should she best manage this situation?

Dilemmas Regarding Patients' Rights

As health care has changed over the years, so too has the nature of relationships between providers and patients. Years ago, healthcare providers, particularly physicians, were considered to have the final word on care decisions and treatment options. Now consumers of health care are increasingly demanding to have a voice in their healthcare decisions. A number of special interest groups have developed and published lists of patient rights. In 1971 the United Nations passed a resolution declaring the rights of persons who have intellectual impairment, an early model that recognized the interests of a particular group of persons with disabilities. In 1990 the Congress of the United States passed the Americans with Disabilities Act, which was amended in 2008. This extensive act has provided a significant improvement in the lives of persons with a variety of psychological/mental health and physical challenges, recognizing their rights to participate fully in all aspects of society.

Other less formal interest groups have written guidelines such as the Dying Person's Bill of Rights, Pregnant Patient's Bill of Rights, and Rights of Senior Citizens. The healthcare system has responded to consumers' awareness of their rights. Many of the rights demanded by patients as consumers of health care are legal rights that have been upheld by the judicial system. The American Hospital Association (AHA) has an extensive website that addresses the wide range of rights of patients in the hospital setting. Replacing the former Patient Bill of Rights, the document "The Patient Care Partnership," published in 2003, is still in use and can be downloaded from https://www.aha.org/system/files/2018-01/aha-patient-care-partnership.pdf. The document describes what patients can and should expect while hospitalized, including a safe, clean environment; quality care; involvement in one's own care that includes a discussion regarding the treatment plan; help with understanding the bill and filing insurance claims; and preparation to leave the hospital (AHA, 2021). Some of the rights described on the website and brochure are the right to privacy, the right to informed consent, the right to die, the right to confidentiality and respectful care, the right to care without discrimination, and the right to information concerning medical condition and treatment (AHA, 2021).

Patient Self-Determination Act

Congress passed the Patient Self-Determination Act (PSDA) in 1990; it was enacted in December 1991. The PSDA is a safeguard for patients' rights, giving patients the legal right to determine how vigorously they wish to be treated in life-or-death situations, and calls for hospitals to abide by patients' advance directives. The PSDA specifies that any organization receiving Medicare or Medicaid funds must inform patients of state laws regarding directives, document the existence of directives in the patient's medical record, educate staff regarding directives, and educate the community about directives. This Act encourages individuals to think about the type of medical and nursing treatment they would want if they were to become critically injured or ill. At the time questions arise, the patient is often unconscious or too sick to make decisions or communicate personal wishes.

Advance directives are designed to ensure individuals the rights of autonomy, refusal of medical intervention, and death with dignity. Advance directives are legal documents that indicate the wishes of individuals in regard to end-of-life issues. Critically ill individuals can remain in charge of their own end-of-life decisions if their advance directives are carried out. Patients should ensure that their advance directives are included in their electronic health record. In addition, copies should be given to significant others and any legal counsel that may be involved with the patient. The best directive is one that has been notarized or developed in conjunction with a legal expert, and the contents of which have been discussed with family or the person with designated healthcare power of attorney who will carry out one's directives in the event of a sudden catastrophic or terminal illness if a patient can no longer communicate their own wishes or expectations of care.

Families should talk about how each member wants critical situations to be handled so that individual preferences are fully expressed. Ideally, family members, caregivers, and courts (in very extreme cases) will not need to make decisions for the patient. Too often the first time a patient learns about advance directives is upon admission to a healthcare facility. The question then arises as to who is responsible for discussing this sensitive issue with the patient. The ideal time for patients to make difficult end-of-life or treatment decisions is well in advance of the need.

Advance directives have not been without controversy. One problem is that states have passed different legislation so there is no guarantee that one state will honor another's advance directives. A trusted person may be appointed to make decisions on behalf of the patient when the patient cannot make them on his or her own. This is known as the *assignment of the healthcare power of attorney*, as mentioned. Rarely, persons have been designated by a family member to hold healthcare power of attorney without their prior knowledge. Ideally, the person making this designation and the trusted person being assigned this important responsibility should have a detailed discussion and prior understanding about what they are to do on behalf of the person. Holding healthcare power of attorney and making decisions based on the unambiguous wishes of the patient is a serious moral obligation, requiring that this designee act as the moral agent for the patient. Prior assignment of one's healthcare power of attorney can minimize, but in some cases not altogether avoid, disagreements among family members. When family members are left to make difficult treatment and end-of-life decisions, conflicts can occur at a time when families are already in distress and are vulnerable. Healthcare providers sometimes convene family meetings to work out these types of difficult situations.

Ethical Issues Related to Immigration and Migration

The movement of people among nations—population migration—has become a topic of great interest across the world. The U.S. is no exception and faces a number of ethical issues that affect health care. Two distinct issues are addressed here that affect nursing and have ethical implications: (1) communication/language problems between patients and healthcare providers and (2) the migration of nurses.

Communication is fundamental to safe, effective health care, the moral commitment to patients. Patients who do not speak English, and who hold a variety of healthcare beliefs and practices to which American healthcare workers may not be accustomed, pose a challenge. Many healthcare institutions, especially larger medical centers, have addressed the issue of language by hiring professional medical interpreters. Interpretation involves the spoken word, and translation refers to the written word.

Medical interpretation is a specialty that requires extensive knowledge of medical terminology, in addition to cultural humility and sensitivity to the needs of the patient. Many American nursing students have some working knowledge of another language, often Spanish. The level of fluency needed for safe interpretation, however, is not typically achieved in language coursework. Nurses who are not bilingual or fluent in medical terminology should defer to a professional medical interpreter for explanations of procedures, diagnoses, obtaining informed consent, and other complex healthcare–related issues. Furthermore, although it is tempting to enlist the assistance of a patient's family member to interpret, this is not a safe practice. Children of patients should never be asked to interpret under any circumstances. The International Medical Interpreters Association (IMIA) works to define educational requirements and qualifications for medical interpreters and to establish norms of practice. IMIA's website (http://imiaweb.org) addresses many issues of interest to nurses.

The second issue with significant ethical implications for healthcare delivery is international nurse migration—that is, the influx of nurses from other countries coming to the United States seeking better pay and working conditions. This poses two distinct ethical problems. First, this exacerbates nursing shortages in other countries. Countries particularly hard hit by this phenomenon include the Philippines, which already loses several thousand nurses a year to the U.S., India, South Africa, and China. The ANA is on record as opposing measures to "uncap" limits on nurses immigrating to the U.S., expressing support instead to increase appropriations to expand nursing programs in this country. This comes at a time when a majority of qualified applicants to American schools of nursing are not admitted because of inadequate numbers of faculty and facilities.

In a statement in 2008 before the Congressional Committee on the Judiciary Subcommittee on Immigration, Citizenship, Refugees, Border Security, and International Law, Cheryl Peterson, MSN, RN, representing the ANA, laid out the ANA's position in opposition of the use of immigration to solve the nursing workforce shortage. Peterson cited these three reasons: (1) Congress had failed to provide adequate funding for domestic schools of nursing; (2) the healthcare industry had failed to establish a workplace environment conducive to the retention of experienced U.S. nurses in patient care; and (3) the United States had failed to engage in active workforce planning to sustain nursing's and other healthcare professions' workforces into the future (ANA, 2008). The ANA was joined by Physicians for Human Rights in opposing any legislation that would increase the United States' reliance on foreign nurses to mediate a shortage of nurses. In a scathing critique of this practice, one physician member of the Physicians for Human Rights described an open-immigration policy as having the potential to "undermine our multibillion-dollar effort to combat AIDS and malaria by potentially worsening the shortage of health workers in developing countries. We're pouring water in a bucket with a hole in it, and we drilled the hole" (Dugger, 2006).

The same problems still affect nursing a decade and a half later. Stokes and Iskander (2021) published a highly informative and detailed paper examining human rights and bioethical considerations associated with global nurse migration. They argue that positive aspects of nurse migration respects nurses' autonomy (they make their own decisions about where to live and work), increased cultural diversity in their destination, and because of improved staffing, leads to better patient satisfaction and health outcomes. Negative effects that they identify are related to issues such as decreasing pay for American nurses related to the lower salaries afforded international nurses, such that the entire pay scale is depressed; lack of respect for the cultural diversity these nurses provide, and the possibilities of coercion and discrimination experienced by nurses who have immigrated to the U.S. Stokes and Iskander assert that ethical challenges of nurse migration are required to enhance the well-being of individual nurses and of patient populations.

The second ethical issue this raises is the documentation of competency to provide safe nursing care, which occurs in the passing of the National Council Licensure Examination (NCLEX®) by graduates of approved American nursing schools. Nurses who may come to the U.S. expecting to find well-paying jobs as professional RNs may find that their education and skills may not be sufficient to practice as a registered nurse. English as a second language for nurses who migrate to the U.S. poses similar communication difficulties, as described previously, and cultural acclimation to the United States healthcare system may pose particular challenges.

Dilemmas Created by Institutional and Social Issues

Healthcare institutions must comply with many governmental regulations that affect both workers and patients. In turn, hospitals and other healthcare institutions implement their own policies and procedures. Nurses may experience moral dilemmas when they disagree with the policies of their institutions. Healthcare organizations are subject to public scrutiny and accountability, and those that receive public funds through the Centers for Medicare and Medicaid Services (CMS) are under particular scrutiny. Ethical dilemmas between nurses and the organizations that employ them may develop over policies dictated by the organizations or mandated by governmental agencies. Nurses experience moral distress when the correct course of action is known, but they are unable to act because of internal or external constraints. If moral distress results for the nurse, it may negatively affect not only patients but the nurse as well (McCarthy and Gastmans, 2015). Thoughtful and conscious action is required to address moral distress, which may lead to greater self-awareness and resilience (McCarthy and Gastmans, 2015).

Ethics committees were created to assist with ethical dilemmas in institutional settings. These committees are multidisciplinary groups charged with the responsibility of providing consultation and emotional support in situations in which difficult ethical choices are necessary. The recommendation from an ethics committee poses no obligation for action; however, they should receive serious consideration by the decision makers. Those desiring help, usually clinical caregivers such as physicians and nurses, refer cases to these committees for additional direction.

Dilemmas Created by Patient Data Access Issues

Digital technologies and EHRs are powerful sources for the storage and transmission of information about patients across healthcare specialties and disciplines. However, these technologies have created a digital portal into patients' confidential medical information (as in the example given earlier about the injured athlete). Those in positions to access healthcare information share a great responsibility to protect this information from unauthorized use.

Information technology, particularly the EHR, places great responsibility in the hands of healthcare providers. Computer ethics have been in existence since the 1970s, but in recent years there has been renewed interest in scholarly inquiry in nursing informatics as the use of technology has become standard in healthcare institutions. The following example illustrates the type of ethical dilemma that can result from the inappropriate access of a patient's EHR.

Tom, a third-year nursing student, observed Susan, a first-year nursing student, sitting at the nurses' station reading patient information about a faculty member's child who was hospitalized with a serious illness in the same hospital. Neither Susan nor Tom was directly involved in the patient's care.

Considering Susan's inexperience, what steps should Tom take? Does Susan's inexperience factor into your thinking about this situation?

TABLE 7.5 The Situational Briefing Model (SBAR)

Situation	Concise statement on the problem/issue. • What is going on?
Background	Provide background detail that is pertinent to the situation/issue. • What is the context?
Assessment	Present subjective and objective data pertinent to the issue. • What do you think is going on? • Analyze options and risks • What are you ruling out (if indicated)?
Recommendation	State the action needed to correct the problem identified in the situation. • What do you want to happen, by when and by whom? • Will the situation need to be reevaluated? Describe.

THE PRACTICE OF MORAL COURAGE

RNs may face a variety of barriers that limit the provision of optimal health care, leading to moral and ethical challenges (McLeod-Sordjan, 2014). Nurses must speak up to address these barriers. Nevertheless, nurses in some situations fail to speak up and are unable to maintain integrity because of fear, resulting from hierarchical organization relationships, or because of uncertainty regarding the best action to take. Nurses have a professional obligation, as emphasized in the Code (ANA, 2015) to speak up, maintaining personal integrity and the integrity of the profession, as well as to advocate for social justice and human rights. There is an ethical mandate for nurses to be prepared to address situations that compromise personal and professional integrity through the use of moral courage (McLeod-Sordjan, 2014).

Moral courage is an individual's capacity to overcome fear and stand up for his or her core values with awareness, despite the potential risk (Lachman, 2010). In other words, moral courage is necessary when moral integrity is in jeopardy, and action to maintain integrity entails risk. Lachman (2010) coined a moral courage model using the acronym *CODE* to signify the necessity to respond to an integrity-compromising situation: ***C***ourage, **O**bligation to honor, ***D***anger management, and ***E***xpression and action. Lachman's (2010) model illustrates the essential elements of being a moral agent.

- **Courage**: The nurse in this step recognizes courage may be necessary to maintain integrity. The nurse analyzes the situation to determine whether an action is required to address the situation.
- **Obligations to honor**: The nurse considers his or her values and beliefs, the ethical principles at stake with the situation, and the ANA (2015) *Code of Ethics for Nurses* provisions to determine what obligations require honoring.
- **Danger management**: The nurse identifies strategies to manage the fear of repercussions when maintaining integrity. Managing danger may include sharing the situation with a trusted nurse or mentor and seeking feedback on how to address the situation. Nurses may also rehearse and practice how they will address the situation and speak up to manage fear. Communicating concerns in an organized manner in an SBAR format guides communication also addressing fear. See Table 7.5, The Situational Briefing Model (SBAR), for additional detail. Another useful tool for managing danger is the CUS Method, coined by the Agency for Healthcare Quality and Research (2014) with Teamstepps. The CUS Method includes first stating the concern ("I am concerned about..."), next sharing why the situation is uncomfortable ("I am uncomfortable with..."), and last if the conflict is unresolved and is a potential safety issue, stating the specific concerns ("this is a safety issue...").
- **Expression and Action**: In the final step, the nurse determines what action is required to maintain integrity considering personal values and beliefs and the obligations to honor. The action may direct (addressing the concern directly with the source) or indirect (addressing the concern with a secondary source such as a manager or supervisor). See Professional Profile Box 7.3 to learn more about a morally courageous modern-day nurse, Alex Wubbels.

The safe practice of nursing is inextricable from ethical challenges. You as students of nursing are encouraged to be aware of your own values, morals, and ethics and to become sensitive to the values, morals, and ethics at work in every nursing situation.

PROFESSIONAL PROFILE BOX 7.3

Modern-Day Morally Courageous Nurse Alex Wubbels

Many nurses such as Florence Nightingale, Mary Eliza Mahoney, and Mary Seacole faced oppression, barriers, and risk when advocating for what is right, demonstrating moral courage. Alex Wubbels is a modern-day nurse who demonstrated moral courage and integrity to advocate for a patient's rights (ANA Enterprise, 2017). On July 26, 2017, Wubbels was ordered by a police officer to allow him to draw blood on an unconscious patient who was a motor vehicle crash victim. The patient's car was struck by a car being chased by police. The patient was not under arrest. Wubbels refused to allow the blood to be drawn, upholding a hospital policy requiring a warrant or the patient's consent. Wubbels protected the patient's privacy and rights and was aggressively arrested as a result. Although no charges were filed, the incident resulted in a national outrage as it was captured on police body cameras. One officer involved in the incident was fired and the other demoted. The hospital also updated its policy regarding obtaining evidence related to a crime scene so that nurses are no longer directly involved with the officers. Wubbels was courageous as she advocated for the patient's rights, and her courage made a national impact. Considering your own practice, what actions would you take to preserve a patient's rights?

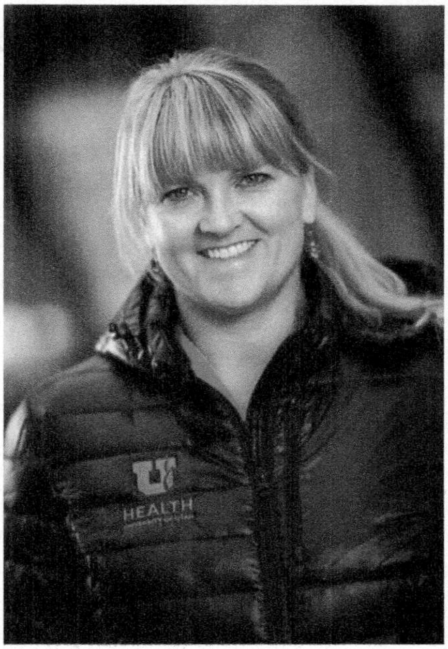

Alex Wubbels, RN
University Hospital, Salt Lake City, Utah

American Nurses Association Enterprise: *American Nurses Association calls for action in wake of police abuse of registered nurse*, 2017. Retrieved from http://www.nursingworld.org/FunctionalMenuCategories/MediaResources/PressReleases/American-Nurses-Association-Calls-for-Action-in-Wake-of-Police-Abuse-of-Registered-Nurse.html

CONCEPTS AND CHALLENGES

- ***Concept:*** Professional ethics override personal ethics in a professional setting.
  Challenge: Patient situations that conflict with a nurse's personal ethics can be very troublesome; however, the ANA's *Code of Ethics for Nurses* is nonnegotiable for nurses regarding ethical behavior.
- ***Concept:*** The terms *morals* and *ethics* are often used interchangeably. Technically, however, morals reflect what is done in a situation, whereas ethics are concerned with what should be done. Values are beliefs, ideals, and attitudes that one uses to guide behavior.
  Challenge: Being familiar with ethical theories and principles, moral development, and decision-making models prepares nurses to participate actively in resolving ethical dilemmas that commonly occur in healthcare settings.
- ***Concept:*** Ethical dilemmas occur in all areas of nursing practice, and in fact, each nursing situation has ethical implications.
  Challenge: Nurses need to understand that even simple decisions such as prioritizing care have an ethical basis.
- ***Concept:*** Respect for humans is the foundation for the six ethical principles of autonomy, beneficence, nonmaleficence, fidelity, veracity, and justice.
  Challenge: These principles are more than a matter of opinion about what constitutes right and wrong. Understanding basic ethical principles involved in a situation can clarify, rather than complicate, how to act ethically and are helpful in determining the best action to take when faced with an ethical dilemma.

- ***Concept:*** Nurses must protect patients' privacy and confidentiality at all times when using social media.
  Challenge: Social media has blurred professional and personal boundaries, making it particularly important for nurses to be vigilant to protect their patients when using social media.
- ***Concept:*** Use of technology such as electronic health records has compounded common ethical dilemmas and created new ones for healthcare providers.
  Challenge: Access to health records are increasingly monitored in healthcare institutions; however, nurses can ensure that they manage digital information correctly by simply asking themselves, "Do I need to know this?"

IDEAS FOR FURTHER EXPLORATION

1. Explain the differences among morals, values, and ethics, using the definitions from this chapter. Describe a patient situation in which you would feel challenged in terms of your own morals, values, and ethics.
2. Compare the ANA's Code of Ethics for Nurses with the ICN's Code of Ethics for Nurses. How are they similar, and how are they different?
3. Select an ethical theory or principle that is most congruent with your approach to ethical dilemmas. Use it as a basis for considering the ethical dilemmas in this chapter. How helpful to you is this particular theory or principle in determining how you would act?
4. Discuss your reactions to the following scenarios and questions in a small group:
   a. Mrs. Otto has recently undergone extensive surgery for gynecologic cancer. The day after surgery, she asks for more pain medication than the physician has prescribed. You call for an order to increase the pain medication dosage, but she still complains every 2 hours that she cannot tolerate the pain. What should be done?
   b. Mrs. Loriz suffers from severe chronic pain, the cause of which has not been diagnosed definitively. Her husband has brought her into the emergency department for the fifth time this month asking for narcotic relief from the pain. In tears she states, "A shot of a narcotic is the only thing that takes the edge off." She threatens suicide if she is sent home without some help. The physician has ordered a placebo. What is the nurse's responsibility?
   c. Mr. Nelson, age 87 years, suffered a serious stroke. His wife of 65 years keeps a constant vigil at his bedside. After 4 weeks, he remains unresponsive and develops pneumonia. He is being fed through a feeding tube and ventilated through a tracheotomy. Mrs. Nelson feels that agreeing to a do-not-resuscitate (DNR) order is letting her husband down but recognizes he has no quality of life. What is the nurse's role and responsibilities when Mrs. Nelson asks for her advice about what to do?
   d. Emily and Michael are parents of a young child dying of Tay-Sachs disease. Emily recently found out she is pregnant again and wants to know whether their second child is affected with the same disease. She undergoes genetic testing and learns that the fetus also has Tay-Sachs disease. Emily and Michael are considering whether to terminate the pregnancy, knowing that their expected baby will have a fatal condition. How can the nurse assist these parents in making their decision?
5. Answer the following questions, basing your answers on identified ethical principles:
   a. When is it acceptable to refuse an assignment?
   b. What is the nurse's duty when a patient confides the desire to self-harm?
   c. Is health care a right?
   d. What should the nurse do when their personal values are in conflict with those of the patient?

REFERENCES

Agency for Healthcare Research and Quality: *Pocket guide: Teamstepps*, 2014. (website). Available at: http://www.ahrq.gov/professionals/education/curriculum-tools/teamstepps/instructor/essentials/pocketguide.html.

American Hospital Association (AHA): *The patient care partnership: what to expect during your hospital stay*, 2021. (website). Available at: https://www.aha.org/other-resources/patient-care-partnership.

American Nurses Association (ANA): *Immigration, citizenship, refugees, border security, and international law*,2008. *(website)*. Available at: www.nursingworld.org/DocumentVault/GOVA/Federal/Testimonies/Testimony061208.pdf, 2008.

American Nurses Association (ANA): *Position statement: the nonnegotiable nature of the ANA code for nurses with interpretive statements*,1994. (website). Available at: http://gm6.nursingworld.org/MainMenuCategories/Policy-Advocacy/Positions-and-Resolutions/ANAPositionStatements/Position-Statements-Alphabetically/prtetcode14446.html.

American Nurses Association (ANA): *Code of ethics for nurses with interpretive statements*, Washington, DC, 2015, American Nurses Publishing.

America Nurses Association (ANA): *Nursing: scope and standards of practice*, 4th ed., Silver Spring, MD, 2021, American Nurses Association.

American Nurses Association Enterprise: *Learn how to cultivate moral courage*, 2017. (website). Available at: https://engage.healthynursehealthynation.org/blogs/8/685.

Baker R: In defense of bioethics, *J Law Med Ethics* 37(1):83–92, 2009.

Bavier A: Holding students accountable when integrity is challenged, *Nurs Educ Perspect*, 30(1):5, 2009.

Beauchamp TL, Childress JF: *Principles of biomedical ethics*, 4, New York, 2001, Oxford University Press.

Brown University: *A framework for making ethical decisions*,2017. (website). Available at: https://www.brown.edu/academics/science-and-technology-studies/framework-making-ethical-decisions.

Buckley WJ, Sulmasy DP, Mackler A, Sachedina A: Ethics of palliative sedation and medical disasters: four traditions advance public consensus on three issues, *Ethics Med* 28(10):35–63, 2012.

Bulger JW:: Principlism, *Teaching Ethics* 8(1):81–100, 2007 https://doi.org/10.5840/tej2007816.

Burkhardt MA, Nathaniel AK: *Ethics and issues in contemporary nursing*, 2, Albany, NY, 2002, Delmar.

Burston A, Tuckett A: Moral distress in nursing: contributing factors, outcomes and interventions, *Nursing Ethics* 20(3):312–324, 2013.

Butts J, Rich K: *Nursing ethics: across the curriculum and into practice*, Sudbury, MA, 2005, Jones & Bartlett.

Cook RI, Woods DD: Operating at the sharp end: the complexity of human error editor. In Bogner ME, editor: *Human error in medicine*, Hillsdale, NJ, 1994, Lawrence Erlbaum Associates, pp 255–310.

de Casterlé BD, Izumi S, Godfrey NS, et al.: Nurses' responses to ethical dilemmas in nursing practice: meta-analysis, *J Adv Nurs* 63(6):540–549, 2009.

Dugger CW: U.S. plan to lure nurses may hurt poor nations, *New York Times*, 2006. May 24Available at www.nytimes.com/2006/05/24/world/americas/24nurses.html?pagewanted=all&_r=0.

Fairchild RM: Practical ethical theory for nurses responding to complexity in care, *Nurs Ethics* 17(3):353–362, 2010.

Giddings L: A theoretical model of social consciousness, *Adv Nurs Sci* 28:224–239, 2005.

Gilligan C: *In a different voice: psychological theory and women's development*, Cambridge, MA, 1982, Harvard University Press.

Gilligan C: Moral orientation and moral development. In Kittay EF, Meyers DT, editors: *Women and moral theory*, Savage, MD, 1987, Rowman.

Guido GW: *Legal and ethical issues in nursing*, 4, Upper Saddle River, NJ, 2006, Pearson Education.

Hardingham LB: Integrity and moral residue: nurses as participants in a moral community, *Nurs Philos* 5(2):127–134, 2004.

Harrison E, Falco SM: Health disparity and the nurse advocate: reaching out to alleviate suffering, *Adv Nurs Sci* 28(3):252–264, 2005.

Haynes L, Boese T, Butcher H: *Nursing in contemporary society: issues, trends, and transition to practice*, Upper Saddle River, NJ, 2004, Pearson Prentice-Hall.

Hines PS: Truth-telling, not telling, and listening, *Cancer Nurs* 31(6):415–416, 2008.

International Council of Nurses (ICN): *The International Council of Nurses code for nurses*, Geneva, Switzerland, 2012, International Council of Nurses.

Jameton A: *Nursing practice: the ethical issues*, Englewood Cliffs, NJ, 1984, Prentice-Hall.

Kirkham SR, Van Hofwegen L, Pankratz D: Keeping the vision: sustaining social consciousness with nursing students following international learning experiences, *Int J Nurs Educ Scholarsh (online)*, 2009 6(1) Article 3.

Kohlberg L: Continuities and discontinuities in childhood and adult moral development revisited editor. In Kohlberg L, editor: *Collected papers on moral development and moral education*, Cambridge, MA, 1973, Moral Education Research Foundation.

Kohlberg L: Moral stages and moralization: the cognitive developmental approach editor. In Lickona T, editor: *Moral development and behavior*, New York, 1976, Holt, Rinehart and Winston, pp 31–53.

Kohlberg L: A current statement on some theoretical issues. In Modgil S, Modgil C, editors: *Lawrence Kohlberg: consensus and controversy*, Philadelphia, 1986, Falmer, pp 485–546.

Lachman V: Strategies necessary for MC, *Online J Issues Nurs*, 2010 15(3). Manuscript 3. Available at http://www.nursingworld.org/MainMenuCategories/EthicsStandards/Courage-and-Distress/Strategies-and-Moral-Courage.html.

McCarthy J, Gastmans C: Moral distress: a review of the argument-based nursing ethics literature, *Nurs Ethics* 23(1):131–152, 2015.

McLeod-Sordjan R: Evaluating moral reasoning in nursing education, *Nursing Ethics* 21(4):473–483, 2014.

Pesut DJ, Herman J: *Clinical reasoning: the art and science of creative and critical thinking*, Albany, NY, 1999, Dell.

Rushton CH, Caldwell M, Kurtz M: CE: Moral distress: a catalyst for building moral resilience, *Am J Nurs* 116(7):40–49, 2016.

Saureland J, Marotta K, Peinemann A, Berndt A, Robichaux C: Assessing and addressing moral distress and ethical climate, part I, *Dimens Crit Care Nurs* 33(40):234–245, 2014.

Stokes F, Iskander R: Human rights and bioethical considerations of global nurse migration, *Bioeth Inquiry*, 2021 https://doi.org/10.1007/s11673-021-10110-6.

Uustal DB: *Clinical ethics and values: issues and insights in a changing healthcare environment*, East Greenwich, RI, 1993, Educational Resources in HealthCare.

Zickmund SL: Care and justice: the impact of gender and profession on ethical decision making in the healthcare arena, *J Clin Ethics* 15(2):176–187, 2004.

8

Conceptual and Philosophic Foundations of Professional Nursing Practice

To enhance your understanding of this chapter, try the Student Exercises on the Evolve site at http://evolve.elsevier.com/Black/professional.

LEARNING OUTCOMES

After studying this chapter, students will be able to:

- Describe the components and processes of systems.
- Explain Maslow's hierarchy of human needs and its relationship to motivation.
- Recognize how environmental factors such as family, culture, social support, social media and the Internet, and community influence health.
- Explain the significance of a holistic approach to nursing care.
- Apply Rosenstock's health belief model and Bandura's theory of perceived self-efficacy to personal health behaviors and health behaviors of others.
- Devise a personal plan for achieving high-level wellness.
- Define and give examples of beliefs.
- Define and give examples of values.
- Cite examples of nursing philosophies.
- Discuss the impact of beliefs and values on nurses' professional behaviors.
- Explain how nurses and organizations educating and employing nurses can use a philosophy of nursing.
- Identify personal beliefs, values, and philosophies as they relate to nursing.

Suppose you were building a house. You would want the most solid, safe, and structurally sound building that you could afford. You would want your house to be built on firm ground, set on a foundation of cinderblocks and concrete. You would want to know that this structure would hold up in high wind, heavy snow, blazing heat, and driving rains. Because of what you are asking of your house—that is, for it to be a place to eat, sleep, be with your family, and protect you from the elements—some parts of your house would be similar to almost all houses: a foundation, framing, walls, windows, rooms, and a good roof. Because you have planned and built your house well, it will provide for you what you need from it.

Anything built well must have a solid foundation for support. Your car has a structure—the chassis—that keeps you safe and gives form to your car. Humans have a skeleton that gives us shape and makes us recognizable. The underlying structure tells us something about the function of the object.

The same holds true for a profession; its foundational principles tell us something about what nursing is and what nursing does. These principles are always in place, even when you are not aware of them. Much like the foundation of your house or your own skeleton, you do not have to think about it doing its work; it is simply there.

The foundation of nursing—its bones—is its basic concepts, the ideas that are essential to understanding professional practice. These concepts are person, environment, and health. Each concept has subconcepts, which are other ideas that are related to the larger concept, but which are also related to nursing (Fig. 8.1). Everything professional nurses do is in response to one of these basic interrelated concepts. You do not say, "I am going to check on Mrs. Bruce's homeostasis." But, in fact, when you check her fluid intake and urine output after her major surgery,

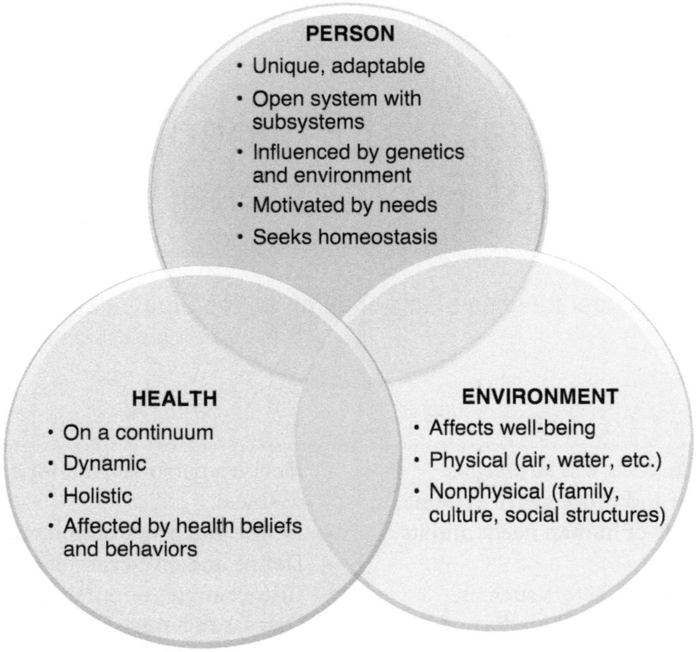

PERSON
• Unique, adaptable
• Open system with subsystems
• Influenced by genetics and environment
• Motivated by needs
• Seeks homeostasis
HEALTH
• On a continuum
• Dynamic
• Holistic
• Affected by health beliefs and behaviors
ENVIRONMENT
• Affects well-being
• Physical (air, water, etc.)
• Nonphysical (family, culture, social structures)

Fig. 8.1 This is the foundation of nursing—its concepts and subconcepts basic to the profession.

you are addressing an element of her *person* (homeostasis—her fluid balance), her *health* (she is in a vulnerable state), and her *environment* (her intravenous line patency, her availability of water), in the context of nursing. You as a nurse are guided by beliefs, values, and a philosophy, which work together to shape your practice.

This is a simple example, but one that will give you an idea of how nursing's concepts are at work in nursing actions. In this chapter we will explore how these concepts relate to each other and to nursing. By the end of this chapter, these abstract ideas will have more meaning to you as you begin to think about your own philosophy of nursing.

UNDERSTANDING SYSTEMS: CONNECTIONS AND INTERACTIONS

An understanding of systems will guide you in understanding the connections and interactions among nursing's basic concepts. A system is a set of interrelated parts that come together to form a whole that performs a function (von Bertalanffy, 1968). General systems theory was developed in 1936 by biologist Ludwig von Bertalanffy, who believed that a common framework for studying several similar disciplines would allow scientists and scholars to organize and communicate findings, making it easier to build on the work of others. Each part of a system is a necessary or integral component required to make a complete, meaningful whole. These parts are input, throughput, output, evaluation, and feedback (von Bertalanffy, 1968).

Components of Systems

Input is the first component of a system—the raw material, such as information, energy, or matter—that enters a system and is transformed by it. For a system to work well, input should contribute to achieving the purpose of the system.

Throughput is the second component of a system. Throughput consists of the processes a system uses to convert raw materials (input) into a form that can be used, either by the system itself or by the environment (also called the *suprasystem*). **Output** is the end result or product of the system. Outputs vary widely, depending on the type and purpose of the system.

Evaluation is the fourth component of a system. **Evaluation** means measuring the success or failure of the output and consequently the effectiveness of the

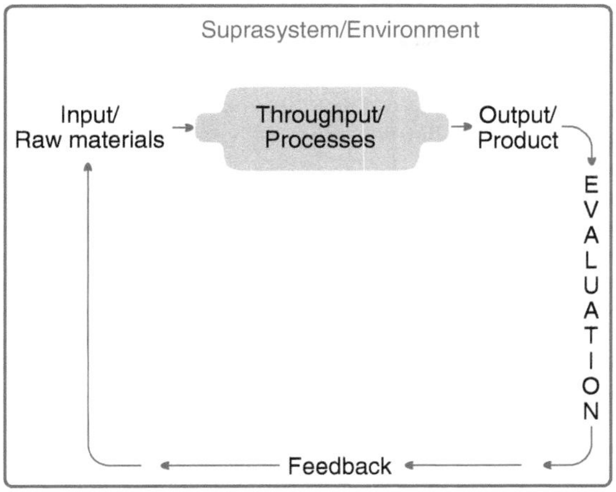

Fig. 8.2 Major components of a general systems model.

system. For evaluation to be meaningful in any system, outcome criteria against which performance or product quality is measured must be identified.

Feedback, the final component of a system, is the process of communicating what is found in evaluation of the system. Feedback is the information given back into the system to determine whether the purpose, or end result, of the system has been achieved. Fig. 8.2 depicts the components of systems and illustrates how they relate to one another.

Examples of Systems

A simple example helps clarify the components of systems. In a school of nursing system, the raw material, or input, consists of students, faculty, ideas, the desire to learn, and knowledge. For high-quality input, students need to be ready to learn, and the faculty should be knowledgeable and well prepared to teach. The processes (throughput) whereby ideas, knowledge, and skills are transmitted must be clear and understandable. In this example, throughput consists of learning experiences such as readings, lectures, discussions, labs, and clinical experiences. The output, or product, of the system is well-educated graduates. For evaluation of the output, the National Council Licensure Examination (NCLEX®) is a good measure of how well the system worked. The passing rate of those taking the NCLEX® on their first try provides feedback to a school's faculty and administrators. If a high percentage of graduates pass on the first try, the system has achieved its purpose. If not, changes need to be made in the input or in the system itself—for example, setting higher admission standards, hiring more talented faculty, and/or designing more effective courses and curricula.

Systems are usually complex and consist of several parts called *subsystems*. Consider a hospital as a system, for example. Technically, it is a system for providing health care, but the success of the system depends on the functioning of many subsystems. The subsystems include many departments: nursing, medicine, imaging, informatics, laboratory, and environmental services, among others. Each of these subsystems is a system itself. All the subsystems function collaboratively to make the healthcare system—the hospital—work.

Open and Closed Systems

Continuing with the example, the hospital and all its subsystems are open systems. An open system promotes the exchange of matter, energy, and information with other systems and the environment. The larger environment outside the hospital is called the suprasystem. A closed system does not interact with other systems or with the surrounding environment. Matter, energy, and information do not flow into or out of a closed system. There are few totally closed systems. Even a completely balanced aquarium, for example, often thought of as approaching a closed system, needs light, air, and additional water and nutrients from time to time.

Two more points are essential to a basic understanding of systems. First, the whole is different from and greater than the sum of its parts (its subsystems). Anyone who has ever been in a hospital, for example, knows that what happens there is different from and more than the sum of the following equation: nurses + pharmacy + physicians + environmental services = hospital. The second point involves synergy. Synergy occurs when all the various subsystems work together to create a result that is not independently achievable. Synergy in the hospital occurs when the people who compose the subsystems collaborate to work with patients and their families, combining efforts to create an outcome that no single group could accomplish alone.

Dynamic Nature of Systems

The final point to be made about systems is that change in one part of the system creates change in other parts. If the hospital admissions office, for example, decided to admit patients only between the hours of 8:00 and 10:00 a.m., that decision would result in changes in the nursing units, environmental services, business office, operating suites, laboratories, and other hospital subsystems. If that change were implemented without prior communication to the other subsystems and coordinated planning, it would likely create chaos in the system.

The exchange of energy and information within open systems and between open systems and their suprasystems is continuous. The dynamic balance within and between the subsystems, the system, and the suprasystems helps create and maintain homeostasis, also known as *internal stability*.

All living systems are open systems. The internal environment is in constant interaction with a changing environment external to the organism. As change occurs in one environment, the other environment is affected. For example, walking into a cold room (change in the external environment) affects a variety of physiologic and psychological subsystems of a person's internal environment. These, in turn, affect a person's blood flow, ability to concentrate, and feeling of comfort, for example (changes in internal environment).

Application of the Systems Model to Nursing

Nurses work within systems every day. Using the hospital example, nurses work within the hospital as a system, the department of nursing's system, within a particular unit's system, and with colleagues in what may be an informal but important system. All are open systems interacting with one another and the environment. If nurses are to work effectively in such complex systems, they need to have an understanding of how systems operate.

At the individual patient level, the openness of human systems makes nursing intervention possible. Understanding systems helps nurses assess relationships among all the factors that affect patients, including the influence of nurses themselves. Nurses who understand systems view patients holistically, including the physiologic subsystems (such as metabolism and the respiratory system) and suprasystem (such as family, culture, and community). These nurses appreciate the influence of change in any part of the system. For instance, when a patient with diabetes has pneumonia (change in subsystem), the infection increases the blood glucose level (metabolic system) and may result in hospitalization. Hospitalization may in turn adversely affect the patient's role in the family and community (change in suprasystem). Key concepts of systems are summarized in Box 8.1. With this brief introduction to systems as a foundation, we can now examine the three basic concepts that are fundamental to the practice of professional nursing: person, environment, and health.

BOX 8.1 Key Concepts About Systems

1. A system is a set of interrelated parts.
2. The parts form a meaningful whole.
3. The whole is different from and greater than the sum of its parts.
4. Systems may be open or closed.
5. All living systems are open systems.
6. Systems strive for homeostasis (internal stability).
7. Systems are part of suprasystems.
8. Systems have subsystems.
9. A change in one part of a system creates change in other parts.

PERSON: AN OPEN SYSTEM WITH HUMAN NEEDS

The term person is used to describe each individual woman, man, and child. There are various approaches to the study of person. This chapter briefly examines the concept of people as systems with human needs.

As mentioned previously, each individual is an open system with numerous subsystems that make up the whole person. For example, the physiologic subsystem is composed of the circulatory, musculoskeletal, respiratory, gastrointestinal, genitourinary, and neurologic subsystems; the psychological, social, cultural, and spiritual subsystems combine with the physiologic subsystem to comprise the whole person. Each person is unique, different from all other people who have been and ever will be. This uniqueness is determined genetically, environmentally, and experientially and is the basis for holistic nursing care, that is, nursing care that takes all the aspects of the person into consideration.

Certain personal characteristics are determined at conception by the genes received from one's biologic parents, such as eye, skin, and hair color; height; sex; and a variety of other features. The environment determines other characteristics. The availability of loving and nurturing parents or parental substitutes, availability of sufficient nutritious foods, cultural beliefs, degree of educational opportunities, adequacy of housing, quality and quantity of parental supervision, and safety are all examples of environmental factors that influence how a person develops.

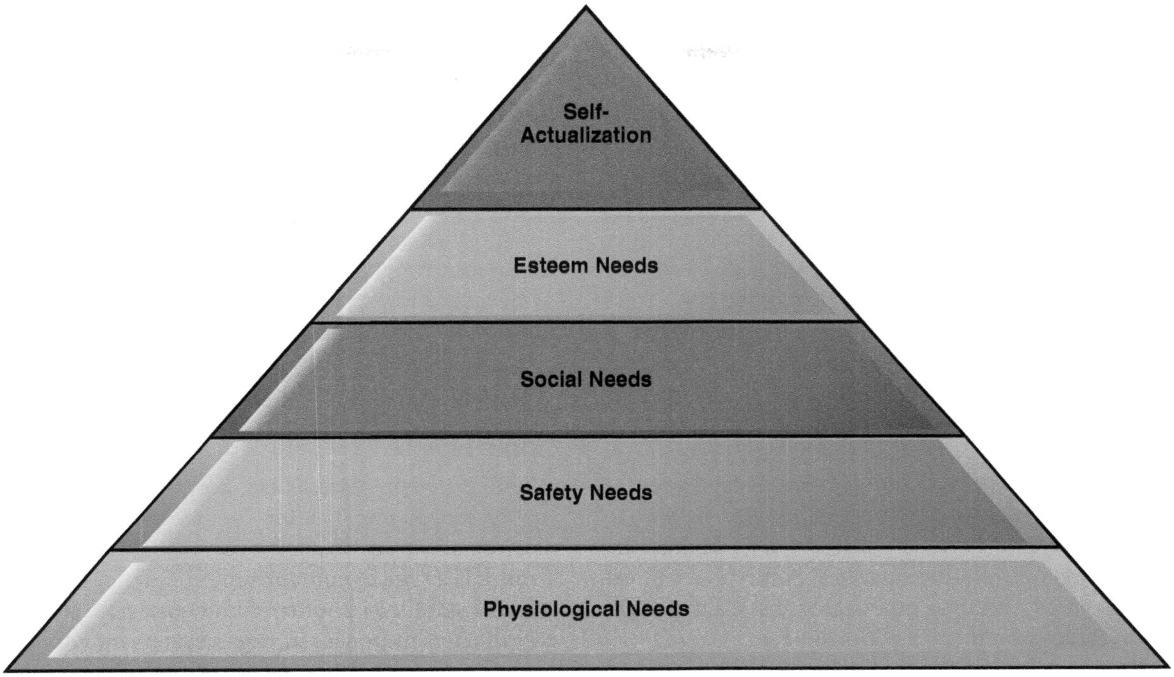

Fig. 8.3 Maslow's hierarchy of needs. Understanding this hierarchy helps nurses prioritize their care. (Maslow AH: A theory of human motivation, Psychological Review 50(4):370-396, 1943.)

Human Needs

In addition to having unique personal characteristics, people have inborn needs. *Human need* refers to something—food, air, social interaction—required for a person's well-being. In 1954 psychologist Abraham Maslow published *Motivation and Personality.* In this classic book, Maslow rejected earlier ideas of Sigmund Freud, who believed that people are motivated by unconscious instincts, and Ivan Pavlov, who believed humans were driven by conditioned reflexes. Instead, Maslow presented his human needs theory and explained that human behavior is motivated by intrinsic needs. He identified five levels of needs and organized them into a hierarchic order, as shown in Fig. 8.3.

Maslow's Hierarchy of Needs

According to Maslow, the most basic level of needs consists of those necessary for physiologic survival: food, oxygen, rest, activity, shelter, and sexual expression. These needs are common to all human beings.

The second level of needs is safety and security. These include physical and psychological safety and security needs. Psychological safety and security include having a reasonably predictable environment with which one has some familiarity and relative freedom from fear and chaos.

The third level of needs consists of love and belonging. To a greater or lesser extent, each person needs close, intimate relationships; social relationships; a place in the social structure; and group affiliations.

Next in Maslow's hierarchy is the need for self-esteem. This includes the need to feel self-worth, self-respect, and self-reliance.

Self-actualization is the highest level of needs. Self-actualized people have realized their maximum potential; they use their talents, skills, and abilities to the fullest extent possible and are true to their own nature. People do not stay in a state of self-actualization but may have "peak experiences" during which they realize self-actualization for some period. Maslow believed that many people strive for self-actualization but few consistently reach that level (Maslow, 1987). He also believed that people are "innately motivated toward psychological growth, self-awareness, and personal freedom. As he saw it, we never outgrow the innate need for self-expression and self-development, no matter how old we are" (Hoffman, 2008, p. 36).

Assumptions About Needs

Maslow's hierarchy is based on several basic assumptions about human needs. One assumption is that basic needs must be at least partially satisfied before higher order needs can become relevant to the individual. For example, people who are starving will not be concerned with issues of self-esteem until their hunger is satisfied.

A second assumption about human needs is that individuals meet their needs in different ways. One person may need 8 or 9 hours of sleep to feel rested, whereas another may require only 5 or 6 hours. Each individual's sleep needs may vary at different stages of life. As people age, they often require less sleep than when they were younger. Individuals also eat different diets in differing quantities and at differing intervals. Some prefer to eat only twice a day, whereas others may snack six or eight times a day to meet their nutritional needs.

Although sleep and food are examples of basic human needs, the manner in which these needs are met, as well as the extent to which any one of them is considered a need, varies according to each individual. It is therefore extremely important to determine a person's perceptions of their own needs to be able to provide appropriate, individualized nursing care. If a patient is uncomfortable eating three large meals, such as those served in most hospitals, nurses can help that person by saving parts of the large meals in the refrigerator on the nursing unit and serving them to the patient between regularly scheduled meals. This is a simple example of what is meant by the term *individualized nursing care,* which recognizes each individual's unique needs and tailors the plan of nursing care to take that uniqueness into consideration.

Adaptation and Human Needs

Another aspect of human needs is the nature of individuals to change, grow, and develop. Carl Rogers, a well-known psychologist, built his theory of personhood based on the idea that people are constantly adapting, discovering, and rediscovering themselves. His book *On Becoming a Person* (Rogers, 1961) is considered a classic in psychological literature. Rogers' idea that a person's needs change as the person changes is important for nurses to remember. The human potential to grow and develop can be used by nurses to assist patients to change unhealthy behaviors and to reach the highest level of wellness possible.

The concept of **adaptation** is also helpful in understanding that people admitted to hospitals and removed from their customary, familiar environments commonly become anxious. Even the most confident person can become fearful when in an uncertain, perhaps threatening, situation. Under these circumstances, nurses have learned to expect people to regress slightly and to become more concerned with basic needs and less focused on the higher needs in Maslow's hierarchy. As you will see in Chapter 9, several nursing theorists based their theoretical models on adaptation.

Homeostasis

When a person's needs are not met, homeostasis is threatened. Remember that homeostasis is a dynamic balance achieved by effectively functioning open systems. It is a state of equilibrium, a tendency to maintain internal stability. In humans, homeostasis is attained by coordinated responses of organ systems that automatically compensate for environmental changes. When someone goes for a brisk walk, for example, heart rate and respiratory rate automatically increase to keep vital organs supplied with oxygen. When the individual comes home and sits down to read, heart rate and breathing slow down. No conscious decision to speed up or slow down these physiologic functions has to be made. Adjustments occur automatically to maintain homeostasis.

Individuals, as open systems, also endeavor to maintain balance between external and internal forces. When that balance is achieved, the person is healthy, or at least resistant to illness. When environmental factors affect a person's homeostasis, the person attempts to adapt to the change. If adaptation is unsuccessful, disequilibrium may occur, setting the stage for the development of illness or disease. How individuals respond to stress is a major factor in the development of illness. Stress and illness are discussed more fully in Chapter 13, and you may wish to review that information now.

ENVIRONMENT: THE SUPRASYSTEM IN WHICH PERSONS LIVE

The second major concept basic to professional nursing practice is environment, or the suprasystem. **Environment** includes all the circumstances, influences, and conditions that surround and affect individuals, families, and groups. The environment can be as small and controlled as a premature infant's isolette or as large and uncontrollable as the weather. Included in environment are the social and cultural attitudes that profoundly shape human experience.

The environment can either promote or interfere with the homeostasis and well-being of individuals. As seen in Maslow's hierarchy of needs, there is a dynamic interaction between a person's needs, which are internal, and the satisfaction of those needs, which is often environmentally determined.

Nurses have always been aware of the influence of environment on people. Florence Nightingale, in particular, stressed the role of a healthful environment in restoration and preservation of health and prevention of disease and injury. Concerns about the health of the public have led governmental entities at local, state, and national levels to establish standards and regulations that ensure the safety of food, water, air, cosmetics, medications, workplaces, and other areas in which health hazards may occur. Environmental systems to be discussed in this section are family systems, cultural systems, social systems, and community systems.

Family Systems

The most direct environmental influence on a person is the family. Families have all types of configurations, from dual-parent homes with children to single parents raising their children on their own; single adults with networks of close friends who constitute their family; extended families with several generations under one roof; or couples without children. These are just a few examples of the many family structures. Families are defined as the patient defines family and do not necessarily involve "blood relatives." The way the family functions with and within the environment and the dynamics among various members of the family constitute the **family system**. The quality and amount of parenting provided to infants and growing children constitute a major determinant of health. Children who are nurtured when young and vulnerable, who are allowed to grow in independence and self-determination, and who are taught the skills they need for social living have a foundation for growing into strong, productive, autonomous adults. Some strong, productive, autonomous adults, however, come from disadvantaged backgrounds where the nurturing was limited. The family background can shape one's adulthood but is not determinative.

Nuclear and Extended Families

For most of the history of humankind, immediate and extended families were relatively intact units that lived together or lived within close proximity to one another. In the **extended family**, children were nurtured by a variety of relatives, as well as by their own parents. Extended family members also cared for elderly people and those with disabilities. This closeness was affected profoundly by industrialization, which fostered urbanization. When families ceased farming, which was a family endeavor, and moved to cities where fathers worked in factories, the first dilution of the influence of extended family began. The **nuclear family** (parents and their children) moved away from former sources of nurturing, as older relatives such as grandparents, aunts, and uncles often stayed in rural areas.

During World War II, more women began to work, taking them out of the home and away from their young children. The increased geographic mobility of families since World War II has changed the extent and nature of relationships of extended family members because nuclear families may live across the continent or the world from their relatives. Currently, digital platforms such as messaging and social media and availability of broadband Internet service are changing the relationships of extended family members yet again. These technologies can allow family members who are geographically separate to interact more intensely and frequently than was possible 20 years ago. For some families, technology allows extended family members to serve as important sources of advice and support without being physically present; however, access to these technologies varies widely among the population of the United States.

Single-Parent Families

Although the majority of children in the United States lives in two-parent households, the percentage of children living in single-parent households increased dramatically over the past 50 years. According to the U.S. Census Bureau (2021), 23% of all households with children under the age of 18 were single-parent households, and most of those were headed by women. For comparison, in 1960, 8% of households were single-parent households. In 2016, 39.8% of all births were to single women (Centers for Disease Control and Prevention

[CDC], 2018), a statistic explaining in part the current high percentage of single-parent homes in the United States. Life is challenging for single parents who must earn a living for the family and fulfill the nurturing roles in the family. Bearing these multiple roles alone over long periods can be extremely stressful, even exhausting, to single parents.

The examples given here represent only a few ways families influence the well-being of individuals: there are many others. A complete nursing assessment includes information about a patient's family and home environment. This information is particularly important when a modification of the home environment is needed, especially when a person is returning home with a disability or a limitation in his or her mobility. Importantly, a complete assessment should include screening for intimate partner violence (IPV), and for signs of neglect and abuse. Signs of neglect or abuse in both adults and children may not be obvious, and survivors often are not forthcoming in the healthcare setting about being abused and by whom. Abuse and neglect are not uncommon, and careful assessment and the development of a trusting professional relationship may be of benefit in helping persons who have been abused disclose their experience.

Cultural Systems

People are deeply entrenched in their culture and may not even recognize the effect of their culture on their lives. **Culture** consists of a population's customs, arts, and social institutions that have been perpetuated across generations. Patterns of language, clothing, eating habits, activities of daily living, attitudes toward those outside the culture, health beliefs and values, spiritual beliefs or religious orientation, recreation and attitudes regarding constructs (e.g., sex, marriage, education, among others), and forms of recreation are influenced by culture.

Significant changes have occurred in the U.S. in the past several decades related to culture. The United States was once known as a "melting pot," referring to the assimilation of persons of varying nationalities, cultures, and languages into one homogeneous culture. Recently however, the melting pot metaphor is being replaced with the "salad bowl" metaphor to describe multiculturalism predominating in the United States today. Multiculturalism has several definitions. The most common usage, however, refers to those with "culturally distinct identities" retaining their cultural identity and with full access to a society's constitutional principles and prevailing shared values (UNESCO, n.d.).

According to the Pew Research Center (2020), 13.7% of people living in the United States were foreign born, translating to more than 40,000,000 persons. The United States has become a multicultural society, with immigrants coming from almost every country in the world. Because basic beliefs about health and illness vary widely from culture to culture, nurses need to develop cultural competence to meet the needs of culturally diverse patients. For example, many Mexican American and Mexican families observe 40 days of recovery in the postpartum period—*la cuarentena* (*cuarenta días* or quarantine)—when traditional behaviors related to diet, clothing, sexual abstinence, bathing, and management of the environment are practiced, and social support is intense. This cultural practice may be misunderstood and even trivialized by providers, leading women to conceal their traditions (Waugh, 2010).

Effective nurses learn to be aware of and to respect cultural influences on patients. Whenever possible, they defer to patients' cultural preferences. They recognize that some cultural groups attribute illness to bad fortune. Individuals from cultures with these beliefs do not see themselves as active participants in their own health status. This belief may pose challenge for American nurses who value the collaboration of patients in their own healthcare planning.

The challenge for nurses in an increasingly diverse world is to understand the risks of **ethnocentrism**—that is, making judgments, often negative, about another's culture relative to one's own. It is tempting to dismiss a cultural tradition or belief because it is not part of one's own experience. Moreover, it is also easy to be blind to one's own deeply entrenched cultural beliefs. In other words, our own traditions will seem strange to others. Astute nurses realize that integration of a patient's cultural health beliefs into planning patient-centered care can make a strong impact on that patient's desire and ability to improve his or her health.

Understanding the relationship between culture and health is the basis for "transcultural nursing," a field of nursing practice initiated by nurse-anthropologist Madeleine Leininger. Additional discussion of the influence of culture on nursing practice can be found in Chapter 13.

Social Systems

In addition to being influenced by family and cultural systems, individuals are influenced by the social system in which they live. Social institutions such as families, neighborhoods, schools, churches, professional associations, civic groups, and recreational groups may constitute a form of social support. Social support also includes such factors as family income; presence in the home of a spouse; proximity to neighbors, children, and other supportive individuals; access to medical care; coping abilities; and educational level.

Social Change

Holmes and Rahe (1967) published a study of the relationship of social change to the subsequent development of illness. They found that people with many social changes that disrupt social support, such as death of a loved one, divorce, job changes, moving, or unemployment, were much more likely to experience illness in the following 12 months than people with few social changes. Both positive and negative changes created the need for social readjustment. In 1995 this study was updated, and the Recent Life Changes Questionnaire (Table 8.1) was devised to reflect more accurately contemporary

TABLE 8.1 Recent Life Changes Questionnaire

The following 74 potential life changes inquire about recent events in a person's life. A 6-month total equal to or greater than 300 Life Change Units (LCUs) or a 1-year total equal to or greater than 500 LCUs is considered indicative of high recent life stress.

Life Change Event	Life Change Units
Health	
An injury or illness that:	
Kept you in bed 1 week or more or sent you to the hospital	74
Was less serious than above	44
Major dental work	26
Major change in eating habits	27
Major change in sleeping habits	26
Major change in your usual type and/or amount of recreation	28
Work	
Change to a new type of work	51
Change in your work hours or conditions	35
Change in your responsibilities at work:	
More responsibilities	29
Fewer responsibilities	21
Promotion	31
Demotion	42
Transfer	32
Troubles at work:	
With your boss	29
With co-workers	35
With persons under your supervision	35
Other work troubles	28
Major business adjustment	60
Retirement	52
Loss of job:	
Laid off from work	68
Fired from work	79
Correspondence course to help you in your work	18
Home and Family	
Major change in living conditions	42
Change in residence:	
Move within the same town or city	25
Move to a different town, city, or state	47
Change in family get-togethers	25
Major change in health or behavior of family member	55
Marriage	50
Pregnancy	67
Miscarriage or abortion	65
Gain of a new family member:	
Birth of a child	66
Adoption of a child	65
A relative moving in with you	59
Spouse beginning or ending work	46
Child leaving home:	
To attend college	41
Because of marriage	41
For other reason	45
Change in arguments with spouse	50
In-law problems	38

Continued

TABLE 8.1 Recent Life Changes Questionnaire—cont'd

Life Change Event	Life Change Units	Life Change Event	Life Change Units
Change in the marital status of your parents:		New close, personal relationship	37
		Engagement to marry	45
Divorce	59	Girlfriend or boyfriend problems	39
Remarriage	50	Sexual difficulties	44
Separation from spouse:		"Falling out" of a close personal relationship	47
Because of work	53		
Because of marital problems	76	An accident	48
Divorce	96	Minor violation of the law	20
Birth of grandchild	43	Being held in jail	75
Death of spouse	119	Death of a close friend	70
Death of a family member:		Major decision regarding your immediate future	51
Child	123		
Brother or sister	102	Major personal achievement	36
Parent	100		
		Financial	
Personal and Social		Major change in finances:	
Change in personal habits	26	Increased income	38
Beginning or ending school or college	38	Decreased income	60
Change of school or college	35	Investment and/or credit difficulties	56
Change in political beliefs	24	Loss or damage of personal property	43
Change in religious beliefs	29	Moderate purchase	20
Change in social activities	27	Major purchase	37
Vacation	24	Foreclosure on a mortgage or loan	58

From Miller MA, Rahe RH: Life changes scaling for the 1990s, *J Psychosom Res* 43 (3):279–292, 1997. Reprinted with permission.

concerns (Miller and Rahe, 1997). Numerous researchers have found additional evidence that social support has a direct relationship to health.

Social Support

Social support is a commonly used, but rarely defined, term. In its largest sense, social support means that a person belongs to a social network, feels cared for, and can count on people for assistance. Social support can be perceived, meaning that individuals recognize that support has been given or is available if needed in the future. *Received support* refers to the actual helpful (supportive) actions that are offered. Social support works in four ways. *Emotional support* comes in the form of concern for, affection, love, caring, encouragement, and conveying a sense of value to the person being supported. *Companionship* is a form of support that gives the supported person a sense of belonging and other persons with whom to share social activities. *Informational support* is advice and guidance, the sharing of useful information. *Material support,* also called tangible support, refers to financial help, providing material goods and/or services. Individuals vary in their need and desire for social support. When doing patient assessments, nurses need to remember that the patient, not the nurse, should determine the adequacy of their social support. For patients who need and desire increased informational support as a form of social support, nurses can be excellent sources of knowledge and direction. Nurses can inform patients about resources for patients and families with specific diagnoses (e.g., cancer support groups, Crohn disease support groups, rare chromosomal disorder support group), parenting classes, religious groups, bereavement and loss support groups, formal and informal educational groups, and self-help groups, among others. These groups may have local meetings or may have a strong online presence as a means of emotional support, companionship, and tangible support.

Poverty

Poverty means living with deprivation and the scarcity of necessities such as food and adequate housing. The

United States is one of the wealthiest nations in the world (International Monetary Fund, 2018; Investopedia, 2017). The poverty level in the United States, however, is high relative to the nation's overall wealth: in 2020 the poverty rate was 11.4% (U.S. Census Bureau, 2020). The U.S. Department of Health and Human Services determines the poverty level annually. In 2021 the poverty threshold was a total income of $12,880 or less for a single person and $26,500 or less for a family of four in the 48 contiguous U.S. states plus the District of Columbia. Alaska and Hawaii have higher costs of living; therefore the poverty threshold income level is somewhat higher (U.S. Department of Health and Human Services: HHS poverty guidelines, 2021).

People living in poverty have diminished access to health care for a variety of reasons. Lack of money means inadequate nutrition and lack of basic health care, adversely affecting the health status of all family members. Specific challenges faced by families at or near poverty levels are food insecurity and hunger; poor transportation; inability to pay mortgage or rent; and inability to pay for utilities such as natural gas, water, and electricity. The World Health Organization considers poverty to be one the most influential determinants of health.

Understanding and appreciating the complex societal forces that contribute to poverty can be challenging for nurses. Some even blame persons living in poverty for their situation. Misconceptions can lead to stereotyping and insensitivity to the feelings and concerns of people in poverty, further alienating them from the healthcare system. Many nursing students have had limited exposure to poverty and may not fully realize the enormous implications of being poor. One student shared her experience:

> *Before I did my community health rotation, I thought that poor meant that someone had to shop for clothes at a "big box" store rather than the mall. Then I made a home visit to a nice woman I had met in the high-risk obstetric clinic. She was pregnant and had the early stages of cervical cancer. She told me that to find her house, I would see a mobile home that looked too run down for anybody to live in. She told me to go past it to the next one that looked even worse, and that was where she lived. I kind of didn't believe her, but she was right. One of the bedrooms was a chicken wire and cardboard addition to the side of the house that her teenager had built. What surprised me was how neat and clean she had tried to make her house, and her children all sat in a line very quietly and responded to my questions politely. This lady's quiet dignity amid this horrible poverty really humbled me, and I cried in my car all the way home.*

Community, National, and World Systems

The health status of people is also influenced by the larger systems in which they live. The types and availability of jobs, housing, schools, and health care, as well as the overall economic well-being, profoundly affect the citizens in a community. Nurses can be instrumental in improving the community systems. Identifying health needs and bringing these to the attention of community planners, offering screening programs, serving on health-related committees and advisory boards, and lobbying political leaders can bring about positive change in a community. Nurses have also become politically active by running for elected offices at local, state, and national levels. They can energetically support political candidates who have sound environmental platforms. More information about political activism in nursing is provided in Chapter 15.

From a broad perspective, environment also includes the nation and the world. A seemingly isolated incident such as an earthquake in Nepal or an outbreak of Ebola in West Africa can have worldwide health repercussions. Similarly, what appeared to be a limited outbreak of COVID-19 in Wuhan, China in 2019 soon spread across the world, and its repercussions are yet to be fully manifested and understood. Nurses can contribute to a healthier world environment by supporting, promoting, and, when possible, participating in humanitarian responses to national and international disasters.

Nurses' Potential Impact on the Environment/Suprasystem

Individual nurses, in the interest of ecological health, can engage in a variety of environmentally sound practices in their personal lives and encourage others to do the same. Most of these simply require paying attention to some of your regular habits—turning off unused lights and computers, recycling household trash and hazardous materials such as batteries and paint, avoiding insecticides and unnecessary use of pest-control chemicals, staying abreast of product and toy recalls, buying energy-efficient appliances and automobiles, carpooling, walking or biking when possible, and using public transportation. Furthermore, nurses need to pay attention to the environmental impact of corporations and avoid buying from or investing in companies that engage in environmentally unsound practices.

Because nurses are interested in the health of the public, they should look for ways to organize their workplaces to contribute to a healthier environment. (Chapter 16 addresses this in more detail.) Healthcare facilities are among the largest producers of waste in the nation. Even as nurses work to promote health, that very work creates all types of pollution, including biohazardous waste, which ultimately adversely affects health.

A decade ago, hospitals were a major source of mercury pollution. This highly toxic substance, once used in thermometers, blood pressure measuring devices, and other medical devices, ultimately flowed into the environment, where it contaminated water. Through the oceans' food chain, mercury in contaminated water becomes concentrated in the bodies of predator fish such as tuna and swordfish, which are eventually consumed by humans. Even in small doses, mercury poses serious health risks to pregnant women and young children. Nurses were instrumental in encouraging their employers to avoid purchasing and using mercury-containing devices and to dispose of them properly. Health Care Without Harm is an organization with the mission to reduce hazardous waste, specifically mercury, produced from healthcare facilities. This organization encourages nurses to become "environmental health activists." You can learn more about Health Care Without Harm at its website: www.noharm.org.

In other efforts to reduce environmental pollution, some healthcare facilities have established committees, sometimes called *green teams,* dedicated to identifying and recommending environmentally sound products and procedures. Nurses can volunteer to serve on these committees or to start one. They can recommend recycling, using compact fluorescent light bulbs, using certified organic foods, reusing or repurposing products safely, and using fewer disposable products and fewer products with wasteful packaging. They can educate themselves about reducing carbon emissions and advocate for sustainable policies in their workplaces. You can join the movement of nurses and other healthcare workers to prevent environmental disease. Health Care Without Harm describes their work as to "transform healthcare worldwide so that it reduces its environmental footprint, becomes a community anchor for sustainability and a leader in the global movement for environmental health and justice" (Health Care Without Harm, 2021). Refer to their website (https://noharm-uscanada.org/) to learn how the organization is addressing this important mission and how you can help.

HEALTH: A CONTINUUM

Health is the third major concept fundamental to the practice of professional nursing. Health is best viewed as a continuum rather than as an absolute state. Each individual's health status varies from day to day depending on a variety of factors, such as rest, nutrition, and stressors; similarly, illness is not an absolute state. People can have chronic illnesses such as diabetes or seizure disorders and still work; take part in recreational activities; and maintain acceptably healthy, meaningful lives. Fig. 8.4 depicts the wellness continuum with six interrelated dimensions contributing to health.

Defining Health

Health "is as hard to define as love or happiness, and even harder to trap and keep" (Zuger, 2008), yet many individuals and organizations have made attempts to define health. Seventy-five years ago, WHO defined **health** as "a state of complete physical, mental, and social well-being and not merely the absence of disease or infirmity" (WHO, 1947, p. 29). This definition was the first official recognition of health as multidimensional. The WHO definition presented a holistic view of health that reflected the interplay among the psychological, social, spiritual, and physical aspects of human life.

A holistic view of health focuses on the interrelationship of all the parts that make up a whole person. Jan Christian Smuts (1926) first introduced the concept of **holism** in modern Western thought by emphasizing the harmony between people and nature. When health is considered holistically, individual health practices must be taken into account. Health practices are culturally determined and include nutritional habits, type and amount of exercise and rest, how one copes with stress, quality of interpersonal relationships, expression of spirituality, and numerous other lifestyle factors. As a profession, nurses embrace a holistic view of health.

Parsons (1959) defined health as an individual's optimum ability to perform his or her roles and tasks

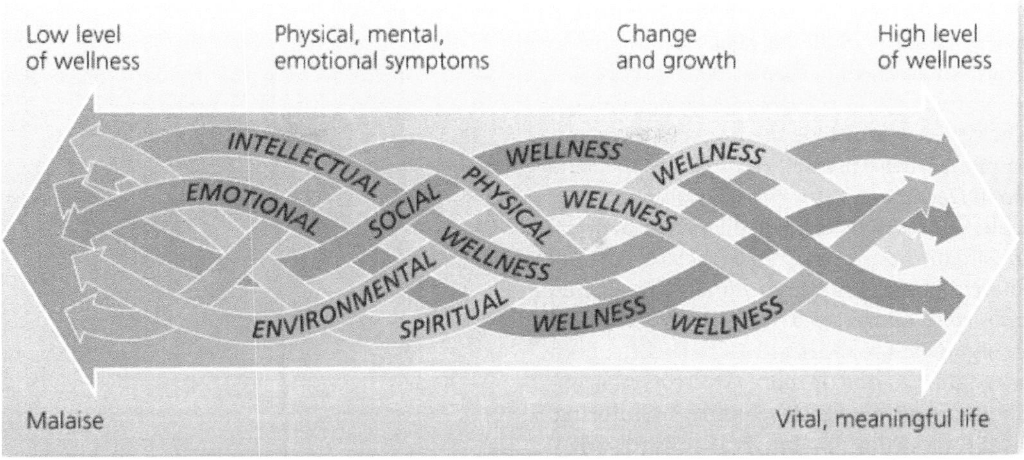

Fig. 8.4 The wellness continuum. The wellness continuum shown here has six interrelated dimensions that contribute to overall wellness. (Used with permission from Fahey T, Insel P, Roth: *Fit & Well: Core Concepts and Labs in Physical Fitness and Wellness, 13e* McGraw Hill.)

effectively. This definition focused on the roles individuals assume in life and the impact health or illness has on the fulfillment of those roles. A few examples of roles that are familiar may include the student role, the parent role, the provider role, and the friend role. One's health influences how well and the extent to which people carry out their roles in life.

Health has been described as the opposite of illness (Dunn, 1959). In his classic text *High-Level Wellness,* Dunn (1961) described health as a continuum with high-level wellness at one end and death at the other. He described high-level wellness as functioning at maximum potential in an integrated way within the environment. An example of maximizing the potential for health under extreme conditions occurred in Chile, where miners were trapped deep in a collapsed mine for 70 days from August to October 2010. Believed to be dead for 17 days, the men were discovered alive by rescuers who drilled a narrow-bore hole, which became the way that food, water, letters from families, Bibles, and other materials were delivered. Under horribly hot and dark conditions, these men supported each other, got exercise, and kept to a routine for more than two months as a rescue operation was implemented. The world celebrated as, one by one, they were brought to the surface, surprisingly vigorous and in good health. Only one miner, the oldest and who also had silicosis (lung fibrosis from inhaling silica dust), needed oxygen as he emerged. After short hospitalizations for observation, all the men returned home. Using Dunn's definition, and considering the environment in which these men were confined, they may have attained high-level wellness.

Pender and colleagues (2006) described health promotion as "approach behavior," whereas prevention is "avoidance behavior" (p. 5). This may be a useful concept for nurses to keep in mind when seeking to help patients expand their positive potential for health.

A National Health Initiative: *Healthy People*

Healthy People is a remarkable national initiative to improve the health of the nation. National objectives are introduced every 10 years, providing the agenda for improving the health of Americans. The *Healthy People* initiative was an unprecedented cooperative effort that grew out of the 1979 U.S. Surgeon General's report on health promotion and disease prevention titled *Healthy People.* That report laid the foundation for a national prevention agenda. Federal, state, and territorial governments, as well as hundreds of private, public, and not-for-profit organizations and concerned individuals, worked together for the first time ever. These partnerships resulted in *Healthy People 2000,* an effort designed to stimulate a national disease prevention and health promotion agenda to improve significantly the health of all Americans in the last decade of the 20th century. On

September 6, 1990, former U.S. Secretary of Health and Human Services Louis W. Sullivan released a report to the United States titled *Healthy People 2000.* He reported that progress on priority areas was mixed, but enough success was achieved to continue the project.

The third phase of the project, *Healthy People 2020,* was launched in December 2010. It was developed by the Healthy People Consortium, a huge alliance of national membership organizations and state health, mental health, substance abuse, and environmental agencies. *Healthy People 2020* addresses a set of forty-two topic areas that are significant to the health of the public. Each topic area is assigned to one or more government agencies, which are responsible for developing, monitoring, and periodically reporting on progress toward objectives. The initiative has partners from all sectors. The next edition, *Healthy People 2030,* is now published, and includes 355 measurable objectives (U.S. Department of Health and Human Services: Healthy People 2030, 2021).

Healthy People offers a simple but powerful idea: provide health objectives in a format that enables diverse groups to combine their efforts and work as a team. It is a road map to better health for all and can be used by many different people, states, communities, professional organizations, and groups to improve health. Partners across groups are encouraged to integrate *Healthy People* objectives into their programs, special events, publications, and meetings. When federal, state, and local health entities combine their efforts, improvements in the health of citizens can be made. However, convincing individual Americans to change their lifestyles, even when doing so would result in improved health, is a challenge. Changing health beliefs and health behaviors is a slow process. You can learn more about *Healthy People 2020* and *Healthy People 2030* online at https://www.healthypeople.gov/.

Another effort to improve health, the Institute for Alternative Futures, founded in 1977, created the *Public Health 2030* project and published a report in 2014 with recommendations for making sure that public health agencies continue to fulfill their mission to protect the health of the public. Challenges to public health include chronic disease and obesity, climate change, and cuts in spending at the state and federal levels. This report noted that 70% of the variance in individuals' health is explained by socioeconomic and environmental determinants, whereas only 15% to 20% of longevity can be attributed to clinical care. This report made a compelling case for addressing other determinants of health than simply access to health care. The Institute closed at the end of 2019, but its work is stored and available publicly in an Internet archive at https://archive-it.org/home/alt-futures.

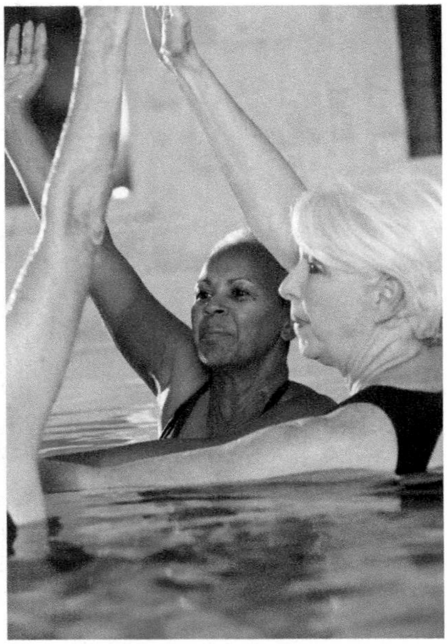

Fig. 8.5 People of all ages are recognizing the benefits of regular exercise. (Photo used with permission from iStockphoto.)

Health Beliefs and Health Behaviors

Health is affected by health beliefs and health behaviors. **Health behaviors** include those choices and habitual actions that promote or diminish health, such as eating habits, frequency of exercise, use of tobacco products and alcohol, sexual practices, and adequacy of rest and sleep (Fig. 8.5). Much is known about health-promoting behaviors, and this information has been available to the public for many years. Yet people do not easily change behaviors even when they know they should. Several theories help explain why people change their health behaviors, or why they do not.

Health Beliefs Model

Rosenstock (1966, 1990) was one of the first scholars interested in determining why some people change their health behaviors whereas others do not. For example, when the surgeon general's report on smoking first came out in 1960, some people immediately quit smoking. Over the years, evidence of the health risks of smoking has accumulated and been widely communicated, yet individuals still smoke. Rosenstock wondered why. He formulated a model of health beliefs that illustrates how people behave in relationship to health maintenance activities and has worked to refine it for three decades. Rosenstock's health beliefs model included three components:

1. An evaluation of one's vulnerability to a condition and the seriousness of that condition
2. An evaluation of how effective the health maintenance behavior might be
3. The presence of a trigger event that precipitates the health maintenance behavior

Using Rosenstock's health beliefs model, smokers choose to participate in a stop-smoking program depending on their perception of smoking-related heart disease and their personal susceptibility to it. If, because of family history, they believe that they are susceptible to heart disease and that it may cause premature death, and if they believe that not smoking will substantially reduce that risk, they are likely to participate in the program. If, however, the stop-smoking program is at an inconvenient location, scheduled at an inconvenient time, or not affordable, they are less likely to participate. If a sibling who also smokes has a massive heart attack, they may be motivated to attend the stop-smoking program despite the inconvenience and cost. The illness of their sibling is what Rosenstock called *a cue to action,* or a trigger event. A trigger event propels a previously unmotivated individual into changing health behaviors. You can see that decisions made about whether to take the COVID-19 can be at least in part explained by the health beliefs model.

Self-Efficacy and Health-Related Behaviors

Albert Bandura (1997), a cognitive psychologist, developed an approach designed to assist people to exercise influence over their own health-related behaviors. He observed that whether people considered altering detrimental health habits depended on their belief in themselves as having the ability to modify their own behavior. He labeled this belief "perceived self-efficacy." High belief in one's self-efficacy leads to efforts to change, whereas low perceived self-efficacy leads to lack of effort to change.

Bandura identified four components needed for an effective program of lifestyle change: information, skill development, skill enhancement through guided practice and feedback, and creating social supports for change (Bandura, 1992). Using Bandura's model, a man wishing to stop smoking needs knowledge of the potential dangers of smoking; guidance on how to translate concern into action; extensive practice and opportunities to perfect new, nonsmoking skills; and strong involvement in a social network supportive of nonsmoking.

Locus of Control and Health-Related Behaviors

The locus of control concept proposed that people tend to be influenced by either an internal or external view of control. People who believe that their health is internally controlled—that is, by what they themselves do—are said to have an internal locus of control. Those who believe their health is determined by outside factors or chance are said to have an external locus of control. A number of studies have hypothesized that internally controlled people tend to see themselves as responsible for their own health status and are therefore more amenable to change. Research findings have been inconsistent, however.

Nurses and Health Beliefs Models

Many other models of health beliefs and health behaviors exist, ranging from simple to complex. Identifying the key to motivating people to improve their health choices and behaviors remains a mystery. No single theory of behavior has yet fully explained the way people make decisions about their own health, nor is a single theory likely to. Nurses, however, should recognize the following:

1. Health is relative, constantly changing, and affected by genetics, environment, behaviors, personal beliefs, and cultural beliefs.
2. Health affects the entire person—physically, socially, psychologically, and spiritually.
3. Individuals' health beliefs are powerful and influence how they respond to efforts to change their health behaviors.
4. Individuals needing or desiring change may lack knowledge, motivation, sense of self-efficacy, and support to implement change.
5. Increased knowledge does not always help change health behavior, which may persist in spite of increased knowledge.

6. Various models of health beliefs can be used to assess individual, family, and group readiness to change.
7. Change is often incremental and usually very slow. Multiple interventions may be necessary to bring about behavior change, and even then only modest changes may result.
8. Patients, healthcare providers, and population-focused entities such as public health programs mutually share the burden of action.

"Dr. Google" and the Influence of the Internet

In early 2012 the Canadian newspaper *Edmonton Journal* ran a headline that read: "Dr. Google not always best source, Edmonton parents advised" (Withey, 2012). This newspaper feature described the challenges of sorting through the numerous studies and health information "floating around" on the Internet. One mother cited in this article bemoaned the amount of health information and opinions available online, describing it as "crippling."

In 2017 more than 4.1 billion people—54.4% of the world's population—were Internet users; in the United States alone, 345 million people were Internet users—more than 95% of the population (Internet World Stats, 2018). The Build America Act, passed by the 117th Congress and signed into law by President Joe Biden in November, 2021, included specific language to improve access to broadband Internet in rural areas, for low income families and tribal communities.

Virtually every aspect of life has a presence on the Internet. People shop, make travel and restaurant reservations, and download music, movies, and books. Social media dominates the Internet to the extent that the verbs "follow," "unfollow," and "block" are now commonly associated with social media. In addition, the venerable *Oxford Dictionary* added words such as "hyper-connected," "binge-watch," and "tech-savvy" that reflect the language that has sprung up around digital technology and viewing habits.

With tens of thousands of health information websites and social media platforms where individuals post their own health experiences and opinions with just a few clicks, Americans have access to more information than has ever before been available to consumers. With this additional information, patients are demanding to be equal partners in making healthcare decisions once decided only by their providers. Providers encounter patients every day who come to appointments with printed results of online research and advice or with links or apps on smartphones, and which include widely divergent information that can be hard for patients to decipher. Some of it is excellent; some is, at best, worthless; some is reckless; and some is dangerous. This phenomenon was particularly in focus during the COVID-19 pandemic, when it became difficult to decipher wave after wave of information and to discern accurate information from disinformation.

"Cyberchondria" is a new word that some use to refer to the propensity of certain people to believe that they suffer from a variety of diseases they read about online, a form of hypochondria. *Cyberchondria* literally means "online concern about health." Mathes and colleagues defined cyberchondria as a "clinical phenomenon in which repeated Internet searches regarding medical information result in excessive concerns about physical health" and is associated with health anxiety symptoms (2018, p. 204). Box 8.2 contains some information to improve the likelihood of obtaining valid health information from online sources.

Nurses can help patients determine which sites are useful and provide sound information and safe advice. Sharing legitimate websites and guidelines for assessing the quality of information is a way to help patients become better consumers of online health data. This means that nurses themselves must be knowledgeable and stay up-to-date on both helpful and unhelpful websites specific to their practice setting and patient population. Nurses also should be supportive of patients when they question traditional advice, citing the Internet as their source. This means that they have an interest in their health and are asserting their autonomy in managing at least some aspects of their own care. These conversations are opportunities to correct misinformation, if needed.

Visit Evolve for WebLinks related to the content of this chapter (http://evolve.elsevier.com/Black/professional).

Devising a Personal Plan for High-Level Wellness

Each individual nurse has a personal definition of health, certain health beliefs, and individual health behaviors. How nurses view health behaviors in their own lives affects nursing practice, both directly and indirectly. The personal health practices of nurses play a direct role in their effectiveness in counseling patients on health-related matters. Patients are more likely to adopt

BOX 8.2 Assessing Health-Related Sites on the Internet

1. Determine who sponsors the site. This should be disclosed on the site itself.
2. Be skeptical. Evaluate the source to determine whether there is self-interest on the part of the sponsor. Example: a drug company promoting one of its products.
3. Make sure the author's name is clearly indicated, including credentials. Is the author qualified on this topic? For whom does the author work?
4. What is the purpose of the site—to inform or to sell something? This is a very important distinction to make.
5. Does the site include a date and information about its last revision?
6. Is there editorial review of the content by a reputable authority or professional peers?
7. Does the material consist of scientific information rather than testimonials?
8. Determine who operates the website. University, government, and reputable medical organization sites may be more objective and less commercial than those run by companies or individuals trying to make a profit.
9. Is the information unbiased, and are you referred to other sources that can validate it?
10. For chat rooms and message boards, go online and "lurk" before getting involved. Monitor conversations and read posts before deciding whether you want to participate.
11. Determine whether the group has a moderator who controls those who monopolize the site or make commercial pitches. A moderated board will usually monitor inappropriate behavior and offensive language.
12. For interactive sites, be sure to read and understand the privacy policy.
13. Until you are confident about the quality of information, cross-check it with print and electronic sources, and discuss it with your healthcare provider.
14. Use the U.S. Department of Health and Human Services' Healthfinder site to find online support groups(www.healthfinder.gov). Note that the .gov indicates a site operated by the government. Its content is typically of high quality.
15. Be highly suspicious of reports of "miracle" cures. Rumors and unsupported claims are rampant online and can cause tremendous harm. Remember that a claim that is too good to be true usually is.

Adapted from Chase M: Health journal: a guide for patients who turn to the Web for solace and support, *Wall Street Journal, Sept. 17, 1999,* p. B1; Beyea SC: Evaluating evidence found on the Internet, *AORN J* 72 (5):906–910, 2000; and Ahmann E: Supporting families' savvy use of the Internet for health research, *Pediatr Nurs* 26 (4):419–423, 2000.

health-related behaviors such as exercising regularly and maintaining a healthy weight when the healthcare provider promoting these behaviors also engages in them. Yet nurses' own health behaviors are far from exemplary. In 2011 researchers reported that in a sample of 2103 nurses, 55% had a BMI in the overweight/obese range, and was in part attributed in job stress and difficult work schedules, including long hours (Han, Trinkoff, Storr and Geiger-Brown, 2011).

Nurses have a professional responsibility to model positive health behaviors in their own lives and, like everyone, have a personal responsibility to take care of their health to the best of their ability. The American Nurses Association (ANA) has a *Healthy Nurse, Healthy Nation™ Grand Challenge* (https://www.healthynursehealthynation.org) that encourages nurses to identify and act on personal and workplace health risks (ANA, 2021). Being or becoming a healthy role model may require some effort. If you are not the positive role model for health that you would like to be, Box 8.3 can help you get started.

NURSING: FORMING THE MEANINGFUL WHOLE

Nursing integrates concepts from person, environment, and health to form a meaningful whole. See Fig. 8.1 for a depiction of the relationships among nursing's major concepts and how they overlap. This overlap creates nursing's sphere of interest and influence. This is termed the *holistic approach* to nursing.

Holistic Nursing

Holistic nursing care nourishes the whole person, that is, the body, mind, and spirit. Not surprisingly, the root for *nurse* and *nurture* is the same Latin word, *nutrire*, which means "to nourish." Eight factors contribute to a holistic approach to nursing:

1. Nursing is an example of an open system that freely interacts with, influences, and is influenced by external and internal forces.
2. Nursing is the provision of healthcare services that focuses on assisting people in maintaining health,

BOX 8.3 Self-Assessment: Developing a Personal Plan for High-Level Wellness

Nurses' personal health behaviors send a powerful message to consumers of nursing care. By answering the following questions, you can assess how well you are meeting your responsibilities in this area of nursing.

1. I am at a healthy weight for my height and age. yes/no
2. I eat a balanced diet, including breakfast, most days. yes/no
3. I limit my intake of saturated fats. yes/no
4. I get exercise regularly. yes/no
5. I try to sleep at least 7 hours most nights. yes/no
6. I do not smoke or use other forms of tobacco. yes/no
7. I drink alcohol in moderation or not at all and take mood-altering medication only as prescribed for me personally. yes/no
8. I work to identify and manage the sources of stress in my life. yes/no
9. I try to balance work and recreation because both are important. yes/no
10. I have friends, neighbors, and/or family members who are sources of social support for me. yes/no

Directions for scoring: If you could not honestly answer yes to all questions, you may need to set goals to work on one or more of these items.

1. On a piece of paper, begin your personal plan for high-level wellness. Write down at least two things you can do to address the "no" answers you gave to the self-assessment questions.
2. Share your health goals with one other person in your class. Make a contract with that person to serve as your "health coach."
3. Review your progress with your health coach at least once a week for the remainder of the term.

avoiding or minimizing disease and disability, restoring wellness, or achieving a peaceful death.

3. Nursing involves collaborating with patients and their families to help them cope with and adapt to situations of disequilibrium in an effort to regain homeostasis.
4. Nursing is integrally involved with people at points along the health-illness continuum.
5. Nursing care is provided regardless of diagnosis, individual differences, age, beliefs, gender identity, sexual orientation, or other factors. As a profession, nursing supports the value, dignity, and uniqueness of every person and takes their culture and belief system into consideration when planning care.
6. Nurses require advanced knowledge and skills; they also must care about their patients.
7. Nursing requires concern, compassion, respect, and warmth, as well as comprehensive, individualized care planning to facilitate patients' growth toward wellness.
8. Nursing links theory and research in an effort to answer difficult questions generated during nursing practice.

With an understanding of nursing's major concepts as a backdrop, it is important to examine the relationship of nurses' attitudes, beliefs, values, and philosophies to the way they practice. It is also useful for readers to explore philosophies of nursing developed by individuals, by divisions of nursing in hospitals, and by schools of nursing; and for readers to begin to develop their own philosophies of nursing.

BELIEFS: GUIDING NURSING BEHAVIORS

Certain beliefs have evolved during the development of professional nursing. Specific statements of beliefs have been published for more than half a century. The most recent code was generated by the members of the ANA and published in the *Code of Ethics for Nurses with Interpretive Statements* (ANA, 2015). Statements such as the *Code* exist to affirm the beliefs of the profession and to guide the practice of nursing.

A **belief** represents the intellectual acceptance of something as true or correct. Beliefs can also be described as convictions. Groupings of beliefs form codes and creeds. Beliefs are opinions that may be, in reality, true or false. They are based on attitudes that have been acquired and verified by experience. Beliefs are generally transmitted from generation to generation, are stable, and are resistant to change.

Beliefs are organized into **belief systems** that serve to guide thinking and decision making. Individuals are not necessarily aware of how their beliefs interrelate or how their beliefs affect their behavior.

Although all people have beliefs, relatively few have spent much time examining their beliefs. In nursing, it is important to know and understand one's beliefs, because the practice of nursing often challenges a nurse's beliefs. Although this conflict may create temporary discomfort, it is ultimately good because it forces nurses to consider their beliefs carefully. They have to answer the question: "Is this something I really believe, or have I accepted it because some influential person [such as a parent or teacher] said it?" Reproductive choice and abortion, advance directives, the right to die, the right to refuse treatment, and similar issues confront all members of contemporary society, most recently in issues surrounding infection mitigation practices, such masking and vaccines for COVID-19. Professional nurses must develop and refine their beliefs about these and many other issues. This is often difficult to do, but the self-awareness that follows grappling with your beliefs helps you to identify when your own opinions may be influencing the way you view a patient's situation rather than accepting the patient's point of view.

Beliefs are exhibited through attitudes and behaviors. Simply observing how nurses relate to patients, their families, and nursing peers reveals something about those nurses' beliefs. Every day nurses meet people whose beliefs are different from, or even diametrically opposed to, their own. Effective nurses recognize that they need to adopt nonjudgmental attitudes toward patients' beliefs. A nurse with a **nonjudgmental** attitude makes every effort to convey neither approval nor disapproval of patients' beliefs and respects each person's right to his or her beliefs (Fig. 8.6).

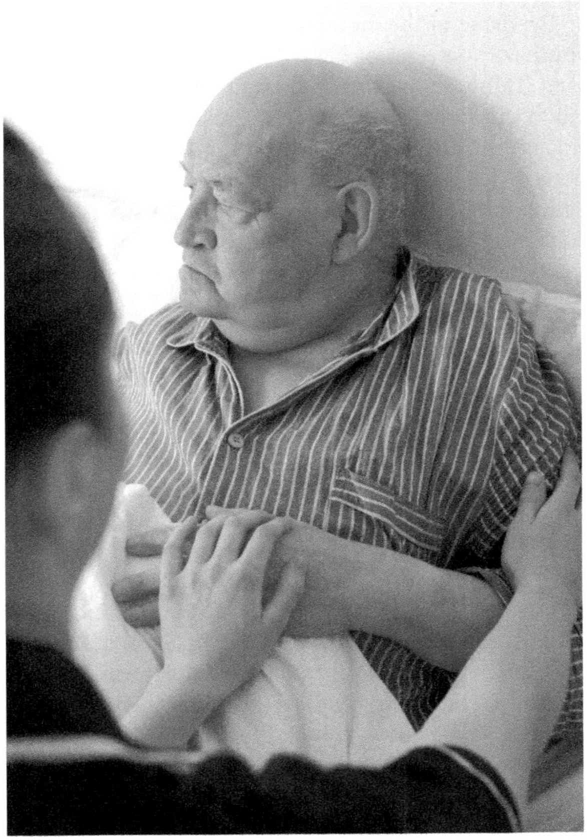

Fig. 8.6 Professional nurses maintain a posture of acceptance and calm, even when patients appear to be angry or upset. This man may simply be very sad or anxious. (Photo used with permission from iStockphoto.)

An example of differences in beliefs that directly affect nursing is the position taken by some religious groups that all healing should be left to a divine power. For members of such groups, seeking medical treatment, even lifesaving measures such as blood transfusions, insulin for diabetes, or chemotherapy for cancer, is not condoned. From time to time, there have been news reports of parents who are charged with criminal acts because they did not take a sick child to a physician. According to the advocacy group Children's Healthcare Is a Legal Duty (CHILD), about 300 children have died in this country over the past 25 years after parents withheld medical care because of religious beliefs (Johnson, 2009). After an 11-year-old girl died of untreated diabetic ketoacidosis in Wisconsin (Sataline, 2008), her parents were charged with reckless endangerment despite their claim that the charges violated their constitutional right to religious freedom. In October 2009, both parents were convicted of second-degree reckless homicide, sentenced to 10 years of probation, and ordered to spend 30 days in jail in each of the first 6 years of probation (Fitzsimmons, 2009). Even prior to the COVID-19 pandemic, a rancorous debate related to childhood vaccinations had been featured in the media, with individuals on both sides of the issue having strong opinions and beliefs. Issues such as this have an effect on patients, families, healthcare providers, public health authorities, and the court system, often creating a frenzy of media coverage and much debate on social media, usually rife with misinformation and mistrust.

By virtue of the fact that you are becoming a nurse, you have some set of beliefs about the value of health care. Think about your beliefs about issues related to blood administration, vaccines, and/or parental decisions regarding seeking or avoiding healthcare institutions. What feelings might you have if assigned to work with a family whose beliefs differ from yours? Even in your imagination, you may be able to see how difficult it can be to maintain a nonjudgmental attitude toward the beliefs of patients.

Three Categories of Beliefs

People often use the words *beliefs* and *values* interchangeably. Even experts disagree about whether they differ or are the same. Although they are related, beliefs and values are differentiated in this chapter and discussed separately.

Theorists studying belief systems have identified three main categories of beliefs:

1. Descriptive or existential beliefs are those that can be shown to be true or false. An example of a descriptive belief is "The sun will come up tomorrow morning."
2. Evaluative beliefs are those in which there is a judgment about good or bad. The belief "Advanced life support for a 90-year-old is immoral" is an example of an evaluative belief.
3. Prescriptive (encouraged) and proscriptive (prohibited) beliefs are those in which certain actions are judged to be desirable or undesirable. The belief "Every citizen of voting age should vote in every election" is a prescriptive belief, whereas the belief "People should not have sex outside of marriage" is a proscriptive belief. These two types of beliefs are closely related to values.

VALUES

Values are the freely chosen principles, ideals, or standards held by an individual, class, or group that give meaning and direction to life. A value is an abstract representation of what is right, worthwhile, or desirable. Values define ideal modes of conduct and reflect what the individual or group endorses and tries to emulate. Values, like beliefs, are relatively stable and resistant to change.

Although many people are unaware of it, values help them make small day-to-day choices, as well as important life decisions. Just as beliefs influence nursing practice, values also influence how nurses practice their profession, often without their conscious awareness. Diann B. Uustal, EdD, RN, is a prominent contemporary nurse who has written and spoken extensively about values and ethics. Dr. Uustal noted in her early work, "Everything we do, every decision we make and course of action we take is based on our consciously and unconsciously chosen beliefs, attitudes and values" (Uustal, 1985, p. 100). She wrote that nurses must give "caring attentiveness and presence" to their patients and that to do otherwise "is equivalent to psychological and spiritual abandonment" (Uustal, 1993, p. 10). Notably, Dr. Uustal survived two severe accidents that left her in pain every day; however, she is now a triathlon coach and world record setter in swimming for her age group. She is also the 2013 winner of the Growing Bolder Inspiration Award (Growing Bolder: Rebranding Aging, 2018).

Nature of Human Values

Values evolve as people mature. An individual's values today are undoubtedly different from those of 10, or even 5, years ago. Rokeach (1973, p. 3) made several assertions about the nature of human values:

1. Each person has a relatively small number of values.
2. All human beings, regardless of location or culture, possess basically the same values to differing degrees.
3. People organize their values into value systems.
4. People develop values in response to culture, society, and even individual personality traits.
5. Most observable human behaviors are manifestations or consequences of human values.

Values influence behavior; people with unclear values may lack direction, persistence, and decision-making skills. Professional nurses must have clear values because the work of nursing requires direction, persistence, and excellent decision-making skills. A number of professional nursing values are listed in Box 8.4.

Process of Valuing

Valuing is the process by which values are determined. There are three identified steps in the process of valuing: choosing, prizing, and acting.

1. *Choosing* is the cognitive (intellectual) aspect of valuing. Ideally, people choose their values freely from all alternatives after considering the possible consequences of their choices.
2. *Prizing* is the affective (emotional) aspect of valuing. People usually feel good about their values and cherish the choices they make.

BOX 8.4 Professional Nursing Values

1. Accountability and responsibility for own actions
2. Altruism
3. Balancing cure and care
4. Benevolence
5. Caring as a foundation for relationships
6. Collaborative multidisciplinary practice
7. Compassion
8. Competence
9. Concern
10. Continuous improvement of service
11. Cooperative work relationships
12. Courage
13. Dependability
14. Empathy
15. Ethical conduct
16. Flexibility
17. Focus on patient-defined quality of life
18. Health promotion
19. Holistic, person-centered care
20. Honesty and authenticity in communication
21. Humaneness
22. Humility
23. Illness prevention
24. Individualized patient care
25. Integrity—personal and professional
26. Involvement with families
27. Kindness
28. Knowledge
29. Listening attentively
30. Nonjudgmental attitude
31. Objectivity
32. Openness to learning
33. Partnerships with patients
34. Patient advocacy
35. Patient education
36. Presence (being fully present)
37. Promotion of health
38. Promotion of patient self-determination and patient preferences
39. Providing care regardless of patient's ability to pay
40. Quality care—physical, emotional, spiritual, social, intellectual
41. Reliability
42. Respect for each person's dignity and worth
43. Responsibility
44. Responsiveness
45. Sensitivity
46. Sharing decision making
47. Sharing self through nursing interventions
48. Stewardship; responsible use of resources
49. Subordination of self-interest
50. Support of fellow nurses
51. Teamwork
52. Trust in self, others, and the institution

Courtesy Diann B. Uustal, personal communication, 2006.

3. *Acting* is the kinesthetic (behavioral) aspect of valuing. When people affirm their values publicly by acting on their choices, they make their values part of their behavior. A real value is acted on consistently in behavior.

All three steps must be taken, or the process of valuing is incomplete (Uustal, 2009). For example, a professional nurse might believe that learning is a lifelong process and that nurses have an obligation to keep up with new developments in the profession. This nurse would choose to take continuing education beyond the minimum required for license renewal and appreciate the consequences of the choice. If the nurse follows through consistently with behaviors such as reading journals, attending conferences, and seeking out other learning opportunities, continuing to learn can be seen as a true value in their life.

Values Clarification

Nurses, as well as people in other helping professions, need to understand their values. This is the first step in self-awareness, which is important in maintaining a nonjudgmental approach to patients.

Considering your reactions to the following statements can help in beginning to identify some nursing values you hold:

1. Patients should always be told the truth about their diagnoses.
2. Nurses, if asked, should assist terminally ill patients to die.
3. Infants with severe congenital defects should be kept alive, regardless of their future quality of life.
4. Nurses should never accept gifts from patients.
5. A college professor should receive a heart transplant before a homeless person does.
6. Nurses should be role models of healthy behavior.

BOX 8.5 Clarifying Your Values

Once you have identified a value, it is important to assess its significance to you and to clarify your willingness to act on the value. The following clarifying questions are organized based on the steps of the valuing process and can help you answer questions about what you value. First, identify a value (or values) that is (are) important to you. Write your value(s) below:

1. ______________________________
2. ______________________________
3. ______________________________
4. ______________________________

Next, use the questions below to assess the importance of a belief or attitude and to determine whether it is a value. Rephrase the questions to suit your own style of conversation.

1. Choosing Freely
   1. Am I sure I have thought about this value and chosen to believe it myself?
   2. Who first taught me this value?
   3. How do I know I am "right"?
2. Choosing Among Alternatives
   1. What other alternatives are possible?
   2. Which alternative has the most appeal for me and why?
   3. Have I thought much about this value/alternative?
3. Choosing After Considering the Consequences
   1. What consequences do I think might occur as a result of my holding this value?
   2. What "price" will I pay for my position?
   3. Is this value worth the "price" I might pay?
4. Complement to Other Values
   1. Does this value "fit" with my other values, and is it consistent with them?
   2. Am I sure this value does not conflict with other values I deem important to me?
5. Prize and Cherish
   1. Am I proud of my position and value? Is this something I feel good about?
   2. How important is this value to me?
   3. If this were not one of my values, how different would my life be?
6. Public Affirmation
   1. Am I willing to speak out for this value?
7. Action
   1. Am I willing to put this value into action?
   2. Do I act on this value? When? How consistently?
   3. Is this a value that can guide me in other situations?
   4. Would I want others who are important to me to follow this value?
   5. Do I think I will always believe this? How committed to this value am I?
   6. Am I willing to do anything about this value?
   7. How do I know this value is "right"? Are my values ethical?

From Uustal DB: *Clinical ethics and values: issues and insights in a changing healthcare environment,* East Greenwich, RI, 1993, Educational Resources in Healthcare. Reprinted with permission.

As you react both emotionally and intellectually to these statements, something about your personal and professional values is revealed. Determining where you stand on these and other nursing issues is an important step in clarifying your values. A variety of values clarification exercises have been developed to stimulate self-reflection and help people understand their values. Box 8.5 contains a values clarification exercise you may want to complete to assist you further in understanding the valuing process.

Values Undergirding Nursing's Social Policy Statement

Professional groups, such as nursing, have a collective identity that is fostered by professional organizations. The ANA sets forth the values that undergird the profession through the document *Nursing's Social Policy Statement: The Essence of the Profession*, last revised in 2010 (ANA, 2010). This document is published from time to time and is designed to serve as a resource for nurses in various practice settings, in education, and in research. It guides nursing practice and informs others, including the public, about nursing's social responsibility. The social policy statement sets forth several underlying values and assumptions on which the statement is based:

1. Humans manifest an essential unity of mind, body, and spirit.
2. Human experience is contextually and culturally defined.
3. Health and illness are human experiences. The presence of illness does not preclude health, nor does optimal health preclude illness.
4. The interaction between the nurse and patient occurs within the context of the values and beliefs of both persons.

5. Public policy and the healthcare delivery system influence the health and well-being of society and professional nursing.

Chapter 7 contains more about values and their relationship to nursing practice.

PHILOSOPHIES AND THEIR RELATIONSHIP TO NURSING CARE

Philosophy is defined as the study of the principles underlying conduct, thought, and the nature of the universe. A simple explanation of philosophy is that it entails a search for meaning in the universe. You may have learned about philosophers such as Plato, Aristotle, Hypatia, Bacon, Kant, Hegel, Kierkegaard, Nietzsche, Descartes, Arendt, and others in general education courses. These philosophers were searching for the underlying principles of reality and truth. Nursing philosophies and theories often derive from or build on the concepts identified by these and other philosophers.

Philosophy begins when someone contemplates, or wonders about, something. If a group of friends sometimes sits and discusses the relationship between men and women and ponders the differences in men's and women's natures and approaches to life, one might say that they were developing a philosophy about male and female ways of being. It is important to remember that philosophy is not the exclusive domain of a few individuals identified as "philosophers"; everyone has a personal philosophy of life that is unique.

People develop personal philosophies as they mature, usually without being aware of it. These philosophies serve as blueprints or guides and incorporate each individual's value and belief systems. Nurses' personal philosophies interact directly with their philosophies of nursing and influence professional behaviors.

Branches of Philosophy

Before examining professional philosophies, consider the discipline of philosophy itself. Philosophy has been divided into specific areas of study. This section reviews six branches: epistemology, logic, aesthetics, ethics, politics, and metaphysics.

1. Epistemology is the branch of philosophy dealing with the theory of knowledge itself. The epistemologist attempts to answer such questions as "What can be known?" and "What constitutes knowledge?" Epistemology attempts to determine how we can know whether our beliefs about the world are true.
2. Logic is the study of proper and improper methods of reasoning. In logic, the nature of reasoning itself is the subject. Logic attempts to answer the question, "What should our thinking methods be in order to reach true conclusions?" Chapter 11 presents a method of logical thinking that nurses use to plan and implement effective patient care, called the *nursing process*.
3. Aesthetics is the study of what is beautiful. It attempts to answer the question, "Why do we find things beautiful?" Painting, sculpture, music, dance, and literature are all associated with beauty. Judgments about what is beautiful, however, differ from individual to individual and culture to culture. For example, Eastern music may be difficult to understand or appreciate by Western listeners and vice versa.
4. Ethics is the branch of philosophy that studies standards of conduct. It attempts to answer the question, "What is the nature of good and evil?" Moral principles and values make up a system of ethics. Behavior depends on moral principles and values. Ethics, therefore, underlies the standards of behavior that govern us as individuals and as nurses. Bioethics is a term describing the branch of ethics that deals with biologic issues. Bioethics and nursing ethics are complex areas of study that are explored in Chapter 7.
5. Politics, in the context of a discussion of philosophy, means the area of philosophy that deals with the regulation and control of people living in society. Political philosophers study the conditions of society and suggest recommendations for improving these conditions. They work to answer the question, "What makes good governments?"
6. Metaphysics is the consideration of the ultimate nature of existence, reality, human experience, and the universe. Metaphysicians believe that through contemplation we can come to a more complete understanding of reality than science alone can provide. They ask the question "What is the meaning of life?" and explore the fundamental nature of all reality.

Philosophies of Nursing

Philosophies of nursing are statements of beliefs about nursing and expressions of values in nursing that are used as bases for thinking and acting. Most philosophies of nursing are built on a foundation of beliefs about people, environment, health, and nursing. Each of these four foundational concepts of nursing is discussed in some detail earlier in this chapter.

Individual Philosophies

If asked, most nurses could list their beliefs about nursing, but it is doubtful that many have written a formal philosophy of nursing. They are influenced daily, however, by their unwritten, informal philosophies. It is useful to go through the process of writing down one's own professional philosophy and revising it from time to time. Comparing recent and earlier versions can reveal professional and personal growth over time. It is also helpful to read one's philosophy of nursing from time to time to make sure daily behaviors are consistent with deeply held beliefs. Box 8.6 contains one nurse's philosophy of nursing and contains a guide for you to develop your own philosophy.

Collective Philosophies

Although few individuals write down their nursing philosophies, it is common for hospitals and schools of nursing to express their collective beliefs about nursing in written philosophies. In fact, both hospitals and schools of nursing are required by their accrediting bodies to develop statements of philosophy. Philosophic statements should be relevant to the setting. They are intended to guide the practice of nurses employed in that setting. Examining some of these statements clarifies what constitutes a collective philosophy of nursing.

BOX 8.6 Developing Your Own Philosophy of Nursing

This is an example of one nurse 's philosophy of nursing. Read it carefully, and then- use the following guide to develop your own philosophy.

1. I believe that the essence of nursing is caring about and caring for human beings who are unable to care for themselves. I believe the core of nursing is the nurse-patient relationship and that through that relationship I can make a difference in the lives of others at a time when they are most vulnerable.
2. Human beings generally do the best they can. When they are uncooperative, critical, or otherwise difficult, it is usually because they are frightened; therefore I will remain professional and nondefensive and try to understand the patient's perception of the situation. I will be a trustworthy advocate for my patients.
3. I realize that my cultural background affects how I deliver nursing care and that patients' cultural backgrounds affect how they perceive and receive my care. I try to learn as much as I can about each individual's cultural beliefs and preferences and individualize care accordingly.
4. My vision for myself as a nurse is that I will provide the best care I can to all patients, regardless of their financial situation, social status, lifestyle choices, or spiritual beliefs. I will collaborate with my patients, their families, and my healthcare colleagues and work cooperatively with them, valuing and respecting what each brings to the situation.
5. I am individually accountable for the care I provide, for what I fail to do and to know; therefore I will be a lifelong learner and actively seek opportunities to stay current in my practice.
6. I will strive for a balance of personal and professional responsibilities. This means I will take care of myself physically, emotionally, socially, and spiritually so I can continue to be an effective nurse.

Use This Guide to Write Your Own Your Philosophy of Nursing

Purpose: To write a beginning philosophy of nursing that reflects the beliefs and values of ____________

____

____________________ [your name and date]

I chose nursing as my profession because nursing is ____

____________________.

I believe that the core of nursing is ____________

____________________.

I believe that the focus of nursing is ____________

____________________.

My vision for myself as a nurse is that I will ________

____________________.

To live out my philosophy of nursing, every day I must remember this about:

My patients: ____________________

____

My patients' families: ____________________

____

My professional colleagues: ____________________

____

My own health: ____________________

____

Philosophy of Nursing in a Hospital Setting or School of Nursing. When considering applying for a professional nursing position in a hospital or health-care agency, you can ask for a copy of the philosophy of nursing of that institution or find it online. Read it carefully, and make sure you accept the beliefs and values it contains, because they will influence nursing care in that setting.

An important point about philosophies of nursing is that they are dynamic; they change over time. When a collective philosophy is written, it reflects the existing values and beliefs of the particular group of people who wrote it. When the group members change, the philosophy may also change. Therefore once a collective philosophy is written, it should be "revisited" regularly and modified to reflect accurately the group's current beliefs about nursing practice.

DEVELOPING A PERSONAL PHILOSOPHY OF NURSING

Your philosophy of life, whether or not you can articulate it, is the basis of your day-to-day behavior. It consists of the principles that underlie your thinking and conduct. Developing a philosophy of nursing is not merely an academic exercise required by accrediting bodies. Having a written philosophy can help guide nurses in the daily decisions they must make in nursing practice.

Writing a philosophy is not a complex, time-consuming task—it simply requires that you write down your beliefs and values about nursing, answering the questions: "What is nursing?" and "Why do I practice nursing the way I do?" Whether individual or collective, a philosophy should provide direction and promote effectiveness.

CONCEPTS AND CHALLENGES

- ***Concept:*** Knowledge of systems and human motivation can be used to understand nursing's major concepts. Persons are unique open systems who are motivated by needs.
  Challenge: Maslow's hierarchy of needs consists of five levels that range from basic physiologic needs, which are common to all people, to self-actualization, which is attained by few. This is a useful framework to understand human motivation.
- ***Concept:*** Environment consists of all the circumstances, influences, and conditions that affect an individual. The physical environment and family, cultural, social, and community systems all affect one's health.
  Challenge: In addition to understanding the effects of the environment on an individual's health, nurses recognize that health affects the way one interacts with his or her environment.
- ***Concept:*** The Internet has become a significant source of health information, the quality of which varies widely.
  Challenge: In a respectful way and with appreciation for patients' desire to be involved in their own care, nurses need to help patients filter factual information from disinformation they read on websites.
- ***Concept:*** Nursing integrates person, environment, and health into a meaningful whole in an open system.
  Challenge: This holistic integration of person, environment, and health does not explain patients' health experiences but rather gives nurses a way of considering the wide variety of factors that affect persons' health at any one time.
- ***Concept:*** Beliefs and values influence how nurses practice their profession and form the basis of one's philosophy of nursing.
  Challenge: Identifying one's beliefs and values will help shape one's philosophy of nursing, which in turn shapes and guides practice.
- ***Concept:*** As they develop and progress professionally, nurses are likely to change their views about patients, care, and nursing, and their values and beliefs may change.
  Challenge: Philosophies are not static; they are changed and adapted as nurses mature and become more experienced.

IDEAS FOR FURTHER EXPLORATION

1. Consider your own family system. What are the family equivalents of inputs, throughputs, subsystems, suprasystems, outputs, evaluation, and feedback? Does your family tend to be an open or a closed system?

2. Describe Maslow's hierarchy of needs, and place yourself on the hierarchy today, on your first day of college, and when you were in middle school. Were you at a different level each time? Consider what factors—internal and external—may have been involved in your placement at each of these times. If possible, compare and discuss your findings with at least one other person.
3. What are the factors that influence your personal health behaviors? Make a list of your health behaviors, including those that promote health and those that do not. Think about the reasons you continue both healthy and not-so-healthy behaviors. Identify factors that could influence you to make decisions that support good health.
4. Select a chronic or acute illness or health condition and do an online search. Examine websites generated by your search, assessing them for accuracy and safety. What items on the site do you consider safe, and why? Why do you consider others as not safe?
5. Conduct an assessment of your community in terms of one of the following factors that affect health: availability of jobs, quality of public education, availability of health services, environmental hazards, and quality of air and water. What is the effect of this factor on the health of the community's citizens? What can you do to improve the health of your community?
6. Find out what your state and community are doing to link their health objectives to those of the *Healthy People* initiatives.
7. Name two of your health-related values. How did these become your values? Describe how you expect these values to influence your nursing practice.
8. Read "Developing Your Own Philosophy of Nursing" in Box 8.6. Then identify at least 10 of that nurse's professional values, using the list in Box 8.4, "Professional Nursing Values." Can you identify other values that are not listed?
9. Obtain the philosophy statement of the faculty of your school of nursing. What concepts are included? Which beliefs do you agree with and disagree with? (Your school may have a vision and mission statement rather than a philosophy. Although they are not usually as detailed, they can be useful in identifying a school's priorities.)
10. Using the work sheet in Box 8.6, write a beginning personal philosophy of nursing. Share your philosophy with one other person.
11. How does articulating one's philosophy of nursing influence a nurse's practice? What if a nurse has never thought about a philosophy?

REFERENCES

American Nurses Association (ANA): *Code of ethics for nurses with interpretive statements*, Washington, DC, 2015, American Nurses Publishing.

American Nurses Association (ANA): *Healthy Nurse, Healthy Nation*, 2021. [website]. Available at https://www.healthynursehealthynation.org.

American Nurses Association (ANA): *Nursing's social policy statement: the essence of the profession*, Washington, DC, 2010, American Nurses Publishing.

Bandura A: A social cognitive approach to the exercise of control over AIDS infection editor. In DiClemente RJ, editor: *Adolescents and AIDS: A Generation in Jeopardy*, Newbury Park, CA, 1992, Sage Publications.

Bandura A: *Self-Efficacy: Exercise of Control*, New York, 1997, WH Freeman.

Beyea SC: Evaluating evidence found on the Internet, *AORN J*, 72(5), 2000.

Centers for Disease Control and Prevention (CDC): Births: final data for 2016, *CDC Natl Vital Stat Rep* 67(4):2018.

Dunn HL: High-level wellness for man and society, *Am J Public Health* 49(6):786–792, 1959.

Dunn HL: *High-Level Wellness*, Thorofare, NJ, 1961, Slack.

Fitzsimmons EG: *Wisconsin couple sentenced in death of their sick child*, Oct 7, 2009, New York Times A–16.

Growing Bolder: *Rebranding aging: Diann Uustal*, 2018. [website]. Available at www.growingbolder.com/diann-uustal-892799/.

Han K, Trinkoff AM, Storr CL, Geiger-Brown J: Job stress and work schedules in relation to nurse obesity, *J Nurs Adm* 41:488–495, 2011. doi:10.1097/NNA.0b013e3182346fff.

Health Care Without Harm: *Mission and goals*, 2021. [website]. Available at https://noharm-uscanada.org/content/us-canada/mission-and-goals.

Hoffman E: The Maslow effect: a humanist legacy for nursing, *Am Nurs Today* 3(8):36–37, 2008.

Holmes TH, Rahe RH: The social readjustment rating scale, *J Psychosom Res* 11(2):213–218, 1967.

International Monetary Fund: *World economic outlook database*, 2018. [website]. Available at https://www.imf.org/external/pubs/ft/weo/2017/01/weodata/index.aspx.

Internet World Stats: *Usage and population statistics: world internet usage and population statistics*, 2018. [website]. Available at https://www.internetworldstats.com/stats.htm.

Investopedia: *The world's top 10 economies*, 2017. [website]. Available at https://www.investopedia.com/articles/investing/022415/worlds-top-10-economies.asp.

Johnson D: *Trials for Parents Who Chose Faith Over Medicine*, 2009, New York Times A–23.

Maslow AH: *Motivation and Personality*, 3, New York, 1987, Harper & Row.

Mathes BM, Norr AM, Allan NP, Albanese GJ, Schmidt NB: Cyberchondria: overlap with health anxiety and unique relationships with impairment, quality of life, and service utilization, *J Psychiatry Res*:204–211, 2018. doi:10.1016/j.psychres.2018.01.002 MarEpub.

Miller MA, Rahe RH: Life changes scaling for the 1990s, *J Psychosom Res* 43(3):279–292, 1997.

Parsons T: Definitions of health and illness in light of American values and social structure editor. In Jaco EG, editor: *Patients, Physicians and Illness*, New York, 1959, Free Press, pp 165–187.

Pender NJ, Murdaugh C, Parsons MA: *Health Promotion in Nursing Practice*, 5, Upper Saddle River, NJ, 2006, Prentice-Hall Health.

Pew Research Center: *Key finding about U.S. immigrants*,2020. (website). Available at: https://www.pewresearch.org/fact-tank/2020/08/20/key-findings-about-u-s-immigrants/.

Rogers C: *On Becoming a Person*, Boston, 1961, Houghton Mifflin.

Rokeach M: *The nature of human values*, New York, 1973, Free Press.

Rosenstock IM: Why people use health services, part II, *Milbank Mem Fund Q* 44(3):94–124, 1966.

Rosenstock IM: The health belief model: explaining health behavior through expectancies. In Glans K, Lewis FM, Rimer BK, editors: *Health behavior and health education: theory, research, and practice*, San Francisco, 1990, Jossey-Bass, pp 39–62.

Sataline S: A child's death and a crisis for faith, *Wall Street J our*, 2008 June 12D–1.

Smuts JC: *Holism and evolution*, New York, 1926, Macmillan.

UNESCO: *Migration and inclusive societies*, n.d. (website). Available at: https://en.unesco.org/themes/fostering-rights-inclusion/migration

U.S. Census Bureau: *National single parent day*, Press Release Number: CB21–SFS.035, 2021. (website). Available at: https://www.census.gov/newsroom/stories/single-parent-day.html.

U.S. Census Bureau. *Income and poverty in the United States: 2020*,2020. (website). Available at: https://www.census.gov/library/publications/2021/demo/p60-273.html.

U.S. Department of Health and Human Services: *Healthy People 2030*, 2021. Available at: https://www.healthypeople.gov/.

U.S. Department of Health and Human Services: *HHS poverty guidelines for 2021*,2021. (website). Available at: https://aspe.hhs.gov/poverty-guidelines.

Uustal DB: *Caring for Yourself, Caring for Others: The Ultimate Balance*, 2, East Greenwich, RI, 2009, Educational Resources in Healthcare.

Uustal DB: *Clinical Ethics and Values: Issues and Insights in a Changing Healthcare Environment*, East Greenwich, RI, 1993, Educational Resources in Healthcare.

Uustal DB: *Values and Ethics in Nursing: From Theory to Practice*, East Greenwich, RI, 1985, Educational Resources in Nursing and Holistic Health.

von Bertalanffy L: *General Systems Theory: Foundations, Development, Applications*, New York, 1968, George Braziller.

Waugh LJ: Beliefs associated with Mexican immigrant families' practice of La Cuarentena during postpartum recovery, *J Obstet Gynecol Neonat Nurs* 40:732–741, 2010.

Withey E: *Dr. Google Not Always Best Source, Edmonton Parents Advised*, 2012. (website). Retrieved from: www.edmontonjournal.com/life/Google+always+best+-source+Edmonton+parents+advised/6288462/story.html.

World Health Organization (WHO): *Constitution*, Geneva, 1947, World Health Organization.

Zuger A: *Healthy right up to the day you're not*, 2008, New York Times, Sept 30.F–3.

9

Nursing Theory: The Basis for Professional Nursing

ⓔ To enhance your understanding of this chapter, try the Student Exercises on the Evolve site at http://evolve.elsevier.com/Black/professional.

LEARNING OUTCOMES

After studying this chapter, students will be able to:

- Define philosophy, conceptual frameworks, theory, and middle-range theory.
- Consider how selected nursing theoretical works guide the practice of nursing.
- Understand how nursing philosophy or theory shapes the curriculum in schools of nursing.
- Delineate the role of nursing theory for different levels of nursing education.
- Describe the function of nursing theory in research and practice.
- Describe the need for current nursing theory to be examined critically in light of the rapid evolution of health care.
- Understand the importance of generating nursing knowledge that both applies to practice and cuts across the boundaries of disciplines.

Theory is a word often used in daily conversation, such as "I have a theory about that" or "In theory, this should work." The word *theory* in this context means the person has some idea about a phenomenon and the way this phenomenon works in the world. When people say, "I have a theory…" about a certain phenomenon or situation, they are demonstrating something about their own distinct orientation or way of seeing the world. The word *theory* is derived from the Latin and Greek word for "a viewing" or "contemplating."

Nursing as a profession has a distinct theoretical orientation to practice. This means that the practice of nursing is based on a specific body of knowledge built on theory. This body of knowledge shapes and is shaped by how nurses see the world. Parsons (1949) described theory as important because it makes a distinction between what we know and what we need to know. The word **theory** has many definitions, but generally it refers to a group of related concepts, definitions, and statements that describe a certain view of nursing **phenomena** (observable occurrences) from which to describe, explain, or predict outcomes (Chinn and Kramer, 1998). Theories represent abstract ideas rather than concrete facts. New theories are always being generated, although some theories are useful for many years. When new knowledge becomes available, theories that are no longer useful are modified or discarded. You will be reading about Sister Callista Roy's adaptation model, one that has "stood the test of time" since the 1970s; its use expanded from its origins as a curriculum framework for Bachelor of Science in Nursing (BSN) education to its current use as an organizing framework for nurses (Alligood, 2011).

So why is theory important? First, nursing as a profession is strengthened when nursing knowledge is built on sound theory. As seen in Chapter 3, one criterion for a profession is a distinct body of knowledge as the basis for practice. Nursing began its transition from a vocation to a profession and academic discipline in the 1950s (Bond et al., 2011). Nursing has knowledge distinct from but related to other disciplines such as medicine, social work, sociology, and physiology, among others. The development of nursing knowledge is the work of nurse researchers and scholars. The evolution of the profession of nursing depends on continued recognition of nursing as a scholarly academic discipline that contributes to society. In today's research environment where theory is developed and tested, collaboration across disciplines is now considered a critical approach to the development of knowledge.

Second, theory is a useful tool for reasoning, critical thinking, and decision making (Alligood, 2018). The ultimate goal of nursing theory is to support excellence in practice. Nursing practice settings are complex, and a large amount of information (data) about each patient is available to nurses. Nurses must analyze this information to make sound clinical judgments and to generate effective interventions. From organization of patient data to the development and evaluation of interventions, theory provides a guide for nurses in developing effective care. Box 9.1 shows how theory guides nursing practice.

Several words are used to describe abstract thoughts and their linkages. From the most to least abstract, these include *metaparadigm*, *philosophy*, *conceptual model* or *framework*, and *theory*. *Metaparadigm* refers to the most abstract aspect of the structure of nursing knowledge (March and McCormack, 2009). The **metaparadigm** of nursing consists of four major concepts of the discipline—person, environment, health, and nursing—discussed in Chapter 8 and addressed again in Chapter 11. In the past two decades, some scholars have suggested that caring is a major concept of the discipline central to nursing knowledge development and practice and should be included as a concept in the metaparadigm. (The arguments for and against this are beyond the scope of this chapter; however). Simply stated, these concepts comprise the metaparadigm of nursing; that is, these are the **concepts** (abstract ideas) of most importance to nursing practice and research. Nursing philosophies, models, and theories contain most or all of these concepts.

BOX 9.1 Nursing Theory and the Professional Nurse

Theory guides the professional nurse in:

1. Making sound clinical judgments based on evidence by
   a. Determining which data are important
   b. Organizing, analyzing, and understanding connections in patient data
2. Planning appropriate nursing interventions
3. Evaluating outcomes of interventions

As you read in Chapter 8, a **philosophy** is a set of beliefs about the nature of how the world works. A nursing philosophy begins to put together some or all concepts of the metaparadigm. For instance, Florence Nightingale, whose work will be considered in more detail later in this chapter, wrote *Notes on Nursing: What It Is and What It Is Not*, in which her basic philosophy of nursing is described in detail. A **conceptual model** or **framework** is a more specific organization of nursing phenomena than philosophies. As the words *model* or *framework* imply, models provide an organizational structure that makes clearer connections between concepts.

Theories are more concrete descriptions of concepts embedded in propositions. **Propositions** are statements that describe linkages between concepts and are more prescriptive; that is, they propose an outcome that is testable in practice and research. For example, Peplau's (1952/1988) book *Interpersonal Relations in Nursing* contains a theory describing very specific elements of effective interaction between the nurse and patient. Using concepts from nursing's metaparadigm, Peplau created a theory delineating elements of excellent and effective practice in psychiatric nursing. She linked abstract concepts such as health and nursing to create a concrete, useful theory for practice. Peplau's theory will be described later in this chapter.

The **primary source**—the original writings of the theorist—is the best source for in-depth understanding of the theory. In the original writings, the theorist will describe exactly what he or she is thinking and how the concepts go together. Articles written by other scholars can be helpful in explaining and interpreting primary sources. Explanatory or interpretive articles introduce students to the historical development of the philosophy, model, or theory and specify **criteria** (standards) by which to analyze, critique, and evaluate them. Articles such as these were first published in the early 1980s with a completely different purpose than the theorists' original articles. Explanatory or interpretive articles are written to contribute to the general understanding of nursing theory and theoretical developments in nursing in a unique but complementary way. Undergraduate and graduate students, faculty, and practicing nurses have found that these explanatory and interpretive articles on nursing theory make a significant contribution to their knowledge and understanding of nursing science in its own right. Many of the articles and books cited in this chapter were texts written to clarify, describe, and interpret theorists' work.

In this chapter, four types of nursing theoretical works will be presented: philosophies, conceptual models, theories, and middle-range theories. Selected works from each of these four types provide a broad overview of theory within the discipline of nursing. Then you will read about emerging contemporary thinking about nursing theory. This thinking points to the need for a shift so that nursing theory—and hence the body of knowledge that grows from theory—accounts for the increasing importance of a transdisciplinary approach to knowledge development. In other words, nurses cannot be content to develop its body of knowledge using the singular lens of nursing. This introduction is designed to help you develop a beginning understanding of nursing theory on which to build as you pursue your nursing education and career in the profession of nursing.

TABLE 9.1 Three Philosophies of Nursing: Three Different Responses to the Same Patient Situation

Florence Nightingale	What needs to be adjusted in this environment to protect the patient?
Virginia Henderson	What can I help this patient do that they would do for themselves if they could?
Jean Watson	How can I create an environment of trust, understanding, and openness so that the patient and I can work together in meeting their needs?

PHILOSOPHIES OF NURSING

Chapter 5 provided several definitions of nursing, and Chapter 8 introduced nursing philosophy and discussed its function in nursing practice and educational institutions. A philosophy provides a broad, general view of nursing that clarifies values and that expands on the definition of nursing to answer broad disciplinary questions, such as "What is nursing?" "What is the profession of nursing?" "What do nurses do?" "What is the nature of human caring?" "What is the nature of nursing practice and the development of practice expertise?" Three philosophies representing different positions in the development of nursing theory are presented here. Table 9.1 contains questions that represent the different views of the same patient situation among nurses who subscribe to the philosophies of Florence Nightingale, Virginia Henderson, and Jean Watson, whose work is presented here.

Nightingale's Philosophy

Florence Nightingale was born in 1820, in Florence, Italy. Her father was William Edward Nightingale, a wealthy English landowner; her mother was Frances Smith Nightingale, who considered it her responsibility to find suitable husbands for her daughters. Florence was close to her father, and he undertook the responsibility for her education, teaching her a classical curriculum of Greek, Latin, French, German, Italian, history, philosophy, and mathematics. At 25 years old, after deciding to remain unmarried, Florence announced her decision to go to Kaiserswerth, Germany, to study nursing, over the strong objections of her parents. At that time, nursing was considered the pursuit of working-class women. Her persistence in the face of her parents' opposition proved to be a defining characteristic across her life. This trait enabled her to accomplish work that many women of the time would have had neither the education nor willingness to achieve.

Nightingale's work represents the beginning of professional nursing as we know it today. In *Notes on Nursing: What It Is and What It Is Not* (1969; originally published in 1859), Nightingale explained her philosophy of health, illness, and the nurse's role in caring for patients. Importantly, she made a distinction between the work of nursing and the work of physicians by identifying health rather than illness as the major concern of nursing. Her writing about nursing reflected the sociohistorical context in which she lived, making a distinction between the work of nursing and the work of household servants, who were common in her day and often cared for the sick.

Nightingale's unique perspective on nursing practice focused on the relationship of patients to their surroundings. She set forth foundational principles for nursing that remain relevant to nursing practice today. For example, her description of the importance of observing the patient and recording information accurately and her principles of cleanliness still shape nursing practice today. Although unintentionally, Nightingale focused on what we now understand are the primary concepts of the metaparadigm of nursing: person (patient), health (as opposed to illness), environment (how the environment affects health and recovery from illness), and nursing (as opposed to medicine).

Using Nightingale's Philosophy in Practice

Nightingale believed that the health of patients was related to their environment. She recognized the importance of clean air and water and of adequate ventilation and sunlight and encouraged the arrangement of patients' beds so they were in direct sunlight. In her writing, she described both the necessity of a balanced diet and the nurse's responsibility to observe and record what was eaten. Cleanliness of the patient, the bed linens, and the room itself was essential. Nightingale recognized the problem of noise in hospital rooms and halls, which foreshadowed the attention given to excess noise in inpatient settings in recent years. (Historical note: in the 1960's it was common to see "Quiet: Hospital Zone" signs on roadways in the vicinity.) Rest is important in the restoration of health; Nightingale believed the sudden disruption of sleep was a serious problem. The relationship of health to the environment seems obvious today, but for nursing in the second half of the 19th century, Nightingale's work was radically different.

Nightingale recognized nursing's role in protecting patients. Nurses were newly responsible for shielding patients from possible harm by well-meaning visitors who may provide false hope, discuss upsetting news, or tire the patient with social conversation. Nightingale even suggested the nurse's responsibility for patients did not end when the nurse was off duty. This view underpins the system of primary nursing found in some settings today. Interestingly, Nightingale suggested that patients might benefit from visits by small pets, an idea that has been incorporated today in both long-term and some acute care settings.

The nurse whose practice is guided by Nightingale's philosophy is sensitive to the effect of the environment on the patient's health or recovery from illness. This philosophy provided the foundational work for theory development that proposed changing patients' environments to effect positive changes in their health. Nightingale promoted the view that nurses' primary responsibility was to protect patients by careful management of their surroundings.

Henderson's Philosophy

Virginia Henderson, whose photo is featured in Professional Profile Box 9.1 of this chapter, was born in 1897 in Kansas City, Missouri, and was named for her mother's home state to which her family returned when Henderson was 4 years old. Although she received an excellent education from a family friend who was a schoolmaster and from her father who was a former teacher, Henderson did not receive a traditional education that awarded a diploma, which delayed her entry into nursing school. During World War II, she studied under Annie Goodrich at Teachers College, Columbia University, where, after numerous interruptions, she received her bachelor's and master's degrees. By the time she died in 1996, Virginia Henderson was internationally known and regarded by many as "the Florence Nightingale of the 20th century."

Virginia Henderson's work first was published 100 years after Nightingale, at a time when efforts to clarify nursing as a profession emphasized the need to define nursing. Henderson's philosophical approach to nursing is contained in her comprehensive definition: the "unique function of the nurse … is to assist the individual, sick or well, in the performance of those activities contributing to health or its recovery (or a peaceful death) that he would perform unaided if he had the necessary strength, will or knowledge" (Henderson, 1966, p. 15). Although Henderson was recognized for many contributions to nursing throughout her long career, her early work remains particularly noteworthy and relevant, defining nursing and specifying the role of the nurse in relation to the patient. Henderson's relationship with one of her former students, who recognizes the ongoing contributions of Henderson's work to nursing, is described in Professional Profile Box 9.1.

Henderson's philosophy linked her definition of nursing that emphasized the functions of the nurse with a list of basic patient needs that are the focus of nursing care. She proposed an answer to questions similar to those addressed by Nightingale a century earlier: "What is the nursing profession?" and "What do nurses do?" Henderson described the nurse's role as that of a substitute for the patient, a helper to the patient, or a partner with the patient.

Henderson identified 14 basic needs (Box 9.2) as a general focus for patient care. She proposed that these needs shaped the fundamental elements of nursing care. The function of nurses was to assist patients if they were

PROFESSIONAL PROFILE BOX 9.1

Remembering Virginia Henderson

Although I had known Virginia Henderson from the time I was a graduate student at Yale, geography later brought us more closely together. Knowing her family lived in Virginia (mine was in Connecticut), whenever I traveled by car from North Carolina to Connecticut I called and asked if she wanted a ride back home with me, because I could drop her off in Virginia en route to North Carolina. Six times we made the 8-hour ride together. Our conversations were wide-ranging because we were both world travelers. We talked much about politics; most about nurses—"see a nurse before you go to a doctor"—as a solution to healthcare cost, quality, and access problems; some about patients—"give them their records"—as a most important patient education tool; and some about our large extended families. I was introduced to two of Virginia Henderson's sisters when they were all in their 90s. Four brothers and a sister had predeceased them, but Frances (Fanny) had maintained the old family homestead so all who could come were welcomed to stay. Come they did for over two generations of reunions, weddings, funerals, and holidays, especially Christmas.

What was most amazing to me about our time together was that Virginia Henderson never said anything to me about our profession that she had not written down somewhere for all nurses to read. Yale's School of Nursing asked me to address the topic of her writing in their Bellos Lecture the year they celebrated her 90th birthday. I read her textbook, *Principles and Practice of Nursing*, sixth edition, and discovered any number of conversations I had experienced with her over the years. In preparing the *Virginia Henderson Reader: Excellence in Nursing*, I discovered even more. Her writings are conversational, that is, completely without the jargon of the medical and nursing professions. Her description of nursing is best used by nurses to tell patients what can be expected, to paraphrase: I am here to help you do what you would do for yourself if you had the strength, will, or knowledge, and to do so for you to become free of my help as rapidly as possible. It is quite reassuring for a patient to know what the nurse is going to do.

Virginia Henderson's writings are timeless. The information in *The Nature of Nursing* and *Basic Principles of Nursing Care* is as relevant today as the day the books were written. *The Nature of Nursing* is the most important document written about nurses and nursing in the 20th century because it provided evidence of effective and efficient nursing. If you read her work, you can have a conversation with her too.

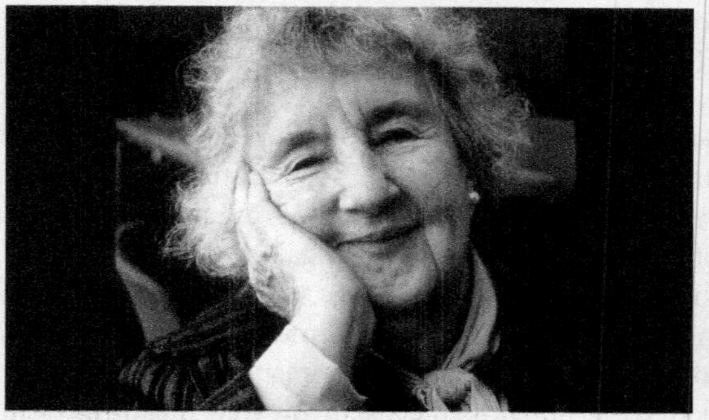

Virginia Henderson

Edward J. Halloran, PhD, RN, FAAN

BOX 9.2 Henderson's 14 Basic Needs of the Patient

1. Breathe normally.
2. Eat and drink adequately.
3. Eliminate body wastes.
4. Move and maintain a desirable position.
5. Sleep and rest.
6. Select suitable clothes—dress and undress.
7. Maintain body temperature within normal range by adjusting clothing and modifying the environment.
8. Keep the body clean and well groomed and protect the integument (skin).
9. Avoid dangers in the environment and avoid injuring others.
10. Communicate with others in expressing emotions, needs, fears, or opinions.
11. Worship according to one's faith.
12. Work in such a way that there is a sense of accomplishment.
13. Play or participate in various forms of recreation.
14. Learn, discover, or satisfy the curiosity that leads to normal development and health and use the available health facilities.

Data from Henderson, V. (1966). The nature of nursing: a definition and its implications for practice, research, and education. New York: Macmillan.

unable to perform any of these 14 functions themselves. Although these needs could be categorized as physical, psychological, emotional, sociologic, spiritual, or developmental, thoughtful analysis reveals that they represent a holistic view of human development and health.

The first nine needs emphasize the importance of care of the physical body: breathing, eating and drinking, elimination, movement and positioning, sleep and rest, suitable clothing, maintenance of suitable environment for the body temperature, cleanliness, and avoidance of danger or harm. Next, she included psychosocial needs such as communication and spirituality, including worship and faith. She concluded with three developmental needs: the need for work and the sense of accomplishment; the need for play and recreation; and the need to learn, discover, and satisfy curiosity. Henderson believed that all 14 basic needs are amenable to nursing care. They continue to be used today in philosophical statements of schools and departments of nursing.

Using Henderson's Philosophy in Practice

Nurses whose practice is consistent with Henderson's philosophy adopt an orientation to care from the perspective of the 14 basic needs. Henderson's clarity about the role and function of the nurse is a strength of her work. This philosophy is easily applied to a variety of patient care settings, from brief outpatient encounters in which a limited number of needs are addressed to a complex setting such as intensive care where patients are extremely vulnerable. Henderson used her definition of nursing and the basic needs approach in her well-known case study of a young patient who had undergone a leg amputation. Using this case, Henderson (1966) demonstrated how the nurse's role changes on a day-to-day, week-to-week, and month-to-month basis in relation to the patient's changing needs and the contributions of other healthcare providers.

Watson's Philosophy

Jean Watson is a more recent contributor to the evolving philosophy of nursing. Born in West Virginia, she earned her BSN degree from the University of Colorado in 1964, her Master of Science (MS) degree from the University of Colorado in 1966, and her doctor of philosophy (PhD) from the University of Colorado in 1973. Six years later, she published her first book, *The Philosophy and Science of Caring*. In this initial work, she called for a return to the earlier values of nursing and emphasized the caring aspects of nursing. Watson's work is recognized as human science. Caring as a theme is reflected in her other professional accomplishments, such as the Center for Human Caring at the University of Colorado in Denver, where nurses can incorporate knowledge of human caring as the basis of nursing practice and scholarship. Watson proposed 10 factors that she initially labeled as "carative" factors, a term she contrasted with *curative* to differentiate nursing from medicine. The term *Caritas Processes* replaced *carative factors* as Watson's work continued to be refined, and these processes taken together were found to be a measure of the concept of caring (DiNapoli et al., 2010). Watson's Ten Caritas Processes are listed in Box 9.3.

Watson's work (1979, 1988, 1999) addressed the philosophical question of the nature of nursing as viewed as a human-to-human relationship. She focused on the relationship of the nurse and the patient, drawing on philosophical sources for a new approach that emphasized how the nurse and patient change together through transpersonal caring. She proposed that nursing be concerned with spiritual matters and the inner knowledge of nurse and patient as they participate together in the transpersonal caring process. She equated health with harmony, resulting from unity of body, mind, and soul, for which the patient is primarily responsible. Illness or disease was equated with lack of harmony within the

BOX 9.3 Watson's 10 Caritas Processes

1. Embrace altruistic values and practice loving kindness with self and others.
2. Instill faith and hope and honor in others.
3. Be sensitive to self and others by nurturing individual beliefs and practices.
4. Develop helping-trusting-caring relationships.
5. Promote and accept positive and negative feelings as you authentically listen to another's story.
6. Use creative scientific problem-solving methods for caring decision making.
7. Share teaching and learning that addresses the individual needs and comprehension styles.
8. Create a healing environment for the physical and spiritual self which respects human dignity.
9. Assist with basic physical, emotional, and spiritual human needs.
10. Open to mystery and allow miracles to enter.

From Jean Watson, Caritas Processes refined from Inova Health. Boulder, CO. Available at www.watsoncaringscience.org.

mind, body, and soul experienced in internal or external environments (Watson, 1979). Nursing is based on human values and interest in the welfare of others and is concerned with health promotion, health restoration, and illness prevention.

Using Watson's Philosophy in Practice

Watson's caritas processes guide nurses who use transpersonal caring in practice. Caritas processes specify the meaning of the relationship of nurse and patient as human beings. Nurses are encouraged to share their genuine selves with patients. Patients' spiritual strength is recognized, supported, and encouraged for its contribution to health. In the process of transpersonal relationships, nurses develop and encourage openness to understanding of self and others. This leads to the development of trusting, accepting relationships in which feelings are shared freely and confidence is inspired. Even a core element of practice such as patient teaching can be carried out in an interpersonal manner true to the philosophy and nature of the caring relationship.

The nurse guided by Watson's work has responsibility for creating and maintaining an environment supporting human caring while recognizing and providing for patients' primary human requirements. In the end, this human-to-human caring approach leads the nurse to respect the overall meaning of life from the perspective of the patient. Watson's (1988) work formalized the theory of human caring from this philosophy. Key aspects of nursing's metaparadigm evident in Watson's work are environment (one that supports human caring), person (both the patient and the nurse), health (in terms of health promotion and illness prevention), and nursing (what nurses contribute to the encounter with the patient). Importantly, Watson's work on caring has contributed another aspect to the metaparadigm of nursing, because caring itself is now considered by many scholars to be a central concept of the discipline of nursing.

Clinical Example: Watson's Philosophy of Caring

Understanding how philosophy guides practice can be hard, but an example drawn from a nurse's clinical practice may help.

Anna, a hospice nurse, was working with a patient who was very ill with lung cancer and who had received both chemotherapy and radiation with the hope of achieving a long remission. The patient, a 60-year-old woman named Mavis, was what some people would call a "character," full of opinions that she would share with anyone who came close, still smoking, still cursing. Mavis' cancer did not respond to the various therapies and metastases developed in her brain, causing occasional seizures. Mavis was terminally ill. Her abrasive personality did not allow many people to get near her, but she was very fond of Anna, who understood Mavis in a way that few did. They connected on a deep level, and, although they never talked in great depth about Mavis' impending death, Mavis revealed that one of her unfulfilled plans was to be baptized. She did not remember her baptism from childhood and did not want to die without having that memory.

Although nothing in the nursing texts says it is a good idea to take a terminally ill patient into the cold of January to church for an immersion baptism, it was Anna's human-to-human caring approach that allowed her to respect the meaning of this event from Mavis' point of view.

On a bitterly cold night with a howling wind, Mavis was baptized by a friend who was a minister, her family in attendance, her turban covering her bald head. Mavis told Anna that she was free to die now, and within days her family reported that Mavis had "taken to her bed." On one of her final days, the family called Anna frantically because Mavis had called for her all day. The on-call nurse covering the hospice service that weekend could not console her, and Mavis' cries for her hospice nurse made the family muster the courage to call Anna on her day off. Anna, knowing Mavis as she did, responded, and when she arrived at the bedside, she asked Mavis what she could do to help her. Mavis' response was what Anna knew as "vintage Mavis": "I just wanted to see if you would come." Anna said simply, "I am here." Mavis lapsed into a peaceful coma that evening. Her last words had been to Anna.

Anna practiced nursing with the philosophy that human-to-human relationships are primary in professional practice. In the confines of this deeply caring relationship, Mavis found acceptance and peace from her nurse and was guided into a calm death. Although the nurse whose guiding philosophy is based on human relationships must set clear professional boundaries, this philosophical approach to the practice of nursing raises the possibility of exquisite experiences between humans that transcend the nurse-patient relationship, just as Anna and Mavis experienced.

CONCEPTUAL MODELS OF NURSING

Conceptual models (or conceptual frameworks) are the second type of theoretical work that provides organizational structures for critical thinking about the processes of nursing (Alligood, 2014; Fawcett and DeSanto-Madeya, 2013). These are broad conceptual structures that provide comprehensive, holistic perspectives of nursing by describing the relationships of specific concepts. Models are less abstract and more formalized than the philosophies in this chapter; models are more abstract, however, than theories of nursing, which you will read about later. Theories are built from conceptual models much as buildings are constructed from blueprints. The blueprints show the general relationships between parts of the building and are adaptable; conceptual models provide a preliminary view of the relationship between concepts of nursing that can be used to build theory.

Three conceptual models will be presented in the following section. These models represent different decades in the development of nursing theory; they are models developed by Dorothea Orem, Imogene King, and Sister Callista Roy. The focus and perspective of each model are discussed, followed by a brief overview of how that model guides nursing practice. Table 9.2 contains questions that represent how the same patient situation is viewed differently by nurses whose practices are based on the models of Orem, King, or Roy.

Orem's Self-Care Model

Dorothea Orem, born in 1914 in Baltimore, Maryland, first received her diploma in nursing in the 1930s, soon followed by a BS in nursing education in 1939. Six years later, she earned an MS in nursing education (Sitzman and Eichelberger, 2004). Working as a nurse in a number of roles, Orem first published her concept of self-care in 1959. She continued to develop her conceptual model over several decades, with the sixth edition of her work *Nursing: Concepts of Practice* published in 2001. Over the years, Orem formalized three interrelated theories: the theory of self-care, theory of self-care deficit, and theory of nursing system. Her model focuses on the patient's self-care capacities and the process of designing nursing actions to meet the patient's self-care needs. In this model the nurse prescribes and regulates the nursing system on the basis of the patient's self-care deficit, which is the extent to which a patient is incapable of providing effective self-care. An underlying assumption of Orem's model is that "ordinary people in contemporary society want to be in control of their lives" (Pearson et al., 2005, p. 104). Nursing is needed in the presence of an actual or potential self-care deficit (Orem, 2001) when patients cannot provide their own care adequately. Orem's work is widely used in nursing education and practice, providing a comprehensive system for nursing practice in a variety of clinical settings.

TABLE 9.2 Three Models of Nursing: Three Different Responses to the Same Patient Situation

Dorothea Orem	What deficits does this patient have in providing his or her own self-care?
Imogene King	What goals can we set together to restore the patient to health?
Callista Roy	How can I modify this patient's environment to facilitate his or her adaptation?

Orem and Nursing Practice

In Orem's model, appropriate care for the patient is developed through a series of three operations: diagnostic, prescriptive, and regulatory. To determine the patient's ability to provide effective self-care, the nurse initiates a diagnostic operation that begins with the establishment of the nurse-patient relationship. This includes contracting with the patient to explore current and potential self-care demands. Factors such as age, gender identity, and developmental status, as well as sociocultural and environmental factors, are examined in relation to universal, developmental, and health requirements and related self-care actions of the patient. In other words, the patient's baseline ability to provide adequate self-care is assessed by the nurse to determine the extent to which the patient is limited in providing their own effective care. These limitations are self-care deficits.

Prescriptive operations occur when therapeutic self-care requisites (based on deficits) are determined and the nurse reviews various methods, actions, and priorities with the patient. This is a planning stage in which the nurse confirms with the patient the nurse's assessment of the patient's needs and begins to formulate a plan of care. In regulatory operations, the nurse designs, plans, and produces a system for care (Berbiglia, 2014). Systems of care range from wholly compensatory, which is the most comprehensive form of care for patients with few (if any) abilities to provide care for self, to supportive-educative in which the patient has the ability to provide effective self-care but needs to work with the nurse to further develop these abilities or acquire additional information to promote self-care (George, 2002).

King's Interacting Systems Framework and Theory of Goal Attainment

Imogene King was born in 1923 and received her basic nursing education from St. John's Hospital School of Nursing in St. Louis, Missouri, in 1945. Three years later she completed her BS in nursing education from Saint Louis University; in 1957 she earned her MSN degree from Saint Louis University. In 1961 she completed her doctor of education (EdD) degree from Teachers College, Columbia University, in New York City. Much of her career was spent in academic settings, including Ohio State University, Loyola University, and the University of South Florida (Johnson and Webber, 2005).

Although King first published early forms of her theoretical work in 1971, *A Theory for Nursing: Systems, Concepts, Process*, published 10 years later in 1981, contained her first claim to a nursing theory (King, 1981). This complex theory focused on people, their interpersonal relationships, and social contexts, with three interacting systems: personal, interpersonal, and social. Within each of these three systems, King identified concepts that provide a conceptual structure describing the processes in each system. Significantly, the focus of the nurse is on phenomena of importance to the patient; unless attention is paid to concerns of the patient, mutual goal setting is unlikely to happen (Sieloff et al., 2006).

King's interacting systems form a framework to view whole people in their family and social contexts: the personal system identifies concepts that provide an understanding of individuals, personally and intrapersonally (within the person); the interpersonal system deals with interactions and transactions between two or more people; and the social system presents concepts that consider social contacts, such as those at school, at work, or in social settings. King's work is unique because it provides a view of people from the perspective of their interactions (or communications, both verbal and nonverbal) with other people at three levels of interacting systems.

Using King's Model in Practice

When using King's work, nurses focus on goal attainment for and by the patient. The traditional steps of the nursing process—assessment, planning, goal setting, intervention, and evaluation—are augmented in several ways. The steps of the process describe the type of action the nurse is taking, and at each step the nurse gathers and uses information to provide care. Like the nursing process, King's model is not linear: steps occur simultaneously as the nurse and patient work to identify goals and the best means to attain those goals.

The focus of nursing care is guided by concepts at each of the system levels. For example, the personal system leads the nurse to pay close attention to the patient's perceptions; the interpersonal system guides the nurse to explore the patient's roles and the stresses in each role; and the social system cues the nurse to consider influences on the patient's decision making. In this model, for instance, the nurse providing care for a young woman who is a mother will recognize that the patient's maternal role will influence her decisions regarding her health, keeping the best interests of her children in addition to her own health in mind as she makes health-related decisions.

Interaction with the patient is an important component of King's goal attainment model. Nurses are aware of their communication with patients, identifying steps from the first encounter to the attainment of the specified goal. King describes these steps as a progression from perception, judgment, action, reaction, and interaction to transaction (King, 1981). These steps involve increasing involvement between the nurse and the patient, requiring a deep understanding of the goals of the patient within the various contexts of the patient's life to plan and provide effective nursing care. King emphasized the importance of joint goal setting by nurse and patient, reminding nurses that this relationship involves mutuality. King's process provided a structure for the nurse to monitor the relationship's progress. King specified clearly that the goal of nursing is attaining or regaining health.

Roy's Adaptation Model

Sister Callista Roy was born in Los Angeles, California, in 1939. Her first degree was a Bachelor of Arts degree in nursing from Mount St. Mary's College in Los Angeles. She then earned a master's degree in pediatric nursing and sociology, followed by a PhD in sociology from the University of California, Los Angeles. She is a member of the order of Sisters of Saint Joseph of Carondelet. Roy is currently on the faculty of the William F. Connell School of Nursing at Boston College. Although the Roy adaptation model has been in use for 45 years, Sr. Roy continues to update, revise, and refine it for use in practice, research, theory, and administration (Roy and Zhan, 2006; Roy and Andrews, 2008).

Roy first presented her model as a conceptual framework for a nursing curriculum in 1970 (Pearson et al., 2005). In 1976 she published *Introduction to Nursing: An Adaptation Model* and followed with a second edition in 1984 (Roy, 1976; Roy, 1984). Roy updated all of her writing in a comprehensive text in 1999 (Roy and Andrews, 1999). Her model is widely used for education, research, and nursing practice today. She focused on the individual as a biopsychosocial adaptive system and described nursing as a humanistic discipline that emphasizes the person's adaptive or coping abilities. Roy's work is based on adaptation and adaptive behavior, which is produced by altering the environment. According to Roy, the individual and the environment are sources of stimuli that require modification to promote adaptation in the patient. Roy viewed the person as an adaptive system with physiologic, self-concept, role function, and interdependent modes.

Roy's model provides a comprehensive understanding of nursing from the perspective of adaptation. When the demands of environmental stimuli are too high or the person's adaptive mechanisms are too low, the person's behavioral responses are ineffective for coping. Effective adaptive responses promote the integrity of the individual by conserving energy and promoting the survival, growth, reproduction, and mastery of the human system. Nursing promotes the patient's adaptation and coping, with progress toward integration as the goal (Phillips, 2002).

Using Roy's Model in Practice

The nurse using Roy's model focuses on the adaptation of the patient and on the environment. Adaptation, specifically patients' adaptation behavior and stimuli in the internal and external environments, is assessed and facilitated. Based on these assessments, the nurse develops nursing diagnoses to guide goal setting and interventions aimed at promoting adaptation. Simply stated, the nurse modifies the environment to facilitate patient adaptation.

Observable behavior is recognized and understood in the context of Roy's physiologic, self-concept, role function, and interdependent modes. Descriptions of the behaviors included in each mode provide the nurse with a means of making evaluative judgments about the patient's progress toward the goal of adaptation (Phillips, 2002). Roy's model is extensively used in nursing practice and has been described comprehensively in the literature (Wood, 2014; Phillips, 2002; Roy and Andrews, 1999).

Clinical Example: Roy's Adaptation Model

A clinical example of Roy's model will help you understand her work in a real-world context.

Mr. Elderd was referred to a home health agency for wound management. He had a very large open surgical (as opposed to trauma-induced) wound on his forehead as a result of a wide excision of several deep basal cell carcinomas, a form of skin cancer. Dean, his nurse, was surprised to see that the wound extended completely to Mr. Elderd's skull. Mr. Elderd was out of work as a result of this wound, saw friends infrequently, and was somewhat depressed. His wife, although well meaning, spent hours each day fixing him high-calorie treats because she liked to cook and found it was a good way to release her own anxiety about her husband's condition.

Dean's nursing practice was shaped by Roy's adaptation model. In his initial assessment of the home environment, he noticed the cleanliness of the home, the evidence of supportive family and social ties, adequacy of income, availability of good nutrition, and other indicators of health. What Dean did not understand at first was why Mr. Elderd's wound was not healing. After Dean's assessment, he believed that there was some "missing link" in Mr. Elderd's adaptive abilities, but he was not sure whether the ineffective coping was psychological, environmental, or physiologic.

Dean visited Mr. Elderd daily for 3 weeks and, although the wound did not become infected, it showed little evidence of closure. Dean expressed his concern to Mr. Elderd and questioned him again about his basic health practices, including nutrition, activity, sleep, and elimination. Mr. Elderd commented almost offhandedly that he was sleeping fine except that he had to get up to go to the bathroom several times each night. His wife chimed in from the kitchen, "But that's no different than from the day. He is always going to the bathroom. I told him to quit drinking so much water all the time!" Dean, being an experienced nurse and seeking ways to assist patients with all forms of adaptation, realized the likely problem. He called Mr. Elderd's surgeon and asked for an order to draw blood for a random glucose level, which was 180 mg/dL. Because a random glucose reading is a screening mechanism for diabetes but is not diagnostic, Mr. Elderd's physician had him come in for glucose and A1C tests the next morning after fasting overnight. Dean's suspicion was correct: Mr. Elderd had undiagnosed type 2 diabetes. Eating Mrs. Elderd's stream of cookies and other treats from the kitchen aggravated the problem to the point that Mr. Elderd was experiencing polyuria and polydipsia, both signs of diabetes. With aggressive blood glucose level management with an oral hypoglycemic agent, strict adherence to a new way of eating, and increased exercise, Mr. Elderd's wound began to heal almost immediately. He did not require a skin graft as had been anticipated.

The use of Roy's adaptation model allowed Dean to see Mr. Elderd's situation as a function of a variety of maladaptive coping efforts. Correcting the problem—diet and exercise habits resulting in hyperglycemia—became the foundation for Mr. Elderd's eventual healing and resumption of his usual life activities.

THEORIES OF NURSING: FROM GRAND TO MIDDLE RANGE

Nursing theories are the third type of theoretical work in the structure of nursing knowledge to be reviewed in this chapter. Fawcett and DeSanto-Madeya (2013) classified theories according to their breadth and depth. For example, a **grand theory** is a broad conceptualization of nursing phenomena, whereas a **middle-range theory** is narrower in focus and makes connections between grand theories and nursing practice (Parker, 2006). Theories are less abstract than models and usually propose specific outcomes. Three theories are presented here that are well known and commonly used to shape nursing practice. Table 9.3 contains questions that represent the differing foci of care of nurses whose practices are shaped by the theories of Hildegard Peplau, Ida Orlando, and Madeleine Leininger.

TABLE 9.3 Three Theories of Nursing: Three Different Responses to the Same Patient Situation

Hildegard Peplau	Within the relationship with my patient, how can I best help him or her understand his or her health problems and develop new, healthier behaviors?
Ida Orlando	How can I best figure out what my patient needs through my interaction with him or her?
Madeleine Leininger	What are the best ways to provide care to my patient that are culturally congruent?

Peplau's Theory of Interpersonal Relations in Nursing

Peplau, born in 1909, was one of the earliest nurse theorists who recognized the importance of the work of nursing rather than continuing to define and delineate nursing (Pearson et al., 2005). After receiving her basic nursing training at the Pottstown, Pennsylvania, Hospital School of Nursing in 1931, Peplau studied interpersonal psychology at Bennington College in Vermont, receiving a Bachelor of Arts degree. Later she received a Master's of Arts degree in teaching and supervision of psychiatric nursing, followed by an EdD from Teachers College, Columbia University, in New York City. Although Peplau's first book, *Interpersonal Relations in Nursing*, was published in 1952, it was published again in 1988, reflecting both the value of her work and nursing's continuing focus on interpersonal relationships. Peplau drew from developmental, interactionist, and human needs theories in developing her work (Pearson et al., 2005), which grew from her interest in nursing care of psychiatric patients. Peplau believed, however, that all nursing is based on the interpersonal process and the nurse-patient relationship (Forchuk, 1993).

Peplau's theory is based on the premise that the relationship between patient and nurse is the focus of attention, rather than the patient only as the unit of attention (Forchuk, 1993, p. 7). Nursing care occurs within the context of the patient-nurse relationship. The goals of a therapeutic interpersonal relationship are twofold: first is the survival of the patient; second is the patient's understanding of his or her health problems and learning from these problems as he or she develops new behavior patterns. As the nurse assists the patient in developing new behavior patterns, the nurse also grows and develops a greater understanding of the effect of universal stressors on the lives and behaviors of individual patients (Pearson et al., 2005).

Using Peplau's Theory in Practice

Although Peplau's theory grew from her experience as a psychiatric nurse, her work is applicable to a wide variety of practice settings. Peplau describes a four-pronged process similar to the nursing process by which the nurse assists the patient in achieving personal growth. Completion of this process involves six roles by the nurse: counselor, resource, teacher, technical expert, surrogate, and leader (Pearson et al., 2005). Depending on the setting, the nurse will spend more or less time in each of these roles. For instance, a nurse in a critical care unit will likely spend more time as a technical expert and less time as a counselor, whereas a nurse on a postpartum unit may act as a surrogate, guiding a new mother into independent care of her newborn infant, with less time spent as a leader.

Peplau's theory is complex. Its importance lies in the focus on what happens between the nurse and patient in a therapeutic relationship. Furthermore, Peplau was visionary in recognizing the importance of the relationship between nurse and patient, publishing her ideas early and continuing to refine and expand her work over several decades.

Orlando's Nursing Process Theory

Ida Orlando was born in New York in 1926 and, like many early nurse theorists, received her basic nursing education in a diploma program. She attended nursing school at the New York Medical College School of Nursing, and in 1951 she graduated with a BS in public health nursing from St. John's University in Brooklyn, New York. Three years later, she completed her MSN from Columbia University. Her early practice settings included maternity, medicine, and emergency department nursing (Gess et al., 2006).

Orlando first proposed her theory of effective nursing practice in 1961 in her first book, *The Dynamic Nurse-Patient Relationship: Function, Process, and Principles*. She later revised it as a nursing process theory (Orlando, 1990). Her work actually proposed both: it is a theory about how nurses process their observations of patient behavior and about how they react to patients based on inferences from patients' behavior, including what they say. Orlando's early research revealed that processing observations as specified in her theory led to effective nursing practice and good outcomes.

Orlando's theory is specific to nurse-patient interactions. The goal of the nurse is to determine and meet patients' immediate needs and to improve their situation by relieving distress or discomfort. Orlando emphasized deliberate action (rather than automatic action) based on observation of the patients' verbal and nonverbal behavior, which leads to inferences. Inferences are confirmed or disconfirmed by the patient, leading the nurse to identify the patient's needs and provide effective nursing care.

Using Orlando's Theory in Practice

In terms of nursing practice, Orlando's theory specified how patients are involved in nurses' decision making. When used in practice, Orlando's theory guides interactions to predictable outcomes, which are different from outcomes that occur when the theory is not used. Nurses individualize care for each patient by attending to behavior, confirming with the patient ideas and inferences the nurse draws from interactions, and identifying pressing needs.

Use of Orlando's theory improves the effectiveness of the nurse by allowing the nurse to get to the "bottom line" more quickly when observing, listening to, and confirming with patients. Therefore use of this theory saves time and energy for both the patient and the nurse.

Leininger's Theory of Culture Care Diversity and Universality

Born in 1924 in Sutton, Nebraska, Madeleine Leininger received her diploma in nursing at St. Anthony's School of Nursing in Denver, Colorado, followed by a BS in biologic science from Benedictine College in Atchison, Kansas, 2 years later. She received her MSN from Catholic University in Washington, D.C., in 1954 and her PhD in anthropology from the University of Washington in Seattle in 1965 (Reynolds and Leininger, 1993).

The work of Madeleine Leininger (1978, 1991) in cultural care grew out of her early nursing experiences. She observed that children of different cultures had widely varying behaviors and needs. After discussing the parallels between nursing and anthropology with the noted anthropologist Margaret Mead, Leininger pursued doctoral study in cultural anthropology. Through her doctoral work she became more convinced about the relationship of cultural differences and health practices. This led her to begin developing a theory of cultural care for nursing. Leininger's work is formalized as a theory rather than as a conceptual model. It has stimulated the formation of the Transcultural Nursing Society, transcultural nursing conferences, newsletters, and the *Journal of Transpersonal Nursing*, as well as the awarding of graduate degrees, including the DNP, in the specialty area known as transcultural nursing.

The goal of transcultural nursing involves more than simply being aware of different cultures. It involves planning nursing care based on knowledge that is culturally defined, classified, and tested, and then used to provide care that is culturally congruent (Leininger, 1978). Leininger described theory as a creative and systematic way of discovering new knowledge or accounting for phenomena in a more complete way (Leininger, 1991). She encouraged nurses to use creativity to discover cultural aspects of human needs and to use these findings to make culturally congruent therapeutic decisions. Her theory is broad because she considers the impact of culture on all aspects of human life, with particular attention to health and caring practices. Leininger's theory has become increasingly relevant as global migration continues and societies become more diverse.

Using Leininger's Theory in Practice

Leininger specified caring as the essence of nursing, and nurses who use Leininger's theory of cultural care in their practices view patients in the context of their cultures. Practice from a cultural perspective begins by respecting the culture of the patient and recognizing the importance of its relationship to nursing care. Use of the "sunrise model" (Fig. 9.1) guides the assessment of cultural data for an understanding of its influence on the

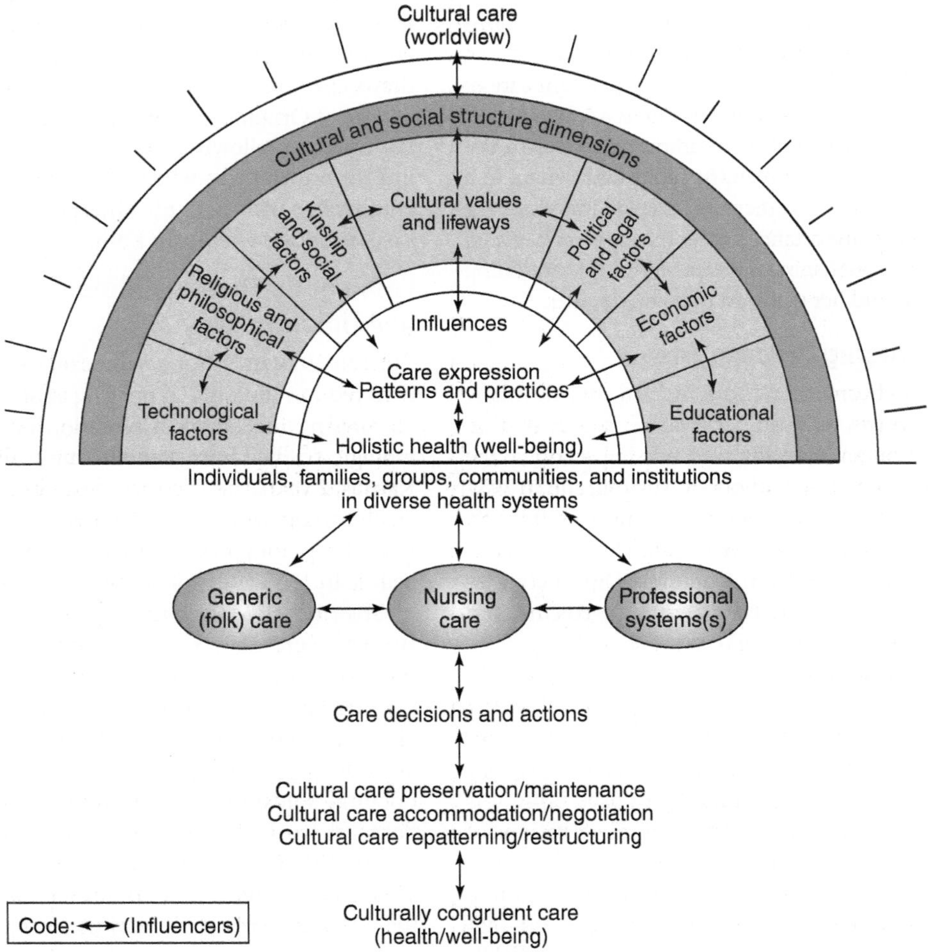

Fig. 9.1 Leininger's sunrise model, created to facilitate the application in practice of the Theory of Culture Care Diversity and Universality. (Courtesy Dr. Madeleine Leininger.)

patient's life (Leininger, 1991). The nurse plans nursing care, recognizing the health beliefs and folk practices of the patient's culture, as well as the culture of traditional health services. To this end, nursing care is then focused on culture care preservation, accommodations, or repatterning, depending on the patient's need. The nursing outcome of culturally congruent nursing care is health and well-being for the patient.

Clinical Example: Leininger's Theory of Culture Care Diversity and Universality

No matter how expert a nurse is in clinical practice, sometimes failure to recognize and appreciate cultural differences can undermine even the best intentions. The following case is an example of what happens when this occurs.

Jan, a nurse with many years of experience providing care for patients with human immunodeficiency virus (HIV) in a large urban hospital, decided that she would move to a less chaotic environment. Jan applied for a job with an agency providing nursing care in the homes of women with HIV who lived in rural areas, and whose incomes were below the poverty line. Jan had grown up and gone to college in a large metropolitan area in the U.S. Northeast; her new home was in a rural county in the Deep South.

Almost immediately Jan ran into some unanticipated situations that posed problems for her. She complained at team meetings that her patients were always late for their appointments. Members of the team, each of whom had grown up nearby, explained to her that this was not unusual and that she should plan "waiting time" into her daily schedule. Jan was always surprised when the rest of the team reported good visits and outcomes with their patients, and almost all seemed to be caught up with their work consistently. Jan always felt like she was running behind. She began to question her nursing skills, her knowledge, and time management behaviors that had served her well in her previous work. Jan described herself as a "fish out of water." She decided that she would spend her "waiting time" by sitting in her car and catching up on documentation and other work until the patient arrived home.

One day she was invited by the patient's grandmother to wait inside but she declined, saying she would wait in the car and "get some work done." Her patient arrived home after 20 minutes and Jan met with her, reporting to the team later that day that she had a productive visit with the patient in which several care goals were addressed. Jan's satisfaction with the visit was short-lived. Her patient called, demanding that she be assigned another nurse because "Jan insulted my grandma." In this community where being invited into the home was considered an honor, Jan's decision to instead wait in the car was interpreted as rude and uncaring. No amount of discussion dissuaded the patient from her insistence that she have a new nurse who "knew how to act." The care team met with Jan, but they too, as products of the culture, did not understand at first that Jan did not mean to be insulting or rude. Because the other members of the team were deeply acculturated, they knew the meaning behind the grandmother's invitation: Jan was an honored, trusted guest who was welcomed in their home.

Jan soon realized that her feelings of being a "fish out of water" in this setting were accurate; in fact, she did not understand the culture and was not eager to learn about the cultural norms that bothered her. Importantly, she recognized that this prevented her from providing the effective patient care that she desired. She left the position and moved to an urban area out of state in which she knew the cultural terrain. Although this was a sad chapter in Jan's professional life, she grew from the experience in her understanding of the substantial influences of culture and its effects on the nurse-patient relationship.

Middle-Range Theories of Nursing

Middle-range theories are those that are neither overly broad nor narrow in scope, usually incorporating a limited number of concepts and focus on a specific aspect of nursing. Middle-range theories are more focused than the theories described earlier and typically merge practice and research. These theories are based in empirical research and are often embedded within a larger theory. Sometimes middle-range theories are developed from theory from disciplines other than nursing. Some well-known middle-range theories include Swanson's Caring Theory, which was developed from her work with couples experiencing miscarriage (Swanson, 1991). Mishel's Uncertainty in Illness Theory was developed from studying men with prostate cancer who were "watchfully waiting" for disease progression rather than seeking aggressive treatment (Mishel, 1988). Jezewski's Cultural Brokering Theory was developed from her qualitative research on the politically and economically powerless or those who were vulnerable as a function of advanced disease (Jezewski, 1995). You can see how close to practice each of these theories are; they were each developed from a specific population and grew from the theorists' research and experiences.

Dobratz (2011) published a description of a new middle-range theory of Psychological Adaptation in Death and Dying. Dobratz had noted that death and dying is a social phenomenon involving a wide range of human responses across a variety of settings from intensive care to hospices. She defined psychological adaptation in death and dying as "using spiritual and social resources, and managing physical symptoms to maintain self-regulation" (p. 373). Importantly, Dobratz tied her middle-range theory back to the more theoretical and conceptual structure of the Roy adaptation model and has continued to develop her work in the context of the Roy model (Dobratz, 2014). More recently, continuing to use the Roy adaptation model, Dobratz developed a new middle-range theory of Adaptive Spirituality, based on a synthesis of published literature on religion/spirituality (Dobratz, 2016).

Nursology: Contemporary Thinking About Nursing Theory

A new energy has developed about nursing theory and the importance of the knowledge nurses own that defines the discipline of nursing. In Chapter 5, you read that a purpose of nursing school is to socialize you in thinking like a nurse. That means that you learn to combine the knowledge you have from all your education and life experience to this point and through your nursing education will learn to synthesize it into a new knowledge that will guide your practice and for many of you, your graduate studies. You have already learned (and been surprised) that nursing school is not just learning psychomotor skills but is a means of teaching you to think in a disciplined way about phenomena of interest to nursing.

Nursology is a word you may have yet to encounter, but assuredly you are familiar with "ologies" such as sociology (study of groups and their interactions, societies and social interactions); anthropology (study of human societies and cultures and their development); and psychology (study of the mind and behavior). In fact, it is likely that you were required to take courses in one or more of these disciplines for admission to your school of nursing. Across your career, you will use your basic knowledge from those established disciplines in many ways that you may not even understand yet.

The suffix *-ology* is a combined with the names of disciplines as a way of naming their science and claiming a body of knowledge. *Nursology* refers to the science and body of knowledge created by and for the discipline of nursing. It is important to understand that nursology is not the study of nurses; it is study by nurses of phenomena of concern to nursing. The word nursology is not new; nurse scholars were using the term in the 1970s, and its use has seen a recent revival.

In 2018, a group of nurse scholars committed to nursology launched the website www.nursology.net, a highly informative, comprehensive and up-to-date site that is easy to use and contains a wealth of information about nursing theory, theorists, and the discipline of nursing. Site content is updated frequently by a management team on whom responsibility of content rests. The site includes the mission and vision statements of nursology.net, definitions of key terms, and a much more thorough and clear description of their work than space allows here. Seventeen nurse scholars comprise the management team currently, three others are bloggers, and there is one emerita member. The website serves as a "repository for resources about nursing conceptual models, grand theories, middle-range theories, and situation-specific theories, philosophies and methodologies" (nursology.net, 2019). The evolution of nursing requires that the discipline's body of knowledge specific to our field be enlarged through robust, meticulous and meaningful inquiry leading to the development of knowledge. The next section will help you understand this more clearly.

USING THEORY FOR NURSING EDUCATION, PRACTICE, AND RESEARCH

The examples of nursing theoretical works you have read about earlier illustrate the vital position of theory in nursing education, practice, and research. To continue the forward movement of nursing and to improve the quality of nursing care, nurses must engage in theory-based practice, theory-testing research, and theory-generating research. Planning educational curricula based on nursing knowledge and theory is essential to further solidifying the foundations of nursing science.

Theory-Based Education

The curricula (courses of study) of schools of nursing are usually built on one or more specific conceptual models or concepts. In 1989 and then again in 2000, Bevis and Watson published a book detailing their view of nursing curricula, with the goal "to create a new curriculum-development orientation for nursing education" (p. 1) to humanize nursing education by recognizing that there are many different modes of knowing shaped by experience and learning (Lewis et al., 2006). Later, Lewis and colleagues (2006) published their description of the development of a nursing curriculum that expanded the earlier theoretical work of Bevis and Watson. Sometimes students wonder why their coursework is set up a particular way, sometimes asking, "Why do we have to take this class?" or "What use will this be later?" It is important that nursing students understand that a philosophy or a conceptual model shapes the curriculum of their school and the coursework they are undertaking.

The nursing profession has evolved from an applied vocation dependent on knowledge from other disciplines to its current stage of development, with its own knowledge base. This period of growth has stimulated—and been stimulated by—the development of the nursing PhD degree, a research degree that generates new, discipline-specific knowledge. In PhD work, nurses are concerned with the philosophy of science—that is, the nature of knowledge and how it is known; the philosophy of nursing science and the generation of nursing knowledge; theory testing; and the development of new theory through research. The nurse who has earned the Doctor of Nursing Practice (DNP) or an MSN degree may be a primary provider in advanced practice, going beyond the generic nursing process. These advanced practice nurses use theoretical perspectives focused on the patient for specific nursing outcomes. Many nurses conduct their first research studies as graduate students, focusing on nursing practice and the testing of nursing interventions with specific patient groups.

The BSN nurse is introduced to the research process, evidence-based practice, and the use of theory to guide it. The research emphasis for bachelor's-level students is on learning to critique nursing research, becoming informed consumers of research relevant to evidence-based practice. BSN nurses are also introduced to theory through the curriculum at their school. Many curricula of BSN programs are based on a particular nursing theoretical perspective; others introduce students to a variety of nursing theoretical perspectives (Thinking Critically Box 9.1). Whether the curriculum is built around one or many nursing theoretical works, the focus for the BSN level is utilization and application of nursing theory as a guide for nursing practice. Associate degree nursing education programs may also use nursing theory to teach the unique perspectives of nursing. Nurses with associate degrees often find middle-range theories, which are specific to patient care, useful in their practice. The importance of theory in four levels of nursing education is noted in Box 9.4.

THINKING CRITICALLY BOX 9.1

Philosophies of Schools of Nursing

Many schools of nursing in colleges and universities describe the philosophic basis for their curriculum on their websites. Others include a mission statement that may indicate the school's philosophical orientation. This information gives potential students at all levels of study an idea about the focus and goals of nursing education at that institution. Look up the website of your school and other colleges and universities, and compare their philosophies and mission statements.

Theory-Based Practice

Practice becomes theory-based when nurses intentionally structure their practice around a particular nursing theory and use it to guide them as they use the nursing process to assess, plan, diagnose, intervene, and evaluate nursing

BOX 9.4 Use of Theory at Four Levels of Nursing Education

PhD in nursing: Conducts theory testing and theory development research for nursing science development; frames practice, administration, or research in nursing works

Doctor of nursing practice (DNP) or master of science in nursing (MSN): Frames advanced practice with a nursing model or theory; uses theory to guide research with practice questions

Bachelor of science in nursing (BSN): Learns the nursing perspective in a nursing model or theory-based curriculum or courses; uses models, theories, and middle-range theories to guide nursing practice

Associate degree in nursing (ADN): May have a nursing model or theory-guided curriculum or courses; may be introduced to middle-range theories for nursing practice

care. (You will learn more about the nursing process in Chapter 11.) Theory provides a systematic way of thinking about nursing that is consistent and guides the decision-making process as data are collected, analyzed, and used in the planning and administration of nursing practice. Theory provides nurses with the tools to challenge the conventional views of patients, illness, the healthcare delivery system, and traditional nursing interventions.

This introduction to some classic nursing theoretical works can lead you to identify one or more theories that are consistent with your values. There are many other nurse theorists whose works are more recent and complex. In addition, substantial numbers of nurse theorists have developed middle-range theories that may be useful to you in specific areas of your practice as you develop your competence as a practitioner. With increased understanding and education, you can integrate the use of nursing theory in your practice.

Nurses and, by extension, their patients, reap many benefits from theory-based practice. First, a function of understanding your theoretical orientation to practice, you will be able to explain your practice to other members of the healthcare team, sometimes as simply as "This is the way that I view this problem/situation." Nursing theory provides language for you to explain what you do, how you do it, and why you do it. Second, this language of practice facilitates the transmission of nursing knowledge to you as students who are new to the profession, as well as to other health professionals. Third, theory contributes to professional autonomy by providing a nursing-based guide for practice, education, and research. Finally, nursing theory develops your analytical skills, challenges your thinking, and clarifies your values and assumptions.

Many nurses have developed their own ideas about nursing and continue to develop nursing assumptions based on education, experience, observation, and reading. Most nurses do not develop their own personal theories formally, even though their ideas influence the way they practice nursing. When you rely on your personal ideas or beliefs as a basis for practice, or when faculty members use their own ideas as a "framework for curricula," the outcome is ineffective. Each of the philosophies, models, theories, and middle-range theories presented in this chapter has been critiqued, analyzed, and evaluated. Application of these works in your practice with specific patient groups is an opportunity to further develop and test middle-range theories.

CONSIDERING CULTURE BOX 9.1

Caring for Persons Who Have Immigrated: Using Nursing Theory to Bridge the Cultural Gap

The issue of immigration is important in today's world. Persons who have emigrated from other nations may pose challenges for providing nursing care to persons with whom you may share no language and have little understanding of the context of their lives. Yet your professional nursing ethic demands that you provide the same level of care as you do with other patients with whom you have more in common. How can the philosophies/frameworks/theories presented in this chapter be adapted to your practice in a way that will assist you in providing excellent care under these circumstances? What cultural barriers do you anticipate may be the hardest for you to overcome as you work with patients of varying cultural backgrounds?

As you engage in theory-based practice, remember to provide feedback to nurse researchers and theorists concerning your experiences. You can do this through a variety of social media sites and blogs where you will find groups of nurses using, discussing, and refining the theoretical works that have been discussed in this chapter. The Internet can be a powerful tool to keep you involved with nurses in practice far removed from your own location and practice setting. You can also assist these scholars and the discipline of nursing by developing manuscripts and submitting your experiences for publication, joining the many nurses who have discovered the benefits of theory-based practice. Considering Culture Box 9.1 gives you the opportunity to consider how nursing philosophies, conceptual models, and theories may be helpful in addressing the complicated issues of care of immigrants whose language and culture may be different from yours.

Theory-Based Research

Great strides have been made in nursing research since the 1970s (Alligood, 2018). The expansion of graduate nursing education at the master's level and the proliferation of PhD and DNP programs have played a major role, as more nurses than ever before are equipped with the knowledge and skills to conduct research and implement its use in practice. Nursing research tests and refines the knowledge base of nursing. Ultimately, research findings enable nurses to improve the quality of care and understand how evidence-based practice influences improved patient outcomes.

Research is vital to the future of nursing, and theory is integral to research. Historically, an emphasis on method has overshadowed the subject of nursing research. In addition, many nurses have continued to use theories developed to address phenomena of interest in other disciplines, theories that do not view persons holistically or provide a nursing perspective. However, nurse scholars are recommitting to the vital role of nursing theory in their mission to develop knowledge for their own discipline. You will be reading more about this in Chapter 10.

CONCEPTS AND CHALLENGES

- ***Concept:*** Nursing philosophies, models, theories, and middle-range theories offer many perspectives on nursing, varying in their levels of abstraction and their definitions of four major concepts known as nursing's metaparadigm: person, environment, health, and nursing.
  Challenge: Theory development is not a mysterious activity restricted to a few nursing scholars. It is an activity that combines education, knowledge, and skill. Theories provide an excellent basis for practice.
- ***Concept:*** As nurses develop theories and test theories of nursing, the discipline moves forward in the development of its unique knowledge base.
  Challenge: The use of theory in practice creates opportunity for the best outcomes for patients because a guiding framework that makes sense supports care.
- ***Concept:*** Nurses at every level of educational preparation make scholarly contributions to the development and use nursing knowledge by questioning, reading, studying, networking, and writing about nursing practice.
  Challenge: Nurses can get caught up in the tasks of their practice and forget that nursing has a specific knowledge base and theoretical orientation that shapes their practice.
- ***Concepts:*** Nurses in practice settings have invaluable insights and observations, thereby contributing to the knowledge base for nursing. Nursing theorists' early work grew out of their clinical observations and experiences.
  Challenge: Theorists rely on practicing nurses to test clinical interventions and explore the usefulness of their theories.
- ***Concept:*** Nurse theorists whose works were reviewed in this chapter, as well as others too numerous to include, have made significant contributions to the development of the unique body of nursing knowledge.
  Challenge: The development of theories continues. Nurses in practice add to the development and refinement of theory by being willing to write about their experiences and perspectives and to communicate with the researchers who continue to expand, clarify, and refine original theories.
- ***Concept:*** Nursology is the word for the study of phenomena central to the discipline (practice, research, theory) of nursing.
  Challenge: Contemporary thinking about nursing requires that nurses develop and maintain their own knowledge and science as a function of the discipline of nursology, but some nurse faculty may not yet embrace that point of view.

IDEAS FOR FURTHER EXPLORATION

1. Which philosophy/conceptual framework/theory/middle-range theory introduced in this chapter appeals to you the most? Which ones describe nursing similar to the way you think about nursing? What is it about these theories that makes sense to you?
2. In thinking about the different examples of philosophy, conceptual frameworks, theories, and middle-range theories, which will be the most useful to help you organize your thoughts for critical thinking and decision making in nursing practice?
3. Describe the use of nursing theory for nurses at your current level of nursing education and how you can begin to shape your practice even during early clinical experiences.
4. Spend time on the nursology.net website, and become familiar with how the scholars who have produced the site think about the importance of nursing having its own science and body of knowledge.

REFERENCES

Alligood MR: *Nursing theorists and their work*, 9, St. Louis, 2018, Elsevier.

Alligood MR: Philosophies, models and theories: critical thinking structures. In Tomey AM, Alligood MR, editors: *Nursing theory: utilization and application*, 5, St. Louis, 2014, Mosby, pp 40–62.

Alligood MR: The power of theoretical knowledge, *Nurs Sci Q* 24(4):304–305, 2011.

Berbiglia V. Orem's self-care deficit theory in nursing practice. In: Alligood MR, Tomey AM, eds. *Nursing theory: utilization and application*. 5; 2014:222–244.

Bevis EO, Watson J: *Toward a caring curriculum: a new pedagogy for nursing*, New York, 1989, National League for Nursing.

Bevis EO, Watson J: *Toward a caring curriculum: a new pedagogy for nursing*, Boston, 2000, Jones & Bartlett.

Chinn P, Kramer M: *Theory and nursing: a systematic approach*, 5, St. Louis, 1998, Mosby.

DiNapoli PP, Turkel M, Nelson J, Watson J: Measuring the caritas processes: caring factor survey, *Int J Human Caring* 14(3):16–21, 2010.

Dobratz MC: Life closure with the Roy adaptation model, *Nurs Sci Q* 27:51–56, 2014.

Dobratz MC: Toward development of a middle-range theory of psychological adaptation in death and dying, *Nurs Sci Q* 24:370–376, 2011.

Dobratz MC: Building a middle-range theory of adaptive spirituality, *Nurs Sci Q* 29:146–153, 2016.

Fawcett J, DeSanto-Madeya S: *Contemporary nursing knowledge: analysis and evaluation of nursing models and theories*, 3, Philadelphia, 2013, FA Davis.

Forchuk C, Hildegard E: *Peplau: interpersonal nursing theory*, Newbury Park, Calif, 1993, Sage Publications.

George JB: *Nursing theories: the base for professional nursing practice*, 5, Norwalk, Conn, 2002, Appleton & Lange.

Gess T, Dombro M, Gordon SC, et al.: Part one: twentieth-century nursing: Wiedenbach, Henderson, and Orlando's theories and their applications editor. In Parker ME, editor: *Nursing theories and nursing practice*, 2, Philadelphia, 2006, FA Davis.

Henderson V: *The nature of nursing: a definition and its implications for practice, research, and education*, New York, 1966, Macmillan.

Jezewski MA: Evolution of a grounded theory: conflict resolution through cultural brokering, *Adv Nurs Sci* 17(3):14–30, 1995.

Johnson BM, Webber PB: *An introduction to theory and reasoning in nursing*, 2, Philadelphia, 2005, Lippincott Williams & Wilkins.

King IM: *A theory for nursing: systems, concepts, process*, New York, 1981, John Wiley & Sons.

Leininger M: *Transcultural nursing: concepts, theories, and practices*, New York, 1978, John Wiley & Sons.

Leininger M: *Culture care diversity and universality: a theory of nursing*, New York, 1991, National League for Nursing.

Lewis S, Rogers M, Naef R: Caring-human science philosophy in nursing education: beyond the curriculum revolution, *Int J Human Caring* 10(4):31–37, 2006.

March A, McCormack D: Nursing theory-directed healthcare, *Holist Nurs Pract* 23(2):75–80, 2009.

Mishel MH: Uncertainty in illness, *Image J Nurs Sch* 20(4):225–232, 1988.

Nightingale F: *Notes on nursing: what it is and what it is not*, New York, 1969, Dover Publications [originally published in 1859].

nursology.net: *About,*2019. (website). Available at: https://nursology.net/about/.

Orem D: *Nursing: concepts of practice*, 6, St. Louis, 2001, Mosby.

Orlando I: *The dynamic nurse-patient relationship: function, process and principles*, New York, 1990, National League for Nursing [originally published in 1961].

Parker M: *Nursing theories and nursing practice*, Philadelphia, 2006, FA Davis.

Parsons T: *Structure of social action*, Glencoe, Ill, 1949, The Free Press.

Pearson A, Vaughan B, FitzGerald M: *Nursing models for practice*, Edinburgh, United Kingdom, 2005, Butterworth Heinemann.

Peplau HE: *Interpersonal relations in nursing*, New York, 1952/1988, GP Putnam's Sons.

Phillips KD, Harris R: Roy's adaptation model in nursing practice. In Alligood MR, Tomey AM, editors: *Nursing theory: utilization and application*, 5, St Louis, 2014, Mosby, pp 263–284.

Phillips KD: Roy's adaptation model in nursing practice. In Alligood MR, Tomey AM, editors: *Nursing Theory: Utilization and Application*, 2, St Louis, 2002, Mosby, pp 289–314.

Reynolds CL, Leininger M: *Madeleine Leininger: cultural care diversity and universality theory*, Newbury Park, Calif, 1993, Sage Publications.

Roy Sr C: *Introduction to nursing: an adaptation model*, Old Tappan, NJ, 1976, Prentice Hall.

Roy Sr C: *Introduction to nursing: an adaptation model*, 2, Englewood Cliffs, NJ, 1984, Prentice Hall.

Roy Sr C, Andrews HA: *The Roy adaptation model*, 2, Norwalk, Conn, 1999, Appleton & Lange.

Roy Sr C, Andrews HA: *The Roy adaptation model*, 3, New York, 2008, Pearson.

Roy Sr C, Zhan L: Sister Callista Roy's adaptation model and its applications editor. In Parker ME, editor: *Nursing theories and nursing practice*, 2, Philadelphia, 2006, FA Davis.

Sieloff CL, Frey M, Killeen M: Part two: Applications of King's theory of goal attainment editor. In Parker ME, editor: *Nursing theories and nursing practice*, 2, Philadelphia, 2006, FA Davis, pp 244–267.

Sitzman K, Eichelberger LW: *Understanding the work of nurse theorists: a creative beginning*, Sudbury, Mass, 2004, Jones & Bartlett.

Swanson KM: Empirical development of a middle range theory of caring, *Nurs Res* 40:161–166, 1991.

Watson J: *Nursing: the philosophy and science of caring*, Boston, 1979, Little, Brown.

Watson J: *Nursing: human science and human care*, New York, 1988, National League for Nursing.

Watson J: *Postmodern nursing and beyond*, Edinburgh, UK, 1999, Churchill Livingstone/Saunders/Harcourt Health Sciences.

Watson J: *Caring science theory—10 caritas processes*,2018. (website). Available at: https://www.watsoncaringscience.org/jean-bio/caring-science-theory/.

Wood AF: Nursing models: normal science for nursing practice. In Alligood MR, Tomey AM, editors: *Nursing theory: utilization and application*, 5, St Louis, 2014, Mosby, pp 13–39.

10

The Science of Nursing and Evidence-Based Practice

ⓔ To enhance your understanding of this chapter, try the Student Exercises on the Evolve site at http://evolve.elsevier.com/Black/professional.

LEARNING OUTCOMES

After studying this chapter, students will be able to:

- Differentiate among bench, clinical, and translational science.
- Describe the historical development of the scientific method.
- Give examples of inductive and deductive reasoning.
- Discuss the limitations of the scientific method when applied to nursing.
- Differentiate between problem solving and research.
- List the steps in the research process.
- Discuss contributions nursing research has made to nursing practice and to health care.
- Describe the relationship of nursing research to nursing theory and practice.
- Identify sources of financial support for nursing research.
- Discuss the roles of nurses in research at various levels of education.
- Define *evidence-based practice.*

The word *science* comes from the Latin word *scire*, meaning "to know," and refers to knowledge gained by systematic study: research. Although science and research can be imposing concepts, they actually form the base of the discipline and profession of nursing. The purpose of this chapter is to help you understand nursing's scientific base—the science of nursing—and the links among nursing practice, research, and science. Many of you who are studying this chapter are working toward completion of a bachelor's degree of science in nursing (BSN); each of you is using nursing science to shape your practice.

Mature professions have a strong scientific base, which both defines and is defined by the purposes of a profession. Florence Nightingale, whose work is detailed in Chapter 2, advanced the practice of nursing by both defining it clearly and providing scientific evidence of the outcomes of excellent nursing care in the Crimea. Fig. 10.1 shows her careful documentation of the improvement in morbidity and mortality rates among soldiers in Bulgaria and the Crimea over a course of a year. In the mid-20th century, scholars and researchers realized that nursing could achieve a high level of professional status only to the extent that the discipline was based on a scientific body of knowledge unique to nursing. As a result, nursing researchers began developing knowledge unique to nursing, and nursing theorists began developing theories and testing them. Theory and research are the foundations of scientifically based nursing practice.

At the same time, nurses realized that professionalization of patient care practices was also needed. Until that time, nurses relied on traditional techniques to manage common patient problems. More unusual problems were often managed by trial and error or intuition. However, these were no longer acceptable ways to care for patients. The momentum toward evidence-based practice was developing, which required nurses to base their care and activities on research-based knowledge, in addition to their clinical

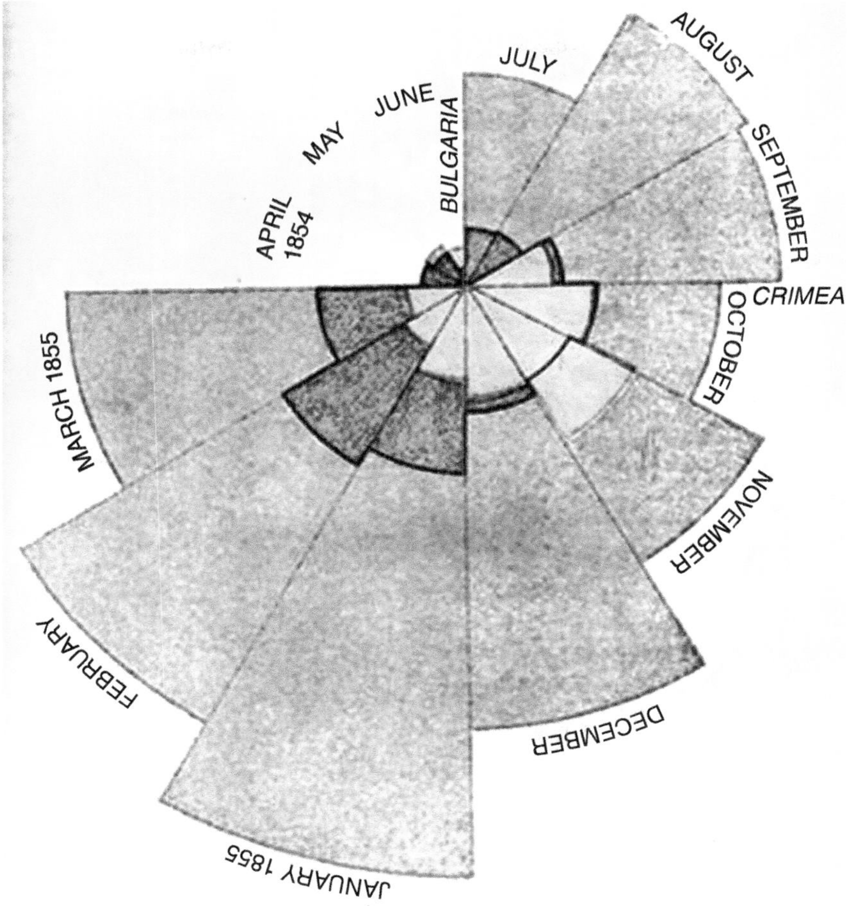

Fig. 10.1 Florence Nightingale's careful detailing of mortality statistics in the Crimean War demonstrated the effectiveness of nursing care in 1855. The area of each wedge is proportional to the statistic being represented. The wedges closest to the center (appearing as yellow) represented deaths from wounds; the largest wedges (appearing as green) represented deaths from contagious diseases such as cholera and typhus; and middle wedges (brown) represented deaths from other causes. (Originally from Nightingale's book *Notes on Matters Affecting the Health, Efficiency and Hospital Administration of the British Army,* published in 1858.)

expertise and patient preferences. The development of evidence-based practice necessitated a strong link between the work of nurse researchers and nurses in practice. The development of the nursing process became a means of adapting a scientific framework to the management of patient care so that nurses were no longer depending on hit-or-miss techniques but were shaping care in direct response to the individual needs of the patient. The nursing process is presented in depth in Chapter 11.

Furthermore, the American Nurses Credentialing Center (ANCC) Magnet Recognition Program, described in Chapter 3, includes in its Magnet Model a requirement for "New Knowledge, Innovation, and Improvements." Inclusion of this requirement for hospitals seeking Magnet status underscores the importance for nursing to be responsible for the development, maintenance, and application of its own professional scientific knowledge base. The Magnet Model requires that initiatives and leadership for nursing research reside with clinical nurses, not nurse managers or others in administrative positions.

SCIENCE AND THE SCIENTIFIC METHOD

Science is research based on one or more past scientific achievements or accomplishments that are acknowledged by the scientific (academic) community as providing a foundation for further study or practice (Kuhn, 1970). Good science—that which contributes to the knowledge bases of a discipline—requires that research be based on the previous work of others in the same academic discipline or be related to work of others from other disciplines. This is a safeguard to ensure that knowledge development is based on sound principles and theory rather than simply the product of a creative idea that is not based on any known science. Sound science and creativity are not mutually exclusive; creativity has led to many interesting and useful research developments that in turn guide nursing practice.

Science has three distinct divisions: natural, social, and formal sciences. Natural sciences include disciplines such as biology, chemistry, and physics. Social sciences such as economics, sociology, anthropology, and history are focused on aspects of the human experience. Formal sciences include logic, systems theory, statistics, and mathematics and are concerned with formal systems—sets of axioms, definitions, and rules—to create knowledge.

Each academic discipline has its own specific scientific community, meaning that nurse researchers and scholars acknowledge and judge scientific developments in nursing. Common to research in all disciplines, however, is the use of an orderly, systematic way of thinking about and solving problems. This systematic way of thinking is traditionally known as the **scientific method**, used by scientists for centuries to discover and test facts and principles. The history of the development of the scientific method is complex; however, Sir Francis Bacon (1561–1626) is widely considered the father of today's scientific method.

The traditional form of "doing science" requires standardized experimental designs with hypotheses, measurable variables and outcomes, and statistical analyses. This form of inquiry is sometimes referred to as **quantitative research** because variables are measurable (quantifiable). This type of research requires that subjectivity and bias are minimized. *Bias* refers to the systematic distortion of a finding from the data, often resulting from a problem with the sample—that is, the persons being studied. For instance, if you wanted to test an intervention focusing on the benefits of early mobility after abdominal surgery, your sample should include a wide age range of patients. If you included, for instance, only young patients—who, because of their age, are likely to be in otherwise good health and thus are likely to get out of bed soon after surgery—your results may be biased; that is, they show more benefit than the intervention actually delivers because your sample is narrowly confined to younger patients. You introduced bias through your sampling strategy.

Because nursing is interested in human phenomena (events or circumstances) that might not be best studied using traditional quantitative research techniques, a significant number of noted researchers in nursing use a different approach to explore human responses in health and illness. This approach is known as **qualitative research** because there are no variables being manipulated; rather, qualities of the human experience are described and interpreted. Manipulation of variables is not a goal in this type of research; the systematic and detailed description and interpretation of phenomena are the goals.

Qualitative research, also known as *naturalistic inquiry* or *interpretivism*, relies on data collection techniques such as narrative interviews and participant observation, among others. These techniques are known as "field work," where the researcher spends much time in the setting where the phenomenon occurs. Examples of phenomena studied by qualitative researchers include women's responses to intimate partner violence, fatigue related to HIV infection, women's experiences of pregnancy when the fetus has a serious congenital condition, and the adjustment by older persons to living in a skilled nursing facility. Qualitative methods are commonly used in the social sciences, where measurement of phenomena may not be possible or even acceptable in terms of understanding the human experience. Several types of inquiry are commonly identified with naturalistic inquiry; ethnography, phenomenology, and grounded theory are the most familiar.

A combination of quantitative and qualitative methodologies is known as **mixed-methods research**, a means of examining phenomena of interest using a variety of data collection techniques and analyses. Regardless of type of methods, all good research has a theoretical basis and is carried out in a systematic, disciplined way that furthers the development of a discipline's knowledge base.

Basic, Clinical, and Translational Science

Traditionally, scientists divided scientific knowledge into two categories: pure and applied. Pure science or pure research, sometimes referred to as bench science, summarizes and explains the universe without regard for whether the information is immediately useful. When Joseph Priestley discovered oxygen in 1774, he did not have an immediate use for that information. Therefore that discovery could be classified as pure science—that is, information gathered solely for the sake of obtaining new knowledge. Applied science is the practical application of scientific theory and laws. Applied science is usually referred to as clinical science now—taking to the patient's bedside those findings that may be useful in curing, managing, or preventing diseases or managing symptoms. For instance, when Priestley discovered oxygen almost 250 years ago, he had no idea that one day this elemental substance would be used as a therapy under pressure (as hyperbaric oxygen therapy) in the treatment of air emboli, decompression sickness, myonecrosis (gangrene), and other wounds.

More recently, however, scientists have recognized the importance of a third type of research—translational research—that serves as a conduit between "bench and the bedside." Translational research takes the findings in the laboratories and develops them for use at the bedside. In turn, translational research takes the findings from clinical research done at the bedside to ask new questions and to direct new research at the bench level.

In 2006 the National Institutes of Health (NIH), an agency of the U.S. Department of Health and Human Services and the largest source of public funding for health-related research, launched an initiative known as the NIH Common Fund. The Common Fund supports "short-term, goal-driven strategic investments" that are "transformative, catalytic, synergistic, cross-cutting across NIH centers and institutes, and unique" (NIH, 2021). The Common Fund has supported a series of high-impact programs across the NIH in an effort to enhance the way that American biomedical research is conducted, making it more streamlined and flexible in responding to the health needs of society, while still maintaining the high standards required of excellent scholarship and science.

Inductive and Deductive Reasoning

Research requires the use of one of two kinds of logic: inductive reasoning or deductive reasoning. In inductive reasoning, the process begins with a particular experience and proceeds to generalizations. Repeated observations of an experiment or event enable the observer to draw general conclusions. For example, a researcher may be interested in the experiences of women who participated in centering, a form of group prenatal care. After interviewing 25 women who had this form of care and finding a generally positive response, inductive reasoning may lead the researcher to infer that this is an acceptable intervention for pregnant women, based on the responses from this small sample of women. Note that the research did not address the effectiveness of centering prenatal care, but determined that at least for this sample of women, their responses to centering were generally positive. This type of inferential reasoning leads to the development of probabilities but not certainties, unless every single woman who received centering prenatal care was included in the research, a study that would be impossible to conduct.

One of the important uses of research that uses an inductive approach is that inferences are made that lead to further research. For instance, the researcher studying centering prenatal care finds that most women experienced this form of care as acceptable, but also that several mentioned they would appreciate some one-to-one time with a provider to discuss more personal matters. From the findings in the original study, the researcher can develop an intervention and test it against the usual standards of care. In this case three different forms of care could be tested: centering only, centering with provider time (based on the responses of several women in the original qualitative study), and usual care as typically provided in the clinical setting. Note that the research still is focused on the acceptability of care, not the effectiveness of care. The extent of acceptability can be measured and have meaningful results.

Scientists also use deductive reasoning, a process in which conclusions are drawn by logical inference from given premises. Deductive reasoning proceeds from the general case to the specific. For example, if the premises "All pregnant women benefit from centering prenatal care" and "Ms. Foster is a pregnant woman" are accepted, the conclusion "Ms. Foster will benefit from centering prenatal care" can be drawn. It may be entirely possible, however, that Ms. Foster, although pregnant and needing prenatal care, may have specific needs not amenable to centering care and will not benefit from receiving care in a group setting. In deductive reasoning, the premises used must be correct or the conclusions will not be. The faulty premise in this example is that "All pregnant women will benefit from centering prenatal care."

Conclusions drawn through deductive processes are called *valid* rather than *true. Valid* is a term meaning "soundly founded," whereas *true* means "in accordance with the fact or reality" (Flexner et al., 1980). It is possible for a conclusion to be solidly founded without being true for everyone. There is a subtle but real difference between the words *valid* and *true.* For example, the premise that women benefit from centering care may be valid; this is soundly founded in the original findings of the researcher who interviewed 25 women. What is not true, however, is that *all* women benefit from centering care. The premise is valid but not true in all cases.

As seen by these examples, neither inductive nor deductive processes alone are adequate. If scientists used only deductive logic, experience would be ignored. If they used only inductive logic, relationships between facts and principles could be overlooked. A combination of both types of reasoning processes in science unifies the theoretical and the practical, which is the basis for the scientific method and research.

Limitations of the Strict Definition of Scientific Method in Nursing

The traditional scientific method used by quantitative researchers has considerable value, and it has been used by nurse researchers to address a wide range of nursing problems. However, the scientific method as implemented exclusively with quantitative techniques has limitations when applied to phenomena of interest to nursing.

The first and most obvious drawback is that healthcare settings are not comparable with laboratories. Certain phenomena of interest to nurses are not amenable to study in a laboratory setting and in fact are not amenable to study in tightly controlled circumstances. For instance, in the discussion of inductive/deductive logic regarding centering prenatal care, measurement of women's experiences and reactions to this method of care is not possible in the laboratory setting by conventional measures. The phenomenon of pregnancy care may be of great interest to perinatal nurses; however, the systematic examination of this intervention and the measurement of outcomes may not be a particularly good fit with the laboratory setting. Women's reaction to this form of care is a human response that occurs in real-world settings. Research techniques associated with qualitative research may be more appropriate to the aims of this research. Note that the term *naturalistic inquiry* is sometimes used in place of *qualitative research* to refer to the examination of phenomena that occur in the "real world" as opposed to the laboratory setting or in research where variables are controlled.

Second, humans are far more than collections of parts to be dissected and subjected to examination or experimentation. A criticism of methodology that relies solely on measuring attributes of people is that it is "reductionistic"; that is, the richness of human experience is reduced to variables that can be measured. Conversely, a strength of nursing is its holistic view of patients. Because humans are complex organisms with interrelated parts and systems, the effectiveness of the scientific method is reduced in the examination of complex human phenomena.

A third limitation of the scientific method as the only approach to solving patient problems is its claim to objectivity (freedom from bias); it fails to consider the meaning of patients' own experiences—that is, their subjective view of reality. Nurses are keenly aware, however, that patients' perceptions of their experiences (subjective data) are just as important as objective data and may have significant effects on their health behaviors. Again referring to the centering prenatal care example, assume that a well-designed, reliable, and valid instrument (such as a questionnaire) can measure Ms. Foster's satisfaction with this form of care. One month after giving birth, her satisfaction scores are higher than they were when she was pregnant, thus it appears that she is satisfied from the centering care. However, this approach fails to take into consideration the complex changes one undergoes when becoming a mother, and Ms. Foster's higher scores may represent something completely different from her satisfaction with her care—her happiness in being a new mother or her relief that she is not pregnant anymore. There may be many reasons she is now scoring higher on satisfaction with this form of prenatal care. The questionnaire by itself may not capture in its entirety the nuances of the experience of Ms. Foster's centering prenatal care in light of her new motherhood.

NURSING RESEARCH: IMPROVING CARE OF PATIENTS

If you are a college or university student, you may have been introduced to research through your basic psychology or sociology courses, or you may have participated in professors' research on your campus. Although sometimes these projects involve interesting experiments, in some cases the only type of research to which you may have been exposed used surveys or questionnaires to collect data. This kind of introduction to research may lead you to wonder what research has to do with your ability to care for patients.

The rest of this chapter describes some basic concepts of nursing research. The purpose is to introduce nursing research, demonstrate its merit, and provide a basic vocabulary. The ultimate goal is for nurses to participate in the research process and apply research findings to clinical practice. This is a key component of what is known as evidence-based practice.

Nursing research is the systematic investigation of phenomena related to improving patient care. Ideas for nursing research often arise from nurses' clinical observations. Although a research topic may be new and innovative, much can be gained from choosing research problems that are connected to work already done, thereby building the body of knowledge of nursing. A problem may be amenable to being addressed by research if these criteria are met:

1. A conceptual framework exists or can be constructed from research that already has been done; that is, the researcher's ideas about the problem fit logically and align with what is already known about the topic.
2. The proposed research project is based on related research findings published in professional peer-reviewed journals or is supported by similar ongoing research in other settings or disciplines, thereby building nursing knowledge.
3. The proposed research is carefully designed so that the results will be applicable in similar situations or will generate hypotheses for further research and testing.

In addition to building nursing knowledge, studies building on previous work are more likely to receive financial support. Research can be expensive and sometimes requires funding beyond what one nurse, hospital, or university can supply. Small projects such as survey research may not be prohibitively expensive, especially if the sample (the persons in the study) is not large or if the survey can be completed online. Many hospitals and professional nursing organizations have funds available for small projects to encourage nurses in practice to do research.

Nurses who want to do large, expensive research studies will find it necessary to obtain outside (external) funding or compete with other aspiring researchers for limited internal (from within the agency) funding. Therefore, to receive funding, nurses must do research that interests others, has demonstrated significance, and has support from reviewers who examine the proposed research for the specific funding agency and make recommendations about whether or not to fund it.

Furthermore, research that is not based on or is not related to previous foundational work may have inadvertent violations of human participants' rights. In other words, it is hard to justify asking people to participate in research if there is no real connection to previous work or theory that supports the idea that an intervention works or a problem is significant. Researching or testing an intervention in humans just to see whether it works or that "seemed like a good idea" ignores potential shortcomings or may fail to anticipate problems if adequate foundational work is not done before instituting the research. In fact, such research will not receive approval from a federal human participants' review board if significant linkages with previous research are not demonstrated. This review board (commonly known as the IRB: institutional review board) approval must occur before any research involving humans is undertaken.

Thus although nursing research may be broadly defined as anything that interests nurses and helps them provide better care, controversy exists over what can legitimately be included. When considering a research question, nurse researchers consider the practical issues of background and financial support. An important source of funding and support for nursing research is the NIH's National Institute of Nursing Research (NINR), which in 2020 celebrated its 35th year of existence. NINR has been developing its 2022-2026 Strategic Plan Framework. The guiding principles of the framework state that's NINR supports research that is innovative; advances equity, diversity and inclusion; addresses today's health challenges and anticipates tomorrow's challenges, and discovers solutions for improving health at the clinical, community and policy levels (NINR, 2021). Specifically, the strategic plan framework will have these priorities: health equity, social determinants of health, community and population health, prevention and health promotion, care models and systems (NINR, 2021). In Nurses Doing Research Box 10.1, you will read about Dr. Hudson Santos, who early in his nursing career noted depressive symptoms in new Latina mothers. These observations sparked an interest that has led to his cutting edge, innovative work on how early life stressors interact with the genome and manifest differently in high-risk populations, as well as across socioeconomic status levels and culturally, racially, and ethnically diverse communities.

NURSES DOING RESEARCH BOX 10.1

How Early Life Stressors Interact With the Genome in Latina Mothers and Across Diverse Communities

I started my education and career as a nurse in Brazil, first graduating from a 2 year LPN program and then working as a nurse in mental health settings. Like many nurse researchers, my early clinical experiences, first as an LPN and then as an RN, sparked an interest that influenced my later research. I became interested in postpartum depressive symptoms in Latino families. Perinatal mental health issues have been overlooked in the Latino community. After a year, I returned to school to study at State University of Paraiba in Campina Grande to earn my BSN to become an RN. Immediately after graduation, I enrolled at the University of São Paolo PhD program focusing on nursing research.

I first completed research on postpartum depressive symptoms in Latina mothers and primary healthcare providers' knowledge and approaches to prevent or manage these symptoms. I found that providers were insecure about identifying and treating women with postpartum affective symptoms and needed training. Findings from my early work were used in the implementation of a training program for screening of postpartum depressive symptoms in primary health care.

My early publications addressed an initiative from the Brazilian Ministry of Health to define new policies and production of community-based services to achieve effective deinstitutionalization from psychiatric hospitals and reintegration of low-income people with severe mental illness into the community. By providing evidence and clinical approaches in the implementation of halfway houses for people with chronic mental illness, this work has helped change the standards of mental health services in Brazil and other Latin American countries. The Brazilian Ministry of Health highlighted this work in the implementation of halfway houses to replace psychiatric hospitalizations.

Near the end of my doctoral studies, I had the opportunity to study for a year with two significant North American scholars and spent six months studying in the U.S. and six months in Canada. After completing my PhD, I had the opportunity to complete a postdoctoral fellowship at the Duke University School of Nursing. The fellowship gave me the opportunity to focus my interest on perinatal mood symptoms, and I gained expertise in genomics and early life stressors related to perinatal and child health outcomes in high risk populations. I have since developed a program of research focusing on the psychosocial and biologic dimensions of early life adversity and its effects on perinatal and child developmental health outcomes.

My work builds on research on the developmental origins of health and disease, as well as research examining how development is programmed in utero. We know there can be devastating effects of prenatal stress on women's early and late-stage pregnancies, and on birth outcomes for their infants, including children's neurodevelopment, and that these poor outcomes can continue to affect young children in their first few years and maybe longer. Because we are not yet sure how this occurs, or how to minimize these effects, I am now studying how early life stressors interact with the genome and manifest differently in high-risk populations, as well as across socioeconomic status (SES) levels and culturally, racially, and ethnically diverse communities.

I am the principal investigator of three studies funded by the NIH. My funded research has focused on placental epigenetic mechanisms and neurodevelopmental outcomes in children born extremely preterm; on placental origins of positive child health outcomes using multiomics approaches; and on genetic and epigenetic predictors of childhood cognitive trajectories in children born extremely preterm. I have also done research on gene–environment interactions that regulate social stressors and birth outcomes in high-risk families, and I am part of a research team working on the landmark Extremely Low Gestational Age Newborns (ELGAN) Cohort study, which is part of the Environmental Influences of Child Health

Outcomes (ECHO) Consortium. Together, these studies are helping us identify protective and risk factors that can affect the developmental trajectory of children's cognition from birth to 17 years of age. In addition, we are identifying genes as well as mechanisms that can be used for risk-stratification, allowing the development and/or optimization of early risk-mitigating interventions to improve quality of life for children.

My research team was the first to report a crucial finding: how ethnic discrimination affects biologic changes in DNA methylation in pregnant and postpartum women. Moving forward, my ultimate goal is to prevent or minimize neurodevelopmental impairment through intervention and precision health approaches and sustain well-being in children and families, despite early life exposure to adversity in Latina women. It is important to remember that my research career now started with observations I made about new mothers' depressive symptoms while I was working as an LPN in my first nursing job. You never know what may inspire you in your work as a nurse.

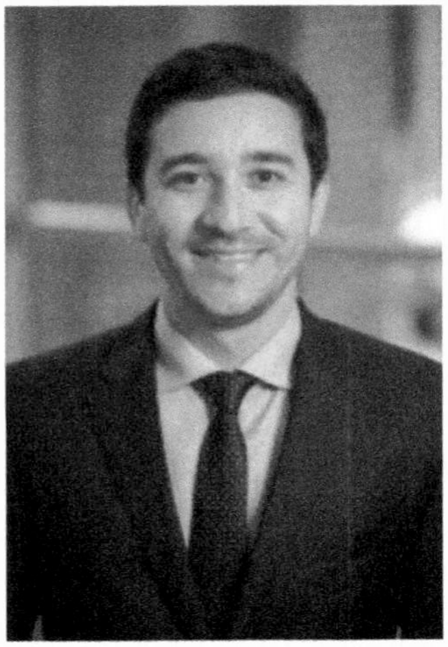

Hudson Santos, PhD, RN, FABMR, FAAN
Professor,
Dolores J. Chambreau Endowed Chair in Nursing
University of Miami School of Nursing and Health Studies

Research is different from problem solving. Problem solving is specific to a given situation and is designed for immediate action, whereas research is generalizable or transferable to other situations and deals with long-term solutions rather than immediate ones. For example, Mrs. Abney, an 80-year-old woman with Alzheimer's disease, is a resident in a skilled nursing facility and is often found wandering the halls unable to find her way back to her room. This is distressing to her and time consuming for the nursing staff who help her find her way "home." A nurse notices that Mrs. Abney has no difficulty recognizing her daughter, so she tapes a photograph of the daughter to Mrs. Abney's door. Now Mrs. Abney can find her room easily. She is less agitated, and the nursing staff time can be spent elsewhere.

Mrs. Abney's case is an example of problem solving, an effective intervention in one set of circumstances that has immediate application. However, the solution that worked for Mrs. Abney may not work for all confused patients. In fact, it may not continue to work for Mrs. Abney as her cognitive abilities decline further. Remember that nursing research was developed in response to the professional and scientific mandate that nursing care be based on evidence and not simply on trial and error. Occasionally, creative problem solving such as that of the nurse caring for Mrs. Abney is required on a per-case, situational basis. But this sort of trial-and-error problem-solving approach is not adequate to base one's professional practice in a substantial and sustained way. Table 10.1 contrasts research and problem solving.

EVIDENCE-BASED PRACTICE: EVIDENCE, EXPERTISE, PATIENT PREFERENCE

The best efforts of nurse researchers are pointless unless nurses make use of their research findings to improve patient care in their day-to-day practices. Patients have become more knowledgeable consumers of health care, and nurses must ensure that they provide the latest and best available care. One way to ensure positive patient outcomes is through evidence-based practice.

Evidence-based practice (EBP) is defined as an approach to the delivery of health care that "integrates the best evidence from [research] studies and patient care data with clinician expertise and patient preferences and values" (Melnyk et al., 2009, p. 49). The development of EBP is credited to the work of Archie Cochrane, a British epidemiologist. His work ultimately was reflected in the development of the Cochrane Library, which holds the *Cochrane Database of Systematic Reviews*. Systematic

TABLE 10.1 Comparison of Research and Problem Solving

Characteristic	Research	Problem Solving
Type of problems addressed	Significant number of people affected or significant impact on smaller number of people	Situation specific
Conceptual basis	Theoretical framework; keys to researching the problem found in previous research	Often none; trial and error
Knowledge base needed	Extensive review of literature to determine latest thinking and research	Practical knowledge, common sense, and experience
Scope of application	Generalizable or transferable to similar situations	Useful in immediate situation; may or may not be useful in other situations

reviews are important means of reviewing data collectively across a number of studies. Clinicians and scholars recognized that practice was improved when critical appraisal of the best evidence is the foundation for practice (Cleary-Holdforth and Leufer, 2008).

In nursing, EBP requires that you are knowledgeable about research that supports specific interventions. Basing one's practice on peer-reviewed work or reliable texts is an element of critical thinking and a good means of improving clinical judgment. Focusing on evidence of effective interventions is a good means of preventing one's practice from deteriorating into routine or traditional care without concern for advances in care. Taking continuing education courses, attending professional conferences, reading journals, and maintaining membership in professional organizations are professionally responsible ways of staying current and keeping aware of new evidence of best practices.

Evidence-based practice, however, requires more than simply knowing what research shows. Clinician expertise and patient preferences are equally important in determining best practices. Sometimes nurses do not realize the importance of these two prongs of the requirement for practice to be evidence based. The issue of patient preference became an important one in the early days of human immunodeficiency virus (HIV) antiretroviral treatments, which at the time were very complicated regimens that sometimes required patients to set an alarm clock to wake themselves in the middle of the night to take their scheduled medications. These were highly effective medications; there was a great deal of scientific research to demonstrate they worked to decrease the patient's viral load and extend survival.

BOX 10.1 National Institute of Nursing Research: Strategic Plan

The mission of the National Institute of Nursing Research (NINR) is to promote and improve the health of individuals, families, communities, and populations. The Institute supports and conducts clinical and basic research and research training on health and illness across the life span to build the scientific foundation for clinical practice and to improve persons' quality of life in all stages of life, and spanning populations and settings. NINR seeks to advance nursing science by supporting research on the science of health, which focuses on the promotion of health and quality of life.

The current areas of scientific focus by NINR are:

- Symptom science: Promoting personalized health strategies
- Wellness: Promoting health and preventing illness
- Self-management: Improving quality of life for individuals with chronic conditions
- End-of-life and palliative care: The science of compassion.

From the National Institute of Nursing Research: *The NINR strategic plan: Advancing science, improving lives.* Bethesda, MD, 2016. National Institutes of Health (NIH). Available at https://www.ninr.nih.gov/sites/files/docs/NINR_StratPlan2016_reduced.pdf [Note: At the time this edition was written, the 2016 NINR Strategic Plan shown here was in effect; the new version is due to be published in 2022.]

Furthermore, infectious disease providers had tremendous expertise in managing HIV and prescribing effective medication regimens.

So what happened? Many patients simply could not follow the complex routines these regimens required. It was not that they did not want to get better; it was

TABLE 10.2 PICOT as a Tool for Evaluating Interventions

You are concerned by the lack of adequate pain management for preschool children on your pediatric surgery unit:

P	Population of interest (patient group with which you want to intervene)	Children aged 2–5 after uncomplicated abdominal surgery
I	Intervention (a new idea or practice that you are interested in implementing)	Quiet environment; presence of a parent or other family member; scheduled pain medicine administration rather than as needed (PRN)
C	Comparison (what is already being done)	No accommodations in environment; parental presence is common; pain medication given on PRN basis as evidenced by child crying or parent report that child is in pain
O	Outcome (the goal of interventions with the population)	Patients will have better pain management, which allows them improved sleep, increased mobility, and faster healing
T	Time (the time frame in which the patient problem is relevant)	For 48 hours postsurgery

simply that the regimens altered the way they lived their lives so much that sustaining these complex schedules was untenable. This reality led to the development of drugs in which doses could be given at longer intervals and in combination. Research evidence, clinician expertise, and patient preference for more manageable treatment regimens meant that HIV could be managed much more effectively. Patient preference had been the "missing link" in the equation. In Evidence-Based Practice Box 1.2 (Chapter 1) you were introduced to clinically expert community health nurses who initiated aggressive and successful COVID-19 testing in Native Alaskan communities, an evidence-based intervention that took patient (community) preference into consideration.

Questions regarding best practices are often raised by nurses in direct patient care roles. Nurses in practice commonly question procedures and routines, asking whether there is a better way to achieve the outcomes of patient care. Most nurses in bedside practice are not equipped to study those questions; however, answers may already be available in the nursing literature. An important focus of professional nursing education is to learn how to seek out and critique research findings to implement best practices in one's own nursing practice. One way to streamline the process of examining research literature is a process known as PICO, an acronym for a four-step process: *P*—population of interest, *I*—intervention, *C*—comparison, *O*—outcome (Cleary-Holdforth and Leufer, 2008). Often *T*—time is added to the acronym. By using PICOT as a framework, you can eliminate research that is not specific enough to the particular problem or intervention you are interested in. Table 10.2 details the elements of the PICOT process with an example of pain management in preschool children after uncomplicated abdominal surgery. By using the PICOT format, evidence addressing pain management in other populations could be eliminated, such as pain management in older patients after hip fracture. PICOT is a way of focusing your search for evidence.

Some research carries more weight than others in terms of immediate change in practice. Well-executed randomized controlled trials (RCT), long considered the gold standard in research, carry much weight in determining a change in practice; however, descriptive or qualitative studies may inform practice. This means that the findings from a descriptive study may suggest that further research needs to done or an intervention needs to be developed and tested. For example, suppose a hospice nurse notes that the families of terminally ill patients appear to become increasingly anxious about pain symptoms in the evenings, evidenced by an increase in phone calls to the on-call nurse after 7:00 p.m. Interestingly, the patients do not seem to be reporting increased pain. The hospice nurse consults the research literature and finds numerous descriptions of this same phenomenon described several times, but no tested interventions are reported. The nurse, who happens to be a graduate student in a local school of nursing, has identified an interesting topic for her Doctor of Nursing Practice (DNP) project: identifying ways to decrease families' anxiety so that they may spend quality time with their family member.

BOX 10.2 Sigma Theta Tau International Position Statement on Evidence-Based Nursing

As a leader in the development and dissemination of knowledge to improve nursing practice, the Honor Society of Nursing, Sigma Theta Tau International, supports the development and implementation of evidence-based nursing. The society defines EBN [evidence-based nursing] as an integration of the best evidence available, nursing expertise, and the values and preferences of the individuals, families, and communities who are served. This assumes that optimal nursing care is provided when nurses and healthcare decision-makers have access to a synthesis of the latest research, a consensus of expert opinion, and are thus able to exercise their judgment as they plan and provide care that takes into account cultural and personal values and preferences. This approach to nursing care bridges the gap between the best evidence available and the most appropriate nursing care of individuals, groups, and populations with varied needs.

The society, working closely with key partners who provide information to support nursing research and EBN around the world, will be a leading source of information on EBN with an integrated cluster of resources, products, and services that will foster optimal nursing care globally. The society, along with its strategic partners, will provide nurses with the most current and comprehensive resources to translate the best evidence into the best nursing research, education, administration, policy, and practice.

From Sigma Theta Tau International (STTI): *Position statement on evidence-based nursing,* 2005. Available at https://www.sigmanursing.org/why-sigma/about-sigma/position-statements-and-resource-papers/evidence-based-nursing-position-statement.

Sigma, formerly Sigma Theta Tau International, has a long history of support of nursing research and dissemination of research findings. This association has adopted a position statement on evidence-based nursing (EBN) that demonstrates the importance of EBP to its members. Although this position statement was approved in 2002, it still appears on the Sigma website as one of their active positions. Note that this statement refers to EBN, as opposed to evidence-based practice. This reflects early discussion about semantic differences between EBN and EBP. *EBP* is now typically used in nursing, which is consistent with other practice disciplines; you can read this position statement in Box 10.2. Drs. Bernadette Melnyk and Ellen Fineout-Overholt have written extensively about EBP in nursing. The *American Journal of Nursing (AJN),* starting in November 2009, published a series of articles every two months, "Evidence-Based Practice: Step by Step," from the Arizona State University College of Nursing and Health Innovation's Center for the Advancement of Evidence-Based Practice. The purpose of this series was to give nurses in practice the tools they need to implement EBP and remains applicable to today's nurses (Melnyk et al., 2009).

THE RESEARCH PROCESS

The research process used by nurses is the same process used in any other scientific endeavor; nursing research, however, focuses on patients' responses amenable to nursing care. Research starts with a problem: an observation that something related to practice or patients' responses needs to be addressed. This may be a newly recognized problem that needs an innovative solution. The problem may have been addressed by researchers previously, but the research is insufficient or the findings are inconsistent, unclear, or conflicting. When the need for more information exists, or information is unclear or conflicting, research is the means to resolve, clarify, or inform.

Regardless of method a researcher uses, all research must be rigorously planned, carefully implemented, and analyzed meticulously. Therefore most research follows a formal order known as the research process. Students in BSN programs often take a semester-long course in nursing research in which types of methods are described, so this chapter will attempt only a brief introduction to the research process. Steps in the research process will be presented briefly and include the following:

1. Identification of a researchable problem
2. Review of the literature
3. Formulation of the research question or hypothesis
4. Design of the study
5. Implementation of the study
6. Drawing conclusions based on findings
7. Discussion and/or clinical implications
8. Dissemination of findings

Identification of a Researchable Problem

Researchable problems generally come from three sources: clinical situations, the literature, or theories. The word *researchable* is used specifically because not all problems are researchable; sometimes a problem may occur too infrequently or pose such ethical challenges that conducting research on the problem is not feasible. Clinical situations are rich sources for researchable problems, and nurses are in a prime position for identifying problems and issues for research. For instance, a common issue among nurses in gerontologic settings is the propensity for some older persons to wander and risk getting lost or injured. There are several issues related to this problem, including characteristics of patients who tend to wander, time of day this occurs, staffing issues, and medications. Is the nurse seeking to identify patients at high risk for wandering, or is the nurse more interested in preventing nighttime wandering, specifically? A nurse who has identified a clinical problem that may be amenable to research will have a number of questions to consider while formulating the research. Streamlining the problem into a researchable question is a primary goal early in the research process.

Second, sometimes researchers become interested in a problem because someone else has published research findings about the problem from their own study. The researchers may decide to **replicate** (repeat) the published study or may design a similar one to test part of the original study in a new way. For example, suppose that the nurses in the previous scenario read an article in a professional journal reporting findings from a research study testing an innovative intervention to minimize wandering among older persons, and the intervention was found to be effective. In a discussion at their staff meeting about the article, one of the nurses suggests that this approach may not work on this unit for several reasons. The nurses decide to consult with a nurse researcher at the local university to discuss replicating the study on their unit to determine whether, in fact, this innovative intervention will work under the conditions in place locally or to determine what prevents the intervention from working.

The third source of research problems—theory—relates to testing theoretical models. In Chapter 9, you read about several types of nursing theory that have been developed. Theoretical models are designed to predict patients' responses to nursing actions; whether a model actually does predict patients' responses can be tested through research. The researcher can create certain conditions and determine whether, in fact, the events happen as predicted by the theoretical model. Again, consider the nurses on the gerontology nursing unit. Suppose that one of the nurses who has a psychiatric nursing background noted that some psychiatric patients will wander, but using Peplau's theory of interpersonal relations as the basis for their psychiatric practice, the nurses on the unit found that patients who formed excellent relationships with their primary nurses were the least likely to wander. The gerontology nursing staff decided to test this theory in their older patients, using Peplau's theoretical model as a basis for their intervention, predicting that the formation of a trusting relationship between patient and primary nurse would result in less nighttime wandering among patients without cognitive impairment.

Review of the Literature

Once a problem is identified, researchers must review the current literature to see what has been published about the topic. A review of the literature (ROL) is comprehensive and covers all relevant research and supporting documents to support the research. Completing a thorough ROL requires a great deal of searching and detective work, made much easier with sophisticated search engines and tools. A major study with many parts requires huge review efforts, usually involving multiple investigators (researchers) in the work to make sure that the literature review is comprehensive and reflects the current state of the science. A research librarian can be extremely helpful in determining search terms to ensure that the literature review is thorough and comprehensive.

The ROL is essential to locate similar or related studies that have already been completed and on which a new study can build. The review is helpful in creating a **conceptual framework**, or organization of supporting ideas, on which to base the study. The ROL addresses the question, "What have other researchers and theorists written about this problem?" Sometimes the literature review causes the researcher to rethink or reconceptualize the initial problem, especially if the problem has been studied a variety of ways or if findings in other work are unclear, statistically insignificant, or ambiguous.

Nursing as an academic discipline is relatively young in comparison with other disciplines such as medicine, and the humanities and social sciences, such as history, sociology, and anthropology. Because nursing has a holistic view of patients and problems, and the nursing literature may not be sufficiently broad, often the ROL includes research outside of the discipline of nursing.

For instance, if a researcher is interested in a phenomenon such as perinatal loss, an ROL must include what has been written in nursing about the phenomenon of perinatal loss, including all aspects such as early and late miscarriage, stillbirth, and elective termination. However, because this is a research topic that has many social, ethical, and psychological issues at stake, a thorough ROL would also include literature from sociology, anthropology, ethics, and psychology. In addition, the researcher would review literature from the medical field, such as maternal-fetal medicine and reproductive genetics.

As the researcher reviews the literature, they will find that other researchers commonly cite some specific papers. These "classics" in research, despite being older papers, have a place in a new ROL. Otherwise, most researchers find that literature published within the past five years tends to be adequate. Although reviewing literature can seem tedious, it is a crucial step in ensuring that the planned research will be scientifically sound and theoretically congruent with work that has already been completed.

A caveat is in order here about the use of Internet resources for scholarly work. Although much information is available on the Internet about almost any topic you can imagine, much of this work is not peer-reviewed and should be used with caution. The Internet is best used as a tool for disciplined, organized searches of established databases such as CINAHL, Web of Science, PsycINFO, and PubMed. Your school, college, or university may have licenses for these databases so that you have them available to you as a student. These online databases will lead you to peer-reviewed articles that have earned a place in scholarly work. Increasing your ability to use database searches well strengthens your ROL by allowing you increased access to scientific publications that have met the challenges of peer review.

In your research, you are likely to find that some websites, older references, papers and other digital resources are no longer available or links to these sources no longer work. Remember in Chapter 6 the caveat that nothing in digital form is ever really gone. You may find that https://archive.org/ is useful for retrieving online material that appears to be gone. This huge public site archives countless documents, versions of sites, videos, and other digital material. Although many nursing faculty subscribe to the "five year" rule as the cut-off for citing research and other sources, excellent scholarship may require that you build a foundation for your work that requires archived sources. This site is especially useful in finding original sources.

Keep in mind that by citing secondary sources (those who cite another's work, and in turn you cite that source secondarily), you are depending on the scholarship and accuracy of the person who cites the original source. Reliance on secondary sources is akin to the "whisper game" in which a message gets changed or misinterpreted in subsequent sharing from one person to the next. The Internet archive site is extremely useful in finding original sources, thus ensuring that your review of the literature and other scholarly work is consistent with an author's original meaning.

Formulation of the Research Question or Hypothesis

Once researchers have identified a research problem, are thoroughly knowledgeable of the relevant literature, and have chosen or created a conceptual framework that helps focus and support the topic, they will formulate the **research question**. If the researcher is interested in determining and describing certain characteristics of a situation, he or she may simply pose the situation as a question. For example, "What are the characteristics of mothers who have difficulty initiating breastfeeding with their newborns?" is a research question asking about specific characteristics of a population (mothers with breastfeeding difficulties). If comparing the relationship of two or more variables, a different type of question might be asked, such as "What are the relationships among maternal age, number of previous children, and difficulty in initiating breastfeeding?" This question demonstrates that the researcher has some idea that these variables are related (and that the literature supports this idea), but the exact nature of the relationship is not known or hypothesized.

If conducting an experiment, researchers must have a **hypothesis** (educated or informed speculation as to what the outcome will be) so that hypothesis-testing statistics may later be applied. For example, "Younger, inexperienced mothers giving birth for the first time will demonstrate later initiation of breastfeeding than older, experienced mothers who have given birth previously" is a testable hypothesis. The form and content of the research question are key to the development of the rest of the study. Larger, more complex studies will have multiple questions or hypotheses to address.

In the example on breastfeeding, the challenge to the researcher is to define the variables such as "younger" versus "older." The researcher might establish a cutoff in age, defining "younger" as younger than 30 years old and "older" as equal to or older than 30. Defining "experienced" versus "not experienced" might be more challenging: a mother might have previous children but may be breastfeeding for the first time; is she experienced or not? Researchers have to define their variables in a way that makes sense and is consistent with what has been shown in the literature. In other words, the researcher must be able to defend how the variables are defined.

Design of the Study

Once the research questions are identified or hypotheses are generated, the researcher then designs the study. Numerous forms of research designs exist, but experimental and nonexperimental designs are the two major categories. If the purpose of the research is to determine the effect of an intervention or to compare the responses of participants to two or more differing treatments, for example, the research will have an experimental design. If not, the research will have a nonexperimental design. The main difference between experimental and nonexperimental research is whether the researcher manipulates, influences, or changes the participants in any way by the testing of an intervention or medication or other substance.

True experimental designs provide evidence of a cause-and-effect relationship between actions. For example, testing the hypothesis "Patients who receive preoperative anxiolytics need less pain medication in the first 24 hours postoperatively than those who do not receive preoperative anxiolytics" could provide evidence of a significant relationship between preoperative anxiolytics and perception of pain. Experimental designs require quantitative measures to determine whether there are statistically significant differences between the conditions being tested.

Sometimes it is impossible to conduct a true experimental study with humans because to do so might endanger them in some way. In those instances, modified experimental studies are used. In this case a new intensive form of preparation for discharge home might be compared with the usual form of discharge teaching. Because discharge teaching is standard care and an expected nursing action, denying discharge teaching to patients would be unethical and inappropriate. The experimental design could, however, test a new intervention against the usual care received by patients who are preparing for discharge home.

Nonexperimental designs are sometimes referred to as "descriptive" or "exploratory" research because the investigator is seeking to increase the knowledge base about a nursing phenomenon by doing careful, disciplined research. There are many types of nonexperimental designs: surveys, descriptive comparisons, evaluation studies, and historical-documentary research, among others. Nonexperimental designs may be either quantitative or qualitative, or they may use a combination of both. Nurses Doing Research Boxes 10.2 and 10.3 feature researchers who are doing nonexperimental research in their drive to understand factors that affect the health of their communities. In Box 10.2, Dr. Jada Brooks describes her innovative work on racial disparities in health outcomes among American Indians, specifically the Lumbee Tribe, using culturally appropriate methods to gather data. Dr. Cheryl Woods-Giscombé's work is featured in Box 10.3. Her research on African American women has resulted in a clearer understanding of the stresses of the Superwoman Role that pose challenges to their health.

Whether the researcher chooses an experimental or nonexperimental design influences the data collection process. The data collection process includes selection of data collection instruments, design of the data collection protocol, the data analysis plan, participant selection and informed consent, and institutional review plans.

Data Collection Instruments

When designing a study, researchers must consider how the data will be collected. Data collection instruments, sometimes called *data collection tools,* range from simple survey forms to complex gene sequencing instruments. The selected instrument used must be reliable, or consistently accurate. A reliable instrument is one that yields the same values dependably each time the instrument is used to measure the same thing. The tool must also be valid, which means that it must measure what it is supposed to be measuring. The ideal instrument is highly reliable and provides a valid measure of the condition under study, such as weight, temperature, depression, or anxiety.

If body temperature is being measured, a thermometer is an obvious data collection tool—meaning that

NURSES DOING RESEARCH BOX 10.2

Addressing Racial Disparities and Environmental Factors in Health Outcomes among American Indians

Growing up as a young Indigenous girl of the Lumbee Tribe in North Carolina, I was intrigued by the complex health issues I saw in my community. Belonging to one of the most historically understudied populations in the United States, I became interested in research when working in a local pediatric clinic as an undergraduate student. I noticed that Native children experienced more ear infections than children from other racial and ethnic backgrounds—this sparked my curiosity and drove me to pursue a career in science. My first foray into research was on a statewide project in North Carolina to improve mammography use and breast pathology outcomes for American Indian women by designing culturally tailored materials about the potential benefits of breast cancer screening. Because this work showed me the importance of accurately identifying population-specific disparities, I pursued a master's degree in epidemiology. I conducted a statewide project involving seven tribes recognized in North Carolina and four American Indian urban organizations to study the cancer-related inequalities in American Indian women.

Because of a negative experience with a research mentor early in my career, I contemplated other career options. After considering several health professions, I selected nursing because of the endless opportunities it seemed to offer. Immediately after graduating, I worked as a public health nurse trainee with the Robeson (NC) County Health Department. In this role, I provided care to diverse families, many living in impoverished conditions. Seeing how the environment largely influenced families' health motivated me to pursue a doctoral degree in nursing. As a doctoral student, I studied the interactive behaviors of Lumbee mothers and their premature infants. I also examined their perceptions of birthing and parenting a premature infant over the first year of life. After graduating, I completed a postdoctoral fellowship to examine Lumbee mothers' capacity to manage asthma in their children. After completing my fellowship, I accepted a tenure track faculty position at the UNC School of Nursing.

As a nurse scientist, I created a research program that describes and addresses racial disparities in health outcomes among American Indians. To achieve this, I conduct community-engaged research to understand and address environmental factors contributing to health inequalities in the American Indian population. In my work, I use Indigenous methodological approaches, such as Talking Circles—a group method of communication designed to elicit personally meaningful stories rooted in orality and the lived experience—to collect data that embodies the traditional culture of Indigenous people.

I am fortunate but also disheartened to be one of few doctorally prepared American Indian nurse researchers in the nation. My unwavering resolve is to reclaim American Indian health and to see my community flourish.

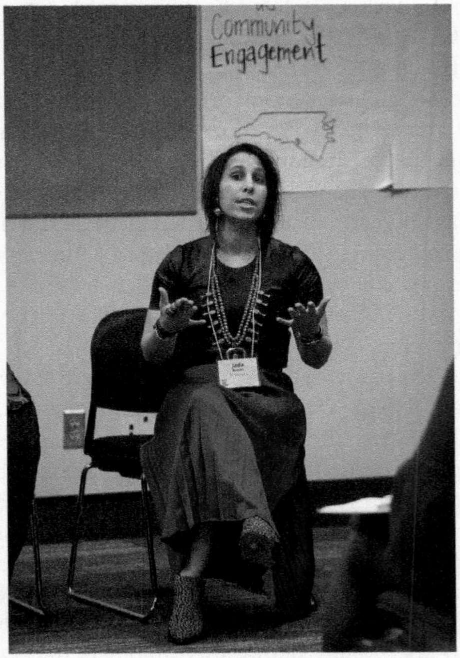

Jada Brooks, PhD, RN, FAAN
Associate Professor
UNC at Chapel Hill School of Nursing

Photo by Ben McKeown, Carolina Center for Public Service

it is known to be a valid measure of temperature—and a scale is the appropriate (valid) measure for weight. Importantly, a valid measure may not be reliable. A scale that varies widely between measurements is not reliable; anyone who has stepped on and off a scale several times to (eventually) get it to show an acceptable weight understands what "unreliable" means (Fig. 10.2). The regular bathroom scale is a valid tool to measure weight; its fluctuation, however, means that it is not reliable.

NURSES DOING RESEARCH BOX 10.3

Understanding How Stress and Coping Contribute to Psychological and Physical Health Outcomes in African American Women

I was always perplexed by health disparities and the contribution of stress to health behaviors and overall well-being. I learned in health classes that African Americans had disproportionately high rates of chronic illness and experienced a shorter life span, yet I never heard any explanation for these disparities. In eighth grade I set the goal of earning my doctor of philosophy (PhD) degree in psychology. My grandmother, a licensed practical/vocational nurse, reminded me that as a young child I had wanted to be a nurse; as a teenager, I did not yet connect nursing with a career in psychology.

As an undergraduate psychology major, I witnessed a psychiatric intake interview with an elderly African American woman admitted to the hospital for "psychotic symptoms." As the only other African American in the room among a team of well-intentioned medical personnel, I thought that no one seemed to "get her." The patient seemed overwhelmed by us. The medical team's labeling of her behavior as bizarre overshadowed her humanity; her explanation of her religious faith was interpreted as delusional. Yet to me she was not so different from other older African American women I knew: optimistic and faithful, yet worn down by chronic stress and familial commitments. I realized then that communication gaps and limited understanding of sociocultural context could not only limit the delivery of health care but also contribute to worsening symptoms and disparities.

While working on my PhD in psychology, I collected data for a clinic-based study that allowed me to observe the work of a nurse practitioner (NP). After a short time of observing how the NP engaged with her patients, their positive responses, and the NP's delight and commitment to providing the best interpersonal and clinically sound strategies to promote health, I was sold! I became a nurse and a psychiatric NP to achieve my career goal of being a national leader in health disparities research and having a clinical practice focusing on the influence of stress on mental and physical health outcomes and on culturally relevant stress management interventions.

Currently my research incorporates sociohistorical and biopsychosocial perspectives to investigate how stress and coping strategies contribute to psychological and physical health outcomes. My Multi-Dimensional Stress Model and Superwoman Schema (SWS) Conceptual Framework show how race- and gender-related factors specifically influence stress, coping, and health inequities among African American women. The SWS Conceptual Framework posits that African American women are at increased risk for health disparities as a result of perceived obligations to remain silent about feelings of distress in order to project an image of strength for their families and communities. These obligations may result from sociohistorical patterns of marginalization, oppression, and stress exposure related to African American women's interconnected race, gender, and socioeconomic status and contribute to the development of resilience, fortitude, and a sense of invulnerability.

The potential contributions of nursing to science and evidence-based health care are practically limitless. I am so proud to be a nursing scholar!

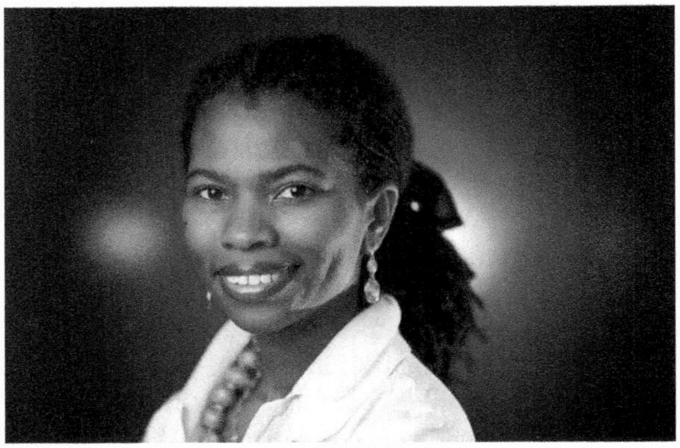

Cheryl Woods-Giscombé, PhD, PMHNP
Professor and Associate Dean of the PhD Division & Program
UNC at Chapel Hill School of Nursing

When measuring psychological phenomena such as anxiety or depression, or constructs (conditions) such as satisfaction or quality of life, researchers face a challenge to determine the best data collection tool. To minimize measurement errors, beginning researchers should choose instruments with established reliability and validity that have been published and widely used rather than designing their own. Inexperienced researchers will occasionally make the mistake of designing a questionnaire they believe is a valid measure of the construct they want to study; doing this, however, constitutes a serious flaw in the research and must be avoided.

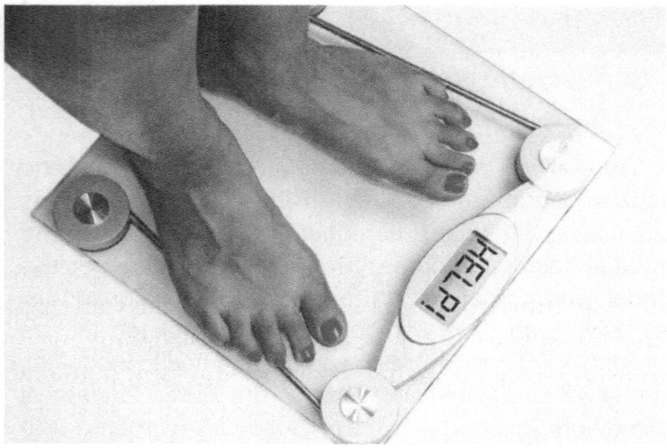

Fig. 10.2 A scale may not always be a reliable way to measure your weight, although it is a valid measure.

Data Collection Protocol

Another aspect of designing the study is deciding on the data collection protocol. The quality of the data depends on strict adherence to the protocol. If, for example, the protocol calls for administering a questionnaire to patients with cancer two days after their first cycle of chemotherapy, the data collectors must be sure to give the questionnaire to all participants on time. The protocol for data collection must be explicit and used by everyone who is collecting data for the study. Data collected in the wrong way or at the wrong time introduces errors into the study.

Data Analysis Plan

It may seem premature to decide how the data will be analyzed before they are even collected, but careful planning for the analysis is important. The research design is developed with data analysis in mind. The analysis must be part of the planning process because the data and the protocols for collecting them depend on how the data will be analyzed. Unless the nurse researcher is an expert in statistics or a statistician is on the research team, consultation with a statistician well versed in human research is recommended in designing the data analysis plan, which answers the question, "What will we do with the data once we collect them?"

Qualitative analysis, notably, begins immediately with the collection of data, because the data themselves often drive the shape and design of the research. Qualitative analysis is a difficult and exacting procedure requiring extensive training. Although some researchers believe that qualitative research may be less challenging to execute than quantitative research, in fact they are similar in the disciplined approach to data analysis required to produce usable, meaningful results.

Participant Selection

A key part of planning research is determining specifically the population to be studied. The individuals enrolled in a study are participants (formerly "subjects"). If the researchers plan to study pain management in patients with traumatic injuries in the emergency department, for example, they have to decide the specific type and severity of traumatic injury and will likely consider the age, gender, ethnicity, and geographic location of the patients, as well as a variety of other factors, in planning the participant selection. Qualitative studies use different sampling strategies; that is, the participants are selected for study in a different manner than is typically used in quantitative studies. Qualitative researchers often use a strategy known as "purposeful sampling"; potential participants are selected for the study specifically rather than randomly, as is sometimes used in quantitative studies. These participants exhibit a trait or have had an experience that the researcher is studying.

Informed Consent and Institutional Review

Next, researchers who want to enroll humans in their study must protect the rights of participants. This involves the use of the informed consent process, which includes having participants sign an informed consent document detailing the study and what participation in the research means. Any risks must be explained. A basic principle of informed consent is that participation in research is *always voluntary*—no one may be pressured in any way to enroll in the study or to continue in the study once enrolled. Confidentiality (privacy) of participants must be ensured. Considering Culture Box 10.1 addresses the difficulties of enrolling participants in research when they do not speak English.

A related step when studying humans is the submission of the proposal to the institution, such as a hospital or clinic, where the research will take place, for review by a federally approved board known as an institutional review board (IRB). An IRB is composed of individuals from the community and different academic disciplines and exists to ensure that research is well designed and does not violate the policies and procedures of the institution or the rights of the participants. Only after

CONSIDERING CULTURE BOX 10.1

The Challenge of Informed Consent: When the Participant Does Not Speak English

Researchers studying humans must protect the rights of their participants by asking them to sign a detailed consent form that describes the study and what participation in the study means. With an increasing number of potential participants who may not speak English or for whom English is a second language, what measures would researchers need to consider when planning to recruit and enroll these potential participants? What are the risks to these persons? How can these risks be minimized? How might researchers ensure that these participants do not feel pressured to participate?

the IRB approves the proposal can the study begin. Persons conducting research or assisting with the management of data must demonstrate evidence that they have taken an online course on the protection of the rights of human participants (www.citiprogram.org). The protection of the rights of participants is the primary consideration of all research involving humans. Modification of any aspect of the research requires that the IRB be notified and approval procured before the change is implemented.

Implementation of the Study

Up until this point, only planning has taken place. Careful planning is, however, the key to a successful study. In the implementation phase, the actual study is conducted. The two main tasks during this phase are data collection and data analysis.

Data Collection

Data (research-generated information) should be collected only by persons (usually research assistants) thoroughly familiar with the study. All research assistants should understand the purpose of the data and the importance of accuracy and careful record keeping. No matter who is collecting the data, the integrity of the project is ultimately the responsibility of the primary researcher.

Data Analysis

If all goes well, data are analyzed exactly as proposed. In analyzing data, most researchers use the same statistician with whom they consulted in planning the study. The researcher works closely with the statistician in interpreting, as well as analyzing the data. The nurse researcher is in charge, however, and they have the final word on what interpretations are made from the data.

Analyzing the findings of qualitative research presents formidable challenges for several reasons. First, the data sets are huge, often consisting of lengthy dialogues between researchers and participants. Next, dialogues must be transcribed verbatim, yielding long transcripts. The investigator then faces the task of organizing the transcripts, identifying themes, and arranging the themes into meaningful patterns. Software is available to assist in this process; however, nothing substitutes for contemplation in determining the nuances of meanings in narrative data.

Findings, Discussion, and Clinical Implications

In writing the research report, the findings directly related to the research question are presented first. Findings are presented objectively, without value judgments. The findings must speak for themselves. Accurate presentation of the facts is the only requirement. After findings related to the research question are reported, unexpected findings can be reported. The researchers address the question, "What do these findings mean?" In discussion sections, researchers can be more reflective about the findings, discussing what was anticipated versus what was found in the study, suggesting alternative explanations for their findings and further research to clarify findings.

Researchers are always alert to the implications of their studies. Implications are suggestions for actions that can be taken as a result of the research findings in the future. Every good study raises more questions than it answers. In nursing studies there may be indications for modifications in nursing education or nursing practice. Nearly every study has implications for further research, and if the findings turn out as expected, almost all studies should be carefully replicated. Replication can answer these and other questions: What needs to be known to develop more confidence in the findings? Will the research instrument produce similar results in a similar population in a different geographic location? Will the procedure be effective with patients having a slightly different diagnosis, condition, or type of surgery? Will age make a difference? Will cultural beliefs make a difference? What else do we need to know to improve the care of patients?

Dissemination of Findings

Findings from a research study must be disseminated so that others can learn from the work that was done. **Dissemination** refers to the process of publication and presentation of findings. Most funding agencies want to know in advance how the researcher plans to disseminate findings because letting others know about the findings is essential. The two major vehicles for dissemination of knowledge are articles published in professional journals and presentations given at conferences. Prominent nursing research journals include *Research in Nursing & Health (RINAH)*, *Nursing Research (NR)*, *Journal of Nursing Scholarship* (published by Sigma), *Nursing Inquiry*, *Journal of Advanced Nursing*, and *Advances in Nursing Science (ANS)*. These journals are not specific to any particular type of nursing but publish articles of wide interest in nursing. Professional nursing organizations are likely to have their own research journals targeting specific interests, such as *JOGNN: Journal of Obstetric, Gynecologic, & Neonatal Nursing*, published by the Association of Women's Health, Obstetric and Neonatal Nurses (AWHONN), and *Journal of the Association of Nurses in AIDS Care (JANAC)*, published by the Association of Nurses in AIDS Care (ANAC).

A review process, called **peer review**, is the method most journals use to determine whether to publish a research report. During peer review, a manuscript is circulated, usually but not always anonymously, to a review panel consisting of two to three experts in the area of study. Reviewers evaluate its scientific soundness, appropriateness of design and data analysis, and accuracy and recommend that it be published, that it be revised and then resubmitted with changes, or that it be rejected. Most research that is carefully conceived, conducted, and presented can get published, although the researcher must be persistent and resilient in taking criticism and revising manuscripts.

A somewhat easier, yet still discriminating, route to dissemination is presentation at one or more of the numerous nursing research conferences. Many research conferences also use the peer-review process. In general, however, the proportion of **abstracts** (summaries of research) selected for presentation at conferences is higher than the proportion of manuscripts chosen for publication. In addition to oral presentation of research papers, conferences offer the opportunity for nurses to present their findings in poster sessions, especially appropriate when work is preliminary or still in progress. Posters allow for brief explanations of the research method and findings in written form, usually a 3- × 4-foot poster. Poster presentations are often the first way that students doing research disseminate their findings.

Whether research is published or presented at conferences, it is important to disseminate research results to other nurses, who may choose to use the results either to improve patient care practices directly or to replicate the study.

THE RELATIONSHIP OF RESEARCH TO THEORY AND PRACTICE

Relationships among nursing research, practice, and theory are circular. As mentioned earlier, research ideas are generated from three sources: (1) clinical practice, (2) literature, and (3) theory.

Questions about how best to deal with patient problems regularly arise in clinical situations. As shown in the earlier example of Mrs. Abney, the woman who could not find her room, problems often can be "solved" for the present. However, when the same questions recur, long-term answers may be needed. Research develops solutions that can be used with confidence in different situations.

Published articles about nursing research often generate interest in further studies. If there is published research on a particular nursing care problem, other researchers may be stimulated to investigate the subject further and refine the solutions. This is how nursing knowledge builds.

Nursing theorists also generate research ideas. They piece together postulates or premises that explain what has been discovered. The explanation is tested via research to determine whether it is robust or strong enough to be useful. If so, there may be more implications for applications in clinical practice. Nursing research journals are filled with clinical studies that have made a difference in patient care. A few examples of changes in nursing practice stimulated by research include decreasing light and noise in critical care units to prevent sleep deprivation; using caps on newborns to decrease heat loss and stabilize body temperature; and proper positioning of patients after chest surgery to facilitate respiration.

Nursing research findings not only improve patient care but also affect the healthcare system itself. For example, research studies have demonstrated the cost effectiveness of nurses as healthcare providers. This is discussed further in Chapter 14.

A final point about the influence of research on practice is a reminder about the relationship of research and professionalism. In Chapter 3, you learned about the characteristics of professions. One of the hallmarks of a mature profession is a scientific body of knowledge that is expanded through research. Nursing research enhances the status of nursing as a profession by expanding nursing's scientific knowledge base. Researchers in other disciplines can then use the sound research produced by nurse researchers as part of a foundation for their own work.

FINANCIAL SUPPORT FOR NURSING RESEARCH

Research of any kind is expensive, and support takes many forms. It can include encouragement, consultation, digital and library resources, money, and release time from researchers' regular teaching responsibilities. Each of these forms of support is important, but none alone is adequate. Early in the development of nursing research, encouragement was often the only support available, and not all nurse researchers had that. Gradually, more sources of funding have been developed, but financial support can still be difficult to obtain, particularly for inexperienced researchers.

Many federal agencies accept proposals that meet their funding guidelines when submitted by qualified nurse researchers. These include the 27 centers and institutes of the NIH, including NINR. Competition with researchers from other disciplines is strong, however, and generally funding is limited to experienced nurse researchers with PhDs.

Nursing associations also fund nursing research. The American Nurses Foundation, Sigma, and clinical specialty organizations provide research awards, even for beginning researchers. State and local nursing associations sometimes have seed money for pilot projects. Universities, schools of nursing, and large hospitals also may provide some research funds. In general, however, finding adequate funding for large-scale studies continues to be a problem faced by researchers.

ADVANCING THE PROFESSION THROUGH THE USE OF RESEARCH

The American Nurses Association's *Code of Ethics*, Provision 7.3, states: "The nursing profession should engage in scholarly inquiry to identify, evaluate, refine, and expand the body of knowledge that forms the foundation of its discipline and practice. ... All nurses working alone or in collaboration with others can participate in the advancement of the profession through the development, evaluation, dissemination, and application of knowledge in practice" (American Nurses Association, 2015). Ideally, every nurse should be involved in research, but practically, as a minimum, all nurses should use research to support and improve their practices. EBP requires staying informed about current research literature, especially studies done in one's own specific area of clinical practice.

As shown in Table 10.3, in addition to using research to improve practice, all professional nurses can contribute to one or more aspects of the research process. From the time nurses begin their basic nursing education, they become consumers of research. BSN-prepared nurses can read, interpret, and evaluate research for use in supporting their evidence-based practice. Through clinical practice they can identify nursing problems that need to be investigated. They can also participate in the implementation of scientific studies by helping principal researchers collect data in clinical settings or elsewhere. These beginning researchers must know enough about the purpose of

TABLE 10.3 Levels of Educational Preparation and Participation in Nursing Research

Level of Preparation	Level of Research Participation
Nursing student	Learning about research; doing honors projects and/or assisting in laboratories
Bachelor of science in nursing (BSN)	Identifies problems that can be studied; may do data collection for research studies
Master of science in nursing (MSN)	Replicates earlier research; beginning independent research
Doctor of nursing practice (DNP)	Connect research to practice; do research in collaboration with a PhD-prepared colleague
Doctor of philosophy (PhD)	Generate and test theory; establishing independent research career with external funding (e.g., National Institutes of Health, foundation grants)

Note: Nurses at all levels are assumed to be consumers of research.

PROFESSIONAL PROFILE BOX 10.1

A Career Helping Others With Their Research

After earning my bachelor of science degree in nursing (BSN) with a major in nursing at Villa Maria College in Erie, Pennsylvania, I first worked as a staff nurse in a surgery intensive care unit in Pittsburg, Pennsylvania, but within a short time I moved to Chapel Hill, North Carolina, to work in the cardiothoracic intensive care unit.

To be truthful, I got into clinical research by accident for my first position as a cardiology research nurse, an experience in which I learned—unfortunately—what the term *soft money* means. It means that funding for research is not permanent or guaranteed, and after 1½ years, we lost our funding. But even after learning what it meant to be working on soft money, I knew I wanted to continue working as a clinical research nurse. Soon hired as a pediatric intensive care unit (PICU) research nurse, I managed all aspects of a research study (screening for participants, completing the informed consent process, collecting data, responding to queries, negotiating budgets, and eventually closing out the study).

Most recently, I was a research nurse consultant with North Carolina Translational and Clinical Sciences Institute (NC TraCS). I facilitated a study group for persons interested in preparation for the clinical research certification examination and 29 people who participated in the study group passed the examination. I am a member of the Association of Clinical Research Professionals (ACRP) and have been a Certified Clinical Research Coordinator (CCRC) for 10 years.

I have done many local and national presentations on the protection of the rights of human subjects in research. Through the ACRP I met Eva Mozes Kor, a survivor of Mengele's experiments at Auschwitz, touring Auschwitz with her during the 65th anniversary of its liberation. This relationship fueled my passion for research ethics.

Being a nurse is a real asset in my role. One of the PICU researchers asked me, "When did you quit being a real nurse?" I responded, "I am still a nurse." The role of the nurse is not limited to bedside patient care. There are other ways to be a nurse! In both roles, the first priority is protection—of your patient or your research participant.

Because I am a nurse, I can review a medical record to see if someone qualifies for a study, understand the participant's disease process, and recognize adverse events. As a research nurse I have to *assess* the situation, participant, or protocol; *plan* how the study would be implemented; *implement* the study; and *evaluate* the extent to which it is being implemented correctly. That sounds like the nursing process to me. Critical thinking is central in the role of the research nurse.

While completing my Master of Science in Nursing (MSN), I developed an interest in four areas: research, ethics, legal, and quality. As a clinical research nurse, I found a role where I could be involved in all four.

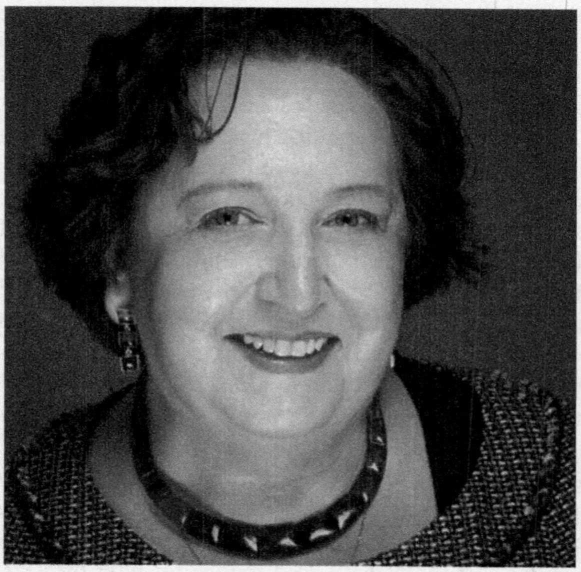

Claudia Christy, MSN, RN, CCRC, FACRP

the research to follow the research protocols explicitly or know when it is necessary to deviate from the protocol for a patient's well-being. BSN-prepared nurses also can help disseminate research-based knowledge by sharing useful research findings with colleagues.

The master's-prepared nurse may be ready to work with experienced nurse researchers to replicate studies that have been previously conducted. Depending on education, clinical and research experiences, and interests, some nurses at the master's level are better prepared to conduct research than others. In addition to education and experience, a crucial factor is the support system the nurse has available. To do research, nurses need time, money, consultation, and participants. With rich resources in a research environment, master's degree–prepared nurses can and do make vital research contributions.

Nurses with doctor of philosophy (PhD) or other doctoral degrees (e.g., doctor of nursing practice [DNP], doctor of education [EdD], doctor of public health [DrPH]) are more favorably positioned to receive research funding than are nurses without doctorates. Researchers across the United States in all professions and academic disciplines compete for a limited pool of research dollars available each year. Only those nurses with strong academic and experiential backgrounds and carefully conceptualized and well-written proposals succeed in obtaining federal funding. Currently, only nurses with PhDs may receive funding from the NIH, although other funding sources are open to nurses with other doctoral degrees.

Research in nursing provides the avenue for creative, scholarly endeavors driven by a desire to improve the care for patients. Professional Profile Box 10.1 contains a description of the work and career of Claudia Christy, MSN, RN, CCRC, FACRP, whose work demonstrates ways other than conducting studies that nurses can be involved in the development and implementation of research. You will find research to be an important part of your professional practice both as a consumer of research and as an adherent to evidence-based practice. And someday you may confront a question or situation in practice so compelling that you respond by starting your own research career to improve patient outcomes by improving nursing practice.

CONCEPTS AND CHALLENGES

- ***Concept:*** Nursing research is defined as the systematic investigation of phenomena of interest to nursing with the goal of improving care.
  Challenge: Nurses must value research as an important means of optimizing patient outcomes, in addition to clinician expertise and patient preferences, in having practices that are evidence based.
- ***Concept:*** The scientific method is a systematic, orderly process of solving problems. It has been used for centuries and is applicable in many different situations.
  Challenge: There are several types of research; laboratory (bench) research and bedside (clinical) research are two traditional types. Translational research is a means of connecting more efficiently the work that is generated in laboratories and directly within patient populations, a connection that is not always easy to make.
- ***Concept:*** For safety and ethical reasons, there are limitations on research with human participants.
  Challenge: It can be difficult to determine all of the ways that research may pose a threat to participants; therefore all research involving humans must go through a process of approval by an institutional review board.
- ***Concept:*** The major steps in the research process are identification of a research problem, review of the literature, formulation of the research question, design of the study, implementation, drawing conclusions based on findings, discussion of implications, and dissemination of findings.
  Challenge: Assessing research for its usefulness requires that nurses recognize the presence of each of these steps. Well-executed research has followed these steps carefully.
- ***Concept:*** Nursing research is related to and informed by nursing theory and nursing practice.
  Challenge: The relationship among theory, research, and practice can be difficult to understand; however, each depends on the others for clarity and direction.
- ***Concept:*** Nurses of all educational backgrounds are consumers of research and have a role in carrying out research either directly through the implementation of a study or through the use of research in informing practice.
  Challenge: Envisioning oneself as a nurse researcher can pose a challenge; however, the use of research must be a priority for students and nurses to continue to advance the profession and discipline of nursing, and to continue to build the body of nursing knowledge.

IDEAS FOR FURTHER EXPLORATION

1. Define *inductive* and *deductive reasoning.* Why is neither adequate to advance knowledge alone? Are you more likely to change practice using research that uses an inductive or a deductive approach to reasoning?
2. Go to your college or university library or online site and determine what nursing research journals are available to you. Scan through some recent issues and notice the types of studies reported. Compare them with studies done 20 years ago. What similarities and differences do you note?
3. Read a research article on a topic of interest to you. See whether you can identify each of the steps in the research process. Is the article one that makes you consider practicing in a different way?
4. Find out what research is being done in your school of nursing or patient care setting. Talk to the nurses who are involved in the research for their perspectives about their role in the study and what the research will accomplish.
5. Consider what it means to have your nursing practice based in evidence. What are the implications for a new nurse who lacks the clinical expertise that is required for EBP? Can a nurse without much experience have a practice that is evidence based?

REFERENCES

American Nurses Association: *Code of ethics*, Washington, DC, 2015, American Nurses Publishing. [website]. Available at https://www.nursingworld.org/practice-policy/nursing-excellence/ethics/code-of-ethics-for-nurses/coe-view-only/.

Cleary-Holdforth J, Leufer T: Essential elements in developing evidence-based practice, *Nurs Stand* 23(2):42–46, 2008.

Flexner SB, Stein J, Su PY: *The Random House dictionary*, New York, 1980, Random House.

Kuhn TS: The structure of scientific revolutions. In Nurath O, editor: *International Encyclopedia of Unified Science, vol. 2*, 2, Chicago, 1970, University of Chicago Press.

Melnyk BM, Fineout-Overhold E, Stillwell SB, et al.: Igniting a spirit of inquiry: An essential foundation for evidence-based practice, *Am J Nurs* 109(11):49–52, 2009.

National Institutes of Health: *Office of strategic coordination: the common fund*, 2021. (website). Retrieved from: www.commonfund.nih.gov.

National Institute of Nursing Research (NINR): *The NINR strategic plan: advancing science, improving lives*, Bethesda, Md, 2016, National Institutes of Health (NIH). [website]Available at https://www.ninr.nih.gov/sites/files/docs/NINR_StratPlan2016_reduced.pdf.

National Institute of Nursing Research (NINR): *Mission & strategic plan*, 2021. (website). Available at: https://www.ninr.nih.gov/aboutninr/ninr-mission-and-strategic-plan.

11

Developing Nursing Judgment Through Critical Thinking

To enhance your understanding of this chapter, try the Student Exercises on the Evolve site at http://evolve.elsevier.com/Black/professional.

LEARNING OUTCOMES

After studying this chapter, students will be able to:

- Define *critical thinking,* and describe its importance in nursing.
- Contrast the characteristics of "novice thinking" with those of "expert thinking."
- Explain the purpose and phases of the nursing process.
- Explain the differences between independent, interdependent (collaborative), and dependent nursing actions.
- Describe evaluation and its importance in the nursing process.
- Define *clinical judgment in nursing practice* and explain how it is developed.
- Devise a personal plan to use in developing sound clinical judgment.

Almost every encounter a nurse has with a patient is an opportunity for the nurse to assist the patient to a higher level of wellness or comfort. A nurse's ability to think critically about a patient's particular needs and how best to meet them will determine the extent to which a patient benefits from the nurse's care. A nurse's ability to use a reliable, consistent cognitive approach is crucial in determining a patient's priorities for care and in making sound clinical decisions in addressing those priorities. This chapter explores important and interdependent aspects of thinking and decision making in nursing. Some of these aspects include critical thinking, the nursing process, and clinical judgment.

CRITICAL THINKING: CULTIVATING INTELLECTUAL STANDARDS

Defining *critical thinking* is a complex task that requires an understanding of how people think through problems. Educators and philosophers struggled with definitions of critical thinking for several decades. Two decades ago, the American Philosophical Association published an expert consensus statement (Box 11.1) describing critical thinking and attributes of the ideal critical thinker. This expert statement, still widely used, was the culmination of 3 years of work by Facione and others who synthesized the work of numerous persons who had defined critical thinking. More recently, Facione (2013) noted that giving a definition of critical thinking that can be memorized by the learner is actually antithetical to critical thinking. This means that the very definition of critical thinking does not lend itself to simplistic thinking and memorization.

The Paul-Elder Critical Thinking Framework (Paul and Elder, 2015) is grounded in this definition of critical thinking:

Critical thinking is that mode of thinking—about any subject, content, or problem—in which the thinker improves the quality of his or her thinking by skillfully

BOX 11.1 Expert Consensus Statement Regarding Critical Thinking and the Ideal Critical Thinker

We understand critical thinking (CT) to be purposeful, self-regulatory judgment that results in interpretation, analysis, evaluation, inference, as well as explanation of the evidential, conceptual, methodological, criteriological, or contextual considerations upon which that judgment is based. CT is essential as a tool of inquiry. As such, CT is a liberating force in education and a powerful resource in one's personal and civic life. Although not synonymous with good thinking, CT is a pervasive and self-rectifying human phenomenon. The ideal critical thinker is habitually inquisitive, well-informed, trustful of reason, open-minded, flexible, fair-minded in evaluation, honest in facing personal biases, prudent in making judgments, willing to reconsider, clear about issues, orderly in complex matters, diligent in seeking relevant information, reasonable in the selection of criteria, focused in inquiry, and persistent in seeking results that are as precise as the subject and the circumstances of inquiry permit. Thus educating good critical thinkers means working toward this ideal. It combines developing CT skills with nurturing those dispositions that consistently yield useful insights and that are the basis of a rational and democratic society.

From American Philosophical Association: *Critical thinking: a statement of expert consensus for purposes of educational assessment and instruction,* The Delphi report: Research findings and recommendations prepared for the committee on pre-college philosophy, 1990, Newark, ERIC Document Reproduction Services, pp 315–423.

taking charge of the structures inherent in thinking and imposing intellectual standards upon them.

Paul and Elder (2015) describe the "well-cultivated critical thinker" as one who does the following:

1. Raises questions and problems and formulates them clearly and precisely
2. Gathers and assesses relevant information, using abstract ideas for interpretation
3. Arrives at conclusions and solutions that are well reasoned and tests them against relevant standards
4. Is open-minded and recognizes alternative ways of seeing problems and has the ability to assess the assumptions, implications, and consequences of alternative views of problems
5. Communicates effectively with others as solutions to complex problems are formulated

We live in a "new knowledge economy" driven by information and technology that changes quickly. Analyzing and integrating information across an increasing number of sources of knowledge require that you have flexible intellectual skills. Being a good critical thinker makes you more adaptable in this new economy of knowledge (Lau and Chan, 2012). An excellent website on critical thinking can be found at http://philosophy.hku.hk/think/ (OpenCourseWare on critical thinking, logic, and creativity).

So what does this have to do with nursing? The answer is simple: excellent critical thinking skills are required for you to make good clinical judgments. You will be responsible and accountable for your own decisions as a professional nurse. The development of critical thinking skills is crucial as you provide nursing care for patients with increasingly complex conditions. Critical thinking skills provide you with a powerful means of determining patient needs, interpreting physician orders, and intervening appropriately. Box 11.2 presents an example of the importance of critical thinking in the provision of safe care. The nurse in this example takes several sources of data about her patient, uses her clinical expertise, advocates for her patient, and thus gets the patient help for a serious postoperative complication.

CRITICAL THINKING IN NURSING

You may be wondering at this point, "How am I ever going to learn how to make connections among all of the data I have about a patient?" This is a common response for a nursing student who is just learning some of the most basic psychomotor skills in preparation for practice. You need to understand that, just like learning to give injections safely and maintaining a sterile field, you can learn to think critically. This involves paying attention to how you think and making thinking itself a focus of concern. A nurse who is exercising critical thinking asks the following questions: "What assumptions have I made about this patient?" "How do I know my assumptions are accurate?" "Do I need any additional information?" and "How might I look at this situation differently?" Schneider (2015) noted that "basic nursing care encompasses a responsibility for correct interpretation of assessment data using critical thinking" (p. 60).

Nurses just beginning to pay attention to their thinking processes may ask these questions after

BOX 11.2 Using Critical Thinking Skills to Improve a Patient's Care

Ms. George has recently undergone bariatric surgery after many attempts to lose weight over the years have failed. She is to be discharged home on postoperative day 2, as per the usual protocol. Although she describes herself as "not feeling well at all," the physician writes the order for discharge and you, as the nurse who does postoperative discharge planning for the surgery practice, meet with Ms. George to go over dietary guidelines that should help her lose weight successfully. You note that Ms. George does not seem as comfortable or pleased with her surgery as most patients with whom you have worked in the past.

Ms. George has to wait three hours for her husband to drive her home, and you note that she continues to lie on the bed passively, and her lethargy is increasing. You take her vital signs, and note that her temperature is 37.8°C and her pulse is 115. You listen to her chest, and note that it is difficult to appreciate breath sounds because of the patient's body habitus. Ms. George points to an area just below her left breast where she notes pain with inspiration. You call her physician to report your findings; she responds that Ms. George's pain is "not unusual" with her type of bariatric surgery and that her slightly increased temperature is "most likely" related to her being somewhat dehydrated. She instructs you to have Ms. George force fluids to the extent that she can tolerate it and take mild pain medication for postoperative pain. You ask the surgeon to consider delaying Ms. George's discharge home, but she refuses.

You give Ms. George acetaminophen as ordered, but her pain on inspiration continues. Her temperature remains at 37.8°C, and her pulse is 120. You measure her O_2 saturation with a pulse oximeter, and it is 91%. Her respirations are 26 and somewhat shallow. Her surgeon does not respond to your page, so you call the nursing supervisor, explaining to him that you are concerned with Ms. George's impending discharge. Because Ms. George's surgeon has not been responsive to your concerns, you call the hospitalist (a physician who sees inpatients in the absence of their attending physician), who orders a chest x-ray study. Ms. George has evidence of a consolidation in her left lower lobe, which turns out to be a pulmonary abscess in its early stages. She is treated on intravenous antibiotics for five days, and the abscess eventually has to be aspirated and drained.

Your critical thinking skills and willingness to advocate for your patient prevented an even worse postoperative course. You recognized that Ms. George's lethargy was unusual, and the location and timing of her pain were of concern. You also realized that although her temperature appeared to be stable, she had been given a pain medicine (acetaminophen) that also reduces fever, so in fact, a temperature increase may have been masked by the antipyretic properties of the acetaminophen. You demonstrated excellent clinical judgment in measuring her O_2 saturation, noting that her respiratory rate and pulse were consistent with decreased oxygenation. Furthermore, you sought support through the nursing "chain of command" when you engaged the nursing supervisor, who supported you in contacting the hospitalist. The specific, detailed information that you were able to provide the hospitalist allowed him to follow a logical diagnostic path, determining that Ms. George did indeed have a significant postoperative complication. Two days later, Ms. George reports that she is "feeling much better" and is walking in the hallways several times a day.

nurse-patient interactions have ended. This is known as **reflective thinking**, an active process valuable in learning and changing behaviors, perspectives, or practices. Nurses can also learn to examine their thinking processes during an interaction as they learn to "think on their feet." This is a characteristic of expert nurses. As you move from novice to expert, your ability to think critically will improve with practice. In Chapter 5 you read about Dr. Patricia Benner (1984; Benner et al., 1996), who studied the differences in expertise of nurses at different stages in their careers, from novice to expert. So it is with critical thinking: novices think differently from experts. Box 11.3 summarizes the differences in novice and expert thinking.

Critical thinking is a complex, purposeful, disciplined process that has specific characteristics that make it different from typical problem solving. Critical thinking in nursing is undergirded by the standards and ethics of the profession. Consciously developed to improve patient outcomes, critical thinking by the nurse is driven by the needs of the patient and family. Nurses who think critically are engaged in a process of constant evaluation, redirection, improvement, and increased efficiency. Be aware that critical thinking involves far more than stating your opinion; critical thinking is not the same as being critical. You must be able to describe how you came to a conclusion and support your conclusions with explicit data and rationales. Becoming an excellent

BOX 11.3 Novice Thinking Compared With Expert Thinking

Novice Nurses

1. Tend to organize knowledge as separate facts. Must rely heavily on resources (e.g., texts, notes, preceptors). Lack knowledge gained from actually doing (e.g., listening to breath sounds).
2. Focus so much on actions that they may not fully assess before acting.
3. Need and follow clear-cut rules.
4. Are often hampered by unawareness of resources.
5. May be hindered by anxiety and lack of self-confidence.
6. Tend to rely on step-by-step procedures and follow standards and policies rigidly.
7. Tend to focus more on performing procedures correctly than on the patient's response to the procedure.
8. Have limited knowledge of suspected problems; therefore they question and collect data more superficially or in a less focused way than more experienced nurses.
9. Learn more readily when matched with a supportive, knowledgeable preceptor or mentor.

Expert Nurses

1. Tend to store knowledge in a highly organized and structured manner, making recall of information easier. Have a large storehouse of experiential knowledge (e.g., what abnormal breath sounds sound like, what subtle changes look like).
2. Assess and consider different options for intervening before acting.
3. Know which rules are flexible and when it is appropriate to bend the rules.
4. Are aware of resources and how to use them.
5. Are usually more self-confident, less anxious, and therefore more focused than less experienced nurses.
6. Are comfortable with rethinking a procedure if patient needs require modification of the procedure.
7. Have a better idea of suspected problems, allowing them to question more deeply and collect more relevant and in-depth data.
8. Analyze standards and policies, looking for ways to improve them.
9. Are challenged by novices' questions, clarifying their own thinking when teaching novices.

From Alfaro-LeFevre R: *Critical thinking in nursing: a practical approach,* ed 2, Philadelphia, 1999, Saunders. Reprinted with permission.

critical thinker is significantly related to increased years of work experience and to higher education level; moreover, nurses with critical thinking abilities tend to be more competent in their practice than nurses with less well-developed critical thinking skills (Chang et al., 2011). Box 11.4 summarizes these characteristics and offers an opportunity for you to evaluate your progress as a critical thinker.

An excellent continuing education (CE) self-study module designed to improve your ability to think critically can be found online at http://ce.nurse.com/course/ce168-60/improving-your-ability-to-think-critically/. (Note that there is a modest fee for this course.) Continuing one's education through lifelong learning is an excellent way to maintain and enhance your critical thinking skills. The website http://ce.nurse.com has more than 500 CE opportunities available online and may be helpful to you as you seek to increase your knowledge base and improve your clinical judgment. Being intentional about improving your critical thinking skills ensures that you bring your best effort to the bedside in providing care for your patients.

THE NURSING PROCESS: A UNIVERSAL INTELLECTUAL STANDARD

Critical thinking requires systematic and disciplined use of universal intellectual standards (Paul and Elder, 2015). In the practice of nursing, the **nursing process** represents a universal intellectual standard by which problems are addressed and solved. The nursing process is a method of critical thinking focused on solving patient problems in professional practice. The nursing process is "a conceptual framework that enables the student or the practicing nurse to think systematically and process pertinent information about the patient" (Huckabay, 2009, p. 72). This process combines the "art of nursing" (creativity) with systems theory and the scientific method to produce high level care for your patients that is both interpersonal and interactive (Doenges et al., 2013).

You engage in problem solving daily. Suppose your favorite band is performing in a nearby city the night before a big exam in pathophysiology. Your exam counts as 35% of your final grade. But you have wanted to see

BOX 11.4 Self-Assessment: Critical Thinking

Directions: Listed below are 15 characteristics of critical thinkers. Mark a plus sign (+) next to those you now possess, mark IP (in progress) next to those you have partially mastered, and mark a zero (0) next to those you have not yet mastered. When you are finished, make a plan for developing the areas that need improvement. Share it with at least one person, and report on progress weekly.

Characteristics of Critical Thinkers

1. ______ Inquisitive/curious/seeks truth
2. ______ Self-informed/finds own answers
3. ______ Analytic/confident in own reasoning skills
4. ______ Open-minded
5. ______ Flexible
6. ______ Fair-minded
7. ______ Honest about personal biases/self-aware
8. ______ Prudent/exercises sound judgment
9. ______ Willing to revise judgment when new evidence warrants
10. ______ Clear about issues
11. ______ Orderly in complex matters/organized approach to problems
12. ______ Diligent in seeking information
13. ______ Persistent
14. ______ Reasonable
15. ______ Focused on inquiry

this band since you were 15, and you do not know when you will have another chance. You are faced with weighing a number of factors that will influence your decision about whether to go see the band: your grade going into the exam; how late you will be out the night before the exam; how far you will have to drive to see the band; and how much study time you will have to prepare for the exam in advance. You are really conflicted about this, so you decide to let another factor determine what you will do: the cost of the ticket. When you learn that the only seats available are near the back of the venue and cost $120.00 each, you decide to stay home and get a good night's sleep before the big exam; the next day you make a grade of 98% on the exam. You then realize that because you made such a good grade on this exam, you will have much less pressure when studying for the final exam at the end of the semester. You have identified a problem (not a particularly serious one, but one with personal significance), considered various factors related to the problem, identified possible actions, selected the best alternative, evaluated the success of the alternative selected, and made adjustments to the solution based on the evaluation. This is the same general process nurses use in solving patient problems through the nursing process.

For individuals outside the profession, nursing is commonly and simplistically defined in terms of tasks nurses perform. Many students get frustrated with activities and courses in nursing school that are not focused on these tasks, believing that the tasks of nursing *are* nursing. Even within the profession, the intellectual basis of nursing practice was not articulated until the 1960s, when nursing educators and leaders began to identify and name the components of nursing's intellectual processes. This marked the beginning of the nursing process. In today's evolving health care environment, the use of the nursing process streamlines the processes of care that are entered into the electronic health record (EHR). Furthermore, the use of the nursing process provides a means of determining the economic contributions of nursing to patient outcomes, so nursing care can be cost effective yet still be consistent with the goals and perspectives of the profession (Doenges et al., 2013).

In the 1970s and 1980s, debate about the use of the term *diagnosis* began. Until then, diagnosis was considered to be within the scope of practice of physicians only. Although nurses were not educated or licensed to diagnose medical conditions in patients, nurses recognized that there were human responses amenable to independent nursing intervention. Using diagnoses gave nurses a universal terminology, "standardizing the 'what' and 'how' of the work of nursing" (Doenges et al., 2013, p. 10). A nursing diagnosis, then, is "a clinical judgment about individual, family or community responses to actual or potential health problems or life processes which provide the basis for selection of nursing interventions to achieve outcomes for which the nurse has accountability" (NANDA-I, 2012). These responses could be identified (diagnosed) through the careful application of specific defining characteristics. On its website, NANDA-I notes that "Nursing diagnoses communicate the professional judgments that nurses make every day to our patients, colleagues, members of other disciplines, and the public. Nursing diagnoses define what we know—they are our words" (nanda.org, 2021).

In 1973 the National Group for the Classification of Nursing Diagnosis published its first list of nursing diagnoses. This group later became known as NANDA, founded in 1982, and is now known as NANDA International, Inc. (NANDA-I; NANDA was the acronym for the now obsolete name North American Nursing Diagnosis Association). Its mission is to "facilitate the development, refinement, dissemination and use of standardized nursing diagnostic terminology" with the vision to "improve the health care of all people" (nanda.org, 2021). NANDA-I's 2021-2023 12th edition of *Nursing Diagnoses: Definitions and Classifications* contains 267 diagnoses approved for clinical testing, 46 of which are new in this edition, and 67 are diagnoses that have been revised since the previous edition. Diagnoses are retired if it becomes evident that their usefulness is limited or outdated.

A diagnosis is "a clinical judgment concerning a human response to health conditions/life processes, or susceptibility to that response, by an individual, family, group or community" (NANDA-I, 2021, sec. 5.1). NANDA-I's work is more than a list of accepted diagnoses: it is a taxonomy (classification system) with 13 domains, such as health promotion, nutrition, elimination and exchange, self-perception, among others. Under each domain are classes, for example, in Domain 1 Health promotion, Class 1 is health awareness, defined as recognition of normal function and well-being. In this class, there are three associated diagnoses: decreased diversional activity engagement, readiness for enhanced health literacy, and sedentary lifestyle. Each diagnosis has a definition and associated defining characteristics, related factors, at-risk populations, and associated conditions.

A diagnosis is approved for use by NANDA-I based on up-to-date evidence and the guidance from researchers, expert diagnosticians, and educators. Here is an example of how a nurse would develop a diagnosis:

Three days after a surgery under general anesthesia for a large but benign abdominal mass, Mr. Stevens, 55 years old, 104 kg (229 lb), is getting oxycodone (an opioid) every 5–6 hours for pain. His Foley (indwelling) catheter had been removed at 8:00 a.m., and by 4:00 p.m. he still had not urinated despite feeling the urge. By 5:00 p.m. he was very uncomfortable and reported that "I have to pee, but it just won't come out." The nurse is aware that opioids can cause urinary retention, and recognizes that he has an elimination and exchange (domain 3) urinary function (class 1) diagnosis: impaired urinary elimination. This definition of this diagnosis is "dysfunction in urinary elimination" and Mr. Stevens has a defining characteristic of urinary retention. Although opioid use is not listed in the NANDA taxonomy as a factor related to urinary dysfunction, the nurse knows from her pharmacology course and clinical experience that this may be the cause of Mr. Stevens' urinary retention. She explained this to him, and he said he was "ready to get off that stuff anyway" and took ibuprofen and acetaminophen the next time he needed pain medication and reported good relief. After getting an order from Mr. Stevens' surgeon, the nurse did an in-and-out catheterization, removing 800+ cc of urine. He immediately felt better, and by 9:00 p.m. was able to urinate on his own without retention.

A more detailed discussion of making diagnoses is located in the next section of this chapter.

The nursing process as a method of addressing clinical problems is taught in schools of nursing across the U.S., and many states refer to it in their nursing practice acts. Ideally, the nursing process is used as a creative approach to thinking and decision making in nursing. Because the nursing process is an integral aspect of nursing education, practice, standards, and practice acts nationwide, learning to use it as a mechanism for critical thinking and as a dynamic and creative approach to patient care is a worthwhile endeavor. The nursing process has sometimes been the subject of criticism among nurses. In recent years, some nursing leaders have questioned the use of the nursing process, describing it as linear, rigid, and mechanistic. They believe that the nursing process contributes to linear thinking and stymies critical thinking. Despite reservations among some nurses about its use, the nursing process remains the cornerstone of nursing standards, legal definitions, and practice and, as such, should be understood by nurses.

STEPS OF THE NURSING PROCESS

Like many frameworks for thinking through problems, the nursing process is a series of organized steps, the purpose of which is to impose some discipline and critical thinking on the provision of excellent care. Identifying specific steps makes the process clear and concrete but can cause nurses to use them rigidly. Keep in mind that this is a process, that progression through the process may not be linear, and that it is a tool to use, not a road map to follow rigidly. More creative use of the nursing process may occur by expert nurses who have a greater repertoire of interventions from which to select. For example, if a newly hospitalized patient is experiencing a great deal of pain, a novice nurse might proceed by asking family members to leave so that the patient could rest in a quiet environment. An expert nurse would realize that the family may be a source of distraction from the pain or may be a source of comfort in ways that the nurse may not be able to provide. The expert nurse, in addition to assessing the patient, is willing to consider alternative explanations and interventions, enhancing the possibility that the patient's pain will be relieved.

Phase 1: Assessment

Assessment is the initial phase or operation in the nursing process. During this phase, information or data about the individual patient, family, or community are gathered. Data may include physiologic, psychological, sociocultural, developmental, spiritual, and environmental information. The patient's available financial or material resources also need to be assessed and recorded in a standard format; each institution will have its distinct method of collecting and recording assessment data.

Types of Data

Nurses obtain two types of data about and from patients: subjective and objective. Subjective data are obtained from patients as they describe their needs, feelings, strengths, and perceptions of the problem. Symptoms are a form of subjective data, such as a patient noting they are "in pain" or "don't have much energy." The only source for these data is the patient. Subjective data should include physical, psychosocial, and spiritual information. Subjective data can be very private. Nurses must be sensitive to the patient's need for confidence in the nurse's trustworthiness when collecting subjective data.

Objective data are the other types of data that the nurse will collect through observation, examination, or consultation with other healthcare providers. These data are measurable, such as pulse rate and blood pressure, and include observable patient behaviors. Objective data are often called *signs*. An example of objective data that a nurse might gather is the observation that the patient, who is lying in bed, is diaphoretic, pale, and tachypneic, clutching his hands to his chest.

Objective data and subjective data are often congruent; that is, they usually are in agreement. In the situation just described, if the patient told the nurse, "I feel like a rock is crushing my chest," the subjective data would substantiate the nurse's observations (objective data) that the patient has signs consistent with a heart attack (myocardial infarction). Occasionally, subjective and objective data are in conflict. In this example, the patient may deny having chest pain (subjective data) despite evidence of signs of a myocardial infarction, including characteristic changes associated with a heart attack on the patient's electrocardiogram (objective data). A stark example of incongruent subjective and objective data unfortunately well known to labor and delivery nurses is that of a pregnant woman in labor who describes ongoing fetal activity (subjective data); however, there are no fetal heart tones (objective data), and it is determined that the fetus has died in utero. Incongruent objective and subjective data require further careful assessment to ascertain the patient's situation more completely and accurately. Sometimes incongruent data reveal something about the patient's concerns and fears—such as the fear of a heart attack or that one's baby will be stillborn. To get a clearer picture of the patient's situation, the nurse should use the best communication skills they possess to increase the patient's trust.

Methods of Collecting Patient Data

A number of methods are used when collecting patient data. The patient interview is a primary means of obtaining both subjective and objective data. The interview typically involves a face-to-face interaction with the patient that requires the nurse to use the skills of interviewing, observation, and listening (Fig. 11.1).

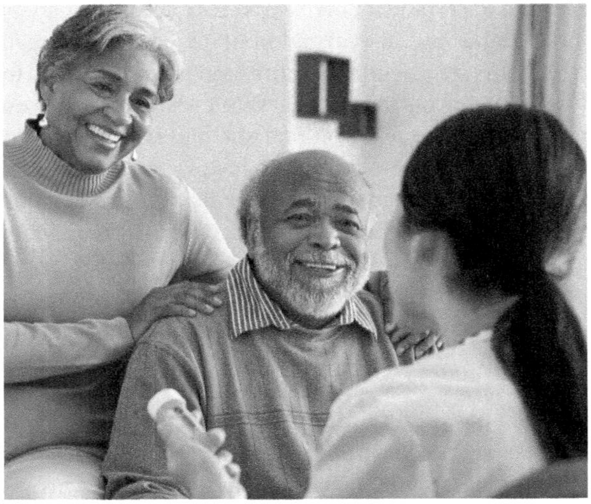

Fig. 11.1 A face-to-face interview with a patient is a primary means of collecting data and requires good interviewing skills, observation, and listening. (Photo used with permission from iStockPhoto.)

Many factors influence the quality of the interview, including the physical environment in which the interaction occurs. If the patient is not in a private room, the open exchange of information may not occur easily. Sometimes the presence of family members constrains the flow of information from a patient, especially when dealing with sensitive or private issues. Similarly, if an interview takes place in a cold, noisy, or public place, the type and quality of data obtained may be affected by environmental distractions. Internal factors related to the patient's condition may influence the amount and the type of data obtained. For example, when interviewing a patient who is experiencing shortness of breath, the verbal data obtained in the interview may be limited, but careful observation and attentive listening can yield much information about the patient's condition.

Physical examination is the second method for obtaining data. Nurses use physical assessment techniques of inspection, auscultation, percussion, and palpation to obtain these data, in addition to technology such as a bladder scan to detect or confirm urinary retention. A third method of obtaining data is through consultation. Consultation is discussing patient needs with healthcare providers who are directly involved in the care of the patient. Nurses also consult with patients' families to obtain background information and their perceptions about the patients' needs; however, nurse should remember that the patient's family may be unaware of certain concerns or situations of the patient. For example, an 18-year-old young woman is brought to the emergency department's urgent care facility for dysuria (pain on urination). While her mother is out of the room, she tells you that she had intercourse two days earlier, a useful piece of history in determining the patient's likely medical diagnosis of a urinary tract infection. You note that she has waited until her mother is absent before telling you this important piece of information; recognizing that this is sensitive and private information, you do not mention it in front of the patient's mother.

Organizing Patient Data

Once patient data have been collected, they must be sorted or organized. A number of methods have been developed to assist nurses in organizing patient data. Abdellah's 21 nursing problems, Henderson's 14 nursing problems, Yura and Walsh's (1983) human needs approach, and Gordon's (1976) 11 functional health patterns are commonly used frameworks for collecting and organizing patient data. Contemporary nursing theorists continue to develop other organizing frameworks, including those of Madeleine Leininger, Sister Callista Roy, Dorothy Orem, and others that you read about in Chapter 9.

Confidentiality of Patient Data

A word of caution is needed concerning patient data. Earlier it was noted that patients confide personal information to nurses if they believe the nurse is trustworthy. It can seem obvious when to avoid sharing sensitive information with patients' families. However, nurses must limit the sharing of information to only the other providers directly involved in the patient's care. Nurses must respect patients' privacy rights and should never discuss patient information with anyone who does not have a work-related need to know. This is not only an ethical issue but also a legal issue. Patients' privacy is protected by federal law (see Health Insurance Portability and Accountability Act of 1996 [HIPAA] in Chapter 6). Conversations about patients in public places or consulting with other providers on a mobile phone in a hallway or elevator are other ways in which patients' privacy is breached.

Ensuring patients' privacy is complicated in that vast amounts of patient data are stored digitally and retrieved relatively easily. Although the issues of confidentiality and access to digital data have yet to be fully resolved, each nurse should be entrusted never to violate a patient's privacy by revealing patient information except to other members of that patient's treatment team on a need-to-know basis.

Phase 2: Analysis and Identification of the Problem

During the data-gathering phase of the nursing process, nurses obtain a great deal of information about their patients. These data must first be validated and then compared with norms to sort out data that might indicate a problem or identify a pattern. Next, the data must be clustered or grouped so that problems can be identified and their cause discerned. Knowledge from the science of nursing, biologic sciences, and social sciences enables nurses to observe relationships among various pieces of patient data. This process is known as data analysis and results in the identification of one or more problems that are amenable to nursing intervention. The problems are often then characterized as nursing diagnoses.

Here is an example of how a nurse will take information from a variety of sources, analyze it, and adjust the plan of care accordingly:

Ms. Wills is a 62-year-old woman with a four-year history of stage 4 breast cancer who is admitted to your unit for paracentesis to remove the large volume of ascites that has accumulated in her abdomen, making it very uncomfortable for her to breathe and move. Ms. Wills is a trustworthy historian: she tells you in detail about her cancer diagnosis and treatments, her abundant family support, her religious faith, and her decision to enter hospice care after the cancer was found to have metastasized to her brain.

Ms. Wills' hospice nurse calls to check on her and gives you some important information: although Ms. Wills is receiving end-of-life care, she insists that her cancer will be cured because she and others have been praying for a cure. The hospice nurse shares this information because she believes that you need to know this may be a factor in Ms. Wills' care. You read part of the patient's medical record and note that it is consistent with Ms. Wills' account of her illness. The paracentesis removes 4 liters of ascites. Afterward, Ms. Wills tells you that she feels so much better that she plans to contact her hospice nurse and tell her she will not be needing their services any longer because she is cured. Ms. Wills' physician believes that she needs a psychiatric consultation because he believes that she is "in denial" about still having cancer.

What had appeared to be a short admission for the management of a common occurrence (ascites) may have become a bit more complicated when Ms. Wills—the excellent historian who chronicled her cancer progression in such detail—makes a statement that may have surprised you had you not been given specific information about Ms. Wills' hope for a cure from her hospice nurse. This is the type of behavior you may see in certain settings, and although it seems inconsistent and even alarming, having the right information about a patient can be very useful in analyzing the patient's responses.

Distinctions Between Medical and Nursing Diagnosis

Nursing diagnosis is different from medical diagnosis and was never intended to be a substitute. Rather than focusing on what is wrong with the patient in terms of a disease process, a nursing diagnosis identifies the problems the patient is experiencing as a result of the disease process, that is, the human responses to the illness, injury, or threat.

An important difference between nursing diagnosis and medical diagnosis is that nursing diagnoses address patient problems that nurses can treat within their scope of practice. The medical diagnosis becomes a platform from which nursing diagnoses are developed. For example, a patient with a new medical diagnosis of diabetes will have some very specific nursing diagnoses and interventions based on the requirements of the medical condition (diabetes) that caused the patient to seek care.

All nursing diagnoses must be supported by data, which NANDA-I refers to as defining characteristics (i.e., signs and symptoms). Accurate diagnosis of human responses is very important. Effective interventions depend on an accurate diagnosis. Lunney (2008) wrote an appeal to nurses in practice and education to address this issue of diagnostic accuracy. Lunney based the appeal on research findings that there is a need for more diagnostic consistency among nurses, that the issue of accuracy will always be present because of the complexities of nursing, and that EHRs make the issue of accuracy of diagnosis even more significant. Paans and colleagues (2011) found four domains of factors that affect nurses' accurate documentation of diagnoses: (1) nurses themselves as effective diagnosticians; (2) how nurses are educated about nursing diagnoses; (3) the complexity of a patient's situation; and (4) the degree to which a hospital's policy and environment supports the use of nursing diagnosis.

A format formerly used to write the diagnostic statement, called the PES format (problem, etiology, signs/symptoms), was developed by Marjory Gordon (1987), a founder of NANDA-I. Once commonly used, NANDA-I no longer uses this format and now refers to the component parts of the nursing diagnosis as related factors and defining characteristics. Several countries and nursing publications, however, still use the PES format, which is shown in Box 11.5 so that you can become familiar with it when you run across it in journals and settings that still use this format. NANDA-I continues to work to align its mission for a nursing diagnostic system to the demands of today's healthcare environment.

BOX 11.5 Writing Nursing Diagnoses

1. **P** = Problem (NANDA-I diagnostic label)
2. **E** = Etiology (causal factors)
3. **S** = Signs and symptoms (defining characteristics)

Prioritizing Nursing Diagnoses

After diagnoses are identified, the nurse must put them in order of priority. Two common frameworks are used to establish priorities. One of these considers the relative danger to the patient. With use of this framework, diagnoses that are life threatening are the nurse's first priority. Next are those that have the potential to cause harm or injury. Last in priority are those diagnoses that are related to the overall general health of the patient. Thus a diagnosis of "impaired gas exchange" would be dealt with before "sleep deprivation," and "readiness for enhanced sleep."

Another framework used to prioritize diagnoses is Maslow's (1970) hierarchy of needs (refer to Chapter 8, Fig. 8.3). When this framework is used, inverse relationship exists between high-priority nursing diagnoses and high-level needs. In other words, highest priority is given to diagnoses related to basic physiologic needs. Diagnoses related to higher-level needs such as love and belonging or self-esteem, although important, have priority only after basic physiologic needs are met.

Except in life-threatening or other emergency situations, nurses should take care to involve patients in identifying priority diagnoses. Because varied sociocultural factors have a great impact on the manner in which patients prioritize problems, nurses must be aware of these factors and take them into consideration when planning patient care. The nurse's own cultural perspective must not take priority over that of the patient in determining priorities. For example, many maternity nurses are strong proponents of breastfeeding and consider it one of their priorities to assist new mothers to establish effective breastfeeding patterns. However, for some women, breastfeeding is not a cultural norm or a desirable behavior of new motherhood. Although it may be difficult to understand for the maternity nurse who has expertise in the benefits of breastfeeding, imposing the nurse's cultural and professional perspective on the patient is unacceptable and can lead to diminished effectiveness of nursing care in other domains in which the new mother needs assistance.

Phase 3: Planning

Planning is the third phase in the nursing process. Planning begins with identification of patient goals and determination of ways to reach those goals. Goals are used by the patient and the nurse to guide the selection of interventions and to evaluate patient progress. Bloom's taxonomy (as described by Spring, 2010) in Box 11.6 provides a simple description of domains of learning that drive the development of patient goals: psychomotor, cognitive, and affective goals. This taxonomy identified domains of educational activities well suited to nursing.

BOX 11.6 Bloom's Taxonomy

A taxonomy is a classification system. Bloom, an educator, described types of learning in terms of domains of educational activities. This taxonomy is helpful for nursing:

1. **Psychomotor domain:** Involves physical movement and increasingly complex activities in the motor-skill arena. Learning in this domain can be assessed by measures such as distance, time, and speed.
   1. *Nursing goal:* Patient will move from bed to chair three times today without assistance.
2. **Cognitive domain:** Involves knowledge and intellectual skills. Cognitive skills range from simple recall to complex tasks such as synthesis and evaluation.
   1. *Nursing goal:* Maternity patient will list five signs of illness in her newborn infant by the time she is discharged.
3. **Affective domain:** Involves the emotions, such as feelings, values, and attitudes.
   1. *Nursing goal:* Pregnant patient will describe willingness to consider breastfeeding her newborn infant.

Setting nursing goals using Bloom's taxonomy is a simple way to address the three important domains of the patient's needs. A single patient is likely to have goals in each of these domains.

Modified from American Philosophical Association: The Delphi report: research findings and recommendations prepared for the Committee on Pre-college Philosophy, Milbrae, Calif, 1990, The California Academic Press.

Just as nursing diagnoses are written in collaboration with the patient, goals should also be agreed on by both nurse and patient unless collaboration is impossible, such as when the patient has an altered mental status, is a young child, or is incapacitated in some way, or if the nurse and patient do not speak the same language. In the event of a cognitive problem, family members or significant others can collaborate with the nurse. In the case of the nurse whose patient speaks another language, a qualified medical interpreter can be instrumental in helping the nurse collaborate with the patient; in fact, it is not acceptable to use a patient's family members or friends to interpret. Goals give the patient, family, significant others, and nurse direction and make them active partners.

Writing Patient Goals and Outcomes

The terms *goal* and *objective* are often used interchangeably. Note that the word *objective* is used differently here than its earlier use, when it was used as an adjective describing observable and measurable data. In terms of outcomes, the word *objective* is a noun and means a goal or specific aim of intervention. Goals or objectives are statements of what is to be accomplished and are derived from the diagnoses. Because the problem or diagnosis is written as a patient problem, the goal should also be stated in terms of what the patient will do rather than what the nurse will do. The goal begins with the words *the patient will* or *the patient will be able to*. The goal sets a general direction, includes an action verb, and should be both attainable and realistic for the patient.

Outcome criteria are specific and make the goal measurable. Outcome criteria define the terms under which the goal is said to be met, partially met, or unmet. Each diagnosis has at least one patient goal, and each patient goal may have several outcome criteria. Effective outcome criteria state under what conditions, to what extent, and in what time frame the patient is to act. For the postoperative patient who had an abdominal procedure, a sample patient goal with outcome criteria might be, "The patient will be able to walk three blocks a day with a cane within one month after hip replacement surgery." It is easy to see that this goal is written in terms of what the patient will do (walk), is measurable (three blocks), gives conditions (with a cane), and has a specified time frame for accomplishment (one month after surgery).

Establishing a time frame for patient goals to be met is important. **Short-term goals** may be attainable within hours or days. They are usually specific and are small steps leading to the achievement of broader, long-term goals. For example, "The patient will limit his smoking to a half-pack per day within a week" is a short-term goal, and the time limit for accomplishment can be brief, perhaps a week or ten days. **Long-term goals**, however, usually represent major changes or rehabilitation. A goal such as "The patient will stop smoking entirely" may take months or perhaps even years to accomplish, and the time frame should be set accordingly. Setting realistic goals in terms of both outcomes and time is extremely important. Frustration and discouragement can occur when goals are unrealistic in outcomes or time.

The nurse can be a good resource for helping patients in determining accessible goals. For example, assume that your patient is a young man with a severe compound fracture of his thigh and several torn ligaments in his knee from a single-car automobile accident. The injury will require several orthopedic surgeries. To complicate matters, he has a nosocomial (hospital-acquired) infection in his surgical site. One day, he mentions to you that his goal is to run a marathon within a year. Running a marathon is a worthy goal and is reachable eventually for this young man. It is immaterial whether you believe he can reach his goal; however, as his nurse on the orthopedic and trauma unit, you recognize the importance of setting short-term goals right now that will improve his health and better the chances of achieving his goal of running a marathon. Your care plan should reflect the short-term, attainable goals (such as walking with a walker the length of the hallway twice a day) that he needs to reach in the meantime that will move him toward his long-term, personal goal.

Cultural congruency is an important consideration in setting patient goals and selecting interventions. A culturally congruent intervention is one that is developed within the broad social, cultural, and demographic context of the patient's life. The patient is more likely to benefit from an intervention that is tailored to his or her specific sociocultural needs and interests. Although cultural congruency is an important element to effective intervention, the nurse must take care not to stereotype patients or assume that "all ________" (fill in the blank) like the same things, will react the same way, or respond to the same intervention. In Considering Culture Box 11.1, you will be introduced to a research report explaining the importance of having culturally appropriate educational materials to prepare African American women for their breast biopsies. Read the paper carefully, and then address the questions.

Selecting Interventions and Planning Care

After short- and long-term goals are identified through collaboration between nurse and patient, the nurse develops a plan of care that contains actions designed to assist the patient in achieving a stated goal. Every goal has a specific intervention, which may be carried out by an RN or delegated to other members of the nursing staff.

The nursing care plan is part of the whole plan of care by the healthcare team. Nursing interventions are designed to treat the patient's response to an illness or

CONSIDERING CULTURE BOX 11.1

Challenge: Culturally Appropriate Interventions—Impact of Culture on Nursing Interventions

From the Association of Black Nursing Faculty website (www.abnf.net): "The purpose of the Association of Black Nursing Faculty, Inc. (ABNF) is to form and maintain a group whereby Black professional nurses with similar credentials, interests, and concerns may work to promote certain health-related issues and educational interests for the benefit of themselves and the Black community."

An example of the interests and work that have developed from the ABNF is found in *The ABNF Journal,* published six times each year. Volume 17, issue 1 in 2006 was dedicated to the issue of breast cancer in African American women. The research article "Getting Ready: Developing an Educational Intervention to Prepare African American Women for Breast Biopsy" describes the efforts to produce intervention materials for African American women preparing to undergo breast biopsies. African American women are more likely to die of breast cancer than are White American women, although fewer Black women than White women have a diagnosis of breast cancer. This is a source of great concern in the African American community and among researchers, who are trying to determine why this is the case.

In the Implications section at the end of the article, the authors refer to the cultural appropriateness of study materials to be used in an intervention. As you read this article, consider these questions:

1. In addition to ethnicity, can you think of other ways that interventions should be made culturally appropriate?
2. What might happen if an intervention is not culturally appropriate?
3. Who determines what is and is not culturally appropriate?
4. You can find the article here: Bradley PK, Berry A, Lang C, Myers RE: Getting ready: developing an educational intervention to prepare African American women for breast biopsy, *ABFN J* 17(1):15–19, 2006.

medical treatment, whereas the physician or an advanced practice nurse will prescribe treatments for the specific illness or disease. Nursing interventions can and should begin before diagnostic testing or surgery, common reasons why patients are admitted to inpatient units. For example, before surgery patients are taught about pain management and pulmonary care that they will face after surgery. These activities are designed to manage pain and prevent postoperative respiratory problems caused by immobility. They are appropriate because prevention of complications resulting from immobility is a nursing responsibility. Nurses may consult with other healthcare providers, such as the dietitian, physical therapist, or pharmacist, to adequately prepare their patient for upcoming surgery or other invasive procedures.

Types of nursing interventions. Nursing interventions are of three basic types: independent, dependent, or interdependent. **Independent interventions** are those for which the nurse's intervention requires no supervision or direction by others and are within their scope of practice as defined by their state nursing practice act. Nurses have the knowledge and skills to carry out independent actions safely. An example of an independent nursing intervention is teaching a patient how to breastfeed her newborn infant.

Dependent interventions require instructions, written prescriptions, or supervision of another health professional with prescriptive authority. These actions require knowledge and skills on the part of the nurse but may not be done without explicit directions. An example of a dependent nursing intervention is the administration of medications. Although a physician or advanced practice nurse must prescribe medications in inpatient settings, it is the responsibility of the nurse to know how to administer them safely and to monitor their effectiveness. The nurse also must question prescriptions they think are inconsistent with safe care or are not within accepted standards of care.

The third type, **interdependent (or collaborative) interventions**, includes actions in which the nurse must collaborate or consult with another health professional before carrying out the action. One example of this type of action is the nurse implementing prescriptions or treatments that have been written by a physician in a protocol. **Protocols** define under what conditions and circumstances a nurse is allowed to treat the patient, as well as what treatments are permissible. They are used in situations in which nurses need to take immediate action without consulting with a physician, such as in an emergency department, a critical care unit, or a home setting.

Writing the Plan of Care

Once interventions are selected, a written plan of care is devised, often in the EHR. Some healthcare agencies use individually developed plans of care for their patients. The nurse creates and develops a plan for each patient. Others use standardized plans of care that are based on common and recurring problems. The nurse then individualizes these standard plans of care. An advantage of using standardized plans is that they can decrease the time spent in generating a completely new plan each time a patient is seen. These plans are easily generated in the EHR, with the nurse making selections from menus to individualize the plan to the particular patient. The amount of time needed to update and document these plans is then minimized.

Because of the decreasing average length of stay for patients in healthcare facilities, the increasing focus on achieving timely patient outcomes in the specific time frame permitted by reimbursement systems, and the emphasis by accrediting bodies on multidisciplinary care, many agencies have adopted the use of multidisciplinary plans of care known as critical pathways, collaborative care plans, or care maps. Critical pathways have been replaced with other types of multidisciplinary care plans in some settings. Multidisciplinary care plans are written in collaboration with physicians and other healthcare providers and establish a sequence of short-term daily outcomes that are easily measured. This type of care planning facilitates communication and collaboration among all members of the healthcare team. It also permits comparisons of outcomes between treatment plans, as well as among healthcare facilities. As with the nursing process, unyielding adherence to the critical path without considering a patient's idiosyncratic responses can negatively affect patient outcomes and is a detriment to successful nursing care.

The development of appropriate plans of care depends on the nurse's ability to use critical thinking. Nurses must be able to analyze information and arguments, make reasoned decisions, recognize many viewpoints, and question and seek answers continuously. At the same time, nurses must be logical, flexible, and creative and take initiative while considering the holistic nature of each patient.

Phase 4: Implementation of Planned Interventions

Implementation, the fourth phase or operation of the nursing process, occurs when nursing orders are actually carried out. Most people think of nursing as "doing something" for or to a patient. Notice, however, that in using the nursing process, nurses do a great deal of thinking, analyzing, and planning before the first actual nursing action takes place.

Professional nurses understand the crucial nature of the first three phases of the nursing process in ensuring that safe and appropriate care occurs. Nurses who forgo these essential phases and move immediately into action are not providing care in a responsible, professional manner. Patients feel a greater sense of trust in nurses who are providing care when dependent, independent, and interdependent orders are planned and carried out in an orderly, competent manner. Common nursing interventions include such actions as managing pain, preventing postoperative complications, educating patients, and monitoring certain aspects of the patient's physiologic care. As the nurse carries out planned interventions, they continually assess the patient, noting responses to nursing interventions, and modifying the care plan or adding nursing diagnoses as needed. Documentation of nursing actions is an integral part of the implementation phase.

Let's refer back to the case of Ms. Wills, who appears to believe after her paracentesis that she is cured of cancer and no longer needs hospice care; remember that her physician believes that she needs a psychiatric consultation.

You have done a thorough assessment of Ms. Wills and have no reason to believe, given what you have noted about her from both her objective and subjective data, that she has developed a psychiatric problem. You do know, however, that she has been praying a lot for a cure and that as a person of faith, she wants to trust that this will happen. You also know that she had in fact agreed to enter hospice care rather than to continue to seek medical treatment. Furthermore, you know that she truly feels better after having a gallon or more of fluid removed from her abdomen. As you are doing her 4:00 p.m. assessment, she says, "I feel so good, I'm going to call my hospice nurse right now." Without judgment or further questioning, you sit at her bedside, take her hand and simply say, "It must feel so good to have all that fluid gone." Ms. Wills says with a sigh, "You can't imagine. I just wish it was that easy to drain away all the cancer." You ask Ms. Wills if she would like for you to help her call her hospice nurse to tell her how much better she feels.

You acted in a caring, professional way by addressing the specific reason Ms. Wills feels better—the fluid removal—without confronting her with harsh fact that her cancer was not gone. You correctly surmised that she in fact knew that. Helping her call her hospice nurse is a good way to help connect Ms. Wills to her substantial supportive network in hospice. The simple act of affirming her relief without judgment or trying to correct a momentarily hopeful thought gave you time to assess that Ms. Wills in fact does understand her situation. Sometimes the intervention itself becomes a means of assessment. You can tell Ms. Wills' physician after your assessment that you do not recommend a psychiatric consultation. (You will read about SBAR communication—**s**ituation, **b**ackground, **a**ssessment, **r**ecommendation—in Chapter 12.)

Phase 5: Evaluation

Evaluation is the final phase of the nursing process. In this phase the nurse examines the patient's progress in relation to the goals and outcome criteria to determine whether a problem is resolved, is in the process of being resolved, or is unresolved. In other words, the outcome criteria are the basis for evaluation of the goal. Evaluation may reveal that data, diagnosis, goals, and nursing interventions were all on target and that the problem is resolved.

Evaluation may also indicate a need for a change in the plan of care. Perhaps inadequate patient data were the basis for the plan, and further assessment has uncovered additional needs. The nursing diagnoses may have been incorrect or placed in the wrong order of priority. Patient goals may have been inappropriate or unattainable within the designated time frame. It is possible that nursing actions were incorrectly implemented.

Evaluation is a critical phase in the nursing process and one that is often slighted. The best nursing care plan is one that is evaluated frequently and changed in response to the patient's condition. Sometimes a care plan will reflect all the most common nursing interventions used to treat specific diagnoses; it is not enough, however, to continue to do the "right things" if the patient is not improving in the expected manner. If, on evaluation, the problem is not resolving in a timely way or will not resolve at all, the nursing care plan must be revised to reflect the necessary changes.

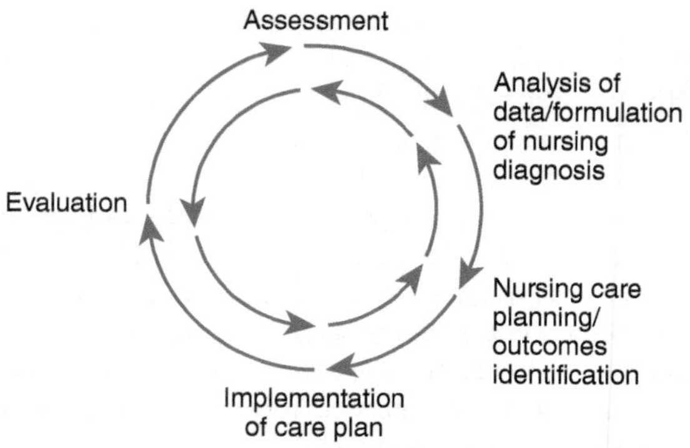

Fig. 11.2 The nursing process is a dynamic, nonlinear tool for critical thinking about human responses.

THE DYNAMIC NATURE OF THE NURSING PROCESS

The next morning Ms. Wills is leaving for home with her daughter after a restful night. She asks you if there is anything she can do to keep her ascites from coming back, such as limiting her fluid intake. Even as she is preparing to walk out the door, you understand that she is still your patient and has a specific need for knowledge. You tell her that the fluid—ascites—is happening because of the cancer and that there is really no way to prevent it from recurring. You also assure her, "We are always here to take care of you if you need us again."

A good plan is a flexible, responsive one; however, a care plan is only as effective as the nurse who carries it out.

Although the phases in the nursing process are discussed separately here, in practice they are not so clearly delineated, nor do they always proceed from one to another in a linear fashion. The nursing process (Fig. 11.2) is dynamic, meaning that nurses are continuously moving from one phase to another and then beginning the process again. Often a nurse performs two or more phases at the same time—for instance, observing a wound for signs of infection (assessment) while changing the dressing on the wound (intervention) and asking the patient the extent to which pain has been relieved by comfort measures (evaluation).

Now that you have read about the phases of the nursing process, we will look back at the scenario in which you tried to determine whether you should go see your favorite band. The problem that was identified was the choice between studying for a pathophysiology exam or

BOX 11.7 Nursing Process Case Study of a High-Priority Diagnosis

You have just received a report from the day shift about Mr. Burkes. You were told that he had been admitted with a diagnosis of cancer of the tongue and that he had a radical neck dissection yesterday. He has a tracheostomy and requires frequent suctioning of his secretions. He is alert and responds by nodding his head or writing short notes.

When you enter his room, you note that he is apprehensive and tachypneic and is gesturing for you to come into the room. You auscultate his lungs and note coarse crackles and expiratory wheezes. You can see thick secretions bubbling out of his tracheotomy. He has poor cough effort.

Based on these data, you realize that a priority nursing diagnosis is ineffective airway clearance. You immediately prepare to perform tracheal suctioning. As you are suctioning, you watch the patient's nonverbal responses and note that he is less apprehensive when the suctioning is completed. You also auscultate the lungs and note that there are decreased crackles and that the expiratory wheezes are no longer present. Mr. Burkes writes "I can breathe now" on his note pad.

1. Assessment
   A. Subjective data
      (i) None because of inability to speak
2. Objective data
   A. Tracheostomy with copious, thick secretions
   B. Tachypnea
   C. Gesturing for help
   D. Coarse crackles and expiratory wheezes
   E. Poor cough effort
3. Analysis
   A. Ineffective airway clearance related to copious, thick secretions
4. Plan
   A. Short-term goal: Patient will maintain patent airway as evidenced by absence of expiratory wheezes and crackles, decreased signs of anxiety, and air hunger.
   B. Long-term goal: Patient will have patent airway as evidenced by his ability to clear the airway without the use of suctioning by the time of discharge.
5. Implementation
   A. Assess lung sounds every hour for crackles and wheezes.
   B. Suction airway as needed.
   C. Elevate head of bed to 45 degrees.
   D. Teach patient abdominal breathing techniques.
   E. Encourage patient to cough out secretions.
6. Evaluation
   A. Short-term goal: Achieved as evidenced by decreased crackles and absent wheezes when auscultating the lungs; patient appears less anxious, indicated by writing that he "can breathe now"
   B. Long-term goal: Will be evaluated before discharge

going to see the band. Data, both objective (the schedule of the exam and the concert, the distance to be driven, the percentage of the final grade the exam represents, the cost of the ticket, the location of the available seats) and subjective (the long-term desire to see your favorite band, your hope to make a good grade on the exam), were gathered. Selection was made and implemented, and an evaluation of the implementation was carried out when you got your grade on your exam. Problem solving is something each person does every day. The use of the nursing process provides professional nurses with a patient-centered framework with which to solve clinical problems to optimize the opportunity for excellent patient outcomes.

An example of using the nursing process in a high-priority clinical situation is described in Box 11.7. This case study demonstrates how using the nursing process becomes so natural that experienced nurses go through the phases fluidly and automatically. Although no responsible nurse would take the time to write out this care plan in advance of acting on a diagnosis of "ineffective airway clearance," you should understand that the nursing process is exactly the same for those high-priority nursing situations that require immediate action and those that will evolve over time.

DEVELOPING CLINICAL JUDGMENT IN NURSING

Becoming an effective nurse involves more than critical thinking and the ability to use the nursing process. It depends heavily on developing excellent clinical judgment. Clinical judgment consists of informed opinions and decisions based on empirical knowledge and experience. Nurses develop clinical judgment gradually as they gain a broader, deeper knowledge base and clinical experience. Extensive direct patient contact is the best means of developing clinical judgment.

Critical thinking and clinical reasoning used in the nursing process are both important aspects of clinical judgment. A nurse who has developed sound clinical

BOX 11.8 Clinical Judgment: Nine Key Questions

1. What major outcomes (observable beneficial results) do we expect to see in this particular patient, family, or group when the plan of care is terminated? Example: The patient will be discharged without complications, able to care for himself, three days after surgery. Outcomes may be addressed on a standard plan, or you may have to develop these outcomes yourself. Make sure any predetermined outcomes in standard plans are appropriate to your patient's specific situation.
2. What problems or issues must be addressed to achieve the major outcomes? Answering this question will help you prioritize. You may have a long list of actual or potential health problems needing to be structured to set your priorities.
3. What are the circumstances? Who is involved (e.g., child, adult, group)? How urgent are the problems (e.g., life-threatening, chronic)? What are the factors influencing their presentation (e.g., when, where, and how did the problems develop)? What are the patient's values, beliefs, and cultural influences?
4. What knowledge is required? You must know problem-specific facts (e.g., how problems usually present, how they are diagnosed, what their common causes and risk factors are, what common complications occur, and how these complications are prevented and managed), nursing process and related knowledge and skills (e.g., ethics, research, health assessment, communication, priority setting), and related sciences (e.g., anatomy, physiology, pathophysiology, pharmacology, chemistry, physics, psychology, sociology). You must also be clearly aware of the circumstances, as addressed in question 3 above.
5. How much room is there for error? In the clinical setting, there is usually minimal room for error. However, it depends on the health of the individual and the risks of interventions. A healthy, young postoperative patient with no chronic illnesses may tolerate early mobility after surgery better than an elderly person with a history of multiple chronic problems requiring numerous medications. Although their orders for postoperative ambulation may be identical and your commitment to their safe care exactly the same for these two patients, excellent clinical judgment based on your assessments allows you to conclude that the young patient is safe walking in the hallway with a family member, whereas the elderly patient needs your assistance and guidance during early ambulation.
6. How much time do I have? Time frame for decision making depends on (1) the urgency of the problems (e.g., there is little time in life-threatening situations, such as cardiac arrest) and (2) the planned length of contact (e.g., if your patient will be hospitalized for only two days, you have to be realistic about what can be accomplished, and key decisions need to be made early).
7. What resources can help me? Human resources include clinical nurse educators, nursing faculty, preceptors, experienced nurses, advanced practice nurses, peers, librarians, and other healthcare professionals (e.g., pharmacists, nutritionists, physical therapists, physicians). The patient and family are also valuable resources (usually they know their own problems best). Other resources include texts, articles, other references, computer databases, decision-making support, national practice guidelines, and facility documents (e.g., guidelines, policies, procedures, assessment forms).
8. Whose perspectives must be considered? The most significant perspective to consider is the patient's point of view. Other important perspectives include those of the family and significant others, caregivers, and relevant third parties (e.g., insurers).
9. What is influencing my thinking? Identify your personal biases and any other factors influencing your critical thinking and therefore your clinical judgment.

From Alfaro-LeFevre R: *Critical thinking in nursing: a practical approach,* ed 2, Philadelphia, 1999, Saunders. Reprinted with permission.

judgment knows what to look for (e.g., elevation of temperature in a surgical patient), draws valid conclusions about possible alternative meanings of signs and symptoms (e.g., dehydration, atelectasis, postoperative infection), and knows what to do about it (e.g., assess for dehydration, listen to breath sounds, check incision for redness and drainage, seek another opinion, notify the surgeon). Developing sound clinical judgment requires recalling facts, recognizing patterns in patient behaviors, putting facts and observations together to form a meaningful whole, and acting on the resulting information in an appropriate way.

Knowing the limitations of your expertise is an important aspect of clinical judgment. Most nurses have an instinctive awareness of when they are approaching the limits of their expertise and will consult with other

BOX 11.9 Self-Assessment: Developing Sound Clinical Judgment

Answer the following questions honestly. When finished, make a list of the items you need to work on in your quest to develop sound clinical judgment and review it often. Seek opportunities to practice activities you have identified that you need.

1. Use high-quality references and resources.
   - Do I look up new terms when I encounter them to make them part of my vocabulary?
   - Do I familiarize myself with normal findings so that I can recognize those outside the norm?
   - Do I use research findings and base my practice on scientific evidence?
   - Do I learn the signs and symptoms of various conditions, what causes them, and how they are managed?
2. Use the nursing process.
   - Do I always assess before acting, stay focused on outcomes, and make changes as needed?
   - Do I always base my judgments on fact, not emotion or speculation?
3. Assess systematically.
   - Do I have a systematic approach to assessing patients to decrease the likelihood that I will overlook important data?
4. Set priorities systematically.
   - Do I evaluate both the problem and the probable cause before acting?
   - Am I willing to obtain assistance from a more knowledgeable source when indicated?
5. Refuse to act without knowledge.
   - Do I refuse to act when I do not know the indication, why it works, and what risks there are for harm to this particular patient?
6. Use resources wisely.
   - Do I look for opportunities to learn from others, such as teachers, other experts, my colleagues, and continuing education?
   - Do I seek help when needed, being mindful of patient privacy?
7. Know standards of care.
   - Do I know facility policies, professional standards, school policies, and state board of nursing rules and regulations with regard to my legal scope of practice?
   - Do I know the clinical agency's policies and procedures affecting my particular patients?
   - Do I attempt to understand the rationales behind policies and procedures?
   - Do I follow policies and procedures carefully, recognizing that they are designed to help me use good judgment?
   - Do I recognize that no workplace policy or procedure can override my state's limits on scope of practice?
8. Know technology and equipment.
   - Do I routinely learn how to use patient technology such as intravenous pumps, patient monitors, and other equipment?
   - Do I learn how to check equipment for proper functioning and safety?
9. Give patient-centered care.
   - Do I always remember the needs and feelings of the patient, family, and significant others?
   - Do I value knowing my patients' health beliefs and values within context of their own culture?
   - Am I willing to "go the extra mile" for patients?
   - Do I demonstrate the belief that every patient deserves my very best efforts?

Modified from Alfaro-LeFevre R: *Critical thinking in nursing: a practical approach,* ed 2, Philadelphia, 1999, Saunders, pp. 88–92. Used with permission.

professionals as needed. Your state's nursing practice act, health agency policies, school of nursing policies, and the profession's standards of practice all provide guidance in making the decision about nursing actions within your scope of practice. Nursing students, whether new to nursing or RNs in baccalaureate and master's programs, must consider policies and standards in determining their scope of practice in any given nursing situation.

Box 11.8 contains a list of nine key questions to consider as you seek to improve your clinical judgment. Because the goal of nursing is to provide the best care to patients based on research and clinical evidence, the development of excellent clinical judgment is a professional responsibility. As you work to gain clinical experience and improve your own clinical judgment, these questions will help focus your thinking.

Nurses are responsible for developing sound clinical judgment and are accountable for their decisions and nursing practice that arises from those decisions. Your current level of clinical judgment can always be improved, and you may want to devise a personal plan for improving your own clinical decision making. Working thoughtfully through the self-assessment in Box 11.9 will help you begin.

CONCEPTS AND CHALLENGES

- ***Concept:*** In nursing, critical thinking is a purposeful, disciplined, active process that improves clinical judgment and thereby improves patient care.
  Challenge: Critical thinking is a skill that can be learned and requires that one continues to "think about thinking" to sustain high-level critical thinking ability.
- ***Concept:*** The nursing process is a systematic problem-solving framework that ensures that care is developed in an organized, analytic way.
  Challenge: Properly used, the nursing process is cyclic and dynamic rather than rigid and linear.
- ***Concept:*** Consistent, comprehensive, and coordinated patient care results when all nurses use the nursing process effectively.
  Challenge: Nurses may initially find that using the nursing process feels awkward or slow. With experience, however, most find that it becomes a natural, organized approach to patient care.
- ***Concept:*** Both the scientific basis of nursing and professionalism are advanced when nurses resolve patient problems through development of sound clinical judgment.
  Challenge: Sound clinical judgment is developed when nurses use critical thinking, apply the nursing process, stay current with developments in practice and research, understand their scope of practice, and acquire substantial clinical experience.

IDEAS FOR FURTHER EXPLORATION

1. Describe the characteristics of critical thinkers, and explain why critical thinking is important in nursing.
2. List at least four ways in which novice thinking and expert thinking differ, and give an example that illustrates each.
3. Describe the phases in the nursing process, and explain the activities of each phase.
4. Describe the debate related to the use of nursing diagnosis. Which side do you agree with and why?
5. Describe what is meant by the statement, "The nursing process is a cyclic process."
6. Using what you learned about yourself from Self-Assessment: Developing Sound Clinical Judgment (see Box 11.9), set short-term goals for improvement in each of the nine areas. Make a checklist to take to your next clinical experience, and consciously work on improving your clinical judgment.

REFERENCES

Alfaro-LeFevre R: *Critical thinking in nursing: a practical approach*, ed 2, Philadelphia, 1999, Saunders.

American Philosophical Association: *Critical thinking: a statement of expert consensus for purposes of educational assessment and instruction,* The Delphi report: research findings and recommendations prepared for the committee on pre-college philosophy, *ERIC Document Reproduction Services pp,* 315–423, 1990.

Benner P: *From novice to expert*, Menlo Park, Calif, 1984, Addison-Wesley.

Benner P, Tanner CA, Chesla CA: *Expertise in nursing practice: caring, clinical judgment, and ethics*, New York, 1996, Springer.

Bradley PK, Berry A, Lang C, et al.: Getting ready: developing an educational intervention to prepare African American women for breast biopsy, *ABFN J* 17(1):15–19, 2006.

Chang MJ, Chang Y-J, Kuo S-Het, et al.: Relationships between critical thinking ability and nursing competence in clinical nurses, *J Clin Nurs* 20:3224–3232, 2011.

Facione PA: *Critical thinking: what it is and why it counts, Insight Assessment*, 2020. [website]Available at https://www.insightassessment.com/article/critical-thinking-what-it-is-and-why-it-counts-pdf.

Doenges M, Moorhouse MF, Murr AC: *Nursing diagnosis manual: planning, individualizing, and documenting client care*, Philadelphia, 2013, FA Davis.

Gordon M: Nursing diagnosis and the diagnostic process, *Am J Nurs* 76(5):1298–1300, 1976.

Gordon M: *Nursing diagnosis: process and application,* ed 2, New York, 1987, McGraw-Hill.

Huckabay LM: Clinical reasoned judgment and the nursing process, *Nurs Forum* 44(2):72–78, 2009.

Lau J, Chan J: OpenCourseWare on critical thinking, logic, and creativity, 2012. (website). Available at: http://philosophy.hku.hk/think.

Lunney M: Critical need to address accuracy of nurses' diagnoses, *Online J Issues Nurs*, 2008 13(3). [website] Available at www.nursingworld.org/MainMenuCategories/ANAMarketplace/ANAPeriodicals/OJIN/TableofContents/vol132008/No1Jan08/ArticlePreviousTopic/AccuracyofNursesDiagnoses.aspx.

Maslow AH: *Motivation and personality*, New York, 1970, Harper & Row.

NANDA International (NANDA-I): *Nursing diagnoses: definitions and classification*, 12th edition, New York, 2021, Thieme Publishers –2023.

nanda.org: *Our story*, 2021. [website] Available at https://nanda.org/who-we-are/our-story/.

Paans W, Nieweg RMB, van der Schans CP, et al.: What factors influence the prevalence and accuracy of nursing diagnoses documentation in clinical practice? A systematic literature review, *J Clin Nurs* 20(17–18):2386–2403, 2011.

Paul R, Elder L: Paul-Elder critical thinking framework, 2015. (website). Available at: www.louisville.edu/ideastoaction/about/criticalthinking/framework.

Schneider MA: Fundamentals: still the building block of safe patient care, *Nursing* 45(6):60–63, 2015.

Spring H: Learning and teaching in action, *Health Info Libr J* 27:327–331, 2010.

Yura H, Walsh MBThe nursing process: assessing, planning, implementing, evaluation, Norwalk, Conn, 1983, Appleton-Century-Crofts.

12

Communication and Collaboration in Professional Nursing

ⓔ To enhance your understanding of this chapter, try the Student Exercises on the Evolve site at http://evolve.elsevier.com/Black/professional.

LEARNING OUTCOMES

After studying this chapter, students will be able to:

- Describe therapeutic use of self.
- Identify and describe the phases of the traditional nurse–patient relationship.
- Differentiate between social and professional relationships.
- Explore the role self-awareness plays in the ability to use nonjudgmental acceptance as a helping technique.
- Explain the concept of professional boundaries.
- Discuss factors creating successful or unsuccessful communication.
- Evaluate helpful and unhelpful communication techniques.
- Identify strategies in providing care to patients who do not speak English.
- Understand the roles of professional interpreters and translators.
- Identify their own communication strengths and challenges.
- Demonstrate components of active listening.
- Identify key aspects of collaboration.
- Explain the effects of gender, cultural, and generational diversity on nurse–patient and nurse–colleague relationships.

The name Joseph Priestley may be familiar to you; if you were reading carefully, you will remember his name from Chapter 10 as the scientist who discovered oxygen, an example of "pure science." Priestley was an interesting figure in 18th-century England, in addition to being a chemist, he was also a theologian, philosopher, educator, and political theorist. He once wrote, "The more elaborate our means of communication, the less we communicate." Priestley's words have particular relevance now because even as excellent communication is highly valued in health care, the many forms and avenues of communication create opportunities for communication to break down.

In nursing, breakdowns in communication can have significant, even dire consequences. Developing excellent communication skills is important in your education as a nurse because much of what you do as a professional nurse requires the ability to express yourself clearly and to understand another person. Note that communication does not involve simply being able to talk, but to listen to and engage with another person nonverbally, because much of the way that humans express themselves is through nonverbal communication.

The skill set that includes communication is often referred to as *interpersonal skills*. Nurses interact with many people every day regardless of their role or the setting in which they work. The way in which they relate to patients, families, colleagues, and other professionals and nonprofessionals determines the level of comfort and trust others feel and, ultimately, the success of their interactions. This chapter includes information that can enhance the development of self-awareness, nonjudgmental acceptance of others, communication skills, and collaboration skills, all of which are essential components of effective interpersonal skills in nursing.

THE THERAPEUTIC USE OF SELF

Hildegard Peplau, a pioneer in nursing theory development, first focused on the importance of the nurse–patient relationship in her 1952 book *Interpersonal Relations in Nursing*. She referred to the use of one's personality and communication skills to help patients as the "therapeutic use of self" (Peplau, 1952), a strategy that you can develop with practice. Therapeutic use of self can be helpful to you in relating effectively to patients, patients' families, and other healthcare professionals.

The Therapeutic Nurse–Patient Relationship: A Traditional Model

The nursing process can begin only after the nurse and patient establish their initial therapeutic nurse–patient relationship. Awareness of the three identifiable phases of the nurse–patient relationship helps nurses to be realistic in their expectations of this important relationship. Each of three phases—orientation, working, and termination—is sequential and builds on previous phases.

The Orientation Phase

The **orientation phase**, or introductory phase, is the period often described as "getting to know you" in social settings. Relationships between nurses and their patients have some commonalities with other types of relationships. The chief similarity is that there must be trust between the two parties for the relationship to develop. Nurses cannot expect patients to trust them automatically and to reveal their innermost thoughts and feelings immediately.

During the orientation phase, the nurse and patient assess each other. Early impressions made by the nurse are important. Some people have difficulty accepting help of any kind, including nursing care. Putting the patient at ease with a calm, unhurried approach is important during the early part of any nurse–patient relationship.

During the orientation phase, the patient has a right to expect to learn the nurse's name, credentials, and extent of responsibility. The use of simple orienting statements is one way to begin: "Good morning, Mr. Davis. I am Jennifer Carter, and I am your nurse until 7 this evening. I am responsible for your care while I am here."

Developing trust. The orientation phase includes the initial development of trust. Notice the use of the phrase "initial development." Full development of trust is slow and may take months of regular contact. A fact of contemporary nursing practice is that patient interactions may be brief, sometimes lasting only minutes. However, even in the most abbreviated contacts, nurses must orient patients and help them feel comfortable and as trusting as possible.

Certain behaviors help patients develop trust in the nurse. A straightforward, nondefensive manner is important. Answering all questions as fully as possible and admitting to the limits of your knowledge also facilitate trust. Patients accept a simple explanation, such as "I don't know the answer to your question, but I will find out for you," more readily than an evasive response. Promise to find out the answers to all questions, and report the information to the patient as soon as possible. If you tell a patient that you will check on them at 11:30 a.m., make every attempt to follow through on that promise, even if it means that you send someone else in to explain that you are otherwise occupied and will be in as soon as possible. In addition, and most importantly, withhold judgments about patients and their situations. Use active listening, and accept the patient's thoughts and feelings without passing judgment on what they are telling you.

Listen carefully to your own responses, because it is easy to fall into the habit of using platitudes and clichés in response. Imagine your patient telling you, "I am really worried about my surgery tomorrow." Then imagine yourself responding with, "That's silly, you will be fine," as you take their blood pressure and then leave the room. Even as a student, you recognize the harm that this dismissive response will have for the frightened patient awaiting surgery.

Congruence between verbal and nonverbal communication is a key factor in the development of trust. Communicating in a congruent manner requires that nurses be aware of their own thoughts and feelings and be able to share those with others in a nonthreatening manner. Developing an initial understanding of the patient's problem or needs also starts in the orientation phase. Because patients themselves often do not clearly understand their problems or may be reluctant to discuss them, nurses must use their communication skills to elicit the information needed to make a nursing diagnosis. Communication skills useful in nurse–patient interactions are discussed later in this chapter.

Tasks of the orientation phase. By the end of a successful orientation phase, regardless of its length, several things will have happened. First, the patient will have developed enough trust in the nurse to continue to participate in the relationship. Second, the patient and nurse will see each other as individuals. Third, the patient's perception of major problems and needs will have been identified. Fourth, the approximate length of the relationship will have been estimated, and the nurse and patient will have agreed to work together on some aspect of the identified problems. This agreement, whether formalized in writing or informally agreed on, is sometimes called a *contract*. An example of a contract that might emerge from the orientation phase of the relationship with a patient with newly diagnosed diabetes is an agreement to work together on the patient's ability to monitor glucose levels and to manage diet using specific guidelines.

The Working Phase

The second phase of the nurse–patient relationship is called the working phase, during which the nurse and patient address tasks outlined in the previous phase. Because the participants in this relationship now know each other in a professional context, a sense of interpersonal comfort in the relationship may be possible.

Nurses should recognize that in the working phase patients may exhibit alternating periods of intense effort and of resistance to change. Continuing the example of the patient with diabetes, the nurse can anticipate that the patient will experience some degree of difficulty in accepting the lifestyle changes that managing diabetes requires. The patient may show progress one week but not be able to sustain the appropriate diet the following week. This "two steps forward and one backward" approach to behavior change is common; it is not a reflection on one's skill as a nurse, nor is it an indictment of the patient's desire to manage their own care. This is a phenomenon known as regression, a psychological device that occurs as a reaction to stress and that can precede positive changes in behaviors.

Making and sustaining change are very difficult. Patience, self-awareness, and maturity are required of nurses during the working phase. Continued building of trust, use of active listening, and other helpful communication responses facilitate the patient's expression of needs and feelings during the working phase.

The Termination Phase

The **termination phase** includes those activities that enable the patient and the nurse to end the relationship in a therapeutic manner. The process of terminating the nurse–patient relationship begins in the orientation phase when participants estimate the length of time it will take to accomplish the desired outcomes. This is part of the informal contract.

As in any relationship, positive and negative feelings often accompany termination. The patient and nurse are satisfied about the gains the patient has made in accomplishing goals. They may feel sadness about ending a relationship that has been open and trusting. People tend to respond to the end of relationships in much the same way they have responded to other losses in life. Feelings of anger and fear may surface, in addition to sadness. This is particularly true on the part of the patient who has come to trust and depend on the nurse who tended to their needs at a time of vulnerability. Some patients receive care in their homes from a nurse over a long period of time, and the end of those relationships can be particularly difficult for patients.

Feelings evoked by termination should be discussed and accepted. Summarizing the gains that the patient has made is an important activity during this phase. The importance of the relationship to both patient and nurse can be shared in a caring manner.

The giving and receiving of gifts at termination have different meanings for different people. The meaning of such behavior should be explored in a sensitive manner with the patient. When a nurse has been involved with a family over a long or intense period, such as in an end-of-life setting, it is common for those families to want to give the nurse a gift as a sign of their appreciation and as a remembrance of the patient who has died. Both the agency's policy on gifts and your clinical faculty should be consulted. Even if you are not allowed to accept a gift, you can acknowledge that you wish you could accept their gift and express your gratitude for their thoughtfulness.

Because termination is often painful, participants are often tempted to continue the relationship on a social basis, and requests for screen names for social media, addresses, phone numbers, and e-mail addresses are not uncommon. The nurse must realize that professional relationships are different from social relationships. This is an issue of professional boundaries that has been discussed earlier in this text. Differences between social and professional relationships are outlined in Box 12.1.

BOX 12.1 Differences in Social and Professional Relationships

Social Relationships	Professional Relationships
1. Evolve spontaneously	1. Evolve through recognized phases; interactions are planned and purposeful
2. Not time limited	2. Limited in time with termination date often predetermined
3. Not necessarily goal directed; broad purpose is pleasure, companionship, sharing	3. Goal directed; systematic exploration of identified problem areas
4. Centered on meeting both parties' needs	4. Centered on meeting patient's needs
5. Problem solving is rarely/occasionally a focus	5. Problem solving is a primary focus
6. May or may not include nonjudgmental acceptance	6. Includes nonjudgmental acceptance
7. Outcome is pleasure for both parties	7. Outcome is improved health status of patient

During the course of a professional career, every nurse will develop relationships with a large number of patients, each with its own meaning and duration. If nurses can view each new relationship both as an opportunity to assist another human being to grow and change in a positive, healthful way and as a challenge to grow and change themselves, the rewards of nursing will be rich in and of themselves, allowing the nurse to separate from patients gracefully at the natural end of the therapeutic relationship.

Developing Self-Awareness

Self-awareness is basic to effective interpersonal relationships and is especially important in the nurse–patient relationship. Few people, however, recognize their own emotions, prejudices, and biases and how they are perceived by others. With practice, however, most people can become self-aware, thereby increasing their effectiveness in both professional and personal relationships.

Nurses must get their own emotional needs met outside of the nurse–patient relationship. When nurses have strong unmet needs for acceptance, approval, friendship, or even love, they run the risk of allowing these needs to enter into their relationships with patients at the cost of professionalism. Boundaries get blurred, and relationships become social, not professional. Worse, patients can bear the burden of their nurses' emotional needs. This is a particular risk in settings where the nurse takes care of a patient and family over a long period, such as in home health or hospice/palliative care settings, or in long-term care facilities. Patients come to know their nurses well, and details of nurses' lives are sometimes shared as part of conversation over time. Although it is not necessarily a boundary issue for a patient to learn certain details of nurses' lives, it is always a problem when they depend on patients to meet their own emotional support.

Baca (2011) listed five ways in which self-disclosure becomes problematic: (1) if the nurse's problems or needs are disclosed; (2) if disclosure by the nurse becomes a common, rather than rare, event during interactions with a patient; (3) when the disclosure is unrelated to the patient's problems or experiences; (4) if it takes more than a very short time during a patient care encounter; and (5) when the nurse discloses personal information even if it is clear that the patient is confused by the interaction. Becoming aware of one's needs and making conscious efforts to have those needs met in one's private life keep relationships with patients professional and therapeutic for the patient. When the nurse–patient relationship crosses professional boundaries, role confusion can result, risking harm to both patient and nurse.

Professional Boundaries

Questions of professional boundaries are common in nursing. They were first addressed by Florence Nightingale in the Nightingale Pledge (refer to Box 3.1 to review this statement). The National Council of State Boards of Nursing (NCSBN) detailed the subject of professional boundaries comprehensively in a document available online titled "A Nurse's Guide to Professional Boundaries" (NCSBN, 2014). In this document, the NCSBN defines professional boundaries as "the spaces between the nurse's power and the client's vulnerability. The power of the nurse comes from the professional position and the access to private knowledge about the client" (NCSBN, 2014). Boundary violations occur when "there is confusion between the needs of the nurse and those of the [patient]" (NCSBN, 2014).

According to the NCSBN, nurse–patient relationships can be plotted on a continuum of professional behavior that ranges from underinvolvement (such as distancing, disinterest, neglect) through a zone of helpfulness (the ideal space) to overinvolvement (such as excessive personal disclosure by the nurse, secrecy, role reversal, touching, gestures, money or gifts, special attention, social contact, getting involved in a patient's personal affairs, and/or sexual misconduct). Both underinvolvement and overinvolvement can be detrimental to patient and nurse. A quick way of monitoring yourself with regard to boundaries is to ask yourself, "Would I feel comfortable telling a colleague about my interaction with this patient?" If the answer is no, then you are at least on the edge of a boundary violation and need to take corrective measures. Secretive behavior is a signal that a nurse does not feel comfortable or is unwilling to share with trusted others (Baca, 2011). Box 12.2 describes a case in which a nurse was disciplined by his state board of nursing for failing to honor the professional boundaries between a nurse and patient.

Failure to maintain professional boundaries with a patient is an offense reportable to your employer and/or your state board of nursing and violates nursing's code of ethics. This means that students and nurses in practice must have a thorough understanding of professional boundaries. Box 12.3 contains seven principles to guide nurses in determining professional boundaries across the continuum of professional behavior (NCSBN, 2014). You can find a .pdf file of the popular NCSBN publication explaining professional boundaries by following the links at www.ncsbn.org.

Reflective Practice

Nurses care for a diverse array of patients whose values, beliefs, and lifestyles may challenge nurses' own values. Although nurses sometimes are attracted to patients, conversely, nurses may be repelled by some patients. Nurses who have emotional reactions to patients—positive or negative—sometimes feel guilty or disturbed about these feelings. Being self-aware means recognizing one's feelings and understanding that, although feelings cannot be controlled, behaviors can. Effective nurses conducting themselves professionally take charge of their behavior to prevent their own prejudices, beliefs, and needs from intruding into nurse–patient relationships. This ability arises from self-awareness.

BOX 12.2 Nurse's Relationship With Patient Results in Disciplinary Action

Tapp v. Board of Registered Nursing, 2002 WL 31820206 P2d-CA

This case involved a California registered nurse at a psychiatric facility in Fresno who was accused of having a sexual relationship with his former patient after her discharge. The patient was hospitalized for emotional problems related to sex. She was hospitalized on a unit where the nurse worked the night shift. They became friendly; he brought her small gifts, gave her his phone number, and called her during his off-work hours. After she was discharged, they spoke often by phone, and he began to visit her at her apartment. On one occasion, the nurse gave his former patient a pill containing a controlled substance.

One week after her discharge from the psychiatric unit, they began a sexual relationship that lasted for two weeks. Shortly after the relationship ended, the patient was readmitted "suffering adverse effects from the affair" (p. 4). The California Board of Registered Nursing initiated disciplinary proceedings for "acts of unprofessional conduct." An administrative law judge heard testimony, made a determination of misconduct, and recommended that the nurse's license be revoked, but stayed the revocation and recommended that the nurse be placed on probation for 5 years on multiple conditions. The California Board of Registered Nursing disagreed and ordered the revocation of his license. There were subsequent appeals, dismissals, and further appeals.

Nurses must realize that there can be no socialization between themselves and patients, particularly when sexual in nature. The ruling noted that not only was the nurse's behavior with this patient during her hospitalization "highly improper, but his socialization with the patient after her discharge from the hospital, not to mention the fact that he provided the patient with a controlled substance, was ample reason to impose strict disciplinary action" (p. 5).

Abstracted from Nurse's relationship with patient results in disciplinary action, *Nurs Law Regan Rep* 43(8):4–5, 2003.

Developing self-awareness requires individuals to engage in personal reflection. This requires taking time to focus on their own thoughts, feelings, actions, and beliefs. Finding the time and space for **reflective practice** can be a challenge to busy students and practicing nurses alike. Reflection can produce discomfort as nurses become aware of the tensions and anxieties

BOX 12.3 Principles for Determining Professional Boundaries

1. Establishing and maintaining professional boundaries is the nurse's responsibility.
2. The nurse's relationship with the patient should be therapeutic within those established professional boundaries.
3. Combining a professional and a personal or business relationship should be avoided.
4. The nurse is responsible for monitoring for deviations outside of those boundaries and modifying behaviors accordingly.
5. Termination of the professional relationship is the nurse's responsibility, but that may be difficult when the patient needs ongoing care such as in a home care situation.

Modified from National Council of State Boards of Nursing (NCSBN): *Professional boundaries: a nurse's guide to the importance of appropriate professional boundaries,* Chicago, 1996, National Council of State Boards of Nursing.

within themselves about their everyday activities. Nurses and nursing students may find that their personal values are challenged by the realities of practice. Importantly, nurses may recognize in themselves a desensitization to the needs of their patients because of time constraints, the need to create emotional space, or a personal dislike for a particular patient.

It can be hard for you when you recognize that you may have thoughts that are less than kind about patients entrusted to your care. This makes the need for reflection more, not less, important. No human being is immune from emotional responses to others, both positive and negative. Despite the difficulty in coming to terms with your emotional responses to patients and to your work, becoming self-aware allows you to understand your responses and to look past your own negative (and positive) responses to particular patients in order to create and maintain a healthy professional space in which you can provide care most effectively. Box 12.4 contains a model for structured reflection that will be helpful to you reflecting on your practice and becoming more self-aware.

BOX 12.4 Model for Structured Reflection

1. Write a description of an experience was significant in some way.
2. What issue seemed significant to pay attention to?
3. How was I feeling and what influenced the way I felt?
4. What was I trying to achieve?
5. Did I respond effectively and in a way consistent with my values?
6. What were the consequences of my actions on the patient, others, and myself?
7. How were others feeling?
8. What made them feel that way?
9. What factors influenced the way I was feeling, thinking, or responding?
10. What knowledge did or might have informed me?
11. To what extent did I act with best intentions?
12. How does this situation connect with previous experiences?
13. How might I respond more effectively given this situation again?
14. What would be the consequences of alternative actions for the patient, others, and myself?
15. How do I now feel about this experience?
16. Am I now more able to support myself and others as a consequence?
17. Am I now more available to work with patients/families and staff to help them meet their needs?

From Johns C: *Guided reflection: advancing practice,* Oxford, 2002, Blackwell Science, p. 10. Reprinted with permission of Wiley-Blackwell.

Avoiding Stereotypes

Stereotypes are simplistic, distorted images used to describe or characterize groups. Stereotypes result in prejudices and negative attitudes developed through social and cultural interactions. It is unfortunately easy to develop stereotyped views of groups of people different from themselves and to have expectations of those groups based on these distorted images. Stereotypes are established through a lifetime of experiences and negatively affect relationships with people in the stereotyped group. Because stereotypes and prejudices tend to persist despite contrary experiences, they are irrational or illogical beliefs. Stereotypes may be based on ethnicity, gender, nationality, or political affiliation, among others; for instance, portrayals or descriptions of nurses as sex objects, physicians' handmaidens, or not bright enough to attend medical school are all stereotypes affecting the profession of nursing negatively.

A subtle form of stereotyping that affects nursing is related to expectations of others based on one's distorted view of the other. This in turn causes problems relating to patients who are stereotyped. For example, if a nurse expects that older people are irritable and demanding, the nurse may seek to avoid caring for older patients or may treat their complaints as unimportant: "just another grumpy old person." Moreover, some nurses demonstrate lack of respect to older patients, using names such as "sweetie," "dear," and "honey," among others. These types of names are actually inappropriate in any professional nursing setting, especially with adult patients; these types of names diminish the patient by demonstrating a lack of respect for the patient as a person.

Professional nurses deliver high-quality care to all patients regardless of the patients' ethnicity, age, sex, gender identity, sexual orientation, religion, lifestyle, or diagnosis. The ANA's Code of Ethics for Nurses requires nurses to do this. Nurses are prone to stereotyping just like anyone else; however, the nature of the nurse–patient relationship requires that nurses become aware of how their stereotyped views of certain patients negatively affect the delivery of care. Every professional nurse's goal is to accept all patients as individuals of dignity and worth who deserve the best nursing care possible.

Becoming Nonjudgmental

Prejudices are simply what the word implies: judging a person in advance of knowing him or her, based on stereotypes and biases. Prejudices are strong and are often outside our awareness, which in turn makes acceptance of others difficult. Prejudging others as "good" or "bad," "right" or "wrong," is usually unconscious, hence the need for nurses to examine their prejudices and become aware of when prejudices are operating. Nonjudgmental acceptance means that nurses acknowledge all patients' rights to be who they are and to express their uniqueness. Acceptance conveys neither approval nor disapproval of patients and their personal beliefs, habits, expressions of feelings, or lifestyles.

Therapeutic use of self begins with the ability to convey acceptance to patients and requires self-awareness and nonjudgmental attitudes on the part of nurses. Ongoing examination of attitudes toward others is both a lifelong process and an essential part of self-awareness, maturation, and personal growth.

Thinking Differently about Nurses and Patients: Caring and Human Relatedness

Fundamentals of the traditional nurse–patient relationship model as described earlier have been taught and practiced since the middle of the 20th century; however, several assumptions on which it is based no longer hold true in many of today's practice settings. For instance, this older model assumes that the development of the nurse–patient relationship is linear, is incremental, and requires trust-building in the earliest phases of the relationship, and, importantly, it assumes that patients desire relationships with nurses, wish to receive services from them, and will cooperate and comply with those nurses (Hagerty and Patusky, 2003).

Although the traditional nurse–patient relationship is still appropriate in some settings, the assumptions on which it is based are being challenged by the fact that hospitalized patients today are more acutely ill, nurses' workloads have increased, and the time nurses spend with patients may be limited. This raises the question of how we can rethink the nurse–patient relationship and find ways to modify it to suit today's contexts of healthcare delivery.

Patient-Centered Care

Patient-centered care has been proposed as an approach to alleviating some of the problems that currently trouble the U.S. healthcare system, such as poor care quality, limited access to care, and dehumanization of care (Hobbs, 2009). In a detailed analysis, Hobbs (2009) found that alleviating vulnerabilities (e.g., feeling alienated, lack of control) experienced by the patient is central to patient-centered care in acute care settings. Furthermore, the process of therapeutic engagement is the key process in alleviating vulnerabilities, and one of the mechanisms by which this occurs is by the nurse's caring presence (p. 55).

Theories of caring and human relatedness provide a powerful basis for practice. Many theorists have written about the nature of the nurse–patient relationship, with several writing about caring as the central concept in nursing, through which effective nursing practice occurs. Swanson (1991) defined caring as "a nurturing way of relating to a valued other, toward whom one feels a personal sense of commitment and responsibility" (p. 165). Five caring processes are germane to nursing practice: (1) knowing, (2) being with, (3) doing for, (4) enabling, and (5) maintaining belief (Swanson, 1991). Others have written about caring in nursing, including Watson (1988), whose theory is discussed in Chapter 9, and Roach and Maykut (2010), who described the essential elements of comportment central to professional caring.

Hagerty and Patusky (2003) proposed an interesting theory of human relatedness through which to conceptualize the nurse–patient relationship. Each nurse–patient contact holds the potential for connection and goal achievement, as opposed to one step in a lengthy relationship-building process. They also recommended that nurses approach their patients with a sense of the patient's autonomy, choice, and participation (p. 147), putting the relationship on a more equitable basis than the traditional nurse–patient relationship, which gives much of the power to the nurse.

The Quality and Safety Education for Nurses (QSEN) project identified patient-centered care as one of six competencies required of all prelicensure nurses and defines patient-centered care as fully engaging the patient or designee in all care decisions, respecting the values, needs, and preferences of the patient or designee in all care coordination. Communication is a key component in realizing patient-centered care. A basic understanding of communication theory is a necessary component of becoming a more effective communicator and therefore a better nurse.

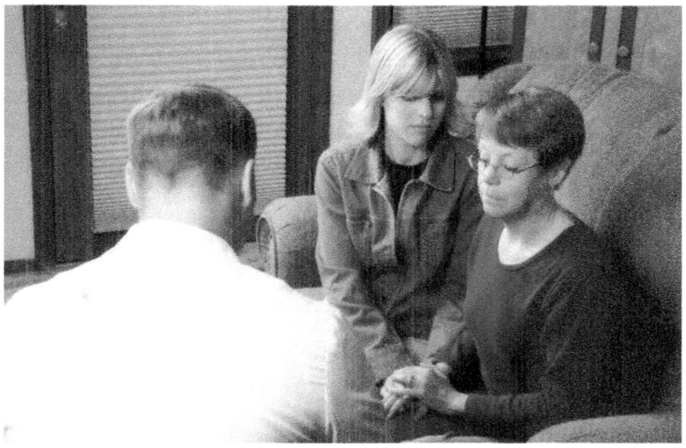

Fig. 12.1 Nonverbal communication consists of grooming, clothing, gestures, posture, facial expressions, tone and volume of voice, and actions. Simply from the visual cues in this picture, you can form an idea of what is happening. (Photo used with permission from iStockPhoto.)

COMMUNICATION THEORY

Communication is the exchange of thoughts, ideas, or information and is at the heart of all relationships. Jurgen Ruesch (1972), a pioneer communications theorist, defined communication as "all the modes of behavior that one individual employs, conscious or unconscious, to affect another: not only the spoken and written word, but also gestures, body movements, somatic signals, and symbolism in the arts" (p. 16).

Communication begins the moment two people become aware of each other's presence. Communication occurs when one is in the presence of another person, even if no words are spoken. Even when alone, people routinely engage in "self-talk," which is an internal form of communication.

Levels of Communication

Communication exists simultaneously on at least two levels: verbal and nonverbal. **Verbal communication** consists of all speech and represents the most obvious aspect of communication. Much of one's message, however, consists of nonverbal communication. **Nonverbal communication** includes grooming, clothing, gestures, posture, facial expressions, eye contact, tone and volume of voice, and actions, among other things (Fig. 12.1). Words can be used to mask feelings, but individuals are less able to exercise conscious control over nonverbal communication than verbal communication, therefore the nonverbal component may be a more reliable expression of feeling. Nurses must pay attention to nonverbal messages as closely as they do to verbal ones.

Consider this example: A nurse who is helping a patient prepare for a breast biopsy notices that the patient keeps her head turned away, has tears in her eyes, and will not look at the nurse. When the nurse says, "I know this is hard. Is there anything you would like to talk about or ask?" the patient responds, "No, I'm fine." The sensitive nurse would pay closer attention to her nonverbal communication than to the spoken word. If the nurse pays attention only to the patient's words, her underlying feelings would be ignored. The nurse's job in evaluating this patient's needs is made more difficult by the incongruence between her verbal and nonverbal messages.

When **congruent** communication occurs, the verbal and nonverbal aspects match and reinforce each other. In **incongruent** communication, the words and nonverbal communication do not match. Incongruent communication creates confusion in receivers, who are unsure which level of communication they should respond to. Nurses should be alert to incongruent communication for clues to patients' unexpressed feelings. Nurses need to understand that patients are vulnerable, and expressions such as "I'm okay" or "No, I'm fine," despite their incongruent nonverbal cues, do not mean that your patient is lying. It may simply mean that the patient is not ready or willing to share verbally what their nonverbal communication is relaying.

Elements of the Communication Process

Five major elements must be present for communication to occur: a sender, a message, a receiver, feedback, and a context (Ruesch, 1972). The sender is the person sending the message; the message is what is actually said plus accompanying nonverbal communication; the receiver is the person acquiring the message. A response to a message is termed feedback. The setting in which an interaction occurs, including the mood, relationship between sender and receiver, and other factors, is known as the context. All these elements are necessary for communication to occur.

Consider the classroom situation. During a lecture, the professor is the sender, the lecture is the message, and students are the receivers. The professor (sender) receives feedback from the students (receivers) through their facial expressions, alertness, posture, attentiveness, and comments/questions. The atmosphere in the classroom is the context. If the atmosphere is a relaxed one of give-and-take discussion between students and professor, the feedback is different from feedback in a more formal context of professor as lecturer and students as note takers. Fig. 12.2 shows the relationships among the elements of communication.

Operations in the Communication Process

In addition to the five elements of communication, three major operations occur in communication: perception, evaluation, and transmission (Ruesch, 1972).

Perception

Perception is the selection, organization, and interpretation of incoming signals into meaningful messages. In the classroom situation just described, students select, organize, and interpret various pieces of the professor's message or lecture. Each student perceives the information differently; their perception is based on a variety of factors such as personal experience, preparation before class, alertness, fatigue, sensitivity to subtleties of meaning, and sociocultural background. This is sometimes referred to as an individual's perceptual screen, through which all incoming messages are filtered.

Evaluation

Evaluation is the analysis of received information. Students will evaluate the content of their professor's lecture: Is it useful? Is it important or relevant? Does it make sense? Is it likely to be on the next test? Each student evaluates the same message (what the sender transmitted) differently.

Transmission

Transmission refers to the expression of information, verbal or nonverbal. As you read this, certain professors of yours may come to mind—those whose nonverbal behaviors spoke "louder than words," indicating their

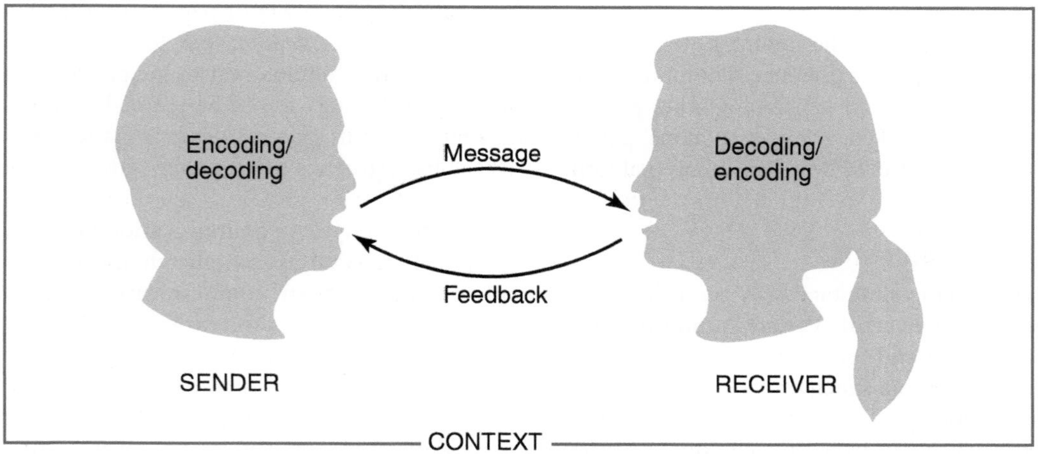

Fig. 12.2 The five major elements of the communication process.

own level of engagement with the subject matter. While the professor is transmitting verbal messages to the students, the nonverbal behavior of excitement, uncertainty, confusion, or boredom with the subject matter also transmits a message to the class.

Factors Influencing Perception, Evaluation, and Transmission

Perception, evaluation, and transmission are influenced by many factors. Gender identity, age, and culture of the sender and receiver; the interest and mood of both parties; the value, clarity, and length of the message; the presence or absence of feedback; and the context all are powerful influences. Also involved are individuals' needs, values, self-concepts, sensory and intellectual abilities or deficits, and sociocultural conditioning. Clearly, communication is a complex human activity to which nurses must pay careful attention.

THE DEVELOPMENT OF HUMAN COMMUNICATION

Humans learn to communicate through a certain developmental sequence, which begins in infancy. Infants use somatic language to signal their needs to caretakers. Somatic language consists of crying; changing skin color; fast, shallow breathing; facial expressions; and flexing of their arms and legs. The sequence progresses to action language in older infants. Mothers describe knowing the difference in their infants' cries: the "hungry" cry, the "mad" cry, the "pick me up!" cry. Understanding somatic language can be learned with close attention. Action language consists of reaching out, pointing, crawling toward a desired object, or closing the lips and turning the head when an undesired food is offered. Even without a sound, an infant's intention or desire has been clearly communicated. Verbal language develops last, beginning with repetitive noises and sounds and progressing to words, phrases, and complete sentences.

In normal child development, any one or combination of these forms of communication can be used. Somatic language usually decreases with maturity, but, because it is not under conscious control, some somatic language may persist past childhood, such as blushing when one is embarrassed or angry. The development of communication is determined by both inborn and environmental factors. The amount of verbal stimulation an infant receives can enhance or delay the development of language skills. The extent of a caretaker's vocabulary and verbal ability can be influential on the infant's language development. Some families simply talk a lot, thereby providing intense verbal stimulation, whereas others are quieter and less verbal.

Nonverbal communication development is similarly influenced by environment. Most families have their own nonverbal gestures such as touch or facial expressions, which children learn to interpret at young ages. The ability to communicate effectively is dependent on a number of factors. The quantity and quality of verbal and nonverbal stimulation received during early development are keys to one's ability to communicate.

CRITERIA FOR SUCCESSFUL COMMUNICATION

Everyone has had the experience of being the sender or receiver of unsuccessful communication. A simple example is arriving for a coffee date with a friend at the wrong time or wrong place because of a problem in communication. Unsuccessful communication in certain social circumstances creates little harm. In nursing situations, however, accurate, complete communication is vitally important. Nurses can achieve successful communication on most occasions if they plan their communication to meet four major criteria: feedback, appropriateness, efficiency, and flexibility.

Feedback

When a receiver relays to a sender the effect of the sender's message, feedback has occurred. It is also a criterion for successful communication. In making the social appointment mentioned earlier, if the receiver of the message had said, "Looking forward to getting caught up —12:30 on Tuesday April 4th at the Looking Glass Café for coffee," that feedback would be successful as an effective way to ensure that both persons were at the same place at the same time. Or, in today's context, a quick confirmation by text message or calendar invitation can also serve the same purpose.

In a nurse–patient interaction, a nurse can give feedback to a patient by saying, "If I understand you correctly, you are saying that you have pain in your lower abdomen every time you stand up." The patient can then either agree or correct what the nurse has said: "No, the pain is there only when I stand up the first time every morning." Effective nurses do not assume that they fully understand what their patients are telling them until they confirm their understanding with the patient.

Appropriateness

Appropriateness refers to the correct "fit" of a reply, that is, when it matches the message, and the size of the reply is neither too lengthy nor too brief. In day-to-day conversation among casual acquaintances passing in a hallway or in public, most people recognize the question asked in passing "How are you?" as an expression of greeting in brief social interaction and not as a genuine inquiry into one's health and well-being. The individual who launches into a lengthy, detailed description of how their morning has gone has responded inappropriately to the casual question, "How are you?" The reply does not fit the circumstances, and the reply is too expansive for casual discourse. The expected response to the casual greeting is usually, "Fine, how about you?" or other short colloquialism.

Conversely, when you go into a patient's room and ask, "How are you?" your intention is to inquire about your patient's health and well-being as a professional interest, and the patient may respond accordingly; however, because this question is so pervasive in everyday discourse, the patient may simply answer, "Fine, how are you?" You will need to ask the question more specifically if your patient responds in that manner. If a patient asks, "When is my doctor coming to see me?" just after the physician has visited the patient, the nurse will be alert to other inappropriate messages by this patient that may signal a variety of problems or misunderstandings. In this instance the inappropriate message does not appear to match the context; however, in a large medical center where a team of providers are involved, the patient may simply be asking about the person they know as "their doctor" as opposed to a member of the care team, such as a resident physician or nurse practitioner making rounds. Knowing the context serves to clarify these kinds of questions.

Efficiency

Efficiency means using simple, clear words that are timed at a pace suitable to participants. Explaining to an adult that she will have "an angioplasty" tomorrow morning may not result in successful communication. Telling her she will have "an angioplasty, a procedure in which a small balloon is threaded into an artery and inflated to open up the vessel so more blood can flow through," will more likely improve her understanding. This message would not be an efficient one for a small child, however. Messages must be adapted to each patient's age, verbal level, and level of understanding.

Oversimplification is a risk in trying to adapt one's language style and word choice to a particular patient. What may seem to be useful simplicity and efficiency may be perceived as "dumbing down" or patronizing language to the patient. One cannot tell with any certainty a patient's communication level, and to assume that a patient cannot understand may also cause problems. For instance, a nurse (the author of this text) once heard a physician tell a teenager with a urinary tract infection that she had "bugs in [her] bladder." The physician's attempt to make the language efficient and simple was misguided; the young woman took his words at face value and became upset to the point of almost fainting at the thought that she had insects in her body. The nurse immediately intervened, explaining to the patient that sometimes providers refer to bacteria or germs as "bugs"; she had bacteria in her bladder causing an infection. The patient immediately calmed down, asking, "Why didn't he just say that? I need some antibiotics." The physician made a significant misjudgment related to the patient's level of understanding. He came across as patronizing, and the patient was unnecessarily upset by his simplistic explanation. He followed up with the nurse, asking, "What just happened in there?" The nurse explained to him what had gone wrong.

Some examples of patients who require special assistance in evaluating and responding to messages are young children; people with certain mental illnesses, neurologic deficits, or autism spectrum disorders and other manifestations of neurodivergence; those with significant developmental delays; and those recovering from anesthesia or receiving pain medication. Although it may seem obvious that people with hearing loss will require special assistance in communication, those with impaired vision do not have the ability to note nonverbal cues, an important element of communication. For efficient communication to occur, nurses must recognize patients' needs and adjust messages accordingly.

Flexibility

Flexibility is the fourth criterion for successful communication. The flexible communicator bases messages on the immediate situation rather than preconceived expectations. When a nursing student who plans to teach a patient about managing diabetes with diet enters the patient's room and finds the patient crying, the student must be flexible enough to regroup and deal with the feelings the patient is expressing. Pressing on with the teaching plan in the face of the patient's distress may be interpreted by the patient as a lack of empathy or caring, as well as inflexibility in communicating.

Nurses can learn to use these four measures of successful communication to enhance their effectiveness with patients. If any of these four criteria are missing, communication can be disrupted and hamper the successful implementation of the nursing process. The following is a true story of what happens when communication breaks down and a rigid reliance on a bureaucratic system prevails. Details are changed to protect the privacy of the patient and family.

Mr. Lewis came to the local emergency department (ED) accompanied by his wife, who was a nurse. Mr. Lewis, who had advanced cancer, was occasionally confused and had tried to retrieve a Popsicle stick stuck on the roof of his large dog's mouth. In the process, he caught the back of his hand on an upper canine tooth, resulting in a deep gash. Mrs. Lewis had witnessed the accident and gave details to the triage nurse, including her first-person account that the dog did not bite her husband and that his skin was fragile and prone to tearing. The nurse noted "dog bite" on her intake form over Mrs. Lewis' objection that the injury was clearly not a bite and that the dog was not at fault. The triage nurse did not acknowledge Mrs. Lewis' account of the accident, continued to get vital signs, and complained about "getting slammed," meaning that the ED was busy.

Mr. Lewis was soon escorted to the urgent care room, where his wound was cleaned and sutured. Both the nurse practitioner and resident physician asked questions about how the "dog bite" happened, and Mrs. Lewis again protested that it was not a bite and pointed out the lack of tooth marks, crushing, or other signs of a bite. The attending physician told the couple that he had no choice but to report "the bite" to the county emergency medical services (EMS) per protocol, because the triage nurse had documented it as a "dog bite," although the couple had never said it was a bite and the wound was not consistent with a bite. The unit secretary called 911 and asked Mrs. Lewis to tell the dispatcher about the "dog that bit your husband." Mrs. Lewis explained what had happened to the dispatcher, who said that he had no discretion in the matter and that he had to report this to the local police.

Within a half hour of arriving home at 12:30 a.m., Mrs. Lewis received a call from a police officer who said he was "initiating an investigation about the dog attack at this address." At that point, Mrs. Lewis burst into tears in frustration and explained one more time to the police officer that there was no attack, no bite, just an accident by her sick and confused husband. The officer said he had no discretion in the case and had to make a report to animal control, who would have the final say about whether their beloved dog would have to be quarantined or worse. He said he would make his report in a way that was sympathetic to the Lewises, although he could not promise what animal control would do. For more than a week, the Lewises were nervous and upset, and every time the phone rang or someone came to the door, they feared it was animal control. Gratefully, they never heard anything else about the matter. But the triage nurse's failure to listen carefully created a cascade of bureaucratic procedure that caused avoidable pain and distress for this couple who were already dealing with devastating illness.

Consider the many ways that communication went wrong in this scenario. Identify points where you believe that this cascade of events could have been interrupted.

DEVELOPING EFFECTIVE COMMUNICATION SKILLS

People are not born as good communicators, although it is hard to argue that a screaming infant is not communicating something. Exactly what the baby is communicating, however, needs to be deciphered by an attentive parent or other caregiver. As the baby grows into a toddler, he or she learns that "no" is a particularly useful word. Anyone who has responded to a petulant 2-year-old, however, knows that the child has much to learn about the other side of communication: being a good listener. The child must learn to increase his or her repertoire of responses.

Communication skills can be developed with time and practice. Becoming a better listener, learning a few basic helpful responding styles, and avoiding common causes of communication breakdowns can put you on the path to becoming a better communicator. To begin evaluating your communication skills, refer to the Communication Patterns Self-Assessment in Box 12.5.

Listening

Listening is hard work, yet it is the only way to get to know patients and understand what is important to them.

BOX 12.5 Communication Patterns Self-Assessment

Directions: Answer the following Yes/No questions as honestly as possible; then review your answers, and draw at least two conclusions about your communication patterns. Check your conclusions for accuracy with a friend who knows your style of communicating well. Then score yourself using the key below.

1. I find it easier to start conversations by talking about myself. Yes/No
2. I usually listen about as much as I talk. Yes/No
3. I tend to be long-winded. Yes/No
4. I rarely interrupt others. Yes/No
5. When people hesitate or speak slowly, I try to complete their sentences for them. Yes/No
6. I pay close attention to what others say, as well as to body cues. Yes/No
7. I find it difficult to make eye contact with the person I am talking with. Yes/No
8. I can usually tell if someone is angry or upset. Yes/No
9. I find it difficult to express myself assertively. Yes/No
10. I expect others to read my mind. Yes/No
11. I hesitate to interrupt someone to ask for clarification. Yes/No
12. People often tell me personal things about themselves. Yes/No
13. I find it is best to change the subject if someone gets too emotional. Yes/No
14. If I cannot "make things better" for a friend with a problem, I feel uncomfortable. Yes/No
15. I am comfortable talking with people much older or much younger than I am. Yes/No
16. I have difficulty saying no. Yes/No
17. I speak to others the way I like to be spoken to. Yes/No
18. I get irritated easily. Yes/No
19. I tend to withdraw from conflict or remain silent. Yes/No
20. I try to evaluate when someone will be most receptive to my message. Yes/No

Key: If you answered Yes to questions 2, 4, 6, 8, 12, 15, 17, and 20, you are on your way to becoming an effective communicator. If you answered Yes to other questions, think about how you might improve on those. Set a realistic goal and seek help from a trusted friend or faculty member.

A requirement of successful communication is listening, but too often we hear without listening or engage in a task while not fully listening. (This was a problem with the triage nurse in the earlier example.) **Active listening** involves focusing solely on a person and acknowledging feelings in a nonjudgmental manner. In active listening, the nurse is communicating interest and attention. It is best accomplished without background distractions, such as the television or chatting visitors. Using an intentionally unrushed manner, making good eye contact, nodding, and encouraging the speaker ("Go on" or "Tell me more") also help communicate interest. Facing the speaker squarely and using an **open posture** (sitting up straight, relaxed, arms uncrossed) also communicate interest. Sit, bend, or stoop to be at eye level of the patient, and repeat (reflect) what you hear, including feelings, checking to be sure you heard correctly. These indications of interest and active listening will help you focus on patients and tune into the meanings behind their words. These same behaviors and practices are just as important when communicating with a patient's family member or friend who may be relaying information to you because the patient cannot communicate effectively themselves (e.g., medicated for pain; aftermath of a stroke; shyness; among others).

Having someone listen to concerns, even if no problem solving takes place, may be therapeutic. **Venting** is the term used to describe the verbal "letting off steam" that occurs when talking about concerns or frustrations. In today's complex healthcare system, the risk is high that patients feel ignored or anxious on occasion. Because nurses are available to patients more than any other healthcare provider, they are likely to hear patients' complaints. It is important that nurses understand these complaints and frustrations as a professional, realizing that they are rarely personally directed at the nurse.

Nurses may have difficulty listening for a variety of reasons. They may be intent on accomplishing a task and be frustrated by the time it takes to be a good listener. They may be planning their own next question or response and not truly hear what the patient is saying. They may be distracted by a colleague, a mobile phone, or worries about another patient. Like all people, nurses have their own personal and professional problems that sometimes preoccupy them and interfere with effective listening. No message can be received if the receiver (the nurse) is not listening. In the context of care, being listened to meets the patient's emotional need to be respected and valued by the nurse. Hospitalized patients

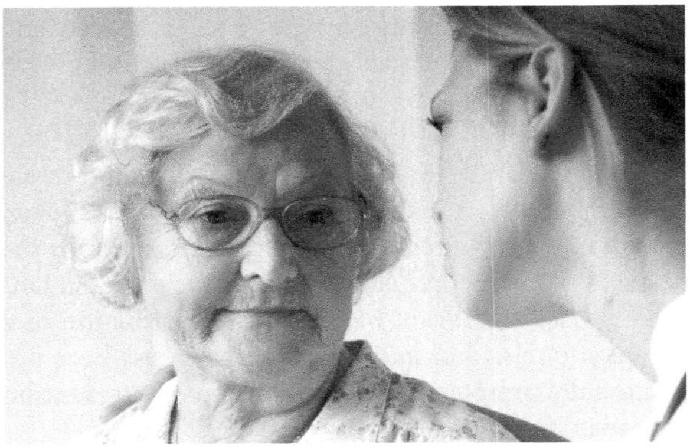

Fig. 12.3 Being an active listener is an important part of communication. Identify behaviors in this photograph that may demonstrate active listening by the nurse. (Photo used with permission from iStockPhoto.)

particularly may feel that their lives are out of control and that they are isolated or invisible. They may need to discuss those feelings with someone who will listen without judgment or defensiveness (Fig. 12.3). Listening is a skill that can be developed; properly used, it can be an essential part of a nurse's communication repertoire.

Using Helpful Responding Techniques

A variety of helpful responding techniques demonstrate respect and encourage patients to communicate openly with their nurses. Helpful responses that have already been discussed in this chapter include being nonjudgmental, observing body language, and using active listening. Other useful responses, detailed in the following five sections, include demonstrating empathy, asking open-ended questions, giving information, using reflection, and being silent.

Empathy

Empathy consists of awareness of, sensitivity to, and identification with the feelings of another person. Nurses can empathize with patients even if they have not experienced an event in their own lives exactly like the one the patient is experiencing. If nurses have had a similar or parallel experience, empathy is possible. For example, the feeling of loss is familiar to most nurses, even though they may not personally have lost a close family member. The nurse, however, must avoid the temptation to overidentify with patients when the patient's situation is very similar to one that the nurse has experienced. "I know exactly how you feel" is not helpful in good communication, because human experience varies widely.

Empathy is different from sympathy in that the sympathetic nurse enters into the feeling with the patient, whereas the empathetic nurse appreciates the patient's feelings but is not swept along with the feelings. "You seem upset about the upcoming procedure" is an example of a nursing statement that demonstrates empathy.

If you find yourself overcome by emotions related to a patient, you will need to seek out a colleague to assist you or even replace you in providing care for your patient, because you cannot be effective under these circumstances. You will learn what situations are the most likely to cause you to feel highly emotional and will develop strategies to deal with them. Nurses might "cover" for each other as a matter of collegiality by switching patient assignments or volunteering to work with a particular patient if it is overly burdensome for a colleague.

Open-Ended Questions

An open-ended question is one that causes the patient to answer fully, giving more than a "yes" or "no" answer. Open-ended questions are very useful in data gathering and in the opening stages of any nurse–patient interaction. For example, asking a patient, "Are you in pain?" may elicit only a confirming yes. Saying to the patient, "Tell me about any pain you may be having." is more likely to elicit information about the site, type, intensity, and duration of the pain, therefore making the nurse–patient interaction more useful.

Giving Information

An essential part of nursing is providing information to patients and as appropriate, with a family member or other person accompanying them. Giving information includes sharing knowledge that the recipients are not expected to know. Nurses provide information when they tell patients what to expect during diagnostic procedures; inform them of their rights as patients; and teach them about their conditions, diets, or medications.

An important distinction every nurse needs to make is the difference between providing information and giving opinions. Although providing information is a helpful aspect of the nursing role, giving opinions is unhelpful. Instead, nurses should encourage patients to consider their own values and opinions as primary in importance. Nurses are occasionally asked about other providers, especially physicians, with questions such as "Is Dr. Charles a good surgeon?" or "Would you go to see Dr. Adams if you had cancer?" The nurse will need to refocus the patient's question, for instance, responding, "I am wondering if you have a concern about your care." This deflects the question asked of the nurse and returns the focus of the interaction back to the patient.

Reflection

The nurse using **reflection** is serving as a mirror for the patient. Reflection demonstrates understanding and acceptance. It is a method of encouraging patients to think through problems for themselves by directing patient questions back to the patient. Reflection implies respect because the nurse believes the patient has adequate resources to solve the problem without outside assistance. In response to the patient's question, "Do you think I should go through with this surgery?" the nurse can reflect the question: "What *you* think is most important. Do you think you should go through with this surgery?" Note that the patient's exact words are used. Reflection helps clarify the patient's thoughts and feelings and helps the nurse obtain additional information that may assist in developing the plan of care.

Silence

Although silent periods in social conversations may feel uncomfortable, using silence in nurse–patient relationships can be helpful. Using silence means allowing periods of quiet thought during an interaction without feeling pressure to fill the silence with conversation or activity. For example, when a patient has just been given upsetting news, sitting quietly without making any demands for conversation may be the most therapeutic response a nurse can make at that time. Being with patients (presence) is just as valuable as doing for them and conveys respect for the patient's feelings in distressing circumstances. Be aware, however, of the patient's nonverbal language because they may need privacy and space to deal with the news they have received. The nurse can ask, "Would like some privacy or is it helpful for me to be here with you? If you would rather be alone, I can step out. If you need anything, all you need to do is ring your call light and I'll be right in." A key here is that you need to be available if the patient asks for you, or have a colleague on "stand by" in case you are not available.

Nurses have at their disposal many more helpful responding styles to use in their interactions with patients. The five discussed here, once practiced and mastered, can be a foundation on which to build.

Communication Across Differing Languages

Nurses in the United States are encountering an increasing number of patients whose command of spoken English may be limited. Because communication is the means by which people connect, speaking different languages poses significant barriers to the formation of a therapeutic relationship. The nursing process becomes additionally complex when assessment and intervention must span two languages.

Spanish is the second most prevalent language spoken in the United States today, and many nurses are achieving increased fluency in Spanish. Some nurses are bilingual, a significant advantage in the context of today's healthcare system. Most larger healthcare systems now provide interpreter services for patients on nursing units and in clinics. An **interpreter** is a professional who is fluent in two or more languages or is bilingual and is trained to translate orally from one language to another. A **translator** is a professional who works with written documents, moving words and meaning from one document into another. Patient education materials are usually offered in a variety of languages, although you should not assume that a patient is literate regardless of their ability to speak English. Some persons will work to hide their limited reading skills.

Note that the word *professional* is attached to both these definitions. It is tempting to have a patient's family members interpret for you if a family member speaks both English and the patient's primary language; however, this is not good practice and in fact is not within acceptable standards of care. Interpreters have special training in medical language and in how to do this work most effectively. Similarly, it may be tempting to have a colleague translate teaching materials and other patient information into a second language that your colleague speaks. Again, this is not good practice. Translators are specially trained in how to maintain meaning as closely as possible across languages using the written word. The command of a conversational level of a foreign language, such as what one obtains in high school and basic college courses, is not adequate; very specific technical language required in healthcare settings. Also, fluency in spoken language does not mean that one's written skills are adequate to translate patient materials correctly.

Working with an interpreter takes practice, and you will become more comfortable with doing so over time. You will notice that having a third person present can both enhance and inhibit communication. The helpfulness of having an interpreter with you may allow you to be more relaxed and assured that your patient is getting high quality care. Some patients may find that having an interpreter present may be inhibiting, especially in relation to very sensitive topics. For instance, some women may feel very shy about discussing issues related to childbirth and reproduction in the presence of a male interpreter, regardless of his professional conduct and demeanor. You may have to make some decisions about issues related to gender on occasion if the interpreter and the patient are not of the same gender. Some patients do not have any problem and welcome the assistance by these trained professionals. Your careful guidance may help your patients feel more comfortable, especially when they are reminded that you can provide better care when you can communicate more clearly. The Professional Profile Box 12.1 contains

PROFESSIONAL PROFILE BOX 12.1

Minimizing Language Barriers: Working With a Medical Interpreter

The goal of the medical interpreter is to facilitate patient care by minimizing language barriers; as a nurse, it is important to know how to best use an interpreter's services so that the patient who speaks limited English may receive proper care. The first step is to call the interpreter. It is obvious: if a patient does not understand the provider, an interpreter must be called. What is less obvious: even if your patient seems to speak English as a second language fairly well, the stress of being sick is likely to inhibit his or her ability to understand you. You will reduce a huge burden for your patient by calling an interpreter.

Your patient may confuse you, however, by using body cues such as nodding in agreement or even verbal cues such as the repetition of words of assent ("yes," "okay") that may lead you to believe he or she understands English well. A quick assessment using open-ended questions might reveal that the patient is only showing respect for you but does not understand the content of the interaction. If the patient cannot answer your open-ended questions, or if a family member offers to interpret, an interpreter should be called to give expert assistance in this situation.

When the interpreter arrives, brief them about any delicate situations that might be at play with the patient. For example, if you need to ask about domestic violence or substance abuse, the interpreter should be warned in advance. Once the interpreter has been briefed and you and the interpreter have entered the room together, you should approach the patient as you would any other patient, without hiding behind the interpreter.

Make eye contact with the patient, not the interpreter. Despite the popular image of the triangular positioning of patient-interpreter-provider, to ensure adequate facilitation of the conversation, the interpreter should be positioned behind you or behind the patient. The interpreter's position may change depending on environmental factors such as the availability of space or seating options.

The medical interpreter uses transparency to mitigate communication factors that contribute to health disparities; the ultimate goal is to ensure equal care for those patients for whom English represents a significant barrier. The principle of transparency dictates that anything the nurse says, or other provider or party says, stays within the confines of the patient's room. All of the patient's verbal expressions will, in turn, be repeated to the provider. The interpreter will use the first person to relay the information between the parties. If the interpreter feels the need to intervene, whether to explain a cultural gap or to clarify word choice to either party, she or he will advise both parties that the correction or clarification is taking place.

Your rhythm of speech should be adjusted so that the interpreter can keep pace. This means stopping every few sentences so as not to present too much content for the interpreter to relay at once. If the pace is too fast, the interpreter may indicate the need for a break between sentences. The interpretation should be consecutive, not simultaneous, meaning that the interpreter waits for you or the patient to stop speaking before interpreting your words.

Whenever possible, all applicable paperwork that has previously been translated (consent forms, patient forms, informational brochures) should be gathered before the interpreter arrives. If a form has not yet been translated, the interpreter may use sight translation to read the form aloud to the patient. A form must be completely understood by the patient in order to serve as a legal document.

The expertise of a professional interpreter is essential when you and your patient do not speak the same language. Although you may feel awkward at first when working with an interpreter, you will soon realize that the interpreter is a great ally in your nursing practice.

Amanda M. Black, MA
Professional Interpreter and Translator

CONSIDERING CULTURE BOX 12.1

The Challenge: When You Don't Speak the Patient's Language

Mrs. Reyes gave birth by cesarean section to her first child, a baby boy she named Carlos, yesterday, and she is recovering well. She speaks Spanish only. On the previous shift, she had received a mild narcotic twice for incisional pain. Her nurse on that shift had learned Spanish through high school and then two semesters in college, so she felt that she was able to communicate basic information with Mrs. Reyes, who will be your patient today.

When you go in to take care of Mrs. Reyes, you find her lying on her side, weeping brokenheartedly. You know only a few words of Spanish, so you ask her if she has pain, and point to your lower abdomen. She replies, "No, no, *aquí*" and puts her hand on her chest. You are wondering if she is having some problem with breastfeeding or if she is having chest pain, so you take her pulse and blood pressure, which are both a little elevated but within normal limits. You know she is upset, and her pain appears to be emotional. You realize that she has said something about *"mi niño"* [my baby boy] and *"cirugía"* [surgery]; you decide it is time to call in a medical interpreter, because you know that her baby is healthy and is in the newborn nursery.

The interpreter arrives and you explain briefly what you understand Mrs. Reyes to have said. Mrs. Reyes is still crying when you go back in her room with the interpreter, and you tell Mrs. Reyes through the interpreter that the interpreter speaks Spanish and will be assisting you in figuring out what is wrong. Mrs. Reyes begins a very animated narrative to the interpreter who tries to get her to slow down and let her tell you what she (Mrs. Reyes) has said.

Mrs. Reyes tells you through the interpreter that the nurse on the previous shift had awakened her to sign a paper giving permission for a doctor to "do surgery—to cut" on her baby, and now she is afraid something is wrong with the baby and no one has told her. You realize the nurse had gotten Mrs. Reyes to sign a consent form for circumcision, a common procedure in newborn males, and that the nurse had not explained it properly, nor had she used an interpreter to help. You explain through the interpreter, carefully, about circumcision and Mrs. Reyes calms down quickly, because she understands what circumcision is. You realize that a serious, preventable communication problem has occurred.

As you think about this situation, address these questions:

1. What were the errors that occurred in this situation?
2. How could they have been avoided?
3. What are the ethical considerations in this situation?
4. What are your next steps in helping manage this situation?
5. What should you do regarding your co-worker?

information from a professional interpreter on how to best work with an interpreter. Once you have learned about working with an interpreter, use this knowledge to analyze the scenario in Considering Culture Box 12.1.

Communication practices are unique for each individual and vary widely, even for people from the same cultural backgrounds. Nurses must become skilled in assessing various elements of communication: dialect, style, volume, use of touch, emotional tone, gestures, stance, space needs, and eye contact of individual patients. Note that this requires you to recognize your stereotypes and biases and to avoid making assumptions about how any individual patient is likely to communicate.

Nurses who are sensitive to culture recognize that even when individuals speak the same language, the sender and receiver may perceive different meanings because of life experiences unique to each person. Patients may be unwilling to share certain information with nurses because of cultural constraints. In turn, nurses may inadvertently offend patients or family members by violating cultural norms concerning touch, space, and eye contact. Because nursing involves much hands-on work, it is imperative that nurses be aware of the impact of cultural issues that may affect patients' responses to their care.

Avoiding Common Causes of Communication Breakdown

Unsuccessful communication can occur for many reasons. A sender may send an incomplete or confusing message. A message may not be received, or it may be misunderstood or distorted by the receiver. Incongruent messages may cause confusion in the receiver. In nursing situations, there are several common causes of communication breakdown. These include failing to see each individual as unique, failing to recognize levels of meaning, using value statements, using false reassurance, and failing to clarify unclear messages.

Failing to See the Uniqueness of the Individual

Failing to see the uniqueness of each individual is a common cause of communication breakdown. This failure is caused by preconceived ideas, prejudices, and stereotypes, illustrated by the following interchange between a 65-year-old patient and a nurse:

Patient: "My back is really hurting today. I can hardly turn over in bed."

Nurse: "I guess we have to expect these little problems when we get older."

This nurse has categorized the patient into a specific group, "older people," and therefore does not respond to the patient as an individual. The likelihood that the nurse will get any more information from the patient has been significantly decreased. The nurse could have promoted continued communication by responding to the patient as an individual:

Nurse: "Tell me more about your back pain, Mrs. Jameson."

Failing to Recognize Levels of Meaning

When nurses recognize only the overt level of meaning, communication breakdown can occur. Patients often give verbal cues to meanings that lie under the surface content of their verbalizations, a form of symbolic communication:

Patient: "It's getting awfully warm in here."

Nurse: (Responding only to surface meaning) "I'll adjust the air conditioning for you."

This response does not help this patient express himself fully. A different type of response focuses on the symbolic level of meaning:

Nurse: "I haven't noticed that it is getting warm. I am wondering if perhaps there is something about our conversation that is making you uncomfortable."

Although it takes a lot of experience to know when and how to respond to symbolic communication, nurses should be aware of its existence. It is incumbent on the nurse, however, not to "psychologize," that is, to make more of a comment than is necessary. Sometimes, in fact, it does get warm. When patients begin to evade you, their body language may be a better indicator than their words. For instance, they may make less eye contact, become distracted by the television or phone, or feign fatigue or sleep. These are common ways in which people strive to create space in their communication when they are vulnerable.

Using Value Statements and Clichés

Using value statements and clichés is another communication problem. **Value statements** indicate that the nurse has made a judgment, either positive or negative. The use of value statements indicates that the nurse is operating out of their own set of values without considering that the patient might feel differently. The use of clichés, which are trite, stereotyped expressions, is common in social conversation but should be used carefully in professional relationships. Consider the prevalence of the cliché "Have a good day." This statement has come to have little real meaning. This common error can cut off communication by showing the patient that the nurse does not understand the patient's true feelings.

Patient: "My mother is coming to see me today."

Nurse: "How nice. There's nothing as comforting as a mother's love."

This nurse has used a value statement ("how nice") and a cliché ("there's nothing as comforting as a mother's love"). They have made an assumption that the patient welcomes a visit from their mother and has failed to verify what the patient's actual wishes are. In fact, the patient and their mother may have a difficult relationship, and the patient may dread the impending visit. By assuming otherwise, the nurse has contributed to communication breakdown. This patient probably will not attempt to discuss their relationship with their mother any further with this nurse. A more helpful response would be: "How are you feeling about your mother's visit? This allows the patient to express their feelings about their mother's visit, whether positive or negative. The nurse has conveyed a genuine interest in the patient's true feelings and has avoided a "yes" or "no" answer by asking the patient a "how" question.

Giving False Reassurance

Using **false reassurance** is another communication pitfall. Although the nurse (and patient) may feel better temporarily, this strategy impedes communication and does not help the patient.

Patient: "I'm so afraid the biopsy will show cancer."

Nurse: "Don't worry. You have the best doctor in town. Besides, cancer treatment is really good these days."

For a fearful patient, this type of glib reassurance does not help. The patient has stated very clearly a legitimate concern as they face a biopsy and may indeed have cancer. A more sensitive response would be:

Nurse: "I regret that you are having to go through this. Let's talk about your concerns."

Note that in the first sentence, the nurse did not offer any reassurance, but expressed human feelings of regret, which indicates concern to the patient. The nurse then gave the patient an opportunity to talk about his concerns. Note that when you say, "Let's talk about...," you are indicating that you are available to your patient for this kind of in-depth conversation. If you are in the middle of your early shift assessments, you may need to follow this up by setting a time at which the patient knows you will return to continue this conversation. These types of patient needs are common; not honoring your offer to talk to him about his fears is dehumanizing for the patient. Also, note the use of the word "regret" as opposed to the word "sorry" here. It is common to say, "I'm sorry you are having to go through this." Sometimes patients will take this as an apology, and respond accordingly: "It's not your fault." By using "regret" instead, you are avoiding having to explain that you mean that you are regretful and can move the conversation forward more efficiently.

Failing to Clarify

Failing to clarify the patient's unclear statements is a fifth common communication pitfall.

Patient: "I've got to get out of the hospital. They have found out I'm here and may come after me."

Nurse: "No one will harm you here."

This nurse has responded as if the patient's meaning was clear. A clarifying response might be:

Nurse: "Who are 'they,' Mrs. Johnson?"

Patients who are confused or those with a mental health condition may communicate in ways that are difficult to understand. Although it is unlikely, sometimes patients' meanings are quite clear in the initial sentence, and their fears are based in reality. It is reassuring to patients to know that nurses are trying to understand them, even if they are not always successful. Communication is facilitated by clarification responses.

Practicing Helpful Responses

Nurses can practice using helpful responses and avoiding common communication pitfalls with family members, friends, and co-workers, as well as in patient contacts. Being a good communicator takes practice and often feels unnatural at first. Any new behavior takes time to integrate into habitual patterns. By practicing new skills, nurses soon find themselves feeling more natural responding in a therapeutic manner. They find these newly acquired skills are beneficial both professionally and personally. Thinking Critically Box 12.1, Helpful and Unhelpful Responding Techniques, compares the helpfulness of different types of responses in a nurse–patient interaction.

EFFECTIVE COMMUNICATION WITH OTHER PROVIDERS

SBAR: Structured Communication Across the Healthcare Team

This chapter has focused on communication as the core of the nursing process and foundation of the therapeutic use of self. In addition to communicating with patients and their families, however, nurses must also communicate effectively with an array of professional and unlicensed personnel, including other nurses, physicians, phlebotomists, pharmacists, respiratory and physical therapists, and others. Traditionally, socialization in healthcare professions tended to be discipline specific, and what providers in other disciplines offered to patients was not always clear. This resulted in territoriality in which each discipline defended its own domain of influence rather than promoting collegiality and collaboration. Healthcare delivery becomes fragmented under those conditions, and the old hierarchy that values the contributions of some disciplines over others flourishes. The problem, however, is that patients suffer when the members of the healthcare team fail to use the resources and interdisciplinary knowledge available to them.

SBAR/I-SBAR-R: Standardizing Communication in Health Care

The Joint Commission has standardized health care communication within and across disciplines through the practice of **SBAR—Situation Background Assessment Recommendation**. SBAR is a structured way of relaying critical information in spoken form. It is a means of establishing a culture of quality, reliability, and patient safety because individuals—regardless of discipline—communicate with each other through a shared set of expectations. SBAR means that information is clear, complete, concise, and structured and is therefore more efficient and accurate. SBAR

THINKING CRITICALLY BOX 12.1

Helpful and Unhelpful Responding Techniques

Directions: Critique both of the following interactions, identifying each helpful and unhelpful response used by the nurse. Describe how you imagine the patient might feel at the close of each interaction. Identify what the nurse has accomplished in each instance.

Mr. Goodman has been admitted to the hospital for coronary bypass surgery. During the admission process, the following interactions might take place.

Interaction One

- *Nurse:* Mr. Goodman, I'm Cora. May I get some information about you now?
- *Patient:* Okay.
- *Nurse:* You're here for bypass surgery?
- *Patient:* Yes, that's what they tell me.
- *Nurse:* (Taking blood pressure) Do you have any allergies to foods or medications?
- *Patient:* Not that I know of. I've never been in a hospital before.
- *Nurse:* Well, your blood pressure looks good. (Silence while patient has thermometer in mouth.) This is a really nice room—just remodeled. I know you'll be comfortable here. Will your wife be coming to see you tonight? (Removes thermometer.)
- *Patient:* My wife is sick. She hasn't been able to leave home for 2 years. I don't know what will happen to her while I am here.
- *Nurse:* Gosh, I'm so sorry to hear that. I guess having you back home healthy is what she wants though, isn't it? And you've got a great surgeon. Well, I've got to run now. Check on you later.

Interaction Two

- *Nurse:* Good afternoon, Mr. Goodman. I'm Cora Scott, and I'll be your nurse this evening. If this is a good time, I'd like to ask you some questions and complete your admission process.
- *Patient:* Okay.
- *Nurse:* First, I'll get your temperature and blood pressure, and then we'll talk. (Silence while nurse takes vital signs.) Everything looks good. Do you have any allergies to foods or medications?
- *Patient:* Not that I know of. I've never been in a hospital before.
- *Nurse:* Hospitals can be a little overwhelming, especially when you've never been a patient before. Now, would you please tell me in your own words why you are here?
- *Patient:* Well, the doc tells me I have a clogged artery and I need a bypass. I guess they'll open up my heart.
- *Nurse:* What exactly do you know about the surgery?
- *Patient:* Not too much, really. He told me yesterday that I need it right away—and here I am.
- *Nurse:* It sounds like you need some more information about what will happen. Later this evening I will come back, and we'll talk some more. Are you expecting to have visitors tonight?
- *Patient:* No, my wife can't leave home. I don't know what she will do without me while I'm here. This came up so suddenly.
- *Nurse:* I can see that this is a serious concern for you. We can explore some possibilities when I come back this evening. I'll plan to come around 7:15, if that suits you.
- *Patient:* Sure, I can use all the help I can get.

was originally developed by the U.S. Navy for use on nuclear submarines; it was introduced into health care in the late 1990s and has been adopted in healthcare facilities around the world to standardize communication among care providers. The SBAR format was later revised to I-SBAR-R, which starts with the **I**ntroduction and ends with a **R**eadback to improve communication even further (QSEN, 2008).

In using I-SBAR-R, you filter quickly through irrelevant data so that the most relevant and important data are featured. You then present your briefing on the situation to colleagues who understand and expect the SBAR format, which gets to the problem—and hence solution—sooner. Your colleagues respond with questions to confirm or clarify what you have presented. Here is an example of a nurse in the neonatal intensive care unit (NICU) calling the neonatal nurse practitioner regarding a premature infant:

- (**I**ntroduction): Hello, this is Katherine Mischew. I am the RN taking care of Jeremy Benton.
- (**S**ituation): Here's the situation: Jeremy's latest arterial blood gas showed a Po_2 of 68, Pco_2 of 64, and pH of 7.32.
- (**B**ackground): Jeremy is a male born 22 hours ago at 32 weeks' gestation, weighing 1550 g. He has been on CPAP [continuous positive airway pressure] since birth and is now at 40% O_2, up from 35% 8 hours ago. In the past 2 hours, his respiratory rate has increased from 60 to 88 and his O_2 saturation has decreased from 96% to 92%.

- (**A**ssessment): My assessment is that Jeremy is developing respiratory failure.
- (**R**ecommendation): I recommend that you or one of the neonatal fellows come see him and that I call for a respiratory therapist to be in the NICU in case Jeremy needs to be intubated.
- Nurse Practitioner: I will be there shortly, but in the meantime, call a respiratory therapist to adjust the CPAP as necessary, and I will also order a chest x-ray STAT. Recheck blood gases in 15 minutes.
- (**R**eadback—nurse): I will call respiratory therapy and request adjustment to CPAP, and I will confirm that radiology will perform a chest x-ray STAT. I will recheck ABG [arterial blood gases] in 15 minutes.

The information the nurse has communicated is clear, appropriate, and without tangential details that obscure the problem. The nurse practitioner has clear data from a professional registered nurse who has captured the most salient issues related to the care of a premature infant. No time is wasted in filtering out extraneous information such as, "Jeremy's mother came in for a visit this afternoon. She is really worried about him, but she has a lot of family support." Is this helpful information? No, not in this circumstance. However, if the nurse was responding to a call from a social worker assigned to the Benton family, this may be useful background information.

Safety is the key issue behind I-SBAR-R as a communication format. This format decreases the inherently unsafe and dysfunctional hierarchy of providers. In his introduction to John Nance's (2009) important book *Why Hospitals Should Fly: The Ultimate Flight Plan to Patient Safety and Quality Care*, Lucian Leape, MD, a physician and professor at the Harvard School of Public Health, noted that "an authoritarian structure that devalues many workers, lacks of a sense of personal accountability, autonomous functioning and major barriers to effective care stymies progress" in creating a safe culture of health care (p. viii). A culture of safety requires teamwork, Leape argued, the "common denominator" in safe cultures, which are "rarely found in health care organizations" (p. viii).

As you gain more experience clinically, develop your critical thinking skills, and improve your clinical judgment, you will become increasingly comfortable in communicating using the I-SBAR-R format.

Effective Use of Electronic Communication

An unprecedented proliferation of ways to communicate exist today: mobile phones; smart phones; e-mail; messaging on apps such as iMessage, WhatsApp, and WeChat; and services such as Skype and FaceTime, among others. Nurses are often interrupted in their care by the ringing of their mobile phones or unit communication devices, consulting with other staff members even as they care for patients. This behavior is insensitive and sends a message to patients that they and their needs are secondary.

The use of e-mail in professional settings can lead to misunderstanding because the facial expression, tone of voice, and other contextual cues are not visible to message recipients and are therefore subject to misinterpretation (everyone knows someone who appears to be yelling on e-mail because they type in all capital letters). A few commonsense guidelines are useful to prevent the use of communication devices from becoming a barrier to nurse–patient or nurse-colleague communication:

- Give your full attention to the person you are with. Avoid checking your phone for messages while conversing with others.
- If you are interrupted by a call that you must take, go into the hallway to have your conversation; you may need to leave the patient area completely to avoid having your personal business overheard in a professional setting.
- Adopt a courteous tone in e-mail and voicemail messages regardless of how rushed you are; remember that the recipient cannot see your nonverbal communication. Emoticons or emojis, however, are rarely appropriate. If you have to use a ":)" to show that you are not really upset or to take the edge off criticism, you probably need to reword your e-mail rather than resort to smiley faces. Like all communication, they too can be misconstrued or seem incongruent with the message.
- Avoid the use of jargon in verbal and written communication; use acronyms only when you are confident of their universal understanding.
- Keep messages short; include only necessary useful details, but avoid being abrupt.
- When leaving your return phone number in a voicemail, make sure that you enunciate the number slowly and clearly. It is helpful to repeat at the end of your message: "Again, this is [first name, last name] at 111-555-4321."
- When receiving a message, read, listen, and evaluate the entire message before reacting. This is particularly important when you are feeling pressed for time or if your first response to the message is one of irritation or anger.

Communication in Today's Multicultural Workplace

Sensitivity to cultural differences in communication is essential in today's culturally diverse workplace. The composition of the healthcare workforce is being rapidly transformed by the population demographics of the nation. Diversity in age, race, ethnicity, country of origin, gender identity, sexual orientation, and levels of abilities creates opportunities for nurses to develop skill in transcultural communication.

One's culture determines the lens through which most aspects of life are viewed and experienced and includes an individual's health beliefs and practices. Culture also dictates the meaning of work, such as caring for the sick. Some cultures see caring for the sick to be a sacred responsibility, whereas others place care for the sick with no significance beyond an occupation or means of income. The meaning of work in a given culture also affects how people of that culture communicate.

Attention is now being paid to the cultural differences among different generations of nurses, all of whom can be found working side by side. Even when race and ethnicity are similar, the ages of nurses in a single setting may range from early 20s to middle 60s, a 40-year span. This can create interpersonal challenges in the workplace. Although it is risky to make generalizations about groups, anecdotal evidence and research studies reveal differing opinions among age-groups about what is important to them professionally and personally.

Each generation experiences political and historical events and social trends during their formative years that influence their values, and hence become part of a cohort similarly affected by historical and sociocultural events. Known as the sociohistorical context of one's life, these influences cut across racial and ethnic lines. Different age groups may have differing work ethics, means of communication, manners, and views of authority; more superficial issues such as habits of speech, modes of dress, and even hairstyles and music choices can be the source of tension and friction (Siela, 2006).

Three generations currently occupy the workforce. Two-thirds of today's workforce in all occupational groups consists of Baby Boomers, people born between 1946 and 1959; many in this group are now at the age of retirement. Those born between 1960 and 1980 make up Generation X. Generation Y, also known as Millennials, were born between 1981 and 2000. Generation Y overlaps with a newer group born since 1990 known as the Net Generation, or N-Geners, who have grown up with an unprecedented high level of interconnectivity in the digital age.

The characteristics and attitudes of the various groups may differ; however it is simply another form of stereotyping to attribute beliefs or behaviors simply to one's age group. Professional nurses strive to understand colleagues of different generations and capitalize on the strengths each group brings to the workplace, rather than viewing these varying attitudes toward life and work as problems. Siela offers this insight: "Knowing the characteristics and core values of each generation can help nurses of diverse ages understand colleagues who are much younger or older than they are. However, take care not to stereotype anyone. Each person is a unique individual with distinctive traits, which may or may not be typical of [their] generation as a whole" (2006, p. 47).

Astute nurses use their communication skills throughout their personal and professional lives. Using clear, simple messages and clarifying the intent of others constitute a positive goal in all personal and professional communication.

INTERPROFESSIONAL COLLABORATION: PRESCRIPTION FOR IMPROVED PATIENT OUTCOMES

Interprofessional collaboration is central to excellent patient outcomes (Rose, 2011). **Collaboration** is a complex process that builds on communication. Collaboration in healthcare settings is far more than simply cooperation, negotiation, or compromise. It implies working jointly with other professionals, all of whom are respected for their unique knowledge and abilities, to improve a patient's health status or to solve an organizational problem. Furthermore, interprofessional collaboration implies interdependency, rather than autonomy, and roles among providers are understood as complementary and require mutual respect and power sharing (Rose, 2011). The Institute of Medicine (IOM; now the National Academy of Medicine) (2003) made interdisciplinary learning a core educational requirement, with the assumption that education across healthcare disciplines will improve communication, increase collaboration, and decrease errors (Reese et al., 2010).

Interdisciplinary learning provides the setting for professionals to learn specific roles of others in health care and to understand clearly delineated professional contributions of each member of the healthcare team (Suter et al., 2009). Currently, most healthcare providers are taught similar core content, skills, knowledge, and values; however, this education occurs in isolation (Angelini, 2011) or "professional silos" (Margalit et al., 2009). In addition, interdisciplinary learning may serve to reduce stereotypes and alleviate misconceptions regarding the value of other professional roles (MacDonald et al., 2010). Furthermore, MacDonald and colleagues (2010) found that knowledge of the professional role of others is related to successful interprofessional practice and that the development of this core competency should ideally begin during nurses' basic education. Box 12.6 contains a checklist of key components necessary for effective collaboration. You can check your own readiness for interprofessional collaboration by referring to this list. At this point in your education, you will probably have most of these components mastered.

Successful collaboration entails several steps (Gardner, 2005):

- Identification of those who have stake in the outcome of the collaboration
- Identification of the problem(s) to be solved
- Identification of barriers to creating a solution
- Clarification of the desired outcomes (agree on criteria for success)
- Clarification of the process (How will we approach the task?)
- Identification of who will be responsible for each step in the task
- Evaluation (Have we met our criteria for success?)

BOX 12.6 Key Components Necessary for Effective Interprofessional Collaboration

- Respect for other collaborators
- Confidence in own knowledge
- Willingness to learn
- Cooperative spirit
- Belief in a common purpose
- Value contributions of other disciplines
- Willingness to negotiate
- Excellent communication skills
- Self-awareness (e.g., biases, values, goals, agendas)
- Tolerance of differing opinions
- Not threatened by conflict
- Knowledge of one's own limits

Collaboration is a positive process that benefits the people involved, as individuals and as a group; the organization in which they work; and healthcare consumers. Increased feelings of self-worth; a sense of accomplishment; enhanced collegiality and respect; and increased productivity, retention, and employee satisfaction are positive benefits of collaboration (LeTourneau, 2004). Despite these positive benefits and potential for improved patient outcomes, interprofessional collaboration can be difficult to institute. Rice and colleagues (2010) found that even though a well-planned and well-implemented intervention to increase interprofessional communication and collaboration was received with enthusiasm by various stakeholders on general internal medicine units, no changes in behaviors were noted over the year after the intervention. This was attributed to several causes, including deeply entrenched interprofessional hierarchies.

One of the most deeply entrenched hierarchies in health care today is that of nursing in relation to medicine. Weinberg and colleagues (2009) noted that this hierarchy is dominated by physicians, in which they see their role in part as one of giving orders that nurses carry out; nurses, however, typically prefer collaborative interactions that are more egalitarian. In their study of the quality of the nurse-physician relationship, Weinberg and colleagues found that 19 of 20 resident physicians reported instances of poor communication or troubled relationships with nurses, which, unfortunately, was not seen as a threat to patient care. The nurses' role was limited, in their opinion, to following the physicians' orders. The findings of this research are troublesome in light of the directives by the IOM to foster interprofessional collaboration that would include the disciplines of nursing and medicine.

Recent strategies to increase interprofessional collaboration through interprofessional education (IPE) will require what is sometimes called a "sea change," a reference to Ariel's song in the Shakespeare play *The Tempest*. A sea change is a progressive transformation over time during which the substance of a structure is changed, although its form remains. A hospital may still look like a hospital, but what goes on within that structure will be required to change in response to substantial reform in the healthcare system. Change is difficult, however, and is usually accompanied by conflict. Conflict resolution requires constructive conflict negotiation skills that can be developed (Gerardi and

Morrison, 2005). Examples of these conflict resolution skills include the following:

- Acknowledge the conflict.
- Recognize and affirm that positive outcomes can result from conflict.
- Facilitate debate over task issues while redirecting concerns away from the personal level.
- Promote expression of varying perspectives.
- As conflict is worked through, explore alternative positions, taking opportunities to synthesize several ideas to create a new position.
- Be willing to change your position on an issue.
- Share power: elicit everyone's opinions and look for win-win situations.
- Stay focused on the desired outcome.

A caveat is in order, however. More than two decades ago, David (2000) wrote a powerful treatise on the gender politics of nursing; among many important arguments, David noted that nurses' ongoing self-deception in terms of the location of power in health care has served to "perpetuate professional mediocrity . . . and preserve the borderline status of nurses" (p. 83). This means that nurses take a secondary role to physicians and others in the healthcare hierarchy, making true interprofessional collaboration impossible under these conditions. There are no simple fixes for this deeply entrenched view of nursing for which nurses are ultimately responsible. A good first step for you is to consider the negative effects of gender politics on you as a nurse (regardless of your own gender identity) and on the profession of nursing.

You have been exposed to a great deal of material in this chapter, from the therapeutic use of self in one-on-one professional relationships with patients to the effect of gender politics on the profession of nursing. The "take-home message" of this chapter is an important one, however, and one not to be lost in the wide range of topics to which you have been exposed. The message: How you communicate as a professional nurse matters. Whether you are sitting at the bedside consoling a frantic mother of a sick infant, addressing a group of citizens concerned about environmental issues in your community, or writing a letter to your representative in Congress about healthcare coverage, you are never "not a nurse."

CONCEPTS AND CHALLENGES

- ***Concept:*** The "therapeutic use of self" means using one's personality and communication skills effectively while implementing the nursing process to help patients improve their health status.
  Challenge: Although it is difficult, nurses can learn new skills to improve their communication.
- ***Concept:*** In long-term nurse–patient relationships, each phase (orientation, working, and termination) has specific tasks that should be accomplished before progressing to subsequent phases.
  Challenge: Short-term patient contacts in today's streamlined care delivery system also present opportunities for connection and goal achievement.
- ***Concept:*** Acceptance of others is important for effective nursing practice.
  Challenge: Developing awareness of biases can help nurses to prevent the intrusion of these biases into nurse–patient relationships.
- ***Concept:*** Professional nurses are aware of the boundaries of the therapeutic relationship and strive to stay within the "zone of helpfulness" at all times.
  Challenge: Boundaries can be difficult to ascertain, especially in the use of social media. Nurses have to be vigilant in identifying professional boundaries and setting limits to prevent crossing a boundary.
- ***Concept:*** Communication is the core of all relationships; it is both verbal and nonverbal and consists of a sender, a receiver, a message, feedback, and context.
  Challenge: Effective communication meets four major criteria: feedback, appropriateness, efficiency, and flexibility.
- ***Concept:*** Professional medical interpreters are your best resource in providing care for patients for whom English is their second language or who do not speak English.
  Challenge: Conversational skills in a second language are inadequate in the provision of healthcare, and asking a family member to interpret is inappropriate and can be unsafe.
- ***Concept:*** SBAR is an excellent means of communication to transmit important data effectively across healthcare disciplines and all members of the healthcare team.
  Challenge: Effective communication both requires and reflects excellent critical thinking and clinical judgment.

IDEAS FOR FURTHER EXPLORATION

1. Explain what is meant by the expression "therapeutic use of self." What challenges, if any, do you anticipate encountering in learning this important communication technique?
2. Describe professional boundaries and what the implications are in crossing professional boundaries.
3. Think about why nonverbal communication may be more reliable than verbal communication. Consider your own nonverbal communication style and what you might be communicating unintentionally.
4. Identify a recent interaction you have had in which communication was incongruent. Analyze the effect of the incongruence on the communication. When are people most likely to use incongruent communication?
5. Think of a person with whom you have experienced difficult communication. Identify the barriers to successful communication between you and the other person, and critique your responses to that person.
6. Think about a collaborative experience you have had with another health care professional. What are the features of that collaboration in which collaboration improved the outcome for the patient? Were there features of the collaboration with which you were uncomfortable?

REFERENCES

Angelini D: Interdisciplinary and interprofessional education: What are the key issues and considerations for the future? *J Perinat Neonatal Nurs* 25(2):175–179, 2011.

Baca M: Professional boundaries and dual relationships in clinical practice, *J Nurs Pract* 7(3):195–200, 2011.

David BA: Nursing's gender politics: reformulating the footnotes, *Adv Nurs Sci* 23(1):83–93, 2000.

Gardner DB: Ten lessons in collaboration, *Online J Issues Nurs* 10(1):1–6, 2005. [website]. Available at https://ojin.nursingworld.org/MainMenuCategories/ANAMarketplace/ANAPeriodicals/OJIN/TableofContents/Volume102005/No1Jan05/tpc26_116008.aspx.

Gerardi DS, Morrison F: Managing conflict creatively, *Crit Care Nurs*:31–32, 2005.

Hagerty BM, Patusky KL: Reconceptualizing the nurse-patient relationship, *Image J Nurs Sch* 35(2):145–150, 2003.

Hobbs JL: A dimensional analysis of patient-centered care, *Nurs Res* 58(1):52–62, 2009.

Institute of Medicine (IOM): *Health professions education: a bridge to quality*, Washington, DC, 2003, National Academies Press.

Johns C: *Guided reflection: advancing practice*, Oxford, 2002, Blackwell Science.

LeTourneau B: Physicians and nurses: friends or foes? *J Healthc Manag* 49(1):12–14, 2004.

MacDonald MB, Bally JM, Ferguson LM, et al.: Knowledge of the professional role of others: a key interprofessional competency, *Nurs Ed Prac* 217:238–242, 2010.

Margalit R, Thompson S, Visovsky C, et al.: From professional silos to interprofessional education: campuswide focus on quality of care, *Qual Manag Health Care* 18:165–173, 2009.

Nance JJ: *Why hospitals should fly: the ultimate flight plan to patient safety and quality care*, Bozeman, MT, 2009, Second River Health Care Books.

National Council of State Boards of Nursing (NCSBN): *Professional boundaries: a nurse's guide to the importance of appropriate professional boundaries*, Chicago, 2014, National Council of State Boards of Nursing. [website]. Available at www.ncsbn.org.

Nurse's relationship with patient results in disciplinary action, *Nurs Law Regan Rep* 43(8):4–5, 2003.

Peplau H: *Interpersonal relations in nursing*, New York, 1952, GP Putnam's Sons.

Quality and Safety Education for Nurses: *Reformulating SBAR to I-SBAR-R*,2008. (website). Retrieved from: http://qsen.org/reformulating-sbar-to-i-sbar-r/.

Reese CE, Jeffries PR, Scott AE: Learning together: using simulations to develop nursing and medical student collaboration, *Nurse Ed Perspec* 31(1): 33–37, 2010.

Rice K, Zwarenstein M, Conn LG, et al.: An intervention to improve interpersonal collaboration and communications: a comparative qualitative study, *J Interprof Care* 24(4):350–361, 2010.

Roach MS, Maykut C: Comportment: A caring attribute in the formation of an intentional practice, *Int J Hum Caring* 14(4):22–26, 2010.

Rose L: Interprofessional collaboration in the ICU: how to define? *Nurs Crit Care* 16(1):5–10, 2011.

Ruesch J: *Disturbed communication: the clinical assessment of normal and pathological communicative behavior*, New York, 1972, WW Norton.

Siela D: Managing the multigenerational nursing staff, *Am Nurse Today* 1(3):47–49, 2006.

Suter E, Arndt J, Arthur N, et al.: Role understanding and effective communication as core competencies for collaborative practice, *J Interprof Care* 23(1):41–51, 2009.
Swanson KM: Empirical development of a middle range theory of caring, *Nurs Res* 40:161–166, 1991.
Watson J: *Nursing: human science and human care*, New York, 1988, National League for Nursing.
Weinberg DB, Miner DC, Rivlin L: It depends: medical residents' perspectives on working with nurses: a qualitative study shows that residents don't necessarily view nurses as colleagues and collaborators, *Am J Nurs* 109(7):34–43, 2009.

13

Nurses, Patients, and Families: Caring at the Intersection of Health, Illness, and Culture

ⓔ To enhance your understanding of this chapter, try the Student Exercises on the Evolve site at http://evolve.elsevier.com/Black/professional.

LEARNING OUTCOMES

After studying this chapter, students will be able to:

- Differentiate between acute and chronic illness.
- Describe the stages of illness and how patients move among the stages.
- Explain behavioral responses to illness and what influences these behaviors.
- Discuss the influence of culture on illness behaviors.
- Describe the characteristics of the culturally competent nurse.
- Explain the physical, emotional, and cognitive effects of stress.
- Discuss how family functioning is altered during illness.
- Explain the necessity of and strategies for self-care by nurses.
- Explain how current efforts to increase diversity and inclusion actually perpetuate systems of oppression.

Joyful partners stand at the altar or before a magistrate on their wedding day, vowing to "have and to hold … in sickness and in health …" On a day of robust health and exuberant energy, couples rarely envision the specter of illness as they celebrate their marriage. It is a day of hope and expectation. Sickness, and all it means, has little place at the wedding. Yet as the anniversaries of this beautiful day come and go, the meaning of sickness becomes clearer. A part of life, illness affects not just the sick person, but the people providing care—the spouse, the partner, their children. Illness changes lives (Fig. 13.1). In Chapter 8 you were introduced to systems theory in depth. Remember, a key concept of systems theory is that a change in one part of a system results in changes in other parts. A family is a system; a change in one member affects the other members.

Supporting health, managing illness, and addressing the complex changes and human responses to illness are central to nursing. A key characteristic of nursing is the emphasis on viewing patients holistically. Nurses recognize that humans are complex beings with physical, mental, emotional, spiritual, social, and cultural dimensions. Each of these dimensions may be challenged by illness. In this chapter the stages of illness, illness behaviors, and cultural factors influencing responses to illness are explored, as is the impact of illness and culture on patients, families, and nurses. Developing strategies to maintain your own health and learning to develop balance in your life—care of self—is also explored.

ACUTE AND CHRONIC ILLNESS

Illness is a highly personal experience. Culture plays a significant role in health beliefs and behaviors; it also determines how individuals and families react to illness. Nurses can be more effective in providing care when they understand some of the factors that affect how people cope with illness.

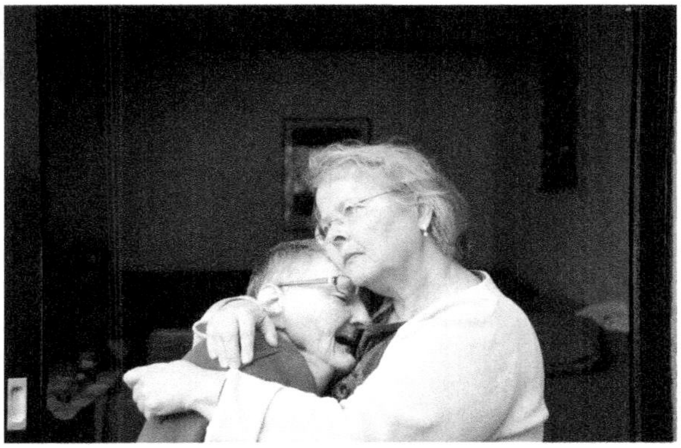

Fig. 13.1 In times of illness, roles in families change. An adult daughter is caring for and comforting her mother. (Photo used with permission from iStockphoto.)

Acute Illness

Acute illness is characterized by severe symptoms that are relatively short lived. Symptoms tend to appear suddenly, progress steadily, and subside quickly. Depending on the illness, the patient may or may not require medical attention. Most viral infections such as the common cold are acute infections that do not usually require the attention of a healthcare provider. Others, however, as recently demonstrated during the COVID-19 pandemic, can become life-threatening quickly. Unless complications arise, people with acute illness usually return to their previous level of wellness. Some acute illnesses, such as acute myocardial infarction, may lead to chronic conditions, such as congestive heart failure. "Long COVID" is a newly recognized chronic condition in which patients deal with sequelae of the acute COVID infection long after their acute illness.

Individuals with sudden, catastrophic injuries, such as a spinal cord injury or major stroke, experience dramatic and extensive changes. They face physical limitations, challenging modifications in daily living, and changes in social roles for which they had no preparation. Persons use a variety of their own idiosyncratic coping mechanisms.

Chronic Illness

A chronic illness usually develops gradually, requires ongoing attention, and may continue for the duration of the individual's life. Symptoms associated with chronic illness are often manageable through a combination of medical surveillance, prescription medications, nutrition and lifestyle support.

Chronic illnesses have a significant social and economic impact, being one of the fastest-growing health problems in the United States. In 2018, 51.8% of U.S. adults had at least one chronic illness, and 27.2% had more than one (Centers for Disease Control and Prevention [CDC], 2020). Factors such as sedentary lifestyles, obesity, and the aging of the population are expected to contribute to a continued increase in the number of chronically ill Americans for the foreseeable future. Arthritis (diagnosed by a provider, not self-diagnosis) is the most common disabling illness, then cancer, chronic obstructive pulmonary disease, coronary heart disease, and asthma. Diabetes, the sixth most prevalent chronic condition, can result in another set of chronic conditions including kidney disease, vascular disease, and diabetic eye disease.

Chronic illnesses vary in severity and outcomes, and can be well-managed. Some chronic illnesses are progressively debilitating and result in premature death, whereas others are associated with a normal life span. Certain chronic illnesses go through periods of remission, when symptoms subside, and exacerbation, when symptoms reappear or worsen, sometimes often a long period of dormancy.

Chronic illnesses can be pervasive and life altering, and lead to altered individual functioning and disruption of family life. Long-term medical management of chronic illness can create financial hardship as well. Patients with chronic illness may need to make substantial alterations in the way they live, often making many changes simultaneously. As a matter of self-care, patients may need to do surveillance, such as monitoring blood glucose levels, and incorporate changes their dietary habits, and increase their exercise. Box 13.1 presents the similarities and differences between acute and chronic illnesses.

The diagnosis of an acute or chronic illness can be a major life crisis. The emotional reactions of the patient and family sometimes present a greater challenge than dealing with the physical aspects of the disease. Despite the prevalence of emotional responses to illness, most medical and nursing attention is focused on physical aspects of the disease process rather than emotions. Box 13.2 describes how one patient experiences a chronic illness—systemic lupus erythematosus (SLE)—and describes its effect on her feelings, family

BOX 13.1 Types of Illness

Acute	Chronic
• Sudden onset of symptoms	• Gradual onset of symptoms
• Symptoms progress quickly from mild to severe	• Symptoms may be mild or vague; once illness is resolved may have remissions and exacerbations
• Patient usually returns to former level of functioning	• Illness continues throughout the life span
• Changes often not permanent but may progress to chronic illness	• Changes are permanent and progressive
• Does not usually require long-term behavioral change/treatment	• Requires long-term behavioral change/treatment
• May represent a life crisis	• Often represents a life crisis

BOX 13.2 Comments of a Patient With a Chronic Illness: Systemic Lupus Erythematosus

If there is one thing I want to say to nurses who work with patients with chronic disease, it is "Be patient and understand our problems and feelings." When I go to the doctor's office or to the hospital, I usually leave feeling guilty because I have been impatient with everyone I saw. Guilt and anger are the two feelings I seem to have had since I was diagnosed with this illness. I alternate between being angry that I got lupus and feeling that I should be grateful for the fact that I have something I can at least live with when others are not so fortunate.

I guess the thing that bothers me most is that the nurses keep telling me what changes I need to make to take better care of myself. They never seem to understand that I am doing the best I can do. I can't possibly get the amount of rest they seem to think I need, and I can't avoid as much stress as they seem to think I should avoid. Both my husband and I work hard at our jobs, and I hate asking him and my sons to take over my responsibilities at home when I am feeling sick, so I wind up compromising. I ask them to help some and I do more than I should. When I get the lecture from the nurses on how I should take better care of myself, I usually just nod and say that I will, even when I know that I won't. They don't seem to "get" that my life and decisions are driven by more than just managing my physical health. I have to consider the effects on my family too, and I can't miss work too much because my family's health insurance depends on me keeping my job. It's like they have tunnel vision and all they see are my labs and blood pressure.

Sometimes I leave my appointments wishing that a nurse would just look at me and say, "I know this is hard. You have a lot going on." Then I would feel like someone really understood. But that hasn't ever happened. I don't know that it ever will.

responsibilities, and relationships. As you read her narrative, pay attention to her reaction to her nurses' focus on her physical condition at a time when her emotional responses were her greatest concern. Consider what this narrative says about quality care and if this woman is getting the help that she needs.

Chronically ill people can become acutely ill with something not related to their chronic illness, which will still need management even while the acute condition is being treated. For instance, a 28-year-old man comes to the emergency department (ED) with a severely sprained ankle from a skiing accident. His electronic health record indicates that he is HIV+, although his viral load is nondetectable because of his strict adherence to his highly active antiretroviral therapy (HAART) regimen. What are the implications for the ED providers of his HIV status? If you were giving an SBAR (see Chapter 12) update at your end-of-shift handoff to the next nurse, would you include his HIV status in your report?

ADJUSTING TO ILLNESS

Adjusting to illness is a process. Although the responses are different for each person, people who are ill typically progress through somewhat predictable states. Experts from medicine, sociology, psychology, and nursing have described the states that people experience in adjustment to illness as stages: disbelief and denial, irritability and anger, attempting to gain control, depression and despair, and acceptance and participation. Remember that there are many influences on the way a person responds to an illness and that these states are fluid, meaning that the patient's responses to their own condition are likely to fluctuate, even as they move forward into learning to live with and manage their condition. Human responses to illness are rarely if ever linear.

Disbelief and Denial

People have difficulty believing that signs and symptoms are caused by illness. They may believe that the symptoms will go away. Fear of illness often leads to the mistaken belief that the symptoms will subside without treatment and can delay seeking a diagnosis.

Denial is a psychological defense mechanism that people sometimes use to avoid the anxiety associated with illness. People who place great value on their robust health may downplay the significance of symptoms, therefore avoiding diagnosis and treatment or attempt inappropriate self-treatment. Extended denial can have serious consequences, because some illnesses, left untreated, may become too advanced for effective treatment. (Note: the word *denial* is often used in a way that is incorrect. For instance, someone getting very bad news, such as the sudden death of a loved one, may be in shock such that they cannot take in the reality of trauma. "Denial" in this sense works to protect them from being overwhelmed.) A nurse described her own prolonged denial of the significance of a lump in her breast:

> *I thought it would go away. I thought it was anything but cancer. But I would lie awake at night and run my fingers over the lump and in the dark, I would know it was growing. I would tell myself, "I will call the doctor in the morning." But when morning came, I would make myself believe that the lump was smaller. Then it began to hurt, a little, then a lot. I didn't tell anyone, including my partner. One morning she asked me, "What is that?" and to my horror, I realized that the tumor had broken through my skin and was oozing through my nightgown. She took me to the doctor. I think that my denial will cost me my life. I am a nurse practitioner, and I am dying of breast cancer that could have been treated.*

Irritability and Anger

Some patients get irritable as their ability to function declines, and prolonged irritability may be an indication that the patient is depressed. Anger may be directed at specific people or simply be general, being "mad at the world." Anger may also be directed toward others, such as spouse, family members, coworkers, or healthcare providers. Anger may be directed inward, and guilt feelings may occur for failing to prevent the illness. This is one nurse's experience of a patient's anger directed at her:

> *I dreaded my daily visits to Mr. Kaman. He had pancreatic cancer and a surgical wound that was really slow to heal. It wasn't that he was mean to me, exactly. It was more like I didn't exist to him, or that he had contempt for me. I just couldn't reach him, which was pretty rare in my experience. At first, I would try to chat with him just to draw him out, but he withdrew further and further. I finally got a response from him one day when I commented on a photograph on his dresser. He responded by lashing out at me for "meddling" and told me to mind my own damn business. I was stunned and apologized (although I didn't know exactly what for). When I told Mrs. Kaman what had happened, she explained that the photo was of their son who had died in an accident a few years ago and that her husband had "never been the same" since. I felt like I at least understood a bit more about Mr. Kaman and felt compassion for him.*

Attempting to Gain Control

In the stage of attempting to gain control, people may consult their healthcare provider or use over-the-counter medications, folk practices, or home remedies. They are aware that they are ill and usually experience some concern or even fear about the outcome. These fears usually stimulate treatment-seeking behavior as a way of gaining control over the illness, but fears may also lead to further denial and avoidance, such as the nurse with breast cancer in the earlier example. As in her case, family members may become involved, encouraging or insisting that the person to seek treatment or follow medical advice. Here is another nurse's experience:

> *I was admitting a patient to hospice and per routine, I asked about medications. The patient's oncologist had given me a list of medications when he made the referral for this patient, but I wanted to see what else the patient was taking. I knew that sometimes patients took supplements. This patient brought out a bag, literally a paper grocery bag, full of supplements, vitamins, many that he had bought online that were not adequately labeled. I had no idea what he was taking and neither did he. When I asked him if he was concerned that some of these may be harmful, he laughed and said that he was dying anyway, so what did he have to lose? His husband said that he had tried to talk him out of taking all of these "potions," but in the end, it was not his call to make.*

Depression and Grief

Depression is perhaps the most common mood disorder that occurs with illness. The ability to work is altered, daily activities must be modified, and the sense of well-being and freedom from pain may be lost. Illness results in many types of losses. The difficulty is figuring out the difference between grief—the normal and expected response to any loss, including one's health—and depression, a treatable mental health condition. Immediately after diagnosis, patients may grieve the loss of their previous state of good health. As time goes on and functional limitations add up, persons with chronic illnesses may undergo cycles of depression as remissions and exacerbations occur. Remember that it is beyond the scope of practice for a nurse to diagnose a condition such as depression, which is a psychiatric diagnosis that needs treatment. A careful assessment, however, of the patient's mood states may give the observant nurse an indication that the patient is depressed and can help get him or her the care that he or she needs.

Consider Mr. Kaman's story. How would you assess further to determine whether he was grieving or depressed?

Acceptance and Participation

At this point, the patient has acknowledged the reality of illness and may be ready to participate in decisions about treatment. Active involvement and the hope attached to pursuing treatment usually lead to increased feelings of mastery of the illness. Patients with long-term chronic illnesses become experts in their own care and management of their condition. From the nurse practitioner with breast cancer:

> *I didn't have time to waste getting upset or angry. My partner was doing that for the both of us. I felt horribly guilty at first, but I couldn't spend time on "what ifs" and wishing that I could have a do-over. I had to focus on what to do next. My oncologist set out a plan of care based on where I am now, not what might have been. He has been great. I am getting radiation and chemotherapy as palliative treatment because I have some metastasis in my spine, and there is no point in going through surgery. I feel pretty well, although I am tired. I am eating well and getting some exercise and taking one day at a time.*

Remember that these states are described as a means of understanding how patients work through their illness. Patients do not move through these states in a linear way, nor should these states be used by the student or nurse to characterize a patient's particular response at any one time. Doing this ignores the complex changes that an illness brings to almost every element of a patient's life. One's response to illness is highly idiosyncratic, and it should be treated as such. Acute illness may be experienced differently from chronic illness.

ILLNESS BEHAVIORS

Although illness is highly subjective and is experienced differently by each individual, a number of factors influence how a particular person will respond. One important factor is the cultural expectation about how people should behave when ill. Children learn the part they are expected to play as an ill person through modeling, that is, by observing how their parents or significant adults in their lives respond to major and minor illnesses. These responses can vary from stoic, uncomplaining independence to very passive dependence, with many variations in between. Stoicism in the face of illness should not be confused with strength of character; it may simply mean that the sick person is not comfortable sharing his or her symptoms and does not want to appear to be complaining.

Each culture generally requires that certain criteria be met before people can qualify as "sick." Sociologist Talcott Parsons (1964) identified five attributes and expectations of the sick role that guided the view of illness among White Americans for decades. These attributes and expectations included behaviors that are dependent, passive, and submissive. Over time, Parsons' sick role expectations were taught in medical and nursing schools and guided the way healthcare providers viewed patients' reactions to pain and illness. Today, however, patients have become increasingly likely to engage actively in their health and health care, challenge providers, and seek information regarding their care from sources other than their providers.

From what you read in Chapter 2, and from what you experience in your everyday life, it should come as no surprise that nursing as a profession, and nurses individually, are confronted with issues related to culture and the various ways culture influences health, health practices, illness beliefs and behaviors. Much of the current discourse around culture in health professions has focused on the concepts of cultural humility and cultural competence, often described as if they are discrete approaches to addressing issues of culture.

In 1998, Tervalon and Murray defined cultural humility as "a lifelong commitment to self-evaluation and critique, to redressing power imbalances . . . and to developing mutually beneficial and nonpaternalistic partnerships with communities on behalf of individuals and defined populations" (p. 123). In 2008 the AACN defined cultural competence as having the attitudes, knowledge and skills necessary for providing quality care to diverse populations (AACN, 2008). Culturally competent nurses are prepared to provide patient-centered care with a focus on the patient's specific needs that are shaped by culture. Being culturally competent means that nurses are more likely to be attuned to the significant problem of health disparities. Cultural competence does not mean, however, that nurses learn every facet in detail of each culture's practices. In fact, mastering the subtleties of every culture is impossible. Importantly, no normative illness response based on culture exists. *Normative* means that there is one standard by which all others are judged and valued.

In 2020, Greene-Moton and Minkler described the significant and inextricable link between cultural competence and cultural humility: "*Cultural competence* is not something we achieve or fail to achieve but rather a reminder to continue to strive to know more about communities of all types with which we work or interact. Together with the concept and embodied practice of deep *cultural humility*, it provides health educators and other public health professionals with some of our most important tools in working with diverse individuals, groups, and communities in today's complex world" (Greene-Moton & Minkler, 2020, p. 142).

A cultural expectation that prevails among some White persons in the U.S. is that sick people should want to get well and return to their normal activities as quickly as possible, which means that patients should cooperate in the treatment process and, to defer to the advice of their healthcare providers. Recall the response, however, of the woman with SLE whose nurses demanded more of her than she knew she could do in context of her life circumstances. She understood that to defer to their advice, no matter how much she understood its importance, was not an option for her in context of her life and responsibilities. People who refuse to take medications as ordered or who refuse to perform prescribed activities, such as an exercise program or therapeutic diet, are often viewed negatively. Their friends and family members may become irritated at their lack of participation in getting well again. Their providers may refer to them as "noncompliant" or "disengaged." Often what is missing is an understanding of the patient's perception of the illness. Illnesses and their treatments have great meaning to patients. One patient with HIV describes the meaning of taking antiretroviral medications:

> *Every time I look at those pills, I am reminded all over again that I have HIV. Every day I am reminded. I feel good, and I sometimes think that if I just didn't have to take these pills, I wouldn't even think about having HIV. So now and then I skip a dose to take a little vacation from HIV. It's not about the pills, really. It's about what they mean, and about what having HIV means.*

Working with patients with chronic illnesses can be particularly challenging for nurses, who sometimes feel hopeless, powerless, overwhelmed and inadequate when facing severely ill patients for whom their illness has no cure. Self-aware nurses recognize these feelings and seek to address them outside of the clinical setting where it is safe to work through them (reflective practice). It will help to remember that patients are autonomous and are (typically) fully competent to make healthcare decisions on their own.

Responses to illness vary widely and are, of course, idiosyncratic. Each person in whom diabetes, for example, is newly diagnosed behaves differently from other people with the same condition. Both internal and external variables affect how an individual acts when ill (Box 13.3). An individual's personality has a great deal

BOX 13.3 Internal and External Influences on Illness Behavior

Internal Influences	External Influences
• Dependence/independence needs • Coping ability • Hardiness • Learned resourcefulness • Resilience • Spirituality	• Past experiences • Culture • Communication patterns • Personal space norms • Role expectations • Values • Reaction to prescribed medications • Ethnocentrism

of influence on the response to illness. Past experiences with illness and cultural background also influence illness behaviors.

Internal Influences on Illness Behaviors

One's personality is an internal variable that determines, to a large extent, how one manages illness. Personality characteristics the nurse should consider when assessing the person with an illness are dependence/independence, coping ability, hardiness, learned resourcefulness, resilience, and spirituality.

Dependence and Independence

Patients' needs for **dependence** may be unrelated to the severity of their illnesses. Some patients may be more passive, relying completely on others to take care of them. Others may simply ignore their illness or do not like the idea of being dependent; therefore they may try to live as independently as they did before becoming sick.

People who perceive themselves as helpless may be more willing to submit to advice and treatments suggested by their healthcare providers. Those who are used to being in charge and see themselves as independent may resent the enforced dependency of hospitalization and illness. These two different attitudes are illustrated in Case Study 13.1.

Both overly dependent and overly independent behavior can be frustrating to nurses, who sometimes become angry with patients who request help with activities they are physically capable of doing themselves. Patients who are too dependent require encouragement to assume more responsibility. Highly independent patients may have problems relying on caregivers and may inadvertently put themselves in danger of falls or other accidents. Independent patients need assistance in recognizing limitations and using available resources to meet his or her needs. For instance, Mr. Johnson in Case Study 13.1 risks a fall and injury by not recognizing that his recent surgery will require him to be temporarily more dependent than he is comfortable with, whereas Mrs. Pierce becomes increasingly dependent on the nurses for assistance with activities of daily living even though she is physically capable.

Because nurses most often focus on promoting patient independence, they may react negatively to patients who are exhibiting dependent behavior. Keep in mind that these behaviors may be the patient's way of signaling an increased need for security or support. Sometimes independence may not be the desired outcome. For patients with chronic illnesses who must rely on others for assistance in meeting their needs, too much independence may actually be problematic, even dangerous.

CASE STUDY 13.1

Dependence vs. Independence

Example 1: Dependence

Mrs. Pierce has been in the hospital for several days after major abdominal surgery. Even after she progressed to the point at which she could feed herself, turn over in bed, and go to the bathroom unaided, she continued to call for assistance with these activities of daily living. She now calls the nurse every few minutes, making some small request that she is capable of performing for herself. She is communicating to the nurse that she needs a great deal of assistance and is demonstrating overly dependent behavior.

Example 2: Independence

Three hours ago, Mr. Johnson returned to his room after surgery. The nurse found him trying to get out of bed by himself. He did not call to ask for assistance and, although he still has some pain even after being medicated, he says that he is used to doing things for himself and does not like asking the nurses for help. Mr. Johnson is demonstrating independent behavior that places him at risk for falling and injury given his recent surgery and need for pain medication.

Coping Ability

An individual copes with disease or illness in a variety of ways. **Coping** is a term that describes the strategies a person uses to assess and manage demands. With an acute illness, coping is generally short term and leads to a return to the preillness state. With chronic disorders, coping behaviors must be used continuously.

Sick people use coping strategies to deal with the negative consequences of the disorder, such as pain or physical limitations. Each individual has a unique coping repertoire that is formed across previous illness episodes, modeling coping by others, and by significant factors in the context of their life over which they has little or no control, such as poverty, concurrent losses, tenuous employment, and unstable relationships, among others. Higher levels of life stresses are associated with patients' perceptions of severe consequences of illness and less control over the illness (Karademas et al., 2009).

Resourcefulness

Resourcefulness refers to the use of cognitive skills that one uses to adapt to the world around him, often in very creative ways. Throughout life, individuals acquire a number of skills that enable them to cope effectively with stressful situations. Resourceful people may have an attitude of self-mastery that can be particularly helpful in reducing the feelings of despair and helplessness that can accompany the numerous stressors of chronic illness. Note that *resource* does not refer to material belongings but involves the ability to make the most out of what one has.

Resourcefulness can be taught as a form of coping. Self-regulation, problem solving, conflict resolution, and emotion management are examples of the types of educational interventions the nurse may implement.

Resilience

Scholars studying human behavior have often noted that some children do well in spite of difficult circumstances that are troubling for others. They attributed the differing reactions as a function of the personality trait of resilience. Resilient persons adapt successfully despite challenges or threats to their way of life or routines. Resilient responses are thought to be a result of three factors:

1. Disposition (i.e., temperament, personality, overall health and appearance, and cognitive style)
2. Family influences (e.g., warmth, support, and organization)
3. Outside support factors, such as a supportive network and success in school or work

Resilience can be developed over a person's lifetime and can be taught, modeled, and learned.

The study of resilience has broadened to include adolescents and adults who face difficult, traumatic, or adverse circumstances. It has also been applied to adults with critical illness, persons who experience intimate partner violence, survivors of sexual abuse, and others. You can expect to see much more about resilience as this phenomenon continues to be studied and better understood. The American Psychological Association has a document called "The Road to Resilience" (http://www.apa.org/helpcenter/road-resilience.aspx) that may be useful to you personally as you work to improve your own set of coping skills as you enter the profession of nursing. You may have occasion to use the content in caring for a patient who is struggling with a serious illness.

Spirituality

Spirituality is commonly defined in terms of belief in a higher power, interconnectedness among living beings, and an awareness of life's purpose and meaning. The way one's spirituality manifests itself varies widely from person to person. Religion differs from spirituality in that *religion* refers to a codified way of organizing rituals and beliefs to create meaning. Spirituality is a larger concept of which religion is one of its many expressions. Spirituality is less differentiated than religion and can include concepts and beliefs from many religions and philosophies. Spiritual growth occurs over the life span and is an internal process; as such it cannot be directly observed. Spiritual growth consists of increasing awareness of meaning, connectedness, purpose, and values in life.

The role of spiritual beliefs in health and illness has only recently been formally investigated. A growing number of scholars and health professionals think that spiritual beliefs have psychological, medical, and financial benefits that can be demonstrated scientifically. Questions about the effects of intercessory prayer (prayer by others on behalf of a sick person) have been debated. A scientifically rigorous, privately funded study of more than 1800 patients who had heart surgery was conducted over nearly a decade. To the disappointment of many, it found that intercessory prayer had no effect on recovery (Carey, 2006). In fact, 59% of participants who knew that someone was praying for them had postoperative complications, as opposed to 51% who were uncertain about whether they were being prayed for. The debate will undoubtedly continue.

One of the leading proponents of the spirituality and healing movement in American medicine is Dr. Herbert Benson. He originated the "relaxation-response" therapy to reduce stress in patients with hypertension, chronic pain, and other stress-related illnesses. Many people use prayer as part of the relaxation response (Benson and Klipper, 2000). Massachusetts General Hospital, a large medical center associated with the Harvard School of Medicine, is the home of the Benson-Henry Institute for Mind Body Medicine (https://bensonhenryinstitute.org). Their website describes one of their missions as "helping people build personal resiliency: the ability to rise above or bounce back from stressful situations." Furthermore, mind/body medicine incorporates the relaxation response, positive coping strategies, physical activity, good nutrition, and social support (Massachusetts

General Hospital Benson-Henry Institute for Mind Body Medicine, 2015).

Another indication of the importance of meeting patients' spiritual needs in healthcare settings is the increase in chaplain presence in some inpatient and outpatient settings. Chaplains are typically ordained clergy who have training and experience in pastoral care in healthcare settings and who have special skills in helping patients and their families with spiritual matters. Chaplains are usually on call around the clock, and in large medical centers they have a presence in the hospital at all hours.

The Joint Commission, the International Council of Nurses, the American Association of Colleges of Nursing, and the National Council of State Boards of Nursing all acknowledge that spiritual nursing care is a responsibility that goes beyond calling the chaplain. Yet many nurses are reluctant to render spiritual nursing care. This reluctance may grow from feelings of inadequacy, lack of knowledge, embarrassment, their own spiritual uncertainty, lack of preparation, lack of privacy, lack of time, or failure to see it as a nursing role (McEwen, 2005).

Nurses are encouraged to view spirituality as one aspect of the whole human person and to assess patients for spiritual distress. They should recognize the individuality and value of each patient's spiritual beliefs and encourage their use in coping with illness. Spiritual distress is a NANDA International (NANDA-I) diagnosis meaning "impaired ability to experience and integrate meaning and purpose in life through connectedness with self, others, art, music, literature, nature, and/or a power greater than oneself" (Doenges et al., 2014, p. 758). Patients who question the meaning of suffering and the meaning of life, who express anger at God or other deity, or who view illness as punishment from their deity are experiencing spiritual distress. Spiritual distress can be painful and can hinder a patient's progress.

Nurses with strong religious faith or deeply entrenched religious rituals have to pay attention to how they may use these beliefs with regard to spiritual care of their patients. As with every other domain of care, being nonjudgmental is key. You may have very significant disagreements with your patient's religious beliefs, but it their belief, not yours, and it is not your role to change your patient's view. Proselytizing by nurses can be very upsetting for patients and can increase their spiritual distress. Your role is to help your patient access whatever higher power he or she may believe in. This can be done as simply as providing the patient privacy, quiet, an open window shade, music, or your caring presence. If a patient asks you to read to him or her from his or her religious text, you can do this without risking your own faith if yours is different from your patient's.

Sometimes patients ask nurses to pray with them or for them. If you are not comfortable with this, you can simply say, "Would you like for me to sit with you while you pray?" You can simply sit in silence, and, if the patient agrees, hold their hand while they pray (Fig. 13.2). If you are not someone for whom prayer is part of your spiritual practice, you can simply tell patients who ask you to pray for them that you will have good thoughts for them. If patients trust you enough to engage you in their spiritual practices, they have demonstrated that they trust you. In addition, it is always appropriate to ask your patients if they would

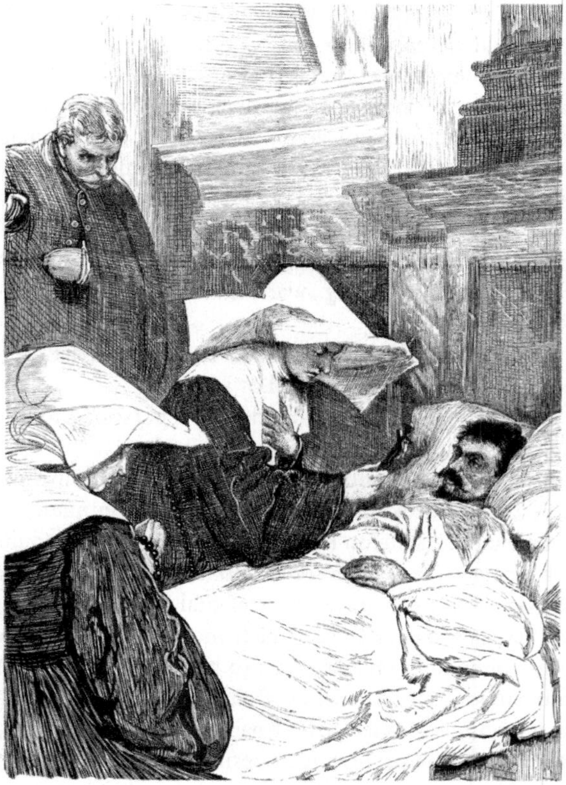

Fig. 13.2 In this illustration of a hospital scene during the Siege of Paris in 1870, two nuns pray for a dying man. Religion and nursing have intersected for centuries. (Photo used with permission from iStockphoto.)

like for you to call a imam, minister, priest, rabbi or other clergy for them if they have deep spiritual needs that you cannot meet.

Sometimes nursing education takes the path of least resistance in the discussion of deeply important and even divisive issues. A "one size fits all" approach to care for patients whose faith is different from yours usually means a feel-good bromide (like the two previous paragraphs), giving the illusion that all is well because nurses learn to "take patients where they are." But healthcare settings are not immune from the injustices and bigotry related to race, ethnicity and religion. In Professional Profile 13.1, Tarteel Suliman, BSN, RN poses a perspective and a challenge related to current inclusion and diversity efforts, based on what she learned in completing her senior honors thesis in 2021, in which she explored racism and oppression encountered by Black Muslim women in healthcare settings. As a Black Muslim woman herself, she is sharing her view on current diversity and inclusion work, and who it serves to benefit. Her words are powerful and unapologetic, and may make some readers uncomfortable. But discomfort often points to a place where rehabilitation and healing need to occur.

External Influences on Illness Behaviors

External factors that affect illness behaviors include past experiences and cultural group membership. Both directly influence how an individual perceives and responds to illness. The values that guide feelings about illness and steer a person toward particular methods of treatment are acquired primarily in the family of origin and in the culture.

Past Experiences

Some adults may accept being ill fairly easily and will accept care easily. Some adults, however, may have difficulty accepting illness and the restrictions that accompany. It is possible that as children, they received signals from their parents or adult caretakers that "it is weak to be ill" or "one must keep going even when not feeling well." Other adults who experienced traumatic hospitalizations as children or who were threatened with injections for misbehaving may see hospitals and nurses as threatening. They are understandably affected by their early negative experiences. Nurses should determine the patient's past experiences with illness and the healthcare system during a careful admission assessment. These findings can be used to individualize care.

Culture

Culture has been discussed several times throughout this book and chapter, because it is difficult to discuss almost any topic related to health care without mentioning culture. Culture is a pattern of learned behavior and values that are reinforced through social interactions, shared by members of a particular group, and transmitted from one generation to the next. Culture exerts considerable influence over most of an individual's life experiences. Meanings attached to health, illness, and perceptions of treatment are affected to a large degree by a person's culture. Culture determines when one seeks help and the type of practitioner consulted. It also prescribes customs of responding to the sick. Culture defines whether illness is seen as a punishment for misdeeds or as the result of inadequate personal health practices. It influences whether one goes to an acupuncturist, an herbalist, a folk healer, or healthcare providers such as physicians and nurse practitioners.

Beginning in the early 1970s, schools of nursing began including cultural concepts in their curricula. Increasing numbers of universities and colleges offered graduate programs in transcultural nursing. The Transcultural Nursing Society was incorporated in 1981, and in 1988 it began certifying nurses in transcultural nursing. Through oral and written examinations and evaluation of educational background and working experiences, a qualified nurse can become a certified transcultural nurse (CTN). More information about this interesting certification can be found at https://tcns.org/tcncertification/.

The Transcultural Nursing Society began publishing the *Journal of Transcultural Nursing* in 1989. In the decades since transcultural nursing was first emphasized in educational programs, the cultural makeup of the U.S. population has undergone rapid change. In the 2020 census, 50% of all children under age 18 years were members of ethnic minority groups and the growth of ethnic minority groups has accelerated at rates faster than were predicted a decade ago (Brookings Institution, 2021). These cultural shifts mean that changes in the nursing workforce are needed to deal more effectively with commonalities and differences in patients. Significant disparities exist between the health status of Whites and non-Whites in the United States. For example, the death rate for heart disease is more than 40% higher in African Americans than in the White population.

PROFESSIONAL PROFILE 13.1

Beyond Diversity and Inclusion Efforts: The Need for Anti-Racism Work Across Nursing

I once believed that I had to be a part of a system if I had any intention to change it. Yet it is still difficult to pinpoint why I chose health care—specifically, nursing—as my career path. I see life in two main forms: brilliant and dreadful. Brilliant in the sense that we are born, we grow up, we develop livelihoods, and we find happiness in whatever form that may be. Dreadful in the sense that we fall ill, we suffer, and we experience trauma. I find great pain in knowing that some of us experience the latter. More so, I find pain knowing that some experience this alone. I only hope to provide solace for those who are enduring that dread.

For many of my patients, I know I cannot completely repair their struggles. Yet in the event that I can alleviate even an atom's weight of pain, I hope they know that I am glad to be of use. So, for my patients whose needs are vast or miniscule, arduous or simple, challenging or light; it does not matter to me. My goal is to help them experience those brilliant parts of life again, no matter how trivial some parts may be. Again—returning to that brilliant part of life—if nursing allows me to do this, then what a beautiful career I have chosen.

I often reflect among the possibilities of what I am capable of doing for my patients but in the same breath I am pained by what I cannot do. Being a Black Muslim means I am no stranger to the inequity that those who share my identity face in health care. However, being in this White-dominated field means I will never have the power to change this system if we continue to coddle what has left us stagnant in the fight for equity—White supremacy. In my honors thesis, *Islamophobia and the Healthcare System*, I explored the experiences of three Black Muslim women and their encounters in health care, where they faced questioning to the point of argument and derision by their providers and, for one who was a medical student, singling out by a physician during rounds related to her religious beliefs. I came to the conclusion that diversity and inclusion work in curricula today is simply not enough to mitigate negative outcomes. The focus must shift into antiracism work should we anticipate any radical change.

Diversity and inclusion work in curricula seems to have been shaped into a performance, centering around giving those who are oppressed a seat at the table. At these tables we discuss the same script—what harms our communities, frustrations, and expressions of contempt—without any mention of White supremacy. This is not unity. It is strategic violence. If we continue to fail to be explicit in naming White supremacy as the source of inequity, then these tables must be eradicated. They are unjust. I assert that diversity and inclusion work is redundant and has become a means to assuage White guilt. Further, current diversity and inclusion work exists to benefit White people more than anyone else. Inviting us to a seat at the table is not allyship. It is theater. It is disingenuous to be in solidarity with the oppressed with one hand and cater to White supremacists with the other. Institutions—educational, health, and political, among others—have grown comfortable in maintaining a moderate position and these very institutions are the source of my rage. So much work is left to be done, and if we continue to ignore the roles our colleagues hold in the face of White supremacy as we fight for equity, years from now, I expect to see us all in the same dormant position in which we are in today.

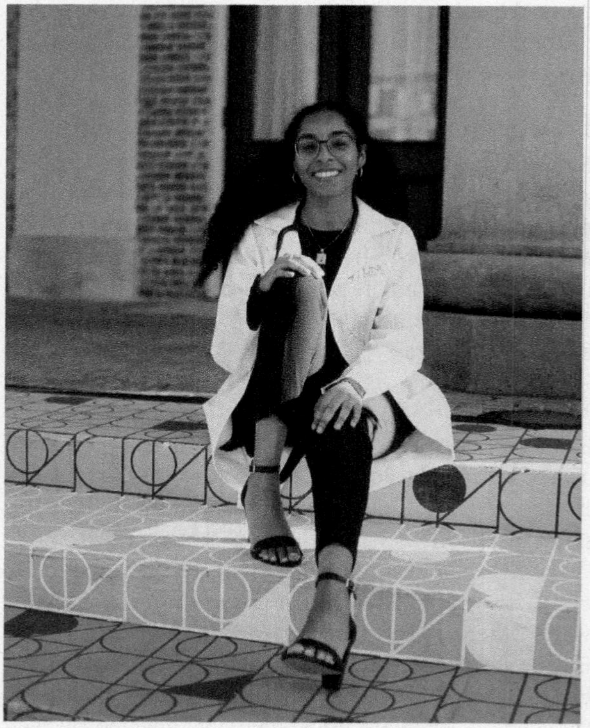

Tarteel Suliman, BSN, RN
Highest Honors, UNC at Chapel Hill, 2021

Courtesy Tarteel Suliman, BSN, RN

Similarly discouraging disparities exist in death rates for cancer and HIV/acquired immunodeficiency syndrome (AIDS), among other diseases. Although these disparities may partly result from education, poverty, and lifestyle factors, there is a growing recognition among health professionals that racism may play a role. As a result, professional associations such as the American Nurses Association, The Joint Commission, and the federal government have all endorsed standards for culturally appropriate healthcare services.

The Joint Commission developed and revised accreditation standards for hospitals to incorporate diversity, cultural, language, and health literacy issues into patient care processes. In 2010 The Joint Commission published a monograph, *Advancing Effective Communication, Cultural Competence, and Patient- and Family-Centered Care: A Roadmap for Hospitals,* to set standards for quality, safety, and equity for hospitalized patients. This document is available at http://www.jointcommission.org/assets/1/6/ARoadmapforHospitalsfinalversion727.pdf. Some states have passed legislation requiring healthcare professions to include cultural competence training in their educational and continuing education programs. The profession of nursing is largely White, whereas the nation is racially more diverse than ever before, which underscores the need for culturally competent nurses. Clearly, transcultural nursing is an important field of study, practice, and research and an essential one in today's increasingly diverse society.

The culturally competent nurse. Cultural competence, defined earlier, guides the nurse in understanding behaviors and planning appropriate approaches to patient needs. Conversely, culture will also guide the patient's response to healthcare providers and their interventions. The U.S. Office of Minority Health defined culturally competent health care as "services that are respectful of and responsive to the health beliefs and practices and cultural and linguistic needs of diverse patient populations" (U.S. Department of Health and Human Services, 2001, p. 131), a definition still being used today. Understanding a patient's cultural background can facilitate communication and support establishing an effective nurse-patient relationship. Conversely, lack of understanding can create barriers that impede nursing care.

The shared values and beliefs in a culture enable its members to predict each other's actions. They also affect how members react to each other's behavior. When nurses work with patients from cultures different from their own and about which little is known, they lack these familiar guidelines for predicting behavior. This can cause anxiety, frustration, and feelings of distrust in both patient and nurse. Some of the issues that can arise when nurses care for patients from other cultures include stereotyping, communication difficulties, misperceptions about personal space, differing values and role expectations, ethnopharmacologic considerations, and ethnocentrism.

Stereotyping. In an effort to predict behavior, nurses may stereotype or make prejudgments about patients from different cultures. It is important that nurses refrain from **stereotyping** members of cultures or ethnic groups that are different from their own. When providing nursing care, one size does not fit all. *Cultural conditioning* is a term that means people are culture bound. They are unconscious of their own innate values and beliefs and assume that all people are basically alike, that is, that all people share their values and beliefs.

It is important to recognize that the healthcare professions create **cultural conditioning** in their practitioners during school. Nursing is no exception. Nurses tend to hold their knowledge and beliefs about health in high regard and may devalue people who do not possess similar knowledge and beliefs. Individualized planning is always the best basis for care, whatever the patient's culture or ethnic group. Care that is not individualized can result in nonadherence to treatment plans, dissatisfaction with care, and suboptimal outcomes.

Ethnocentrism. Nurses respond to sick people based not only on their formal education but also on their own socialization and culture. All persons can be unaware of their own biases and tend to be ethnocentric. **Ethnocentrism** is the inclination to view one's own cultural group as the standard by which to judge the value of other cultural groups. One nurse describes her embarrassment when a patient challenged her ethnocentric view of dining customs:

> *My patient was from another country, and her family brought in the most delicious smelling food. When I went into the room, I was surprised to see them all eating with their fingers. I left right away and brought them some knives and forks. They refused them, nicely. I regret that I mentioned how messy this probably was. My patient asked me, "Do you use a fork when you eat?" I answered, "Of course," and the patient laughed and pointed out that I had a good portion of salad dressing down*

the front of my scrubs. The patient and her family, on the other hand, were immaculate. I was a little embarrassed, but I learned a good lesson. I didn't have any choice except to laugh too, and apologize.

The nurse who identifies how personal beliefs and expectations can influence care is better able to recognize and deal with any prejudices that may impede patient care. Cultural assessment therefore begins with self-assessment. To begin a cultural self-assessment, examine your own values. The nurse who is frustrated by the difficulty of caring for a patient from a different culture may benefit from taking a few minutes to imagine what it would be like to be hospitalized in a foreign country. Candidly answering the questions in Considering Culture Box 13.1 will help you begin the important process of self-assessment.

CONSIDERING CULTURE BOX 13.1

The Challenge of Understanding Your Own Cultural Beliefs: Sociocultural Self-Assessment

Directions: Use your answers to these questions to better understand your own social and cultural beliefs and expectations.

1. To what groups do I belong? What is my cultural heritage? My socioeconomic status? My age-group? My religious affiliation?
2. How do I describe myself? What parts of the description come from the groups to which I belong?
3. What kinds of contact have I had with people from groups different from mine? Do I assume that others have the same values and beliefs that I have?
4. How am I ethnocentric in my attitudes and behavior? What would I change about my group affiliations if I could? Why?
5. Have I ever experienced the feeling of being rejected by another group? Did this experience heighten my sensitivity to other cultures or cause me to denigrate others different from myself?
6. When I was growing up, what messages did I get from parents and friends about people from groups different from mine? Do these attitudes cause me any difficulty today?
7. What are the stereotypes I hold about people from groups different from mine? Do these biases help or hinder me in developing cultural sensitivity?
8. To work more effectively with people across cultural groups, what do I need to work on?

Cultural assessment. An important step in meeting the challenge of providing nursing care to diverse patients is the cultural assessment. Cultural assessments are used to identify beliefs, values, and health practices that may help or hinder nursing interventions. Dr. Madeleine Leininger, an iconic figure in nursing—anthropologist, theorist, and founder of transcultural nursing—advocated that nurses routinely perform cultural assessments to determine patients' culturally specific needs (Leininger, 1999).

A cultural assessment is really as simple as asking patients their preferences, what they think or believe about their illness, their family structure, who providers should talk to in making a decision, and what the illness and its treatments mean to them (Fig. 13.3). Numerous cultural assessment instruments have been developed. Some of them require in-depth interviews and comprehensive data gathering, which may prove to be challenging for busy nurses. However, patients often find themselves "a stranger in a strange land" just by virtue of entering the healthcare setting with its own language, routines, and culture. A careful assessment is warranted, and if there is any question that about a language barrier, consult a professional interpreter (see Chapter 12). Remember that under stress, as patients often are, one's second language, even if otherwise conversant, may not be adequate for medical circumstances.

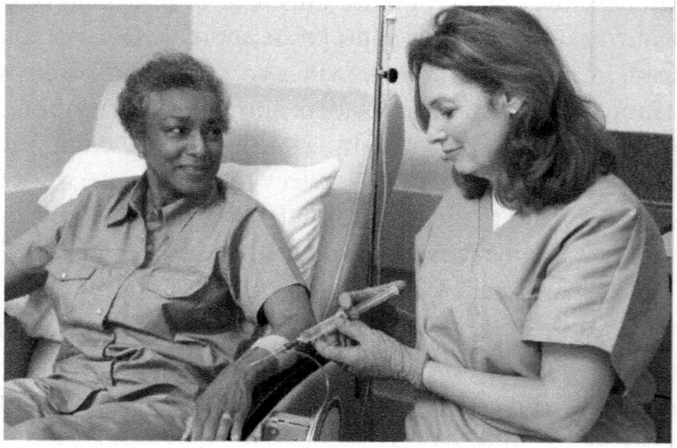

Fig. 13.3 Nurses administering chemotherapy in an outpatient setting often see the same patients over time. A cultural assessment at the onset of treatment can be useful in helping the patient feel accepted and supported as she faces the challenges of having cancer. (Photo used with permission from iStockphoto.)

Culturally competent nurses take cultural differences between themselves and their patient into consideration, are aware of where potential misunderstandings may occur, usually interpret patient behavior accurately, and, importantly, recognize when issues arise that need to be addressed. They realize that cultural norms must be included in the plan of care to prevent conflicts between nursing goals and patient/family goals.

In addition, being knowledgeable about other cultures promotes feelings of respect and enhances understanding of attitudes, behaviors, and the impact of illness. The accompanying interview with Dr. Madeleine Leininger provides insights into her vast experience and strongly held beliefs about cultural competence in nursing. Becoming culturally competent is a process. Nurses must remember that continuous learning and sensitivity to and respect for cultural differences are qualities required of culturally competent nurses (Interview Box 13.1).

THE IMPACT OF ILLNESS ON PATIENTS AND FAMILIES

Across all cultures, illness forces change in patients and their families: behavioral and emotional changes, role changes, and unpredictable changes in family dynamics. Illness creates stress and other emotional responses. The suddenness and seriousness of an acute illness affect responses to illness and can disrupt almost all aspects of family life. Illnesses that result in enduring lifestyle adjustments have serious effects on the family. Responses to illness are usually affected by the patient's stage of human development. For instance, an elderly widowed family member who has previously enjoyed good health may elect not to seek treatment for cancer, but a younger member with a spouse and children may elect aggressive treatment for the same illness. Religious faith also plays a role in responses to illness.

Severe illnesses that profoundly affect physical appearance and functioning can result in high levels of anxiety and extensive behavioral changes than are short-term, non–life-threatening illnesses. These effects are significant and may continue for the patient's lifetime. When planning holistic nursing care, the nurse must take into consideration how the family both influences and is influenced by the illness of a family member.

Impact of Illness on Patients

Illness creates a variety of emotional responses, some of which have been described briefly earlier in this chapter. Among the more common responses are guilt, anger, anxiety, and stress.

Guilt

Guilt is not uncommon when a person becomes ill, particularly if the illness is related to behavioral choices. Persons may feel guilty when they are unable to perform usual activities because of illness. Parents who are unable to take care of their children as they would prefer, or a who have to cut back work hours and hence decrease their income because of illness may experience considerable guilt. Nurses who identify and encourage patients to talk about their feelings of guilt may help assuage these uncomfortable feelings that may impede the patient's ability to participate in their care.

Anger

Anger is another common emotional response to illness. When patients must make significant changes to manage their illnesses, such as giving up favorite foods or activities, they may experience anger about the changes. Anger may also be directed toward healthcare providers for their inability to produce a cure, reduce pain, or prevent negative consequences of the illness. Nurses must be prepared to accept such angry feelings, to refrain from rejecting or avoiding patients who express their fears through anger, and to encourage the adaptive expression of feelings of anger. Angry patients can be difficult to deal with, and the nurse must be very careful not to further incite the patient by becoming upset or angry too. In the example of Mr. Kaman earlier in this chapter, the nurse appropriately sought out some explanation from Mrs. Kaman, who was able to help her understand the source of at least some of Mr. Kaman's anger.

Anxiety

Anxiety is a common and universal experience. It is also a common emotional response to illness and hospitalization. **Anxiety** is an ill-defined, diffuse feeling of apprehension and uncertainty. Anxiety occurs as a result of some threat to an individual's selfhood, self-esteem, or identity. A number of threats are associated with illness. Illness may alter the way people view themselves. Some illnesses result in a change in physical appearance.

INTERVIEW BOX 13.1

Dr. Madeleine Leininger, Founder of Transcultural Nursing

Interviewer: Dr. Leininger, please tell us what you mean by the term *culturally competent.*

Dr. Leininger: Culturally competent care has been defined as the culturally based knowledge with a care focus that is used in creative, meaningful, and appropriate ways to provide beneficial and satisfying care to individuals, families, groups, or communities or to help people face death or disabilities. I coined this term in 1962 as the goal of my theory of culture care diversity and universality. The term has caught hold today and is being used by many healthcare providers. It is now used as a requirement for The Joint Commission accreditation and with other organizations as essential to work effectively with cultures and their healthcare needs.

Interviewer: Please describe how a culturally competent nurse's patient care differs from that of one who is not culturally competent.

Dr. Leininger: A culturally competent nurse demonstrates the following attributes and skills: (1) uses transcultural nursing concepts, principles, and available research findings to assess and guide care practices; (2) understands and values the cultural beliefs and practices of designated cultures so that nursing care is tailor-made or fits individuals' needs in meaningful ways; (3) knows how to prevent major kinds of cultural conflicts, clashes, or hurtful care practices; (4) demonstrates reasonable confidence to work effectively and knowingly with clients of different cultures and can also evaluate transcultural nursing care outcomes.

The nurse who is unable to demonstrate these culturally competent attributes often shows signs of being frustrated and impatient with people of different cultures. Moreover, the nurse who does not practice cultural competencies often shows signs of excessive ethnocentrism, biases, and related problems that impede client recovery and well-being.

Interviewer: How do patients respond differently when nurses take their cultural patterns into consideration when planning and implementing care?

Dr. Leininger: It is most encouraging to observe and listen to clients who have received culturally based nursing care. These clients often exhibit the following behaviors: (1) They show signs of being satisfied and very pleased with nurse's actions and decisions. (2) They make comments such as, "This is the best care I or my family members have received from healthcare providers." Frequently they say, "How did you know about my values, my culture, and how to use these ideas in my care? You anticipated my needs well." (3) They appreciate the different ways the nurse incorporates their cultural needs. They express their gratitude to the nurse. (4) Clients appreciate respect for their culture shown by the nurse in care decisions and practices. (5) The clients do not experience racial biases and negative comments about their cultures or familiar lifeways.

Interviewer: With so many cultural groups in this country, knowing all one needs to know about other cultures seems overwhelming. How do you advise nurses to begin the process of becoming culturally competent?

Dr. Leininger: The nurse should first enroll in a substantive transcultural nursing course to learn the basic and important concepts, principles, and practices of transcultural nursing. This knowledge base is essential so the nurse becomes aware of common cultural needs and ways to work with a few cultures that are different. A few cultures are studied in depth, focusing on common and unique cultural features. The most frequently occurring cultures in the nurse's home or local region are studied first, and then one learns about other cultures over time, becoming sensitive and knowledgeable about these cultures. The nurse can greatly increase her or his knowledge of several cultures or subcultures by reading the literature, or by studying specific cultures when caring for people under transcultural mentors. Gradually, the nurse learns several cultures in a general way and a few in depth. As the nurse becomes increasingly knowledgeable about several cultures, comparative knowledge and competencies become evident.

There is no expectation that professional nurses can know all human cultures, as this would be impossible. An open learning attitude and mind with a sincere desire to learn as much as possible about a few cultures will help the nurse in becoming culturally knowledgeable, competent, and sensitive.

Interviewer: What signs can students look for to determine whether their nursing programs are preparing them to provide culturally competent care?

Dr. Leininger: Nursing students will find they are able to provide culturally competent care when (or if) the following signs are evident:

- They consistently know, understand, and respect specific cultures and appreciate commonalities and differences among cultures.
- They feel a sense of confidence, creativity, and competence in their nursing care practices, see how their care fits specific cultures, and accommodate cultural differences in meaningful and creative ways.

INTERVIEW BOX 13.1—cont'd

Dr. Madeleine Leininger, Founder of Transcultural Nursing

- They go beyond common sense to actual use of culture-specific knowledge in patient care as shown in the Sunrise Model (see Chapter 9, Fig. 9.2).
- They creatively use the clients' beliefs, values, and patterns along with appropriate professional knowledge and skills that meet clients' needs.
- They prevent racial discrimination practices in nursing and in other places; they avoid cultural imposition, ethnocentrism, cultural conflicts, cultural pain, and related negative practices.
- They value and know how to use Leininger's Culture Care Theory and basic transcultural care concepts, principles, and research findings in their nursing practices to provide culturally congruent care for people's health and well-being.
- They appreciate a global perspective of nursing and value transcultural nursing to meet a growing and intense multicultural world.
- They markedly grow in their professional knowledge and sensitivities, developing a global worldview of transcultural nursing. They reach out to help cultural strangers in different living contexts.

Courtesy Dr. Madeleine Leininger.

Often, ability to function is affected, altering relationships, work performance, and abilities to meet others' expectations. In addition, there may be concern about pain and discomfort associated with illness or treatment. Because of real and potential threats and changes arising from illness, nurses must develop skills that enable them to help patients recognize and manage anxiety.

Although the responses are similar, anxiety and fear are different. Fear results from specific known causes, whereas anxiety is more unfocused. For example, if you are home alone at night and you hear an unusual noise outside, your heartbeat and respirations may increase, your stomach tightens, and you perspire. The emotion in this situation is fear of an intruder. If you begin to have the same feelings but have heard no noises and cannot identify a source of fear, you may be experiencing anxiety. Both emotions may be present at the same time. The patient who is in the hospital for surgery or invasive testing may experience anxiety about the unknown consequences of the surgery and fear in anticipation of pain, a long recovery, or a diagnosis of a life-limiting illness.

Symptoms of anxiety. Nurses should be familiar with the numerous symptoms of anxiety. They are classified as physiologic, emotional, and cognitive. Signs and symptoms include increased heart rate, respirations, and blood pressure; insomnia; nausea and vomiting; fatigue; sweaty palms; and tremors. Emotional responses include restlessness, irritability, feelings of helplessness, crying, and depression. Cognitive symptoms include inability to concentrate, forgetfulness, inattention to surroundings, and preoccupation.

Responses to anxiety. Responses to anxiety occur on a continuum. The continuum is along four levels of anxiety: mild, moderate, severe, and panic. A mild level is characterized by increased alertness and ability to focus attention and concentrate. There is an expanded capacity for learning at this stage.

A person with a moderate level of anxiety is able to concentrate on only one thing at a time. Commonly, there is increased body movement (restlessness), rapid speech, and a subjective awareness of discomfort.

At the severe level, thoughts become scattered. The severely anxious person may not be able to communicate verbally, and there is considerable discomfort accompanied by purposeless movements such as handwringing and pacing.

At the panic level, the person becomes completely disorganized and loses the ability to differentiate between reality and unreality. There are constant random and purposeless movements. The individual experiencing panic levels of anxiety is unable to function without assistance. Panic levels of anxiety cannot be continued indefinitely because the patient will become exhausted. Box 13.4 lists the characteristics of each level of anxiety.

Because anxiety is such a common response to illness and hospitalization, nurses often encounter patients who are experiencing mild or moderate anxiety and, occasionally, patients who are severely anxious. When interacting with an anxious patient, the nurse should carefully assess the level of anxiety before attempting to develop the plan of care. Because anxiety can cause an increase in heart and respiratory rates and

BOX 13.4 Levels of Anxiety

Mild Anxiety
- Increased alertness, increased ability to focus, improved concentration, expanded capacity for learning

Moderate Anxiety
- Concentration limited to one thing, increased body movement, rapid speech, subjective awareness of discomfort

Severe Anxiety
- Scattered thoughts, difficulty with verbal communication, considerable discomfort, purposeless movements

Panic
- Complete disorganization, difficulty differentiating reality from unreality, constant random movements, unable to function without assistance

blood pressure, the nurse may need to consult with the patient's primary provider for an order for an anxiolytic if needed. It is important, however, to talk with the patient first before administering a medication to decrease their sense of anxiety. Anxiolytics can make a person groggy or otherwise less alert, and the patient may prefer the symptoms of anxiety rather than the way these medications can make them feel.

Anxiety tends to be transferred between persons. For this reason, nurses must be aware of and manage personal anxiety so that it is not inadvertently transferred to patients. Conversely, self-awareness is essential to avoid responding to a patient's anxiety by becoming anxious.

Stress

Stress is another internal variable that affects patients. **Stress** is both a response to illness and may be a factor in the development of illness. Because illness and hospitalization involve so many alterations in a patient's routine and environment, they cause a great deal of stress.

Stress is an unavoidable and essential part of life. To survive and grow, individuals must cope adaptively with constantly changing demands. The stress related to examinations, for example, motivates most students to grow by studying and learning. Although stress is unavoidable, and even sometimes desirable, some control can be exerted over the number and types of **stressors** (factors that create stress) encountered, and responses to the stressors can often be managed.

Hospitalized patients are removed from their usual routines and support systems. They lose much of their control because nurses and other care providers make decisions for them. Often, being ill means that they are no longer able to perform activities as they did before the illness occurred. Some patients find themselves in the role of comforting other family members rather than being comforted, to avoid increasing family members' distress.

Differentiating between stress and anxiety. Stress and anxiety have some characteristics in common. The physiologic responses are similar. Anxiety is a response to a real or perceived threat to the individual, whereas stress is an interaction between the individual and the environment. Stress includes all the responses the body makes while striving to maintain equilibrium and deal with demands.

Internal, external, and interpersonal stressors. Selye (1956) defined *stress* as the nonspecific response of the body to any demand made on it. He named this response the *general adaptation syndrome* and identified three stages through which the body progresses while responding to stress.

Stressors trigger the body's stress response. Stressors are agents or stimuli that an individual perceives as posing a threat to homeostasis. Stressors may come from external, interpersonal, or internal sources. External stressors include such things as noise, heat, cold, malfunctioning equipment (such as an intravenous pump that keeps alarming), or organizational rules and expectations. Interpersonal sources of stress include the demands made by others and conflicts with others. Placing unrealistic expectations on oneself is an example of an internal stressor. For example, a patient with a traumatic injury to his lower extremity begins making plans to take part in a race within a month. Although his rehabilitation advances well, he becomes discouraged and experiences stress because it is not at a pace that he would like, and it becomes clear that racing will not be part of his life in the near future.

Responses to stress. Outward responses to stress are determined by the individual's perception of the stressor. Cognitive appraisal, or the way one thinks about a specific situation, determines the degree to which the situation is considered stressful. Loud music at a concert, for example, might seem less stressful to adolescents than it would to their parents.

Another factor related to the assessment of threat is whether the individual feels capable of handling the threat, that is, whether the person exhibits hardiness. The person who feels capable can be expected to feel less stress than the person who does not generally feel competent.

Stress affects the physical, emotional, and cognitive areas of functioning just as anxiety does. Physically, there can be a feeling of fatigue with muscular tightness and tension. Heart rate and respirations are increased. The person who is under prolonged or serious stress may be unable to sleep or eat, or he or she may sleep or eat excessively in an attempt to avoid or cope with the stress.

Emotionally, people under stress feel drained and unable to care for themselves or others. This can result in social isolation and distancing from others. They experience difficulty enjoying life. They may have feelings of hopelessness and of being out of control. Irritability and impatience often occur.

Cognitively, stress causes decreased mental capacity and problem-solving skills; therefore there is a tendency to have difficulty making decisions. Someone who is under a great deal of stress may be experiencing *distress*, a response to environmental, physical, or cognitive stressors in which the person may find it difficult to function and cope.

Stress and illness. Constant stress plays a role in the development of illness. Recent research has provided better understanding of the links between prolonged stress and body functioning.

The person who is under stress for long periods is at risk for a number of physical problems. The body produces cortisol when a person is under stress. Cortisol, a steroid hormone, can affect both the metabolism and immune response and lead to susceptibility to weight gain and poor healing. Disorders such as hypertension, certain skin disorders, and autoimmune disorders have been termed *stress-related diseases* because they commonly occur in individuals who have been severely stressed.

Coping with stress. Nurses have a role in helping patients modify their stressors. They should assess patients' abilities to recognize symptoms of stress and their usual methods of coping.

Coping with stress can be direct or indirect. In assisting patients to use direct coping, nurses help patients to identify those situations that can be changed and to take responsibility for changing them. The focus is on using problem-solving skills and planning to eliminate or avoid as many stressors as possible. Completely eliminating stress from one's life is neither possible nor desirable.

In helping patients use indirect coping, nurses' actions are aimed at reducing the affective (feelings) and physiologic (body) disturbances resulting from stress. Patients are sometimes taught techniques such as deep breathing, muscle relaxation, and imagery, which may help them cope more effectively with stress. It is crucial, however, for nurses to understand that these exercises do not address the actual sources of stress, but may be effective in the moment to manage uncomfortable physical and psychological manifestations of stress.

To help patients manage stress, nurses must be skilled in assessing and managing their own personal stress. Nurses who are feeling stressed themselves have difficulty assisting patients in dealing with similar problems. The statements in Table 13.1 can help you identify your own sources of stress and develop self-awareness so that you can be effective in helping patients deal with their stress.

Coping with stress through education. Patient education is a major part of the practice of nursing, and nurses have a professional responsibility to ensure that their patients' learning needs are met. When patients are competent in the knowledge and skills they need to manage their illnesses, they tend to feel more masterful and less stressed.

As a first step, nurses must identify factors that can create barriers to learning (Box 13.5). One factor is anxiety. Mild anxiety improves learning by increasing the ability to focus on the task. As anxiety increases, however, the ability to listen, focus, and concentrate decreases. Information is not retained, and the patient is unable to make the cognitive connections required for learning to take place.

Physiologic factors may also impede learning. For instance, visual or hearing deficits must be addressed. Unmet physiologic needs, such as fatigue, shortness of breath, hunger, and thirst, decrease the patient's attention to learning. Pain dramatically impairs the ability to learn, and pain medication may make the patient drowsy and unable to focus. Learning requires energy so a fatigued patient may not learn well. Nurses who assess and ensure that patients' physiologic needs are met enhance these patients' readiness to learn.

Patient teaching is an important part of the culture of nursing; however, culture also can influence patients'

TABLE 13.1 Personal Stress Inventory

	Very Often	Sometimes	Rarely or Never
1. I feel tense and anxious and have uncomfortable physical symptoms sometimes.			
2. People at home, school, or work make me feel tense.			
3. I eat, drink, or smoke in response to feeling tense or anxious.			
4. My neck or shoulders are tense and it is painful.			
5. I have headaches and/or insomnia.			
6. I have trouble turning off my thoughts long enough to feel relaxed.			
7. I find it difficult to concentrate on what I am doing because I worry about other things.			
8. I use alcohol, tranquilizers, or other medications to relax or sleep.			
9. I feel a lot of pressure at work or school.			
10. I do not feel that my work is appreciated.			
11. My family does not appreciate what I do for them.			
12. I feel I do not have enough time for myself.			
13. I have difficulty saying "no."			
14. I wish I had more friends with whom to share experiences.			
15. I do not have enough time for physical exercise.			

Scoring: Give yourself 2 points for every check in the Very Often column, 1 point for every check in the Sometimes column, and 0 points for every check in the Rarely or Never column. Total the number of points. A score of 20 to 30 represents a high level of stress. If you scored in this range, you should take steps to reduce your stress level. A score from 10 to 19 means that you are experiencing midlevel stress. You should monitor your stress and begin relaxation exercises. A score of 9 or less means that you are experiencing relatively low stress at present.

responses to teaching by nurses. Understanding the meaning of illness in the patient's culture is an early step that will help the nurse determine the educational needs of the patient and family and effectively provide culturally congruent patient education. When the nurse works toward a learning goal that is not seen as desirable by a patient, their cultural values may be in conflict. In fact, this is not really a patient goal but a reflection of the nurse's ingrained cultural expectation that patients need or want to be taught.

BOX 13.5 Barriers to Patient Learning

- High anxiety
- Sensory deficits (e.g., vision, hearing)
- Pain
- Fatigue
- Hunger/thirst
- Shortness of breath
- Cultural expectations
- Language barriers
- Differing health values
- Low literacy
- Lack of motivation
- Environmental factors (e.g., noise, lack of privacy)

Self-awareness on the part of the nurse is essential to avoid allowing cross-cultural barriers to occur. In all patient teaching, and especially in a cross-cultural situation, individualizing patient teaching is essential. Learning appropriate greetings and phrases in the patient's language and obtaining the services of an interpreter also show sensitivity to cultural differences. Always show respect for folk remedies and traditions valued by the patient and family and make every effort to incorporate them into the patient's healthcare treatment plan. Nurses must recognize that low literacy rates are a problem among patients of all cultures. This may require communicating in simple language both orally and with printed materials that the patient can understand.

Lack of motivation and readiness are often significant barriers to education. The patient may still be upset from an unexpected serious diagnosis and are thus unable to focus on learning or simply may not be motivated to learn what the nurse believes is important to teach. Patients with an external locus of control, for example, believe that nothing they can do will make a difference and may not be motivated to learn about their own illnesses. Often nurses believe that simply pointing out what patients need to know is sufficient to motivate

BOX 13.6 Principles of Adult Learning

- Prior experiences are resources for learning.
  - *Example:* If the patient enjoys gardening, try to link health maintenance suggestions to preventive maintenance of indoor/outdoor plants.
- Readiness to learn is usually related to a social role or developmental task.
  - *Example:* New parents are usually eager to learn how to care for their first infants.
- Motivation to learn is greater when the material is seen as immediately useful.
  - *Example:* The same new parents are more motivated to learn care of the small infant than they are to learn about disciplining toddlers.
- The learning environment must be arranged to facilitate learning.
  - *Example:* The room is quiet and kept at a comfortable temperature, with adequate lighting, privacy, and seating.
- Physical needs are met before the teaching session.
  - *Example:* The patient has his or her reading glasses and/or hearing aid, has been given the opportunity to go to the bathroom, and is relatively pain free.

them. When nurses help the patients make their own decisions about the knowledge they need, teaching is usually more effective. This approach may require greater effort initially, but it is ultimately more efficient to assess patient motivation and readiness first, before engaging in patient teaching.

The nurse who is preparing to teach should also assess and manage the environment. A setting that is private, comfortable, and free of distractions is beneficial to the learning process. Once barriers have been identified and removed to the extent possible, nurses must plan patient education using sound principles of learning and teaching-learning concepts. Although it goes beyond the scope of this text to review all the complexities of learning, certain basic ideas should be considered. The patient's prior experiences, culture, cognitive style, and motivation are all important determinants of learning. The nurse-teacher's knowledge, flexibility, creativity, communication skills, confidence in the patient's ability to learn, and ability to motivate all facilitate or impede learning. Boxes 13.6 and 13.7 include simple principles of adult learning and teaching-learning concepts that are useful in working with patients.

BOX 13.7 Basics of Teaching Patients and Families

- Identify and remove, if possible, barriers to learning.
- Evaluate what the patient and family already know and what they want to know.
- When possible, frequent, short sessions work better than long ones.
- Goals for each session must be realistic.
- Be respectful of cultural differences, for example, in diet planning.
- Avoid medical jargon, acronyms such as "PRN," and slang.
- The presentation should proceed from simple to complex concepts.
- Present complex concepts only after there is mastery of simpler ones.
- Patients learn best when they are actively engaged.
- Learning is enhanced when multiple senses are used: seeing, hearing, telling, and doing make the best combination.
- Practice, or frequent repetition, reinforces skill acquisition.
- Reinforce learning with return demonstrations of skills.
- When you give feedback, be sure to include positives, as well as negatives.
- Written materials should be at a fourth-grade reading level and, if possible, in the patient's first language to make reading easier for the patient.
- Evaluate patient's understanding of the information presented; provide time to clarify misunderstandings and answer questions.
- Remember to document the teaching session and your evaluation of the outcome.

Impact of Illness on Families

Families are best understood as systems, which means that change in one member changes the functioning of the total family. The entire family system is affected by a member's illness. Whether the ill family member is hospitalized or cared for in the home, illness drastically increases stress in a family and disrupts usual family function.

The most important factor in how a family tolerates stress is the individual and group coping abilities. Families already experiencing difficulties may find that their problems are intensified to the point of disruption when acute or chronic illness occurs.

A sick family member has to give up responsibility to other family members. The family must continue to fulfill its usual functions while dealing with the alterations imposed by the illness or absence of a member. Family members who are able to be flexible and assume different roles, who can share their feelings, and who seek assistance may adjust better to changes than those who are inflexible. Some persons are simply resilient and adapt more readily in stressful situations.

Both acute and chronic illnesses cause changes in family functioning and create stress. Chronic illness can be particularly stressful because it is never completely cured. Families experience emotional highs and lows as the patient has remissions and exacerbations. They may experience resentment and other negative feelings. Family members may feel angry too—and often will explain that they are angry "at the situation" and not the person who is sick. Guilt often accompanies the anger of family members. If they cannot deal directly with feelings of anger, they may displace them onto nurses by becoming critical and demanding. Similarly, patients may feel guilty about creating hardships for loved ones. They may become convinced that they are no longer essential because others are capably taking over their roles. Family members sometimes withdraw from each other because they fear that their negative feelings may not be understood and accepted. This mutual withdrawal leads to feelings of isolation for both patients and family members.

Families are often confused or uncertain about how to treat the sick person. They may have problems accepting and responding appropriately to the patients' dependency needs. As discussed earlier, patients may react to illness with either dependent or independent behaviors that sometimes become problematic. Nurses need to monitor whether family members foster dependence, thereby keeping the patient from becoming more independent. Here is a home health nurse's extreme and sad example:

I was taking care of a 37-year-old patient in his own home, where he lived with an older sister who was taking care of him. He was morbidly obese, weighing over 400 pounds and had a lot of health problems. I was doing wound care of deep stasis ulcers on his lower legs. I knew it was going to be hard for them to heal. I did a lot of teaching with him and his sister, who seemed to understand that her brother's healing was going to require that he lose a lot of weight and eat a high-quality diet. Well, we went nowhere fast. No matter what I did, the ulcers got worse and although my patient said that he was trying to lose weight, he did not seem to be making progress. One day I came to her house earlier than usual and his sister was in the kitchen, cooking a tall stack of French toast with syrup for her brother. She laughed a little about "being caught in the act." I realized that I was caught in the middle of a complex relationship where the sister enjoyed "taking care of" her brother, even though this care was not helping him, and that her brother enjoyed being taken care of. I am not sure that "enjoyed" is the right word, but he was very dependent on his sister. One morning a few weeks later, the sister found him dead in his recliner, where he had died watching TV the night before. It was just so sad. I had to come to terms with the fact that I was powerless to change their dynamic and had done the best job I could to help.

As opposed to this tragic situation, nurses should also be aware that some families are uncomfortable with the ill person being dependent and do not allow the necessary "down time" for recovery. For example, if a man who is very much in control in a family has a heart attack and is in the coronary care unit, family members may have difficulty seeing the usually strong father in a helpless position. They may continue to bring family problems to him. Other families may find it difficult to shift responsibilities back to the formerly ill member when they become able to resume role functions, thereby prolonging dependence.

The nurse needs to recognize the anxiety in the family and take steps to reduce it. Talking with family members, explaining what is happening and what to expect, and teaching them how to participate in their family member's care can be helpful. During hospitalizations, it may be helpful to allow family members to be present during invasive procedures such as central line placements and chest tube insertions. Their presence can comfort and support the patient and allay family members' anxiety about such procedures. Some family members of course cannot tolerate seeing procedures being done or hearing expressions of discomfort or pain and should feel free to leave the room. As in any case, the patient's safety comes first.

Some families find that becoming active in seeking information, such as through the Internet, helps them manage their anxieties. Support groups and chat rooms where family members can express their concerns and hear from others with similar issues are also helpful. Nurses can help family members use these adaptive coping activities effectively by assisting them to find credible websites and evaluate the information they find online. The Internet, however, can make things worse. Here is an example from a young man's experience of seeking information on the Internet about a severe birth defect that had been diagnosed in his expected child:

I wrote down the word "anencephaly" on a piece of paper and put it in my pocket. That night after my wife went to bed, I got the paper out and went online to see what I could find out. I saw pictures that I couldn't have imagined and I never want to see again. I got really upset about what my baby might look like. I felt like I had to hide what I had seen from my wife. I wish I hadn't looked.

Nurses must be prepared to accept the anger and distrust that often is directed toward care providers who are unable to cure disease or relieve the negative consequences of illness. Understanding that anger expressed by patients and families is not personally directed can enable nurses to assess patients objectively and respond to feelings expressed in a nondefensive manner. Box 13.8 summarizes common examples of family feelings and behaviors that nurses need to recognize, acknowledge, and explore in a sensitive manner with the family.

Caregiver stress is common in families of patients with prolonged, progressive illnesses, such as Alzheimer's disease and amyotrophic lateral sclerosis (ALS). Caregiver stress looks very much other stressful responses—anxiety symptoms, sleeplessness, fatigue, irritability, and so on. Many associations and support networks are dedicated to the care of persons with progressive illnesses. Caregivers can often find support from people going through the same experience, or who have had the same experience in the past. Nurses who work with patients with progressive illnesses and their families should be aware of which websites are useful and provide substantial support and information.

Despite the numerous stresses, role strains, and adjustments necessitated by illness of a family member, many families find that there are also positive experiences in illness. Finding new activities to share and working together to meet challenges can lead to feelings of closeness and affiliation that were not present before. Previously unrecognized individual strengths may be identified as new roles and responsibilities are assumed. New meanings for the entire family may emerge as values are reassessed, priorities are shifted, and roles become more flexible.

BOX 13.8 Potential Reactions to Illness in a Family Member

- Frightened
- Resentful
- Angry
- Guilty
- Exhausted
- Feelings of uselessness
- Feelings of hopelessness
- Distrust of healthcare providers
- Critical and demanding behavior
- Withdrawal from the situation
- Confusion
- Denial of seriousness of patient's illness
- Promotion of dependence by patient

THE IMPACT OF PROFESSIONAL CAREGIVING ON NURSES

Caring is the foundation of professional nursing practice. Caring meets the essential human need for love and belongingness and assists nurses to provide high-quality nursing care. A caring attitude toward patients, their families, and colleagues begins with the caregiver: the nurse. Many nurses are not accustomed to caring for themselves, tending to put the needs of others before their own. Finding a balance between caring for others and self-care can be a challenging, lifelong pursuit.

Caring for Self While Caring for Others

Nurses can experience **compassion fatigue,** a condition in which one experiences loss of physical energy, burnout, accident proneness, emotional breakdowns, apathy, indifference, poor judgment, and disinterest in being introspective (Coetzee and Klopper, 2010). Nurses often report that the needs of patients and families, as well as their own spouses and children, take priority over their own needs. They are left feeling stretched, overwhelmed, frustrated, unappreciated, and resentful.

Negative feelings interfere with the ability to maintain a caring attitude and drain caring out of our interactions with others. One nurse described his episode with compassion fatigue:

> *I didn't realize how tired and disinterested I had become about my work until one day my wife noted that I never talked about work anymore. Actually, she said that I never really talked about anything anymore. I had no energy, and I felt like every time I walked into the emergency department where I worked that I would scream if I saw one more drop of blood or heard one more patient crying. But I just "turned it off" and quit caring. It was a bad time in my career.*

Although the NANDA-I diagnosis "caregiver role strain" refers to family caregivers and not professional nurses, some of the defining characteristics of this diagnosis are the same for nurses: anger, stress, lack of sleep, increased nervousness, frustration, lack of time to meet personal needs, low work productivity, gastrointestinal upset, impatience, difficulty performing/completing required tasks, lack of support, and insufficient time (Doenges et al., 2004, p. 139). These descriptors could also be applied to nurses who feel overwhelmed with competing demands in their work and professional lives.

Nursing theorist Jean Watson described caring as the essence of nursing practice. Caregivers who are filled with stress and negativity cannot provide an atmosphere conducive to healing. We must learn to care for ourselves to truly care for others. Watson, who is mentioned elsewhere in this text, is founder of the Center for Human Caring in Colorado and a renowned nurse theorist, speaker, and author. She has identified the consequences of caring and noncaring for nurses (Watson, 2005). The consequences of caring for nurses include the following:

- Emotional: spiritual sense of accomplishment, satisfaction, purpose, and gratification
- Preserved integrity, fulfillment, wholeness, and self-esteem
- Living own philosophy
- Respect for life and death
- Reflective; increased knowledge
- Love of nursing

The consequences of noncaring for nurses include the following:

- Hardened attitude
- Oblivious to needs of patients and co-workers
- Robotlike manner
- Depression
- Fear
- Fatigue; worn-down feeling

Watson's work also includes the consequences of caring and noncaring for patients. She identified the consequences of caring for patients as follows:

- Emotional-spiritual: well-being, dignity, self-control, personhood
- Physical: enhanced healing, saved lives, safety, energy, fewer costs, more comfort, less loss
- Trust relationships; decrease in alienation, closer family relationships

The consequences of noncaring for patients, according to Watson, include the following:

- Humiliation, fear, feeling out of control, despair
- Helplessness, alienation, vulnerability
- Lingering bad memories
- Decreased healing, lack of trust, detachment

Professional nurses must stay attuned to themselves to avoid the consequences of noncaring for themselves and their patients. This is a lifelong challenge. How does one go about maintaining the ability to be caring? Diann Uustal (2009), an early proponent of work-life balance, recommended "creating a balanced life rather than merely maintaining a balancing act" (p. 7). She uses the analogy of the announcement heard before every flight departure: "Put on your own oxygen mask first, before assisting others who may need it" (p. 13). That announcement has a lot of relevance to our lives as professional caregivers. Just as airline passengers in an emergency depressurization need oxygen before they can help others, nurses need to meet their own needs so that they will have the physical and emotional energy to care for others.

Choosing to work in a setting that supports caring and professional nursing practice is an important strategy to reduce the stress nurses feel while at work. Hospitals are very stressful working environments for nurses today. Because of the nursing shortages and the expense involved in hiring and orienting new staff, nursing leaders in hospitals are focusing on retention—that is, keeping the nurses that they have. They realize that the work environment can help nurses cope with stress in the workplace, thereby enhancing retention. In the early 2000's, some hospitals were intentional in creating work setting based on principles of caring, involving the input of nurses to determine the best ways to ensure a good work environment.

Magnet Recognition Program

Another program that supports nurses is the American Nurses Credentialing Center's (ANCC's) Magnet Recognition Program. This program formally recognizes healthcare organizations that have a proven level of excellence in nursing care. Achieving Magnet designation demonstrates the importance of nursing and nurses to the entire organization and signals the importance of quality care and a positive practice environment for nurses. It recognizes the caliber of the nursing staff, which validates nurses for their hard work and elevates the self-esteem of the entire nursing staff. These facilities strive to be "nurse friendly," have low turnover and vacancy rates, and provide opportunities for professional and personal growth. All these factors lead to better patient care and greater career satisfaction.

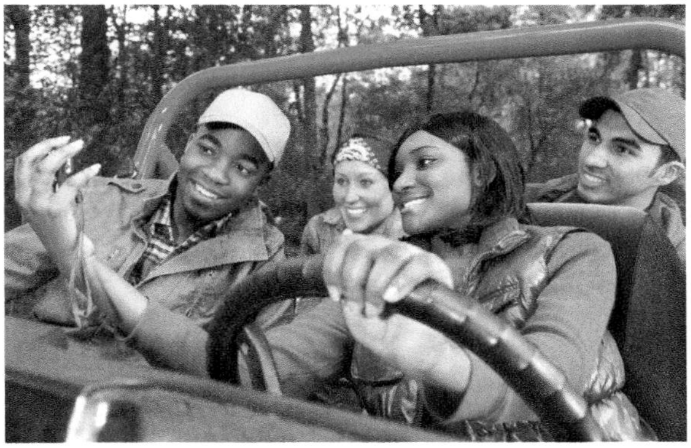

Fig. 13.4 By spending time having fun outside of the hospital, these nurses are taking care of themselves. Self-care is crucial in creating a long and healthy nursing career. (Photo used with permission from iStockphoto.)

Developing and Maintaining a Life-Work Balance

Nurses who feel chronically exhausted and irritable at home and at work; who worry more than usual, cannot seem to complete tasks, lack concentration, and/or are forgetful; and who have diminished self-confidence should be aware that these symptoms indicate a need for more self-care. Keeping the balance between work and personal responsibilities takes conscious and continuous effort. To remain energized and fully engaged in your profession, however, you can learn strategies to help you develop and maintain a life-work balance. Just as nurses use treatment plans to organize how they care for patients, they can also identify how to create balance in their own lives. Taking time to be with your friends and colleagues outside of work is an important strategy to reenergize yourself and prepare for the demands at work (Fig. 13.4).

Diann Uustal, in her book *Caring for Yourself, Caring for Others: The Ultimate Balance* (2009), recommended taking stock periodically using the guidelines listed in Box 13.9. Read these guidelines, and think about how you can begin now to apply them in your busy life. This can be the beginning of a lifelong effort to maintain balance so that you can continue to be the caring person you want to be in all aspects of your life.

BOX 13.9 Create a Balanced Life Care Plan for Yourself

Read the following ideas and reflect on their practical application in your life.

- Taking personal responsibility for your health—physically, emotionally, intellectually, socially, and spiritually—is not easy, but it is the first step. Like it or not, there is no one who can do a better job of taking care of yourself than you.
- Start today with the changes you know are healthful. Make your choices one meal at a time or one day at a time. Do not beat yourself up if you do not always stick to the care plan.
- Balance. Try to stay in balance from a holistic perspective. What this means is different to each of us and different at various stages in our own lives.
- Increase your happiness quotient. Identify the things that bring you happiness and joy and enhance your quality of life. Try to do something pleasurable or satisfying each day.
- Identify and decrease the stressors in your personal and professional life. Develop strategies for decreasing the overall level of stress in your life. Some situations and habits can be corrected easily; others will take a real commitment and time to change.
- Make sure your goals and expectations are realistic. Unrealistic goals are self-defeating. Make sure the goals are measurable, manageable, and meaningful to you, not to please somebody else.

BOX 13.9 Create a Balanced Life Care Plan for Yourself—cont'd

- Give yourself permission to relax and take some time for yourself each day. Learn to take "mental health breaks," no matter how brief. Enjoy the time without thinking about what you should be doing, so you can return refreshed.
- Prioritize your commitments based on your values. Make sure you give appropriate time and attention to the relationships that have stability and meaning over time.
- Learn to say "no" if you are pressured and overcommitted. Learn to say no without feeling guilty. Practice thinking that every problem is not your sole responsibility.
- Treat yourself like you treat your best friend. Do something special and befriend yourself.
- Be a person of encouragement—to yourself. Be affirming to yourself. Do not criticize yourself harshly.
- Make your physical fitness a priority. Commit to a balanced fitness program that includes stretching, aerobic exercise, and strength exercises. Work exercise into your daily life and exercise with a friend if possible.
- Nutrition. Eat a balanced diet, drink lots of water, and limit refined sugar intake. Practice portion control. If necessary, consult a dietitian.
- Sleep. Know how much you need and plan to get it. A pattern of too little sleep can affect your health negatively. Avoid trying to be more productive by sleeping less. That can be counterproductive.
- Pay attention to your spiritual growth. If you have a specific religious faith, is your faith a first resort or a last resort when all else fails? What does it mean to be "spiritual"? Is being a part of a faith community important to you? Remember that being "spiritual" and "religious" are not the same.
- Challenge yourself intellectually and develop your intellectual curiosity. Try to learn something new every day, no matter how small or insignificant it may seem.
- Stay connected with healthy people. Set time aside and plan for fun with people who can help you lighten up and enjoy some free time. Get out and do things you enjoy doing.
- Spend as little time as possible with people who affect you negatively.
- Make sure you get enough time alone. How much time alone each of us needs varies, so find out what is right for you. Most caregivers spend very little time alone. Check out your balance.
- Express your creativity through music, painting, needlework, sports, decorating, acting, or whatever lets you share yourself from the inside out.
- Don't be afraid to talk with a friend or a professional counselor to help you clarify your direction and put you back in balance again.

From Uustal DB: The ultimate balance: caring for yourself - caring for others. *Orthopedic nursing,* 11(3), 11–15, 1992.

CONCEPTS AND CHALLENGES

- ***Concept:*** Illness is a highly personal experience and reactions to illness are affected by one's culture.
  Challenge: Culture is not always determinative of a person's responses to illness; explaining a response in terms of culture only can lead to stereotyping.
- ***Concept:*** Persons with illness may experience disbelief and denial, become irritable and angry, attempt to gain control, become depressed, and, eventually, come to accept their circumstance and participate in their own care.
  Challenge: Responses to illness are not encountered in a linear way. Patients will move back and forth between these reactions.
- ***Concept:*** Because of the stress and anxiety involved with illness, patients' abilities to cope may be tested.
  Challenge: Resourcefulness and resilience are characteristics of some persons who may cope with change and stress well, but coping skills can be taught to those who are not naturally as resourceful or resilient.
- ***Concept:*** Providing holistic care means that nurses must consider their patients' physical, mental, emotional, spiritual, social, cultural, and family strengths and challenges to personalize care.
  Challenge: Recognizing that family is a system in which a change in one member affects all the other members helps nurses anticipate ways in which a family may be affected by illness.
- ***Concept:*** Illness causes alterations in usual family functioning that results in emotional responses such as anger and guilt; old patterns such as fostering dependence can become very entrenched during illness.
  Challenge: The nurse needs to assess both how the family is influencing the patient and how the

family is being influenced by the member who is ill.

- ***Concept:*** An understanding of the cultural factors that affect behaviors associated with illness can provide a better framework for the provision of nursing care that is both effective and satisfying to patients, families, and nurses.

Challenge: Understanding that culture influences health behaviors and responses is not the same as understanding a particular culture. Effective nurses have cultural humility.

- ***Concept and Challenge:*** Creating a work-life balance, in which caring for self has a high priority, is the key to sustaining a caring approach to others.

IDEAS FOR FURTHER EXPLORATION

1. If you or someone close to you has been hospitalized, how did the nurses and family members encourage or discourage dependent behaviors? Independent behaviors?
2. Try to identify your own cultural group's response to illness. What are your family's characteristic responses to illness of a family member?
3. In a small group, discuss aspects of spiritual nursing care that you have been exposed to, feel comfortable using, or do not feel comfortable using. Appoint a group member to monitor those interventions or behaviors that primarily benefit the patient and those that primarily benefit the nurse. What stands out to you in terms of your response to providing spiritual care?
4. Identify the ways you show a caring attitude toward patients and toward yourself. Who do you treat better: your patients or yourself? In what ways can you provide better care for yourself?
5. Plan a nurse-friendly work setting. What would make it nurse-friendly? Would being nurse-friendly affect the level of care your patients would receive?

REFERENCES

American Association of Colleges of Nursing: Cultural competency in baccalaureate nursing education, 2008. (website). Available at: www.aacn.nche.edu/leading-initiatives/education-resources/competency.pdf.

Benson H, Klipper MZ: *The relaxation response, twenty-fifth anniversary update*, New York, 2000, HarperCollins.

Brookings Institution: The nation is diversifying even faster than predicted, according to new census data, 2021. (website). Available at: https://www.brookings.edu/research/new-census-data-shows-the-nation-is-diversifying-even-faster-than-predicted/

Carey B: *Long-Awaited Medical Study Questions the Power of Prayer*, 2006, New York Times. [website]. Available at www.nytimes.com/2006/03/31/health/31pray.html?ex=;1145937600&en=3cd622f0fc1f109b&ei=5070.

Centers for Disease Control and Prevention: Prevalence of multiple chronic conditions among US adults, 2020 (website). Available at: https://www.cdc.gov/pcd/issues/2020/20_0130.htm.

Coetzee SK, Klopper HC: Compassion fatigue within nursing practice: a concept analysis, *Nurs Heal Sci* 12:235–243, 2010.

Doenges ME, Moorhouse MF, Murr AC: *Nursing care plans: guidelines for individualizing client care across the life span*, Philadelphia, 2014, FA Davis.

Greene-Moton E, Minkler M: Cultural competence or cultural humility? moving beyond the debate, *Health Promot Pract* 21(1):142–145, 2020. doi:10.1177/1524839919884912.

Karademas EC, Karamvakalis N, Zarogiannos A: Life context and the experience of chronic illness: is the stress of life associated with illness perceptions and coping?, *Stress Heal* 25:405–412, 2009.

Leininger M: *Personal communication,* 1999.

Massachusetts General Hospital Benson-Henry Institute for Mind Body Medicine, 2015. (website). Available at:. https://bensonhenryinstitute.org

McEwen M: Spiritual nursing care: state of the art, *Holist Nurs Pract* 19(4):161–168, 2005.

Parsons T: *The social system*, New York, 1964, Free Press.

Selye H: *The stress of life*, New York, 1956, McGraw-Hill.

U.S. Department of Health and Human Services: *Office of Minority Health: National Standards for Culturally and Linguistically Appropriate Services in Health Care, [Final report]*, Washington, DC, 2001, U.S. Department of Health and Human Services.

Uustal DB: *Caring for yourself, caring for others: the ultimate balance*, 2, Jamestown, RI, 2009, Sea Spirit Press.

Uustal DB: The ultimate balance: caring for yourself – caring for others, *Orthopedic Nurs* 11(3), 11–15, 1992.

Watson J: *Caring science as sacred science: caritas/love and caring-healing*, King of Prussia, Penn, 2005, presentation at the American Holistic Nurses Association 25th Annual Conference.

14

Health Care in the United States

ⓔ To enhance your understanding of this chapter, try the Student Exercises on the Evolve site at http://evolve.elsevier.com/Black/professional.

LEARNING OUTCOMES

After studying this chapter, students will be able to:

- Describe the four basic categories of services provided by the healthcare delivery system.
- Describe the shared governance model, and explain its use in nursing.
- Relate two major mechanisms used to maintain quality in healthcare agencies.
- Explain how disparities in healthcare disproportionately affect minority and poor populations.
- Identify the key members of the interprofessional healthcare team, and explain what each contributes.
- Explain the economic principles of supply and demand, free-market economies, and price sensitivity, and discuss their relevance to healthcare costs.
- Describe current methods of payment for healthcare.
- Discuss the possibility of universal healthcare as an outcome of healthcare reform.

TODAY'S HEALTHCARE SYSTEM

Healthcare reform continues to be a hot topic in American life and across the political scene. How healthcare is delivered, how it is accessed, and how it is paid for have become polarizing issues. The complexities and detail cause misunderstanding and confusion. This complicated debate mirrors the system of healthcare in place in the United States today.

The term *healthcare system* as it is used in the U.S. is a misnomer. Rather than providing healthcare, the system has traditionally provided illness care, focusing on treating health problems once they have occurred rather than encouraging wellness through healthy habits. The complexity of the system has resulted in fragmentation that is difficult to understand and navigate. Although the U.S. has some of the most cutting edge healthcare technologies, sophisticated procedures, and well-educated healthcare providers, many people do not have access to basic care and even fewer to care focused on wellness.

In 1979 the federal government initiated the *Healthy People* program, a science-based program that sets forth national objectives focusing on health promotion and disease prevention every 10 years. *Healthy People* sets new national health objectives for each decade and monitors the progress of these objectives, building on lessons learned in the previous decade. Input is sought from both experts and the general public through a collaborative process. The *Healthy People* campaign was instituted in the late 1990s to establish health benchmarks and monitor progress toward these benchmarks. The intention was to encourage collaborations across communities and sectors; empower persons to make informed health decisions; and measure the impact of prevention activities (www.healthypeople.gov). *Healthy People 2030* is a more streamlined version: there are 335 main objectives, as opposed to the more than 1000 in the 2020 version (Healthy People 2030 Framework, 2021). This was done to avoid overlap and confusion among workgroups charged with assessing movement toward the objectives. Despite this decrease in objectives, the 2030 campaign provides a comprehensive plan to move Americans toward better health by the end of the decade. The full plan with objectives can be found at https://health.gov/healthypeople.

The *Healthy People* initiative encourages individuals, agencies, communities, and states to participate in its programs, but it does not mandate change in the healthcare system. The passage of the State Children's Health Insurance Program (SCHIP) reauthorization legislation in 2009 and the Affordable Care Act (ACA) in 2010 were crucial steps in addressing systemic problems in the healthcare system, particularly with regard to the financing of healthcare by improving access to health insurance coverage for most Americans. The ACA, known colloquially as "Obamacare," has withstood two significant challenges in the U.S. Supreme Court, one in 2012 and the other in 2015. Most recently, in 2017, an effort by Senate Republicans to repeal and replace the ACA failed because of a shortfall of support. There will no doubt be challenges ahead to maintain affordable healthcare insurance coverage for Americans.

You are likely to enter the nursing workforce with much of the current system still recognizable. This chapter will give you basic information about the way health (and illness) care is delivered in the United States and nursing's role within this system; healthcare finance is also addressed.

Major Categories of Healthcare Services

Four major categories of health services make up the current system: (1) health promotion and maintenance, including early detection; (2) illness prevention; (3) diagnosis and treatment; and (4) rehabilitation and long-term care. Even though these services are provided in a wide variety of settings, virtually all care falls into one of these four categories.

Health Promotion and Maintenance

Health promotion and maintenance services assist patients to remain healthy, prevent diseases and injuries, detect diseases early, and promote healthier lifestyles. These services require patients' active participation and cannot be performed solely by healthcare providers. Health promotion and maintenance services are based on the assumption that patients who adopt healthy behaviors are more likely to avoid certain illnesses such as heart attacks, lung cancers, and certain infections than those whose behaviors are not as healthy.

An example of health promotion and maintenance services is prenatal classes. By adopting good nutritional and exercise habits, a pregnant woman may improve the likelihood that she will have a healthy infant born at full term. Other examples of health promotion and maintenance include education about safe driving, alcohol consumption, and responsible sexual activity.

Health promotion also includes the detection of warning signs indicating the presence of a disease in early stages. Early detection may mean minimal and less costly treatment and good patient outcomes. An example of early detection is breast self-examination and mammography, both aimed at detecting breast cancer in its early stages, thereby providing a better chance for successful treatment. Experts disagree, however, about the necessity or wisdom of screening such as mammography or prostate-specific antigen (PSA) that may result in a high number of false-positive results and unnecessary treatment and stress associated with a positive diagnosis. Recommendations about health screenings change as we gain new knowledge from ongoing research studies. It is important for nurses to be aware of the latest recommendations for health promotion and maintenance.

Illness Prevention

With the increasing ability to identify risk factors, such as a family history of disease and genetic predispositions, illness prevention services are now better able to assist patients in reducing the impact of those risk factors on their health and well-being. These services require the patient's active participation.

Prevention services differ from health promotion services in that they address health problems after risk factors are identified, whereas health promotion services seek to prevent development of risk factors. For example, a health promotion program might teach the detrimental effects of alcohol and drugs on health to prevent individuals from using alcohol and drugs. Illness prevention services are used when the patient has been abusing alcohol or drugs and is at risk for developing conditions related to using these substances. The boundaries between health promotion and maintenance, early detection, and illness prevention are often blurred. During the COVID-19 pandemic of the early 2020s, illness prevention efforts took the form of wearing masks, practicing distancing, and vaccine administration. Box 14.1 gives examples of activities in these three areas.

Diagnosis and Treatment

Traditionally, in the U.S. healthcare system, heavy emphasis has been put on diagnosis and treatment.

BOX 14.1 Examples of Health Promotion and Maintenance, Early Detection, and Illness Prevention Activities

Health Promotion/Maintenance

- Health education programs (e.g., prenatal classes)
- Exercise programs
- Health fairs
- Wellness programs (worksite/school)
- Nutrition education

Early Detection

- Mammograms
- Vision and hearing screening
- Cholesterol screening
- Periodic histories and physical examinations
- Blood glucose screening
- Osteoporosis screening

Illness Prevention

- Community health programs
- Promotion of healthy lifestyles to counteract risk factors
- Occupational safety programs (e.g., use of eye protection for work that endangers the eyes)
- Environmental safety programs (e.g., proper disposal of hazardous waste)
- Legislation that prevents injury or disease (e.g., seat belt/child restraint laws; motorcycle helmet laws).
- Vaccine mandates to prevent serious and life-threatening infectious illnesses.

Modern technology has enabled the medical profession to refine methods of diagnosing illnesses and disorders and to treat them more effectively than in the past. Scientific advances permit many noninvasive tests and treatments to be performed. For instance, imaging has become important in diagnosing and following the size and location of solid tumor cancers through sophisticated combinations of positron emission tomography (PET) and computed tomography (CT) images. In addition, three-dimensional (3-D) ultrasonography creates 3-D images of various organs and structures, including fetal development. Another example of advanced technology is called breast tomosynthesis, which is a special mammography technique that provides a 3-D picture that gives a clearer image and makes it easier to detect a breast mass. The future promises more noninvasive visual technologies that will aid in diagnosis and treatment.

Minimally invasive surgery techniques have transformed surgical procedures, allowing incisions of a half-inch or less. This technology has reduced postoperative pain; reduced hospital stays from days to hours, thereby reducing costs; and enabled patients to return to normal function much more rapidly. Surgical procedures that reduce postoperative pain are especially favorable because of the national attention on the issue of addiction and the sense of urgency to reduce the use of prescription opioids.

Unfortunately, high-tech services can lead patients to feel dehumanized. This occurs when caregivers focus on machines and techniques rather than on patients. Even in high-tech settings, nurses must remember that patients benefit most when they understand their diagnoses and treatments and can be active participants in the development and implementation of their own treatment plans, in other words, when care is patient-centered.

Rehabilitation and Long-Term Care

Rehabilitation services help restore the patient to the fullest possible level of function and independence after injury or illness. Rehabilitation programs also deal with conditions that leave patients with diminished functioning, such as strokes or severe burns. Both patients and their families must be active participants in this care if it is to be successful. Rehabilitation services should begin as soon as the patient's condition has stabilized after an injury or illness. These services may be provided in institutional settings such as hospitals, in special rehabilitation facilities, in long-term care facilities such as nursing homes, or in the home and the community. The objectives of rehabilitation are to assist patients to achieve the highest level of functioning possible so that they may have the best quality of life they can.

Rehabilitation services also include **disease management** services. Disease management services deal with chronic diseases, such as congestive heart failure and diabetes, and ongoing conditions, such as low back pain and hypertension, that contribute to higher healthcare costs and a reduced quality of life, particularly for aging populations. Disease management programs focus on helping patients understand and manage their chronic conditions more effectively through phone/telehealth calls or e-mails, coaching and education, symptom prevention and management, and collaboration with their providers. These steps give providers information between office visits so that they can actively manage the patient's condition before emergency or hospital services are required, thus reducing healthcare costs and improving the quality of life for their patients.

Long-term care is provided in residential facilities such as assisted living, intermediate and skilled nursing facilities, and personal care homes. Personal care homes provide housing, food, and one or more personal services for two or more adults who are not related to the owner of the home. Long-term care is defined and regulated by states. Long-term care is tailored to provide services that the patient or family cannot provide but at levels that maintain the individual's independence as long as possible. The population is aging, and with more patients surviving serious trauma and living with illnesses that involve impairments in physical or mental functioning or both, long-term care facilities are expected to experience continuing growth.

Classifications of Healthcare Agencies

There are many agencies involved in the total healthcare delivery system. Organizations that deliver care can be classified in three major ways: as governmental or voluntary agencies; as not-for-profit or for-profit agencies; or by the level of healthcare services they provide.

Governmental (Public) Agencies

Many governmental (public) agencies contribute to the health and well-being of U.S. citizens. All these public agencies are primarily supported by taxes, administered by elected or appointed officials, and tailored to the needs of the public.

Federal agencies. Federal agencies focus on the health of all U.S. citizens. They promote and conduct health and illness research, provide funding to train healthcare workers, and assist communities in planning and evaluating the outcomes of healthcare services. They also develop health programs and services and provide financial and personnel support to staff them. Federal agencies establish standards of practice and safety for healthcare workers and conduct national health education programs on subjects such as the benefits of not smoking, the prevention of acquired immunodeficiency syndrome (AIDS), and the need for prenatal care. Examples of federal agencies are the Centers for Medicare & Medicaid Services (CMS), the National Institutes of Health, the U.S. Department of Health and Human Services, the Occupational Safety and Health Administration, and the Centers for Disease Control and Prevention (CDC). An example of a federally supported agency that provides care at the local level is the Federally Qualified Health Center (FQHC). According to the Health Resources and Services Administration (HRSA, 2018), an FQHC can provide primary care, dental services, and mental health services for underserved populations, such as migrant workers, the homeless, and residents of public housing.

State agencies. State health agencies oversee programs that affect the health of citizens within an individual state. Examples of state agencies include state departments of health and environment; departments of mental health; regulatory bodies that regulate and license health professionals, such as state boards of nursing; and agencies that administer Medicaid insurance programs for families and individuals in poverty. These agencies are not typically involved in providing direct patient care but license and support local agencies that do provide direct care.

Local agencies. Local agencies serve one community, one county, or a few adjacent counties. They provide services to both paying and nonpaying citizens. Public health departments are examples of local governmental agencies found in almost every county in the United States. All citizens, whether or not they can pay, are eligible for certain healthcare services through local public health departments. These services usually include immunizations, prenatal care and counseling, well-baby and well-child clinics, sexually transmitted infection clinics, tuberculosis clinics, and others. Community health nurses sometimes make home visits as well.

Voluntary (Private) Agencies and Nongovernmental Organizations

Citizens often voluntarily support agencies working to promote or restore health. When private volunteers support an agency providing healthcare, it is called a voluntary (private) agency. Support is generally through private donations, although many of these agencies apply for governmental grants to support some of their activities.

Voluntary agencies often begin when a group of individuals bands together to address a health problem. Volunteers may initially perform all their services. Later they may obtain enough donations to hire personnel, staff an office, and expand services. They may be able to secure ongoing funding through grants or organizations such as the United Way. Examples of voluntary health agencies are the American Heart Association, the American Cancer Society, the American Red Cross, and the March of Dimes.

A nongovernmental organization (NGO) is an association of citizens that operates independently of the government with the goal to deliver resources or serve a social or political purpose. Much of the focus of health-related NGOs is international and involves the delivery of direct healthcare, providing drinkable water, mitigating endemic diseases such as malaria, and improving nutrition, among other highly significant causes. Médecins Sans Frontières (Doctors Without Borders) is a well-known NGO, as are the International Committee of the Red Cross, Oxfam, Project Hope, and Save the Children.

Not-for-Profit or For-Profit Agencies

The second major way to classify health service delivery agencies is by what is done with the income earned by the agency. A not-for-profit agency is one that uses profits to pay personnel, improve services, advertise services, provide educational programs, or otherwise contribute to the mission of the agency. A common misconception is that not-for-profit agencies do not ever make a profit. Actually, they may make profits, but the profits are used to further the mission of the agency; there are no partners or shareholders to pay in not-for-profit agencies. Most voluntary agencies, such as the ones listed previously, are also not-for-profit agencies, as are many hospitals. The Joint Commission is an independent, not-for-profit organization that certifies healthcare organizations and programs in the United States.

For-profit agencies distribute profits earned to partners or shareholders. The growth in for-profit healthcare agencies has risen over the past several decades because of the potential for healthcare to be very profitable.

For-profit agencies include numerous home healthcare companies that send nurses and other health personnel to care for patients at home. Several large national chains of for-profit healthcare providers also exist and have demonstrated that it is possible to provide quality patient care and make a profit while doing so. Examples include national nursing home networks, specialty outpatient centers for ambulatory surgery, heart hospitals, urgent care clinics, and rehabilitation centers. A controversial issue related to for-profit healthcare organizations is the possibility that they might not treat nonpaying patients, meaning that these persons must go to publicly funded facilities that may be overburdened with patients who are unable to afford expensive healthcare.

Level of Healthcare Services Provided

The third way in which healthcare services can be classified is by the level of healthcare services they provide. These levels have traditionally been termed *primary care, secondary care,* and *tertiary care.* A new level—*subacute care*—has emerged. These four levels are discussed next.

Primary care services. Care rendered at the point at which a patient first enters the healthcare system is considered **primary care**. This care may be provided in student health clinics, community health centers, emergency departments, physicians' offices, nurse practitioners' clinics, or health clinics at worksites. The major goals of the primary healthcare system are providing the following:

1. Entry into the system
2. Emergency care
3. Health maintenance
4. Management of long-term and chronic conditions
5. Treatment of temporary health problems that do not require hospitalization

In addition to treating common health problems, primary care centers are, for many citizens, where much of prevention and health promotion takes place. Access to primary care in the least costly setting is now mandated by third-party payers such as insurance companies, the government, and managed care organizations.

Secondary care services. **Secondary care** involves the management of a condition or illness by a specialist (e.g., endocrinologist, cardiologist, pulmonologist, oncologist) after having been referred by one's primary care provider. This includes management of patients with suspected or new diagnoses of a complex illness; evaluating patients with chronic illness who may need treatment changes; and providing counseling or other therapies that are not available in primary care settings.

Tertiary care services. **Tertiary care** services are those provided to acutely ill patients, to those requiring long-term care, to those needing rehabilitation services, and to terminally ill patients. Tertiary care usually involves many health professionals working on interdisciplinary teams to design and implement treatment plans. Examples of tertiary agencies are specialized hospitals such as trauma centers, burn centers, and pediatric hospitals; long-term care facilities offering skilled nursing, intermediate care, and supportive care; rehabilitation centers; and hospices, where care is provided to the terminally ill and their families in the hospital, in the home, or in freestanding, independent hospice homes that provide a setting for terminally ill patients to die in comfort. An extension of tertiary care is even more specialized care sometimes referred to as quaternary care, such as at a research facility or very uncommon, highly specialized surgery requiring exceptional levels of training and expertise, such as fetal surgery.

Subacute care services. An additional segment of healthcare—subacute care services—emerged in the 1990s. Subacute care is goal-oriented, comprehensive inpatient care designed for an individual who has had an acute illness, injury, or exacerbation of a disease process. In general, the condition of an individual receiving subacute care is less complex than acute care and does not depend heavily on high-technology monitoring or complex diagnostic procedures. The goal of subacute services is to provide lower-cost healthcare and create a seamless transition for patients moving through the healthcare system.

Subacute care is generally more intensive than skilled nursing facility care and less intensive than acute inpatient care. It requires frequent patient assessment and review of the clinical course and treatment plan for a limited time ranging from several days to several months, until a condition is stabilized or a predetermined treatment course is completed.

In each of the types of healthcare services and agencies presented in this chapter, there is an important role for nurses to fulfill.

Organizational Structures Within Healthcare Agencies

The healthcare delivery system in the United States consists of a variety of agencies such as hospitals, clinics, associations, long-term care facilities, and home health services that provide any of the four major types of health services just discussed. Although the mission, category, and level of healthcare services provided vary, the organizational structures within them may be similar.

Organizational Structure

Organizational structure refers to how an agency is organized to accomplish its mission. The organizational structure of most agencies includes a governing body or board of directors, which may also be called a board of trustees.

Board of directors. In the past, board members were often chosen from two groups: community philanthropists, who were expected to donate generously to the facility; and physicians, who practiced in the institution. Boards were large, met infrequently, and had mainly ceremonial functions such as "rubber stamping" executive decisions or attending fundraising events.

As the healthcare environment has become more complex, board members are now chosen to represent various business and political interests of the community. They are expected to bring knowledge and expertise from the business world, as well as to have an appreciation and understanding of healthcare agencies and how they operate. Because nurses have particular expertise and perspectives about healthcare, they are often sought out to serve on boards.

Boards now carry significant responsibility and accountability for the mission of the organization, the quality of services provided, and the financial stability of the organization. Boards are not involved in the day-to-day running of the agency, but they are legally responsible for establishing policies governing operations and for ensuring that the policies are executed. They delegate responsibility for running the agency to the chief executive officer (CEO). Boards of directors may or may not be paid for their services. Box 14.2 is a list of the primary responsibilities of the board of directors of a healthcare organization. In Professional Profile Box 14.1, the author of this text describes her role and activities as a director on the board of a large not-for-profit end-of-life care organization.

Chief executive officer. The chief executive officer (CEO) is the individual responsible for the overall daily operation and the strategic planning for the organization. They usually have a minimum of a master's degree in business or hospital administration. Responsibilities

BOX 14.2 Board of Directors Responsibilities in Healthcare Organizations

- Establish mission, visions, goals, and strategic plan
- Ensure the organization's financial health
- Ensure quality patient care
- Select and evaluate the CEO
- Board self-evaluation

From www.ache.org.

PROFESSIONAL PROFILE BOX 14.1

A Member of the Board: Using the Lessons of Nursing

As a lifelong resident of the Triangle area of North Carolina (Raleigh-Durham-Chapel Hill), I had always known that Hospice of Wake County (HOWC) was the primary provider of end-of-life care in the area. Several close family members received expert care from this agency at the end of their lives. When I was nominated and then elected to serve a 3-year term on the 23-member Board of Directors (BOD), I was both humbled and pleased for the chance to give back something to HOWC, which is now known as Transitions LifeCare. I was one of the few nurses ever to serve on the board in its 30-plus years of existence. Although I was a former hospice nurse, I will admit I was pretty intimidated by the collective wisdom and expertise of the other directors, who represented a host of other professions, including law, marketing, finance, medicine, clergy, and funeral home management. I couldn't imagine how much I was going to learn about organizational structure, healthcare finance, quality indicators, not-for-profit governance, and strategic planning.

At the start of my second year on the BOD, I made a plea at a board meeting to consider the development and implementation of a pediatric palliative and end-of-life care program. My faculty research and collaboration with local providers had demonstrated the profound need for this service. Planning for and implementing a pediatric program was added to the BOD's strategic plan. At the time, we had five service lines: hospice, palliative care, grief counseling, a caregiver support service, and home health. And in September 2015 we opened our sixth service line, Transitions Kids, a comprehensive palliative and end-of-life-care for children and their families.

In my second term, I was elected president of the board. As I reflect on my long nursing career, I think that my work on the Board of Directors has been among the most meaningful endeavors of my professional life. After a required year off the board after my second 3-year term, I was reelected to the board and am now in my third term and 10th year of service. I am both honored and humbled to continue to serve this organization, using the lessons that nursing taught me to improve the lives of families at their most difficult, vulnerable time.

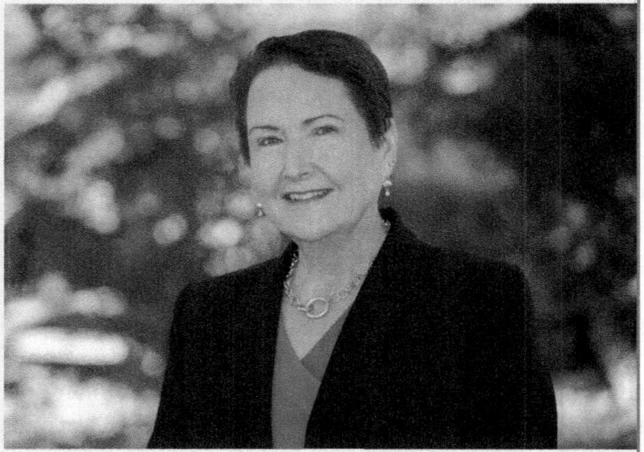

Beth Perry Black, PhD, RN, FAAN

Courtesy Beth Perry Black

include making sure that the institution runs efficiently and is cost effective and carrying out policies established by the board. The CEO also has an important external role addressing healthcare issues in the community and usually sits on the board of directors, as well as reports to it. In larger organizations, a chief operating officer (COO) often assists the CEO to make decisions for the daily operations and leadership of the organization.

Nurses with advanced degrees and experience in administration, business, and healthcare policy increasingly occupy both CEO and COO positions. Boards, which are responsible for hiring CEOs, have found that the broad holistic education and clinical experience of nurses prepare them well for these positions.

Medical staff. A medical staff consists of physicians, who may be either employees of the healthcare organization or independent practitioners. In either case, they must be granted privileges by the board of directors to care for patients at that particular institution. They cannot simply decide to admit patients to an institution. A credentials committee, composed of members of the medical staff, performs the credentialing process. This committee is charged with the responsibility of assuring the board of directors that every physician admitted to the medical staff of that facility is a qualified and competent practitioner and that, over time, each one keeps his or her skills and knowledge updated.

In large medical centers associated with university schools of medicine, the medical staff may include house staff, that is, intern and resident physicians in their first years after completing medical school. Physician residencies are 3 to 4 years and are sometimes followed by fellowships that provide additional training in a specific field such as maternal-fetal medicine, neonatology, and pediatric surgery. Residents and fellows provide much of the hour-to-hour medical care of patients hospitalized in these settings; attending physicians make rounds with the residents and fellows usually once a day. Hospitalists—physicians who work in inpatient settings only—are becoming increasingly visible members of the healthcare team, managing patient care needs when a primary physician is unavailable or needs consultation. Likewise, nurse practitioners, particularly those with acute care certification, are increasingly filling a role in hospitals to provide care for hospitalized patients around the clock.

The medical staff, through its credentials committee, is also charged with the responsibility for credentialing providers such as advanced practice nurses, psychologists, optometrists, podiatrists, and others who admit or consult with patients.

Medical staff governance. In large organizations, medical staffs are usually organized by service (e.g., department of surgery, department of medicine, department of maternal-fetal medicine). The entire medical staff usually elects a **chief of staff**. The chief of staff and the chiefs of the various services work together with the CEO and other administrative representatives through the medical executive committee to make important decisions about medical policy and physician discipline for the institution. The rules and regulations that govern these activities are called bylaws. The board of directors, to which the physicians are responsible, must officially approve the credentialing and disciplinary actions of the medical staff.

Service on committees and leadership positions of the medical staff are time-consuming activities; therefore some institutions pay members of the medical staff a fee for special services or a stipend in recognition that time away from seeing patients reduces their income.

Nursing staff. The senior administrative nurse in an organization is known as the **chief nurse executive** (CNE) or **chief nursing officer** (CNO), vice president for nursing, or in smaller hospitals, director of nursing. Once excluded from broad institutional decision making, nurse executives today are often members of the board of directors. Progressive organizations now recognize that the CNE and the chief of the medical staff are of equal importance, and this is reflected in their organizational charts.

The educational preparation of CNEs typically requires a minimum of a master's degree in nursing, business, or health administration. Some nurse executives hold joint Master of Science in Nursing and master of business administration (MSN/MBA) degrees or joint master of health administration and master of business administration (MHA/MBA) degrees. Many nurse executives are also choosing educational preparation at the doctoral level with a focus on leadership, such as the Doctor of Nursing Practice (DNP) degree.

CNEs are responsible for overseeing all the nursing care provided in the institution and serve as clinical leaders and administrators. Because of the need to coordinate patient care and outcomes among all disciplines, the role may also include administrative responsibilities for departments other than nursing, such as surgery, pharmacy, respiratory therapy, and social services, among others.

The nursing staff consists of all the registered nurses (RNs), licensed practical nurses/licensed vocational nurses (LPNs/LVNs), unlicensed assistive personnel (UAP), and, in some settings, clerical and administrative assistants hired by the department of nursing. These staff members are usually organized according to the units on which they work.

Each patient care unit has its own budget and staff, for which the unit manager is responsible. The manager, who is usually a nurse, is also a communication link between the staff and the next level of management.

In large or networked organizations, there may be an additional level of management between the nurse executive and the manager of a unit. These are middle managers, known as clinical directors or supervisors. In most cases they are also nurses, but they may come from other clinical disciplines or from a business background. These directors are responsible for multiple units or for specific projects or programs. They ensure that nursing and all other services they manage are integrated with other hospital services. They also serve as the communication link between the unit managers and the executive staff.

Other nurses combine direct patient care responsibilities with research, education, and management responsibilities, such as nurse educators, nurse researchers, clinical nurse specialists, and infection control nurses. Nurses in these roles support direct care nurses and serve as expert resources to them in their areas of specialization. Examples of other specialty areas where nurses serve as experts include wound and ostomy care, case management, intravenous (IV) therapy, and quality improvement.

Nursing organization governance. In most healthcare agencies, nurses have a nursing staff organization. In some settings this organization serves mainly as a communication vehicle. In other more progressive settings, nurses govern themselves through the organization, much as the medical staff is expected to govern itself through the medical staff organization.

The concept of shared governance is founded on the philosophy that employees have both a right and a responsibility to govern their own work and time within a financially secure, patient-centered system. Shared governance promotes decentralization and participation at all levels of nursing. In shared governance, the role of the clinical nursing staff is to be responsible for the professional practice of their nursing unit by adhering to standards and benchmarks of quality care. The role of the nurse manager and other nurse leaders is to set expectations, facilitate, coordinate, support, and create partnerships with the staff in achieving the identified goals. The shared governance model promotes improved patient outcomes and enhanced nurse job satisfaction brought about by increased autonomy. Over the past several decades since the concept of shared governance was first introduced, the U.S. healthcare system has become more complex and nurses increasingly share in decisions and responsibilities. Experts have asserted that the time has come for nurses to replace the concept of shared governance with "professional governance" which includes the core attributes of accountability, professional obligation, collateral relationships, and decision making (Clavelle et al., 2016). In a work environment that supports professional governance, nurses function as peers within the healthcare system and have the freedom to innovate and transform their practice, thereby contributing to the profession and the community.

Healthcare organizations are complex entities. The way they are organized may vary, but each has an organizational chart that shows its unique structure and explains lines of authority. When considering employment in a healthcare organization, you can learn a great deal by examining its organizational chart to see how nursing is governed and how it relates to senior management and the board of directors. Fig. 14.1 shows an example of a basic healthcare organizational chart.

Maintaining Quality in Healthcare Agencies

Providing and maintaining high-quality services are goals of healthcare agencies. As pressure increases to control costs, it becomes even more important to ensure that quality is not sacrificed to save money. Accreditation and quality improvement initiatives are two ways to foster quality care.

Accreditation of Healthcare Agencies

Healthcare organizations such as hospitals, home health agencies, and long-term care facilities seek accreditation through one of two accrediting bodies approved by the CMS. They are The Joint Commission, a not-for-profit organization that serves as the nation's predominant standard-setting and accrediting body in healthcare (The Joint Commission, 2018), and the Healthcare Facilities Accreditation Program, authorized by the CMS. The goal of accreditation is to improve patient outcomes. Each year, the Joint Commission sets national patient safety goals to guide hospitals' efforts to improve patient outcomes. In 2018 the national patient safety goals included to identify patients correctly, to improve staff communication, to use medicines and alarms safely, to prevent infection, to identify patient safety risks, and to prevent mistakes in surgery (The Joint Commission, 2018). Accreditation is important and requires that a number of standards be met in every department. Considerable resources of time and money are spent making sure accreditation criteria, set by these external accrediting bodies, are met.

Continuous Quality Improvement and Total Quality Management

An additional strategy through which most organizations choose to work internally toward improvement in patient outcomes is continuous quality improvement (CQI).

The concept of CQI was first developed by management expert W. Edwards Deming in the 1940s, when he suggested that managers in industry should rely on groups of employees, which he called quality circles, as they made decisions about how work was to be done. In today's healthcare systems, CQI, also called total quality management (TQM), is one of the most important concepts borrowed from industry. Rather than trying to identify mistakes after they have occurred, these systems focus on establishing procedures for ensuring high-quality patient care. Using quality improvement concepts, groups of employees from different departments decide

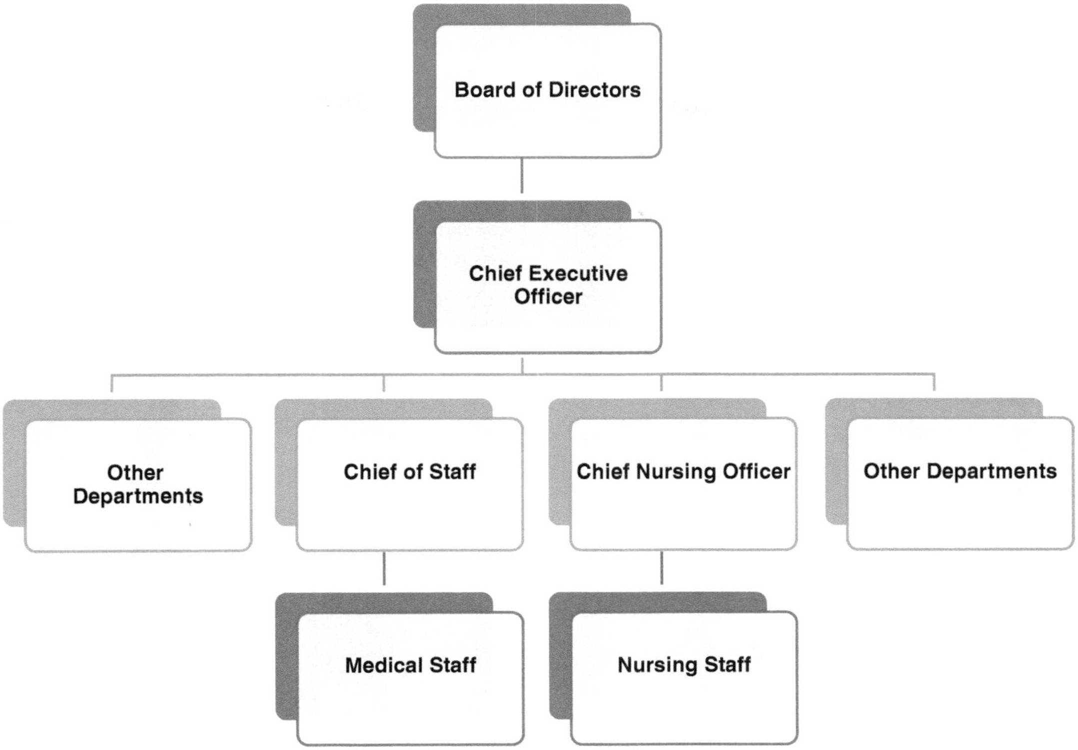

Fig. 14.1 This is a simple version of an organizational chart showing lines of responsibility in a large healthcare setting.

how care will be provided. They decide what outcomes are desired, and they design systems and assign roles and activities to create those outcomes. Every effort is made to anticipate potential problems and prevent their occurrence. Management delegates authority to the providers of services to plan and carry out quality improvement programs. Programs in CQI/TQM reinforce the belief that quality is everyone's responsibility. The Institute for Healthcare Improvement (IHI) is a not-for-profit organization that exists to improve the quality and safety of health care worldwide. The IHI partners with innovative leaders around the world to discover new ideas for improving the health of individuals and population. The IHI provides many practical tools for teaching the concepts of quality improvement and thus is a valuable resource for all nurses (www.ihi.org, 2021).

Performance improvement (PI) is another term used to describe organizational efforts to improve corporate performance. Incorporating aspects of quality management, PI focuses efforts on increasing individual and group competence and productivity. Quality can be compromised in the process of increasing productivity, a situation that is not acceptable in caring for patients.

Nurses are actively involved in leading quality and PI and in accreditation processes, but these activities are not the responsibility of nursing alone. They are institution-wide initiatives, and everyone, at all levels, gets involved. Working together to improve patient care builds cooperation among departments and clinical disciplines and, when done well, fosters an environment of collegiality and cooperation.

A Continuing Challenge: Healthcare Disparities

The phrase *healthcare disparities* refers to the differences in access to and the quality of healthcare provided to different populations. Ethnic or racial disparities receive much attention among those examining healthcare delivery; however, differences also have been found to exist between the treatment and treatment outcomes of men and women, as well as younger and older people. Healthcare disparities may be due to race, ethnicity, gender, age, income, education, disability, sexual

CONSIDERING CULTURE BOX 14.1

This Land We Call America

A Poem by Lucinda Canty, PhD, CNM

I sit in the complexities of life
Wondering if I will ever feel safe
As a Black woman
On this land we call America
You call the land of the free, the home of the brave

Free, Brave
I wish those words could mean the same thing to me
And the sons and daughters I will birth on
This land that my ancestors built
This Land called America

Built on the backs of Black bodies
A forgotten history
Of birth, pain, of suffering
But also of Resilience and determination

It is because of Black women that I am here
I am inflicted with 400 years of harm
Still affecting the treatment of my womb
A black body I am still trying to control today

In a health care system
Where I should feel safe
But we all know I may not survive

You act like you don't see me
You pretend you don't hear me
You turn your head away from the treatment
You know is killing me
Afraid to look in my eyes
Afraid I am going to tell you the truth

You need to know who I am
To understand why I fight
Just to safely give birth
On this land we call America

I am a first-generation college graduate. I attended Columbia University, Yale University and recently received my PhD in Nursing from the University of Connecticut. While my resume is impressive, it is not what I value most about myself. What I value most about who I am, is that I am a Black, African American woman. Being a Black woman is the foundation of everything else that I represent. I am a Black woman first then I am a mother, nurse, nurse-midwife, nurse-researcher and nurse educator. Being a Black woman in this country represents a painful history, but it also represents strength and resilience.

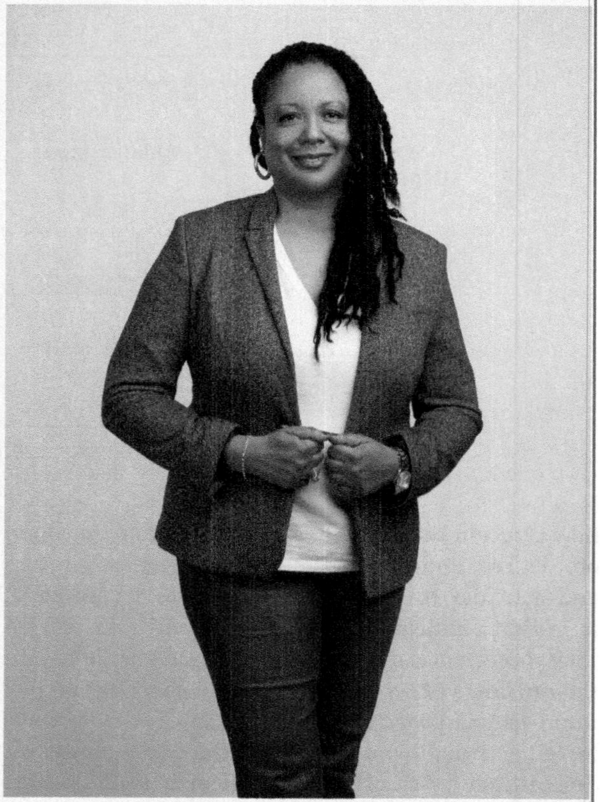

Lucinda Canty, PhD, CNM
Associate Professor
University of Massachusetts Amherst
School of Nursing

Courtesy Lucinda Canty

orientation, and rurality (Healthypeople.gov, 2018). Factors that influence health outcomes, such as the societal and economic influences that people have no power to control, are considered social determinants of health. Access to clean water, healthy food, and unpolluted air are examples of social determinants of health. Other examples include safe work places, quality education, and healthy relationships (Healthypeople.gov, 2018). The powerful influence of social determinants of health makes it difficult to reduce disparities despite increasing attention to their significant negative effect on large segments of the population.

In previous editions of this text, there was a large textbox here featuring "the ongoing challenge of disparities in health care." The box included many statistics and trends that are well-documented and well-known at this point. What was missing what a clear explanation of the human cost of healthcare disparities. Lucinda Canty, PhD, CNM described the struggle "just to safely give birth" as a Black woman in America in a poem she wrote and generously shares in Considering Culture Box 14.1.

The Healthcare Team

A wide array of providers deliver care across the variety and spectrum of healthcare settings presented in this chapter. At one time, physicians and nurses were the central members of the healthcare team, but as health care became complex and technology expanded, a number of other health disciplines developed. Today there are many different healthcare providers who come from a variety of educational backgrounds. Physicians, nurses, and all the other individuals who work with patients are called the healthcare team, or multidisciplinary team. *Multidisciplinary* refers to the presence of more than one discipline (e.g., nursing, medicine, social work) on the team working together. The team is supported in their work by a number of other departments, such as nutrition, environmental services, pharmacy, and laboratory services, among others. The decision about which of these various personnel should be involved in the care of a patient depends on the desired patient outcomes. You may also hear the term *interprofessional* used to refer to different disciplines working together to offer specialized knowledge and skills to collaboratively care for patients. Professional nurses must understand and appreciate the education and skills of all members of the healthcare team and strive to work effectively with them. One approach to help nurses understand how members from other healthcare disciplines are educated is called interprofessional education. Interprofessional education involves students from a variety of disciplines, such as nursing, medicine, and respiratory therapy, learning together during their professional training. Several of the key members who are most likely to be involved in the care of patients are discussed next.

Physicians

Physicians are responsible for assigning medical diagnoses and prescribing interventions designed to restore patient health. Although physicians have traditionally been involved mainly in restorative care and treatment of diseases and disorders, physicians now recognize the value of health promotion and maintenance, as well as illness and injury prevention. Some physicians are also integrating nontraditional or alternative treatment choices such as chiropractic medicine, acupuncture, herbal treatments, and massage therapy into their practices.

Physicians have completed college and 3 or 4 years of medical school and are licensed by a state board of medical examiners. Although a hospital residency is not required to practice medicine in all states, most physicians have completed one, and many do postgraduate work in a specialty area and then take examinations to become board certified in the specialty area.

Physician Assistants

Physician assistants (PAs) have emerged in the past 30 years as members of the healthcare team. According to the American Academy of Physician Assistants (2018), PAs practice medicine, including prescribing medications, as part of a healthcare team with physicians and other providers, working in all 50 states, the District of Columbia, and all U.S. territories.

Prerequisites for entering a PA program vary, depending on the degree offered. Virtually all programs require that applicants have healthcare experience before attending a PA program, which usually lasts approximately 26 months, or three academic years. Beyond graduation from this program, PAs must pass a national certifying examination and are required to be licensed by the state in which they practice. They are required to obtain continuing medical education and regularly be retested on their clinical skills. PAs may also choose to then complete a postgraduate PA program in a clinical specialty area.

Unlicensed Assistive Personnel

Unlicensed assistive personnel (UAP) are unlicensed workers who are key members of the nursing staff. UAP work under the supervision of nurses to assist with basic patient care. Certified nursing assistants (CNAs) are the most well-known of UAP. Their responsibilities include the management of tasks such as assisting with personal hygiene; measuring and recording vital signs, height, weight, and intake and output (I&O); collecting and testing specimens; and reporting and recording patients' conditions and treatments. They also help patients meet their nutritional needs by checking and delivering food trays, assisting with feeding patients when necessary, and replenishing bedside water and ice. Additional duties include assisting patients with their mobility by turning and positioning, performing range-of-motion exercises, transferring patients to and from wheelchairs or bedside chairs, and assisting with ambulation.

To become a UAP, specialized training may be required in a vocational or technical school or a community or junior college. Individuals who become UAP sometimes pursue additional education to become LPNs/LVNs or RNs. Some other types of UAP include medical assistants, home health assistants, doulas (birth assistants), and surgical technologists. Some of these UAP have on-the-job training or short-term courses to learn a specific aspect of health care. UAP who are certified have had more in-depth training and have taken a state-sponsored certification examination; certification is not the same as being licensed, however. In some states, certain UAP such as CNAs are regulated by the nursing practice act.

Licensed Practical Nurses/Licensed Vocational Nurses

Licensed practical nurses/licensed vocational nurses (LPNs/LVNs) care for patients under the direction of physicians and RNs. (LPNs and LVNs are essentially the same—they take the same licensing examination; only Texas and California use the term *LVN*.) The supervision required varies by state and job setting. LPNs/LVNs provide basic bedside care. They measure and record patients' vital signs, such as height, weight, temperature, blood pressure, pulse, and respirations. They also prepare and give injections and enemas, monitor catheters, and perform uncomplicated wound care. They assist with bathing, dressing, personal hygiene, moving in bed, standing, and walking. They might also feed patients who need help eating. LPNs/LVNs collect samples for testing, perform routine laboratory tests, and record food and fluid I&O. They clean and monitor medical equipment. Sometimes they help physicians and RNs perform tests and procedures. Some LPNs/LVNs help care for and feed infants.

LPNs/LVNs monitor their patients and report adverse reactions to medications or treatments. They gather information from patients, including their health history and how they are currently feeling. They may use this information to complete insurance forms, preauthorizations, and referrals, and they share information with RNs and physicians to help determine the best course of care for a patient.

Most LPNs/LVNs are generalists and work in all areas of health care. However, some work in a specialized setting, such as nursing homes or doctors' offices, or in home health care. LPNs/LVNs in nursing home facilities help evaluate residents' needs, develop care plans, and supervise the care provided by nursing aides. In doctors' offices and clinics, they may be responsible for drawing blood, measuring vital signs, making appointments, keeping records, and performing other clinical and clerical duties. LPNs/LVNs who work in home health care may prepare meals and teach family members simple nursing tasks. In some states, LPNs/LVNs are permitted to administer prescribed medicines, start IV fluids, and provide care to ventilator-dependent patients (Bureau of Labor Statistics, 2018).

Training programs for LPNs/LVNs are offered in state-approved vocational or technical schools or community or junior colleges. The programs usually last one year. To become licensed, graduates must pass a national examination, the National Council Licensure Examination for Practical Nurses® (NCLEX-PN®), developed and administered by the National Council of State Boards of Nursing.

Dietitians

Many patients require management of their nutritional intake as part of the healing process. Others need to learn how to shop for and prepare food to maintain a healthy diet. **Registered dietitians (RDs)** understand how what one consumes, whether oral or IV, can affect a patient's recovery and promote and maintain health. They focus on the therapeutic value of foods and on teaching people about appropriate diets and healthy nutrition. Dietitians are especially helpful in assisting patients with specific dietary restrictions (patients with diabetes, patients seeking help with weight management) or those who need extra caloric support (high-risk neonates or people with cancer). Dietitians have bachelor's or higher degrees and may have completed internships in specialty areas, such as pediatrics. Only nutritionists who become registered with the Commission on Dietetic Registration (CDR) may call themselves a dietitian or RD. Not all nutritionists are RDs, but all RDs are nutritionists.

Pharmacists

Pharmacists prepare and dispense medications, instruct patients and other health workers about medications, monitor the use of controlled substances such as narcotics, and work to reduce medication errors. Pharmacists require special education and training to safely and accurately prepare, dispense, and monitor the effects of complex medications on patients. Clinical pharmacists spend time on hospital units working closely with physicians and nursing case managers to coordinate complex drug administration, such as chemotherapy. They assist in monitoring and minimizing the drug interactions resulting from a patient taking multiple medications, and in outpatient settings they are involved in counseling patients about their medications (Fig. 14.2).

Pharmacists must obtain a Doctor of Pharmacy degree, also known as a PharmD, which takes 6 years to complete, and pass a state board of pharmacy's licensure examination (Bureau of Labor Statistics, 2018).

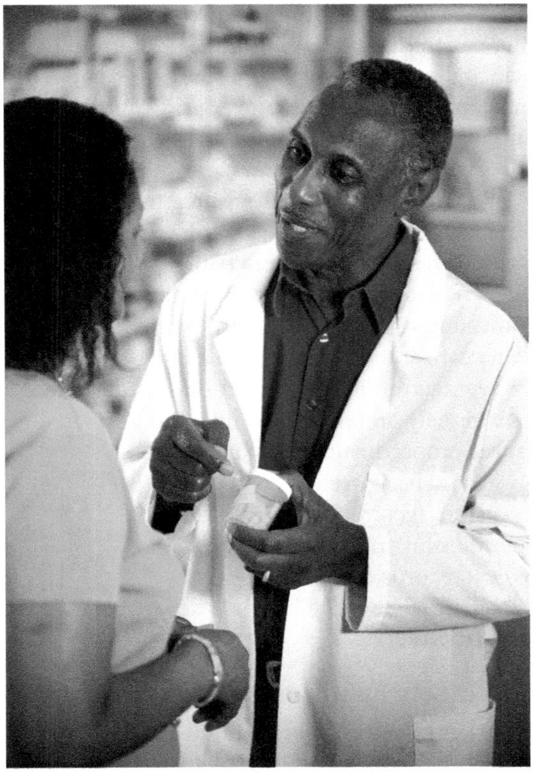

Fig. 14.2 An important part of the work of pharmacists is consulting with patients about their medications. (Photo used with permission from iStockphoto.)

Depending on state licensing requirements, they may also be required to complete an internship. Certified pharmacy technicians, who are certified by state licensing boards, assist them.

Technologists

Technologists are personnel who assist in the diagnosis of patient problems.

Laboratory technologists handle patient specimens—such as blood, sputum, feces, urine, and body tissues—to be examined for abnormalities. They also manage blood banks (Fig. 14.3). Laboratory technologists carefully subject these body substances to various tests to determine deviations from normal ranges. Technologists have at least a bachelor's degree and are often assisted by laboratory technicians, who have 2-year associate's degrees. Technologists must pass a state licensing examination to practice.

Radiology technologists (RTs) perform imaging procedures, assist physicians with procedures such as angioplasty, and administer therapeutic radiation. Although patients still need routine flat-plate radiography studies, technology in this field has become much more sophisticated. Subspecialties such as CT, magnetic resonance imaging (MRI), and PET have developed. All these techniques allow practitioners to see what is occurring inside the body without surgery. They also require specially educated technicians who operate multimillion-dollar equipment. RTs are educated in formal programs lasting from 1 to 4 years. Specific requirements, such as licensing and certification for working as an RT, vary from state to state (see www.arrt.org, 2021).

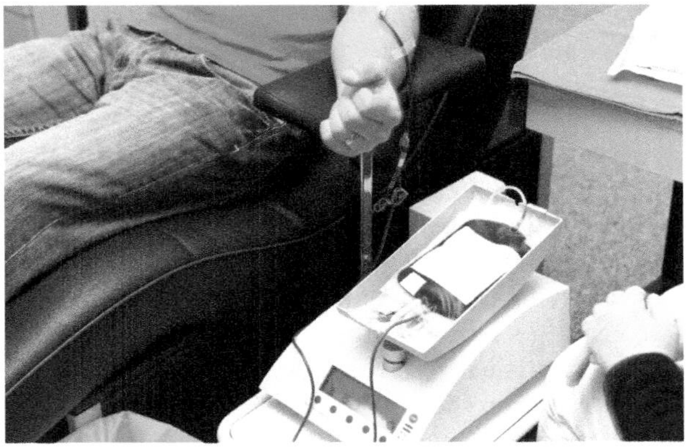

Fig. 14.3 Collection and safe management of blood are critical aspects of care in the hospital. (Photo used with permission from iStockphoto.)

Respiratory Therapists

Acutely ill or injured patients often require assistance in breathing. Respiratory therapists operate equipment such as ventilators, oxygen therapy devices, and intermittent positive-pressure breathing machines. They also perform some diagnostic procedures, such as pulmonary function tests and blood gas analysis. With the increase in respiratory care in the home and community, these healthcare team members work closely with home health agencies and community health centers. Respiratory therapists must complete a 2- or 4-year educational program and obtain state licensure; in some states they must complete an internship. Respiratory therapists take a certification exam to become a certified respiratory therapist (CRT). Once credentialed as a CRT, the respiratory therapist can take an optional voluntary clinical simulation examination to earn the credential of registered respiratory therapist (www.aarc.org/careers/, 2021).

Social Workers

The social worker is specifically educated and trained to assist patients and their families as they face the impact of illness and injury. They serve as liaisons between hospitalized patients and the resources and services available in the community. They help patients and their families deal with financial problems caused by interruption of work or inadequate insurance benefits; they also direct them to the appropriate community support systems or facilities for home health care, long-term care, or rehabilitation. In addition to counseling patients and families, social workers are called on to assist other healthcare personnel to cope more effectively with the stresses associated with caring for patients in crisis. Social workers hold either a bachelor's or a master's degree and are licensed.

Therapists

Therapists help patients with special challenges. Physical therapists, known as physiotherapists in some countries, assist patients to regain maximum possible physical activity and strength. They focus on assessing preillness or preinjury function, current deficits, and potential for recovery. They then develop a long-term plan for gradual return to function through exercise, rest, heat, hydrotherapy, and other measures. The Commission on Accreditation in Physical Therapy Education (CAPTE) mandated that the Doctor of Physical Therapy (DPT) degree is the minimal professional educational qualification for physical therapists (www.apta.org, 2021). Physical therapists also supervise physical therapy assistants, who hold associate degrees.

Occupational therapists work with physical therapists to develop plans to assist patients in resuming the activities of daily living after illness or injury. They may help patients learn to cook, carry out their personal hygiene, or drive a specially equipped car. In addition, they assist patients to learn skills to return to their previous jobs or retrain patients for new employment options. The Accreditation Council for Occupational Therapy Education (ACOTE) has mandated that entry level into occupational therapy be at the doctoral level and programs offering the OT degree must transition to doctoral programs by 2027 (www.aota.org, 2021). Other types of therapists include recreational therapists, art and music therapists, speech therapists, and massage therapists.

Administrative Support Personnel

In all organizations, administrative support staff members are needed for clerical jobs such as admitting patients, answering phones, directing visitors, scheduling patient tests, filing insurance claims, filing forms, paying bills, facilitating payroll, and other support functions. These activities require considerable time. Hiring administrative staff members frees the clinical staff to concentrate on direct patient care.

The administrative staff ensures that the operations of the facility run smoothly and that clinicians have the resources necessary to meet patient needs. These staff members also educate the clinical staff on financial constraints and work with the staff to find ways to provide quality care at the lowest possible cost.

Keeping complete and accurate medical records is an extremely important administrative function that ensures proper insurance billing, eligibility for accreditation, and legal protection of the hospital and its staff. Registered records administrators are vital members of the administrative staff. These professionals staff the medical records department. Many organizations today now refer to the medical records departments as "health information services."

The Nurse's Role on the Healthcare Team

Whatever the setting, nurses fulfill a number of roles on the healthcare team. As the healthcare delivery system changes, the evolving role of the RN requires new competencies and skills in each of the following roles.

Provider of Care

Nurses provide direct, hands-on care to patients in all healthcare agencies and settings. As providers, they take an active role in illness prevention and health promotion and maintenance. They offer health screenings, home health services, and an array of healthcare services in schools, workplaces, churches, clinics, physicians' offices, and other settings. They are instrumental in the high survival rates in trauma centers and newborn intensive care units, among others. Nurses with advanced nursing degrees are increasingly providing care at all levels of the healthcare system. Their breadth and depth of knowledge, their ability to care holistically for patients, and their natural partnership with physicians make nurses some of the most sought after and trusted care providers. A major role of the nurse is to ensure continuity in a patient's transition from inpatient to outpatient care through coordination of home-based services, community services, and discharge teaching.

Educator

As patient and family educators, nurses provide information about illnesses and teach about medications, treatments, and rehabilitation needs. They also help patients understand how to deal with the life changes necessitated by chronic illnesses and teach how to adapt care to the home or community setting. In the current healthcare climate, patients are being discharged from hospitals faster than ever before. Patients and their families must often manage complex treatments, such as central lines or feeding tubes, in the home setting.

Nurses also act as educators in community settings. The major focus of the nurse in the community setting is health promotion and injury and illness prevention. Often nurses teach classes jointly with other healthcare team members. For example, a nutritionist and a nurse may teach a group of expectant parents the benefits of breastfeeding their infants. Nurses also have a responsibility to understand and teach how a healthy or unhealthy environment may affect both the short- and long-term health of the community.

Nurses also serve as patient educators in disease management companies. By educating patients about their chronic diseases and coaching them in effective self-care behaviors, nurses work with the patient and the primary care provider to keep the patient healthier. Thus nurses as patient educators help reduce healthcare utilization and cost.

Nurses often teach other team members about the patient and family and why different interventions may have varying degrees of success. Nurses help other team members find cost-effective, quality interventions that are desired and needed by the patient rather than wasting resources on ineffective, inefficient, undesired, or unneeded services. Importantly, nurses also serve as teachers of the next generation of nurses.

The Internet plays a significant role in health education today, having transformed access to and dissemination of information for millions of Americans. Nurses functioning in the role of educator assist patients to use the Internet as an enhancement to traditional education by teaching them how to select reliable websites and evaluate the health information they find. Therefore nurse educators must keep up to date with technology advances as related to teaching patients.

Manager

In their daily work, all nurses are managers. The bedside staff nurse must manage the care of a group of patients, prioritize how to accomplish patient care activities during an 8- or 12-hour period, and determine staff and patient assignments. Nurses are also involved in reviewing patient cases and coordinating services so that quality care can be achieved at the lowest cost.

In addition, nurses serve in the role of managers of patient care units, outpatient clinics, or home health agencies. The effective management of nursing resources is essential. With budgets ranging from hundreds of thousands to millions of dollars, nurse managers manage "businesses" larger than many small companies. Nurse managers must have clinical and administrative expertise, including leadership, human resources, finance, organizational behavior, system and program design, outcome research, and marketing.

Chief nursing officers, also known as chief nurse executives, may manage more than 1000 employees and multimillion-dollar budgets. They interact with other top executives and community leaders, often sitting on the healthcare organization's board of directors. CNEs must ensure the quality of nursing care within financial, regulatory, and legislative constraints. As noted earlier, nurses often serve as patient care executives, COOs, and CEOs. Key responsibilities of nurse administrators, both as managers and executives, are listed in Box 14.3.

BOX 14.3 Key Elements of the Role of Nurse Administrator

- Nursing practice issues
  - Nursing autonomy
  - Accountability for nursing practice
  - Nursing control of nursing practice
  - Promotion of evidence-based practice
- Oversight of practice environment
  - Safe and healthy workplace
  - Evidence-based practice
  - Adequate numbers of competent staff
- Communication between staff and administration
- Promotion of positive working relationships
- Responsible stewardship of resources

Data from American Nurses Association (ANA): *Nursing administration: scope and standards of practice,* ed 2, Silver Spring, Md, 2016, ANA, p. 11.

Researcher

All nurses should be involved in nursing research whether or not research is a nurse's primary responsibility. According to the ANA's *Scope and Standards of Practice 2015* (ANA, 2015), the RN integrates research findings into practice and engages in evidence-based practice. Nurse researchers investigate whether current or potential interventions work to achieve their expected outcomes, what options for care may be available, and how best to provide care. Nursing research is focused on many aspects of phenomena important to nursing, such as patient outcomes, the nursing process, nursing systems, aspects of patient care, and interventions, in addition to testing theory.

Outcomes research has become an integral part of the healthcare delivery system. Insurers and regulatory agencies require healthcare organizations to report outcome data related to quality of care, which requires research by nurses. Participation in research by all nurses is essential to the growth and development of the nursing profession. The increasing emphasis on evidence-based practice underscores the need for nurses at all levels to know how to evaluate and use research.

Collaborator

With so many healthcare workers involved in providing patient care, collaboration among the professions is increasingly important. The collaborator role is a vital one for nurses to ensure that everyone agrees on the same goals and plan to reach the best patient outcomes. Interprofessional teams require collaborative practice, and nurses play key roles as both team members and team leaders. Collaboration requires that nurses understand and appreciate what other health professionals have to offer. Nurses must also interpret to others the nursing needs of patients.

An often-overlooked collaborative function of nurses is collaboration with patients and families. Involving patients and their families in the plan of care from the beginning is the best way to ensure their cooperation, enthusiasm, and willingness to work toward the best patient outcomes. More in-depth information about collaboration can be found in Chapter 12.

Patient Advocate

The word *advocate* comes from Latin *advocare*, meaning "to call to one's aid." Some nursing experts believe that being a patient advocate is the most important of all the nursing roles. Rules and regulations designed to help a complex healthcare system run efficiently can sometimes get in the way of a patient's treatment, and an impersonal healthcare system may infringe on a patient's rights. This may occur when there is an unsafe patient load, a patient is being discharged too early, a treatment plan needs revision, or the patient's wishes are not being followed. Advocacy is an important part of patient-centered care; therefore it is every nurse's constant responsibility to advocate for patients, that is, to "call to [their] aid" when they cannot do this for themselves.

Nurses who are advocating for patients must know how to cut through the levels of bureaucracy and red tape of healthcare organizations and stand up for the patient's rights, advocating for his or her best interests at all times. They must value patient self-determination—that is, the patient's right to autonomy and therefore independence in decision making.

Nurses advocate more effectively as they mature in their practice. As an advocate, nurses sometimes help patients bend the rules when it is in the patient's best interests and doing so will harm no one. The discussion on Benner's Stages of Nursing Proficiency in Chapter 5 underscores the ability of more experienced nurses to know when it is safe and appropriate to bend rules. Patient advocates are nurses who realize that policies are important and govern most situations well but occasionally can, and should, be stretched or even broken. For example, special care units may have restricted visiting hours. Family members may be allowed to see the patient for only 10 minutes each hour. If a patient's recovery appears to be impeded as a result of his or her separation from family, the nurse, as the patient's advocate, may allow them more generous visitation than the policy provides.

Well-prepared nurses participate both as leaders and as members of the interdisciplinary team, with the best interests of their patients always their first priority.

Nursing Care Delivery Models

Before World War I, nurses usually visited the sick in their homes to care for them. As hospital care improved and nursing education evolved, more sick people were treated in hospitals. Providing care to groups of patients rather than to individuals required nurses to be efficient and use their time effectively. Over the years, various types of care delivery models were designed to meet the goals of efficient and effective nursing care. Organizing patient care today often requires the professional nurse to work through other care providers, such as UAP and LPNs/LVNs, to achieve excellent patient outcomes. Delivery of high-quality patient care does not happen by chance. Each nurse manager, in collaboration with the staff, must select a care delivery model appropriate for the unit, the acuity of the patients, and the type and number of nursing staff members available. There are a number of principles for selecting a care delivery model. Box 14.4 lists 13 principles to consider when selecting a care delivery model.

> **BOX 14.4 Principles for Selecting a Care Delivery Model**
>
> The care delivery model should do all of the following:
> - Facilitate meeting the organization's goals
> - Be cost effective
> - Contribute to meeting patients' outcomes
> - Provide role satisfaction for nurses
> - Allow implementation of the nursing process
> - Provide adequate communication among all health-care providers
> - Support RNs' responsibility for the overall direction of nursing care
> - Be designed to give RNs the responsibility, authority, and accountability for planning, organizing, and evaluating nursing care
> - Ensure that the skills and knowledge of each care provider are used for the best patient outcomes
> - Ensure that communication can occur
> - Ensure that the model advances professional nursing practice
> - Provide for care that is perceived by the patient as a coherent whole (unity of action by a team of RNs, LPNs/LVNs, or others)
> - Provide the work groups of RNs, LPNs/LVNs, and other workers the appropriate knowledge required to meet the nursing care needs of the patient

From Rogers R: Adapting to the new workplace reality: maximizing the role of RNs within a collaborative nursing practice model, *Info Nurs* 39(1):18–20, 2008.

Four patient care delivery models—team nursing, primary nursing, case management nursing, and patient-centered care—are reviewed in this chapter.

Team Nursing

In response to the frustration some nurses felt when using a functional approach to patient care, Lambertson (1953) designed **team nursing**. She envisioned nursing teams as democratic work groups with varying skill levels represented by different team members. They were assigned as a team to a defined group of patients.

Team nursing has been widely used in hospitals and long-term care facilities. The team usually consists of an RN, who serves as team leader; an LPN/LVN; and one or more UAP. The team leader, although ultimately responsible for all the care provided, **delegates** (assigns responsibility for) certain patients to each team member. Each member of the team provides the level of care for which he or she is best prepared. The least skilled and most inexperienced members care for the patients who require the least complex care, and the most skilled and experienced members care for the most seriously ill patients who require the most complex care.

In team nursing the RN team leader supervises and coordinates all care for a particular shift, makes assessments, and documents responses to care. The LPN/LVN team member provides direct care by performing treatments and procedures and reporting patient responses to the team leader. The UAP provides routine, direct personal care. Today, team nursing is still used, but the model is often modified. Many of the patient-focused care models use RNs as team leaders coordinating care for a group of patients and supervising multiskilled workers who have been trained to perform a variety of comfort measures such as positioning and technical procedures such as taking vital signs or drawing blood.

Team nursing has both advantages and disadvantages; these are presented in Box 14.5.

Primary Nursing

Developed in the 1970s as a result of the increased acuity (severity of illness) of hospitalized patients, primary nursing was designed to promote the concept of an identified nurse for every patient during the patient's stay on a particular unit. The goal of primary nursing is to deliver consistent, comprehensive care by identifying one nurse who is responsible, has authority, and is accountable for the patient's nursing care outcomes for the period during which the patient is in a unit.

In primary nursing, each newly admitted patient is assigned to a primary nurse. Primary nurses assess their patients, plan their care, and write the plan of care. While on duty, they care for their patients and delegate responsibility to associate nurses when they are off duty. Associate nurses may be other RNs or LPNs/LVNs.

Patients are divided among primary nurses in such a manner that each nurse is responsible for the care of a group of patients 24 hours a day. Unless there is a compelling reason to transfer a patient, the primary nurse cares for the patient in the unit from the time of admission to the time of discharge. The primary nurse may be assisted by other care providers (such as other nurses, aides, and technicians) but retains accountability, or responsibility, for care outcomes 24 hours a day while the patient is in the unit. The primary nurse communicates effectively with associate nurses caring for the patient on other shifts and with primary nurses in other units if the patient is transferred (e.g., to the operating room or intensive care unit). Fig. 14.4 shows a nurse caring for an infant in the neonatal intensive care unit, where the complex care and the prolonged hospital stays of their tiny patients is amenable to primary nursing.

Primary nursing is used in a variety of settings and is often modified from its original form. Advantages and disadvantages of primary nursing are listed in Box 14.6.

BOX 14.5 Team Nursing Advantages and Disadvantages

Advantages
- Potential for building team identity
- Provides comprehensive care
- Each worker's abilities used to the fullest
- Promotes job satisfaction
- Decreases nonprofessional duties of RNs

Disadvantages
- Ongoing need for communication among team members requires commitment of time
- All team members must promote teamwork, or team nursing is unsuccessful
- Team composition varies from day to day, which can be confusing and disruptive and decreases continuity of care
- May result in blurred role boundaries, resulting in confusion and resentment

Case Management Nursing

A more recent evolution in nursing care delivery is case management nursing. Begun in the late 1980s as an attempt to improve the cost effectiveness of patient care, case management allows the nurse to oversee patient care and manage the delivery of services from all healthcare disciplines throughout a patient's illness. Nursing case management keeps costs down by striving to achieve predetermined daily patient outcomes within a specified period for patients within the same diagnostic group—for example, patients having total knee replacement. The desired daily outcomes are outlined in a plan of care called a care map or critical path. You may also hear these referred to as clinical care plans or tracks.

Two models of case management nursing have evolved over time. These are characterized by either an "internal" focus, in which the case manager works within a treatment facility, or an "external" approach, in which the case manager oversees patients and the

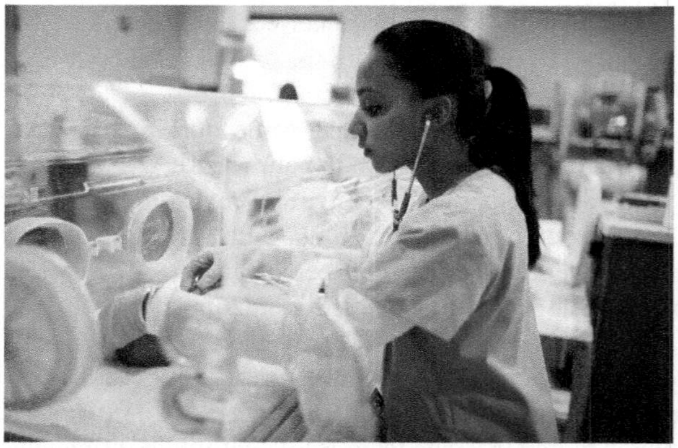

Fig. 14.4 Sick infants and those born prematurely commonly have long stays in neonatal intensive care units, where primary nursing is often practiced. (Photo used with permission from iStockphoto.)

BOX 14.6 Primary Nursing Advantages and Disadvantages

Advantages	Disadvantages
• High patient and family satisfaction • Promotes RN responsibility, authority, autonomy, and accountability • Nurse can care for entire patient—physically, emotionally, socially, and spiritually • Patient knows nurse well, and nurse knows patient well • Promotes patient-centered decision making • Increases coordination and continuity of care • Promotes professionalism • Promotes job satisfaction and sense of accomplishment for nurses	• Difficult to hire all RN staff • Expensive to pay all RN staff • Nurses are not familiar with other patients, making it difficult to "cover" for one another • May create conflicts between primary and associate nurses • Stress of around-the-clock responsibility • Heavy responsibility, especially for new nurses

BOX 14.7 Case Management Nursing Advantages and Disadvantages

Advantages	Disadvantages
• Promotes interdisciplinary collaboration • Increases quality of care • Is cost effective • Eases patient's transition from hospital to community services • Nurse has increased responsibility	• Requires additional training • Requires nurses to be off the unit for periods of time • Is time consuming • Is most useful only with high-risk patients and high-cost/high-volume conditions

delivery of services over the continuum of an illness or chronic disease, whether patients are in a treatment facility or at home. Although different in scope, these two models share the same principles of efficiency and cost effectiveness.

In the internal model of case management, nursing case managers serve as primary nurses for patients in an identified diagnostic group, such as spinal cord injury. They not only care for these patients while on their assigned units but also manage the plans of care from admission to discharge, crossing interdepartmental lines. Although nursing case managers do not physically provide care to the patient group on units other than their own, they actively collaborate with primary nurses assigned to the patients in those units. In this nursing model, critical paths are used for all patients. A critical path is an interdisciplinary agreement showing who will provide care in a given time frame to achieve agreed-on outcomes. The use of critical paths is intended to standardize patient care and allow hospitals to plan staffing levels, lengths of stay, and other factors that heretofore could not be anticipated. Patients whose progress varies from the path are quickly identified. Once the causes for the variation are identified, team members attempt to plan solutions to reduce variances and get the patient back on track. The goal is to treat each patient by using best practices to reduce the length of stay, thereby reducing costs.

In the external model of case management, nurse case managers are part of a large network consisting of, for example, hospitals, clinics, home health agencies, and long-term care settings. They may provide services anywhere in the system, as well as when the patient is at home. They partner with patients and their families to achieve the goal of preventing hospitalizations, thereby reducing costs and minimizing disruptions to the patient's life and family. Nurse case managers play an important role in assuring safe transitions of care as patients move through the healthcare system from hospital to home.

As can be seen from the type of activities in which they engage, case managers perform complex and challenging work. Nurses generally need about 5 years of clinical experience to fill this role effectively. Social workers, psychologists, rehabilitation counselors, or other professionals may also serve as case managers. All case managers, regardless of their discipline, work to reduce the cost of providing services through coordination of providers across the continuum of care. Advantages and disadvantages of case management nursing are shown in Box 14.7.

Patient-Centered Care

Patient-centered care is a contemporary care delivery model implemented by a multidisciplinary team of health professionals. This model of care is based on the patient's right to individualized care that takes his or her values and beliefs into consideration when planning and providing care. Nurses and other providers must be flexible, respect the patient's beliefs and wishes, and negotiate with the patient to meet patient expectations.

Patient-centered care is more an attitude than a particular model of care, and traditional models, alone or in combination, may be used. The attitude of caregivers is that patients' needs have priority over the institution's needs. The model was pioneered by the Planetree Institute in 1978 after its founder experienced several "dehumanizing" hospitalizations. Patient-centered care brings together traditional and nontraditional components of care that work toward optimizing the healing environment. Such components as the architectural design of the facilities; educational programs for patients and families; emphasis on beauty, gardens, art, food, and nutrition; availability of complementary therapies such as massage and aromatherapy; emphasis on spirituality; and community interaction are the hallmarks of patient-centered care. These components are integrated with best medical practices to form a coherent continuum of care characterized by teamwork, communication, and collaboration among professionals and with patients and families. Advantages and disadvantages of patient-centered care are shown in Box 14.8.

BOX 14.8 Patient-Centered Care Advantages and Disadvantages

Advantages
- Expedites care
- Promotes patient convenience
- Capitalizes on professional competence of team members
- Emphasizes continuum of care and reduces fragmentation of care
- Uses resources efficiently
- Fosters teamwork, collaboration, and communication

Disadvantages
- Requires "right staff at right time" to meet patient needs
- Difficult to explain; uses several models of care delivery
- Expensive, requires a high percentage of RNs with both clinical and management skills

Modified from Shirey MR: Nursing practice models for acute and critical care: overview of care delivery models, *Crit Care Nurs Clin North Am* 20:365–373, 2008.

FINANCING HEALTH CARE

The healthcare system in the United States is characterized by high costs and a large number of uninsured citizens, although those numbers have decreased substantially since the individual mandate provision of the ACA was upheld by the U.S. Supreme Court in 2012. The nation's dilemma remains: how to provide high-quality healthcare services to all citizens while keeping costs down.

Among developed nations, the United States has, by far, the largest percentage of its gross domestic product (GDP) spent on health care yet has some of the worst health outcomes. Financial issues profoundly affect nurses and nursing practice. These issues affect nurses professionally, in their nursing practice, and personally, in the type of insurance and health services they and their families are able to afford. Therefore students of professional nursing need to understand the overall economic context in which nursing care is provided. In this section, several concepts necessary to understanding healthcare finance will be explored, including basic economic theory, the economics of nursing care, a brief historical review of the causes of healthcare cost escalation, cost-containment efforts, current methods of payment, and the role nurses can play in managing healthcare costs in their everyday work settings.

Basic Economic Theory

Nursing school curricula do not typically require undergraduates to take courses in economics, yet there is an urgent need for nurses to understand the economic context in which they practice.

Supply and Demand

A basic economic theory is the law of supply and demand. According to this theory, a normal economic system consists of two parts: suppliers, who provide goods and services, and consumers, who demand and use goods and services. In a monetary environment—that is, one in which money is used as a unit of exchange—consumers exchange money for desired goods and services.

In an efficient marketplace, the market price of goods and services serves to create an equilibrium in which supply roughly equals demand, and demand roughly equals supply. When demand exceeds supply, prices rise. When supply exceeds demand, prices fall.

Principles of the Free-Market Economy

In a free-market economy, consumption of any good or service is determined by an individual's ability to pay. In a pure free market, a portion of the population would be denied health care if they were unable to pay. People who support this position consider health care a privilege. Conversely, others believe that everyone should have access to basic health care and consider health care a right, to be administered at the federal and state levels of government. An example of this is the United Kingdom, where the National Health Service (NHS) provides access to basic health care to its citizens.

Despite the United States' general posture favoring a free-market economy, most Americans consider health care a right, not a privilege. Rather than allowing economically disadvantaged citizens to do without health services, the federal government has taken steps to ensure certain groups have access to healthcare services through publicly funded programs such as Medicare and Medicaid. Although this is generally considered an ethical policy, it is nevertheless a policy decision that is inconsistent with free-market principles.

Price Sensitivity in Health Care

In the days before health insurance existed, people paid their own medical bills; providers set their fees with some sensitivity to what patients could afford to pay; and many physicians used sliding-scale payment plans or accepted in-kind payments, for example, exchanging medical care for farm products or a service such as cobbler services. Health insurance created an indirect payment structure known as third-party payment that removed price sensitivity from the concern of most healthcare consumers because they pay only a small portion of the actual costs. A third party (the employer, insurance company, or government) pays the rest. If someone other than the consumer pays, demand can increase because the consumer may be insensitive to or unaware of costs.

Additional Influences on the Healthcare Market

Economists have identified a number of other factors that affect the healthcare market in ways that violate the assumptions surrounding an effective free-market system. For example, consumers cannot always control demand for healthcare services. With ordinary products, a consumer can delay a purchase until there is a sale or forgo the purchase altogether. Health care is different because healthcare needs tend to be immediate. The consumer might suffer serious harm or even death by a delay in seeking services. Certainly in the case of severe traumatic injury, delay of care is not possible, and the costs of the intensive care using sophisticated technologies are enormous in this circumstance. The leading cause of personal bankruptcy in the United States today is medical expenses.

Economics of Nursing Care

Until fairly recently, few efforts were made to determine the actual cost of nursing care. The average hospital bill simply included the cost of nursing services in the general category of "room rate," just as housekeeping services, linens, and food are included in the room rate. It was assumed that the cost of nurses contributed a major portion of overall hospital expenses. During difficult economic times, the first cost-reduction efforts were therefore aimed at reducing the number of nursing personnel, sometimes substituting lower-paid UAP. However, research did not support this prevailing view about the costs of nursing. Instead, research showed that determining the cost of nursing services and developing standardized reimbursements based on costs would enhance the ability of nurse managers to control nursing resources and negotiate for a fair share of hospital financial resources, and many efforts to determine the actual cost of nursing services were conducted.

Not knowing the exact costs of nursing services limits nursing management's ability to calculate the expense required to provide nursing care. Determining the best ratio of RNs to LPNs/LVNs and UAP in each unit is also impaired when the cost of nursing care is unknown. Different patients require different amounts of nursing time, depending in large part on how sick they are. Patient classification systems were developed to identify patients' needs for nursing care in quantitative terms to help hospitals determine the need for nursing resources. However, estimating the cost of nursing services remains an inexact science. Evidence-Based Practice Box 14.1 describes a major study to determine the economic value of professional nursing.

EVIDENCE-BASED PRACTICE BOX 14.1

Demonstrating Nursing's Value

The ANA, with a coalition of other nursing associations, supported a study to improve the understanding of the economic value of the services of RNs. The objective was to quantify the economic value of professional nursing to help shape staffing decisions and policies in the nation's hospitals. A group of researchers from George Mason University in Virginia and a nearby health-care policy research firm, the Lewin Group, conducted the study. They reviewed the research literature on the relationship between RN staffing levels and adverse patient outcomes for a number of nursing-sensitive *nosocomial* (hospital-acquired) complications. Examples of nursing-sensitive complications include urinary tract infections, pressure ulcers, blood infections, post-operative infections, patient falls, and adverse drug events, among others. They used data from a comprehensive literature review, as well as from the 2005 Nationwide Inpatient Sample of more than 1000 hospitals sponsored by the Agency for Healthcare Research and Quality.

The cost of complications—in increased length of stay, healthcare expenditures, and losses of national productivity—were subjected to statistical analyses to determine estimates of the economic value of nursing. The researchers reported that, as a result of increasing nurse staffing levels, patient risk for nurse-sensitive complications and hospital length of stay both decreased, "resulting in medical cost savings, improved national productivity, and lives saved" (p. 97). They concluded that only a portion of professional nurses' services "can be quantified in pecuniary terms, but the partial estimates of economic value presented illustrate the economic value to society of improved quality of care achieved" (p. 97) through higher RN staffing levels.

Modified from Dall T, Chen Y, Seifert R, et al.: The economic value of professional nursing, *Med Care* 47(1):97–104, 2009.

When the drive to provide high-quality nursing care meets the constraints of cost containment head-on, it can create a very difficult situation. What nurses hope, as both providers and consumers of health care, is that quality will not suffer because of the emphasis on "the bottom line." The financial realities that affect the institutions in which most nurses practice—hospitals—cannot be ignored. To stay in business, hospitals must make at least enough money to pay personnel, maintain buildings and equipment, and pay suppliers of goods and services.

The leadership of the ANA has been repeatedly outspoken in their assertion that overzealous cost-containment efforts have led to lower-quality hospital care. A strong boost to their contention that the number and mix of nurses in a hospital make a difference in patient outcomes came early in the 21st century with research that showed an increased patient death rate with higher patient to nurse ratios (see Chapter 1). Peter Buerhaus, PhD, RN, FAAN, of Montana State University, a nurse and a health-care economist, has developed a substantial body of work related to nurse-patient ratios and other matters related to the nursing workforce. As research continues to demonstrate the link between nursing and quality of care, the demand for nurses will continue to increase.

History of Healthcare Finance

Before 1945, more than 90% of Americans either paid directly from their own pockets for health care or depended on charity care. Few had private health insurance. Public insurance programs, such as Medicare and Medicaid, did not exist. After World War II, most industrialized countries began publicly financed healthcare systems that provided care for all citizens. The United States, however, did not adopt a public, universal access system, choosing instead to continue the private, fee-for-service system.

The entire history of healthcare finance in this country is a fascinating study in unintended consequences. As each initiative to improve coverage, access, and quality was implemented, it opened up unforeseen loopholes that have driven costs skyward. Providers, such as hospitals, physicians, insurers, pharmaceutical companies, and others, have learned to "work the system," exploiting loopholes while protecting or enhancing their own bottom lines. All the while, population growth and increases in the number of elderly and chronically ill Americans have further complicated efforts to find solutions.

If you are interested in learning more about the complex history of healthcare finance, including cost-containment initiatives through the years and factors fueling increases in healthcare costs, refer to the Evolve website (http://evolve.elsevier.com/Black/professional).

Current Methods of Payment for Health Care

There are four major methods of payment for health care in use today: private insurance, Medicare, Medicaid, and personal payment, or self-pay. Workers' compensation is an additional mechanism for financing some healthcare services. Each of these is briefly explained in the following paragraphs.

Private Insurance

Private insurance, also called voluntary insurance, is a system wherein insurance premiums are paid by either insured individuals or their employers or are shared between individuals and employers. Periodic payments (premiums) are paid into the insurance plan, and certain healthcare benefits are covered as long as the premiums are paid. Early in the development of private insurance, many treatments were covered only if they were performed in an inpatient (hospital) setting. This feature drove up the cost of services. Today most insurers stipulate that costs of hospitalization are reimbursable only if treatment cannot be performed on an outpatient basis, where costs are typically lower. Most private insurers are heavily influenced by the federal insurance program, Medicare, in determining coverage and amount of reimbursements they will pay.

Medicare

Medicare, or Title XVIII of the Social Security Act, is a nationwide federal health insurance program established in 1965. Medicare is available to people aged 65 years and older, regardless of the recipient's income. It also covers certain disabled individuals and anyone with permanent kidney failure requiring dialysis or a kidney transplant. Medicare has four basic programs.

The first program, known as Part A (Hospital Insurance), helps cover inpatient hospitalization, part-time or intermittent skilled care in nursing facilities, hospice care, and some home health care. Long-term care or custodial care is not covered. Hospice care, available to people with a terminal illness who are expected to live 6 months or less as certified by a physician, is covered under Medicare. People who paid Medicare taxes while working do not pay a Part A premium, but they do pay a deductible, and certain restrictions apply to lengths of stay and benefit periods.

Part B (Medical Insurance) is a supplementary medical insurance program that covers visits to physicians' offices and other outpatient services. It also covers some preventive services. There is a 20% copay for medical and other services and a $233 yearly deductible. Mental health services are covered at 50%. Part B premiums are subject to means testing, meaning that individuals with higher incomes pay more in monthly premiums than do those with lower incomes. In 2022 the monthly premium ranged from $170.10 for individuals with a yearly income less than $85,000 to $578.30 for individuals with a yearly income more than $500,000 (CMS, 2021). The Internal Revenue Service provides tax return information to Medicare to assist in verifying income.

Part C (Medicare Advantage Plans) offers a variety of managed-care options instead of the fee-for-service programs of Parts A and B. Part C plans are run by private companies approved by Medicare. Costs and services vary by plan.

Part D (Prescription Drug Coverage) is an additional supplementary insurance program that helps cover prescription drug costs. Part D has complex regulations including a "gap" period in coverage that many find difficult to understand. In addition to the four basic parts of Medicare, Medigap plans, or supplemental coverage, are available to Medicare-eligible individuals. They are sold by private insurance companies to help fill the "gap" between Medicare and out-of-pocket costs.

Originally intended to be a no-cost or low-cost program for the elderly, the cost of participating in Medicare has risen steadily. Although the program was originally designed to be all-inclusive, many elderly people now find they cannot afford to participate in Medicare. Ironically, some elderly are so poor that they qualify for Medicaid assistance (described next) in paying their Medicare premiums. Medicare regulations and costs change annually. For the most recent updates on Medicare, consult www.medicare.gov.

Medicaid

Medicaid, or Title XIX of the Social Security Act, is a group of jointly funded federal-state programs for low-income, elderly, blind, and disabled individuals. It, too, was established in 1965. There are broad federal guidelines, but states have some flexibility in how they administer the program. People must meet eligibility requirements determined by each state. Eligibility depends on income and varies from state to state. Rates of payment also vary, with some states providing far higher payments than others. The amount the federal government contributes to Medicaid varies from a minimum of 50% of total costs to a maximum of 76.8%.

The differences in eligibility and payment rates lead to wide variations in the level of care provided to the poor in different states and create disparities in care.

TABLE 14.1 Facts about Medicare and Medicaid

	Medicare	Medicaid and State Children's Health Insurance Plan (SCHIP)
Funding	Federal government	Federal and state governments
Administration	Federal government	State governments
Eligibility	≥65 years ≤65 with certain disabilities All ages with end-stage renal disease	*Mandatory eligibility groups:* 133% of the federal poverty level for all Americans ≤65 years based on modified adjusted gross income (MAGI) *SCHIP:* Varies by state, but many states have expanded coverage for children above the federal minimums
Level of benefits	National program with no variation in benefits across states	Varies from state to state
Payment by recipients	Some monthly premiums are required for different parts (A, B, C, D) but varies by plan	States can charge premiums and enrollment fees for certain groups
Coverage	Inpatient care, outpatient care, prescriptions	Comprehensive inpatient and outpatient care, prescriptions with lower copayments for use of generic versus brand-name drugs

Modified from data retrieved from www.medicare.gov and www.medicaid.gov, 2018.

In contrast to those on Medicare, people who receive Medicaid are not required to pay any fees to participate. Table 14.1 highlights the similarities and differences in the Medicare and Medicaid programs.

Personal (Out-of-Pocket) Payment

Personal payment for healthcare services is the least common method. Few people can afford **out-of-pocket payment** for more than the most basic health services. At today's prices, an illness or injury severe enough to require hospitalization can quickly exhaust a family's financial reserves, forcing them into bankruptcy. In general, only those people without access to some form of private group insurance or public insurance rely on personal payment. It can take years for a family to pay a single large medical bill.

Workers' Compensation

Workers' compensation constitutes a small proportion of insurance coverage. The program varies from state to state but generally covers only workers who are injured on the job. It usually covers treatment for injuries and weekly payments during the time the worker is absent from work for injury-related causes. In the case of accidental death, the worker's family receives compensation. Companies are required by law to contribute to a compensation fund from which money is withdrawn when accidental injuries or deaths occur at work.

In Fig. 14.5 you can see what healthcare dollars are spent on in the United States. Note the large percentage that is spent on physician/clinical and hospital care and that 10% is spent on prescription drugs.

Nurses' Role in Managing Healthcare Costs

Staff nurses can play an important role in controlling healthcare costs. They have the most frequent and direct contact with patients and can have a positive impact by reducing unnecessary spending. Reducing spending does not have to mean sacrificing quality patient care. Many small economic changes can lead to large savings.

The first step is to become cost conscious. As a group, nurses tend to have limited awareness of costs. When they are made aware of costs, their supply use patterns can change. Such simple methods as posting the price of supplies on shelves, cutting down on "borrowing" between units, and transferring all patients'

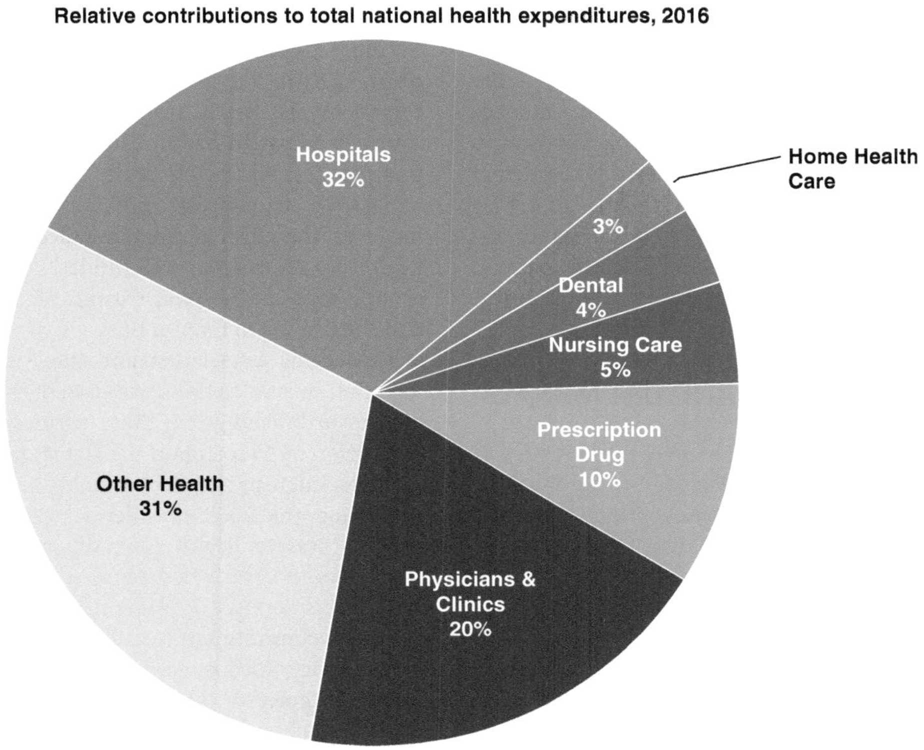

Fig. 14.5 Distribution of health spending: Hospital care and physician/clinical services account for slightly more than half of healthcare expenditures. (From Kaiser Family Foundation analysis of National Health Expenditure (NHE) data from Centers for Medicare and Medicaid Services, Office of the Actuary, National Health Statistics Group, 2018.)

bedside equipment, medications, and supplies carefully can make dramatic changes in per-patient expenditures. Making staff nurses aware of less-expensive alternatives is only one way they can reduce costs. Starting or expanding a revenue-generating recycling program is another measure that all hospital employees can support.

Nurses are positioned to produce even more meaningful savings by providing excellent patient care and being advocates for their patients' personal finances. Nurses must recognize that no matter how well-insured patients may be, they will have to pay some portion of charges personally. Even a small percentage of a healthcare bill can be huge, given the high costs of care. A family's financial resources can be quickly overloaded.

Nurses who question unnecessary or repetitive tests, suggest generic drugs rather than name brands, and teach patients and their families how to monitor their health conditions and detect problems early to avoid repeated hospitalizations all contribute to cost management. Such nursing measures as meticulous handwashing to prevent infections, turning patients on schedule to avoid pressure ulcers, and vigilance to reduce the risk for falls are not usually thought of as cost-containment measures, yet they are. Medicare no longer reimburses facilities for the treatment of certain "reasonably preventable" hospital-acquired conditions ("never conditions") including pressure ulcers, catheter-associated urinary tract infections, falls with injury and burns, and vascular catheter–associated infections, among others, all of which are conditions that can be prevented by nurses. Every day a patient must be hospitalized beyond the length of stay authorized by the payer results in additional charges to the patient and costs to the hospital.

In both inpatient and outpatient settings, organizing and streamlining the flow of patients for maximum efficiency represents a huge savings for the facility and is under the control of nurses and nurse managers. Although nurses can and should look for ways to reduce costs, controlling costs must never take priority over patient care. Remembering the *Code of Ethics for Nurses* will help you maintain your ethical standards: "The nurse's primary commitment is to the patient, whether an individual, family, group, or community" (ANA, 2015).

HEALTHCARE REFORM AND UNIVERSAL ACCESS

The United States and South Africa are the only two industrialized nations that do not provide universal access to health care to all of their citizens. South Africa, however, is implementing a universal system that will be completely phased in by 2026. Despite the fact that U.S. healthcare expenditures by far exceed those of any other country in the world, the U.S. infant mortality rate was an alarming 5.8 in 2017, ranked 170 of 225 ranked nations (Central Intelligence Agency, 2018). Nations with similar rates include Cayman Islands (5.8), Serbia (5.8), and Gibraltar, (5.9); nations with the lowest rates include Monaco (1.80), Japan (2.00), and Iceland (2.10). The infant mortality rate is a sensitive indicator of a nation's healthcare practices. Furthermore, the premature birth rate, another sensitive indicator of a nation's health, remains stubbornly high at 10%, with a disparity in African American/ Black women, who experience a 14% preterm birth rate (CDC, 2018).

Recent History of Healthcare Reform Efforts in the United States

Concerns about healthcare practices in the United States are not new. In the 1992 presidential campaign, candidates in both political parties, as well as nonpartisan groups, advocated some type of healthcare reform. These groups included nursing organizations, the American Association of Retired Persons (now called AARP), labor unions, the American College of Physicians, the National Leadership Coalition for Health Care Reform, and numerous members of the U.S. Congress. Most of these groups put forward specific plans for reform, including *Nursing's Agenda for Health Care Reform* by the ANA, which was endorsed by more than 60 nursing organizations and associations. Early in President Bill Clinton's first term, then–First Lady Hillary Clinton led a bipartisan effort to improve access to health care. For a time, it appeared that progress was being made.

Despite widespread public support for reform, however, the effort ultimately failed. Lobbying against healthcare reform was well funded by powerful interest groups such as the pharmaceutical, health insurance, and medical equipment industries, as well as the American Medical Association and the American Hospital Association, associations with two of the most powerful lobbies in Washington. These entities, as well as others, preferred to maintain the status quo because of the financial interests they had at stake.

During the 2008 presidential campaign, concerns about access to health care, the quality of care, and disparities in care fueled renewed debate about health care in this country. President Barack Obama's administration's commitment to reform health care within his first year in office remained a priority. The economic recession, however, placed severe restrictions on what could be achieved, and partisan politics continues to create stalemates in Congress, where healthcare legislation must be conceived and approved. The same special interest groups that opposed change and defeated the Clinton plan again brought out their forces to oppose the Obama administration's efforts.

An encouraging early sign of President Obama's commitment to change, however, was the passage of the State Children's Health Insurance Program (SCHIP) only a few weeks after he took office. This legislation reauthorized and expanded CHIP coverage to include 4 million additional children. Many, including nursing organizations, applauded this action on behalf of uninsured children. In addition, on March 23, 2010, after very contentious congressional debates and political maneuvering, President Obama signed the ACA into law. This law included comprehensive reforms that improve access to affordable health coverage for everyone and that protect consumers from abusive insurance company practices, such as lifetime limits on coverage and denial of coverage for preexisting conditions. In addition, young people up to age 26 could be added to their parents' insurance policies. Challenges to certain provisions of the ACA, including the individual mandate, were brought before the

U.S. Supreme Court. In 2012 in a 5-4 decision, the Supreme Court upheld these provisions. In 2015 in a 6-3 decision, the Supreme Court ruled that nationwide tax subsidies to help poor and middle-class citizens buy health insurance were not unconstitutional, and hence the ACA remained viable. Despite these positive steps, the issue of affordable health care in the United States remains a significant political and social problem.

Clearly, increasing the number of people covered would increase expenses unless drastic cost-management measures were put in place. In the future, we can expect to see state-by-state efforts to address the specific current issues of concern discussed earlier. Most experts agree that reform efforts must be projected to reduce, or at least not increase, the cost of health care if they are to be supported by Congress. Shortly after President Trump took office, he set about to overturn the ACA in favor of a newly designed plan. The proposed changes were not widely accepted, and the efforts to overturn the ACA failed in 2017. Despite wide-ranging differences of opinion about the specifics of healthcare reform proposals, some general questions should be asked in evaluating reform proposals:

1. Is there a uniform minimum set of benefits for all citizens, otherwise known as universal access?
2. Are coverage and benefits continuous and not dependent on where people live or work?
3. Are there mechanisms for controlling costs, especially administrative expenses?
4. Are provisions made for care to be provided by the most cost-effective personnel, taking quality issues and patient outcomes into consideration?
5. Are the issues of adequate facilities and personnel to ensure access for all addressed?
6. Is there an emphasis on quality care?
7. Are there incentives for healthy lifestyles and preventive care?

Further changes in nursing and healthcare delivery and finance are certain to be on the horizon. These changes will likely be gradual rather than revolutionary. It remains to be seen whether these changes will improve access to and quality of health care for all Americans.

CONCEPTS AND CHALLENGES

- ***Concept:*** Health care in the United States is delivered in a complex system that provides health promotion, illness prevention, diagnosis and treatment, and rehabilitation and long-term care.
  Challenge: Streamlining the healthcare system and focusing on the promotion of health rather than on the treatment of illness can have significant positive effects on the healthcare economy and the health of individuals.
- ***Concept:*** Access to comprehensive treatment and positive treatment outcomes varies among populations, creating disparities that disadvantage certain groups such as minorities and poor people.
  Challenge: Correcting healthcare disparities has proved to be a complex task, with only modest progress reported.
- ***Concept:*** Historically, there have been a number of systems for the provision of nursing care, each of which has advantages and disadvantages.
  Challenge: Many variations and combinations of the major nursing care delivery systems are in use today, and the effectiveness of any one model depends a great deal on the patient population and setting of care.
- ***Concept:*** Medicare and Medicaid programs, begun in 1965, created financial strain on federal and state budgets that continues today. In response, cost-containment efforts were begun by the federal government in the 1970s and persist in various old and new forms.
  Challenge: Regardless of the type of cost-containment efforts used, healthcare costs have continued to increase. Without serious healthcare reform, this will continue.
- ***Concept:*** The ACA, signed into law by President Obama in 2010, was a start in improving access to affordable healthcare coverage for all residents of the United States.
  Challenge: Until the severe problem of healthcare disparities is corrected, the health of a large segment of the American population will continue to suffer.

IDEAS FOR FURTHER EXPLORATION

1. Obtain the organizational chart of a local healthcare facility. Examine it to see how nursing fits into the overall structure. Who reports to the CNE, and to whom does the CNE report? What other administrative staff members are on the same level with the nurse executive?
2. Consider the four types of nursing care delivery systems (team, primary, case management, and patient-centered care) from the viewpoint of the patient. If you were a patient, which system would you prefer? Why?
3. Look at the same issue from the standpoint of the nurse. Which system would you find most satisfying in terms of your practice? Which would you like least?
4. Determine what type of governance structure is used by the nursing staff. What do nurses see as the positive and negative aspects of their governance structure? Do they feel that they are important contributors in this structure?
5. Consider this question: Is access to health care a basic human right or a privilege? Be able to defend your position.
6. What process should be used to determine how healthcare resources are allocated? List criteria you would suggest to determine whether or not a person should receive a kidney transplant, a hip replacement, or a bone marrow transplant.
7. Should people with healthy behaviors pay the same for care or insurance as those whose habits result in a greater likelihood of illness? How could such a differentiation be determined?
8. Consider some things you as an individual nurse can do to become more cost aware and participate in managing healthcare costs.

REFERENCES

American Academy of Physician Assistants: *What is a PA?* 2021. (website). Available at: www.aapa.org/what-is-a-pa/.

American Association for Respiratory Care, *Careers,* 2021. (website). Available at: http://www.aarc.org./careers/.

American Nurses Association (ANA): *Code of ethics for nurses with interpretive statements,* Washington, DC, 2015, American Nurses Publishing.

American Nurses Association (ANA): *Nursing administration: scope and standards of practice,* ed, 2, MD, 2016, Silver Spring. [website]. Available at nursingworld.org.

American Nurses Association (ANA): *Nursing: scope and standards of practice,* ed, 3, Washington, DC, 2015, American Nurses Association.

American Occupational Therapy Association: *Homepage,* 2021.(website). Available at: www.aota.org.

American Physical Therapy Association: *Homepage,* 2021. (website). Available at: www.apta.org.

American Registry of Radiologic Technologists: *Homepage,* 2021. (website). Available at: www.arrt.org.

Bureau of Labor Statistics: *US Department of Labor: Occupational outlook handbook,* 2018. (website). Available at: www.bls.gov/ooh/home.htm.

Centers for Disease Control and Prevention: *Preterm birth,* 2018. (website). Available at: https://www.cdc.gov/reproductivehealth/maternalinfanthealth/pretermbirth.htm.

Centers for Medicare & Medicaid Services (CMS): *Part B costs,* 2021. (website). Available at: www.medicare.gov/your-medicare-costs/part-b-costs/part-b-costs.html.

Central Intelligence Agency: *The world factbook: rank order—infant mortality rate,* 2018. (website). Available at: https://www.cia.gov/library/publications/resources/the-world-factbook/rankorder/2091rank.html.

Clavelle JT, Porter-O'Grady T, Weston MJ, Verran JA: Evolution of structural empowerment: moving from shared to professional governance, *J Nurs Adm* 46(6):308–312, 2016 http://dx.doi.org/10.1097/NNA.0000000000000350.

Dall T, Chen Y, Seifert R, et al.: The economic value of professional nursing, *Med Care* 47(1):97–104, 2009.

Health Resources and Services Administration: *Federally qualified 0020 centers,* 2018. (website). Available at: https://www.hrsa.gov/opa/eligibility-and-registration/health-centers/fqhc/index.html.

Healthy People 2030 Framework: *U.S. Department of Health and Human Services: Office of Disease Prevention and Health Promotion,* 2021. (website). Available at: www.healthypeople.gov.

Institute for Healthcare Improvement: *About us,* 2021. (website). Available at: http://www.ihi.org/about/Pages/default.aspx.

Joint Commission: *The facts about the Joint Commission,* 2018. (website). Available at: https://www.jointcommission.org/about_us/about_the_joint_commission_main.aspx.

Kaiser Family Foundation: *Analysis of national health expenditure (NHE) data from Centers for Medicare and Medicaid Services, Office of the Actuary,* 2018. (website). Available at: https://www.healthsystemtracker.org/indicator/spending/national-spending-services/.

Lambertson E: *Nursing team organization and functioning,* New York, 1953, Columbia University.

Rogers R: Adapting to the new workplace reality: Maximizing the role of RNs within a collaborative nursing practice model, *Info Nurs* 39(1):18–20, 2008.

Shirey MR: Nursing practice models for acute and critical care: Overview of care delivery models, *Crit Care Nurs Clin North Am* 20:365–373, 2008.

15

Political Activism in Nursing: Communities, Organizations, and Government

ⓔ To enhance your understanding of this chapter, try the Student Exercises on the Evolve site at http://evolve.elsevier.com/Black/professional.

LEARNING OUTCOMES

After studying this chapter, students will be able to:

- Differentiate between politics and policy.
- Explain why professions have associations.
- Demonstrate an understanding of the complex role that associations play in the profession and in society.
- Recognize the opportunities that associations offer to increase the leadership capacity of nursing students and registered nurses.
- Explain the concept of personalizing the political process.
- Describe the debate in nursing regarding unionization.
- Cite examples of sources of both personal and professional power.
- Describe how nurses can become involved in politics and policy development at the levels of citizen, activist, and politician.
- Explain how organized nursing is involved in political activities designed to strengthen professional nursing and influence health policy.

The national policymaking stage is close at hand to the American public because of national media networks, 24-hour cable news coverage, and social media. Life "inside the Beltway" of Washington, D.C., is increasingly streamed into American living rooms and to our mobile phones, and thus it is under scrutiny. Interest and involvement of American citizens in governmental processes and accountability are good for democracy. Keeping abreast of events on the national and even the world stage is an important part of good citizenship (Fig. 15.1).

National politics and policy are of great interest; however, much of the politics and policy that affect our daily lives occurs at the state and local levels. The workings of government in your state legislature and local municipalities are likely to be much less familiar to you than what is occurring nationally. Even less conspicuous are the policymaking and policy-influencing activities that occur within the professional organizations that support and shape nursing practice. Yet our day-to-day lives, both professionally and personally, are shaped to a large degree by what happens at the local and organizational levels. This chapter will focus on politics and policymaking in several arenas of importance to nursing. This discussion will start with professional organizations and their roles in setting practice and policy, then will turn to politics and policy in government from both national and local perspectives.

Several chapters of this book cover material that is heavily influenced by government. The content of Chapter 1, the current status of nursing, will be the content of a future edition's Chapter 2, the history and social contexts of nursing. The content of both these chapters reflects policy and politics that affect who nurses are and what we do. Chapter 6 is directly concerned with policy that affects practice. Governmental regulation through

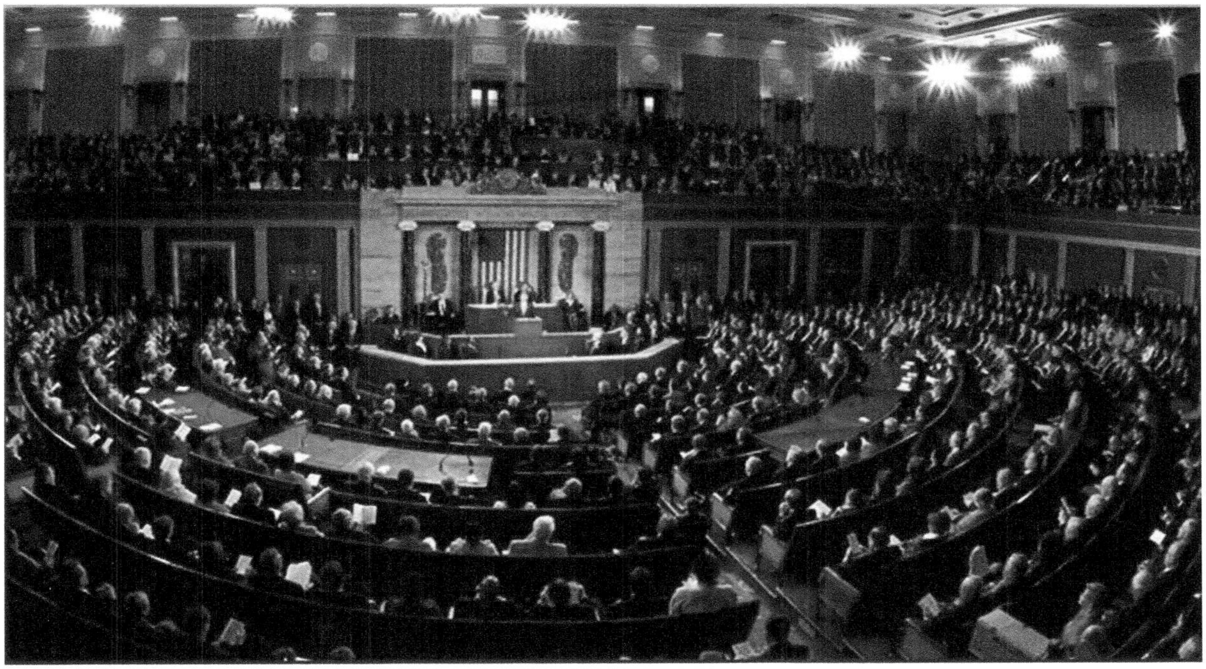

Fig. 15.1 The State of the Union address is delivered once a year by the President of the United States to a joint session of Congress, attended by the Supreme Court justices and the President's Cabinet. All three branches of government are represented at this important address to the nation.

licensure is a function of power, but professional organizations influence how that power is used to set standards and to affect nursing practice acts. The focus on ethics in Chapter 7 describes issues of justice and autonomy, foundational principles in American jurisprudence, which shape how we understand and resolve ethical dilemmas.

Issues of nursing education (Chapter 4) are directly shaped by governmental regulation to ensure that schools of nursing produce graduates who can be entrusted to provide safe care. In Chapter 10, you learned about the National Institutes of Health (NIH) and specifically about the National Institute for Nursing Research (NINR), which are federally funded agencies of the U.S. Department of Health and Human Services. Research is key to the development of the knowledge base of nursing, which in turn protects its status and therefore its influence as a profession and an academic discipline. Chapter 14 introduced the complex issues of healthcare delivery and finance. This is a heavily regulated endeavor with significant implications affecting how and where nurses practice. This completes the circle, leading you back to Chapter 1, the current status of nursing, and where we are going.

Furthermore, you are beginning your practice at the time when health care and its accessibility and affordability continues to be a major focus of the political discourse in the U.S. As the largest single group of healthcare providers in the country, nurses could have significant influence on reforms to our healthcare system.

POLICY AND POLITICS: NOT JUST IN WASHINGTON, D.C

Policy and politics are more than what is happening in Washington, D.C. They encompass what happens to us in our daily lives, in the workplace, and in our organizations, as well as in government. According to the Merriam-Webster dictionary (Merriam-Webster, 2018), the word politics has three meanings. Concise definitions are as follows:

a: the art or science of government

b: the art or science concerned with guiding or influencing governmental policy c: the art or science concerned with winning and holding control over a government

We tend to think of politics in terms of the third definition, the one associated with political parties, campaigns, promises, and wrangling for votes, support, and power. However, the first and second definitions have the more lasting impact on society. The government is the political body that has to do with the regulation and preservation of state and nation. The politics of the third definition is the process by which we determine who will occupy the government in our representative democracy.

Policy, on the other hand, refers to "a definite course or method of action selected from among alternatives and in light of given conditions to guide and determine present and future decisions; a high-level overall plan embracing the general goals and acceptable procedures especially of a governmental body" (Merriam-Webster, 2018).

Policy is formalized by elected officials who describe their agenda before an election to receive support, endorsements, and, ultimately, enough votes to be elected into office. For instance, during the 2008 presidential campaign, the pros and cons of healthcare reform were discussed and debated at length, and as the nominee, then-Senator Barack Obama took a stand in favor of healthcare reform. After his election, legislation known informally as the Affordable Care Act (ACA; "Obamacare") was passed by Congress and signed into law on March 23, 2010. Healthcare reform was debated again in the 2012 campaign, and numerous challenges to the ACA have been unsuccessful, including more than 50 attempts by Congress to have the ACA repealed and two cases argued before the Supreme Court. The first *(National Federation of Independent Business v. Sebelius)* challenged the individual health insurance mandate; the second *(King v. Burwell)* challenged subsidies obtained through HealthCare.gov, claiming that they were illegal. In both cases the Court found for the government. (Sebelius and Burwell were secretaries of the U.S. Department of Health and Human Services when these cases were filed.)

President Obama embarked on a complex and wide-ranging effort to make health care more affordable. The 24-hour cable news outlets both reported and argued the various merits of his healthcare campaign agenda throughout his 2008 and 2012 presidential campaigns. In other words, President Obama used politics

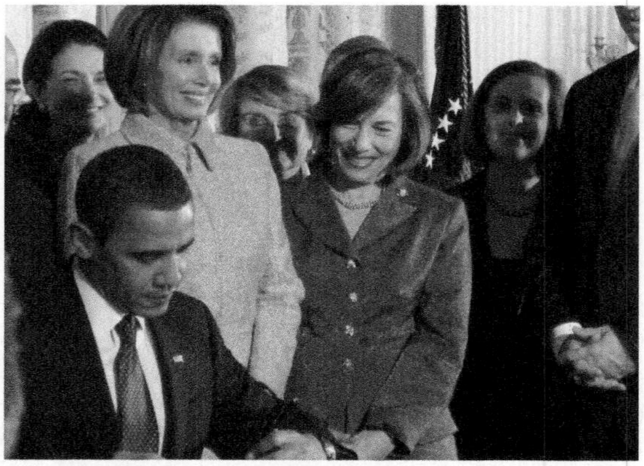

Fig. 15.2 President Barack Obama at a White House signing ceremony of the SCHIP legislation 2 weeks after taking office in January 2009. He said, "I refuse to accept that millions of our children fail to reach their full potential because we fail to meet their basic needs." Used with permission from United Press International.

as a process (the second definition) to achieve a goal of managing the government (first definition) so that he could influence change in healthcare policy with the expectation and hope of improving affordability. One of the first pieces of legislation signed by President Obama during his first term was related to health care, the State Children's Health Insurance Program (SCHIP) reauthorization legislation that extended health insurance coverage to 8 million children whose parents cannot afford health insurance coverage (Fig. 15.2).

Power, Authority, and Influence

A review of the concepts of *power*, *authority*, and *influence* will help focus the discussion of policy and the remainder of this chapter. Power is strength or force that is exerted or capable of being exerted. Power in and of itself is latent.

A person who has authority has legitimacy to exert power—that is, to enforce laws, demand obedience, make commands and determinations, or judge the acts of others. People who have been vested with this power—for instance, through a fair and democratic process—are known as *authorities*, especially a government or body of government officials. Influence is a form of power that is not legitimated through official channels, such as elections or appointments by one in authority, but influence is the action or process of producing effects on the actions, behavior, and opinions of others.

For example, the work of lobbyists is to influence government officials to vote in a certain way that will benefit the constituency that hired the lobbyist to work on its behalf. In other words, lobbyists exist to exert influence.

A simple clinical example will clarify the difference among these three concepts.

Jane Wilson, RN, is an experienced labor and delivery nurse, and her patient is Ms. Gardner. Ms. Gardner has been in labor for several hours but is not making much progress (in SBAR terms, "lack of progress in labor" would be her assessment). Nurse Wilson believes that augmenting Ms. Gardner's labor with oxytocin would be appropriate (in SBAR terms, this would be her recommendation). Nurse Wilson cannot begin this infusion because she does not have the authority to do so without Dr. Martin prescribing it. Dr. Martin has both the power and the authority to prescribe the infusion. Nurse Wilson, because she has extensive experience, understands that she can influence Dr. Martin's decision by giving Dr. Martin her expert opinion on the situation, and in fact SBAR provides her with an excellent structure to provide information necessary for Dr. Martin to make a safe judgment. She calls Dr. Martin, influences Dr. Martin to prescribe the oxytocin, and begins the infusion in a few minutes. Ms. Gardner gives birth to a healthy baby three hours later. Note that Nurse Wilson exerted power through influencing Dr. Martin's decision; Dr. Martin had latent power—that is, power that had not yet been used—and authority as a licensed physician to prescribe the infusion.

This is a common scenario between nurses who need something for their patients and physicians, nurse practitioners and physician assistants who hold (depending on the state) authority to prescribe. You can also see in this example the interdisciplinary collaboration that includes both independent and interdependent actions on the part of Nurse Wilson.

Policy

Policy involves principles that govern actions directed toward given ends; policy statements set forth a plan, direction, or goal for action. Policies may result in laws, regulations, or guidelines that govern behavior in the public arena or in the private arena. *Health policy* refers to public or private rules, regulations, laws, or guidelines that relate to the pursuit of health and the delivery of health services. Policy reflects the choices that an entity (government or organization) makes regarding its goals and priorities and how it will allocate its resources.

Policy decisions (i.e., laws or regulations) reflect the values and beliefs of those making the decisions. As values and beliefs change, so do policy decisions. For instance, laws limiting smoking in public buildings or private restaurants were nonexistent 60 years ago because the harmful effects of smoking and secondhand smoke were not yet well known. As the public became more aware of the dangers of smoking, values about smoking changed. Changes in laws followed the change in values. Laws limiting smoking and the sale and use of tobacco products are common. Elected officials responded to the changing values of the public and recognized that the public supported the passage of laws limiting smoking. In a representative democracy, this is how policy is changed. Officials are elected to represent and then act on the interests of their constituents, that is, the people of their state, congressional district, or municipality.

In professional organizations, policy focuses on the rules and guidelines established by the governing body of the organization, usually a board of directors. Those guidelines or policies also reflect the values of the organization. For instance, one would expect a nursing organization such as the American Nurses Association (ANA) to focus on issues of health promotion, illness prevention, and nursing practice issues. That would be quite different from an organization such as the National Collegiate Athletic Association (NCAA), in which the values of its members would be reflected in policies and recommendations supporting and regulating athletics at the college level across the country.

Politics

Politics is a process that requires influencing the allocation of scarce resources. *Allocation* assumes that there are not enough resources for all who may want them. Those resources might be money, people, time, supplies, or equipment. How those resources are allocated is determined through the political process. Policies are the decisions; politics is influencing those decisions. There are always **stakeholders**—individuals with a vested interest—who try to influence those with the power to make the final decisions.

In organizations, stakeholders are the members, the larger community served by the work of the organization, and other groups or individuals affected by those decisions. For example, Patients Out of Time, an organization started by a nurse, works to educate the public and healthcare professionals about the therapeutic use of cannabis and to advocate for the medicinal use of marijuana (www.medicalcannabis.com). Founded in 1995, stakeholders for Patients Out of Time are patients and their families, healthcare providers, and those who make decisions about the laws and regulations about cannabis use. These include state and federal legislators, as well as the U.S. Food and Drug Administration (FDA), the Secretary of Health and Human Services who oversees the policies of the FDA, and organizations such as the American Public Health Association, which issued a position statement in 1995 supporting patients' safe access to therapeutic marijuana (cannabis) (American Public Health Association, 1995). The ANA issued a position statement in 2016 calling for the development of prescribing standards and evidence-based guidelines for the use of medical marijuana (ANA, 2018).

Politics works similarly in the public arena. For example, to garner support from state legislators to increase funding for nursing scholarships, an organization or coalition of organizations must have a plan to mobilize stakeholders to lobby legislators. Such stakeholders would include administrators of nursing organizations, colleges of nursing, hospitals, nursing homes, and other healthcare organizations, as well as physician groups and others who know the necessity of having a competent and adequate nursing workforce. The more stakeholder support that can be generated, the more likely it is that policymakers will note and respond positively to the broad constituent support for the issue; in this example, this means they would vote for increased funding for nursing education and scholarships.

Linking Practice, Policy, and Politics

Early leaders in nursing, from Florence Nightingale to Lavinia Dock, saw and understood the connection between their work and the larger world in which policy decisions affected what they were able to do. Nightingale could not have been successful in the Crimea without the support of Sir Sidney Herbert, Secretary of War. Lavinia Dock joined with other nurses to found the ANA, pressure hospital administrators to improve working conditions for nurses, and galvanize support for nursing registration (Lewenson, 2007, p. 23). A more recent example of improving the working conditions for nurses can be found in the story of Karen Daley, a nurse who went public with her needlestick injury, from which she contracted human immunodeficiency virus (HIV) and hepatitis C infections (Daley, 2007). She wanted to influence legislation requiring protective devices. In each instance, these leaders knew that nursing practice could be improved only through legislation, regulation, or unification to create a formidable national organization. Daley recognized the power that her story held and the extent to which her experience could influence those with authority to make nursing practice safer. She testified before the House Committee on Education and the Workforce's Subcommittee on Workforce Protection, taking her experience to a large, influential national stage. The larger world of public policy and the work of organizations become the arena in which someone with a vision for improved health or working conditions can change the way health is delivered and improve the health of populations. With these examples in mind, we now turn our attention to professional organizations as a means of activism.

PROFESSIONAL ORGANIZATIONS: STRENGTH IN NUMBERS

Professionals in many domains create organizations to work together on issues that enhance their work and community involvement, to ensure continued learning and competence, and to use political action to influence policymakers to support the organization's mission. The collective strength of a large group of committed persons in a robust organization can be impressive. Professional organizations offer a platform to learn leadership skills, to test ideas, and to follow these ideas to completion. As you know, nursing has a national organization open to all registered nurses (RNs), the ANA (www.nursingworld.org); a national student nurses organization, the National Student Nurses Association (NSNA, www.nsna.org); and many other specialty organizations developed around particular practice areas. Nursing organizations influence public policy in a variety of ways. The following section examines the role and function of organizations, explores why nurses do or do not join organizations, and discusses examples of collective action. Because organizations are often the catalyst for involvement in political action, we will also explore the broader area of political action in the public arena.

Joining a Professional Organization

Nurses join organizations to network with colleagues, to pursue continuing education and certification opportunities, to stay informed on professional issues, to develop leadership skills, to influence health policy, and to work collectively for job security. Despite these benefits of belonging to the ANA, fewer than 10% of the nation's RNs are ANA members and only 20% of nurses belong to one of the many specialty nursing organizations. Nurses cite high cost of dues, lack of time, and lack of interest as reasons they do not join. In some states, complex relationships between the state nurses association, the ANA, and collective bargaining units restrict ANA membership. Professional Profile Box 15.1 contains comments from Megan Williams, MSN, RN, FNP, former President of the North Carolina Nurses Association, on how nurses make a difference through their state nurses associations and the ANA.

PROFESSIONAL PROFILE BOX 15.1

Making a Difference Through the State Nurses Association and the ANA

If you have invested in nursing as your career, the next step is to invest in your profession, and joining a professional association such as the American Nurses Association (ANA) is a great start. As an undergraduate nursing student at the University of North Carolina at Wilmington, I was a member of my school chapter of the Association of Nursing Students (ANS). I attended the National Student Nurses Association (NSNA) annual convention in Atlanta, Georgia. Attending a national convention was a pivotal experience in my nursing career. I heard national leaders in nursing share their passion to improve patient care. I was inspired by those leaders to continue to invest in my career and in the nursing profession as a whole.

I joined the North Carolina Nurses Association (NCNA) and ANA as a new nurse graduate. As a member, I receive monthly publications with up-to-date "best practice" ideas that I can apply directly to my nursing practice, and I participate in continuing education programs with nurses from a variety of practice areas. Another valuable benefit of my membership has been creating professional relationships with nurses across the state and across the nation. I enjoy sharing ideas, asking for advice, and volunteering for leadership opportunities.

In the fall of 2013, I was elected as the 51st president of NCNA. In my role as president, I led the organization in developing a strategic plan to allocate the resources and align the many programs and services that are available to NCNA members with our organizational goals. As president, I provided outreach to the internal nursing community through a variety of communications and I represent NCNA in local, state, and national external venues. One of the most important external communities I communicated with were the state and national elected officials. I have advocated at the state and national level to increase access to care, positively influence the cost and quality of health care, and increase and advance the nursing workforce.

Nurses are in a unique position to share their expertise and knowledge when meeting with legislators. The ability to successfully exert influence in the various arenas where healthcare policy decisions are made and to present nursing's perspective on healthcare issues depends largely on being an engaged member of your professional association. The nursing profession has a rich history of legislative advocacy. Here in North Carolina, Mary Lewis Wyche, founder of NCNA, drafted the first Nurse Practice Act in 1893. In 2015 NCNA collaborated with all Advanced Practice Registered Nurse (APRN) groups and the North Carolina Board of Nursing to support legislation to modernize the Nursing Practice Act in North Carolina. This legislation is necessary to remove barriers to the utilization of nurses at all levels to practice to their full scope of knowledge and expertise in all settings and to receive just payment for their services rendered.

I really believe that the answers to major healthcare issues facing society today can come from a committed group of smart, thoughtful, and connected nursing professionals. It is time that nurses start leaning forward into every critical conversation at every intersection where healthcare decisions are made. Let's keep the conversations forward thinking and solution-oriented. With so many benefits and opportunities awaiting you as a member of a professional nursing organization, what are you waiting for? Join today!

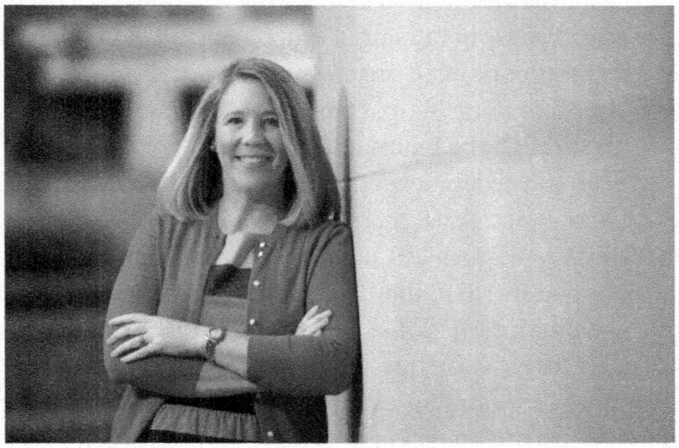

Megan P. Williams, MSN, RN, FNP
Former President, North Carolina Nurses Association

Courtesy Megan P. Williams.

Types of Organizations

There are more than 100 national nursing organizations and many more state and local groups. Nurses often express confusion about which group to join. In general, organizations (associations) can be classified as one of three main types:

1. Broad-purpose professional organizations
2. Specialty practice organizations
3. Special interest organizations

The ANA is an example of a broad-purpose organization. Individual nurses who belong to the ANA typically are members of their state's constituent member association. As the nursing profession's body of knowledge and research grows and diversifies, many nurses limit their practices to specialty practice areas such as maternal/infant care, school or community health, critical care, or palliative and end-of-life care. They often join the specialty organization for their area of clinical interest. Members of specialty practice nursing associations also may choose to belong to the ANA or one of its constituent member associations (at the state level) to support the entire profession because specialty associations focus only on standards of practice or professional needs of the particular specialty. More than 60 specialty organizations and other nursing organizations are represented in the Nursing Organizations Alliance (the Alliance), a coalition of nursing organizations promoting the voice of nursing and cohesive action on issues of concern to nursing (Nursing Organizations Alliance, 2021).

Examples of special interest organizations include Sigma Theta Tau International (the Honor Society of Nursing), which one must be invited to join, and the American Association for the History of Nursing, which focuses on a particular area of study in nursing. Comprehensive and frequently updated lists of nursing organizations are available online at www.nurse.org/orgs.shtml. Nurses are connected internationally through the International Council of Nurses (ICN). The ICN is a federation of more than 130 national nurse associations. The ANA represents U.S. RNs in the ICN, and the NSNA represents U.S. nursing students in the ICN.

Founded in 1899, the ICN is the world's first and widest-reaching international organization for health professionals. Operated by nurses for nurses, the ICN works to ensure quality nursing care for all, sound health policies globally, the advancement of nursing knowledge, the presence worldwide of a respected nursing profession, and a competent and satisfied nursing workforce. For additional details about the ICN's activities in professional nursing practice, nursing regulation, and the socioeconomic welfare of nurses, visit the ICN home page (www.icn.ch).

The Mission and Activities of Organizations

An organization's activities reflect its mission statement. The mission statement is generated by the membership and defines the organization's purpose and goals and who is served by the organization. For instance, the ANA's goals are "fostering high standards of nursing practice, promoting a safe and ethical work environment, bolstering the health and wellness of nurses and advocating on healthcare issues that affect nurses and the public" (ANA, 2018a). These goals are reflected in their concise mission statement: "Nurses advancing our profession to improve health for all" (ANA, 2018a). These goals and mission define the association's areas of focus as practice standards, a code of ethical conduct, continuing education and conferences, and collective action around workplace issues.

Nurses and Unions

Unionization of nurses is a controversial topic. Nurses may choose to join unions to work collectively, to have control over their practice and workplace, and to work to equalize power between management and staff. This can be an effective approach if the healthcare organization is willing to work collaboratively with unions. Union affiliation is a highly complex process, one that is defined by rules and regulations under the National Labor Act and overseen by the National Labor Relations Board. There are limits on the issues for which unions can bargain; for instance, hours, pay, and benefits are included in all contracts for all unionized workers.

For nurses, additional issues are increasingly part of contract negotiations, such as staffing, work assignments, and shared governance responsibilities. The recent nursing shortage created an environment in which both management and nurses themselves aspired to develop work environments that decreased turnover and ensured a competent workforce.

National Nurses United (NNU) is an affiliation of collective bargaining organizations that work to improve working conditions for nurses because this in turn results in better care for patients. The NNU was formed in 2009 when United American Nurses (UAN), which represented only nurses, merged with the California Nurses Association (CNA), the National Nurses Organizing Committee, and the Massachusetts Nurses Association. Some nonnursing unions have nursing units:

the Service Employees International Union (SEIU); the American Federation of Teachers (AFT); the Association of Federal, State, County, and Municipal Employees (AFSCME); and the United Mine Workers (UMW). These organizations all have nursing units but also represent larger, nonnursing constituencies.

Nurses wonder whether they should join unions. Much of that depends on where they work. If seeking a staff position in an institution in which a nursing union already exists, a nurse may be required to join the union as a condition of employment. This is called a "closed shop," meaning that management is required to bargain with the union, and union membership is required as a condition of employment. An "open shop" is one in which employees are not required to join but in which an individual's contract will be dependent on what union and management have negotiated. Most nurses work in nonunion facilities. Some states are more "union friendly" than others. The majority of nursing unions exist in states in which labor unions flourish, such as in the Northeast, Northwest, and Midwest. Other states, particularly in the Southeast (other than Florida) and Southwest, have few or no nurse unions. These are known as "right to work states." Although unions have made numerous attempts to organize nurses in these states, the value system of the work culture is less supportive of union affiliation by nursing professionals. Fig. 15.3

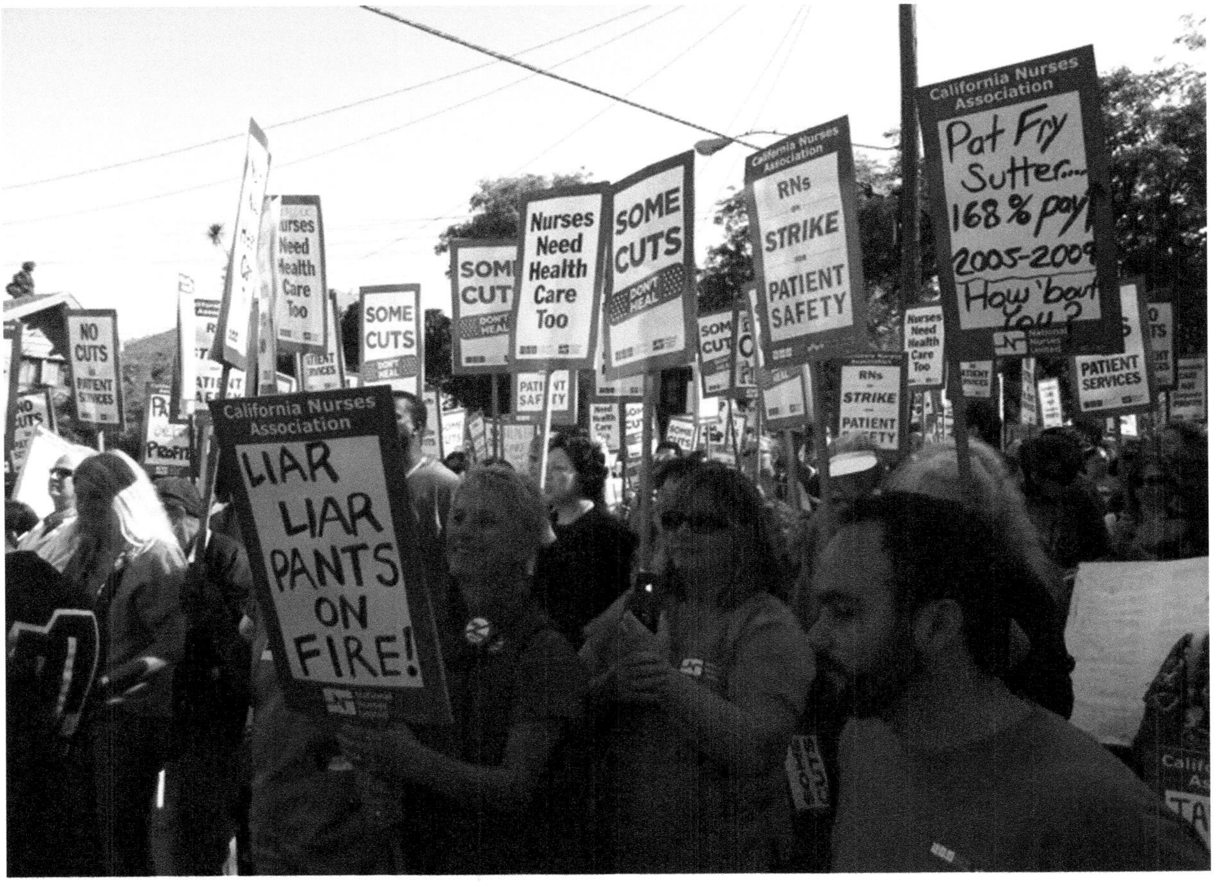
California Nurses Association
Pat Fry
Sutter...
168% pay
How 'bout You?
RNs
STRIKE
PATIENT SAFETY
Nurses Need Health Care Too
SOME CUTS
NO CUTS
PATIENT SERVICES
California Nurses Association
LIAR
LIAR
PANTS
ON
FIRE!

Fig. 15.3 "When nurses are on the outside, there's something wrong on the inside." So noted DeAnne McEwen, Co-President of the California Nurses Association (CNA), at a rally and 1-day RN strike on September 22, 2011. Approximately 23,000 RNs, members of the CNA/National Nurses United, were protesting proposed cuts in nurses' healthcare coverage and retiree benefits and widespread cuts in patient care services. Nurses carried signs that read, "Some cuts don't heal." Courtesy California Nurses Association/National Nurses United.

PROFESSIONAL PROFILE BOX 15.2

United We Stand, Divided We Beg: A Nurse's View of Collective Bargaining

In my workplace, I serve as the chairperson for the faculty union. I am responsible for ensuring that the administration honors the union contract, which describes working conditions, job responsibilities, salaries, and benefits. A contract is negotiated through the bargaining process. Through my experience as a member of the union's bargaining team, I found that negotiating a contract is truly an eye-opening experience because bargaining team members get a glimpse of what administrators would do if they had free reign. Members of the negotiating team begin the process of preparing for negotiations long before the two teams ever meet at the bargaining table. Most unions survey their members to determine which issues are of greatest importance. The negotiating team is then empowered to bargain for the things that matter most to the people in their bargaining unit. At the bargaining table, the union's negotiating team works hard to secure gains for the membership, particularly in the areas cited by the members, which are usually related to salary, benefits, and working conditions. Many strategies are used throughout the negotiating process, and they change from moment to moment. In general, however, one of the most important strategies the team uses is to avoid revealing which items are most important to their members because once the administration knows something is very important to the team, the cost of that item increases significantly. The cost of an item may be a concession in another area or an actual financial trade-off. Successfully negotiating a contract requires give-and-take. Sometimes the process goes smoothly and agreements are procured rather swiftly. Other times, it does not. If the bargaining process becomes stalled, particularly due to intransigence by the administration, union leadership will direct a campaign aimed at pressuring the administration into doing more to ensure that a fair contract is attained. Typically, the union takes actions such as instituting "work to rule," which means that the members do only the minimum required by the contract, or launching a public relations campaign. The contract itself determines what recourse members of the bargaining unit have if those measures are unsuccessful. A strike is an option of last resort and some contracts even include a "no strike/no lockout" clause that prevents union members from going on strike and administrators from locking employees out. The ultimate goal of contract negotiations is to develop a contract that provides fair remuneration, benefits, and work assignments. It should also provide union members with protections against practices that prevent them from doing their job well or create unsafe working conditions. The process works best when union members stick together, support each other, and refuse to settle for unreasonable demands. Unionization ensures that no worker stands alone.

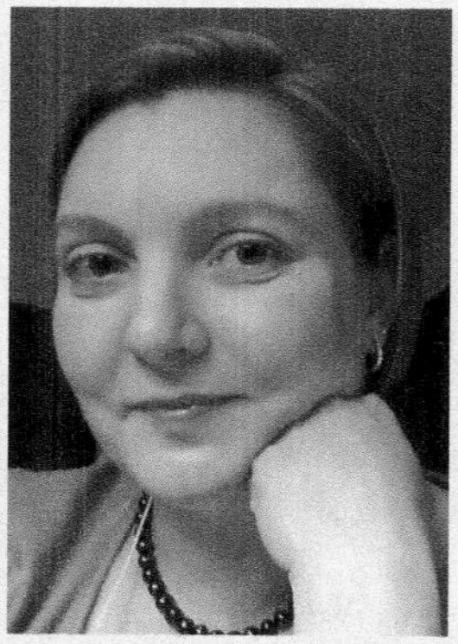

Patricia Moyle Wright, PhD, RN, ACNS-BC, CNE, CHPN
University of Scranton, Scranton, PA

Courtesy Patricia Moyle Wright.

shows nurses protesting during a 1-day strike in California in September 2011. In Professional Profile Box 15.2, you will read comments by Patricia Moyle Wright, PhD, RN, ACNS-BC, CNE, CHPN, who describes her views of the benefits of collective bargaining.

BENEFITS OF JOINING A PROFESSIONAL ORGANIZATION

A variety of benefits result from membership in professional organizations. These range from certification and discounts on travel, products, and services, to opportunities to engage in research projects and learn political action strategies.

Developing Leadership Skills

Students who join the NSNA have opportunities to learn from and socialize with their peers in school and at the state and national levels. As NSNA members, they benefit from developing leadership and organizational skills that can be vital in their professional careers and personal lives. The NSNA embraces the following core values: leadership and autonomy, quality education, advocacy, professionalism, care, and diversity (NSNA, 2018). From the school chapter level to the state and national levels, nursing students learn how to work in shared governance and cooperative relationships with peers, faculty, students in other disciplines, community service organizations, and the public. In addition to preparing students to participate in professional organizations, practicing shared governance also prepares students to work in healthcare delivery settings that incorporate unit-based decision making, such as Magnet hospitals. For complete details about all of the NSNA's programs, visit their website (www.nsna.org).

Leadership skills are foundation blocks for nursing professional practice. Nurses have numerous opportunities to exercise leadership at the bedside, in clinical teams, and in management teams. The Nursing Alliance Leadership Academy (Nursing Organizations Alliance, 2018) was created to help nurses enhance leadership skills and focus on patients and care issues by inspiring and developing future nurse leaders. The academy also focuses on developing political skills and policy awareness (for more information, see https://www.nursing-alliance.org).

Professional associations offer a supportive environment in which members can practice the acquisition of important leadership skills. Speaking publicly, planning projects, managing resources, and developing resolutions and position papers are opportunities to practice skills essential to formal leadership roles. It is no coincidence that nurses who are active in associations also tend to be recognized leaders in their work settings.

Certification and Continuing Education

Practicing nurses want to be recognized, through both compensation and position, for their level of professional expertise. Toward those ends, they may pursue certification in a specialty area. Certification is granted through professional associations. As discussed in Chapter 4, certification is a formal but voluntary process of demonstrating expertise in a particular area of nursing. Certified nurses may receive salary supplements and special opportunities. For information about credentials in nursing, visit the website of the ANA's subsidiary, the American Nurses Credentialing Center, which offers a range of certification credentials (www.nursecredentialing.org).

Political Activism

Nurses depend on activism to protect their interests. For instance, nurses can obtain master's- or doctoral-level preparation to become nurse practitioners and practice independently. These nurses deserve direct reimbursement for their work and need state laws that mandate direct reimbursement. Others work in settings in which there are not enough RNs available to provide the quality of care the residents need. These nurses need laws that ensure appropriate RN staffing and control educational requirements for unlicensed assistive personnel.

In each of these instances, the ANA, labor unions, and specialty organizations are involved in political action with legislators and regulators in the government arena. There are those within these organizations who develop the positions that nursing organizations believe are in nursing's best interests. There are a number of people within these organizations whose responsibilities are to advocate for legislation to support nursing's position. The process of political action and policy recommendations involves both paid staff, usually in the government affairs department, and volunteer members of the organizations, usually practicing nurses. The legislative agenda—that is, the public policy issues the organization supports—is developed by members appointed by the board of directors, as well as by staff who are experts in political and policy issues. The board of directors approves the legislative agenda. Organizations with legislative agendas depend on members to lobby legislators. They provide members with background information and also create "talking points" to use when lobbying for the selected issue. You can read about the ANA's particular legislative interests online in the Policy and Advocacy section (www.nursingworld.org). As part of the process of encouraging nurses to lobby, information is given on the website about specific bills along with talking points for writing or speaking with congressional representatives. Association members can be very influential in lobbying legislators, particularly when the constituency is nationwide and representative of different stakeholders. Learning how to be politically active increases the power of both the individual and the organization represented.

Nursing organizations also work collaboratively through coalitions with other health professional and consumer groups. Such coalitions are focused on specific issues. For example, Health Care Without Harm is a group of hundreds of organizations in 52 countries whose mission is to "transform health care worldwide so that it reduces its environmental footprint, becomes a community anchor for sustainability and a leader in the global movement for environmental health and justice" (Health Care Without Harm, 2018). Hollie Shaner-McRae, DNP, RN, FAAN, founded this organization in 1996 when she became concerned about the waste created by disposable instruments in an operating room. The organization is now a significant national and international force advocating for a healthy climate, safer chemicals, healthy and sustainable food, zero waste from the healthcare sector (including pharmaceuticals), clean air and water, green buildings, and human rights, including access to health care for all (Health care Without Harm, 2018).

Practice Guidelines and Position Statements

Organizations serve an important function by defining practice standards, taking positions on practice issues, and developing ethical guidelines. For example, the ANA has positions on bloodborne and airborne diseases that include statements about HIV infection and nursing students. These positions are consistent with the ANA's recommendation to require educational content about such infections by qualified faculty, mandating universal precautions, and providing postexposure support for students who may sustain a needlestick injury. These statements serve to guide the organization's work in both the practice and the policy arenas and to help individual nurses within workplaces implement the policy. Guidelines and position statements are based on evidence from research, as well as opinions of nurse experts in the field.

Another example is the most recent revision of the *Code of Ethics for Nurses* (ANA, 2015). A task force was appointed by the board of directors to review the previous Code and create revisions and recommendations. The revisions went through a process of approval by many entities within the ANA: the Congress of Nursing Practice, the Board of Directors, and the House of Delegates, which speaks on behalf of all the members. Approval from so many groups within an organization ensures "buy-in" by the membership. Buy-in is important because the Code serves as an ethical standard for all practicing nurses, whether they are ANA members or not, and is therefore of critical importance.

The NSNA also has a Code of Conduct (Box 15.1), which provides guidance for nursing students. This Code serves as the ethical foundation of student practice.

Other Benefits

There are many other benefits of membership, such as access to journals, newsletters, and action alerts about particular topics that need immediate response; eligibility for group health and life insurance; networking with peers; continuing education opportunities; and discounts on products and services, such as car rentals, computers, or books.

Deciding Which Associations to Join

As you decide whether to belong to an association, visit the group's website to find out more about its activities. Then ask yourself the following questions:

1. What is the mission and what are the purposes of this association?
2. Are the association's purposes compatible with my own?
3. How many members are there nationally, statewide, and locally?
4. What activities does the association undertake?
5. How active is the local chapter?
6. What opportunities does the association offer for involvement and leadership development?
7. What are the benefits of membership?
8. Does the association offer continuing education programs?
9. Does the organization lobby for improved healthcare legislation? How successful is it?
10. Is membership in this association cost effective?
11. Even if I am not active, what benefit will I derive from the legislative agenda and other activities that the association undertakes to advocate for nurses and patients?

Answering these questions and speaking with current association members should provide nurses with adequate information to make reasoned decisions.

POLITICAL ACTIVISM IN GOVERNMENT

Now that you understand how professional organizations use collective power to influence policy decisions, let us examine how policy influences the practice of nursing. The ability of the individual nurse to provide

BOX 15.1 National Student Nurses Association Code of Academic and Clinical Conduct

Preamble

Students of nursing have a responsibility to actively promote the highest level of moral and ethical principles and to embody the academic theory and clinical skills needed to continuously provide evidence-based nursing care given the resources available. Grounded in excellence, altruism, and integrity, the clinical setting presents unique challenges and responsibilities while caring for people in a variety of healthcare environments. The Code of Academic and Clinical Conduct is based on an agreement to uphold the trust that society has placed in us while practicing as nursing students. The statements of the Code provide guidance for nursing students in the personal development of an ethical foundation for nursing practice. These moral and ethical principles are not limited to the academic or clinical environment and have relevance for the holistic professional development of all students studying to become registered nurses.

Code of Academic and Clinical Conduct

As students who are involved in the clinical and academic environments, we believe that ethical principles, in adherence with the NSNA Core Values, are a necessary guide to professional development.

Therefore within these environments we:

1. Advocate for the rights of all patients.
2. Diligently maintain patient confidentiality in all respects, regardless of method or medium of communication.
3. Take appropriate action to ensure the safety of patients, self, and others.
4. Provide care for the patient in a timely, compassionate, professional, and culturally sensitive and competent manner.
5. Are truthful timely, and accurate in all communications related to patient care.
6. Accept responsibility for our decisions and actions.
7. Promote excellence and leadership in nursing by encouraging lifelong learning, continuing education, and professional development.
8. Treat others with respect and promote an inclusive environment that values the diversity, rights, cultural practices, and spiritual beliefs of all patients and fellow healthcare professionals.
9. Collaborate with academic faculty and clinical staff to ensure the highest quality of patient care and student education.
10. Use every opportunity to improve faculty and clinical staff understanding of the nursing student's learning needs.
11. Encourage mentorship among nursing students, faculty, clinical staff, and interprofessional peers.
12. Refrain from performing skills or procedures without adequate preparation, and seek supervision and assistance when necessary.
13. Refrain from any deliberate action or omission in academic or clinical settings that create unnecessary risk for injury to the patient, self, or others.
14. Assist the clinical nurse or preceptor in ensuring that adequate informed consent is obtained from patients for research participation, for certain treatments, or for invasive procedures.
15. Abstain from the use of any legal or illegal substances in academic and clinical settings that could impair judgment.
16. Strive to achieve and maintain an optimal level of personal health.
17. Support access to treatment and rehabilitation for students who are experiencing impairment related to substance abuse and mental or physical health issues.
18. Uphold school policies and regulations related to academic and clinical performance, reserving the right to challenge and critique rules and regulations as per school grievance policy.

First adopted by the 2001 House of Delegates, Nashville, TN.
Amended by the House of Delegates at the NSNA Annual Convention on April 7, 2017, in Dallas, TX.
From www.nsna.org.

care is significantly affected by public policy decisions. Yet too few nurses are aware of the importance of their role in influencing such policy outcomes, because they miss the connection between their own practice and the world of public policy.

As discussed in Chapter 6, state licensure of an RN derives from legislation that defines the scope of nursing practice. The defined scope determines what a nurse legally can and cannot do. As a result of changes in education and clinical practice, nursing organizations influence legislators to change state nursing practice acts to reflect what nurses are qualified to do. For instance, at one time the administration of intravenous medications was not within the scope of nursing practice but instead was limited to medical practice. It is difficult to imagine how a hospital or other healthcare setting could function today if this were still the case. Regulations are developed to guide the implementation of legislation. They affect practicing nurses and their work environments. For example, the Food and Drug Administration (FDA), a regulatory agency of the federal government, sets the rules for administering and documenting the administration of narcotics. The FDA is a division of the Department of Health and Human Services. The way in which such regulations are written can greatly affect nursing practice.

The regulations in each state governing nursing practice are contained in the state's nursing practice act. When the regulations change—for example, adding a requirement for continuing education for license renewal—the change affects all nurses in the state. For advanced practice nurses, there are a variety of regulations related to prescription writing and autonomy issues. These change from time to time, and if nurses do not actively participate in changes, new regulations can restrict rather than enhance nursing authority for regulated activities.

Broader issues affecting the nursing profession are also political in nature. Issues of pay equity, or equal pay for work of comparable value, are of concern to nurses because they have been chronically underpaid for their work. One of the earliest cases demonstrating the inequality of nursing salaries involved public health nurses in Colorado. These nurses brought a case against the city of Denver stating that they were paid considerably less than city tree trimmers and garbage collectors. The nurses demanded just compensation for their work by demonstrating that nursing requires more complex knowledge and is of greater value to society than the other occupations (although certainly the value of these other workers is not to be trivialized).

As a result of this suit, recognition of nursing's low pay was brought to public attention, which in turn mobilized public support for increasing nursing salaries. This is an example of political action by nurses that resulted in both policy outcomes (regulations that expanded comparable pay issues to other jobs) and professional outcomes (salary increases for the individual nurse). More recently, the issues of nurse-patient ratios and staffing increasingly have come under scrutiny. Nurses in California mobilized the public and other constituency groups to get the first legislation requiring specific nurse-to-patient ratios passed in 1999; however, the regulations were not implemented until 2004. As of 2018, only 14 states had implemented legislation or adopted regulations related to nurse staffing (California, Connecticut, Illinois, Massachusetts, Minnesota, Nevada, New Jersey, New York, Ohio, Oregon, Rhode Island, Texas, Vermont, Washington) (ANA, 2018b). You can find details of the ANA's principles of nurse staffing and a list of states with staffing laws at www.nursingworld.org/MainMenuCategories/Policy-Advocacy/State/Legislative-Agenda-Reports/State-StaffingPlansRatios. As of 2021, California was the only state requiring minimum nurse-patient ratios to be met at all times by unit. Massachusetts's law requires intensive care unit staffing at a 1:1 or 1:2 nurse-to-patient ratio, depending on stability of the patients.

Becoming Active in Politics: "The Personal Is Political"

Persons involved in the feminist movement in the 1960s coined the phrase "The personal is political." This statement recognized that each individual could use personal experience to understand and become involved in broader social and political issues. This concept enabled individuals who did not consider themselves political to gain insight into what needed to be changed in society and how they could help bring about the change. It gave power to each individual and resulted in people becoming involved in the political process, usually for the first time.

This premise of personalizing the political process has become a fundamental activity for organized nursing. Nurses at the grassroots level become involved in advocating for legislation and supporting candidates for elective office, because they understand the relationship between public policy and their professional and personal lives. Most associations, such as the ANA, American Association of Colleges of Nursing, American Hospital Association, and numerous specialty nursing organizations, actively engage in lobbying to advocate for the professional concerns of their members. Contemporary nursing leaders recognize that "being political," both through professional associations and as individuals, is a professional responsibility essential to the practice and promotion of the nursing profession.

This chapter started with a discussion about national politics because they were the object of intense media coverage and public interest during the past three primary seasons and presidential elections. However, remember that an important premise in the earlier discussion was that much of what affects our day-to-day lives occurs at the state and local levels, in addition to the effects of national legislation. When you work in a practice setting, your scope of practice is set by state law in the nursing practice act and is enacted by your state board of nursing, which also is also the governmental agency that licenses you and certifies your ongoing safety for practice. You may take a detour to work today because of repairs being done on an old bridge from funding awarded your Congressional district through H.R. 3684, The Infrastructure Investment and Jobs Act signed into law by President Joe Biden in late 2021 to fund the improvement of state and local infrastructure. Because you are then in a hurry to get to work, you may be pulled over by your local police officer for speeding, and despite being sympathetic to your need to get to work, they cannot overlook the fact that you were both speeding and driving with an expired license, which you had been meaning to renew but had not gotten around to. You have been busy working extra shifts because your unit is short staffed, and the stagnant economic conditions locally have required a hiring freeze, meaning that you are going to continue to be busy for a while. Later you find a notice in your email account from your state board of nursing reminding you that your nursing license renewal is due in one month. Each of these situations affecting your day-to-day life reflects the notion that you are always, one way or another, in some situation that involves legislation, regulation, or another form of government intervention. The personal is political, and the political is personal.

During the past 50 years of changing national and state health policies, nurses have increased their political astuteness. Through the well-orchestrated efforts of the ANA, other professional organizations, constituent member associations, and political action committees (PACs), nurses are now participating more effectively in both governmental and electoral politics than in the past. Nursing PACs raise and distribute money to candidates who support the profession's stand on certain issues. Nurses' endorsements of candidates have become a valued political asset for many local, state, and national candidates.

Nurses can make a difference in health policy outcomes. Through the political process, nurses influence policy in a variety of ways: by identifying health problems as policy problems; by formulating policy through drafting legislation in collaboration with legislators; by providing formal testimony; by lobbying governmental officials in the executive and legislative branches to make certain health policies a priority for action; and by filing suit as a party or as a friend of the court (an amicus brief) to implement health policy strategies on behalf of consumers. All major nursing professional associations engage in these activities. Because the ANA is the major organization that speaks for all nurses, specific examples of influencing public policy will be drawn largely from ANA's activities.

The ANA reports on the progress of nursing influence with the President, members of Congress and their staffs, and the regulatory agencies that set policy for health programs online on the Policy and Advocacy section of nursingworld.org. Such activity reflects the work of both ANA members and ANA staff. The ANA's political activity in Washington, D.C., is mirrored throughout the United States by other nursing organizations and by ANA constituent member associations conducting similar work with their state governments.

Recognizing the power behind the collective voice of nurses, the ANA declared 2018 as the Year of Advocacy for nurses to "inspire, innovate, and influence." Stories of how nurses have advocated at the bedside, in the boardroom, and even globally are shared through social media as means of inspiring others to action through advocacy. The ANA has created RNAction as a portal to provide the latest updates on health policy developments and advocacy opportunities through regular text messages to those who sign up to receive the notifications. By alerting RNAction members, ANA can rapidly mobilize nurses to lobby their federal representatives to support or oppose particular legislation or rules and regulations. Through the use of digital media and other resources, RNAction members can respond by sending well-timed, well-targeted messages to members of Congress. You can sign up for RNAction at http://p2a.co/Z5pXOHC. Organized activity identifying, financially supporting, and working for candidates who are committed to nursing and "nurse-friendly" issues has dramatically increased in the past two decades. The electoral process is an essential function of the professional association.

Individual nurses can make a difference in policy development and elections. Either by election or by appointment, nurses need to be making health policy decisions, not just influencing them. Getting elected or appointed requires visibility, expertise, energy, risk taking, and a belief that policy and politics are critically important in achieving nursing's goals.

GETTING INVOLVED

To get involved, a nurse must begin to understand the connections between individual practice and public policy. Once that happens, it is easy to get started. Three levels of political involvement in which nurses can participate are as nurse citizens, nurse activists, and nurse politicians.

Nurse Citizens

A nurse citizen brings a health care perspective to the voting booth, to public forums that advocate for health and human services, and to involvement in community activities. For example, budget cuts to a school district might involve elimination of school nurses. At a school board meeting, nurses can effectively speak about the vital services that school nurses provide to children and the cost-effectiveness of maintaining the position.

Nurses tend to vote for candidates who advocate for improved health care. Here are some examples of how the nurse citizen can be politically active.

- Register to vote.
- Vote in every election.
- Keep informed about healthcare issues.
- Speak out when services or working conditions are inadequate.
- Participate in public forums.
- Know your local, state, and federal elected officials.
- Join politically active nursing organizations.
- Participate in community organizations that need health experts.

Once nurses make a decision to become involved politically, they need to learn how to get started. One of the best ways is to form a relationship with one or more policymakers, and clear communication is key in influencing them (Box 15.2).

BOX 15.2 Clear Communication: The Key to Influence

Cultivate a relationship with policymakers from your home district or state. Communicate by visits, phone, e-mail, and letters. When contacting policymakers, do all of the following:

1. State who you are (a nursing student or RN and a voter in a specific district).
2. Identify the issue by a file number, if possible.
3. Be clear on where you stand and why.
4. Be positive when possible.
5. Be concise.
6. Ask for a commitment. State precisely what action you want the policymaker to take.
7. Give your return address, e-mail address, and phone number to urge dialogue.
8. Be persistent. Follow up with calls or letters.
9. If you plan to visit your policymaker, make your appointment in advance in writing and indicate what issue you are interested in discussing.
10. Be quick to thank policymakers when they do something you support.

Nurse Activists

The nurse activist takes a more active role than the nurse citizen and often does so because an issue arises that directly affects the nurse's professional life. The need to respond moves the nurse to a higher level of participation. An early nurse activist, Lillian Wald, featured in Chapter 2, left a notable and lasting legacy after responding to the needs of vulnerable populations in New York City by establishing the Henry Street Settlement, which still is in operation more than a century later. Credited with establishing public health nursing, her tireless work on behalf of impoverished immigrants in New York City embodied her belief that the work of nurses was significant in improving the health of vulnerable people. Wald was also a member of the founding group of the National Association for the Advancement of Colored People (NAACP). Today's nurse activist may respond to a specific need not possibly envisioned in Wald's day. Several nurse activists are presented at various points in the chapter, some of whom became activists in response to a specific issue that became salient to their lives.

Nurse activists can make changes by doing the following:

- Joining politically active nursing organizations
- Contacting a public official through letters, e-mails, or phone calls
- Registering people to vote
- Contributing money to a political campaign
- Working in a campaign
- Lobbying decision makers by providing pertinent statistical and anecdotal information
- Forming or joining coalitions that support an issue of concern

BOX 15.3 Key Questions for Nurses Who Want to Affect Health Policy

1. Know the system. Is it a federal, state, or local issue? Is it in the hands of the executive, legislative, or judicial branch of government?
2. Know the issue. What is wrong? What should happen? Why is it not happening? What is needed—leadership, a plan, pressure, or data?
3. Know the players. Who is on your side, and who is not? Who will make the decision? Who knows whom? Will a coalition be effective? Are you a member of the professional nursing organization?
4. Know the process. Is this a vote? Is this an appropriation? Is this a legislative procedure? Is this a committee or subcommittee report?
5. Know what to do. Should you write, call, arrange a lunch meeting, organize a petition, show up at the hearing, give testimony, demonstrate, or file a suit?

- Writing letters to the editor of local newspapers
- Inviting legislators to visit the workplace
- Holding a media event to publicize an issue
- Providing or giving testimony to legislators and regulatory bodies

Box 15.3 includes guidance on how to affect health policy development.

Nurse Politicians

Once a nurse realizes and experiences the empowerment that can come from political activism, he or she may choose to run for office. No longer satisfied to help others get elected, the nurse politician desires to develop the legislation, not just influence it. Three nurses were elected in 2020 to the 117th Congress of the United States. One of these nurses has been serving in the House of Representatives for 30 years. In 1992 Congresswoman Eddie Bernice Johnson (D-TX-30; Fig. 15.4) was the first nurse elected to the U.S. House of Representatives and has been consistently reelected since. She received her Bachelor of Science in nursing (BSN) from Texas Christian University in 1967 and later earned her master's degree in public administration from Southern Methodist University. At the time of publication, Congresswoman Johnson chaired the House Committee on Science, Space, and Technology. Her Congressional website is https://ebjohnson.house.gov.

Sworn into office in 2019, Congresswoman Lauren Underwood (D-IL-14; Fig. 15.5) is the first woman and person of color to serve in Congress from her district. She is the youngest African American woman to serve in the U.S. House of Representative. In 2021 Underwood introduced the Black Maternal Health Momnibus Act (H.R. 959), a comprehensive package of 12 bills with the goal to end the maternal health crisis in the U.S. Every eligible provision of the Momnibus Act plus

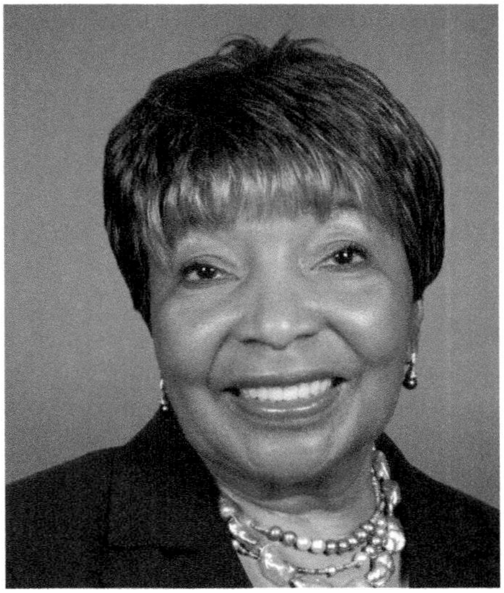

Fig. 15.4 Congresswoman Eddie Bernice Johnson (D-TX-30).

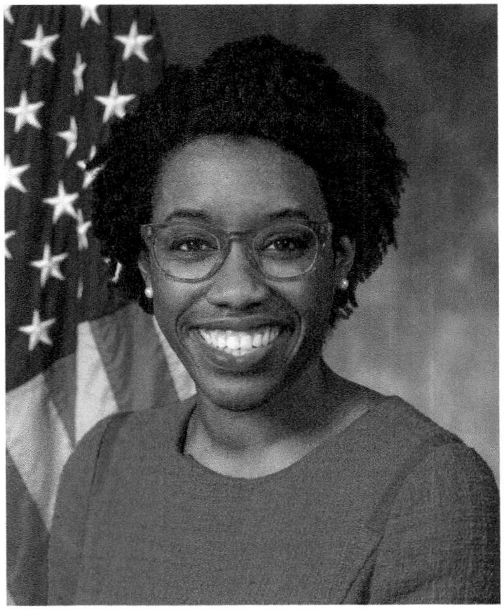

Fig. 15.5 Congresswoman Lauren Underwood (D-IL-14).

permanent expansion of yearlong postpartum Medicaid coverage in every state was included in the Build Back Better Act, which at the time of this writing had been passed by the House of Representatives and had been moved to the Senate for consideration. The Build Back Better Act, the second part of the 2021 infrastructure legislation, proposes legislation related spending on health, climate, childcare, wages and other social programs. The Momnibus provisions are the largest investment in American history to eliminate preventable maternal mortality, end disparate birth outcomes across race and ethnicity, and advance birth equity. After passage in the House of the Build Back Better Act, Congresswoman Underwood responded: "Moms can't wait." Her Congressional website is https://underwood.house.gov.

Elected in 2020, Congresswoman Cori Bush (D-MO-1; Fig. 15.6) was the first Black woman and the first nurse to represent Missouri in Congress and is the first woman to represent her district. In addition to being a nurse, Congresswoman Bush is an ordained pastor and has been a childcare work and a community organizer. She became more politically active after the civil unrest in Ferguson, MO, in 2014. She has been recognized for her advocacy and work in nonviolence, including being a Nonviolence 365 Ambassador with the King Center for Nonviolent Social Change, the Emmitt Till Legacy Foundation, the Hershel Walker Peace and Justice Awards, and the Jefferson City (MO) NAACP. Now serving as the Deputy Whip of the Congressional Progressive Caucus, Congresswoman Bush has introduced a federal bill to decriminalize drug possession, replacing criminalization with a health-centered approach. Her Congressional website is https://bush.house.gov.

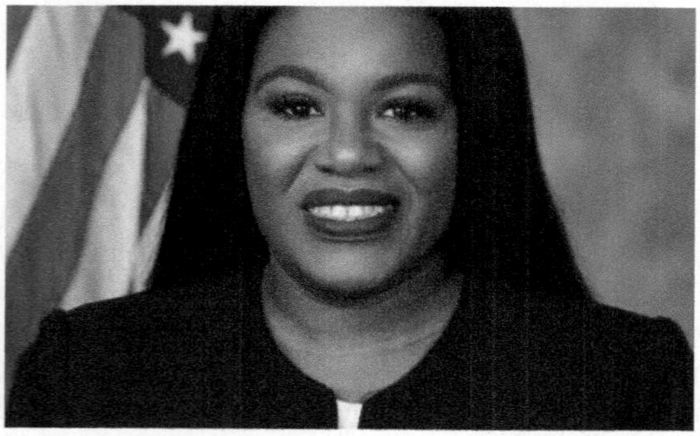

Fig. 15.6 Congresswoman Cori Bush (D-MO-1).

Nurses have shown that they can take on important and public roles in speaking for health care and for the profession of nursing. To be effective agents of change, nurses can do the following:

1. Run for an elected office.
2. Seek appointment to a regulatory agency.
3. Be appointed to a governing board in the public or private sector.
4. Use nursing expertise as a frontline policymaker who can enhance health care and the profession.

Nurses who have achieved success as leaders often started with no knowledge of the political process and no expectations of the greatness they would achieve. Instead, they became involved because some issue, injustice, or abuse of power affected their lives. Instead of complaining or feeling helpless, they responded by taking an active role in bringing about change. The story of nurse and retired Congresswoman Carolyn McCarthy (D-NY) is such an example. McCarthy was a licensed practical nurse who ran for office as a result of her stance on gun control. Her husband was killed and her son critically injured after a lone gunman with a 9 mm semiautomatic pistol walked through a train on the Long Island Railroad and killed 6 people and wounded 19 others. McCarthy was suddenly thrown into the national spotlight when she challenged the incumbent congressman running for office on his stand supporting a repeal on a ban for assault rifles. Her ability to speak passionately about the issue led to her campaign against the incumbent and her election to his seat. For 18 years, McCarthy was a leader in the House of Representatives on gun control, as well as on nursing issues. She retired in 2015.

The mark of a leader is the ability to identify a problem, have a goal, and know how to join others in reaching that goal. A leader must ask the right questions, analyze the positive and restraining forces toward meeting the goal, and know how to obtain and use power. A leader must know how to ask for help and how to give support to those who join the effort. These are the marks of nursing leaders who have become political experts.

NURSING NEEDS YOUR CONTRIBUTION

You no doubt hope to change the world (and you can), but at the same time you hope you pass your upcoming end-of-semester exams, a task that may seem daunting enough without your political aspirations intruding. You can do both. As mentioned throughout this book, mentors can help you become who you want to be. A mentor serves as a role model but also actively teaches, encourages, and critiques the process of growth and change in the learner. You might consider forming a relationship with a political mentor. All nurses who have become political leaders have found mentors along the way to guide and support their growth. Your mentor could be a faculty member, such as the adviser to the nursing student organization or honor society, who can teach you leadership skills. Ask for help in running for a class office or student council position. If elected office does not appeal to you, use your political skills to develop a school or community project with other nursing students. You might find a problem during a clinical experience that inhibits your ability to provide the level of care that you wish to provide. Seek a faculty member or nurse in a clinical facility who can guide you through the process of policy change within the agency or institution.

Seek the help and support of your friends and peers in your activity. The importance of grassroots organization that characterized the most recent election cycles has demonstrated the effectiveness of get-out-the-vote (GOTV) activities and becoming involved in politics at local, state, and national levels. In addition, no matter what your political leanings or positions on issues, it is important that, as a nurse and as a citizen of the democracy, you exercise your right to vote.

CONCEPTS AND CHALLENGES

- ***Concept:*** Professional associations are the vehicle through which nursing takes collective action to improve both the nursing profession and healthcare delivery.
  Challenge: There are many nursing associations from which to choose, offering a variety of benefits to the public, to the nursing profession, and to individual members. Selecting which associations to join can be a challenge.
- ***Concept:*** Professional organizations and professional nurses have much to offer in formulating policy decisions at federal, state, and local levels and in each branch of government.
  Challenge: Becoming politically active is as easy as signing your name in support of an issue, voting, organizing a project, or speaking out on an issue.
- ***Concept:*** Today, organized nursing is involved in politics at many levels in promoting comprehensive health reform and creating a safer workplace.
  Challenge: Political involvement is empowering; one person can make a difference.

IDEAS FOR FURTHER EXPLORATION

1. Look in the media for articles, blog posts, or other communications about legislation that supports nursing's concerns, such as nurse-patient ratio legislation, or other nursing-related or patient-related legislation pending in your state. Contact your representative and/or senators with your opinion about the legislation.
2. Is there a student nurses association on your campus? If there is, consider joining. If there is not a student nurses association, consider establishing one. For resources, go to www.nsna.org.
3. As a student, attend a local or state nurses association meeting to gain a better sense of the issues in the profession so that you can be prepared for what lies ahead when you graduate. How is the association addressing these issues? Do they interest you? How can you get involved?
4. Consider the following hypothetical situation: You are near the end of your final clinical course, a capstone experience in which you have spent almost all of your senior year working with RNs on a medical unit. You have witnessed how working conditions negatively affect patient care, and you are concerned. You learn that the nurses in this hospital are unionized and are planning a 3-day strike in 2 weeks. You support their efforts fully and mention the planned strike to your clinical faculty, who, you discover, is against unionization and collective bargaining. She threatens to fail you for the course if you participate in the nurses' strike. How do you respond? What is at stake if you strike? What is at stake if you do not strike?
5. Register to vote if you are not already registered, and find out what your state laws are regarding voter

identification, early voting, absentee voting, and other issues that may affect your right to cast a ballot. Because some election boards occasionally "purge" voter registration rolls, check to make sure you are registered in your voting district.

6. Because nurses have differing personal and political values, it has been a challenge to get them all united behind a single issue or candidate. If you were the president of the ANA, what techniques would you use to convince the millions of American nurses to use the power of their numbers, their knowledge, and their commitment on behalf of their profession?
7. Find out whether the members of your state board of nursing are elected or appointed. What is the composition of the board (that is, how many RNs, licensed practical/vocational nurses, and consumers are there, for example)? Do nurses hold most of the seats on the state board? Are there any other health professionals, such as physicians, on the board of nursing? If so, are there any nurses on the state board of medicine?

REFERENCES

American Nurses Association (ANA): 2018 *Therapeutic use of marijuana and related cannabinoids,* 2018. (website). Available at: https://www.nursingworld.org/~49a8c8/globalassets/practiceandpolicy/ethics/therapeutic-use-of-marijuana-and-related-cannabinoids-position-statement.pdf.

American Nurses Association (ANA): *About ANA,* 2018a. (website). Available at: http://www.nursingworld.org/FunctionalMenuCategories/AboutANA/.

American Nurses Association (ANA): *Nurse staffing plans and ratios,* 2018b. (website). Available at: www.nursing-world.org/MainMenuCategories/Policy-Advocacy/State/Legislative-Agenda-Reports/State-StaffingPlansRatios.

American Nurses Association (ANA): *Code of ethics for nurses with interpretive statements*, Washington, DC, 2015, American Nurses Publishing.

American Public Health Association: *Endorsement on medical marijuana access to therapeutic cannabis/marijuana,* 1995. (website). Retrieved from: www.drugpolicy.org/docUploads/APHAendorse.pdf.

Daley K: Needlestick injuries in the workplace: Implications for public policy. In Mason D, Leavitt J, Chaffee M, editors: *Policy and politics in nursing and health care*, 5, St. Louis, 2007, Saunders.

Health Care Without Harm: *What we do*, 2018. (website). Available at: https://noharm-uscanada.org/content/us-canada/mission-and-goals.

Lewenson S: An historical perspective on policy, politics and nursing. In Mason D, Leavitt J, Chaffee M, editors: *Policy and politics in nursing and health care*, 5, St. Louis, 2007, Saunders.

Merriam-Webster Dictionary: *Politics,* 2018. (website). Available at: https://www.merriam-webster.com/dictionary/politics.

Nursing Organizations Alliance: *Educating leaders in nursing,* 2021. (website). Available at: https://www.nursing-alliance.org/nursing-alliance-leadership-academy-nala-

National Student Nurses' Association: *Code of academic and clinical conduct*, 2018. (website). Available at: http://www.nsna.org/nsna-code-of-ethics.html.

16

Nursing's Challenge: To Continue to Evolve

To enhance your understanding of this chapter, try the Student Exercises on the Evolve site at http://evolve.elsevier.com/Black/professional.

LEARNING OUTCOMES

After studying this chapter, students will be able to:

- Describe the major challenges facing the profession of nursing.
- List ways that nurses can protect the image of nursing.
- Describe how incivility escalates along a continuum.
- Explain how nursing's role in caring for the environment is related to health.
- Describe four major components of the American Nurses Association's Health System Reform Agenda.

Nursing is a profession steeped in tradition yet responsive to the changing world around us. Nurses Florence Nightingale, Mary Seacole, Lillian Wald, Jessie Sleet Scales, and Isabel Hampton Robb were heroes, and their legacies continue today. Yet the work of nursing today rarely feels heroic; sometimes it just feels like the hard work that it is. Often, nurses are referred to as "unsung heroes" of health care.

Photographer and filmmaker Carolyn Jones has produced a documentary *The American Nurse: Healing America* and a book *The American Nurse* published in 2012. This inspiring film and book chronicle the lives and work of nurses in many settings (Jones, 2015). The faces of the nurses capture America in a way that no pie chart or list of statistics can possibly illustrate. The faces of nursing today stand in stark contrast to those featured in the historical documentary *Sentimental Women Need Not Apply: A History of the American Nurse* (see Chapter 4). Nursing in the United States has come a long way in response to a world changed by war, social movements, and economics.

You have learned about several papers, books, and policy statements that call for nursing to evolve in response to the complex needs of today's world. Evolution means changing in ways that are specific and responsive to changes in the surrounding world. Author George Bernard Shaw once wrote, "Progress is impossible without change, and those who cannot change their minds cannot change anything." Progress is movement forward. In this final chapter, you will be presented with challenges for change and progress in nursing that move from the individual—you—to the global.

THE CHALLENGE: CARING FOR YOURSELF

Nurses have an obligation to care for self as highlighted in the American Nurses Association (ANA) *Code of Ethics for Nurses with Interpretive Statements, Provision 5* (2015a). However, the challenge is that nursing is hard work—physically, mentally, and emotionally—and yet at the end of their workdays, many nurses go home to encounter other demands of adult life, including parenting, care of elderly parents, and economic stresses. Many younger nurses enter the profession at a time when they are of age to become parents. Older nurses face the common situation of the "sandwich" generation, referring to people at midlife who face both the challenges of parenting teens and increasing responsibilities for their own parents. Family is usually one's priority over work and career, although today's economic conditions require many nurses to continue to work even though the demands of their families are high. Balancing the responsibilities of work and family can be stressful, making concentrating on one's work difficult and leaving little time for self-care.

The hard work of nursing lies in the fact that nurses bear heavy responsibilities that they take very seriously. There is no question that nurses affect the lives of their patients in ways that cannot be quantified or fully appreciated. The works of Aiken and of Buerhaus, both mentioned at different points throughout this book, have shown consistently that registered nurses (RNs) make a profound difference in the quality of care of patients in hospitals. Projections show that the supply of nurses is increasing, but with the workforce aging and the demand for professional nurses, there likely will still be shortages of nurses in some states by 2030 (U.S. Department of Health and Human Services, Health Resources and Services Administration, National Center for Health Workforce Analysis, 2017).

These predictions, the hard work of nursing, the working environment, and the economic and family stresses that nurses often experience can lead to any number of responses, some healthier than others. Selye, who described the body's response to stress as the general adaptation syndrome, recognized that unresolved stress over time eventually changes one's body as it attempts to restore homeostasis. Selye noted, "Every stress leaves an indelible scar, and the organism pays for its survival after a stressful situation by becoming a little older" (Selye, n.d.).

You can probably describe the basis of nursing as caring, citing theorists, books, and papers that support this key concept in nursing. However, the caring work that nurses do can have consequences such as secondary traumatic stress or compassion fatigue discussed in Chapter 13.

Caring for yourself is foundational to being able to care for others, whether it is the professional caring characteristic of nursing or the personal caring for your friends and family. More than 20 years ago, Carolyn Cooper, PhD, RN, published a unique book, *The Art of Nursing: A Practical Introduction* (2001), in which she claimed that foundational to caring for others is caring for oneself and her work is just as relevant today. Noting that "Nursing teaches hard lessons" (p. 250), Cooper identified the challenges to self-care for nurses: burnout, professional dynamics, and personal responses to nursing. Notably, what Cooper did not do is create a standard formula for those activities that you can read in self-help books or websites: exercise, sleep, eat well, today's almost clichéd recipe for "taking care of yourself."

Importantly, what Cooper did do was challenge nurses to pay attention to "environmental challenges that may be depleting" (p. 256). By paying attention, you can name specifically what is depleting you, what can be done about it, and then act on it. *What* you do to care for yourself is not as important as doing *something* (p. 256). By acting, you bring to the forefront those parts of your life over which you can take charge. You now are making informed choices—and are taking responsibility for those choices. Here is an example:

Alan is a nurse with 3 years' experience in critical care; he has developed excellent assessment skills and is known for being calm under pressure. He has taken advanced life support training, and at every opportunity attends continuing education courses, conferences, and has joined his professional organization. He has gotten the reputation for being a "superstar" on his unit. His dream job gets posted: there is an opening on the flight team. Alan applies and by his account "aces" his interview. He is not hired for his dream job. He described his response: "I was really mad and took it out on my colleagues for a few days. I was going to quit, I was going to sue, you name it. Then a colleague told me to get over myself and go find out why I wasn't hired. So I did." What he learned was that despite his excellent credentials, he had one fatal flaw: he had developed the reputation for being somewhat arrogant and a "hothead," characteristics noted in each of his reference letters. Alan took this feedback and wrestled with its implications. He could take charge of his responses to stressful circumstances, which he did. Although he found it difficult to change his behavior entirely, he used this humbling experience to take responsibility for his actions.

According to Cooper (p. 257), Alan used this situation to assess his vision of his career and what influenced his career, and he acted accordingly. Knowledge of self is a form of self-care. This allows you to understand changes both in yourself and in the profession of nursing. Change can be difficult, and successful adaptation to change "entails abandoning the hope of always controlling work-related changes, accepting the reality that change is inevitable, tolerating the unpredictability of the future" (p. 257), which can lead to creative

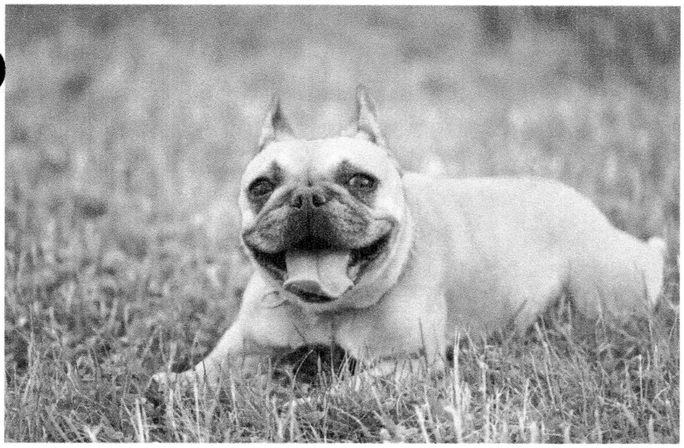

Fig. 16.1 Our pets have a good way of reminding us of the healthful simplicity of eating, sleeping, and playing. (Photo used with permission from iStockphoto.com.)

problem solving rather than being a victim of one's circumstances. Alan refused to be a victim of his circumstances—not getting hired for his dream job—by taking specific steps to change in response to information that was both painful and helpful.

Using this larger view of self-care, exercising, sleeping, and eating well are healthful responses to true caring for oneself. There are other forms of self-care that you may find helpful, including volunteering, becoming involved in a hobby, honoring your spiritual tradition, having a pet, or other source of renewal that keeps you balanced and renews your energy (Fig. 16.1). Achieving balance through a variety of practices and activities is important to your health, which in turn will allow you to be more effective in all of the roles you fulfill in your life as a student, nurse, spouse, parent, daughter or son, and friend.

THE CHALLENGE: CARING FOR THE PROFESSION

Nurses own nursing and nursing practice. Nursing has become a profession with a distinct body of knowledge and self-regulation, with a science that continues to be developed and a central role in the evolving healthcare system of today. This success reflects the tremendous work of nurses who have been relentless in their efforts on behalf of the profession, and ultimately on behalf of our patients. It remains a challenge for today's nurses—including students—to continue to be responsive to the changing landscape of health care and to move nursing into positions of power and influence in the healthcare system. Here are some suggestions.

Join Professional Organizations

You have been introduced in this text to some of the most pressing challenges to nursing today. One of the key problems, and one to which you can respond readily, is the lack of involvement of nurses in professional organizations and the ANA through your constituent state organization. Professional organizations such as the Association of Nurses in AIDS Care (ANAC), American Association of Critical-Care Nurses (AACN), and Association of Women's Health, Obstetric and Neonatal Nurses (AWHONN), among many others, provide up-to-date information about the state of the clinical practice area in which you work or are interested. These organizations provide many outlets for keeping your practice current with the latest developments and research through conferences, webcasts, position papers, websites for members only, and journals. Although there are annual dues, the work of these organizations pays off in keeping you involved and current in your practice, aware of developments in standards of care in your practice area, and advocating for policy change on the behalf of nursing.

The ANA and its constituent state members is the official voice of nursing. The code of ethics, scope and standards of care, and articulation of nursing's social policy are developed and advanced through the ANA. As the official voice for nurses, the ANA publishes position papers on a wide variety of issues and topics and has a political action committee that raises funds from constituent member association members and contributes to political candidates at the federal level whose views of healthcare legislation and regulation are consistent with those of the ANA. regrettably, only about 10% of RNs in the United States are members of the ANA's constituent organizations, meaning that nurses are silencing their own voices by not participating in the work of this organization dedicated to the interests and development of the profession.

Protecting the Image of Nursing

Care of the profession also means that as a nurse, you become aware of the image of nursing in the media and respond appropriately to both negative and positive portrayals of nurses. The Truth About Nursing is a non-profit organization with the mission to "increase public understanding of the central, front-line role nurses play in modern healthcare." The organization asks nurses to take responsibility for its public image by monitoring media images of nursing. Nurses can thereby advocate for accurate images by contacting the organizations/companies with negative or inaccurate images, boycott programs, and applaud efforts of organizations that do portray an accurate image of nursing (www.truthaboutnursing.org). This watchdog organization keeps the image of nursing front and center in its mission, such as by advocating for the halt of a Netflix production *Ratched,* which perpetuated a negative image of nursing first introduced decades ago in the movie *One Flew Over the Cuckoo's Nest* (Truth About Nursing, 2018). A past story included the coverage of the 2014 Ebola outbreak that eventually brought two American nurses into the spotlight: an RN from Texas who contracted Ebola from caring for a patient who eventually died from the virus and a nurse from Maine who was quarantined unnecessarily in New Jersey after returning from her work in Africa with patients with Ebola (Truth About Nursing, 2014). Each nurse was referred to in the media as "Ebola nurse," a designation that trivialized their experiences and ignored their vital work. Truth About Nursing noted that the media consulted chief nurse Susan Mitchell Grant, MS, RN, NEA-BC, FAAN (Emory University Hospital), who explained why her facility accepted the first patients with Ebola brought into the United States. Truth About Nursing also pointed out that otherwise, physicians were heavily featured in accounts about caring for patients with Ebola.

The persistent underreporting or even disappearance of nurses from media coverage of health-related events poses a challenge in getting the media to pay attention to the expertise and work of nursing. For instance, at the height of the COVID-19 pandemic, nurses in ICUs were frequently referred to as "heroes" and in some cities, citizens went outside at 7PM (usual shift change) to clang on pans and otherwise make noise in honor of frontline workers, including healthcare providers. What is missing here was the recognition of the everyday professional efforts of nurses in ICUs and elsewhere to protect patients, families, communities and populations. Nurses are unlikely to describe their work as heroic; unfortunately, they rarely have opportunity to describe their work at all in the public domain.

Another damaging problem for nurses is the highly sexualized images of nurses often portrayed in the media and other venues. In 2012 nurses were outraged over the portrayal of nurses by the Dallas Mavericks of the National Basketball Association, whose dancers performed a halftime routine in revealing "naughty nurse" costumes complete with nursing caps to the tune of the old song that begins, "Doctor, doctor ..." (Truth About Nursing, 2012). Cartoon figures convey and perpetuate this insidious message. For instance, in one cartoon, a very slender White nurse with long blonde hair wearing a cap, a short white uniform, and heels winks and blows a kiss at some unknown recipient of her attention. This image is mild compared with the grotesquely sexualized images of nurses that are easy to find on the Internet and elsewhere. Nurses must protest the use of these images commercially and for entertainment. These images however are not the only kind that can diminish the image of nursing: the message behind many images is subtle. Thinking Critically Box 16.1 guides you through ways to critique common images of nurses.

Maximizing Your Education

Another way of caring for the profession is for nurses to become as educated as possible and to work at the upper limits of their education. From Chapter 4, you learned that nursing education is undergoing significant changes. With the increasing complexity of the healthcare system—and the society in which that system operates—the issue of the requirement of a Bachelor of Science in Nursing (BSN) degree for entry into practice is likely to get significant traction over the next several years. Already, significant numbers of nurses with associate degrees are returning—and in some cases even required to return—to college to complete a BSN. The Doctor of Nursing Practice (DNP) degree may eventually replace the Master of Science in Nursing (MSN) degree for advanced practice nurses, although the MSN will continue to be offered for other purposes.

The Doctor of Philosophy (PhD) degree will remain the degree for nurse scientists, with intense training in research methods and scholarship. PhD-prepared nurses will continue to be needed to advance the science of nursing, and DNP-prepared nurses will join the ranks of other healthcare providers for whom a doctorate is the degree for advanced clinical practice. Nurses have the opportunity at this transformational time in health care to assume their rightful place as leaders in primary care and other forms of practice for which they are well prepared.

THINKING CRITICALLY BOX 16.1

Matters of Image

Images are representations of an external form and provide a general impression of a person or an enterprise. Social media has made persons highly aware of how one "comes across" in photos. Think about how you yourself may have cultivated your best look for posting photos on social media. You may be a careful curator and manager of your own image.

Just as you feel a responsibility to create and protect an excellent representation (image) of yourself in your social media and professional websites, as a member of the nursing profession you have a responsibility to shape and protect the image of nurses and nursing. In earlier editions of this text, a quick search on a well-known search engine using the term "nurse" or "nursing" returned hundreds of thousands of images of nurses, many of which either trivialized nurses as "sexy" or "hot" or reduced the work of nursing to charting or taking orders from physicians, who were typically portrayed as older, distinguished White men. Many of the images returned on these searches were cartoon figures, as described earlier in this chapter. Significantly, many of these images were among the first results of the search.

The COVID-19 pandemic has moved nurses into more prominence in the media, and hence in the public. Members of our highly trusted profession have demonstrated yet again much ingenuity, hard work, compassion and robust advocacy for patients during this enduring public health crisis. A recent search on the same search engine using the terms "nurse" and "nursing" returned notably different results from those described in earlier editions.

Conduct a search for images of nurses and nursing, and consider these ideas as you critique your results:

- Who is in the photo? Consider gender presentation, race/ethnicity and age, and think about cues as to who is in what role. What makes you think a particular person is a nurse, and another is a physician or other provider?
- What is the work of nursing in the photo? How do you distinguish the work of nursing from that of other health care providers? Note that the role of providers in many stock photos are purposefully ambiguous. Again, what makes you think a particular person is a nurse, and another is a physician or other provider?
- Consider alternative interpretations for images. For example, is the older White person in a lab coat who presents as male a nursing student getting additional information from an attending physician who is young, Black and presents as female?

Promoting Civility

Incivility in nursing is a troubling problem that is getting increasing attention, to the extent that in 2015 the ANA published a position statement on incivility, bullying, and workplace violence (2015b). In a profession dedicated to caring for strangers, the spiral of incivility is difficult to explain but crucial to address. In March 2011 Medscape Nurses, a widely read web-based source of information about nursing, featured an interview with Cynthia Clark, PhD, RN, and Sara Ahten, MSN, RN, who addressed several aspects of nursing incivility (Stokowski, 2011). They described a continuum of incivility (Fig. 16.2). Incivility in nursing is manifested as bullying between colleagues and between faculty and students in academic settings. The latter is particularly troubling because nursing school is a potent agent of professional socialization (Luparell, 2011).

The continuum of incivility starts with common behaviors that are distracting, annoying, or irritating to others. Examples of these behaviors are talking on one's phone in a restaurant or sending and reading text messages while someone is talking to you. These behaviors are a matter of poor manners in some cases but that leave the recipient of the behavior feeling ignored and annoyed. Increasingly disruptive behaviors include taunting, using ethnic slurs, and intimidation even without physical contact. At the most extreme of the continuum, bullying, aggression, and violence occur (Stokowski, 2011). Incivility in the workplace has implications for nurses, patients, and healthcare organizations, with poor communication and unprofessional behaviors negatively affecting patient outcomes and safety (Luparell, 2011).

Incivility occurs when people are stressed and feel powerless. Incivility can give one a fleeting sense of control or power, even though it is misplaced and misguided. Furthermore, the widespread use of social media and faceless communication over e-mail, messaging, and so on keeps the other person's humanity at a distance. Talking to or about someone without face-to-face

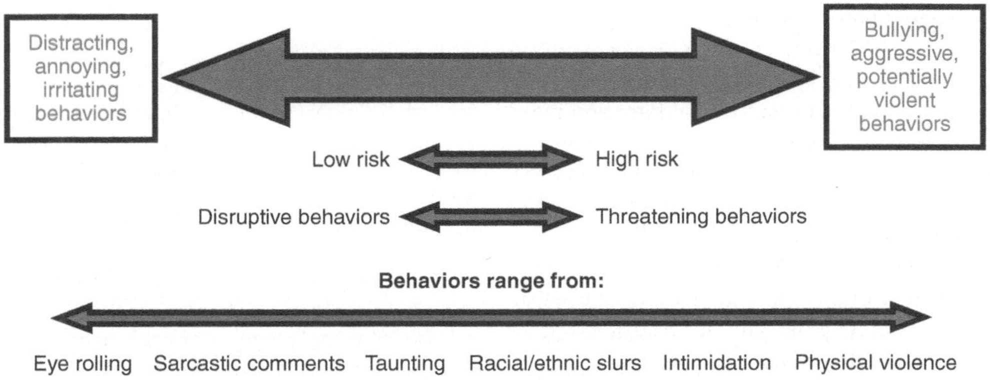

Fig. 16.2 The continuum of incivility goes from simple acts such as being distracting and eye-rolling to aggressive behaviors and bullying. (Courtesy Cynthia Clark.)

communication foments incivility. You are much more likely to express something in an aggressive manner if you are not required to speak directly to the person, even if by phone. Hearing someone's voice is a reminder that you are indeed speaking to a real person.

Cooper's recommendations related to self-care are appropriate to the issue of incivility: you do not have to be victimized by a system that is uncaring and hurtful. You do not have to bully to claim power for yourself, and you do not have to acquiesce to bullying. Valuing others and treating each person with respect are core values in nursing (Fig. 16.3). The disconnection between what is taught and what we do is both alarming and tragic. You will be hearing more about incivility in the workplace as you continue your career in nursing. You do not have to be a part of this disturbing development in our profession. Here is one nurse's experience:

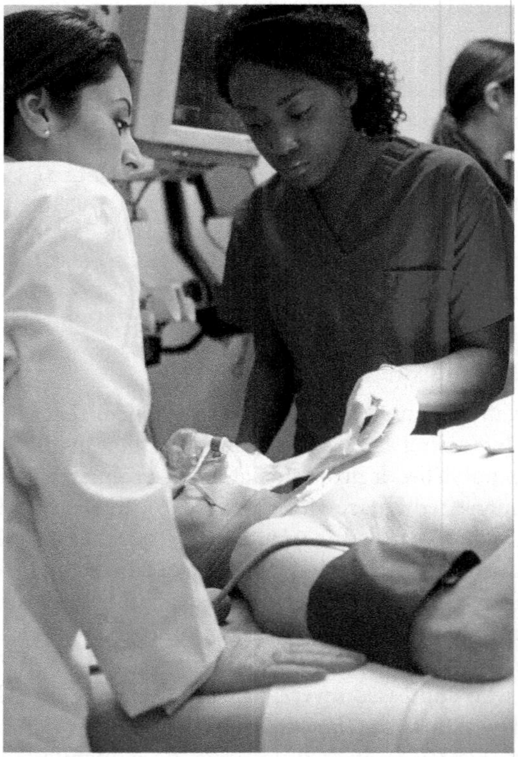

Fig. 16.3 When nurses treat each other with dignity and respect, patients benefit. (Photo used with permission from iStockphoto.)

My stomach hurt every day before I got to work as a new graduate. Everything I suggested was at first just ignored, then later my suggestions were just laughed at, and the older nurses told me that I needed to learn my place. One day I asked for help with a complicated problem that I had not seen before in a patient who had an open wound. The nurse I asked to help me said that maybe all of my "book learning" was not going to help me in nursing, and then she walked off. I could not believe it. It was one thing to be ignored when I suggested that we do shift change hand-off a different way. It was another thing completely to be insulted and then ignored when I needed help with a patient. I finally took a hard look at myself and at the unit where I was working, and I realized that I was not going to be able to change much there. So I put in for a transfer as soon as I could. On my last day, one of the nurses told me that she knew I was not going to be able to "make it" there. It was her parting shot at me, but I was so relieved to be leaving that I did not even care anymore. I loved the new unit that I transferred to. I finally felt like I was going to be a good nurse.

Strategies exist to assist nurses to combat this ongoing issue. Cognitive rehearsal is one approach that can be helpful to nurses when managing situations that are not civil (Longo, 2017). The Passionate About Creating Environments of Respect and Civilities (PACERS) *Civility Tool Kit* developed by Robert Wood Johnson Fellows in 2012 and updated in 2015 is a comprehensive set of resources on how to recognize and address bullying in the workplace. The toolkit is found at http://stopbullyingtoolkit.org (PACERS, 2015).

THE MOST PRESSING CHALLENGE OF OUR TIME: CARING FOR THE ENVIRONMENT

Environmental issues encompass almost every aspect of human life. In its broadest sense, the environment connotes the air, water, organisms, and other natural resources that surround us. It also connotes the social and cultural milieu in which people live. The previous section touched on the social and cultural milieu that has become the breeding ground for incivility, the environment of health care. On its largest scale, the environment is about the world and its resources over which humans are stewards.

The Natural Environment

Reports of the deterioration of the environment are daily occurrences. Catastrophic events such as earthquakes in Haiti and Nepal, and floods in Pakistan will affect those nations for decades, if not centuries. These natural and uncontrollable phenomena sometimes overshadow the less dramatic but insidious gradual decline in the quality of the world's air and water, and the effects of on plant and animal life, including humans.

Acute and chronic respiratory diseases are increasing, as are cancers of all types and debilitating allergic reactions to chemicals in the environment. Increasing evidence supporting climate change as a result of high carbon dioxide levels in the atmosphere; moreover, lead and mercury poisonings; toxic shellfish beds; oil spills in oceans; pesticides and other toxins spilling into streams and rivers; and the collapse of retention ponds, spilling toxic wastewater into the ocean are all-too-common occurrences that barely make mention in the media. Meanwhile, deforestation, destruction of wetlands by development, and relaxing of standards for waste emissions by industries have become common business practices.

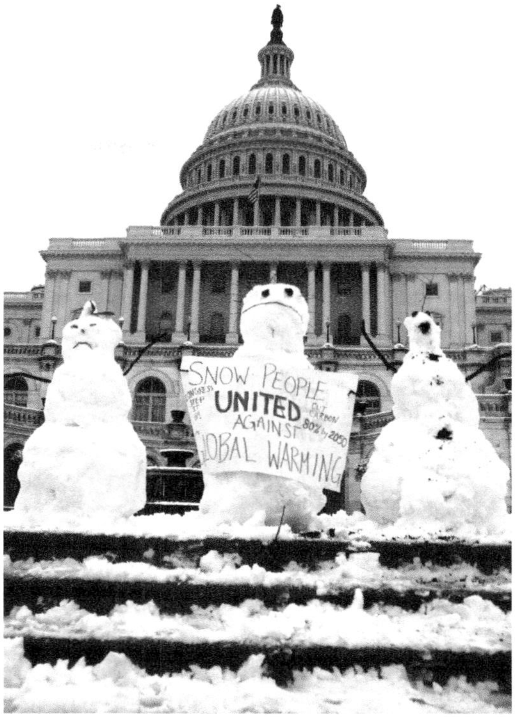

Fig. 16.4 The melting "snow people united against global warming" on the steps of the U.S. Capitol in Washington, D.C., was a protest against policies that do not address climate change and its dire effects. (Photo used with permission from iStockphoto.)

Scientists now overwhelmingly agree that climate change as a result of global warming is accelerating and is attributable to human activity (Fig. 16.4). Much debate continues in the popular media about whether the science of climate change is believable; however, according to scientists across the planet, the evidence demonstrating the relationship between human activity and the trapping of carbon dioxide in the atmosphere is irrefutable.

Failure to care for the environment has health implications beyond the most obvious ones such as lung diseases and the development of certain cancers. Epidemiologists, who study the origins and spread of diseases, believe that there is a relationship between environmental decline and increases in certain diseases, including animal-borne diseases. Emerging diseases and multi-drug-resistant strains of organisms once under control, such as *Mycobacterium tuberculosis* and *Staphylococcus,* will increasingly challenge healthcare resources.

As of mid-January 2017, the world population was estimated to be 7.6 billion and is projected to increase to 8.6 billion by the year 2030 (United Nations, 2017). Feeding, immunizing, providing drinkable water, and caring for this many human beings threaten to overwhelm the environmental, economic, social, and medical systems of the world. In the United States alone, there is one birth every 8 seconds, one person emigrating every 29 seconds, and one death every 11 seconds for a net gain of one person every 15 seconds (U.S. Census Bureau, n.d.).

At the time the previous edition of this text was published, the word "immunizing" in the previous paragraph, while not an afterthought, seemed to be less salient to the world's health than the other items in that list. Now, at the time of this writing, the COVID-10 pandemic is threatening a new "winter wave" in the Northern hemisphere, the issue of whether to vaccinate has been highly politicized in the U.S. and elsewhere, and the threat of the development of a new variant remains high because of continuing widespread infections.

At the Climate Change Conference held in Copenhagen, Denmark, in 2009, the metaphor of the overloaded lifeboat was often used. World overpopulation, overdevelopment, and overconsumption by wealthy nations threaten to deplete the resources and damage the environment of the entire world, not just overpopulated countries. The problems of climate change, the deterioration of the environment, and overpopulation are issues of health care that nurses face now, and these problems will intensify in the future without aggressive efforts to mitigate or reverse them. Immense problems with no easy solutions, they typically affect our most vulnerable populations: elderly, children, pregnant women, and those living in poverty. The Alliance of Nurses for Healthy Environments (AHNE) is dedicated to "promoting healthy people and healthy environments by educating and leading the nursing profession, advancing research, incorporating evidence practice and influencing policy." To discover how these climate changes may be affecting you and the community you are living in, explore the AHNE website https://envirn.org.

Throughout this text, you have been introduced to nurses doing amazing, forward-thinking work in theory, research, and practice. Nursing education tends to socialize students into thinking of nursing practice as primarily in in-patient settings, but the practice of nursing *happens everywhere.* Marla Kasper, BSN, RN is one of those forward-thinking, visionary nurses who has extended her practice of nursing into a commitment to the sustainability and care for the environment. Her work is featured in Professional Profile 16.1.

PROFESSIONAL PROFILE BOX 16.1

A Call to Action for Nurses: Environmental Justice and Sustainability

Unlike some of my colleagues, I did not grow up knowing that I "always wanted to be a nurse." In fact, I thought I wanted to work in the advertising field because I am creative. It wasn't until my senior year in high school, when my older brother suggested that I "should become a nurse," mostly because his college girlfriend at the time was one. I liked the idea of it, and what sold me on nursing was that it was such a dynamic profession. My nursing journey has been just that ... and then some.

I graduated from University of North Carolina at Chapel Hill with my Bachelor of Science in Nursing in 2004. As a fresh "new grad" nurse, I dabbled in med-surg, but found an opportunity to work at UNC's radiology, not a rotation we get in nursing school, but a fantastic foundational experience. Being a radiology nurse then led me to becoming a travel nurse, working short assignments at the nation's top children's hospitals. In addition to pediatrics, another passion of mine was public health, and I served as a Peace Corps Volunteer in Malawi (sub-Saharan Africa) from 2009-2011. After volunteering, I worked as a case manager and later as a clinical research nurse for children with rare neuromuscular disease. However, I experienced caregiver burnout, so I left hospital work for the corporate world. I worked as a medical editor, and most recently a health coach for large insurance company.

When I started working in "corporate America," I was quite shocked and disappointed at the obvious lack of recycling at the workplace, a large campus of nine buildings with about 5000 employees. With this notable lack of corporate sustainability efforts, I decided to take action and start a grassroots employee environmental club. In a year's time, we had tremendous growth in both size and momentum, confirming what I already knew – people care about this topic and need education on how environment

PROFESSIONAL PROFILE BOX 16.1—cont'd

A Call to Action for Nurses: Environmental Justice and Sustainability

and health are inextricably linked. According to the CDC, there will up to 4300 additional premature deaths by 2050 due to ozone and particle health effects (CDC, 2021). In healthcare we talk about "drivers of health," but often environment is the most overlooked of these, especially in my home state of North Carolina.

Since the murder of George Floyd, an even brighter and long-overdue light has been shone on systemic racism and health inequities in America, and the environment is a key link to these as well. The environmental justice movement was sparked in North Carolina in 1982, when a protest started in Warren County, a predominantly black community, was chosen by the state as a landfill site for hazardous waste. Still today, landfills are typically built in black and brown communities. Another huge environmental injustice issue in North Carolina is the hog farms or contained agriculture feed operations (CAFOs) where pig waste is sprayed on crops as "fertilizer," causing respiratory issues to the surrounding residents, who are mostly brown and black communities. According to a 2018 study, "North Carolina communities located near hog CAFOs had higher all-cause and infant mortality, mortality due to anemia, kidney disease, tuberculosis, septicemia, and higher hospital admissions/ED visits of LBW infants" (Kravchenko et al 2018). I became fascinated with this topic of environmental injustice and arranged for an educational speaker series to present at my workplace in 2021.

I was not expecting my niche in corporate world would include starting an environmental revolution there over the last two years, but even senior leadership was noticing. Our CEO personally invited me to present to the executive leadership team about sustainability, which I guarantee had never been discussed at the executive level before. Inspired by this momentum and progress, I started to become more connected with other nurses and clinicians that are also passionate about this topic, educating others on climate and health.

Serendipitously, I received an email invitation to Sigma Theta Tau International's Creating Healthy Work Environments virtual conference, with a special offer: Climate for Health Ambassador training, sponsored by EcoAmerica and Alliance of Nurses for Healthy Environments (ANHE). This training is designed for healthcare professionals to equip them with knowledge, tools, and resources to teach others about the effects of climate and health. During the training, I had a lightbulb moment: I realized that we as nurses have the greatest influence when it comes to teaching about climate and health because we are historically the most trusted profession. The planet needs nurses to help influence policy makers, senior leaders, and other healthcare professionals.

Suddenly, it all made sense ... everything in my past was leading me to this climactic point in my career. In Spring of 2021, I decided to pursue my passion further, so I applied and was accepted to graduate school, an Executive Master's in Sustainability Leadership through Arizona State University. My goal is to become Chief Sustainability Nurse, where I can help hospitals and healthcare companies address sustainability because it influences our customers, patients, costs, and future. According to Johnson & Johnson Learning Institute, in the United States, our hospitals are responsible for 10% of our national greenhouse gas (GHG) emissions.

Sustainability is so much more than "just recycling"; it touches every aspect of business and operations, and affects all of us. Sustainability efforts need more nurses to help lead healthcare through these transitions to a greener, healthier—and more just—planet.

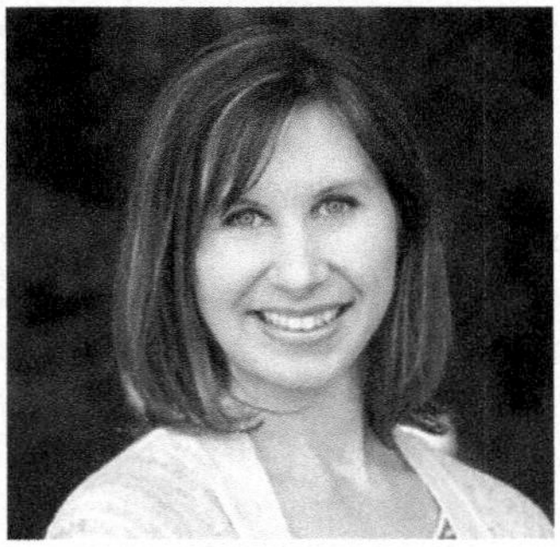

Marla Kasper, BSN, RN
marla.kasper.rn@gmail.com

If you are interested in more information about sustainability and how nurses can take part in sustainability efforts, please reach out via email. You can also find me on LinkedIn.

Courtesy Marla Kasper

The Work Environment

No profession is free from hazards, and no workplace can ever ensure absolute security. Nursing and healthcare settings are no exception. Occupational health hazards in nursing include needlestick injuries and possible infection with bloodborne pathogens; exposure to chemicals such as disinfectants and chemotherapeutic agents; and violence in the workplace, among others.

A major story in the media early in the COVID-19 pandemic was the dire shortage of adequate PPE (personal protective equipment) for nurses and other healthcare providers, especially in ICUs. This posed significant risks to nurses, who resorted to reusing disposable items, and in one photo circulated widely on social media, used plastic garbage bags to cover their clothing. Nurses are resourceful, but the lack of adequate PPE and the yet-to-be-fully-understood modes of transmission for COVID-19 early in the pandemic made for nursing practice that was focused (necessarily) on problem-solving without clear evidence of effectiveness or possible harm that could come from these practices. At a time of great anxiety and extreme stress and distress, the workplace itself posed direct threats to the health of nurses.

The pandemic both exposed and exacerbated the enormous strains on already experienced by nurses in the workplace. Injuries from accidents and back strain are not uncommon, resulting in pain, disability, lost income, absenteeism, and decreased productivity. Shift work itself is a hazard to nurses, causing a variety of physical and psychological problems, including exhaustion, depression, interpersonal problems, and accidents. Sleep deprivation is a significant source of stress in shift workers, including nurses, and its association with an increased risk of breast cancer, obesity, and mortality has been long known (Beccuti and Pannain, 2011; Davis and Mirick, 2006; Gallicchio and Kalesan, 2009). Stress from work overload, inadequate staffing, and the intense feelings generated by caring for acutely ill and dying patients add to the mix of workplace hazards faced by nurses.

Assuring nurses of a healthy work environment is a major challenge over which nurses have some control. Nurses must take positive, effective, united action to ensure the basic dignity and safety of practicing nurses everywhere. They must demand and use safe needlestick devices and disposal containers; high-efficiency ventilation systems; adequate environmental services support; adequate lifting assistance with devices or additional personnel; reduction or elimination of shift rotation and double shifts; and appropriate occupational safety and health training. Many nurses are fortunate enough to work in settings where they can take these practices for granted; however, with the wide variety of settings where health care is provided in the United States, some nurses work without the advantages of up-to-date safety technologies or scheduling practices. The Occupational Safety and Health Administration (OSHA) regulates work environments and has a whistleblower protection program to protect from retribution those workers who believe that their workplace is dangerous.

Genetics and Genomics

Genes are minute nucleotide polymers with huge implications for nurses. The Human Genome Project was the initial mapping and sequencing of a composite set of human genes in 2003. An increasing number of genetic conditions can be identified prenatally, and parents can be aware of some of the genetic conditions of which they may be carriers. Providers can use genomic information to inform their care plan in the areas of screening, monitoring, and treatment decisions; allowing for personalized care. Pharmacogenetics is a developing field in which genetic variants that affect drug metabolism can help providers determine the correct dose of a particular drug and, possibly, whether a particular drug will work at all. As a nurse, it is an important responsibility for you to be able to explain pharmacogenetics and to assist your patients in understanding what these drugs can and cannot do.

Schools of nursing are increasingly offering courses in basic genetics and genomics to prepare graduates for the demands of this increasingly visible field in health care. Competence in genetics is becoming increasingly necessary for nurses.

THE FINAL CHALLENGE: UNITE AND ACT

The call to unite is a loud and constant one. Most of the crucial issues the nursing profession will face in the next decade cannot be resolved by any one group of nurses. These concerns will require the attention of the entire profession, working in a focused, united, active manner through nursing's professional associations. Although collective power is the only way nurses will effectively address and resolve issues affecting their practice, education, and the healthcare system in a time of reform, the lack of organization and involvement in professional organizations is an unfortunate commentary on the lack of priority most nurses place on this vital aspect of professionalism.

As the largest healthcare profession in the United States, nursing can and should have a powerful voice and presence in every setting where substantive healthcare issues are discussed, from the National Institutes of Health to the halls of Congress and the White House. Serious discussions occur in surroundings more accessible than the federal government, and nurses can have a strong presence in many venues where health care is central; however, nursing has let arguments regarding levels of education, political philosophies, and relative importance of practice settings be divisive. The tremendous clinical skills of critical care nurses are no better or worse than the insightful care of psychiatric nurses; the high energy of the emergency department nurse is no better or worse than the calming influence of the nursery nurse rocking a crying baby. Each has his or her own specific and important role. The diversity of skills among nurses should be honored and recognized as a sign of the strength of the profession (Fig. 16.5).

If you think for a moment about other groups to which you belong—for example, a political party, church, or parent-teacher association—you do not expect to agree with every position taken by the organization or its leaders. Nurses seem to have such an expectation of their professional association, however, and use that as a reason for not participating. This is naïve and unrealistic. With nursing and society becoming increasingly diverse, nurses of the future must become more tolerant of differences and work hard to find common ground with their colleagues in the profession. If we fail to do so, nursing will not prosper, nor will its practitioners. In preparing for our future, the four major principles of successful implementation of healthcare reform set forth by the ANA are noteworthy (ANA, 2017):

1. "Ensure universal access to a standardized package of essential healthcare services for all citizens and residents.
2. Optimize primary, community-based, and preventative services while supporting cost effective use of innovative, technology-driven, acute hospital-based services.
3. Encourage mechanisms to stimulate economic use of healthcare services while supporting those who do not have the means to share in costs.
4. Ensure a sufficient supply of a skilled workforce dedicated to providing high quality health care services."

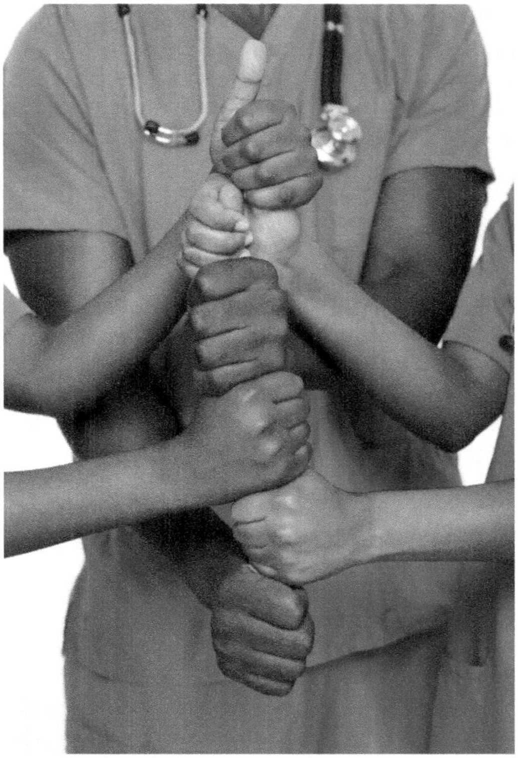

Fig. 16.5 Individual nurses can make positive changes; nurses working together can be even more powerful. (Photo used with permission from iStockphoto.)

This is a time of change in nursing, and you, the readers of this book, are the future of nursing. In Chapter 4 (Professional Profile Box 4.1), you read the first half of a story "From Room to Zoom," in which faculty member Nancy Jo Thompson, DNP, RN gave her account of moving from the bedside (Room) to a faculty position that required her to teach online (Zoom); on her first day of class, Dr. Thompson encountered a student who was a family member involved in one of her most memorable patient experiences as an ICU nurse. In Professional Profile 16.2, you will read the "other side of the story" written by Danielle White, BSN, RN. Ms. White has now moved "From Zoom to Room," specifically, an ICU where she now cares for patients and families during life-threatening illnesses, inspired by Dr. Thompson's care years before.

You represent our best hope for building nursing into an even more powerful force in improving the lives of those entrusted to our care, whether they are individuals, families, communities, or nations. Look around at the other members of your class, all 25 or 125 or 200 of you. You represent an amazing collection of energy and talent—combine those talents and harness that energy and you will accomplish more than you can imagine. So it is with nursing's future: we can accomplish far more by working collectively than alone. All nurses, individually and as a profession, will benefit from the results. Then, most important, so will our patients, families, communities and populations. In the words of anthropologist Margaret Mead, ***"Never believe that a few caring people can't change the world. For, indeed, that's all who ever have."***

PROFESSIONAL PROFILE BOX 16.2

From "Zoom to Room": A Nurse's Move From Online Learning to the ICU Bedside, and an Important Lesson About Acting on Your Inspiration

Caring for others and nursing have always interested me. While working on my first undergraduate degree—a Bachelor of Arts at the University of North Carolina at Greensboro majoring in psychology—I said frequently that if I chose another major, it would be nursing. While working in a corporate job for 3 years after graduation, I contemplated returning to school to pursue nursing. After the illness and death of my sister-in-law Carolyn, I knew that nursing was my calling. I quit my job and started on my journey to become a nurse. I was offered admission to the University of North Carolina at Chapel Hill's accelerated BSN program and graduated 14 months later. Nursing allowed me to combine my passion for helping others with my love of science. I began my nursing career in a Cardiovascular and Thoracic ICU (CTICU) and am working on earning my CCRN certification, with the goal of graduate study to become an Acute Care Nurse Practitioner. I plan to continue to work with our local donor services organization to encourage the public to sign up to be an organ donor and to help dispel misinformation about donation.

One morning during the pandemic when my classes were held online via Zoom, I was attending my pathophysiology/pharmacology class when a faculty member came on to introduce herself. My heart skipped a few beats because I immediately recognized her, Nancy Jo Thompson, the nurse who had cared for my sister-in-law Carolyn during one of life's most difficult moments for my family. I no longer could pay attention to class while I decided whether to reach out to Dr. Thompson. I was worried she would not remember my family, or maybe she would think it was inappropriate for me to reach out. I took the risk and emailed her during class, and she responded that she had time to meet after class over Zoom. I told Dr. Thompson that in 2016, she had cared for Carolyn in the ICU, where after seven days she passed away and became an organ donor. I told Dr. Thompson my specific memories of her caring for not just my sister-in-law but my family. I was surprised to learn that Dr. Thompson remembered Carolyn and all of us. Her words brought a sense of peace, knowing that our loved one made an impact on the care team, just as the care team made an impact on us. We spent the entire hour before my afternoon class talking about our experience and the closure our conversation brought to both of us.

Nothing is easy about having a family member in the ICU. Across seven days, my family and I spent every waking moment with Carolyn, going home only to shower and sleep. The thought of not being there, even for just a moment, left us with terrible feelings of "what if?" and helplessness. I would clean Carolyn's hands with hospital wipes because she was a gardener and always seemed to have dirt under her nails. While this may have seemed silly when my loved one was fighting for her life, it made me feel as if I was helping when otherwise I was utterly, completely helpless. During those seven days, we had amazing physicians, respiratory therapists, nurse aides and of course nurses who cared for Carolyn, each leaving an impact that I'm not sure they fully understand. For families with a loved one who is critically ill, the entire world stops. For the healthcare team, it is a twelve-hour shift, but for the family, it is their lives. The nurses who cared for my sister-in-law gave everything they had each shift, but one stood out. Her name was Nancy, and she was incredibly kind not only to my family, but most importantly to Carolyn. She always spoke to Carolyn before touching her and told her what she was getting ready to do, an effort we sometimes forget in caring for our intubated/sedated patients.

My sister-in-law had long dreadlocks that had taken years to accomplish and were part of her identity. One day while Nancy was caring for Carolyn, she turned to my mother-in-law and told her how much she loved Carolyn's dreadlocks and how well-kept they were. My mother-in-law remembers that comment to this day: it meant so much to her that someone saw her daughter as more than just a patient and who took time to comment on something that was a source of pride for Carolyn. When your loved one is critically ill, you also spend a lot of time in the family conference room, a room we dreaded walking into. After a family meeting where we were given heartbreaking news about Carolyn's prognosis, Nancy approached my mother-in-law and said, "From mother to mother, I am so sorry" and gave her the biggest hug.

She held my mother-in-law as she cried, not as a nurse doing a job, but as a human being who acknowledged our profound pain. Now six years later, I still remember that moment and its impact on me. Six years later, I am starting my career as an ICU nurse, and I take that moment with me. What Nancy showed me was that as an CTICU nurse, the work is not just managing drips and hemodynamics – it is also about caring for the patient and their family as important persons. The care Nancy showed Carolyn and my family truly shaped how I will care for my patients as a nurse. For me, it will be a twelve-hour shift; for them it is a moment in their lives they will never forget.

PROFESSIONAL PROFILE BOX 16.2—cont'd

From "Zoom to Room": A Nurse's Move From Online Learning to the ICU Bedside, and an Important Lesson About Acting on Your Inspiration

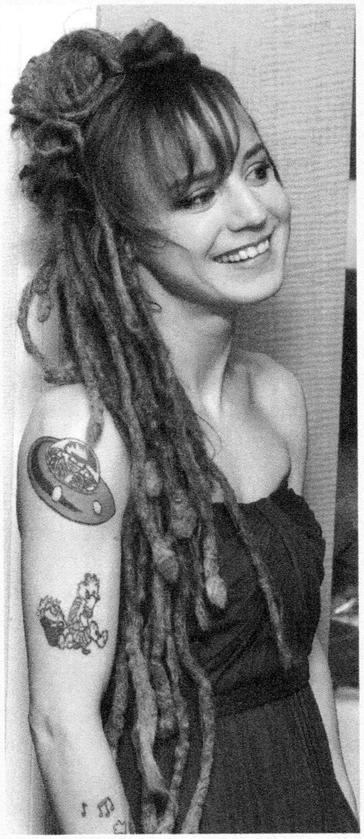

Carolyn's family was generous in sharing this photo of Carolyn, reminding us that there are persons behind each story of nursing, and inspiration to be found where you least expect it. Courtesy Danielle White.

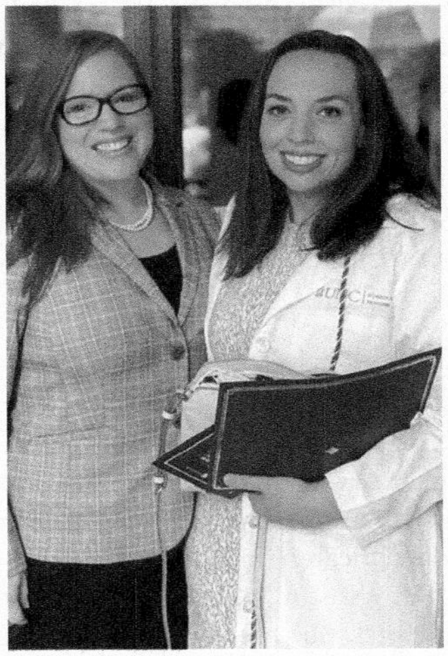

Danielle White, BSN, RN *(right)* with mentor Nancy Jo Thompson.

I never expected to see Nancy again, especially not on a Friday morning in my pathophysiology class, but there she was introducing herself as my faculty for the class. I immediately emailed Nancy and we met after class, via Zoom of course. I told her about the care she provided for Carolyn, and she talked about that time as her nurse. It brought both of us closure and gave me an opportunity to thank her. It felt like a full circle for me, and I was honored to know that such a compassionate, knowledgeable, and caring nurse would be my faculty in nursing school.

Danielle White, BSN, RN

CONCEPTS AND CHALLENGES

- ***Concept:*** Care of the profession begins with care of self.
  Challenge: Working to the extent of your education and seeking to become more educated are important means of caring for the profession and yourself.
- ***Concept:*** Incivility reflects the lack of valuing and respect for others.
  Challenge: Acts of incivility can be small, such as rolling one's eyes; it is important to pay attention to your professional behavior to avoid even small gestures of incivility. Arm yourself with the tools to combat incivility and bullying behaviors.
- ***Concept:*** Nurses must care for the environment, because failure to do so is a direct threat to health.
  Challenge: Notice that your environment includes your home, workplace, and community. Challenges to your health may require attention to your local environment.
- ***Concept:*** You have a significant say in how the profession of nursing evolves. Join forces with those who think and believe like you do, and, collectively, you will make a big difference in the future of nursing.
  Challenge: Do not back down from challenges that seem insurmountable. Nurses are well positioned by their education, experience, creativity, and worldview to improve the health of populations in ways that you cannot yet imagine.

IDEAS FOR FURTHER EXPLORATION

1. Take a position on the following statement: "Nurses of the future will have an impact on the environment that exceeds that of the ordinary citizen." Be prepared to defend your position.
2. What strategies can you use to manage stress? What ideas do you have to ensure that caring for yourself is just as much a priority as caring for others?
3. How have you encountered incivility both in nursing school and in practice? How have you responded?
4. Identify two nursing organizations you are interested in joining. Read their websites, and determine whether they have reduced fees for students. If you can afford it, join one or both. If joining is not yet possible, consult the organizations' websites frequently. Most have some content that is accessible to nonmembers and will be useful to you.

REFERENCES

American Nurses Association (ANA): *Healthcare reform*, 2017. (website). Available at: http://ana.aristotle.com/SitePages/healthcarereform.aspx.

American Nurses Association (ANA): *Code of ethics for nurses with interpretive statements*, Washington, DC, 2015a, American Nurses Publishing.

Beccuti G, Pannain S: Sleep and obesity, *Curr Opin Clin Nutr Metab Care* 14(4):402–412, 2011.

Cooper C: *The art of nursing: a practical introduction*, Philadelphia, 2001, Saunders.

Davis S, Mirick DK: Circadian disruption, shift work and the risk of cancer: a summary of the evidence and studies in Seattle, *Cancer Cause Cont* 17(4):539–545, 2006.

Department of Health and Human Services, Health Resources and Services Administration, National Center for Health Workforce Analysis: *National and regional supply and demand projections of the nursing workforce: 2014–2030*, Maryland, 2017, Rockville.

Gallicchio L, Kalesan B: Sleep duration and mortality a systematic review and metanalysis, *J Sleep Res* 18(2): 148–158, 2009.

Jones C: *American nurse project*,2015. (website). Available at: www.americannurseproject.com/landing-book.

Kravchenko J, Rhew SH, Akushevich I, Agarwal P, Lyerly HK: Mortality and health outcomes in North Carolina communities located in close proximity to hog concentrated animal feeding operations, *N C Med J* 79(5):278–288, 2018.

Longo J: Cognitive rehearsal, *Amer Nurse Today* 12(8):41–42, 2017 Available at https://www.americannursetoday.com/wp-content/uploads/2017/08/cognitive-rehearsal-american-nurses-association-journal.pdf.

Luparell S: Incivility in nursing: the connection between academia and clinical settings, *Crit Care Nurs* 31(2): 92–95, 2011.

PACERS: *Passionate About creating Environments of respects and civilities (PACERS): civility tool kit*, 2015 (website). Available at: http://stopbullyingtoolkit.org.

Selye, H: *General adaptation syndrome*. n.d. (website). Retrieved from: www.essenceofstressrelief.com/general-adaptation-syndrome.html.

Stokowski LA: *The downward spiral: incivility in nursing*, 2011. (website). Available at: www.medscape.com/viewarticle/739328_3.

Truth About Nursing: *Ratched or Wretched?*, 2018 (website). 2018. Available at: http://blog.truthaboutnursing.org/2018/01/marysue-heilemann-on-nurse-ratched/.

Truth About Nursing: *You can smile with your eyes: Ebola and nursing in the news media*,2014.(website). Available at: www.truthaboutnursing.org/news/2014/dec/ebola.html.

Truth About Nursing: *A bad case of loving nurses*,2012. (website). Available at: http://www.truthaboutnursing.org/news/2012/feb/mavericks.html.

United Nations, Department of Economic and Social Affairs, Population Division: *World population prospects: the 2017 revision, data booklet*, 2017. (website). Available at: https://www.un.org/development/desa/publications/world-population-prospects-the-2017-revision.html.

U.S. Census Bureau: *US world and population clock*,n.d. (website). Available at: https://www.census.gov/popclock/.

Epilogue

You are inheriting a rich legacy of achievement and progress in the profession of nursing. At the same time, you are facing challenges related to the global COVID-19 pandemic that, at the time of this writing, still threatens the health and lives of much of the world's population. Some of you will be the names and faces of your generation of nurses, such as Lillian Wald, Jessie Sleet Scales, or Isabel Hampton Robb, persons whose energy, courage, and persistence moved not just nursing but the world forward. Change and evolution are necessary for progress, and although much has been accomplished, there remains much work to be done to transform nursing in ways that make sense in today's complex world. As professional nurses—and as citizens of the world—you will be challenged to be leaders in solving the injustice of health disparities, improving access to health care for the disenfranchised, containing health care costs, and finding solutions for problems that we cannot possibly imagine at the moment. I cannot help but think that, when I wrote the words "we cannot possibly imagine" for the previous edition, the prospect of a global pandemic of the scale of COVID-19 was truly unimaginable, and yet it was right around the corner.

I hope that through reading this book you have been inspired to develop values and beliefs consistent with professional nursing; that you are eager for more knowledge; that you aspire to a high degree of professionalism; and that you understand your potential as a nursing leader of the future and as a positive force for change in the nursing profession and in the world.

— BPB

beth_black@unc.edu

GLOSSARY

A

Acceptance An attitude that conveys neither approval nor disapproval (nonjudgment) of patients or their personal beliefs, habits, expressions of feelings, or chosen lifestyles.

Accountability Responsibility for one's behavior.

Accreditation A voluntary review process of educational programs or service agencies by professional organizations.

Active collaborator One who is engaged as a participant with another person.

Active listening A method of communicating interest and attention using such signals as maintaining eye contact, nodding, and encouraging the speaker.

Acuity Degree of illness.

Acute illness Sudden, steadily progressing symptoms that subside quickly, with or without treatment, such as influenza.

Adaptation A change or coping response to stress of any kind.

Adaptation model A conceptual model that focuses on the patient as an adaptive system, that is, one that strives to cope with both internal demands and external demands of the environment.

Adjudicate To decide or sit in judgment, as in a legal case.

Administrative law Law created by a governmental agency to meet the intent of statutory law.

Advance directives Written instructions recognized by state law that describe individuals' preferences in regard to medical intervention should they become incapacitated.

Advanced degrees Degrees beyond the bachelor's degree; master's and doctoral degrees.

Advanced practice Nursing roles that require either a master's degree or specialized education in a specific area.

Advanced practice nurse A registered nurse who has met advanced educational and practice requirements beyond basic nursing education.

Aesthetics Branch of philosophy that studies the nature of beauty.

Affective domain Field of activity dealing with a person's mood, feelings, values, or belief system.

Alternative therapies Treatments other than traditional Western medical treatments.

Altruism Unselfish concern for the welfare of others.

Ambulatory care Health services provided to those who visit a clinic or hospital as outpatients and depart after treatment on the same day.

American Assembly for Men in Nursing (AAMN) Professional organization that seeks to encourage, support, and advocate for men in nursing.

American Association of Colleges of Nursing (AACN) A national organization devoted to advancing nursing education at the baccalaureate and graduate levels.

American Nurses Association (ANA) Nursing's major professional organization made up of constituent state associations. Addresses issues of policy, ethics, standards of care, and the economic and general welfare of nurses. Membership is limited to nurses.

American Nurses Credentialing Center (ANCC) The organization that deals with certification of individual nurses and approval of organizations as continuing education providers.

American Organization of Nurse Executives (AONE) An organization for high-level nursing managers, such as chief nurses. Leaders in nursing education can be associate members.

Analysis The second step in the nursing process during which various pieces of patient data are analyzed. The outcome is one or more nursing diagnoses.

Anxiety A diffuse, vague feeling of apprehension and uncertainty. Also a psychiatric condition.

Applied science Use of scientific theory and laws in a practical way that has immediate application.

Appropriateness A criterion for successful communication in which the reply fits the circumstances and matches the message, and the amount is neither too great nor too little.

Articulation An educational mobility system providing for direct movement from a program at one level of nursing education to another without significant loss of credit.

Assault A threat or an attempt to make bodily contact with another person without the person's consent.

Assessment The first step in the nursing process involving the collection of information about the patient.

Assisted suicide Suicide by a person with help from another person, such as a health care provider.

Associate Degree in Nursing program A form of basic nursing education program, leading to the Associate Degree in Nursing (ADN), consisting of 3 or fewer years, and usually offered in technical or community colleges.

Association An organization of members with common interests.

Authority Possessing both the responsibility for making decisions and the accountability for the outcome of those decisions.

Autonomy Self-determination. Control over one's own professional practice.

B

Bachelor of Science in Nursing (BSN) Degree offered by programs that combine nursing courses with general education courses in a 4- or 5-year curriculum in a college or university.

Balance of power A distribution of forces among the branches of government so that no one branch is strong enough to dominate the others.

Basic program Any nursing education program preparing beginning practitioners.

Battery The impermissible, unprivileged touching of one person by another.

Belief The intellectual acceptance of something as true or correct.

Belief system Organization of an individual's beliefs into a rational whole.

Beneficence The ethical principle of doing good.

Biases Prejudices, often outside the individual's awareness.

Bioethics An area of ethical inquiry focusing on the dilemmas inherent in modern health care.

Biomedical technology Complex machines or implantable devices used in patient care settings.

Birthrate The number of births in a particular place during a specific time period, usually expressed as a quantity per 1000 people in 1 year.

Burnout A state of emotional exhaustion attributable to cumulative stress.

C

Cadet Corps A government-created entity designed during World War II to rapidly increase the number of registered nurses being educated so that they could assist in the war effort.

Caregiver stress A condition affecting individuals responsible for meeting the needs of others, often a family member, with a chronic condition such as Alzheimer's disease. Consists of feeling overwhelmed and a variety of other emotional and physical symptoms of stress.

Caring A theoretical framework central to nursing that results in a professional form of relating to, attending to, and providing for the needs of others.

Case management Systematic collaboration with patients, their significant others, and their health care providers to coordinate high-quality health care services in a cost-effective manner with positive patient outcomes.

Case management nursing A growing field within nursing in which nurses are responsible for coordinating services provided to patients in a cost-effective manner.

Case manager An individual responsible for coordinating services provided to a group of patients.

Centers for Medicare and Medicaid Services (CMS) Federal cost-containment program that establishes standards and monitors care in the Medicare and Medicaid programs.

Certification Validation of specific qualifications demonstrated by a registered nurse in a defined area of practice.

Certified nurse-midwife (CNM) A nationally certified nurse with advanced specialized education who assists women and couples during uncomplicated pregnancies, deliveries, and postdelivery periods.

Certified registered nurse anesthetist (CRNA) A nationally certified nurse with advanced education who specializes in the administration of anesthesia.

Change agent An individual who recognizes the need for organizational change and facilitates that process.

Chief executive officer (CEO) The senior administrator of an organization.

Chief nurse executive (CNE) The senior nursing administrator of an organization. Also chief nurse officer (CNO).

Chief nurse officer (CNO) The senior nursing administrator of an organization. Also chief nurse executive (CNE).

Chief of staff A physician in a health care facility, generally elected by the medical staff for a specified term, who is responsible for overseeing the activities of the medical staff organization.

Chronic illness Ongoing health problems of a generally incurable nature, such as diabetes.

Civil law Law involving disputes between individuals.

Clarification A therapeutic communication technique in which the nurse seeks to understand a patient's message more clearly.

Cliché An often-repeated expression that conveys little real meaning, such as "Have a nice day."

Clinical director Middle management nurse who has responsibility for multiple units in a health care agency. Also known as a *clinical coordinator.*

Clinical judgment The ability to make consistently effective clinical decisions based on theoretical knowledge, research findings, informed opinions, and prior experience.

Clinical ladder Programs allowing nurses to progress in the organizational hierarchy while staying in direct patient care roles.

Clinical nurse leader A nurse with an advanced degree who is a clinical expert in the care of a distinct group of patients and who may provide direct patient care.

Clinical nurse specialist An advanced practice nurse with an advanced degree who serves as a resource person to other nurses and often provides direct care to patients or families with particularly difficult or complex problems.

Closed system A system that does not interact with other systems or with the surrounding environment.

Code of ethics A statement of professional standards used to guide behavior and as a framework for decision making.

Code of Ethics for Nurses A formal statement by the American Association of Nurses (ANA) of the nursing profession's code of ethics.

Cognitive Pertaining to intellectual activities requiring knowledge.

Cognitive domain Area of activity that affects an individual's knowledge level.

Cognitive rebellion A stage in the educational process wherein students begin to free themselves from external controls and to rely on their own judgment.

Collaboration Working closely with another person in the spirit of cooperation.

Collective action Activities undertaken by or on behalf of a group of people who have common interests.

Collective bargaining Negotiating as a group for improved salary and work conditions.

Collective identity The connection and feeling of similarity individuals in a particular group feel with one another; group identification.

Collegiality The promotion of collaboration, cooperation, and recognition of interdependence among members of a profession.

Commission on Collegiate Nursing Education (CCNE) The accrediting arm of the American Association of Colleges of Nursing (AACN).

Common law Law that develops as a result of decisions made by judges in legal cases.

Communication The exchange of thoughts, ideas, or information; a dynamic process that is a primary instrument through which change occurs in nursing situations.

Community-based nursing Nursing care provided for individuals, families, and groups in a variety of settings, including homes, workplaces, and schools.

Community health nursing Formerly known as *public health nursing*; a nursing specialty that systematically uses a process of delivering nursing care to improve the health of an entire community.

Compassion fatigue A state experienced by those helping people in distress; an extreme state of tension and preoccupation with the suffering of those being helped to the degree that it is traumatizing for the helper.

Competency The capability of a particular patient to understand the information given and to make an informed choice about treatment options.

Complementary therapies Those treatments intended to augment Western medical treatments such as massage therapy or acupuncture.

Concept An abstract classification of data; for example, "temperature" is a concept.

Conceptual model or framework A group of concepts that are broadly defined and systematically organized to provide a focus, a rationale, and a tool for the integration and interpretation of information.

Confidentiality Ensuring the privacy of individuals participating in research studies or being treated in health care settings.

Congruent A characteristic of communication that occurs when the verbal and nonverbal elements of a message match.

Constituent members Organizational members of the American Nurses Association (ANA), such as state nurses associations or specialty nursing organizations.

Consultation The process of conferring with patients, families, or other health professionals.

Contact hour A measurement used to recognize participation in continuing education offerings, usually equivalent to 50 minutes.

Context An essential element of communication consisting of the setting in which an interaction occurs, the mood, the relationship between sender and receiver, and other factors.

Continuing education (CE) Workshops, conferences, and short courses, in which nurses maintain competence during their professional careers.

Continuous quality improvement (CQI) A management concept focusing on excellence and employee involvement at all levels of an organization.

Contracts Documents agreed on by workers and management that include provisions about staffing levels, salary, work conditions, and other issues of concern to either party.

Copayment The portion of a provider's charges that an insured patient is responsible for paying.

Coping The methods a person uses to assess and manage demands.

Coping mechanisms Psychological devices used by individuals when a threat is perceived.

Cost containment An attempt to keep health care costs stable or increasing only slowly.

Criminal law Law involving public concerns against unlawful behavior that threatens society.

Criteria Standards by which something is judged or measured.

Critical paths Multidisciplinary care plans outlining a patient's treatments and expected outcomes, day by day.

Cross-training Preparing a single worker for multiple tasks that formerly were performed by multiple specialized workers.

Cultural assessment The process of determining a patient's cultural practices and preferences in order to render culturally competent care.

Cultural care, theory of A nursing theory focusing on the importance of incorporating a patient's culturally determined health beliefs and practices into care.

Cultural competence The integration of knowledge, attitudes, and skills that enhance cross-cultural communication and appropriate interactions with others.

Cultural diversity Social, ethnic, racial, and religious differences in a group.

Culturally competent education Nursing education that incorporates knowledge, attitudes, and skills that enhance cross-cultural communication and appropriate interactions with others.

Culturally congruent nursing care Care that incorporates knowledge, attitudes, and skills that enhance cross-cultural communication and appropriate interactions with others.

Culture The attitudes, beliefs, and behaviors of social and ethnic groups that have been perpetuated through generations.

Culture of nursing The rites, rituals, and valued behaviors of the nursing profession.

D

Data Information or facts collected for analysis.

Deaconess Institute A large hospital and planned training program for deaconesses established in 1836 by Pastor Theodor Fliedner at Kaiserswerth, Germany.

Decentralization An organizational structure in which decision-making authority is shared with employees most affected by the decisions rather than being retained by top executives.

Deductible The out-of-pocket amount individuals must pay before their health insurance begins to pay for health care.

Deductive reasoning A process through which conclusions are drawn by logical inference from given premises; proceeds from the general case to the specific.

Defining characteristics Signs and symptoms of disease.

Delegate To refer a task to another.

Delegation The practice of assigning tasks or responsibilities to other persons.

Demographics The study of vital statistics and social trends.

Demography The science that studies vital statistics and social trends.

Deontology The ethical theory that the rightness or wrongness of an action depends on the inherent moral significance of the action.

Dependency The degree to which individuals adopt passive attitudes and rely on others to take care of them.

Dependent intervention Nursing actions on behalf of patients that require knowledge and skill on the part of the nurse but may not be done without explicit directions from another health professional, usually a physician, dentist, or nurse practitioner.

Developmental theory A theory in which growth is defined as an increase in physical size and shape toward a point of optimal maturity.

Diagnosis Identification of a disease or condition.

Dietitian Bachelor's or master's degree–prepared nutrition expert who specializes in therapeutic diet preparation and nutrition education. Also known as a *registered dietitian* (RD).

Diploma program The earliest form of formal nursing education in the United States; is usually based in hospitals, requires 3 years of study, and leads to a diploma in nursing.

Disaster An event or situation that is of greater magnitude than an emergency; disrupts essential services such as housing, transportation, communications, sanitation, water, and health care; and requires the response of people outside the community affected.

Disease A pathologic alteration at the tissue or organ level.

Disease management A process of helping patients understand and manage their chronic conditions effectively through coaching and education, symptom recognition and management, and collaboration with the patient's health care provider.

Disenfranchised The state of having no power or voice in a political system.

Disseminate Publish or widely distribute scientific information, such as the findings of a research study.

Dissonance Lack of harmony.

Distance learning The process of taking classes and earning academic credit through technological means such as televised or online classes. The teacher and student may be many miles apart.

Documentation Written communication about a patient's condition, care, and reactions to treatments; found in the patient record/chart.

Dominant culture Mainstream culture that contains one or more subcultures.

Double effect Ethical concept encompassing the belief that there are some situations in which it is necessary to inflict potential harm in an effort to achieve a greater good.

Duty of care The responsibility of a nurse or other health professional for the care of a patient.

Duty to report The requirement, according to state law, for health professionals to report certain illnesses, injuries, and actions of patients.

E

Efficiency A criterion for successful communication that consists of using simple, clear words timed at a pace suitable to participants.

Electoral process The procedures that must be followed to select someone to fill an elected position.

Empathy Awareness of, sensitivity to, and identification with the feelings of another person.

End-of-life care Care aimed at comfort and dignity for patients who are nearing death and for their families and other significant persons in their lives.

Entrepreneur A person who envisions, organizes, manages, and assumes responsibility for a new enterprise or business.

Environment All of the many external and internal factors, such as physical and psychological, that influence life and survival.

Epistemology The branch of philosophy dealing with the theory of knowledge.

Ethical decision making The process of choosing between actions based on a system of beliefs and values.

Ethics The branch of philosophy that studies the propriety of certain courses of action.

Ethnocentrism The belief that one's own culture is the most desirable.

Ethnographic research A type of qualitative research focusing on culture and the phenomena associated with a culture.

Euthanasia The act of painlessly ending the life of a terminally ill individual for whom cure is not possible.

Evaluation Measuring the success or failure of the results or "outputs," and consequently the effectiveness, of a system. It is the final step in the nursing process wherein the nurse examines the patient's progress to determine whether a problem is solved, is in the process of being solved, or is unsolved. In communication theory, it is the analysis of information received.

Evidence-based practice The use of research findings, clinical expertise, and patient preference as the three-pronged basis for practice rather than trial and error, intuition, or traditional methods, such as problem solving.

Exacerbation Reemergence or worsening of the symptoms of a chronic illness.

Executive branch The branch of government responsible for administering the laws of the land.

Experimental design Research design that provides evidence of a cause-and-effect relationship between actions.

Expert witness An individual called on to testify in court because of special skill or knowledge in a certain field, such as nursing.

Extended care Medical, nursing, or custodial care provided to an individual over a prolonged period.

Extended family A term used to describe nonnuclear family members such as grandparents, aunts, and uncles.

External factors Values, beliefs, and behaviors of significant others that have an impact on an individual.

F

Faith community The members of a church, synagogue, mosque, or other entity who worship together and share common beliefs about religion.

Faith community nurse A specialized nurse who focuses on the promotion of health within the context of the values, beliefs, and practices of a church, synagogue, mosque, or other faith community. May also be known as a *parish nurse*.

False reassurance A nontherapeutic form of communication that seeks to convince that everything will turn out well.

Family system The group of individuals who comprise the basic unit of family living and their interactions with one another and the larger society.

Feedback The information given back into a system to determine whether or not the purpose of the system has been achieved. A major element in the communication process.

Fidelity An ethical principle that values faithfulness to one's responsibilities.

Flexibility A criterion for successful communication that occurs when messages are based on the immediate situation rather than preconceived expectations.

Flexible staffing A mechanism whereby nurses may work at times other than the traditional hospital shifts.

Flexner Report A 1910 study of medical education that provided the impetus for much-needed reform.

Formal socialization The process by which individuals learn a new role from the direct instruction of others.

For-profit agency A health care agency established to make a profit for the owners or shareholders.

Frontier Nursing Service Founded in Kentucky in 1925; provided the first organized midwifery service in the United States.

G

General election An election in which all registered voters may vote and choose a candidate from any party on the ballot.

Generalizable Research findings that are transferable to other situations.

General systems theory A theory promulgated by Ludwig von Bertalanffy in the late 1930s to explain the relationship of a whole to its parts.

Generic master's degree An accelerated master's degree in nursing for people with nonnursing bachelor's degrees.

Genetic counseling Health and reproductive advice given to individuals based on their genetic composition.

Goldmark Report A major study of nursing education published in 1923 and named *The Study of Nursing and Nursing Education in the United States.*

Governmental (public) agency An agency primarily supported by taxes, administered by elected or appointed officials, and tailored to the needs of the communities served.

Grand theory A very broad conceptualization of nursing phenomena.

Grassroots activism The involvement of a large number of people, generally widely dispersed, who are concerned about a particular issue.

Growth An increase in physical size and shape toward a point of optimal maturity.

H

Health An individual's physical, mental, spiritual, and social well-being; a continuum, not a constant state.

Health behaviors Choices and habitual actions that promote or diminish health.

Health beliefs Culturally determined beliefs about the nature of health and illness.

Health care network A corporation with a consolidated set of facilities and services for comprehensive health care.

Health Insurance Portability and Accountability Act (HIPAA) Federal law, passed in 1996, designed to protect health insurance coverage for workers and their families when they change or lose their jobs.

Health maintenance Preventing illness and maintaining maximal function.

Health maintenance organization (HMO) A network or group of providers who agree to provide certain basic health care services for a single predetermined yearly fee.

Health promotion Encouraging a condition of maximum physical, mental, and social well-being.

Health promotion model A theoretical nursing model that uses illness prevention and health promotion as a basic framework.

Helping professions Professions such as social work, teaching, and nursing that emphasize meeting the needs of clients.

Henry Street Settlement A clinic for the poor founded by Lillian Wald and her colleague Mary Brewster on New York's Lower East Side.

Heterogeneous Composed of parts of differing kinds.

High-level wellness Functioning at maximum potential in an integrated way within the environment.

Holism A school of health care thought that espouses treating the whole patient—body, mind, and spirit.

Holistic nursing care Nursing care that nourishes the whole person—body, mind, and spirit.

Holistic values The approach to nursing practice that takes the physical, emotional, social, economic, and spiritual needs of the person into consideration.

Home health agency An organization that delivers various health services to patients in their homes.

Home health nursing Field of nursing in which care is provided to patients in their own homes.

Homeostasis A relative constancy in the internal environment of the body.

Homogeneous Composed of parts of the same or similar kinds.

Hospice An agency providing end-of-life care to terminally ill patients and their families.

Hospice and palliative care nursing Specialized nursing care provided at the end of life to patients and their families in homes and residential facilities. Aimed at a comfortable and dignified death that honors the wishes of patients and loved ones.

Hospitalist Hospital-based physicians who care for patients only while patients are hospitalized.

Human Genome Project A scientific project designed to map the genetic structure of composite human DNA, the initial phase of which was completed in 2003.

Human motivation Abraham Maslow's conceptualization of human needs and their relationship to the stimulation of purposeful behavior.

Human needs theory Theory proposed by Abraham Maslow that human motivation is determined by the drive to meet intrinsic human needs.

Hypothesis A statement predicting the relationship among concepts or variables.

I

Illness An abnormal process in which an individual's physical, emotional, social, or intellectual functioning is impaired.

Illness prevention All activities aimed at diminishing the likelihood that an individual's physical, emotional, social, and intellectual functions become impaired.

Implementation A stage of the nursing process during which the plan of care is carried out.

Incongruent Describes a confusing form of communication that occurs when the verbal and nonverbal elements of a message do not match.

Independent intervention Actions on behalf of patients for which the nurse requires no supervision or direction.

Individualized care plan A plan of care designed to meet the needs of a specific person.

Inductive reasoning The process of reasoning from the specific to the general. Repeated observations of an experiment or event enable the observer to draw general conclusions.

Inertia Disinclination to change.

Infant mortality The number of deaths of infants (1 year of age or younger) per 1000 live births.

Informal socialization The process through which individuals learn a new role by observing how others behave.

Informatics nurse A nurse who combines nursing science with information management science and computer science to manage and make accessible the information that nurses need.

Information technology (IT) Hardware and software used to manage and process information.

Informed consent process The process of informing individuals who are scheduled to undergo diagnostic procedures or surgery or who are potential research participants of the procedures and risks. Their consent is indicated by signing a consent form voluntarily once any questions they have are answered and their privacy has been ensured.

Infrastructure Basic support mechanisms needed to ensure that an activity can be conducted.

Input The information, energy, or matter that enters a system.

Institutional review board (IRB) A committee protecting the rights of human participants in the research. Any research involving human participants must have approval of the IRB or the IRB's determination that a study is not human subjects research.

Institutional structure The way in which the workers within an agency are organized to carry out the functions of the agency.

Integrative care Care that combines the best of both standard and nontraditional treatments, for example, pain control through both prescription medication and acupuncture.

Interdependent intervention Actions on behalf of patients in which the nurse must collaborate or consult with another health professional before or while carrying out the action.

Interdisciplinary team Group composed of individuals representing various disciplines who work together toward a common end, blending their expertise in the development of a common goal.

Internal factors Personal feelings and beliefs that influence an individual.

Internalize The process of taking in knowledge, skills, attitudes, beliefs, norms, values, and ethical standards and making them a part of one's own self-image and behavior.

International Council of Nurses (ICN) The federation of national nurses associations, currently representing nurses in more than 100 countries.

Internship An apprenticeship under supervision.

Interpreter A professional who is fluent in a second language or is bilingual who translates the spoken words.

Interprofessional education (IPE) Students across health care disciplines such as nursing, social work, and medicine learning together to address complex health problems collaboratively.

Interprofessionality Teamwork and practice across disciplines using competencies that are central to all health care professions.

J

Jargon Specialized vocabulary used by those in the same line of work to communicate about work-related matters.

Judicial branch The branch of government that decides cases or controversies on particular matters.

Justice An ethical principle stating that equals should be treated the same and that unequals should be treated differently.

K

Knowledge-based power Authority or control based on the way information is used to effect an outcome.

Knowledge technology The use of computer systems to transform information into knowledge and to generate new knowledge; expert systems.

L

Latent power Untapped strength.

Law All the rules of conduct established by a government and applicable to the people, whether in the form of legislation or custom.

Learned resourcefulness An acquired ability to use available resources in one's behalf.

Legal authority A group of people in whom power is vested by law, such as the powers vested in state boards of nursing by nurse practice acts.

Legislative branch The branch of government consisting of elected officials who are responsible for enacting the laws of the land.

Licensure The process by which an agency of government grants permission to qualified persons to engage in a given profession or occupation.

Licensure by endorsement A system whereby registered nurses or licensed practical/vocational nurses can, by submitting proof of licensure in another state and paying a licensure fee, receive licensure from the new state without sitting for a licensing examination.

Lifelong learning Continuing education and increasing knowledge throughout an individual's professional life.

Lobby An attempt to influence the vote of legislators.

Locus of control The place where individuals believes the power in their lives resides, either within or outside of themselves.

Logic The field of philosophy that studies correct and incorrect reasoning.

Long-term care Care provided to individuals, such as people with Alzheimer's disease, who require ongoing assistance in the maintenance of activities of daily living.

Long-term goals Major changes that may take months or even years to accomplish.

Lysaught Report A 1970 report titled *An Abstract for Action* that made recommendations concerning the supply and demand for nurses, nursing roles and functions, and nursing education.

M

Magnet Recognition Program An initiative of the American Nurses Credentialing Center (ANCC) that recognizes excellent patient outcomes, a high level of job satisfaction among nurses, low staff nurse turnover rate, and appropriate grievance resolution, among other factors.

Malpractice An act resulting in injury that occurs when a professional fails to act as a reasonably prudent professional would under similar circumstances.

Managed care A process in which an individual, often a nurse, is assigned to review patients' cases and coordinate services so that quality care can be achieved at the lowest cost.

Managed care organization (MCO) Any of a number of organizations that attempt to coordinate subscriber services to ensure quality care at the lowest cost.

Mandatory continuing education The requirement that nurses complete a certain number of hours of continuing education as a prerequisite for relicensure.

Medicaid A jointly funded federal and state public health insurance that covers citizens below the poverty level and those with certain disabling conditions; established in 1965.

Medically indigent Individuals and families who do not qualify for Medicaid or Medicare but cannot afford health insurance or medical care.

Medicare A federally funded form of public health insurance for citizens 65 years of age and older; established in 1965.

Mentor An experienced nurse who shares knowledge with less experienced nurses to help advance their careers.

Message An essential element of communication consisting of the spoken word and/or nonverbal communication.

Metaparadigm The most abstract aspect of the structure of knowledge; the global concepts that identify the phenomena of interest for a discipline.

Metaphysics The branch of philosophy that considers the ultimate nature of existence, reality, and experience.

Middle-range theory Theory that makes connections between grand theories and nursing practice.

Milieu Surroundings or environment.

Mission The special task(s) to which an organization devotes itself.

Model A symbolic representation of a concept or reality.

Modeling An informal type of socialization that occurs when an individual chooses an admired person to emulate.

Moral development The ways in which a person learns to deal with moral dilemmas from childhood through adulthood.

Moral distress Pain or anguish of a person who unwillingly participates in perceived moral wrongdoing.

Morals Established rules or standards that guide behavior in situations in which a decision about right and wrong must be made.

Mortality rate The number of deaths in a particular population during a specific period of time; usually expressed as a quantity per 1000 people in a specific year.

Mutuality Sharing jointly with others.

Mutual recognition model A system whereby a registered nurse may be licensed in the state of residency yet practice in other states, after being recognized by them, without additional licenses.

N

NANDA International Group working since 1970 to establish a comprehensive list of nursing diagnoses.

National Council Licensure Examination for Practical Nurses (NCLEX-PN®) The examination that graduates of practical nursing programs must take to practice as licensed practical nurses (LPNs) or licensed vocational nurses (LVNs).

National Council Licensure Examination for Registered Nurses (NCLEX-RN®) The examination that graduates of basic nursing programs must take to become licensed to practice as registered nurses (RNs).

National League for Nursing (NLN) National organization that seeks to advance the profession of nursing through advocacy and improving educational standards for nurses. Nonnurses may be members.

National League for Nursing Accrediting Commission (NLNAC) The arm of the National League for Nursing that accredits schools' associate degree, diploma, baccalaureate, and master's programs in nursing.

National Student Nurses Association (NSNA) National organization devoted to developing leadership skills in nursing students.

Negligence The failure to act as a reasonably prudent person would have acted in specific circumstances.

Network A system of interconnected individuals; useful to develop contacts or exchange information to further a career.

Nonexperimental design Research with the intent to describe or clarify a phenomenon. Not intended to test a hypothesis.

Nonjudgmental Describes an attitude that conveys neither approval nor disapproval of patients' beliefs and respects each person's right to his or her own beliefs.

Nonmaleficence The duty to inflict no harm or evil.

Nonverbal communication Communication without words; consists of gestures, posture, facial expressions, tone and loudness of voice, actions, grooming, and clothing, among other things.

Nosocomial Hospital-acquired, as a nosocomial infection.

Not-for-profit agency An organization that does not attempt to make a profit for distribution to owners or stockholders. Any profit made by such organizations is used to operate and improve the organization itself or to extend its services.

Nuclear family Term used to describe a couple, parent, or parents and their children; as opposed to *extended family*.

Nurse activist A nurse who works actively on behalf of a political candidate or certain legislation.

Nurse anesthetist A nurse with specialized advanced education who administers anesthetic agents to patients undergoing operative procedures.

Nurse-based practice A clinic, office, or home practice in which nurses carry their own caseloads of patients with physical and/or psychiatric needs.

Nurse citizen A nurse who exercises all the political rights accorded citizens, such as registering to vote and voting in all elections.

Nurse entrepreneur A nurse who engages in a business undertaking related to health care or nursing, such as owning a traveling nurse agency.

Nurse executive The top nurse in the administrative structure of a health care organization.

Nurse Licensure Compact An agreement among certain states, authorized by legislation, that they will honor licenses issued to registered nurses by other states in the compact.

Nurse manager A nurse who is in charge of all activities in a unit, including patient care, continuous quality improvement, personnel selection and evaluation, and resource (supplies and money) management. Formerly known as a *head nurse*.

Nurse-midwife A nurse with advanced specialized education who assists women and couples during uncomplicated pregnancies, birth, and postbirth periods.

Nurse-patient relationship The mode of connection between a nurse and patient.

Nurse politician A nurse who runs for political office.

Nurse practitioner A nurse with advanced education who specializes in the health care of a particular group, such as children, pregnant women, or the elderly.

Nursing The provision of health care services, focusing on the maintenance, promotion, and restoration of health.

Nursing diagnosis A process of describing a patient's response to health problems that either already exist or may occur in the future.

Nursing goal A statement of the desired long-term or short-term outcome as a result of one or more nursing interventions.

Nursing informatics The branch of nursing that manages knowledge and data through technology with the goal of improving patient care.

Nursing information system A software system that automates the nursing process.

Nursing Outcomes Classification (NOC) A classification system describing patient outcomes sensitive to nursing interventions.

Nursing practice act Law defining the scope of nursing practice in a given state.

Nursing process A cognitive activity that requires both critical and creative thinking and serves as the basis for providing nursing care. A method used by nurses in dealing with patient problems in professional practice.

Nursing research The systematic investigation of events or circumstances related to improving patient outcomes.

Nursing theory A formal statement of related concepts used to explain, predict, control, and understand commonly occurring phenomena of interest to nurses.

O

Obesity A body mass index (BMI) of 30 or more.

Objective data Factual information obtained through observation and examination of the patient or through consultation with other health care providers.

Occupation A person's principal work or business.

Occupational and environmental health nurse A nurse specializing in the care of a specific group of workers in a given occupational setting.

Open-ended question An inquiry that causes the patient to answer fully, giving more than a "yes" or "no" answer.

Open posture Body position, such as squarely facing another person with arms in a relaxed position.

Open system A system that promotes the exchange of matter, energy, and information with other systems and the environment.

Organizational structure How an agency is organized to accomplish its mission.

Orientation phase The beginning phase of a nurse-patient relationship in which the parties are getting acquainted with one another.

Outcome criteria Expected results of nursing intervention.

Out-of-pocket payment Direct payment for health services from individuals' personal funds.

Output The end result or product of a system.

P

Palliative care nursing A rapidly developing specialty in nursing dedicated to management of symptoms and improving the quality of life of seriously, chronically ill patients, patients at the end of their lives, and their families.

Parental modeling A type of socialization that occurs when parents' behavior and responses to various stimuli influence a child's future behaviors and responses.

Participants The individuals who are studied in a research project. Formerly referred to as "subjects."

Patient acuity The degree of illness of a particular patient or group of patients; used to determine staffing needs.

Patient advocate One who promotes the interest of patients. A nursing role.

Patient care technician (PCT) A health technician working under the supervision of a registered nurse, physician, or other health professional to provide basic patient care.

Patient-centered care A system that emphasizes coordinating patient care to maximize patient comfort, convenience, and security.

Patient classification system (PCS) Identification of patients' needs for nursing care in quantitative terms.

Patient interview A face-to-face interaction with the patient in which an interviewer elicits pertinent information.

Patient Self-Determination Act Effective December 1, 1991, this law encourages patients to consider which life-prolonging treatment options they desire and to document their preferences in case they should later become incapable of participating in the decision-making process.

Patients' rights Responsibilities that a hospital and its staff have toward patients and their families during hospitalization.

Pay equity Equal pay for work of comparable value.

Peer review The process of submitting one's work for examination and comment by colleagues in the same profession to ensure scientific and scholarly value.

Perception The selection, organization, and interpretation of incoming signals into meaningful messages.

Performance improvement (PI) Organizational efforts to improve corporate performance, incorporating aspects of quality management.

Person An individual—man, woman, or child.

Personal payment Direct payment for health services from an individual's personal funds.

Personal space The amount of space surrounding individuals in which they feel comfortable interacting with others; usually culturally determined.

Personal value system The social principles, ideals, or standards held by an individual that form the basis for meaning, direction, and decision making in life.

Phenomena Occurrences or circumstances that are observable. The singular form of the word is *phenomenon*.

Phenomenological inquiry/research A qualitative research approach focusing on what people experience in regard to a particular phenomenon, such as grief, and how they interpret those experiences.

Philosophy The study of the truths and principles of being, knowledge, conduct, or nature of the universe.

Planning The third step in the nursing process, which begins with the identification of patient goals.

Policy The principles and values that govern actions directed toward given ends. Policy sets forth a plan, direction, or goal for action.

Policy development The generation of principles and procedures that guide governmental or organizational action.

Policy outcome The result of decisions made by governmental or organizational leaders who choose a certain course of action.

Political action committees (PACs) Groups that raise and distribute money to candidates who support their organization's stand on certain issues.

Politics The area of philosophy that deals with the regulation and control of people living in society; in government, it includes the allocation of scarce resources such as health care resources.

Population The entire group of people possessing a given characteristic; for example, all brown-eyed people older than age 65.

Position paper Statement pertaining to the stance a group or organization takes on an issue; for example, the American Nurses Association's 1965 Position Paper advocated the baccalaureate degree as the entry level into the practice of registered nursing.

Posttraumatic stress disorder (PTSD) An anxiety disorder characterized by an acute emotional response to a traumatic event or situation.

Powers of appointment The authority to select the people who serve in positions such as judges, ambassadors, and cabinet officials.

Practical nurse (LPN/LVN) program A 1-year educational program preparing individuals for direct patient care roles under the supervision of a physician or registered nurse.

Preceptor A teacher; in nursing, usually an experienced nurse who assumes responsibility for teaching a new nurse (novice).

Preferred provider organization (PPO) A form of HMO that contracts with independent providers such as physicians and hospitals for a negotiated discount for services provided to its members.

Premium The amount paid for an insurance policy, usually in installments.

Primary care Basic health care, including promotion of health, early diagnosis of disease, and prevention of disease.

Primary election An election in which voters who are declared members of a political party choose among several candidates of that same party for a particular office.

Primary nursing A system of nursing care delivery in which one nurse has responsibility for the planning, implementation, and evaluation of the care of one or more clients 24 hours a day for the duration of the hospital stay.

Primary source The patient is considered the primary source of data about himself or herself; in a literature review, a primary source is the original writing of a theorist or author.

Principlism Use of multiple ethical principles, such as beneficence, autonomy, nonmaleficence, veracity, justice, and fidelity, in the resolution of ethical conflicts rather than a single principle.

Private insurance Insurance obtained from a privately owned company, as opposed to public or governmental insurance.

Private practice Nursing practice engaged in by some nurses with advanced education; usually provided on a fee-for-service basis, as in most medical practices.

Privileged communications The principle that information given to certain professionals (e.g., attorneys, clergy) is protected and is not to be disclosed even in court.

Problem solving A method of finding solutions to difficulties specific to a given situation and designed for immediate action.

Profession Work requiring advanced training and usually involving mental rather than manual effort. Usually has a code of ethics and a professional organization.

Professional A person who engages in a specific profession, such as law, medicine, or nursing.

Professional accountabilities In the shared governance model, a basic set of responsibilities of all professional nurses regardless of practice setting.

Professional association An organization consisting of people belonging to the same profession and thereby having many common interests.

Professional boundary The dividing line between the activities of two professions. The area in which a professional person functions to avoid both underinvolvement and overinvolvement, maintaining the patient's needs as the focus of the relationship.

Professional outcomes The impact on a profession from political action by its practitioners.

Professional practice advocacy Includes activities such as education, lobbying, and advocating individually and collectively to advance a profession's agenda.

Professional review organization (PRO) Organizations that review Medicare hospital admissions and Medicare patients' lengths of stay.

Professional socialization The process of developing an occupational identity.

Professionalism Professional behavior, appearance, and conduct.

Professionalization A process through which an occupation evolves to professional status.

Proposition A statement about how two or more concepts are related.

Protocol A written plan specifying the procedure to be followed.

Provider A deliverer of health care services—hospital, clinic, nurse, or physician.

Proximate cause Action occurring immediately before an injury, thereby assumed to be the reason for the injury.

Psychomotor domain Area of activity referring to motor skills or actions by an individual; for example, learning to dance is in the psychomotor domain.

Pure science Information that summarizes and explains the universe without regard for whether the information is immediately useful; also known as *basic science*.

Q

Qualitative research A type of inquiry that is characterized by studying phenomena in their natural setting using interviews, observations, and other techniques; includes ethnography, grounded theory, and phenomenology.

Quantitative research Research that uses data-gathering techniques that can be repeated by others and verified. Data collected are quantifiable, that is, they can be counted, measured with standardized instruments, or observed with a high degree of agreement among observers.

Quaternary care Extremely specialized care that may be available in a very few locations, such as a research medical center; a form of very advanced care.

R

Reality shock The feelings of powerlessness and ineffectiveness often experienced by new nursing graduates; usually occurs as a result of the transition from the educational setting to the "real world" of nursing in an actual health care setting.

Receiver An essential element of communication; the person receiving the message.

Reengineering Radical redesign of business processes and thinking to improve performance.

Referendum An election resulting from registered voters being asked by a legislative body to express a preference on a policy issue.

Reflection A communication technique that consists of directing questions back to patients, thereby encouraging patients to think through problems for themselves.

Reflective practice A method of focusing on one's practice, both in the moment and after an event, with an open and curious mind, drawing on all the senses to know oneself more fully.

Reflective thinking The process of evaluating one's thinking processes during a situation that has already occurred, as opposed to evaluating one's thinking during the situation as it occurs.

Registered nurse (RN) An individual who has completed a basic program for registered nurses and successfully passed the NCLEX-RN®.

Rehabilitation services Those activities designed to restore an individual or a body part to normal or near-normal function after a debilitating disease or an accident.

Reliable Yielding the same values dependably each time an instrument is used to measure the same thing.

Remission A period of chronic illness during which symptoms subside.

Replication The process of repeating a research study as closely as possible to the original.

Research process Prescribed steps that must be taken to plan and conduct meaningful research properly.

Research question A statement, question, or hypothesis that a research study is designed to answer.

Resilience A pattern of successful adaptation despite challenging or threatening circumstances.

Resocialized The outcome of a transitional process of giving up part or all of one set of professional values and learning new ones.

Resolution A written position on an issue presented to the voting members of an association for their consideration, discussion, and vote.

Respondeat superior Legal theory that attributes the acts of employees to their employer (Latin term).

Retrospective reimbursement Insurance payment made after services are delivered.

Risk management A program that seeks to identify and eliminate potential safety hazards, thereby reducing patient injuries.

RN-to-BSN in nursing Programs enabling registered nurses who hold associate degrees or diplomas in nursing to acquire baccalaureate degrees in nursing.

Role A goal-directed pattern of behavior learned within a cultural setting.

Role model An individual who serves as an example of desirable behavior for another person.

Role strain Stress created by difficulty experienced in adjusting to a life or occupational role.

S

Salary compression A phenomenon in which pay increases are limited during an individual's career, so that the salary of an experienced nurse may be little higher than that of a recently hired novice nurse.

Sample A subset of an entire population that reflects the characteristics of the population.

School nurse Nurse specializing in the care of school-age children or adolescents and practicing in school settings.

Scientific discipline A branch of instruction or field of learning based on the study of a body of facts about the physical or material world.

Scientific method A systematic, orderly approach to the gathering of data and the solving of problems.

Scope of practice The boundaries of a practice profession's activities as defined by law.

Secondary care An intermediate level of health care performed in a hospital having specialized equipment and laboratory facilities.

Secondary source Sources of data such as the nurse's own observations or perceptions of family and friends of the patient.

Self-actualization A process of realizing one's maximum potential and using one's capabilities to the fullest extent possible.

Self-awareness Understanding of one's own needs, biases, and impact on others.

Self-care The ability to care for oneself, that is, engage in activities of daily living without assistance.

Self-care model Nursing theoretical model based on the concept of ability to care for oneself.

Self-efficacy A belief in self as possessing the ability to perform an activity, such as administering daily insulin.

Sender An essential element of communication; the person sending a message.

Separation of powers Under the U.S. Constitution, each branch of the federal government has separate and distinct functions and powers.

Set A group of circumstances or situations joined and treated as a whole.

Shared governance Incorporation of unit-based decision making in nursing practice models. Generic term used to describe any organization in which decision making is shared throughout.

Short-term goals Specific, small steps leading to the achievement of broader, long-term goals.

Sigma Theta Tau International (STTI) The international honor society for nursing.

Sign Outward evidence of illness visible to others; for example, a rash or bleeding.

Socialization The process whereby values and expectations are transmitted from generation to generation.

Social services Services designed to assist individuals and families in obtaining basic needs, such as housing, food, and medical care.
Somatic language Language used by infants to signal their needs to caretakers; for example, crying; reddening of the skin; fast, shallow breathing; facial expressions; and jerking of the limbs.
Spelman Seminary Site of the first nursing program for Black persons, founded in Atlanta, Georgia, in 1886.
Spirituality Belief in and sense of connectedness with a higher power.
Spiritual nursing care Care that recognizes, respects, and, if appropriate, facilitates the practice of a patient's spiritual beliefs.
Staff nurse The bedside nurse who cares for a group of patients but has no management responsibilities for the nursing unit.
Stage theory A theory that views human development as a series of identifiable stages through which individuals and families pass.
Stakeholders Individuals with an interest in an outcome or process.
Standard of care A guideline stating what the reasonably prudent nurse, under similar circumstances, would have done.
Standards of practice Formal statements by a profession of the accountability of its practitioners.
State board of nursing The regulatory body in each state that regulates and enforces the scope of practice and discipline of the members of the nursing profession.
Statutory law Law established through formal legislative processes.
Stereotypes Simplistic and preconceived image about a person or group.
Stereotyping Erroneous belief that all people of a certain group are alike.
Stress Any emotional, physical, social, economic, or other type of factor that requires a response or change.
Stressors Stimuli that tend to disturb equilibrium.
Subjective data Information obtained from patients as they describe their needs, feelings, strengths, and perceptions of the problem.
Subsystems The parts that make up a system.
Supervision The initial direction and periodic inspection of the actual accomplishment of a task.
Suprasystem The larger environment outside a system.
Symptom An indication of illness felt by the individual but not observable to others, such as pain and nausea.
Synergy Combined action that is greater than that of the individual parts.
System A set of interrelated parts that come together to form a whole.
Systems theory See *General systems theory.*

T

Taxonomy A framework for classifying and organizing information.
Team nursing A system of nursing care delivery in which a group of nurses and ancillary workers are responsible for the care of a group of patients during a specified period, usually 8 to 12 hours.
Technologists Personnel, such as laboratory technologists or radiologic technologists, who assist in the diagnosis of patient problems.
Telehealth The practice of providing health care by means of telecommunication devices, such as telephone lines or televisions; the removal of time and distance barriers for the delivery of health care services and related health care activities through telecommunication technologies such as telephones.
Telehealth nursing The delivery of nursing care services and related health care activities through telecommunication technology, such as telephones, video conferencing, and others.
Termination phase The final phase of the nurse–patient relationship wherein a mutual evaluation of progress is conducted.
Tertiary care Specialized, highly technical level of health care provided in sophisticated research and teaching hospitals.
Tertiary source Sources of data including the medical records and health care providers, such as physical therapists, physicians, or dietitians.
Theory A general explanation scholars use to explain, predict, control, and understand commonly occurring events.
Therapeutic milieu An environment created to foster healing.
Therapist Any of several health care workers with differing educational backgrounds who work with patients with specific deficits; examples include physical therapists and occupational therapists.
Third-party payment Payment for health services by an entity other than the patient or the provider of services, such as the government or insurance companies.
Throughput The processes a system uses to convert raw materials into a form that can be used, either by the system itself or by the environment.
Tort A civil wrong against a person; may be intentional or unintentional.
Total quality management (TQM) Management philosophy and activities directed toward achieving excellence and employee participation in all aspects of that goal.
Transcultural nursing Nursing care that is based on the patient's culturally determined health values, beliefs, and practices.
Transmission In communication theory, the expression of information verbally or nonverbally.

U

Universal health care Provision of health care to all people.
Unlicensed assistive personnel (UAP) Health care personnel, such as nursing assistants and home care aides, who are not licensed but are supervised by licensed individuals, such as nurses or physicians.
Urbanization The process of population migration to cities.
Utilitarianism An ethical theory asserting that it is right to maximize the greatest good for the greatest number of people.

V

Valid Measuring what it is intended to measure, as in a valid test question or research instrument.
Value ethics Ethical beliefs and behaviors that arise from the character of the decision maker.
Value statement A statement regarding the desirability of something.
Values The social principles, ideals, or standards held by an individual, class, or

group that give meaning and direction to behavior.

Veracity Truthfulness.

Verbal communication All language, whether written or spoken; represents only a small part of communication.

Virtue ethics The system of ethics based on a person's natural tendency to act, feel, and judge but developed through training; ethics based on the natural traits of the decision maker.

Voluntariness The degree to which an action is brought about by an individual's own free choice.

Voluntary (private) agency An agency supported entirely through voluntary contributions of time and/or money.

Vulnerable populations Groups who are at risk and unable to advocate for themselves, such as young children, persons with mental illness, developmentally challenged individuals, the frail elderly, or the socially marginalized, such as prisoners.

W

Whistle-blower A person who speaks out against unfair, dishonest, or dangerous practices by a company or agency. Usually an employee of that company or agency.

Woodhull Study on Nurses and the Media A comprehensive 1997 study of nursing in the print media.

Workers' compensation A federally mandated insurance system covering workers injured on the job.

Work ethic A belief on the part of an employee or group in the importance of work; an appreciation for the characteristics employers desire in employees and a commitment to exhibiting them.

Working phase The middle phase of the nurse-patient relationship, wherein goals are achieved.

Working poor Those who, although employed, are unable to earn enough to live at more than a very modest level.

Work-life balance The equilibrium between the amount of time and effort a person devotes to work and that given to other aspects of life.

Workplace advocacy Action ensuring that workers have a voice in the issues that concern them, either through collective action or through other effective means.

Y

Yale School of Nursing The first school of nursing in the world to be established as a separate university department with an independent budget and its own dean, Annie W. Goodrich.

INDEX

Note: Page numbers followed by '*f*' indicate figures those followed by '*t*' indicate tables and '*b*' indicate boxes

D

E

F

G

H

I

O

W